Craniofacial Pain

For Elsevier:

Publisher: Heidi Harrison
Associate Editor: Siobhan Campbell
Production Manager: Emma Riley
Design Direction: Judith Wright
Cover Design: Stewart Larking

Craniofacial Pain

Neuromusculoskeletal Assessment, Treatment and Management

Harry J.M. von Piekartz PhD, MSc, PT, MT

Department of Physiotherapy and Rehabilitation Science, Senior Teacher International Maitland Teacher Association (IMTA), Neuro Orthopaedic Institute (NOI), Cranial Facial Therapy Academy (CFTA)

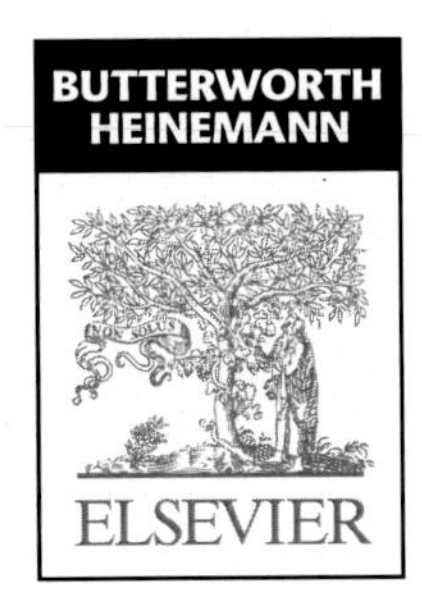

EDINBURGH LONDON NEW YORK OXFORD PHILADELPHIA ST LOUIS SYDNEY TORONTO 2007

BUTTERWORTH
HEINEMANN
ELSEVIER

Translated and updated from German by Pearl Linguistics Ltd, 2006

Original translation by Kerstin Lüdtke

ISBN-13 978 0 7506 8774 4

British Library Cataloguing in Publication Data
A catalogue record for this book is available from the British Library.

Library of Congress Cataloging in Publication Data
A catalog record for this book is available from the Library of Congress.

Note
Neither the Publisher nor the Authors assume any responsibility for any loss or injury and/or damage to persons or property arising out of or related to any use of the material contained in this book. It is the responsibility of the treating practitioner, relying on independent expertise and knowledge of the patient, to determine the best treatment and method of application for the patient.

Printed in China

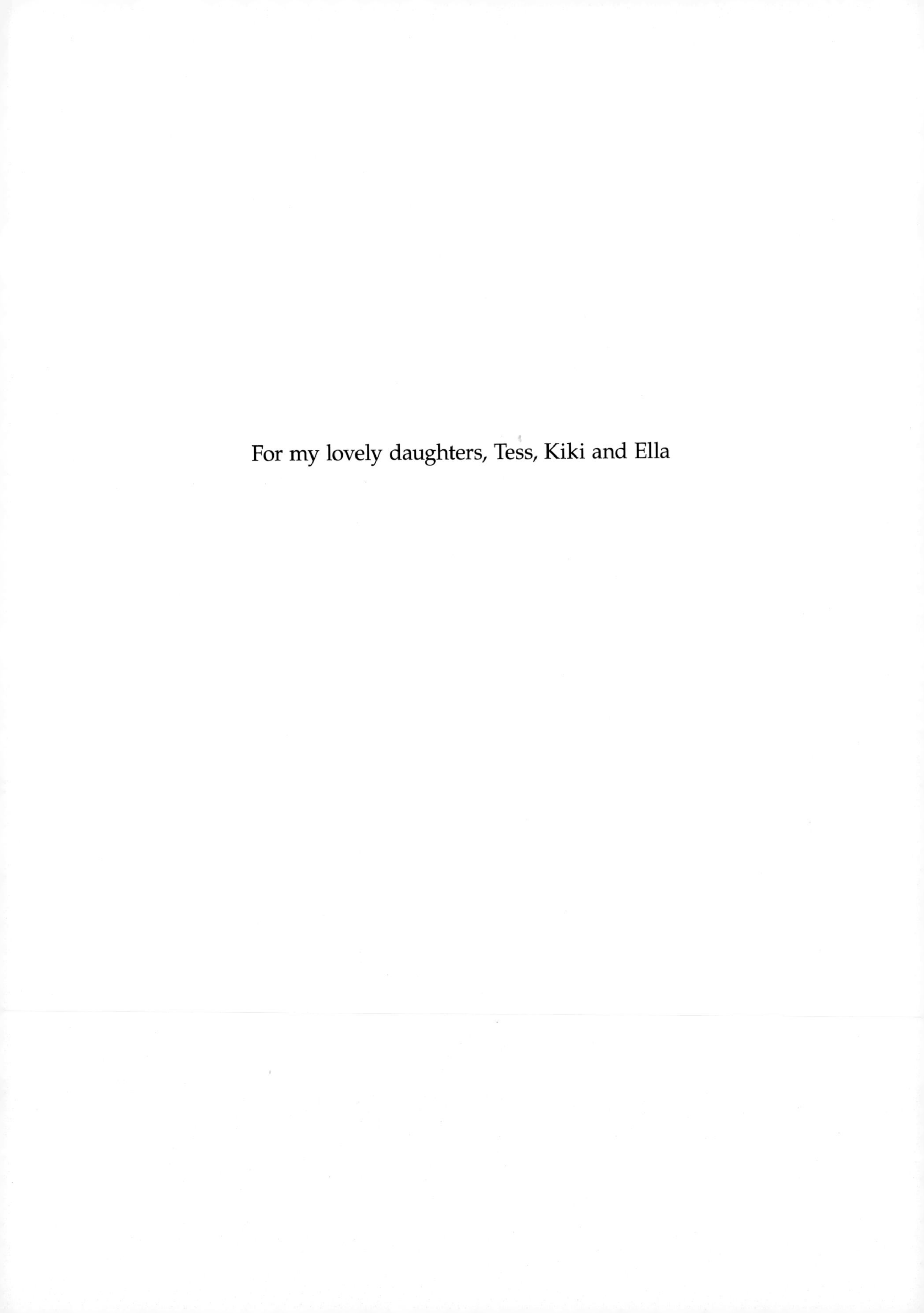

For my lovely daughters, Tess, Kiki and Ella

Contents

Preface

The original idea for a book in this format dates back more than 15 years. The driving forces were my interest in the treatment of patients with craniofacial dysfunction and pain, the great number of patients and the many unanswered questions regarding the treatment of such patients. During my manual therapy training in the Maitland Concept from 1988 to 1992 in Bad Ragaz and Zurzach (Switzerland), and later during my teacher training by the International Maitland Teacher Association (IMTA®), Geoff Maitland asked me to standardize the existing techniques and to classify clinical patterns. In 1994, at the end of teacher training, I was given the opportunity to treat his wife Ann with craniofacial and neural techniques for her persisting headache symptoms. Luckily for me, the final result was satisfying. After one month the frequency and intensity of her headaches were reduced and the symptoms were no longer provoked at night. But I did not understand the mechanisms that improved the symptoms that had for so many years affected her life so severely. I believe that Ann represented a great number of patients that were diagnosed with atypical facial pain, resistant to therapy. Many of these patients seemed to respond positively to a systematic manual therapy approach to the craniofacial region. This was the trigger to publish the book *Craniofacial Dysfunction and Pain: Manual Therapy, Assessment and Management* in 2001. Explanatory models and ideas based on the literature and the resulting suggestions for neuromusculoskeletal treatment techniques abounded. The final aim to standardize manual techniques and to classify clinical patterns relevant for physiotherapists, manual therapists and other clinicians such as dentists and orthodontists could not be realized sufficiently in that first attempt.

It is therefore the intention of this book to provide an overview of the various standardized techniques in the craniocervical, craniomandibular and cranioneural regions for the differential diagnostic process and therapy. The techniques are described in detail and photographs and illustrations are added. Recent biomedical and clinical knowledge from the fields of neurosurgery, plastic surgery, dental medicine and orthodontics is discussed in great detail since most therapists are not familiar with these publications although they may be important for the clinical decision-making process. Furthermore, a great number of references are given, so that the reader may easily gain access to more background information via the internet. However, there is insufficient evidence for the reliability and validity of these techniques.

Generally, this book consists of six main topics:

- The first part (Chapters 1–4) provides the reader with details about the epidemiology, aetiology, classification and models of thinking (Chapter 1), clinical anatomy (Chapter 2), guidelines for assessment and treatment (Chapter 3) and communication strategies that optimize the interaction with patients suffering from craniofacial or craniomandibular dysfunction and pain (Chapter 4).

- Chapters 5–7 focus on the craniocervical region. Two phenomena that I believe are underrated by most physiotherapists and manual therapists are the counteraction of the craniocervical and craniomandibular regions and the commonly unrecognized cervical instability.
- The craniomandibular region is presented in detail in Chapters 8–13. Chapter 8 discusses assessment and differentiation tests, and treatment suggestions for the various myogenic and arthrogenic structures are discussed in Chapter 9. Chapter 10 provides information about the different types of dysgnathia from the orthodontic perspective and the use of neuromuscularly adjusted braces as well as their influence on the movement system, especially the craniocervical region. This is followed by Chapters 12 and 13 that explain the physiotherapy concept.
- Part 4 outlines manual therapy assessment and treatment of the neurocranium and the viscerocranium (Chapters 14 and 15). With an open model of thinking, the various standard techniques and clinical indications are presented.
- The cranial nervous system is the central topic of the fifth part of this book. The evaluation of the cranial nervous system by conduction tests, palpation and neurodynamic tests is presented in Chapter 17, with Chapter 18 suggesting treatment guidelines supported by various examples.
- Due to the increasing incidence of craniofacial problems in children, the last part of the book is focused on the assessment and evaluation of juvenile headache patients and children that show craniofacial and craniocervical dysfunction while suffering from respiratory problems. Some case studies, typical for the daily physiotherapy clinic, conclude this book.

To summarize: the book provides you with ideas and techniques regarding the jaw, face and neck based on current evidence and clinical reasoning. It offers the opportunity to expand the horizon for this group of patients, supported by (new) manual therapy techniques and communication strategies. I hope that it will also stimulate research in this field to increase the amount of reference data for the tests, effect studies and randomized controlled trials. The most important aim is to improve the quality of treatment for the increasing group of patients of all ages that suffer from symptoms in the jaw, face or neck region, which, until now, have not been fully understood.

Harry J. M. von Piekartz
October 2006

Acknowledgements

A book like this cannot be written single handedly. Its realization requires the support of committed others (also in the close environment). I would hereby like to thank various persons for their contributions, always conscious that I may not be able to mention everyone.

Firstly, I would like to thank my co-authors – Prof. Drs G. Bekkering, Dr B. Lossert-Bruggner, Prof. Dr M. Hülse, Dr A. Werres, Dr A. Handrock, P. Westerhuis, E. Hengeveld, D. Andriotti, R. Horst, Dr R. Jordaan – who spontaneously provided their specific contributions and always respected the deadlines. Without them, the book would not have the contents it has now.

Thank you to all the people who helped with the translations and who critically read and corrected the manuscripts: Thomas Horre, Michaela Bulling, Barbara Untersulzer, Renee de Ruyter, Peter Schuster, Christian Voith, Paul Kubben, Hetty Schutman and especially during the final phase: Daniela Doppelhofer, Susi Jacob-Wittling and Paul Kubben.

I owe great thanks to Dr. Anton de Wijer (PT, MT, University of Utrecht), Prof. Drs Geert Bekkering (Saxion University, Enschede), G. Maitland (MSc PT, MT), David Butler (MSc PT, NOI), Pieter Westerhuis (PT, Principal Maitland Teacher IMTA) and Elly Hengeveld (MSc, Senior Teacher IMTA) for their competent support. Conversations and discussions during the past 5 years about their specific knowledge and experience importantly contributed to the structure and the content of this book.

I should also like to thank professional bodies such as the International Maitland Teachers Association (IMTA), the Neuro-Orthopaedic Institute (NOI), the International College of Craniomandibular Orthopaedics (ICCMO)-DE and the Craniofacial Therapy Academy (CRAFTA). In agreement with various colleagues from various organizations, a further education programme was developed that achieved positive feedback from the students. This was a tremendous enrichment and indicated how this book should be structured.

The comprehensive photos in this book are due to Paul Kubben, whose excellent photographic knowledge, combined with his professional skills as a CRAFTA teacher, allowed him to produce material that shows all techniques in the best possible way. The same is true for Dr Geert Bekkering. His insight into the functional anatomy is unique and is reflected by the exceptional anatomical pictures in the book. Thank you also to our colleague Heike Hoos-Leistner, who maintained her good sense of humour and motivation during some long and tedious photo sessions in sometimes strenuous positions.

My sincere gratitude also to all patients and parents who spontaneously agreed to have their photos printed in this book. All understood immediately that this will positively contribute to a better understanding and a better therapy for patients with craniofacial dysfunction and pain.

The book could never have come to fruition so quickly for English-speaking readers without the close collaboration with Kerstin Lüdtke (MSc, PT, MT). Her translation skills combined with her professional knowledge in this field allowed a quick and efficient integration of updates.

Thanks are also due to the Elsevier team, especially to Siobhan Campbell and Heidi Harrison, for their professional attitude. The close cooperation with the German publishers (Thieme-Verlag) greatly enhanced the realization of this project. The final product, the book you are now holding in your hands, is a satisfying result for the publishers as well as for the editor.

Last but not least, the home-front: Tess, Kiki, Ella and Daan. A great amount of family time has been invested in this book during the past year. I thank you for your understanding and the always positive and stimulating input that contributed to the realization of this book.

About the author

Harry J. M. von Piekartz qualified as a physiotherapist in 1984 and completed his manual therapy training in Switzerland (Maitland Concept) in 1988. In 1993 he gained his IFOMT recognition in the Netherlands from the Dutch Manual Therapy Association (NVMT). In 1994 he passed the IMTA (International Maitland Teacher Association) Manual Therapy instructor training and also got involved in the NOI (Neuro-Orthopaedic Institute). His main interests are difficult head, neck and face problems and he treats patients in his practice in Rijssen and Ootmarsum in the Netherlands. This stimulated him to write and edit the book *Craniofacial Dysfunctions and Pain, Manual Therapy, Assessment and Management* that was published by Butterworth-Heinemann in 2001. This book was also translated into German (2001) and Spanish (2003). In 2000 he completed his Master of Science in Physiotherapy at the University of Leuven (Belgium) on the subject 'The neurodynamic test of the mandibular nerve, reliability and normal values'.

In 2002 he was one of the main initiators of the Cranial Facial Therapy Academy (CRAFTA®), an organization that has now developed into three dynamic branches: education, association and a research group. In March 2004 he became Fellow of the International College of CranioMandibular Orthopaedics (ICCMO) in Germany. During this period he published several articles about this subject and was involved in two comparative studies about headache in children. He began to prepare the book about 'head, neck and face pain' and finished his PhD in July 2005. Since 1999 he has spent 50% of his time teaching in different countries in Europe, lecturing at the University of Applied Sciences in Osnabrüch (Germany), 30% working with patients and 20% in research.

Contributors

Dianne Andriotti BSc(PT)
Kinetic Control Accredited Tutor
Physiotherapist, Gordola, Switzerland

Geert H. Bekkering MSc
Professor, Anatomy and Physiology, Saxion Hogeschool Enschede, Academy of Paramedical Studies, Enschede, The Netherlands

Anke Handrock PhD
Dentist, Berlin, Germany

Renata Horst PT OMT
International PNF Instructor
Private Physiotherapist and Manual Therapist, Bad Kvozingen, Germany

Manfred Hülse Prof, PhD
Head of Department of Phoniatry, Paedaudiology and Neurology
University of Heidelberg, Mannheim, Germany

Ronel Jordaan PhD, PT
Lecturer, University of Pretoria, South Africa

Brigitte Losert-Bruggner PhD
Private Dental Practitioner, Lampertheim-Hüttenfeld, Germany

Harry von Piekartz PhD, MSc, PT, MT
Physiotherapist, Ootmarsum, The Netherlands
Teacher, International Maitland Teacher Association, Neuro-Orthopaedic Institute

Antonia Werres PhD
Orthodontist, Neumünster, Germany

Pieter Westerhuis BPT, PTOMTsvomp®
Principal IMTA Teacher, Grenchen, Switzerland

Chapter 1

Craniofacial dysfunction and pain: where are we today?

Harry von Piekartz

CHAPTER CONTENTS

INTRODUCTION

Craniofacial dysfunction and pain (disorders of the head or face) occur in a quarter of the population of the industrialized world. Only a small proportion of cases require treat-ment (De Kanter et al 1993, Carlsson & Magnusson 1999). The majority of symptoms, such as headaches with or without dizziness, tinnitus, atypical toothache of long duration, and unpleasant sensations in the face, are difficult to classify, and diagnoses in this group of patients may vary depending on the clinical knowledge of the treatment provider (Zakrzewska & Hamlyn 1999). As various professions – including dentists, orthodontists, chiropractors, osteopaths and physiotherapists – are involved in the treatment of these disorders, countless clinical approaches exist, but there are no explicit clinical guidelines (Jones & Rivett 2004).

Detailed guidelines for assessment and management of lower back pain and neck disorders are available for physiotherapists and manual therapists (Jull & Moore 2002). National and international guidelines have been published and there is general agreement on standard procedures (Hendriksen et al 2003). This stands in stark contrast to craniofacial dysfunction for which there are no clear guidelines for physiotherapists and manual therapists.

The aim of this chapter, which is in five sections, is to provide a basis for the following chapters of this book. Firstly, the incidence and aetiology of craniofacial dysfunction and pain are dealt with. The most common classification systems are presented and the development of the clinical approaches of various professions is discussed.

This is followed by basic clinical reasoning (thinking and decision-making processes in clinical practice; Jones & Rivett 2004) to support the physiotherapist in day-to-day practice.

Because of the scope of this book, the reader should decide for themselves which chapters are initially most relevant to them and start with those.

The following themes are covered in this chapter:

- Epidemiology, prevalence, incidence
- Aetiology
- Classification and definitions
- Development of clinical approaches
- Clinical reasoning model for the assessment and treatment of neuromusculoskeletal dysfunction by physiotherapists.

EPIDEMIOLOGY, PREVALENCE AND INCIDENCE

It is not the intention of this section to provide unnecessary detail of epidemiological studies, but rather to give the reader an overview of our current state of knowledge. Nevertheless, there are obviously several publications that cannot be overlooked.

When studying publications from the past two decades, the extent to which the incidence of headaches and facial pain in the industrialized world has increased seems surprising (Zakrzewska & Hamlyn 1999). However, care is required in interpreting these results because the majority of studies use variable criteria for (chronic) craniofacial pain and mandibular disorders (Zakrzewska & Hamlyn 1999, Woda & Pionchon 2000).

In a literature review of 24 epidemiological studies (varying substantially in methods and populations) of pain syndromes originating (by criteria of signs and symptoms) from the craniocervical region, LeResche concluded that more than 10% of the population over the age of 18 years experience severe impairment in everyday activities (LeResche 1997). Locker and Slade (1988) investigated facial pain caused by regions other than the craniomandibular area. In a randomized representative population investigated by questionnaire with a 1-month evaluation period, 27% experienced facial pain only, 13% pain and discomfort, and 4.9% experienced severe, acute facial pain. However, it remained unclear whether the symptoms were dental, craniomandibular or facial in origin.

Recently an especially designed questionnaire was distributed to a representative German population (n = 7124) above the age of 18. The prevalence of craniofacial pain was between 7% (for 7 days) and 16% (for 12 months). Conspicuously, quality of life – measured by the SF36 questionnaire – was perceived as significantly reduced for five out of the six subscales. Additional results showed that 43% of the participants who suffered more than 7 days of craniofacial symptoms also experienced pain in five or more areas of the body. The authors concluded that one out of six adults in Western Europe suffers from craniofacial pain once a year (Kohlmann 2002).

A randomized prospective study of 516 subjects between the ages of 20 and 60 showed that 9–10% experienced craniofacial pain. Only 6% of these clearly showed a craniomandibular dysfunction based on the Helkimo-Index (questionnaire) and clinical tests (John & Wefers 1999, Bernhardt et al 2001, John et al 2001). In a similar study, LeResche concluded that 2–6% of all craniofacial pain syndromes derive clearly from mandibular movements (LeResche 1997). Neither study distinguished between specific and non-specific craniomandibular dysfunction and pain.

Men and women

Various studies differentiate between patients with pain due to craniomandibular dysfunction and craniofacial pain that is not directly related to the craniofacial region. Both types of syndrome occur more commonly in women than in men (Lupton 1969, Deubner 1977, von Korff et al 1993, Lemka 1999, McGrath & Koster 2001).

In his literature review, LeResche (1997) stated that pain unambiguously related to craniomandibular dysfunction occurs 1.5–2.5 times more frequently in women than in men, and suggests aetiological investigation of biological and psychological factors that are more common in women than in men and which diminish in older age groups.

Children and adolescents

A cross-sectional study of 2358 schoolchildren (10–17 years) showed that 21% of boys and 26% of girls in elementary school and 14% of boys and 28% of girls in secondary education suffer on average one episode per week of headache or facial pain (Bandell-Hoekstra et al 2001). By comparison to an earlier investigation (Passchier & Orlebeke 1985), the average occurrence of weekly headache in children increased by 6% between 1985 and 2001.

A meta-analysis of 21 studies (Drangsholt & LeResche 1999) found considerable variation of craniomandibular pain in children and adolescents, ranging from 0.7% of all children between the ages of 11 and 16 experiencing severe pain (Sieber et al 1997) to 18.6% in a Finnish group of children aged between 12 and 15 years (Heikinheimo et al 1989). The prevalence of craniomandibular dysfunction in children between 7 and 15 years was estimated at 2–6% (Drangsholt & LeResche 1999).

In a study of 1243 American children between the ages of 10 and 20 years, Lipton et al (1993) showed that the prevalence of craniomandibular pain increases significantly in the second half of the second decade of life. Beyond the age of 20 there is a clear decrease (Lipton et al 1993). The results of similar studies do not show consistent outcomes but methods, population and prevalence vary greatly (Drangsholt & LeResche 1999).

As mentioned above, this is not an extensive list but hopefully it leaves the reader with the impression that craniofacial dysfunction and pain is a serious problem in our society and severely reduces the quality of life of those affected. Further insight into the aetiology of these syndromes might help to explain and understand the prevalence and point towards a more purposeful treatment approach.

ETIOLOGICAL FACTORS

The orthodontic profession has contributed to the idea that aetiology is frequently multidimensional. It is the aim of orthodontists to gently influence cranial and mandibular growth with the aid of braces. Guided by cephalometry, a prognosis of cranial shape can be made (Proffit & Fields 1993, von Piekartz 2001).

As with other disciplines, orthodontistry offers various approaches to problems of occlusion which produce the desired results (Kamann 1999). Despite generally good outcomes, orthodontistry cannot provide clear answers when the desired outcome was not achieved, and it remains unclear whether, in some cases, craniofacial growth guided by braces is identical to that which would have been achieved by natural, physiological growth (Vig et al 1981, Henneberke & Prahl-Andersen 1994).

Until the 1990s craniomandibular dysfunction tended to be explained by joint or muscle deficits based on irregular occlusion patterns or disc lesions (Greene 2001). During this period dentistry and orthodontistry were increasingly challenged by epidemiological studies showing that joint dysfunction such as disc problems does not necessarily directly correlate with temporomandibular and facial complaints (Schiffmann et al 1992, 1995). Although malocclusion was also questioned as a direct cause of pain (Papadopoulos 2003), a number of longitudinal studies showed contradictory results and the long-term outcomes of brace therapy appeared to be only moderately satisfactory (Koh & Robinson 2003, Al-Ani et al 2004).

From a tissue-based to a biopsychosocial approach

Probably only a minority of craniofacial problems are due to a single cause. The majority of problems are multifactorial and may be structural–functional (e.g. occlusion trauma), psychosocial (coping strategies) or systemic (rheumatoid arthritis, fibromyalgia). These factors may interfere with each other (Carlsson & Magnusson 1999). As a result, most recent publications show a shift from local tissue-based explanations to multifactorial biopsychosocial explanatory models (Dworkin & Burgess 1987, Okeson 2005). Consequently, it may be concluded that a number of complex factors lead to the development of the range of symptoms experienced by any particular patient. Oral habits, malocclusion, behavioural factors, muscle dysfunction, hormonal influences and emotional–affective reactions such as stress and fear have all been described as influencing symptoms (Greene 2001).

Due to this new model of thinking (neuromuscular, multistructural, biopsychosocial) and the mounting evidence that contributory factors play an important role, the question of the 'real cause' remains unanswered (Rugh & Davis 1992, Greene 2001). In agreement with the modern physiotherapy paradigm, the old dualistic specification models are replaced by new multistructural and multidisciplinary treatment approaches, individualized to each patient.

No single therapeutic method has been shown to be effective in patients with craniofacial pain syndromes of various aetiological backgrounds (Greene 2001). However, this is not true for specific (aetiologically clearly identified) craniofacial pain (e.g. a patient who suffers from traumatic craniomandibular irritation or from toothache due to a local inflammatory process); in such cases the majority of targeted treatments will be effective and the natural course of the disease will improve (Lobbezoo-Scholte et al 1995).

In-depth studies of the connection between nociceptive mechanisms and neuroplasticity leading to chronic facial pain and headaches are needed (Woda & Pionchon 2000). Reversible, non-invasive treatment procedures that do not injure the tissue are preferred to invasive techniques (Okeson 1996, Woda & Pionchon 2000, Greene 2001). Physiotherapy and manual therapy can make a valuable contribution to this non-invasive approach.

CLASSIFICATION AND DEFINITIONS

Classification problems arise from a lack of agreement regarding aetiological factors and their reciprocal interaction (Mongini 1999).

Various aspects are relevant:

- Different aetiological factors may apply for one patient
- The same aetiological factors may lead to different consequences in different patients
- Symptoms due to craniofacial dysfunction may be influenced by general or systemic factors including hormonal, neural, vascular or psychosocial
- The range of symptoms is due mainly to general/other factors but localized symptoms may either increase or mask the problem (e.g. toothache) (Mongini 1999).

In this section the three most common classification systems are discussed: those of the IHS (International Headache Society), the AAOP (American Academy of Orofacial Pain) and the IASP (International Association for the Study of Pain).

IHS

The International Headache Society uses a classification system of 13 levels (IHS 1988; Box 1.1). This system is most useful for clinical diagnosis (IHS 2004).

AAOP

The AAOP divides temporomandibular pain disorders into physical (Axis I) and psychosocial (Axis II) components. This classification is more useful for research rather than clinical practice. Further factors, such as complexity level and prognosis, are described (Okeson 1995; Box 1.2).

Box 1.1 Classification of headaches, cranial neuralgia and facial pain

1. Migraine headache
2. Tension-type headache (TTH)
3. Cluster headache and other trigeminal autonomic cephalgia
4. Other primary headache
5. Headache attributed to head and/or neck trauma
6. Headache attributed to cranial or cervical vascular disorder
7. Headache attributed to non-vascular intracranial disorder
8. Headache attributed to a substance or its withdrawal
9. Headache attributed to infection
10. Headache attributed to disorder of homeostasis
11. Headache or facial pain attributed to disorder of cranium, neck, eyes, ears, nose, sinuses, teeth, mouth or other facial or cranial structures
12. Headache attributed to psychiatric disorders
13. Cranial neuralgias and central causes of facial pain
14. Other headache, cranial neuralgia, central or primary facial pain

From IHS (2004). For more information or free download of the classification, see www.i-h-s.org.

Box 1.2 Proposed classification of the American Academy of Orofacial Pain (AAOP) in two axes

Axis I

Intracranial disorders

- Neoplasm, aneurysm, abscess, haemorrhage, haematoma, oedema

Primary headache disorders (neurovascular disorders)

- Migraine, migraine variants, cluster headache, paroxysmal hemicranial headache, cranial arthritis, carotodynia, tension-type headache
  - Neurogenic disorders
- Neuralgias
  - Trigeminal, glossopharyngeal, intermedial nerve and superior laryngeal nerve neuralgias
- Continuous pain disorders
  - Deafferentation pain syndromes
  - Peripheral neuritis, postherpetic neuralgia, post-traumatic and postsurgical neuralgia
- Symptomatically maintained pain
  - Intraoral pain disorders
  - Dental pulp, periodontium, mucogingival tissues and tongue
- Temporomandibular disorders
  - Masticatory muscle, temporomandibular joint, associated structures
- Associated structures
  - Ears, eyes, nose, sinuses, throat, lymph nodes, salivary glands and neck

Axis II

Mental disorders

- Somatoform disorders
- Pain syndromes of psychogenic origin

From AAOP and Okeson (1996).

IASP

This classification system is based on an axial 5-figure code system (Merksey & Bogduk 1994).

The five axes represent the regions of pain. The system is constructed as follows:

- Localization of symptoms (axis 1)
- The causative system (axis 2)
- Timing of symptoms (axis 3)
- Intensity (axis 4)
- Aetiology (axis 5).

Craniofacial pain and headache are differentiated on axis 1 into subgroups as shown in Box 1.3.

One important difference between these classification systems is that the IASP classification aims mainly to *describe* symptoms and dysfunction while the AAOP and IHS work on the basis of a structural diagnosis and associated medical tests. For example, the IASP differentiates between classic migraine, general migraine and hybrid headache, while the IHS classifies migraine with or without aura. The 'mixed' headache is listed as 'migraine without aura' and 'chronic tension headache'.

Box 1.3 Classification of headaches and neck pain in various subgroups* on axis I (IASP)

- Group II: neuralgia of the head and the face
- Group III: craniofacial pain of musculoskeletal origin
- Group IV: ear, nose or mouth injury
- Group V: primary headache syndrome, vascular dysfunction, cerebrospinal fluid syndrome
- Group VI: pain of psychological origin in head, face or neck
- Group VII: suboccipital and cervical musculoskeletal dysfunction

* Group I are 'relatively generalized syndromes' and are not mentioned here.

Recently the diagnostic title 'non-specific facial pain' has been used increasingly (Zakrzewska & Hamlyn 1999). In the latest IASP issue (1994) non-specific facial pain is listed as 'temporomandibular joint syndrome'. The same title applies to non-specific odontalgia and otalgia that are unrelated to any specific pathology or syndrome. The latest IHS classification (2004) describes non-specific facial pain as 'facial pain that does not fulfil any of the mentioned criteria' (code 13).

In summary, it can be said that the three above-mentioned classification systems vary widely. Attempts at classification are an important first step to improve the communication between treatment provider and patient. Nevertheless, it is difficult for physiotherapists to decide which classification system to adopt. The therapist should focus on movement and function classifications in which the physiotherapy profession specializes. The most widely known system is the International Classification of Function (ICF) which will be discussed later, but it is also important for interdisciplinary communication and clinimetry to be aware of the other systems.

Classifications and compatibility with diagnoses

If the clinical data do not fit neatly into guidelines and classifications, the concept of 'atypical facial pain' or 'migraine (without aura)' is often used. A number of studies confirm this:

- Solomon et al (1992) assessed the data of 100 patients with headaches and concluded that more than a third fell into the categories of chronic tension type headache or migraine according to the IHS system. Other similar investigations (Manzoni et al 1995, Mongini et al 1997, Mongini 1999) confirmed this.
- Of 251 volunteers with cluster headache, more than half were diagnosed incorrectly using the IHS classification (Nappi et al 1992).
- Of a group of 2691 children, 46% between the ages of 6 and 16 suffered more than two episodes of headache lasting for more than

2 days per year. Of this group, 56% did not meet the IHS diagnostic criteria and the symptoms were classified as 'non-specific headaches' (van Duin et al 2000).
- The IHS system shows high specificity and low sensitivity for migraine (Maytal et al 1997, Viswanathan et al 1998) whereas for tension headaches the opposite is true (Wörter-Bingö et al 1996). (NB: These studies are based upon the first IHS edition from 1988. No comparisons with the new edition are available at present.)

Case study 1.1 illustrates a physiotherapeutic approach.

According to the traditional classification schemes a number of different diagnoses match the described syndrome:

- Post-traumatic headache (IASP), minor craniocerebral trauma without confirming signs (IHS).
  Reason: previous history, prolonged facial pain with vertigo and concentration deficits, post-traumatic stress.
- Ordinary migraine (without aura) (IASP), migraine with aura (IHS).
  Reason: unilateral pulsating pain, photophobia, phonophobia.
- Temporomandibular pain and dysfunction syndrome (IASP) or tension-type headaches with oromandibular dysfunction.
  Reason: unilateral pain, joint clicking, bruxism.
- Atypical odontalgia (IASP), headaches or facial pain in combination with dental, oral or other facial and cranial dysfunctions (IHS).
  Reason: toothache without pathology combined with emotional problems (stress), frequently associated with symptoms deriving from the temporomandibular joint.

Case study 1.1

Jan is a 38-year-old policeman who suffers from facial pain unilaterally on his right side (see Fig. 1.1, p. 14). The symptoms are perceived as a diffuse pressure in the zygomatic region. If the pressure increases and lasts for a couple of hours he also experiences a pulsating headache on the right side of his forehead accompanied by a sensation of dizziness and difficulty concentrating. This severely impairs the performance of his professional duties. To reduce his symptoms he needs to rest in a cool, dark room for a few hours. Stress and prolonged talking increase the symptoms. The mandibular joint occasionally produces a clicking noise and the symptoms seem to worsen when the clicking occurs. The patient has a history of bruxism and still uses a brace at night. Sometimes the brace relieves the symptoms but not always. He has noticed that the bruxism has increased with the facial symptoms.

Four years ago he was hit in the face by an object during an arrest. Trauma was superficial with no fractures and 3 months after the incident the pain had disappeared. One year ago two teeth in his right posterior jaw were extracted and he was provided with a bridge. He then perceived a burning pain in his upper jaw that was referred to the zygomatic region. The symptoms were treated by medication but the pressure/pain in the zygoma remains to this day. Sometimes the toothache increases, for example when he has a cold, after swimming in cold water and during stress. The dentist has excluded pulpitis, periodontitis and abscess. The neurologists did not find a space-occupying lesion.

It should therefore be cautiously concluded that classification of craniofacial dysfunction and pain is not straightforward. This is certainly due at least in part to unknown aetiology. The physiotherapist will need to address this problem and develop an adequate assessment and treatment strategy to cope with the uncertain diagnosis, aetiology and prognosis. The following section will explain a clinical reasoning model that, in the author's opinion, reflects the modern scientific point of view and the latest developments in the field of craniocervical dysfunction and pain (Boxes 1.4, 1.5).

Box 1.4 Synonyms for dysfunction and pain of the craniomandibular region

- Costen syndrome (Costen 1934)
- Dysfunction of the temporomandibular joint (Schwartz 1926)
- Oromandibular dysfunction (IHS 2004)
- Craniomandibular dysfunction (Naeije & Van Loon 1998)
- Craniomandibular interference (Kraus 1994)
- Craniofacial interference (Proffit & Ackerman 1993)
- Stomatognathic system dysfunction (Freesmeyer 1993)
- Chewing dysfunction (Jáger 1997)
- Jaw joint dysfunction (Hansson et al 1992, Perthes & Gross 1995)
- Myoarthropathia of the masticatory system (MAK) (Palla et al 1998)

Box 1.5 Synonyms widely used for headaches and facial dysfunction/pain

- Orofacial pain (Okeson 1996, Lund et al 2000)
- Craniofacial dysfunction and pain (Merksey & Bogduk 1994)
- Facial pain (Mahan & Alling 1991, Mongini 1999)
- Maxillary facial pain (Rocabado & Iglash 1991)
- Idiopathic orofacial pain (Woda & Pionchon 2000)

PHYSIOTHERAPEUTIC DEVELOPMENTS IN THE TREATMENT OF CRANIOMANDIBULAR AND CRANIOFACIAL DYSFUNCTION AND PAIN

Various physiotherapy and manual therapy concepts of the 1960s and 1970s described specific joint and muscle techniques for the treatment of craniomandibular dysfunction (Evjenth & Hamburg 1984, Maitland 1986). Publications by physiotherapists in well-known journals and books about the functional relationship between the craniocervical and the craniomandibular region have had a positive influence on the development of a specialized field within the physiotherapy profession (Kraus 1988, Makosfky et al 1991, Rocabado & Iglash 1991, de Wijer et al 1996). The potential of physiotherapy became increasingly recognized by dentists, and cooperation between physiotherapists, dentists and orthodontists was established. However, the functional assessment and treatment of the cranium itself within the specialized fields of paediatric physiotherapy and manual therapy still seems to be widely ignored.

Although most scientific physiotherapy research is performed in the fields of back and neck pain (Jull & Moore 2002), there is an increasing interest in evidence-based approaches to the craniofacial and craniomandibular region (von Piekartz 2002).

Critically, however, too many efficacy studies are carried out by researchers with no physiotherapy training, and who therefore do not know the clinical concept of modern physiotherapy: a hypothesis-guided model which allows the investigation and analysis of movement disorders (von Piekartz 2002). Based on the results of the physiotherapy and manual therapy assessment, different treatment approaches are chosen. However, studies frequently apply the same method of treatment for every patient. The wrong conclusion, that physiotherapy does not work, is then frequently made (von Piekartz 2002).

Considering the great variability of craniomandibular and craniofacial pain syndromes, and the number of practice uncertainties such as test validity, prognosis and aetiology, it might not be sufficient for the physiotherapist to follow only one model of thinking (Higgs & Jones 1997). The clinical reasoning model is a clinical concept that allows the consideration of various approaches (anatomical, biomechanical, biopsychosocial, etc.) and for which the patient, as an individual, is central. It will be described in detail in the following section.

CLINICAL REASONING: A CLINICAL MODEL OF THINKING FOR THE ASSESSMENT AND TREATMENT OF PATIENTS WITH CRANIOFACIAL DYSFUNCTION AND PAIN*

Introduction

Physiotherapists in many countries work on prescriptions by medical doctors. The doctor decides upon a biomedical diagnosis, whereas the physiotherapist will produce a working diagnosis and treatment plan based upon their own model of thinking. The physiotherapy diagnosis incorporates, initially, a mobility and status diagnosis based on the ICF classification (WHO 2001). The biomedical diagnosis usually does not point towards treatment goals, but remains essential when identifying contraindications, critical situations and prognosis (Jones & Rivett 2004).

The physiotherapist should evaluate the findings of the individual patient regarding movement dysfunction, previous history and personal perception of the problem, before deciding upon a treatment plan (Hengeveld 1998/1999). Particularly among patients with chronic craniofacial pain syndromes of unknown (or partly known) aetiology the assessment and treatment with non-invasive techniques is strongly recommended (Greene 2001).

Where we are today – the job descriptions of the WCPT and the ICF

The physiotherapy profession increasingly follows the biopsychosocial paradigm (Hengeveld 1998a). The profession is currently defined by the World Confederation of Physical Therapy as follows:

> *A health care profession which deals with people to maintain and restore maximum movement and functional ability throughout the life span. Physical therapy is particularly important in circumstances where movement and function are threatened by the process of ageing, or that of injury or disease. It places full and functional movement at the heart of what it means to be healthy.*
>
> *WCPT (1999).*

Furthermore, it is suggested in the description of the physiotherapy profession that the body of knowledge, supported by scientific investigations, should be based upon movement and rehabilitation sciences (Cott et al 1995, de Vries & Wimmers 1997, NPI 1997). A movement continuum accommodating all concepts of physiotherapy is recommended (Hislop 1975, Cott et al 1995).

Physiotherapists and manual therapists will emphasize the analysis and, if appropriate, the treatment of movement disorders for craniofacial dysfunction and pain. This focus on movement makes a unique contribution to the overall management of such symptoms (KNGF 1992). For example, a doctor or dentist refers a patient with the diagnosis 'restricted mouth opening without obvious cause' to the physiotherapist. Analysis by the physiotherapist reveals that acute limitations arose following a (harmless – according to the patient) fall onto the face while playing handball, and that excessive consumption of apples further increases symptoms. According to the specialized physiotherapy assessment this clearly indicates an accident and motion sequence. Accessory movements, especially of the left craniomandibular area, are restricted and painful. There are also trigger points in the masseter and temporal muscles on the left side. Hence, from the physiotherapy point of view there are clear causes for the symptoms.

In addition to the predominantly diagnostic classification systems of the IHS, AAOP and IASP, it is also important to the physiotherapist to identify and classify relevant movement dysfunctions and changes in movement behaviour (Maluf et al 2000).

The movement paradigm of the physiotherapy profession is reflected in the ICF terminology that classifies movement dysfunction at the levels of impairment, activity and participation (WHO 2001).

* This section was written in collaboration with Elly Hengeveld MSc, B.PT, OMTsvomp, SVEB I, M.IMTA.

- Examples of *impairment* include cranial asymmetries, mouth opening deficits and dysfunction found during the assessment of head, neck and face.
- *Activities* are defined as functions that the patient is unable to perform due to their problem, examples of which include speaking, singing, non-verbal facial expressions and concentration.
- *Participation* may encompass social isolation and 'being laughed at' due to difficulties in (non-)verbal communication.

The classification of the clinical problem of movement and behaviour supports the identification of treatment goals and the establishment of priorities (Hengeveld 1998b). This classification is shown in Table 1.1 and clarified using an example.

Although there is a paucity of randomized clinical trials and efficacy studies within the field of craniomandibular/craniofacial dysfunction and pain, physiotherapists may still contribute to the decision as to whether physiotherapy is beneficial for the various craniofacial syndromes. Thorough and conscious clinical reasoning (Higgs & Jones 2000) with subsequent analysis of treatment outcomes (Maitland et al 2001) is needed to decide upon the appropriate treatment technique (Butler

Table 1.1 Classification of the clinical aspects of craniofacial dysfunction: movement and behaviour

Function	Activity	Impairment	Participation
Mouth opening	Limited mouth opening with a shift	Transverse movement of the mandibular caput is restricted and painful	Chewing impaired
Oculomotor movement	Looking to the right/ left impossible	Nerve conduction test of the abducens nerve positive; strabismus	Driving a car is difficult
Speech	Dysphagia	Tongue atrophy	Communication difficulties
Cranial growth	Breathing function impaired; regular sinus infections	Plagiocephaly; various craniofacial techniques are restricted and produce headaches	Concentration deficits due to the headaches
Non-verbal communication problems	Laughing	Restricted neurodynamics of the facial nerve	Finds it difficult to show emotions
Moving the head upwards	Pain and insecure feeling in the upper cervical spine	Instability tests of the apices of the transverse ligament are positive	Work impaired, e.g. overhead activities
Cognition	Belief that any pain-provoking movement causes injury (after whiplash)	Catastrophizing; passive behaviour	Communication difficulties with family and helpers
Affection	Fatigue and passive behaviour	(Unnecessary) feeling of guilt and depressive mood	Cannot share joy of life with friends

2000, Jones & von Piekartz 2001). Even if no 'gold standard' test (with generally accepted high validity) is available, it can still be very valuable in the clinical assessment and treatment procedure.

Clinical reasoning

Physiotherapists, other medical professionals and the research community have paid increasing attention to the clinical reasoning procedure over the past 20 years. The first studies about 'reasoning' were published in the 1950s and initially focused on the differences between expert and novice practitioners (Grant et al 1988, Grant 1995, Gruber 1999). Subsequently, not only the differences in behaviour but also in thinking and organization of knowledge were investigated. Recently researchers investigated the application of various models of thinking and the way the relationship between patient and therapist influences treatment (Hengeveld 1998a, Jones & Rivett 2004).

There are various descriptions and definitions of clinical reasoning. The most common definition for the physiotherapy profession is: 'the process of thinking and decision making that is the basis for clinical action' (Higgs & Jones 1997).

The WCPT definition (1999) includes clinical reasoning as a basic component of physiotherapy practice. Furthermore. Jones (1995) states that conscious clinical reasoning obviates uncritical application of fashionable theories, techniques and models without considering alternative theories and clinical interventions.

Clinical reasoning is therefore a learning process requiring reflection on, and sometimes modification of, thought processes, daily therapeutic decision-making and the therapist–patient relationship (Jones & Rivett 2004). Every patient contact therefore increases the experiential knowledge base of the individual therapist.

Within neuromusculoskeletal physiotherapy, clinical reasoning is applied mainly to treatment procedures. Physiotherapy training concentrates principally on the processes of history taking, physical examination, treatment and reassessment (Maitland et al 2001). In this way the therapist develops a number of hypotheses based on the available information which will then be refined, confirmed or dismissed during the course of treatment. Experienced therapists can generally give a more detailed and conclusive summary of their initial assessment than less experienced colleagues; both groups form hypotheses but only the more experienced therapists will categorize them (Thomas-Edding 1987). These categories of hypotheses are sometimes called *attention directors* (De Bono 1994) because they direct the focus of the physiotherapeutic process. The categories listed in Box 1.6 are common for musculoskeletal physiotherapy and are discussed in the remaining sections of this chapter.

PATHOBIOLOGICAL MECHANISMS*

Tissue healing and pathology

The majority of physiotherapists will find it fairly easy to create a hypothesis about the state of tissue healing and pathology, since this is part of the dominant model of thinking during their training. This also includes hypotheses about the grade of injury, acute vs. subacute, inflammation, wound healing, etc.

A retrodiscal irritation after disc derangement and reposition may cause inflammation with severe localized pain in the mandibular joint together with swelling and eventually lead to restricted movement. Treating this type of problem with a closely supervised exercise regime with several rest periods is recommended (Okeson 2005).

Pain

Classification of pain mechanisms is a fairly new paradigm in physiotherapy and other disciplines. The area where the pain is perceived does not necessarily reflect the injured tissue

* This section was written in collaboration with Elly Hengeveld MSc, B.PT, OMTsvomp, SVEB I, M.IMTA.

Box 1.6 Hypothetical categories frequently applied in neuromusculoskeletal physiotherapy

Pathobiological processes
The therapist forms hypotheses about the potential and dominant neurophysiological pain mechanisms such as nociceptive and peripheral neurogenic processes, the modulation of the pain experience by the central nervous system and autonomous procedures. The therapist further considers whether pathobiological tissue healing processes are important for the revalidation of movement at this stage.

Sources of movement dysfunction
In this category the therapist considers whether movement dysfunction and pain are caused dominantly by muscles, soft tissue, joints, neurodynamics, visceral structures and/or blood vessels.

Contributing factors
Any potential predisposing factor that may be responsible for the development or maintenance of the symptoms is evaluated. These factors may be physical, biomechanical, social, behavioural or affective.

Contraindications and risk factors for functional assessment and treatment
In this category proportionality of the assessment is determined and the therapist makes a decision as to whether physiotherapy is indicated in this particular case. This depends on the severity of the pain, the level of disability, the stability of the problem, the progression of the symptoms, the patient's general health status and their willingness to move.

Individual pain experience and behaviour
This is influenced by thoughts and beliefs, emotions, experience, future perspectives, environmental factors, coping strategies, knowledge and behaviour.

Management
Management depends on short- and long-term goals. These again depend on the limitations and resources according to the ICF (WHO 2001). Once the goals have been set, the best therapeutic interventions and their alternatives are determined. Risk factors are decisive for the intensity of interventions.

Prognosis
To make a prognosis not only for the following three to four sessions but also for the final treatment result is a complex but important process. The prognosis depends on:

- Pain intensity (irritability)
- Level of impairment
- Level of disability (ICF)
- Duration of previous history and progress of the problem
- Previous dysfunction
- Number of components to the problem (e.g. temporomandibular joint only or additional cervical movement dysfunction)
- Whether a unidimensional approach is sufficient or a multidimensional approach is necessary
- The expectations of the patient
- Cognitive, affective, sociocultural aspects and learning processes
- Movement behaviour of the patient
- Patient compliance.

Based on Jones (1995), Hengeveld (1998a), Butler (2000) and Jones & Rivett (2004).

but may depend upon individual central (biological) mechanisms (Butler 2000, Wall 2000). This means that pain may be present in the absence of pathology or dysfunction of the affected area and instead may be due to processes in the neuronal network. Recent years have seen a substantial increase in our understanding of the neurobiological origin of pain and an overview is presented below. Three levels can be differentiated (Gifford 1998a, Shacklock 1999a, 1999b), i.e. symptoms dependent on:

- Input (afferent) mechanisms
- Central mechanisms (central sensitization)
- Output (efferent) mechanisms.

Symptoms related to input (afferent) mechanisms

Two categories can be differentiated: nociceptive pain and peripheral neurogenic mechanisms.

NOCICEPTIVE PAIN

Mechanical, chemical or thermal stimuli in the skin, joints, connective tissue of the nervous system, muscles, etc. may activate A-delta or C-fibres (Mense 1996, Schmidt 1996). This results in pain that behaves in a stimulus–response manner during investigation of movement and function. For example, if the capsule of the temporomandibular joint is irritated, local pain will frequently occur on both palpation and movement.

PERIPHERAL NEUROGENIC MECHANISMS

Pain derives from a process within the cell body of a peripheral nerve outside of the dorsal horn and the brainstem (Devor 1996). A typical example is trigeminal neuralgia due to demyelinization of the nerve or odontalgia after tooth extraction with abnormal impulse generating sites (AIGS) as a result of nerve sprouting (Rappaport & Devor 1994). Pain is often felt locally but may be referred or perceived as paraesthesia.

In contrast to nociceptive pain, peripheral neurogenic pain does not always show typical stimulus–response characteristics, since they frequently cause modulation of the central nervous system (Lavigne et al 2005).

Symptoms related to central mechanisms (central sensitization)

This comprises pain associated with processes within the central nervous system (spinal cord, brainstem, brain). This type of pain shows extrasegmental characteristics, may be independent from movement and behaviour and is often strongly influenced by emotional and cognitive factors. During physical examination multiple tests may be positive, and the range of motion may be unlimited and without any clear clinical (mechanical) pattern.

Examples of diagnoses for which centralization pain is frequently the predominant mechanism include atypical facial pain, atypical odontalgia and some forms of tinnitus. Frequently (and as described above) there is no clear stimulus–response characteristic: particular stimuli may be extremely painful one minute and elicit almost no pain just moments later. This phenomenon may have various causes, including cognitive, pathophysiological and affective; learning processes may also be involved.

SOMATOTOPIA OF THE CRANIOFACIAL REGION

An interesting development of the last few years is an increasing understanding of body projection onto the cortex and its enormous plasticity as a reaction to various movement behaviours (Ramachandran & Blakesee 1998).

This phenomenon will be mentioned frequently in this book since it may explain symptoms and treatment approaches, for example as described in Chapters 11, 12 and 13. There follows some short explanations and examples of how techniques that are described in this book may be applied.

Somatotopia is a feature of somatic field arrangement (Butler 2000). The body is reflected within the central nervous system in an organized way. The somatosensory cortex, the thalamus and the cerebellum (subcortical level) are examples for such central areas (Buonomano & Merzenich 1998, Kaas 1999). Of these, the homunculus in the primary somatosensory cortex is the most investigated area (Ramachandran & Blakesee 1998; Fig. 1.1). Of note are the following.

The size of the projective field does not represent the size of the body part. The orofacial region, for example, covers roughly two-fifths of the whole projection. This explains the discrepancy between the perceived severity of the complaints and the findings of the physical examination. Examples are pain of the inside of the upper lip (half a centimetre towards the

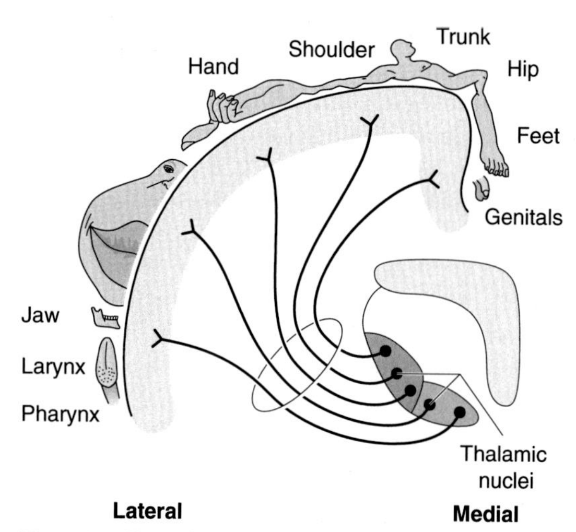

Fig. 1.1 The primary somatosensory homunculus (adapted from Pritchard & Alloway 1999).

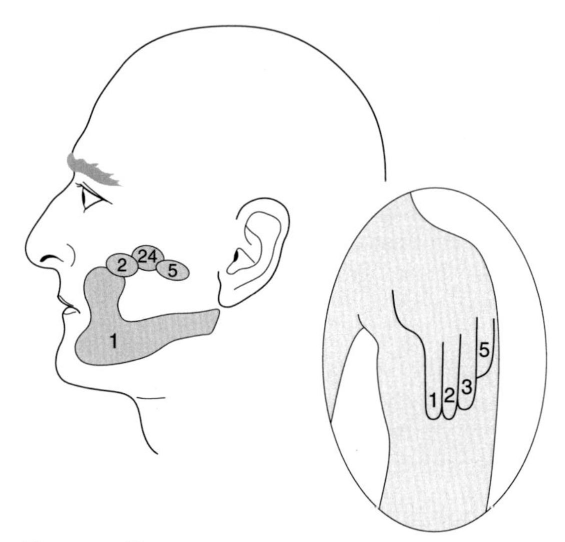

Fig. 1.2 Phantom sensations and hyperalgic zones in the face. Projection pain in the face of a patient, 10 years after a left arm amputation (adapted from Ramachandran & Blakesee 1998).

inside) or a grain of sand between the teeth that may be perceived like a stone. It also partly explains the perceived intensity of pain (Ramachandran & Blakesee 1998). Consider, for example, pain measurements like the visual analogue scale (VAS) that rates higher in migraine or trigeminal neuralgia patients than in low back pain patients (Zakrzewska 1995).

The body is divided into fields that touch or overlap each other, for example the hand is projected next to the face, thus activities in one projective field may cause sensations in a bordering field. Many phenomena were explained after it was discovered accidentally that following an arm amputation the fingers were represented in the projective field of the face (Doetch 1997, Ramachandran & Blakesee 1998, Fig. 1.2). This proved that the projective field of the face may actively be involved in the takeover of the somatosensory projection of the hand (Butler 2000). The result is phantom sensations in the face after amputation of the arm.

Other studies point out that a change of input may influence the projective field (Pascual-Leone & Torres 1993). For example, the projective fields of the fingers are larger in violin players than in non-musicians (Elbert et al 1995). It may be the case that a child with dysgnathia has a less differentiated presentation of the craniofacial region in the homunculus than a normally developed child. Simple movements of the tongue, such as propulsion and lateropulsion, may therefore become difficult manoeuvres for such patients. If these movements are not a problem the phenomenon can be observed when assessing for associated movements in neighbouring regions such as the cervical spine (e.g. mouth opening can only be performed with extension of the upper cervical spine).

SOMATOTOPIA AND CRANIOFACIAL MOVEMENT RE-EDUCATION

Because of the large projective field occupied by the craniofacial region and the changes that occur here, it is important to integrate this knowledge into the rehabilitation procedure. Practical and often simple principles as described below may optimize the rehabilitation of function and control pain.

- Learning similar movements in the same region. If there is a shift on mouth opening try to teach a pain-free laterotrusion to the opposite side.

- Stimulation of the body part that has the largest input to the somatosensory cortex, e.g. the lips or the tongue. If the patient suffers from facial paresis it may be useful to stimulate the tongue papilla and to teach active and passive tongue exercises to stimulate the afferent input of the facial nerve to the facial muscles.
- Try to imagine movements before actively performing them, e.g. 2.5 cm mouth opening.
- Facilitate a body part that is projected in a neighbouring field to the dysfunctional part. You may want to facilitate the hand for facial problems or, correspondingly, the face if the patient suffers from hand dysfunction.
- Change the stimulus (input) that usually shows an output reaction which is impaired, e.g. produce a swallowing reaction (stimulation of the glossopharyngeal and vagus nerves) if the patient suffers from dysarthria with a potential hypoglossal neuropathy. A classic example is to treat facial paresis by laughing or (if possible) tasting a bitter or sour substance.

Symptoms related to output (efferent) mechanisms

Output systems are the sympathetic and parasympathetic nervous system, the motor system, the neuroendocrine system and the neuroimmune system as well as the influence of descending impulses and descending behaviours (Sapolsky 1994, Gifford 1998b, Fink 2000). The type of output depends upon the input, the central processes and time.

If, for example, a patient suffers from pulpitis in the maxilla for more than a few days (nociceptive), the problem may lead to central sensitization. Therefore the surrounding structures may become more sensitive (hyperalgesia). At the same time an increased muscle tone of the masticatory muscles (motor system), sympathetic reactions like blushing of the face and local temperature changes in the innervation area of the maxillary nerve may be observed. This again will influence the input and set off a vicious circle of pain and functional limitations.

Pain mechanism features that influence the interpretation of the clinical situation

- Pain mechanisms do not occur alone: Usually one pain mechanism is dominant. For example, the maxillary region is still red and swollen (input) 2 days after the patient has been hit in the face by an elbow. The surrounding tissues and the opposite side are also slightly sensitive on palpation (processing).
- Pain mechanisms change with time and influence each other: Long-term retrodiscal inflammation (input) may reduce after a few weeks but the oedema of mandibular joint and orbit is still present, and the area is reddened and painful (non-segmentally) (output).
- Pain mechanism diagnosis is independent of the tissue diagnosis: Manual distraction of the mandibular joint may be painful as a result of 'sleeping nociceptor' facilitation (input). The pain reaction may also be connected with processes in the dorsal horn or the brainstem, causing a severe secondary hyperalgesia. The characteristics of these pains largely determine classification of the pain.
- The dominant pain mechanism influences interpretation of the test: While examining the cranium of a whiplash patient with passive techniques, the therapist finds that all the assessed movement directions are painful and that reactions are inconsistent. That the pain mechanism is dominantly central is therefore confirmed by the mainly false-positive test results (Fig. 1.3).

Interpretation of pathobiological mechanisms in children

In children the various pain mechanisms are generally easily observed. A child that has suffered from craniocervical trauma since birth, a so-called KISS child (kinematically induced symmetry stress), shows a change in cerebral processing because of the long-term nociceptive inputs during daily life activities

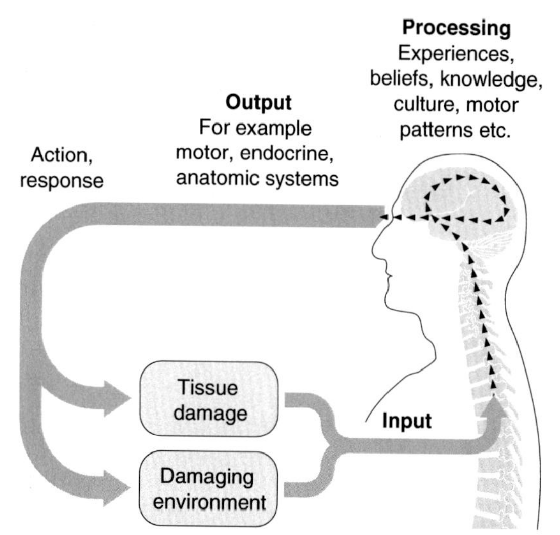

Fig. 1.3 A circular model of health based on pain mechanism: 'the mature organism model'. At the end of the 1990s, Gifford introduced this model with three levels (Input, Processing and Output) which interact with each other in circular fashion. The qualities of the pain mechanisms, as discussed in 'Pathobiological mechanisms', are clarified by this model. Note the importance of the effect of the environment, which during tissue damage influences the individual processing mechanism.

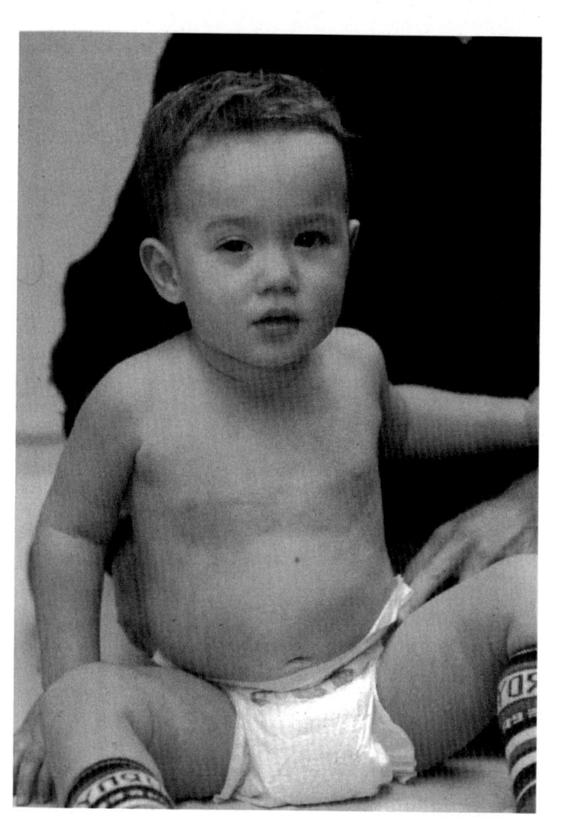

Fig. 1.4 A child with a craniocervical dysfunction. Related to the pain mechanism there may be a disturbance of the input (nociception of the craniocervical region). There is predictive consistent (pain) behaviour during small passive movements of the upper cervical region which can have repercussions for the processing and output mechanisms (long crying periods, extreme sweating, irregular tonus, delayed growth). This is expressed in the neuromusculoskeletal system of this 8-month-old boy. Note the difference in shape and size of the eyes, prominence of the left frontal region and slight upper cervical right lateral flexion.

(e.g. lying, rolling, sitting). An essential basic instinct of young children is security, which implies sensory input without nociceptive input (De Lange 2002). Reactions such as crying, delayed motor development, opisthotonos, swollen arms, red marks of unknown origin on the face and bonding difficulties are the expected output mechanisms. There is clinical evidence that an adequate therapeutic stimulus (e.g. craniocervical or craniofacial treatment) may reduce such output mechanisms within one day (Biedermann 2001, von Piekartz 2001) (Fig. 1.4).

Pathophysiological mechanisms of the craniofacial and mandibular region

Woda and Pionchon summarize:

> *There is a great chance that a patient with long-term headaches or facial pain will not fit into any traditional classification scheme. This is due to the enormous complexity of pain mechanisms and insufficient knowledge about contributing factors. Any unknown (idiopathic) craniofacial syndrome belongs to the neuropathic pain mechanisms that are facilitated by one or more contributing risk factors.*
>
> *Woda & Pionchon (2000)* (Fig. 1.5).

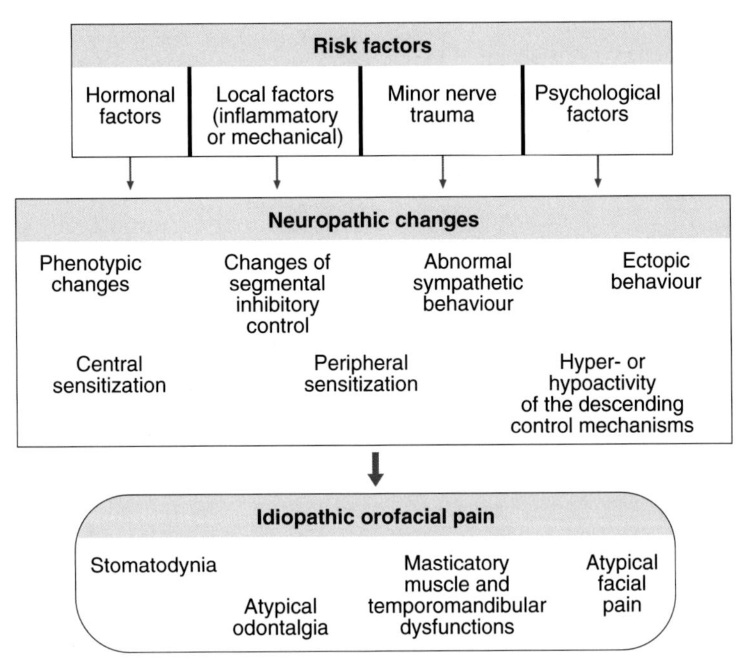

Fig. 1.5 A neuropathic model of craniofacial pain. Symptoms of every craniofacial–mandibular patient are related to tissue damage, activity level and different contributing factors (modified after Woda & Pionchon 2000).

For example, the changes in hormone levels in women (risk factor) may explain a higher prevalence of craniofacial pain (Kopp 2001). Input mechanisms such as a minor infection or a temporary psychological imbalance may influence each other and be facilitating factors for (severe) pain. The individual cause for 'symptoms of unknown origin' depends not only on the sensitization of the structures but also on the level of the contributing factors.

Figure 1.6 shows some potential hypotheses for pain mechanisms. Some explanations for long-term craniofacial pain are added.

- Summation (Fig. 1.6a): Different mechanisms (nociceptive, peripheral neurogenic, processing, output) occur with time and may coexist. Clinically this is typical for patients with an extensive history and several contributory factors for head and neck pain.
- Accumulation (Fig. 1.6b): One mechanism occurs in the presence or absence of another. For example, vasomotor headaches may occur in patients with prolonged retrodiscal pain because of an inflammatory process. This category may be recognized by a previous history where different symptoms occur one after another with location and intensity increasing with time.
- Interference (Fig. 1.6c): Different mechanisms interfere with each other, causing craniofacial pain which again facilitates new mechanisms. This is the case, for example, among patients with a prior history of various events in the head, neck and throat area which, taken together, are a contributory factor for craniofacial pain. Persistent symptoms such as vertigo, tinnitus and poor concentration are examples of this.

The pain classification for which some examples are shown also contributes to the patient's and the therapist's understanding of the complexity of headaches, facial and neck pain, and may assist in the planning of optimum treatment strategies (Gifford 1998a).

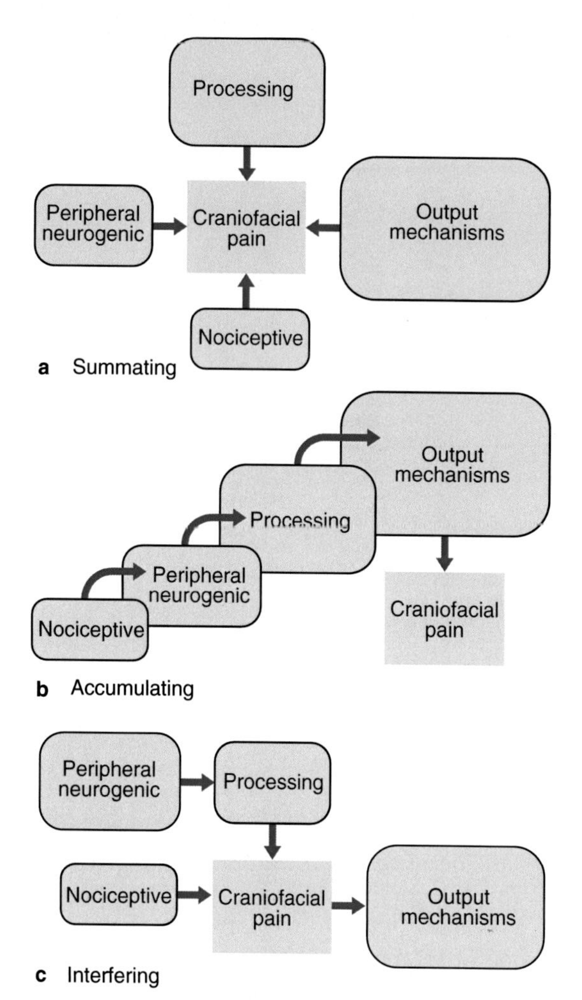

Fig. 1.6 Interference of different pain mechanisms with time which may be related to craniofacial pain.

SOURCES OF DYSFUNCTION

'Sources' are defined as the actual anatomical site or structure that shows pathological mechanisms (Jones & Rivett 2004). Within the tissue-based model, the average therapist will check for dysfunction mainly in peripheral structures such as muscles, capsules, ligaments or peripheral nerves. This is justified as long as the pain derives predominantly from nociceptive input. More complex pain syndromes (e.g. craniofacial pain in fibromyalgia patients) require an understanding of brain function (Septon et al 2003) for adequate assessment and patient management.

The patient's understanding of the source of their symptoms

Patients with craniofacial symptoms often have their own ideas of where their pain comes from. Often this is based on previous doctor or therapist statements or on knowledge from books and the internet. These ideas might have a negative influence on daily life activities or the physiotherapy management (Woda & Pionchon 2000, Jones & Rivett 2004). Therefore treatment always incorporates an element of education adapted to the patient's level of understanding, and which includes the potential source of the symptoms as well as contributing factors.

Classification of potential sources

A potential source is the structure that the therapist assesses first, based on information from case history. The aim is to find dysfunction (impairments) that indicate either a hands-on or hands-off approach. This book intentionally uses the expression 'region' since embryological, anatomical, neurophysiogical and functional criteria do not allow a separation of the structures.

The following regions can be differentiated:

- Craniocervical
- Craniofacial
- Craniomandibular
- Cranial nervous system.

CRANIOCERVICAL REGION

The craniocervical region refers to all anatomical structures that lie between occiput and C3, including zygapophyseal joints, neck muscles, ligaments, capsules, dura, nerve roots and bony structures.

Active and passive physiological tests as well as accessory tests allow an idea to be formed about the function of the upper cervical spine (see also Chapters 5, 6 and 7).

CRANIOFACIAL REGION

This encompasses all anatomical and functional structures of the cranium except for the temporomandibular joint (TMJ), including bony structures of the neurocranium and viscerocranium, blood vessels, intercranial dura, falx, tentorium cerebelli, cranial organs such as eyes, balance organ, etc. This region (which can be divided roughly into neuro- and viscero-cranium by location and phylogeny) is tested by passive movements (see Chapters 14 and 15).

CRANIOMANDIBULAR REGION

This includes all structures that are anatomically and functionally connected with the TMJ. The articular disc, the retrodiscal space, the mandibular nerve and the infrahyoid and suprahyoid muscles are included as well as the hyoid itself. This region can be tested by active and passive examination of the TMJ and the hyoid region, focusing on joint function, muscle function and function of the peripheral nerves (see also Chapter 8).

CRANIAL NERVOUS SYSTEM

This includes all intercranial nervous tissue such as the dura, falx and tentorium cerebelli, brain, brainstem, cranial nerves within the cranium and extracranial nervous tissue (e.g. cranial nerves such as the vagus nerve, accessory nerve, hypoglossal nerve, trigeminal nerve). This region is examined by conduction tests (strength, reflexes, sensory function), palpation and neurodynamic tests (Table 1.2) (see also Chapter 18).

Note on classification of these regions

OVERLAPPING

Some anatomical structures belong to two or more regions (Fig. 1.7). The dura mater, for example, belongs to the craniocervical and the craniomandibular region. After a whiplash injury (whiplash associated disorder, WAD) it is quite common to find the nervous tissue of both regions dysfunctional. Therefore the therapist will find positive tests in both regions on physical examination.

Classification is based not only on traditional anatomical location but also on movement function.

For example, the mandibular nerve belongs to the craniomandibular region *and* to the cranial nervous tissue and, since TMJ movements influence the mandibular nerve and vice versa, a neuropathy of the nerve will influence the range of TMJ movements (von Piekartz 2001).

DIAGNOSTIC INDEPENDENCE

Thinking in 'regions' rather than in 'structures' when examining a patient and interpreting the results helps the therapist to keep an open mind and assists classification of the pain mechanism.

If, for example, anteroposterior movements of the jaw and palpation of the retrodiscal space are painful on examination but the rest of the region around the head of mandible is not, it can be hypothesized that pain is dominantly nociceptive (input). The potential source is a local, retrodiscal structure (see Table 1.2). If the majority of craniofacial and craniomandibular tests are positive, a sensitization process would seem more likely. The focus here is not on one single structure but on pain mechanisms.

COMMUNICATION AND CLASSIFICATION

Classification into regions aims to assist the initial clinical decision-making process. This may be of advantage in the case of severe headache or neck pain. The therapist can now focus on one region and perform initial treatment to test for efficacy. If necessary, the therapist may then 'translate' their knowledge into one of the more common classification systems of the IHS, AAOP or IASP as described earlier in this chapter.

PRECAUTIONS AND CONTRAINDICATIONS

These are defined as risk factors for assessment and treatment. The expression 'red flags' was introduced for the assessment of low back pain (AHCPR 1994). Red flags stand for all traumatic, neoplastic and inflammatory processes that require immediate medical attention.

Table 1.2 Functional categories of the most important neuromusculoskeletal structures in the various regions*

Craniomandibular region	
Bony structures	Mandibular head Articular disc Coronoid process Zygomatic arch External auditory meatus Mandibular bone Temporal bone Styloid process Hyoid
Capsule, ligaments, fascias	Capsule Retrodiscal ligaments Stylomandibular ligament Sphenomandibular ligament
Muscles	Masseter Temporalis Lateral pterygoid muscle Medial pterygoid muscle Supra-/infrahyoid muscles Genioglossal muscle (tongue) Sternocleidomastoid
Nervous system	Intracranial dura Trigeminal ganglion Trigeminal nerve (mandibular nerve) Facial nerve Buccal process Zygomatic process Mandibular process Hypoglossal nerve
Teeth	Maxillary and mandibular teeth
Craniocervical region	
Bony structures	Atlas (C1) Axis (C2) 3rd cervical vertebra Occiput Petrous bone
Capsule, ligaments	Cruciform ligaments Posterior longitudinal ligament Transverse ligament (axis) Nuchal ligament Alar ligaments Dura–atlas ligament Dura Capsule and ligaments of the zygapophyseal joints

Table 1.2—cont'd

Muscles	Deep dorsal muscles Minor rectus capitis posterior muscle Major rectus capitis posterior muscle Inferior oblique capitis muscle Major oblique capitis posterior muscle Semispinal muscle Longissimus muscle Iliocostal muscle Splenius capitis muscle Levator scapula Sternocleidomastoid Ventral neck muscles Longus colli Longissimus capitis
Nervous system	Craniocervical dura Nerve roots C0–C3 Hypoglossal nerve Vagus nerve Glossopharyngeal nerve Accessory nerve Occipital nerve
Craniofacial region	
Bony structures	Neurocranium and viscerocranium Atlas Mandibular head
Capsule, fascias	Sural ligaments Tentorium cerebelli Falx cerebelli Occipital fascia Stylomandibular ligament Sphenomandibular ligament
Muscles	Mimic muscles Muscles that insert at the cranium Rectus capitis posterior major and minor Major oblique capitis posterior Semispinalis muscle Longissimus muscle Splenus capitis Sternocleidomastoid
Nervous system	Cranial and craniocervical dura Tentorium cerebelli Falx cerebelli All cranial nerves that run extracranially through the cranial foramina Nerve roots of C0

Table 1.2—cont'd

Cranial nervous system	
Bony structures	All bones that are connected to the cranial nervous system Neurocranium Viscerocranium Mandible Atlas
Capsule, ligaments, fascias	All non-contractile soft tissues that are connected to the cranial nervous system, e.g.: Dura–atlas ligament Stylomandibular ligament Sphenomandibular ligament Temporomandibular capsule
Muscles	All contractile structures that are connected to the cranial nervous system, e.g.: Medial and lateral pterygoid muscle Masseter Temporalis Mimic muscles Dorsal neck muscles Supra-/infrahyoid muscles Trapezius pars descendens Sternocleidomastoid

* Note that the regions overlap. The therapist needs to decide by subjective assessment and biomedical knowledge which regions is/are principally responsible for dysfunction and pain.

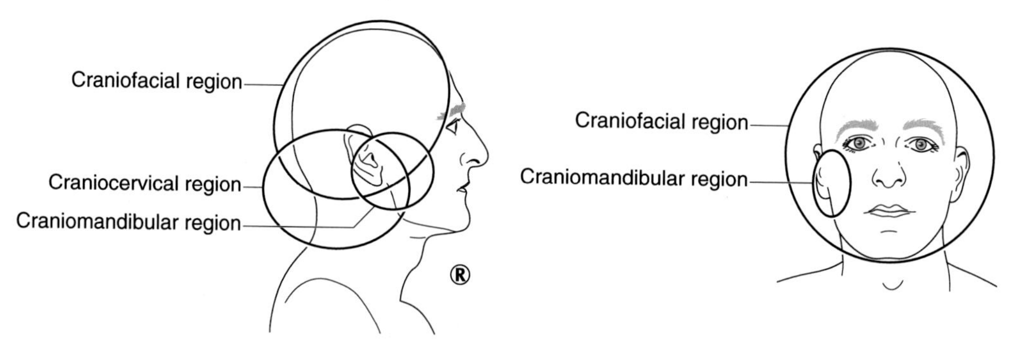

Fig. 1.7 Topographic expression of the different candidate regions:
1. Craniocervical region
2. Craniofacial region
3. Craniomandibular region.

The cranial nervous system is not mentioned as a separate region because this system is in continuity with all three regions (see text). Note the overlap between the different regions (see also Table 1.2).

Therapists that work on prescription will rarely need to assess for red flags since they have usually already been excluded by medical specialists. Sometimes patients are falsely labelled with a simple diagnosis such as tension headache or myalgia of the masticatory muscles; however, if features do not fit the therapist should be alerted and refer patients back to the specialist without delay. The following classic examples from the case history require further attention:

- Unchanged or spreading hyposensitivity of the chin
- Numbness of the palate
- Ongoing nightly headaches and weight loss (Boissonault 1995).

Chapter 3 provides more in-depth information on this topic.

CONTRIBUTING FACTORS

All influences that may be predisposing, that exacerbate, develop or maintain the symptoms fall into this category. Headaches and facial pain often have a range of such factors connected to previous history, mood, emotions, learning processes, previous experiences, knowledge, behaviour and neurobiological features (McGrath & Koster 2001). Insight into these factors may assist the therapist in designing management strategies and establishing a prognosis. An extensive list of such contributing factors for the craniofacial region is presented in Chapter 3.

PROGNOSIS

Prognosis is one of the most difficult but also one of the most important therapeutic tasks (Butler 2000, Maitland et al 2001, Jones & Rivett 2004). Every medical professional knows the patient's main question: 'How long will pain last and when will I regain full function?' It has been shown that unhelpful cognitions, anger, fear, depression and catastrophizing could be reduced to a minimum in patients with low back pain if they are informed early on about the causes and the possible duration of their symptoms (Moseley 2000). Comparable results for patients with craniofacial symptoms are also expected (Woda & Pionchon 2000).

Making a prognosis

After tooth extraction, a multiple sclerosis patient (risk factor) experiences a sudden onset of burning pain (pathobiological process; peripheral neurogenic) along the mandibular nerve (source) that remains unchanged for more than 2 months. The patient has difficulty in opening the mouth (dysfunction) and fears (contributing factor) that opening the mouth will increase the symptoms. Obviously the prognosis in this case is less promising than the prognosis of a patient who experiences acute toothache for the first time and who does not have any other problems.

MANAGEMENT

Ideal management of craniofacial pain patients starts by assessment of all short- and long-term goals regarding pain, dysfunction and participation deficits. Another important aspect is to prevent new episodes of pain by providing the patient with adequate self-management strategies. From a phenomenological point of view the therapist will guide the patient from the individual illness experience and illness behaviour to health experience and health-promoting behaviour (Hengeveld 2003a). Various intervention strategies may contribute to this approach, including manual therapy, exercise therapy and verbal communication. Therapists are strongly advised to use more than one strategy at a time (McIndoe 1995).

During the past few years there has been a somewhat polarized debate about the disadvantages of hands-on strategies (treatment techniques that include direct body contact) and the advantages of hands-off strategies (interventions without direct body contact). The truth probably lies somewhere in between: the therapist should combine targeted hands-on techniques with adequate self-management strategies such as relaxation, stretching, muscle control exercises and self-mobilization. The aim of self-management is for the patient to regain the locus of control and to improve self-efficacy beliefs (Bandura 1977), which have been described as important factors in the secondary prevention of disabilities due to chronic pain (Yoda et al 2003). This is surely also true for craniofacial pain syndromes.

Hence, explanation, information and motivation are used at the same time as manual techniques and exercises such as 'tongue-teeth-breathing-and-swallowing' (TTBS) or 'touch-and-bite' (see also Chapter 9).

CLINICAL REASONING SUPPORTS THE USE OF VARIOUS MODELS OF THINKING

In summary, it can be said that conscious clinical reasoning promotes the development of an open mind. The therapist does not have to rely on a single assessment and treatment method such as an arthrogenic, muscular, neurogenic, biomechanical or psychosocial approach (Jones & von Piekartz 2001, Jones & Rivett 2004). Conscious clinical reasoning integrates the different models of thinking into clinical practice by constantly reassessing the treatment results and evaluating for the most beneficial approach. This way it is not the patient who will have to adapt to the therapist's model of thinking but the therapist who adapts management to the individual patient. A common expression for this process is 'wise action' (Higgs & Jones 1997). This includes the selection of 'the best from science', 'the best available technique' and 'the best from the therapeutic relationship with the patient' (Butler 1998). Considering today's knowledge about aetiology and classification of craniomandibular and craniofacial syndromes, the concept of 'wise action' is a good starting point for therapists who regularly deal with this group of patients.

> **!** Clinical reasoning is the basis of clinical practice for treatment providers and patients and, according to popular knowledge, is one of the best forms of therapy (Butler 1998).

The best from science

For the assessment and treatment of patients with craniofacial dysfunctions and pain a thorough knowledge of these aspects is essential:

- Tissue pathology: For example, pathophysiological knowledge of masticatory muscles including trigger points, disc pathologies and disc derangements as well as their effect on pain and dysfunction (Hathaway 1995, Okeson 1995, Svensson & Graven-Nielsen 2001).
- Cranial growth: For the application of cranial treatment techniques and also for the observation of changes in cranial shape, it is essential to have a thorough knowledge of normal cranial growth. Usually the facial bones develop between the ages of 9 and 15 years, whereas the neurocranium remains unchanged after the age of 5 (Proffit & Fields 1993, Oudhof 2001). This knowledge may assist the interpretation of patient complaints.
- Pain sciences: It is essential for assessment and treatment to differentiate between nociceptive pain, neuropathic symptoms, central modulation aspects and the influence of the sympathetic nervous system. For example, one should know that after tooth extraction it is quite common to develop AIGS that may cause toothache of long duration or facial symptoms (Okeson 1995).

The best from the therapeutic relationship with the patient

This includes a thorough subjective and physical examination with conscious communication processes, that should leave room for individual questions and information giving (May 2001, Hengeveld 2003b). Patients should be left with an impression of involvement in the treatment process and that treatment goals and interventions are agreed in a collaborative process. In the treatment of children it is important to involve parents for optimal success of the treatment strategy (McGrath & Koster 2001, see also Chapters 4, 20 and 21).

The best available technique

The choice of treatment techniques depends on both subjective evaluation and physical examination. Constant re-evaluation of the treatment effects by questioning the patient about their perception of pain and function helps to adapt the technique. This is called 'reassessment' (Maitland 1987).

At present there is no purely clinical approach to determining the most appropriate therapy for any particular clinical syndrome. Thus it has been claimed that anterior disc derangements without reduction of the TMJ respond well to medication, physiotherapy, braces or a combination of these approaches (Stiesch-Scholz et al 2002). Physiotherapy is mentioned as a whole but no particular intervention methods are specifically indicated (von Piekartz 2002). The same is true for migraines, atypical facial pain, non-specific otalgia, etc.

An example for 'wise action'

During craniomandibular examination all indicators point towards an anterior disc derangement. There are no additional myogenic or neurogenic dysfunctions. Assessing joint mobility, limited mouth opening with a shift and painful limitation on posterior–anterior movement are found. In such cases, manual techniques (usually distraction and accessory movements to the left), combined with coordinating and stabilizing exercises, are generally helpful. A brace may be considered although it has been shown in

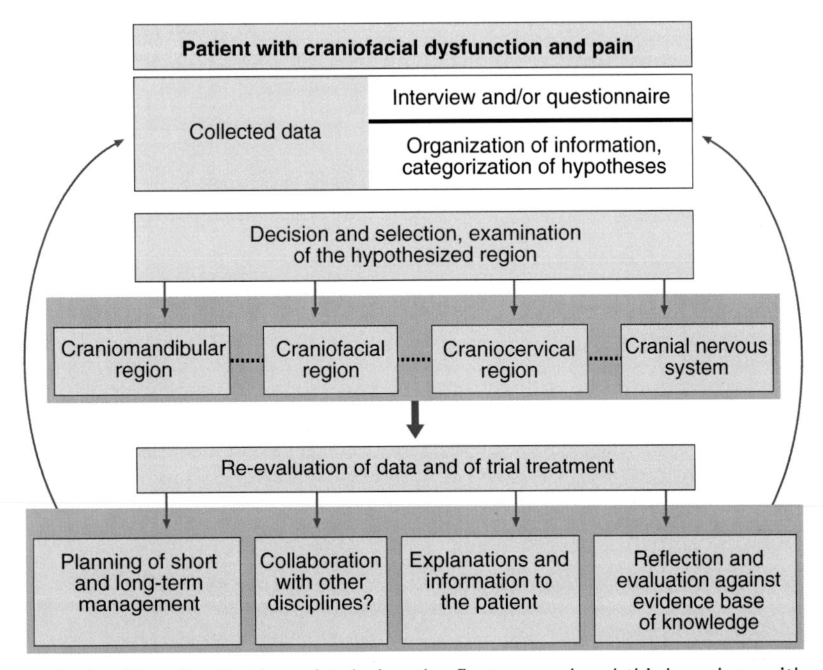

Fig. 1.8 A general algorithm for the therapist during the first, second and third sessions with a patient with craniofacial pain. The dotted line (- - -) between the different regions reflects the functional interrelationships. The arrows from the last boxes backwards to the first box reflect the continuous (re)assessment of the effect of treatment and management.

randomized controlled studies that the effect of braces is no better than placebo (Koh & Robinson 2003, Al-Ani et al 2004). The therapist makes a decision based on the clinical examination and, if possible, supported by information (Medline, Cinahl, Cochrane) from a literature review (evidence-based practice) (Sackett et al 1998).

Using algorithms for support

The algorithm shown in Figure 1.8 can be used to assist in the clinical decision-making process for the individual craniofacial pain patient. This overview includes hypothesis categories as well as possible sources for the symptoms.

SUMMARY

- There is an increasing prevalence of craniofacial dysfunction and pain in the industrialized world.
- The aetiology is unknown in most cases and classification systems are inadequate in their description of clinical syndromes.
- The overall physiotherapeutic thinking changes from a unilateral, linear and biomedical view to a holistic, biopsychosocial movement model. Within this framework, craniofacial pain patients are assessed and treated individually. The physiotherapy (movement) approach contributes greatly to the treatment of craniofacial dysfunction and pain. Clinical reasoning promotes the integration of various models of thinking. A better scientific base for the treatment is urgently required.
- This chapter suggests an approach for the hypothetically dysfunctional region with an easy algorithm. This may contribute to scientific research and may be used as a guideline for clinical decisions in the treatment of headaches, neck pain and facial pain without inventing a new terminology.

References

AHCPR 1994 Clinical Practice Guideline Number 14: Acute low back problems in adults. Agency for Health Care Problems and Research. US Department of Health and Human Services, Rockville MD

Al-Ani M, Davies S, Gray R, Sloan P, Glenny A 2004 Stabilisation splint therapy for temporomandibular pain dysfunction syndrome. Cochrane Database of Systematic Reviews 1:CD002778

Bandell-Hoekstra I, Abu-Saad H, Passchier J et al 2001 Prevalence and characteristics of headache in Dutch schoolchildren. European Journal of Pain 5:145

Bandura A 1977 Self-efficacy: toward a unifying theory of behavioural change. Psychological Review 84:191

Bernhardt O, Bitter K, Schwahn C et al 2001 Das Profil funktioneller Störungen des Kauorgans im vergleich einer populationbasierten Probantengruppe und einer Gruppe mit Tinnitus. Journal of Public Health 9:156–165

Biedermann H 2001 Primäre und sekundäre Schädelassymmetrie bei KISS Kinder. In: Piekartz von H (ed.) Kraniofaziale Dysfunktionen und schmerzen: Untersuchung, Beurteilung, Management. Thieme, Stuttgart, p 45

Boissonault W 1995 Examination in physical therapy practice. Screening for medical diseases, 2nd edn. Churchill Livingstone, Philadelphia

Buonomano D V, Merzenich M M 1998 Cortical plasticity from synapsis to maps. Annual Review of Neuroscience 21:149–186

Butler D 1998 Intergrating pain awareness into physiotherapy – wise action for the future. In: Gifford L (ed.) Topical issues in pain. Whiplash: science and management, fear-avoidance beliefs and behaviour. NOI Press, Adelaide, p 1:27

Butler D 2000 The sensitive nervous system. NOI Press, Adelaide

Carlsson G, Magnusson T 1999 Management of temporomandibular disorders in the general dental practice: epidemiologic studies of TMD. Quintessence, Chicago

Costen J 1934 Syndrome of ear and sinus symptoms dependent upon disturbed function of the temporomandibular joint. Annals of Otology, Rhinololgy and Laryngology 43:1

Cott C, Finch E, Gasner D et al 1995 The movement continuum theory for physiotherapy. Physiotherapy Canada 47:87

De Bono E 1994 Parallel thinking, from Socratic thinking to de Bono thinking. Viking, London

De Kanter R J, Truin G J, Burgersdijk R C et al 1993 Prevalence in the Dutch adult population and a meta-analysis of signs and symptoms of temporomandibular disorder. Journal of Dental Research 72(11):1509–1518

De Lange G 2002 Hechtingsstoornissen – orthopedagogische Behandelingsstrategien. HBO Reeks Gezondheidszorg/Welzijn:dl 2. NUGI: 725

de Vries C, Wimmers R 1997 Is fysiotherapie gevolgengeneeskunde? FysioPraxis 6:10

de Wijer A, Rob J, Leeuw de J, Steenks M H, Bosmans F 1996 Temporomandibular and cervical spine disorders. Self-reported signs and symptoms. Spine 21:1638–1646

Deubner D C 1977 An epidemiologic study of migraine and headache in 10–20 year olds. Headache 17:173–180

Devor M 1996 Pain mechanisms and pain syndromes. In: Campell J (ed.) Pain 1996 – an updated review. IASP Press, Seattle

Doetsch G 1997 Progressive changes in cutaneous trigger zones for sensation referred to a phantom hand: a case report and review with implications for cortical reorganisation. Somatosensory and Motor Research 14:6

Drangsholt M, LeResche L 1999 Temporomandibular pain. In: Crombie I, Croft P, Linton S, LeResche L, von Korff M (eds) Epidemiology of pain. IASP Press, Seattle, p 203

Dworkin S, Burgess J 1987 Orofacial pain of psychogenic origin: current concepts and classification. Journal of the American Dental Association 115:565

Elbert T, Pantev C, Wienbruch C et al 1995 Increased cortical representation of the left hand in string players. Science 270:305

Epstein A 1990 The outcome movement. Will it get us where we want? New England Journal of Medicine 323:266

Evjenth O, Hamburg J 1984 Muscle stretching in manual therapy. Alfta Rehab, Alfta, Sweden

Fink G 2000 Encyclopedia of stress. Academic Press, San Diego

Freesmeyer W 1993 Zahärztliche Funktionstherapie. Hanser, Munich

Gifford L 1998a Pain, the tissues and the nervous system: a conceptual model. Physiotherapy 84:27

Gifford L 1998b Topical issues in pain. Whiplash: science and management, fear-avoidance beliefs and behaviour. NOI Press, Adelaide

Grant R 1995 The pursuit of excellence in the face of constant change. Physiotherapy 81:338

Grant R, Jones M, Maitland G 1988 Clinical decision making in upper quadrant dysfunction. In: Grant R (ed.) Physical therapy of the cervical and thoracic spine. Churchill Livingstone, New York, p 51–80

Greene C 2001 The etiology of temporomandibular disorders: implications for treatment. Journal of Orofacial Pain 15:93

Gruber H 1999 Mustererkennung und Erfahrungswissen. Zwischen Erfahrung und Beweis. Fischer and W. Martens. Hans Huber, Bern

Hansson T, Christensen Minor C, Wagnon Taylor D 1992 Physical therapy in craniomandibular disorders. Quintessence, Copenhagen, p 45

Hathaway K 1995 Bruxism: definition, measurement, and treatment. Orofacial pain and temporomandibular disorders. Raven Press, New York

Heikinheimo K, Salmi K, Myllarniemi S, Kirveskari P 1989 Symptoms of craniomandibular disorder in a sample of Finnish adolescents at the ages of 12 and 15 years. European Journal of Orthodontics 11:325–331

Hendriksen E, van der Wees P, de Bie R 2003 Clinical practical guidelines in the Netherlands. Royal Dutch Society for Physical Therapy (KNGF), Amersfoort

Hengeveld E 1998/1999 Gedanken zum Indikationsbereich der Manuellen Therapie. Teil 1 und Teil 2. Manuelle Therapie 1998; 2.; 1999; 3:176–181

Hengeveld E 1998a Clinical Reasoning in Manueller Therapie – eine klinische Fallstudie. Manuelle Therapie 2:42

Hengeveld E 1998b Theorie der Physiotherapie: Plädoyer für einen Paradigmawechsel. Teil 1 und Teil 2. Physiotherapie (Schweiz) 11:18–28; 12:13–20

Hengeveld E 2003a Compliance und Verhaltensänderung in Manueller Therapie. Manuelle Therapie 7:122

Hengeveld E 2003b Das biopsychosoziale Modell. Angewandte Physiologie, Band 4: Schmerzen verstehen und beeinflussen. F. v.d. Berg. Thieme, Stuttgart, p 1

Higgs J, Jones M 1997 Clinical reasoning: the foundation of clinical practice. Part 1. Australian Journal of Physiotherapy 43:167

Higgs J, Jones M 2000 Clinical reasoning in the health professions. Butterworth-Heinemann, Oxford
Hislop H 1975 The not-so impossible dream. Physical Therapy 55:1069
IHS 1988 Headache Classification Committee of the International Headache Society. Classification and diagnostic criteria for headache disorders, cranial neuralgias and facial pain. Cephalalgia 8(Suppl 7):1–96
IHS 2004 Headache Classification Committee of the International Headache Society. Classification and diagnostic criteria of headache disorders, cranial neuralgias and facial pain. Cephalalgia 24(Suppl 1): 9–160
John M, Wefers K 1999 Orale Dysfunktion bei Erwachsenen. Quintessenz, Berlin
John M, Hirsch C, Reiber T 2001 Häufigkeit, Bedeutung und Behandlungsbedarf kraniomandibulärer Dysfunktionen. Zeitschrift fur Gesundheidswissenschaften 9:136–155
Jones M 1995 Clinical reasoning and pain. Manual Therapy 1:17
Jones M, Rivett D 2004 Clinical reasoning for manual therapists. Butterworth-Heinemann, Edinburgh
Jones M, von Piekartz H 2001 Clinical reasoning – a basis for examination and treatment in the cranial region. In: von Piekartz H (ed.) Craniofacial dysfunction and pain: manual therapy, assessment and management. Butterworth-Heinemann, Oxford
Jull G, Moore A 2002 Are manipulative therapy approaches the same [editorial]. Manual Therapy 7(2):63
Kaas J 1999 Is most of the neural plasticity in the thalamus cortical? Proceedings of the National Academy of Sciences USA 96:7622
Kamann W K 1999 Zur Entwicklung der Okklusionskonzepte. Phillip Journal 1
KNGF 1992 Visie op fysiotherapie. KNGF, Amersfoort, Koninklijk Nederlands Genootschap voor Fysiotherapie
Koh H, Robinson P G 2003 Occlusal adjustment for treating and preventing temporomandibular joint disorders. Cochrane Database of Systematic Reviews CD003812
Kohlmann T 2002 Epidemiology of orofacial pain. Schmerz 16(5):339-45
Kopp S 2001 Neuroendocrine, immune, and local responses related to temporomandibular disorders. Journal of Orofacial Pain 15:1
Kraus S L (ed.) 1988 Cervical spine influence on the craniomandibular region. In: TMJ disorders: management of the craniomandibular complex. Churchill Livingstone, New York
Kraus S 1994 Cervical spine influences on the management of TMD. In: Kraus S (ed.) Temporomandibular disorders, 2nd edn. Churchill Livingstone, New York, p 348
Lavigne G, Woda A, Truelove E, Ship J A, Dao T, Goulet J P 2005 Mechanisms associated with unusual orofacial pain. Journal of Orofacial Pain 19(1):9–21
Lemka M 1999 Headache as the consequence of brain concussion and contusion in closed head injuries in children. Neurologia i Neurochirurgia Polska 33:37
LeResche L 1997 Epidemiology of temporomandibular disorders: implications for the investigation of etiological factors. Critical Reviews in Oral Biology and Medicine 8:291
Lipton J, Ship J, Larach-Robinson D 1993 Estimated prevalence and distribution of reported orofacial pain in the United States. Journal of the American Dental Association 124:115
Lobbezoo-Scholte A M, Lobbezoo F, Steenks M H, De Leeuw J R, Bosman F 1995 Diagnostic subgroups of craniomandibular disorders. Part II: Symptom profiles. Orofacial Pain 9(1):37–43
Locker D, Slade G 1988 Prevalence of symptoms associated with temporomandibular disorders in a Canadian population. Community Dentistry and Oral Epidemiology 16:310–313
Lund J, Lavigne G, Dubner R, Sessle B 2000 Orofacial pain: from basic science to clinical management. Quintessence, Chicago
Lupton D 1969 Psychological aspects of temporomandibular joint dysfunction. Journal of the American Dental Association 79:131–136
Mahan P, Alling C 1991 Facial pain, 3rd edn. Lea and Febiger, Philadelphia, p 311
Maitland G 1986 Vertebral manipulation. Butterworth-Heinemann, Oxford
Maitland G 1987 The Maitland concept: assessment, examination and treatment by passive movement. In: Twomey L T, Taylor J R (eds) Physical therapy of the low back. Churchill Livingstone, New York
Maitland G, Hengeveld E, Banks K, English K 2001 Maitland's vertebral manipulation, 6th edn. Butterworth-Heinemann, Oxford
Makofsky H, Sexton T, Diamond D, Sexton M 1991 The effect of head posture on muscle contact position using the T-Scan system of occlusal analysis. Journal of Craniomandibular Practice 9:316
Maluf K, Sahrmann S, Van Dillen L 2000 Use of a classification system to guide nonsurgical management of patients with low back pain. Physical Therapy 80:1097
Manzoni G C, Granella F, Sandrini G, Cavallini A, Zanferrari C, Nappi G 1995 Classification of chronic daily headache by International Headache Society criteria: limits and new proposals. Cephalalgia 15(1):37–43
May S 2001 Patient satisfaction with management of back pain. Part 1: What is satisfaction? Review of satisfaction with medical management. Part 2: An explorative, qualitative study into patients'

satisfaction with physiotherapy. Physiotherapy 87:4–20
Maytal J, Young M, Shechter A, Lipton R 1997 Pediatric migraine and the international headache society. Neurology 48:607
McGrath P, Koster A 2001 Headache measures for children: a practical approach. The child with headache: diagnosis and treatment. Progress in pain research and management. IASP Press, Seattle, p 9
McIndoe R 1995 Moving out of pain. Hands-on or hands-off. In: Schacklock M (ed.) Moving out of pain. Butterworth-Heinemann, Oxford, p 153
Mense S 1996 Group III and IV nociceptors in skeletal muscle: are they specific or polymodal? In: Kumazawa T, Kruger L, Mizumura K (eds) Progress in brain research. Elsevier, Amsterdam, p 113
Merskey H, Bogduk N 1994 Classification of chronic pain: descriptions of chronic pain syndromes and definitions of pain terms. IASP Press, Seattle
Mongini F 1999 Taxonomy of headache and facial pain. In: Headache and facial pain. Thieme, Stuttgart, p 2–10
Mongini F, Defilippi N, Negro C 1997 Chronic daily headache. A clinical and psychological profile before and after treatment. Headache. 37:83
Moseley L 2000 The effect of neuroscience education on pain attitudes, somatic perception and catastrophising in people with chronic low back pain. Australian Pain Society Annual Conference: Progress of Pain
Naeije M, Van Loon L 1998 Craniomandibulaire functie en disfunctie. Bohn Stafleu Van Lochum, Houten/Diegem
Nappi G, Micieli G, Cavallini A et al 1992 Accompanying symptoms of cluster attacks: their relevance to the diagnostic criteria. Cephalalgia 12:165
NPI 1997 'Evidence-based' paramedische zorg. Een balans tussen 'consensus based evidence' en 'research based evidence'. Issue 4:44
Okeson J 1996 Orofacial pain. Guidelines for assessment, diagnosis, and management: the biopsychosocial model of disease. Quintessence, Chicago
Okeson J 2005 Bell's orofacial pains, 6th edn. Quintessence, Chicago
Oudhof H 2001 Skull growth in relation with mechanical stimulation. In: von Piekartz H, Bryden L (eds) Craniofacial dysfunction and pain, assessment, manual therapy and management. Butterworth-Heinemann, Oxford, p 1–21
Palla S, Koller M, Airoldi R 1998 Befunderhebung und Diagnose bei Myoarthropathien. In: Myoarthropathien des Kausystems und orofaziale Schmerzen. Fotoplast AG, Zurich, p 73
Papadopoulos M A 2003 Meta-analysis in evidence-based orthodontics. Orthodontics and Craniofacial Research 6:112–26
Pascual-Leone A, Torres F 1993 Plasticity of the sensorimotor cortex representation of the reading finger of Braille readers. Brain 116:39–52
Passchier J, Orlebeke J F 1985 Headaches and stress in schoolchildren: an epidemiological study. Cephalalgia 5:167–176
Perthes R, Gross S 1995 Disorders of the temporomandibular joint. In: Clinical management of the temporomandibular disorders and orofacial pain. Quintessence, Chicago, p 69
Prichard T C, Alloway K D 1999 Medical neuroscience. Fence Creek Publishing, Madison, CT, p 112–113
Proffit W, Fields H 1993 Contemporary orthodontics, 2nd edn. Mosby-YearBook, St Louis, section II, p 18
Proffit W, Ackerman J 1993 Orthodontic diagnosis: the development of a problem list. In: Contemporary orthodontics. Mosby, Philadelphia, p 139
Ramachandran V, Blakesee S 1998 Phantoms in the brain. William and Morrow, New York
Rappaport Z, Devor M 1994 Trigeminal neuralgia: the role of self-sustaining discharge in the trigeminal ganglion. Pain 56:127
Rocabado M, Iglash Z 1991 Musculoskeletal approach to maxillofacial pain. J B Lippincott, Philadelphia
Rugh J, Davis S 1992 Temporomandibular disorders: psychological and behavioral aspects. In: Sarnat B, Laskin D (eds) The temporomandibular joint: a biologic basis for clinical practice, 4th edn. Saunders, Philadelphia, p 329
Sackett D, Richardson W, Rosenberg W M C, Haynes R B 1998 Evidence-based medicine – how to practice and teach EBM. Churchill Livingstone, Edinburgh
Sapolsky R 1994 Why zebras don't get ulcers. Freeman, New York
Schiffmann E, Anderson G, Fricton J et al 1992 The relationship between level of mandibular pain and dysfunction and stage of temporomandibular joint internal derangement. Journal of Dental Research 71:1812
Schiffmann E, Haley D, Baker C et al 1995 Diagnostic criteria for screening headache patients for temporomandibular disorders. Headache 35:121
Schmidt R 1996 The articular polymodal nociceptor in health and disease. In: Kumazama T, Kruger L, Mizumura K (eds) Progress in brain research. Elsevier, Amsterdam, p 113
Schwarz A 1926 Kopfhaltung und Kiefer. Zeitschrift für Stomatologie: Organ für wissenschaftliche und praktische Zahnheilkunde
Septon S, Studts J, Hoover K et al 2003 Biological and psychological factors associated with memory

function in fibromyalgia syndrome. Health Psychology 22:592

Shacklock M 1999a Central pain mechanisms: a new horizon in manual therapy. Australian Journal of Physiotherapy 45:83

Shacklock M 1999b The clinical application of central pain mechanisms in manual therapy. Australian Journal of Physiotherapy 45:215

Sieber M, Ruggia G, Grubenmann E, Palla S 1997 The functional status of the masticatory system of 11–16 year-old adolescents: classification and validity. Community Dentistry and Oral Epidemiology 25:256

Solomon S, Lipton R, Newman L 1992. Evaluation of chronic daily headache: comparison to criteria for chronic tension-type headache. Cephalalgia 12:365

Stiesch-Scholz M, Fink M, Tschernitschek H, Rossbach A 2002 Medical and physical therapy of temporomandibular joint disk displacement without reduction. Cranio 20(2):85–90

Svensson P, Graven-Nielsen T 2001 Craniofacial muscle pain: review of mechanisms and clinical manifestations. Journal of Orofacial Pain 15:117

Thomas-Edding D 1987 Clinical problem solving in physical therapy and its implications for curriculum development. Proceedings of the 10th International Congress of the World Confederation of Physical Therapy. Sydney, Australia

van Duin N, Brouwer H, Gooskens R 2000 Kinderen met Hoofdpijn. Een onderschat Probleem. Medisch contact 55:26

Vig P S, Sarver D M, Hall D J, Warren D W 1981 Quantitative evaluation of nasal airflow in relation to facial morphology. American Journal of Orthodontics 79(3):263–272

Viswanathan V, Bridges S, Whitehouse W, Newton R 1998 Childhood headaches: discrete entities or continuum? Developmental Medicine and Child Neurology 40:544

von Korff M, LeResche L, Dworkin S 1993 First onset of common pain symptoms: a prospective study of depression as a risk factor. Pain 55:251

von Piekartz H 2001a Kraniofaziale Dysfunktionen und Schmerzen: Merkmale des Schädelgewebes als Grundlage zur Erkennung, Untersuchung und Behandlung klinischer Muster. Thieme, Stuttgart

von Piekartz H 2001b Kraniofaziale Dysfunktionen und Schmerzen: Schädelwachstum und Einfluss von mechanischer Stimulation. Thieme, Stuttgart

von Piekartz H 2002 Comment on Dr. Stiesch-Sholtz et al´s article in Cranio. Cranio 4:238–240, 240–241

Wall P 2000 The science of suffering. Orion, London

WCPT 1999 Description of physical therapy. World Confederation of Physical Therapy, London

Woda A, Pionchon P 2000 A unified concept of idiopathic orofacial pain: clinical features. Orofacial Pain 13:172–184, discussion 185–195

World Health Organization (WHO) 2001 ICF – International classification of functioning, disablility and health. WHO, Geneva

Wörter-Bingö C, Wober C, Karawautz A et al 1996 Tension-type headache in different age groups at two headache centers. Pain 67:53–58

Yoda T, Sakamoto I, Imai H, Honma Y 2003 A randomised controlled trial of therapeutic exercise for clicking due to disk anterior displacement with reduction in the temporomandibular joint. Journal of Craniomandibular Practice 21:10

Zakrzewska J 1995 Trigeminal neuralgia. Saunders, London

Zakrzewska J, Hamlyn P 1999 Facial pain. In: Crombie I K (ed.) Epidemiology of pain. IASP Press, Seattle

Chapter 2

Functional anatomy of the craniomandibular and craniofacial region: a palpation perspective

G.H. Bekkering

CHAPTER CONTENTS

INTRODUCTION

The skull is one of the most remarkable parts of the skeleton. It is referred to in legends and superstition, and was depicted and studied by Stone Age people. All over the world, people used (and use!) human skulls for many purposes. In modern times, most anatomical books have a large section on this intricate bone assembly (Fig. 2.1).

According to the Greek historian Herodotus, Persians used head coverings but Egyptians did not. Skulls would grow better, it was claimed, when exposed to the air. On the battlefields one could easily discriminate the more commonly fractured Persian skulls from the Egyptian. Herodotus can be considered the first person to have collected scientific data on the thickness of skull bones and the reason for the difference in thickness, though probably not the correct reason.

Since the craniofacial region is the focus of the book, the focus of this chapter will be on the connections, the joints between the cranium's bony parts, the insertions of muscles and ligaments, and the passage of nerves and blood vessels. As clinicians are required to locate the landmarks of the

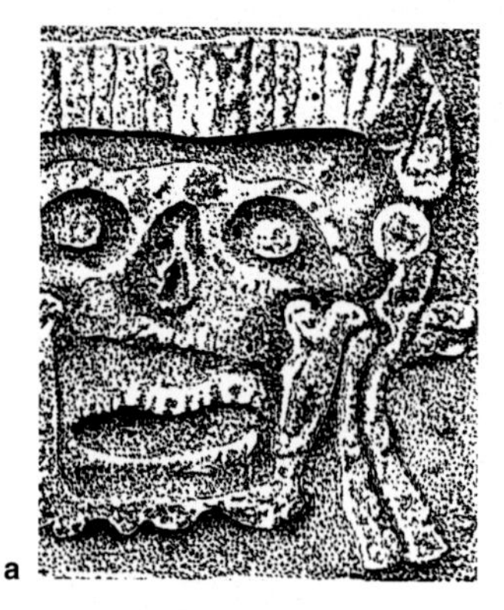

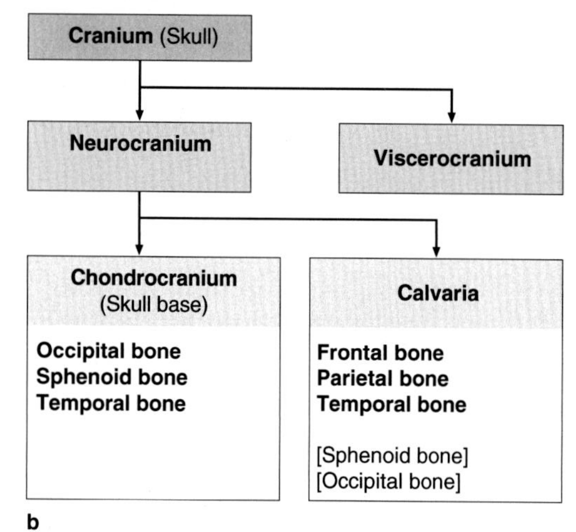

Fig. 2.1 Skulls in ancient cultures:
a Part of a stone Maya altar at Uxmal, Yucatan, probably influenced by Toltekens in the 10th century AD.
b Segments of the cranium.

skull, this chapter contains guidelines for palpation. The nature of this chapter is mainly descriptive.

As this chapter deals with functional anatomy, numerous anatomical atlases have been used for reference (Kahle et al 1975, Pernkopf 1980). Many (slight) differences were found in the skulls represented in their figures, and these were compared with several (Indian and European) skulls to which the author had access. Most figures are drawn from an 'average' Indian skull.

THE ADULT SKULL

In this chapter a skull will be considered to be fully grown after puberty, though relatively small changes in skull shape after puberty are known (Oudhof 2001).

The bony skull envelops the brain and some important sensory organs such as the eyes and ears. It allows nerves and blood vessels to pass through. It supports the facial muscles and forms the entrance to the digestive and respiratory systems. The combination of all these functions makes it very complicated. Sometimes scientists, especially anthropologists, consider the 'skull' to be the bony part of our head without the jaw. To avoid confusion, use of the word 'cranium' is advised.

We usually subdivide the cranium into the following parts (Fig. 2.1c):

- Viscerocranium (or splanchnocranium)
- Neurocranium
- Chondrocranium (or basicranium)
- Calvaria (or cranial vault).

The shape of the skull is, apart from genetic factors, influenced by the pull of muscles, the pressure of the growing brain and the pressure of blood vessels (Oudhof 2001). On the other hand, skull characteristics also influence the developmental potential of muscles and brain. A rapidly enlarging brain, such as occurs in hydrocephalus, may result in a much larger skull, and limited development of the brain can be the result of early fusion of the skull bones (Kahle et al 1975). Similar interrelations exist between the facial skeleton and the use of muscles. The use of the facial muscles, for example, is even said to influence the dura mater inside the skull (Enlow 1986).

To fully understand the peculiarities of the adult skull we have to look at the embryonic development of the skull.

There are basically two different types of ossification:

- *Membranous ossification* (also known as desmal ossification) occurs inside a layer of connective tissue, when fibroblasts convert to osteoblasts and start building bone.

- *Enchondral ossification* is that in which at first a piece of cartilage is formed by mesenchymal cells converting to chondroblasts. Later the cartilage is broken down and gradually replaced by bone, by fibroblasts modifying into osteoblasts (Fig. 2.2).

Both types of ossification occur in functional parts of the skull. Sometimes two embryonic bones – one of membranous origin and the other of enchondral origin – fuse to form one adult skull bone (as in the occipital bone).

In general, enchondral ossification is found in relation to the embryonic chorda dorsalis, and so predominantly in the skull base. Membranous ossification has relations to the subcutaneous skin and the first two embryonic brachial arcs, as well as the calvaria and the viscerocranium.

During membranous ossification a central spongiform compartment, the diploe, develops; this contains well-vascularized connective tissue – red (bone) marrow. From this stage on, the outer sheath of lamellar bone is called tabula externa and the inner sheath, tabula interna. Both tabulae are relatively thick.

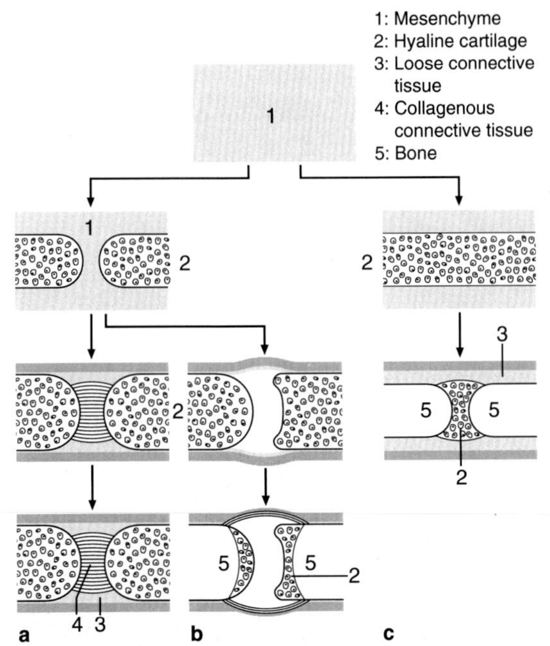

Fig. 2.2 Embryonic development of connections between bones:
a Fibrous junction.
b Synovial junction.
c Cartilaginous junction.

In the enchondral bones the outside is lined with a relatively thin layer of lamellar bone; most of the bone is spongiform and filled with red marrow.

In the nasal region, bones of both types can be 'pneumatized'. They hold cavities, lined with epithelium, in contact with the nasal cavity and the air contained within it.

Membranous ossification usually starts in the centre of a bone and radiates in all directions. This ossification centre can be found in fully grown skull bones and is called the tubercle. Most bones have grown close to each other at the time of birth but the connective tissue between the young bones still allows considerable movement. This connective tissue is considered to be a joint and is called a syndesmosis. The particular form is called a suture.

According to the shape of the joint lines we subdivide the sutures into (Fig. 2.3):

- Serrate suture, also called sutura serrata (like jigsaw pieces), e.g. the coronal suture
- Squamous suture
- Laevis suture, also called sutura plana (smooth and straight), e.g. the internasal and nasomaxillary sutures
- Gomphosis, connecting the teeth with the jaw.

Membranous ossification of the calvaria continues for several years and some of the syndesmoses remain throughout life. As long as sutures are present, growth of the skull bones is possible.

What makes the growth rate of the calvaria bones increase and decrease?

As a general rule in biology, structures that exist have a reason to exist. Orthopaedic surgeons know that if a joint is not allowed to move for some time arthrodesis (fusion of the bones) will occur. So, without any doubt, movements between the skull bones, however small

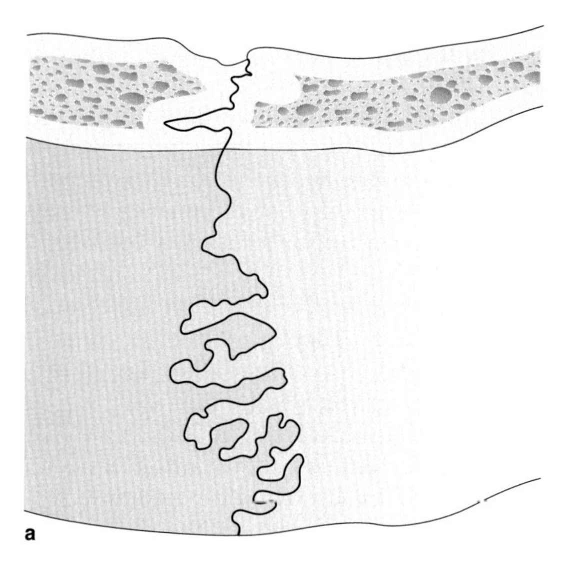

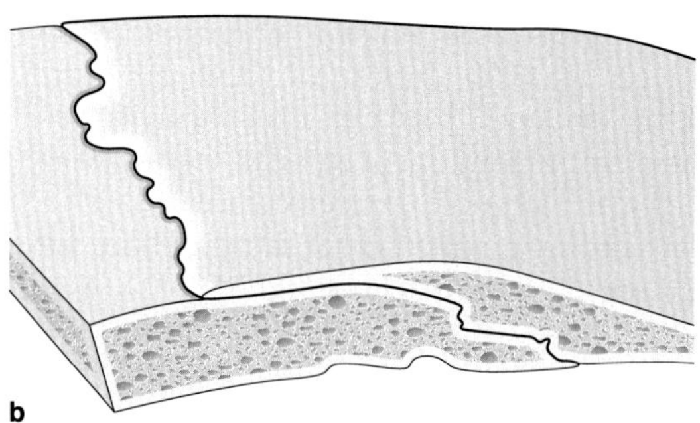

Fig. 2.3 Sutures:
a Serrate suture.
b Squamous suture.

they might be, occur constantly until the suture closes (Oudhof 2001).

As long as there is (dense, fibrous) connective tissue in the sutures there will be nerve fibres, blood vessels and lymphatic vessels. Because free nerve endings have sensory functions (viscerosensory as well as somatosensory) we have to assume that information on tension and pressure within the sutures is sent to the central nervous system (CNS). According to the conversion model most of the sensory information that reaches the CNS is 'assessed' by the 'decision-making stations' of the CNS, such as the dorsal horn, reticular formation and thalamus (van Cranenburg 1993). These gates 'neglect' the afferent information as long as there are no major changes in the enormous stream of information constantly entering the CNS, i.e. we do not become aware of the sensory input. This does not, however, imply that there is no information coming through these stations. The CNS can react to this information on a 'lower level'. The function of these gates, however, is currently unknown. Selection and filtering of impulses, and thus their transmission, depends on many factors such as motor activity, memory, emotions and sensory information.

Apart from the wealth of information about gomphosis innervation, little is known about the importance of the sensory information from the sutures, but its existence can hardly be called speculative (von Piekartz 2001).

It can also be useful to recall that membranous bone is formed within a layer of connective tissue, the inner and outer periosteum and the connective tissue in the sutures being the remnant of the original layer. Furthermore, muscle fascia (especially in the temporal and occipital regions) is continuous with the outer periosteum and the membranes surrounding the brain. The dura mater is (in places) continuous with the inner periosteum. To a small extent, therefore, the pull of muscles can influence the compartments within the skull (Fig. 2.4).

Which factors influence the final closure of some sutures?

A chondral junction (synchondrosis) can be found between skull bones with enchondral ossification. Of practical interest is the spheno-occipital synchondrosis that does not disappear before the 18th year of age (os tribasilare), with the same being true for sphenoethmoidal synchondroses. Intersphenoidal synchondroses, however, fuse early (see Chapter 1).

Growth of the neurocranium and the viscerocranium does not occur at the same pace. It mainly depends on genetic factors, the growth of the brain and the pull of muscles. A slight asymmetry in the calvaria as well as in the face is usually related to asymmetry of the brain, which in turn could be related to functional right/left differences in the brain.

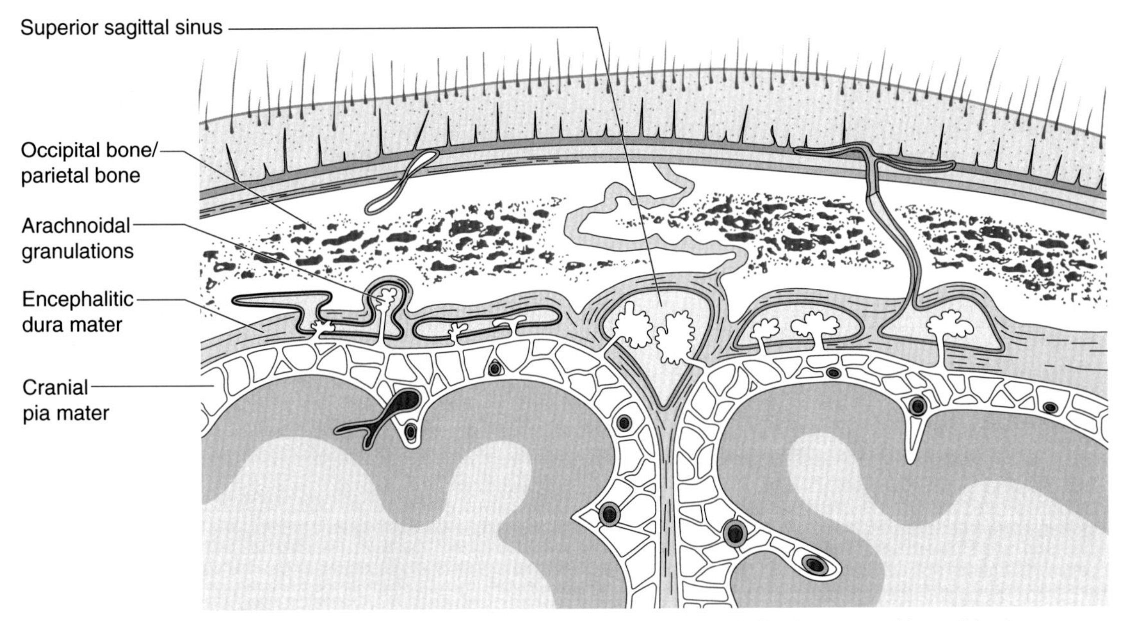

Fig. 2.4 Connective tissue structures derived from the mesoderm which lies between skin and brain.

The viscerocranium is not remarkable in the newborn, because of the lack of teeth, the small size of the mandible and the lack of paranasal cavities. The viscerocranium grows relatively fast shortly after birth and during puberty. On the other hand, the neurocranium is relatively large at the time of birth, because of the enormous prenatal development of the brain, especially the eyes.

The mastoid process is virtually absent in the newborn. It develops in reaction to the pull of (mainly) the sternocleidomastoid muscle (Spermon-Marijnen & Spermon 2001) (Table 2.1).

CRANIAL NERVES

Traditionally, 12 cranial nerves are named. Unlike the first two cranial nerves, which obviously are projections of the brain, the other 10 cranial nerves are essentially spinal nerves. Like the other spinal nerves they may contain several types of fibre:

- Somatosensory
- Somatomotor
- General viscerosensory (parasympathetic)
- Special viscerosensory (taste, artery receptors)
- General visceromotor (parasympathetic)
- Special visceromotor (brachial arch muscles)
- Special sensory (i.e. smell, vision, equilibrium, hearing, taste).

As in the spinal cord, the anterior horn is the origin of the motor fibres, and the dorsal horn the destination of the sensory fibres. The middle part of the spinal cord holds originating nuclei, where efferent (motor) fibres start, and terminal nuclei where afferent fibres end, after passing their pseudounipolar cells in ganglia outside the brainstem (Fig. 2.5).

The somatosensory nuclei are close to the midline. From caudal to cranial they are: hypoglossal nucleus, abducens nucleus, trochlear nucleus and oculomotor nucleus.

Lateral to these the visceromotor nuclei are found: the real parasympathetic visceromotor nuclei, and slightly more lateral the modified brachial arch motor nuclei. From caudal to cranial the parasympathetic nuclei are: the dorsal vagus nucleus (X), inferior salivatorius

Table 2.1 Anatomical terms

Term	Description
Basicranium	Basal part of the neurocranium, formed by enchondral ossification
Calvaria	Cranial part of the neurocranium, formed by membranous ossification
Chondrocranium	See basicranium
Cranial vault	See calvaria
Desmal ossification	Bone formation directly from connective tissue
Diploe	Bone marrow in tabular bone
Endochondral ossification	Bone formation preceded by cartilage
Gomphosis	Fibrous connection between tooth and jaw
Membranous ossification	See desmal ossification
Neurocranium	Part of the skull surrounding the brain
Periosteum	Layer of connective tissue surrounding a bone
Tabula externa	Peripheral layer of tabular bone
Tabula interna	Central layer of tabular bone
Splanchnocranium	Part of the skull surrounding nose, mouth
Suture	Connective tissue between skull bones
Synchondrosis	Cartilage connection between bones
Syndesmosis	Fibrous connection between bones
Viscerocranium	See splanchnocranium

nucleus, superior salivatorius nucleus and Edinger–Westphal nucleus. From caudal to cranial the motor nuclei of the brachial arch are: spinal nucleus, accessory nerve nucleus (XI), ambiguus nucleus (X, IX), facial nerve nucleus (VII) and trigeminal motor nerve nucleus (V).

The sensory nuclei are located most laterally. Their (relatively) most medial nucleus is the solitarius (VII, IX, X). The trigeminal nerve nucleus (V) spreads over a large area: the spinalis nucleus, pontinus nucleus (nucleus principalis) and mesencephalic nucleus.

The vestibular and cochlear nuclei (VIII) are located most laterally.

Several classifications of cranial nerves are given in the literature (e.g. anatomical, embryological or functional) as described in the introduction on cranial nerves of this section of the book. In this book a classification based upon clinical presentation is promoted, because the therapist is often involved with patients without diagnosed pathology after intensive evaluation. In such patients it should be borne in mind that a (minor) dysfunction of cranial nerves may play an undiagnosed role in the problem – one of the reasons for promoting an efficient and easy to use classification system for clinicians:

- Key cranial nerves (innervating a relatively broad spectrum of target tissues, and often involved in clinical settings):
  - Trigeminal nerve
  - Facial nerve
  - Vestibulocochlear nerve
  - Accessory nerve
  - Hypoglossal nerve.
- Particular cranial nerves (innervating a relatively small spectrum of target tissues,

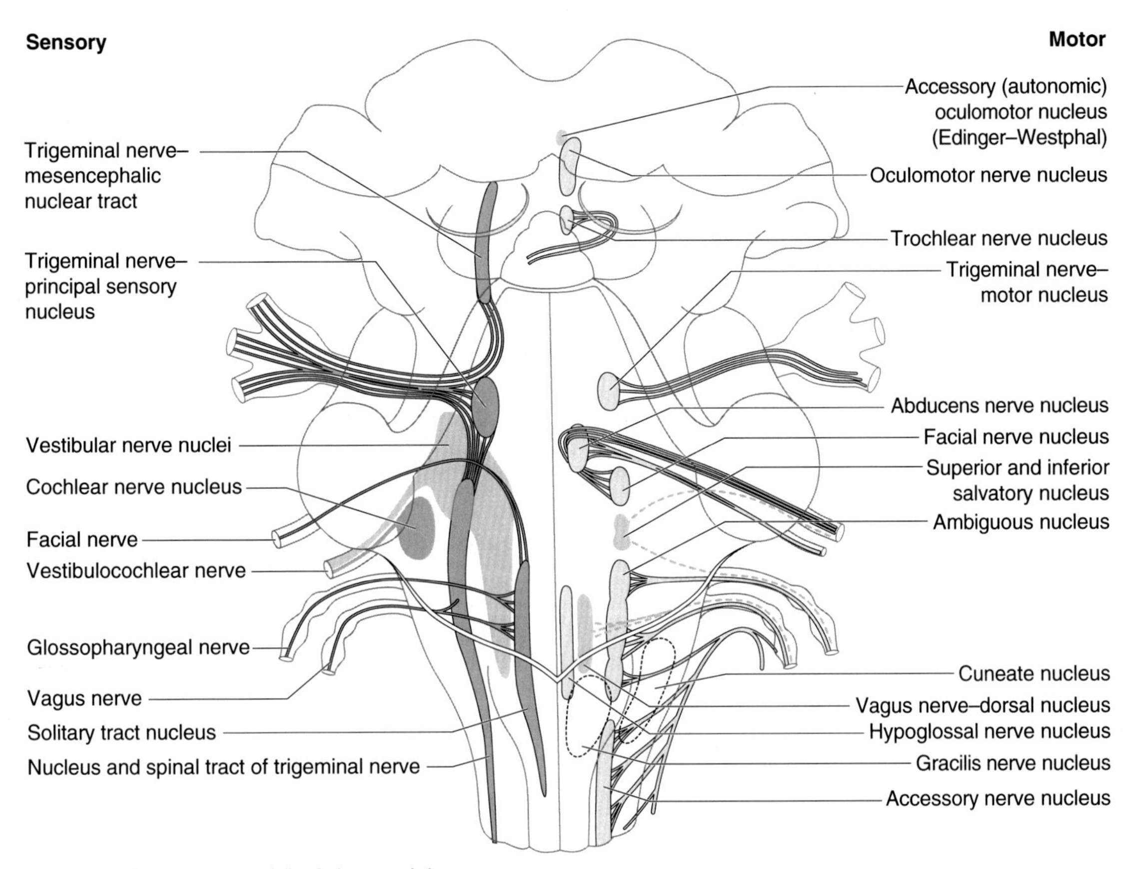

Fig. 2.5 Brainstem nuclei of the cranial nerves.

and mostly involved with specific dysfunctions or pathology):

- Olfactory nerve
- Optic nerve
- The eye muscle nerves:
  - oculomotor nerve
  - trochlear nerve
  - abducens nerve
- Glossopharyngeal nerve
- Vagus nerve.

For more information about tests for these nerves, target tissue examination and management, see Chapters 15–18.

In the next section we introduce a general anatomical overview of the cranial nerves. Their palpation is discussed below in the section on 'The craniofacial region, orientation and palpation'.

KEY CRANIAL NERVES (TABLE 2.2)

Trigeminal nerve (V)

The trigeminal nerve arises from the cranioventral part of the pons and includes the trigeminal ganglion (Gasser's ganglion) in the medial cranial groove, or more precisely in the trigeminal cavity (Meckel's cavity), which is enveloped by a dural cuff. The trigeminal nerve splits into three nerves.

OPHTHALMIC NERVE (V1)

The ophthalmic nerve (Fig. 2.6) is the most cranial branch of the trigeminal nerve and contains somatosensory fibres. It enters the cavernous sinus laterally, splits into three nerves, all of which (separately) enter the orbit through the superior orbital fissure.

Table 2.2 Key cranial nerves

Nerve	Function	Target tissue
V Trigeminal nerve		
V1 Ophthalmic nerve		
Frontal nerve	Somatosensory	Supraorbital nerve: skin of the forehead Supratrochlear nerve: medial corner of the eye
Lacrimal nerve	Somatosensory, with visceromotor fibres of V2	Lacrimal gland
Nasociliary nerve	Somatosensory	Infratrochlear nerve: the skin close to the medial corner of the eye: Communicating branch: the ciliary ganglion (constriction of the pupil) Long ciliary nerves: the cornea of the eye, and with sympathetic fibres, dilation of the pupil Short ciliary nerves: cornea, sclera and iris Posterior ethmoidal nerve: sphenoidal and ethmoidal sinuses Anterior ethmoidal nerve, external nasal branch: medial side of the nose and dorsum of the nose
V2 Maxillary nerve	Somatosensory	
Infraorbital nerve		Skin between upper lip and lower eyelid and the teeth in the maxilla
Zygomatic nerve		Skin of the upper part of the cheek and the temple
Nasopalatine nerve		Several taste sensors and glands at palate, nose and pharynx, accompanied by fibres from the pterygopalatine ganglion
V3 Mandibular nerve	Somatosensory and motor	
Masseter nerve	Motor	Masseter muscle
Deep temporal nerves	Motor	Temporal muscle
Pterygoid nerves	Motor	Pterygoid muscles
Motor fibres	Motor	For the tensor veli tympani muscle and the tensor tympani muscle
Auriculotemporal nerve	Somatosensory	Skin of the temple, the auditory tube and the tympanic membrane
	Visceromotor (from ear ganglion)	Parotid gland
Lingual nerve	Somatosensory	Ventral two-thirds of the tongue and the bottom of the mouth (with N. VII fibres)
Inferior alveolar nerve	Motor	Mylohyoid muscle and the anterior portion of the digastric muscle
	Somatosensory	Inferior dental branches innervate the teeth of the lower jaw ending in the mental nerve for skin of lower lip, chin and over the mandibular body

Table 2.2—cont'd

Nerve	Function	Target tissue
Buccal nerve	Somatosensory	Inner lateral side of the mouth and the skin of the lower half of the cheek
VII Facial nerve	Motor fibres, taste fibres, sensory fibres and visceromotor (secretory) fibres	
Greater superficial petrous nerve	Special sensory and viscerosensory	Peripheral glands and taste sensors (with fibres of maxillary nerve (V2)
Chorda tympani	Special sensory and viscerosensory	Taste of the ventral two-thirds of the tongue and gives preganglionic fibres to the submandibular and sublingual glands
Stapedius nerve	Motor	Muscle that regulates the vibration of the stapes
VIII Vestibulocochlear nerve	Special sensory	Cochlear branch: hearing Vestibular branch: equilibrium
XI Accessory nerve	Somatomotor	Sternocleidomastoid and trapezius muscles
XII Hypoglossal nerve	Somatomotor	Tongue muscles

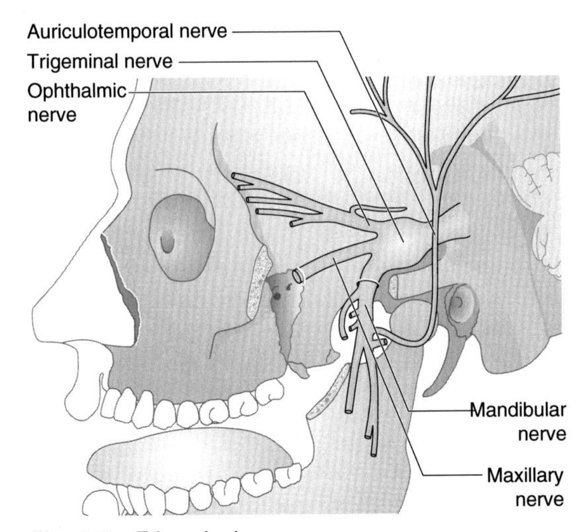

Fig. 2.6 Trigeminal nerve.

Frontal nerve

This nerve follows the superior levator palpebrae muscle. One branch (supraorbital nerve) leaves the orbit by the supraorbital incisure to innervate the skin of the forehead. Another branch (supratrochlear nerve) innervates the medial corner of the eye.

Lacrimal nerve

This nerve follows the orbital portion of the frontal bone laterally towards the lacrimal gland and innervates the skin of the lateral corner of the eye. Visceromotor fibres of the zygomaticotemporal branch of the maxillary nerve (V2) join the lacrimal nerve distally and innervate the lacrimal gland parasympathetically.

Nasociliary nerve

The nasociliary nerve follows the optic nerve and the medial eye muscles towards the mediocranial side of the orbit, where it divides. Its terminal branch (infratrochlear nerve) innervates the skin close to the medial corner of the eye.

Its branches are:

- Communicating branch to the ciliary ganglion (constriction of the pupil)
- Long ciliary nerves to the cornea, and with sympathetic fibres, dilation of the pupil
- Short ciliary nerves to cornea, sclera and iris

- Posterior ethmoidal nerve to sphenoidal and ethmoidal sinuses
- Anterior ethmoidal nerve passes the anterior ethmoidal foramen, into the anterior ethmoidal sinus. It passes the cribrous lamina of the ethmoid bone into the skull, where (still outside the dura) it passes the ethmoid bone, before it enters the nose through the cribrous lamina of the ethmoid bone again. Its final external nasal branch innervates the medial side of the nose and (sometimes after passing through the nasal cartilage) the dorsum of the nose.

MAXILLARY NERVE (V2)

The maxillary nerve is the middle branch of the trigeminal nerve (see Fig. 2.6) and contains somatosensory fibres. It enters the cavernous sinus laterally. After giving off a meningeal branch for the anterior part of the medial cranial groove, it reaches the pterygopalatine fossa through the round foramen (in the greater wing of the sphenoid bone) and splits into three nerves.

Infraorbital nerve

The infraorbital nerve is located at the laterodorsal side of the palate and the maxilla. It reaches the infraorbital canal through the inferior orbital fissure of the maxilla. It innervates the skin in between the upper lip and the lower eyelid. It also innervates the teeth in the maxilla.

Zygomatic nerve

The zygomatic nerve passes the inferior orbital fissure, stays close to the lateral side of the orbit and splits into a zygomaticotemporal branch and a zygomaticofacial branch. These run through canals in the zygomatic bone to innervate the skin of the upper part of the cheek and the temple.

Nasopalatine nerve

This nerve passes the sphenopalatine foramen into the craniodorsal inner part of the nose. It innervates several taste sensors and glands at the palate, nose and pharynx accompanied by fibres from the pterygopalatine ganglion.

MANDIBULAR NERVE (V3)

The large somatosensory part of the mandibular nerve (see Fig. 2.6), along with the much smaller medial motor part, passes the oval foramen of the greater wing of the sphenoid bone. A meningeal branch immediately returns through the spinous foramen to the dura of the medial cranial groove.

The mandibular nerve gives off motor innervations, predominantly of the masticatory muscles:

- Masseter nerve for the masseter muscle
- Deep temporal nerves for the temporal muscle
- Pterygoid nerves for the pterygoid muscles
- Motor fibres for the tensor veli tympani muscle and the tensor tympani muscle.

The mandibular nerve also gives off somatosensory and mixed nerves.

Auriculotemporal nerve

This nerve usually starts with two roots that unite after enveloping the medial meningeal artery. The nerve runs in between the mandibular neck and the sphenomandibular ligament, and crosses craniodorsally towards the parotid gland in between the temporomandibular joint and outer ear opening. The somatosensory fibres innervate the skin of the temple, the ear canal and the tympanic membrane. The visceromotor fibres from the ear ganglion join the nerve innervating the parotid gland.

Lingual nerve

This nerve runs caudoventrally to the base of the tongue. It provides somatosensory innervation to the ventral two-thirds of the tongue and the floor of the mouth. It receives its taste fibres from the chorda tympani (facial nerve).

Inferior alveolar nerve

This nerve (a branch of the mandibular nerve) contains motor fibres for the mylohyoid muscle and the anterior portion of the digastric muscle. The other part of the nerve enters the mandibular body at its medial side through the mandibular foramen. The inferior dental branches innervate the teeth of the lower jaw. The end of the nerve is called the mental nerve as soon as it leaves the mandible through the mental foramen. It innervates the skin of lower lip and chin, and over the mandibular body.

Buccal nerve

This nerve passes the buccal muscle and innervates the inner lateral side of the mouth as well as the skin of the lower half of the cheek.

Facial nerve (VII)

The facial nerve (Fig. 2.7) contains motor fibres for the mimic muscles of the face, and in the intermediate nerve taste fibres, some sensory fibres to the auditory meatus, and visceromotor (secretory) fibres. The nerve emerges from the lateral side of the medulla oblongata, just under the pons. The visceroefferent fibres emerge slightly more caudal to the rest of the nerve (intermediate nerve). Both parts form one nerve in the subarachnoid space and enter the internal acoustic pore. The nerve keeps to the lateral side of the opening before it enters the facial canal, a curving canal in the petrous bone. The canal is outside the middle ear and ends in the stylomastoid foramen. Inside the parotid gland the nerve splits into its motor branches for the mimic muscles (parotid plexus).

Inside the facial canal three nerves originate: the greater superficial petrous nerve, the chorda tympani and the stapedius nerve.

GREATER SUPERFICIAL PETROUS NERVE

This nerve returns into the facial canal and leaves it by the hiatus of the facial canal as the

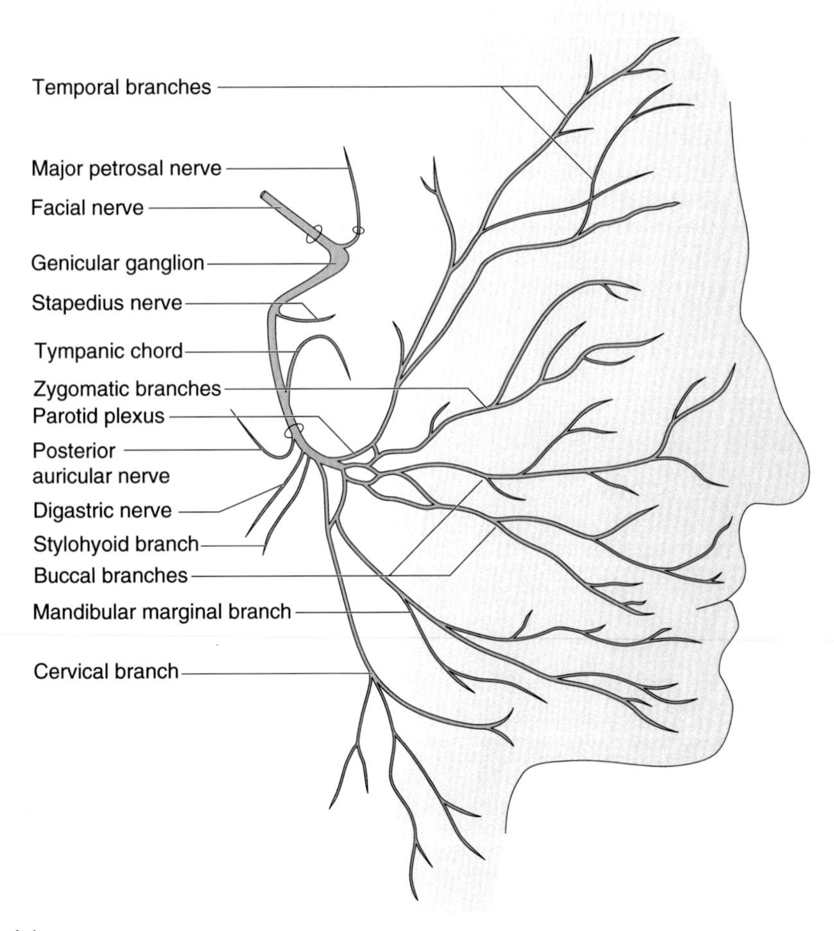

Fig. 2.7 Facial nerve.

greater petrous nerve to enter the skull outside the dura ventrally. It passes the lacerated foramen to unite with the deeper petrous nerve (sympathetic) in the pterygoid canal (Vidian's canal). After redistribution of the fibres in the pterygopalatine ganglion the nerve joins branches of the maxillary nerve (V2) to the peripheral glands and taste sensors.

CHORDA TYMPANI

This nerve is responsible for the taste receptors of the ventral two-thirds of the tongue and gives preganglionic fibres to the submandibular and sublingual glands. This nerve also returns to the facial canal, penetrates the petrous bone and passes through the acoustic bones in the middle. It leaves the tympanic cavity by the petrotympanic fissure. The nerve then joins the lingular nerve of the mandibular nerve (V3).

STAPEDIUS NERVE

This small and short nerve innervates the musculature which regulates the vibration of the stapes.

Vestibulocochlear nerve (VIII)

This special sensory nerve (hearing: cochlear branch, and equilibrium: vestibular branch) emerges from the dorsolateral side of the medulla oblongata, close to the facial nerve. It reaches the internal auditory opening via the subarachnoid space. The nerve is covered with a connective tissue layer and splits inside the petrous bone canal into its two branches.

Accessory nerve (XI)

This is a pure motor nerve (Fig. 2.8), innervating the sternocleidomastoid and trapezius muscles. The central nervous origin of this nerve is in the spinal cord, segments C1–C5 or C6. All motor fibres start laterally at all these levels and ascend to the skull via the foramen magnum. Here they are joined by some cranial fibres which leave the skull along with the cervical fibres via the jugular foramen, but split off immediately after leaving the skull and join the vagus nerve. The accessory nerve enters the sternocleidomastoid muscle, innervates it, crosses the lateral neck region and ends within the trapezius muscle.

Hypoglossal nerve (XII)

This pure somatomotor nerve innervates the tongue muscles (see Fig. 2.8). The nerve fibres emerge from the medulla oblongata in between

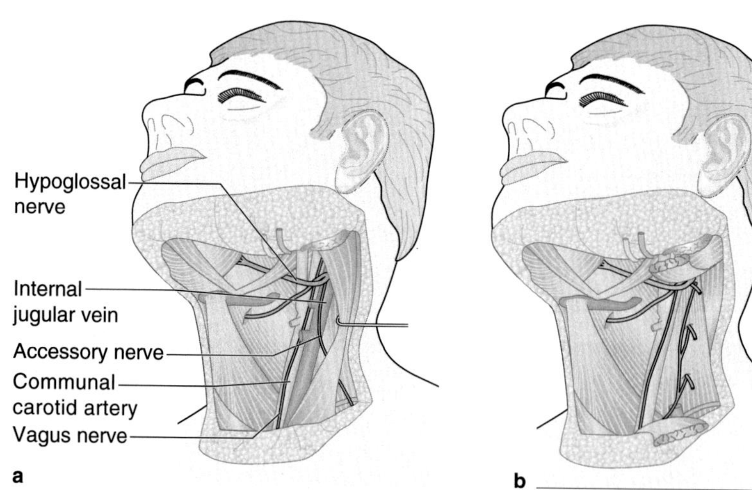

Fig. 2.8 Accessory nerve and hypoglossal nerve.

the pyramid and olive, and enter the hypoglossal canal dorsal to the vertebral artery to leave the skull. The nerve descends in between the vagus nerve and internal carotid artery. The nerve reaches the tongue muscles after passing the tip of the hyoid bone and splits into its final branches in between the mylohyoid and the hypoglossus muscles.

PARTICULAR CRANIAL NERVES (Table 2.3)

Olfactory nerve (I)

The nerve fibres (fila olfactoria) are the proximal parts of the sensory cells in the smell area (regio olfactoria) in the upper part of the nose.

Table 2.3 Particular cranial nerves

Nerve	Function	Target tissue
I Olfactory nerve	Special sensory	Regio olfactoria (olfactory tissue in nose)
II Optic nerve	Special sensory	Optical cortex (vision area in the occipital lobe)
III Oculomotor nerve	Somatosensory	Four of the six external eye muscles and the muscle of the upper eyelid
	Viscerosensory (parasympathetic)	The internal eye muscles
IV Trochlear nerve	Somatosensory	The superior oblique muscle of the eye
IX Glossopharyngeal nerve		
Tympanic nerve	Visceromotor	For the parotid gland and lesser petrous nerve to supply the parotid ganglion
	Viscerosensory	Tympanic cavity and the ear canal
Carotid sinus branch	Viscerosensory	Communal carotid artery split; helps regulation of cardiac output
Pharyngeal branches	Motor branch	Stylopharyngeal muscle
	Sensory	Tonsillar branches: tonsils at the roof of the throat
	Sensory and specialized taste fibres	Lingual branches: the posterior one-third of the tongue
X Vagus nerve		
Auricular branch	Motor	The (mimic) muscles of the ear
	Somatosensory	Skin of the outer auditory pore, some skin of ear and temple
Pharyngeal branches	Motor	Muscles of the soft palate and the throat
	Sensory	To the epiglottis
	With sympathetic fibres and fibres of N. IX	The trachea, oesophagus
Upper laryngeal nerve	Motor	Cricothyroid muscle (vocal cords)
	Sensory	Lining of the throat above the vocal cords
Recurrent laryngeal nerve	Motor	Supplies trachea, oesophagus and larynx
Plexi	Parasympathetic	For the lungs, stomach, liver, intestines and kidneys

They coalesce into olfactory nerves, which pass through the small holes of the cribrous lamina of the ethmoid bone. They synapse in the olfactory bulb. The olfactory bulb passes into the olfactory tract, located under the frontal lobe in the medial cranial groove. The olfactory tract sends fibres to the praepiriform cortical area, to the anterior perforated area and the septal area (subcallosa). The olfactory cortex is in close functional relation to the limbic system (emotions).

While passing the cribrous lamina, the olfactory nerves are accompanied by the paired terminal nerves (autonomic nerve) and the vomeronasal nerves that in humans are present only during embryonic development, and supply the vomeronasal organ.

Optic nerve (II)

The optic nerve and the retina (Fig. 2.9) may be considered embryonic projections of the brain, so that the eyes literally can be seen as windows to the soul.

The optic tract consists of four synapsing nerves. The processing of optic information is in the retina as well as in the lateral geniculate body and in the optic cortex.

The optic nerves run through the optic canal of the sphenoid bone, and thence to the medial cranial groove, where they are medial to the anterior clinoid process. This is where the nerves leave their dura cuff and enter the subdural cavity. From there on the nerves unite in between brain and pineal gland (hypophysis) in the optic chiasma, where the fibres from the medial retina (temporal field of vision) meet. Aside from the infundibulum (stalk of the pineal gland), the optic tract runs laterodorsal to the lateral geniculate body, which is in between the cerebral peduncle (brain stalk) and uncus (hook) of the temporal lobe. The optic radiation (within the brain) brings the optic fibres to the optic cortex in the occipital lobe.

Oculomotor nerve (III)

The oculomotor nerve (see Fig. 2.9) leaves the brainstem at the interpeduncular fossa, just medial to the cerebral peduncle, at the rostral side of the brainstem. After passing the posterior clinoid process, laterally to the sella turcica, it penetrates the dura mater and enters the cavernous sinus. It then passes into the orbit via the superior orbital fissure. Its somatosensory fibres innervate four of the six external eye muscles and the muscle of the upper eyelid. The viscerosensory (parasympathetic) fibres synapse in the ciliary ganglion in the orbit and innervate the internal eye muscles.

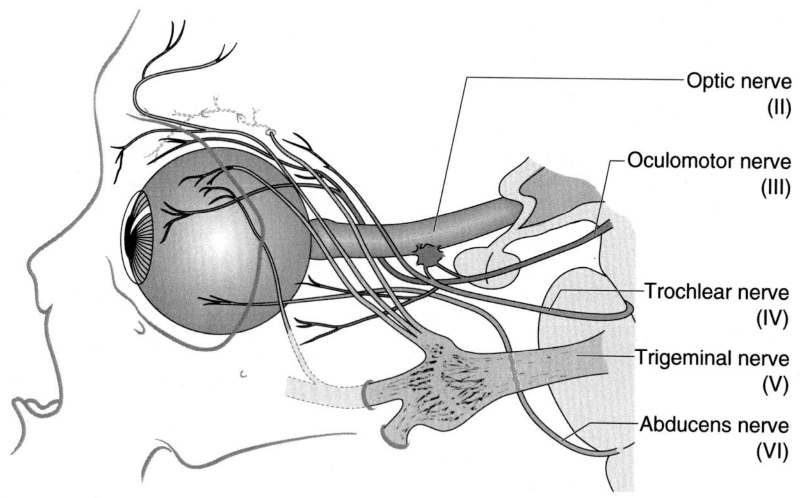

Fig. 2.9 Optic nerve and oculomotor nerves.

Trochlear nerve (IV)

This somatosensory nerve is the only cranial nerve that originates at the dorsal side of the brainstem (see Fig. 2.9). It leaves the brainstem immediately below the inferior colliculus and curves around the brainstem within the subarachnoid space. It penetrates the dura close to the ophthalmic nerve (V1) into the cavernous sinus. It reaches the orbit through the superior orbital fissure to innervate the superior oblique muscle.

Abducens nerve (VI)

This motor nerve originates between the pons and the medulla oblongata at the ventral side of the brainstem (see Fig. 2.9). The nerve runs intradurally (cisterna pontis) to craniorostral in the posterior cranial fossa. The fibres penetrate the dura dorsocaudal of the sella turcica and reach the cavernous sinus after passing the inferior petrous sinus. The nerve innervates the lateral rectus muscle after passing the superior orbital fissure.

Glossopharyngeal nerve (IX)

This nerve emerges from the medulla oblongata dorsal to the olive and cranial to the vagus nerve (Fig. 2.10). It contains motor fibres for the pharynx muscles, visceromotor fibres for the parotid gland, viscerosensory fibres for the tympanic cavity and Eustachian tube, and special sensory fibres (taste) for the posterior third of the tongue and the throat.

The nerve passes the jugular foramen in between the petrous bone and the occipital bone, along with the vagus nerve (X) and the accessory nerve (XI), and leaves it between the internal jugular vein and the internal carotid

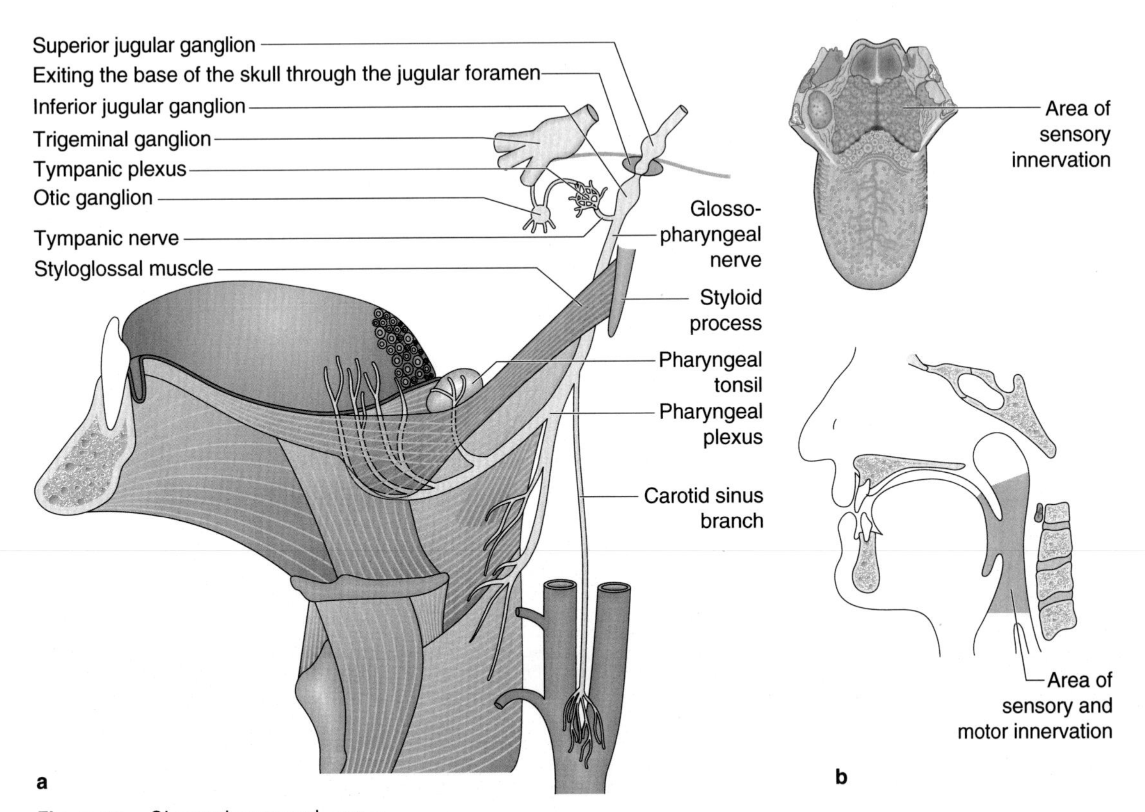

Fig. 2.10 Glossopharyngeal nerve.

artery. It proceeds downwards around the stylopharyngeal muscle and under the hypoglossus muscle where it produces its branches to tongue and throat.

TYMPANIC NERVE

This is its first branch. It has viscerosensory and preganglionic secretory fibres. It passes the inferior tympanic canal to the tympanic cavity. There it receives sympathetic fibres from the caroticotympanic nerve and forms the tympanic sensory plexus innervating the tympanic cavity and the ear canal. The secretory fibres pass the oval foramen as the lesser petrous nerve to supply the parotid ganglion.

CAROTID SINUS BRANCH

This viscerosensory branch innervates the place where the communal carotid artery splits. Its sensors help regulation of cardiac output.

PHARYNGEAL BRANCHES

These comprise the pharyngeal plexus with fibres of the vagus nerve. A motor branch innervates the stylopharyngeal muscle. Some sensory tonsillar branches innervate the tonsils at the roof of the throat. The lingual branches innervate the posterior third of the tongue with sensory and specialized taste fibres.

Vagus nerve (X)

The vagus nerve innervates parts of the head, but is also the most important parasympathetic nerve for the thorax and abdomen (Fig. 2.11). It has motor fibres for the brachial arch muscles, exteroceptive sensory fibres, visceromotor and viscerosensory fibres, and taste fibres.

The nerve starts dorsal of the olive at the medulla oblongata, just caudal to the glossopharyngeal nerve and passes through the jugular foramen along with the glossopharyngeal and accessory nerves (which add some fibres). The vagus nerve descends in between the internal carotid artery and the external jugular vein in a shared sheet of connective tissue (carotid sheath).

AURICULAR BRANCH

This branch returns to the skull via the mastoid canal and the tympanicomastoid fissure for the dura in the posterior cranial groove and supplies the skin of the opening of the external acoustic meatus, some skin of ear and temple, and the (mimic) muscles of the ear.

PHARYNGEAL BRANCHES

These branches, most of which come from the glossopharyngeal nerve, form a pharyngeal plexus with sympathetic fibres and fibres of the glossopharyngeal nerve. They innervate the trachea and oesophagus, and provide a sensory supply to the epiglottis. Motor fibres innervate the muscles of the soft palate and the throat.

UPPER LARYNGEAL NERVE

This nerve runs alongside the internal carotid artery until it penetrates the carotid sheath. Its motor fibres follow the throat towards the cricothyroideus muscles (vocal cords) where it provides sensory fibres to the lining of the throat at the level of the vocal cords.

RECURRENT LARYNGEAL NERVE

This nerve splits off in the thorax after the vagus nerve has passed the aortic arch (left side) or the subclavian artery (right side) and supplies the trachea, oesophagus and larynx with motor fibres.

PLEXI

The vagus nerve then descends into the thorax and abdomen where it innervates the heart and forms plexi for the lungs, stomach, liver, intestines and kidneys.

THE CRANIOFACIAL REGION, ORIENTATION AND PALPATION

CONTOURS OF THE FACE

The interindividual differences in the (relative) proportions of the skull bones are considerable. A marked diversity of faces exists. Genetic factors, age, sex and race all play a role (Oudhof 2001).

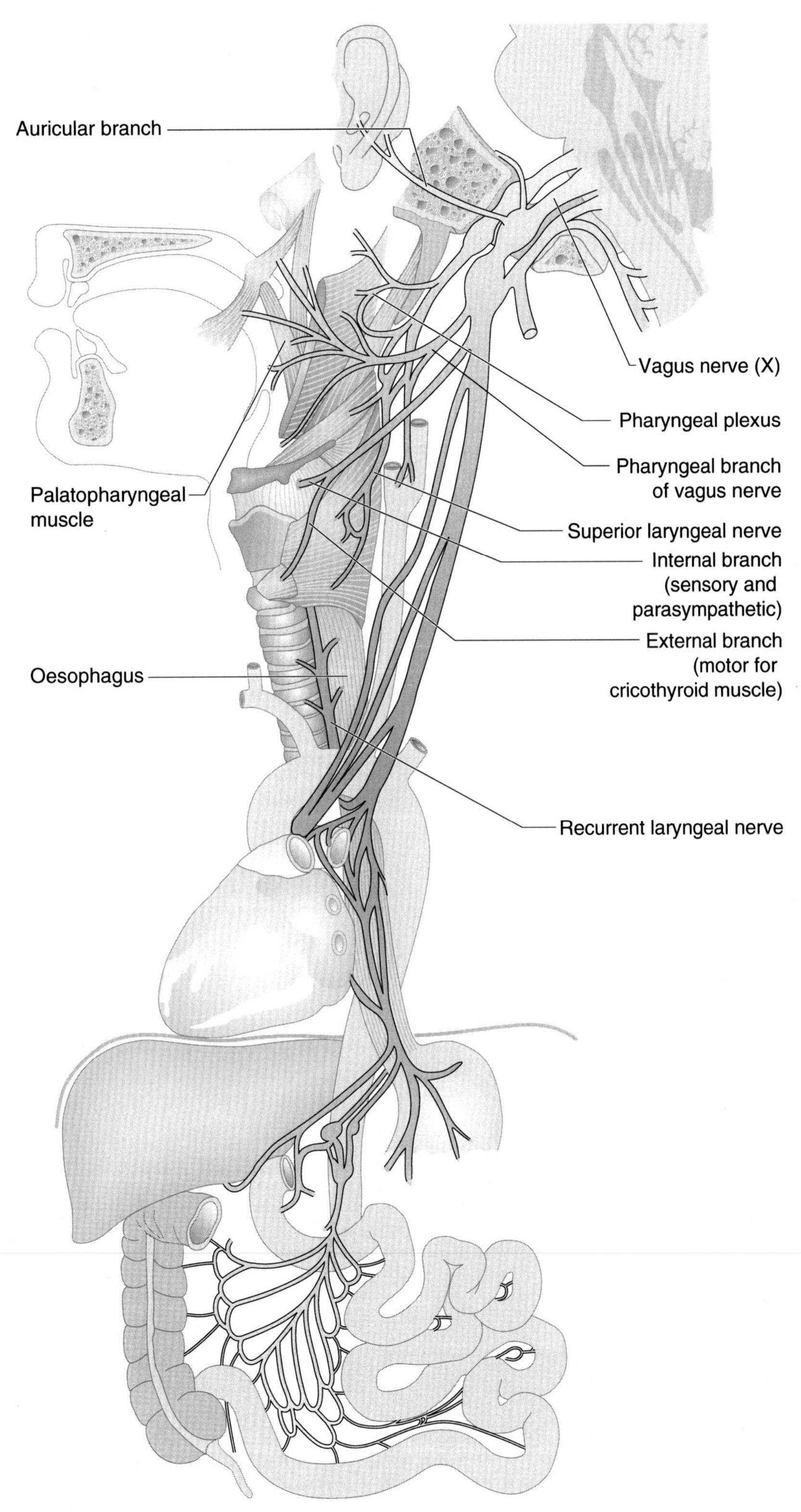

Fig. 2.11 Vagus nerve.

Most important for the contours of the face is the zygomatic arch (the cheek bone) which determines the shape of the cheeks and the mandible, which in turn determines the shape of the chin. Together with the frontal bone they give the face a heart, rectangular or oval/round shape.

The folds of the skin are the result of the activity of the mimic muscles. Although interindividual differences in skin quality are enormous, most skin folds develop between the 25th and 30th years of life. Most marked are the folds at the forehead and around the eyes.

THE NEUROCRANIUM

Cues for palpation of craniofacial bony structures

Interindividual variations in qualities such as shape, form and constitution of the tissues around sutures can be found during palpation (Fig. 2.12).

- Palpate the sutures with the tips of your fingers with the middle and distal phalanxes flexed to about 45°.
- If possible, support your lower arm on the table to create an optimally relaxed position of your hand to give yourself the best prospect of feeling the contours.
- Palpate perpendicular to the suture. That way, the sutures can be recognized more easily, and it is simpler to feel the direction in which the sutures go.
- If possible, palpate the left and right sides at the same time and judge possible differences related to the clinical pattern found before palpation. The coronary and lambdoid sutures can be compared relatively easily.
- Most neurocranial sutures have thickened borders with a gap in between which is normally a little sensitive.

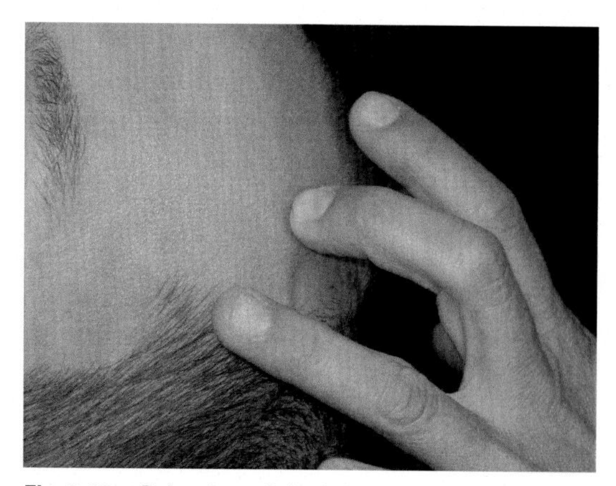

Fig 2.12 Palpation of the left coronal suture with the middle finger.

Localization of the calvarium

Palpation of the calvarial sutures, and thus determining the dimensions of the calvarial bones, is relatively easy. It is of course essential to know where to palpate, but once you try, you will find them. Like the tubercles, they are covered only by the (hair) skin and a very thin epicranial muscle. Figure 2.13 shows an overview of the sutures.

The sagittal suture lies between the parietal bones. The coronal suture is between the frontal bone and the parietal bones. The lambdoid suture is between the occipital bone and the parietal bone. Each parietal bone has a parietal tubercle. The frontal bone has two frontal tubercles because of its double embryonic origin. The tubercle of the occipital bone develops into the external occipital protuberance, the origin of the nuchal ligament, and can grow to considerable proportions.

We know, however, that variations of the sutures are frequent. This is certainly true for small bones that develop like islands within the sutures.

Cues for palpation of immature craniofacial bony structures

- In general, the sutures are not fused but jointed with elastic connective tissue.
- The sutures are slightly broader than in adult bones.
- The margin of the sutures is not yet thickened nor is it as rigid as in mature skulls.
- All in all, the region of the sutures seems considerably broader.

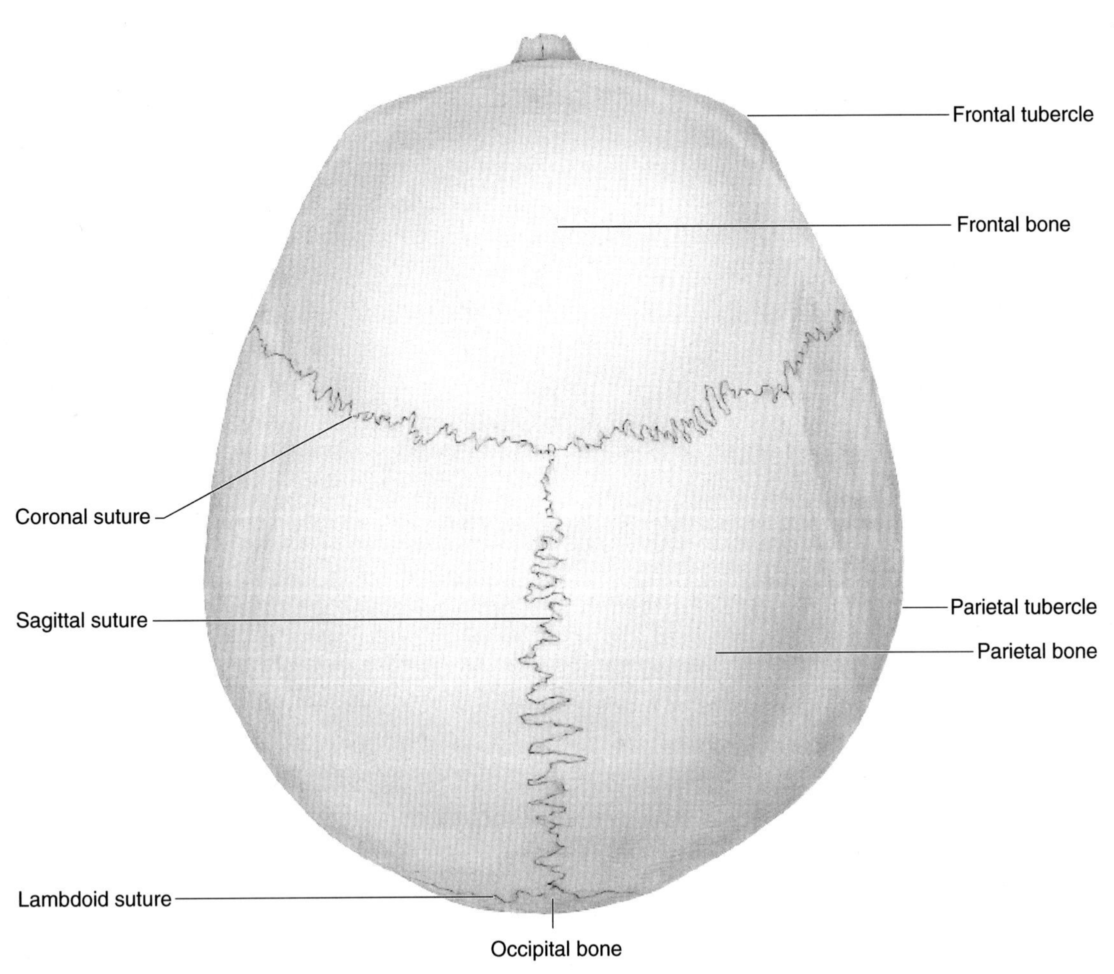

Fig 2.13 View of neurocranium from above.

You may find an extra frontal suture between both embryonic parts of the frontal bone, if they did not fuse. A remnant of this suture right above the base of the nose is regularly found.

You may find an extra transverse occipital suture if the cranial part of a membranous interparietal bone remained apart from the caudal part of that bone. Normally both membranous parts will fuse with the chondral part of the occipital bone and build the squama of the occipital bone. The resulting extra bone (inca bone) got its name because it is found with very high frequency in ancient Peruvian skulls.

All fontanelles may, albeit rarely, contain their own bones (Fig. 2.14).

The anterior fontanelle can develop into the bregmatic bone (os frontoparietale); the posterior fontanelle can develop into the apex bone; the sphenoid fontanelle can develop into the epipteric bone, and can even be split into two separate bones. The mastoid fontanelle can likewise develop into a bone (asterion).

Infrequently one finds a bone isolated within the parietal bone or (even more rarely) within the frontal bone. It is important to realize that all these extra bones can consist of both bone layers (tabulae) of the calvaria, so forming a full joint with their neighbouring bones. It is

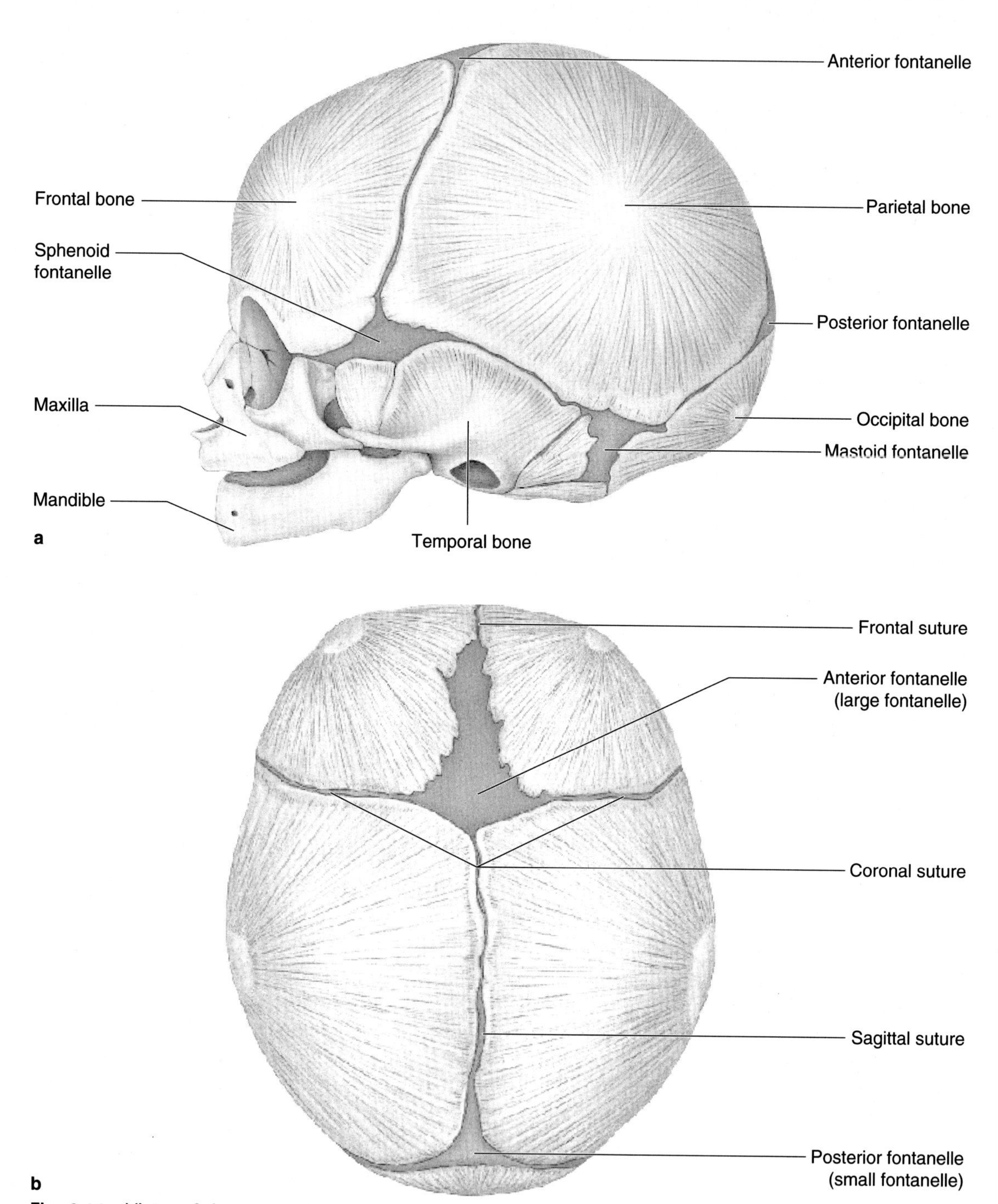

Fig. 2.14 Views of the neonatal cranium.

also possible that these extra bones consist of only the outer or inner layer. In the latter case they have no full joint with their neighbouring bone and you will possibly not discover them by palpating.

The properties of all cranial bones are described below. We advise practising with a real skull and a comparable individual.

The occipital bone

The occipital bone (Fig. 2.15) forms the dorsal side of the skull and the skull base. The spinal cord passes via the foramen magnum in the basal part of this bone. In the midline, at the caudal part of the squama of this bone, you can palpate a marked protuberance: the external occipital protuberance. This well-known structure is called the inion by anthropologists and is used as a measuring point. It is virtually impossible to miss it, from caudal as well as from cranial. From the protuberance, passing laterally, a horizontal ridge is palpable: the superior nuchal line, the origin of the descending portion of the trapezius muscle. Following this ridge further laterally one can find the mastoid process: a large protuberance behind the ear, part of the petrous bone (temporal

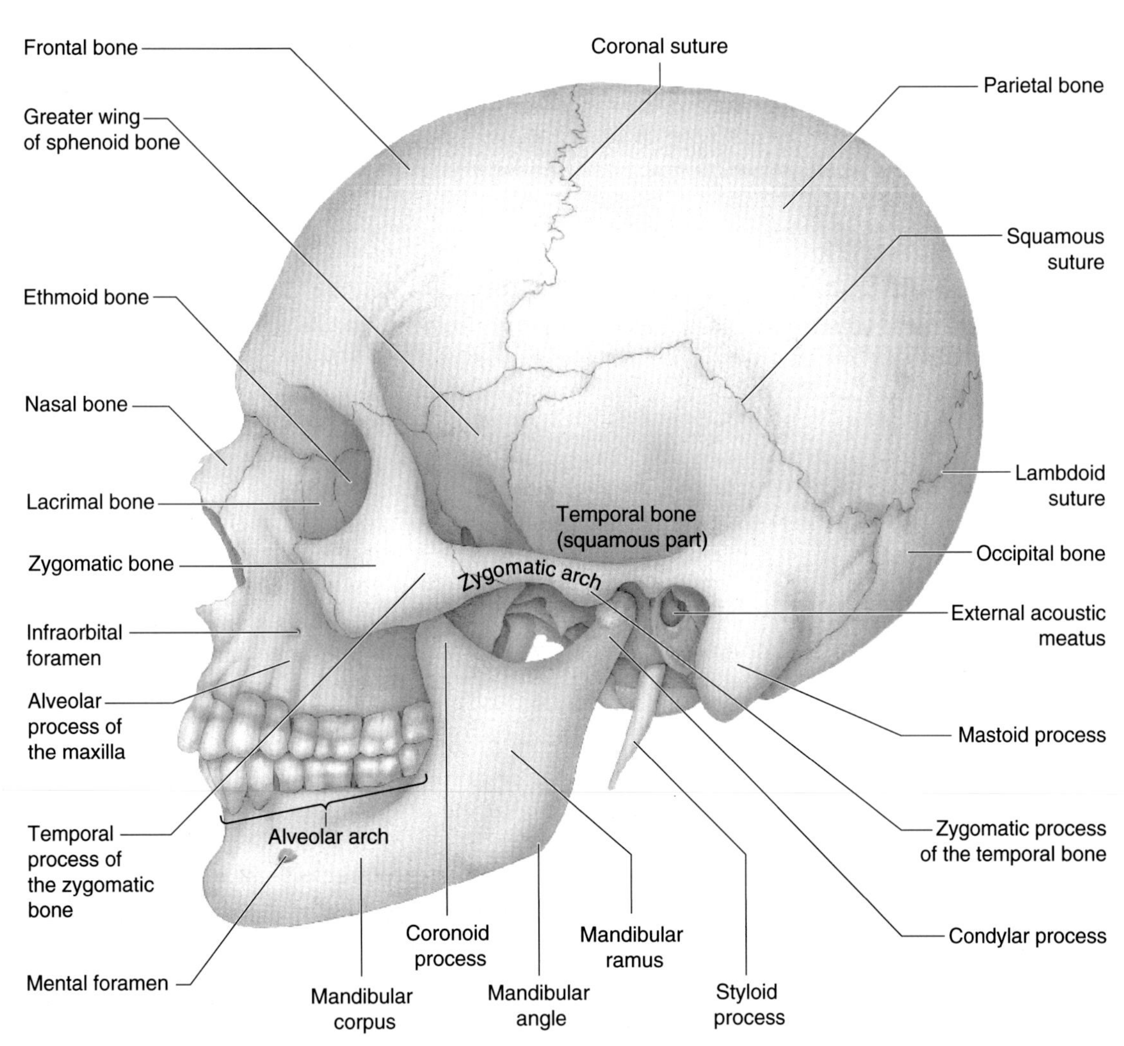

Fig. 2.15 Side view of the skull.

bone) and origin of the sternocleidomastoid muscle. It is possible to palpate the mastoid process by following the muscle cranially towards its origin. The mastoid process is virtually absent in the neonate. It is the pull of the sternocleidomastoid muscle that 'creates' the mastoid process.

The lambdoid suture joining this bone with the temporal bones is not easy to palpate, but can be found in a slight dent of the skull.

The temporal bone and the temporomandibular joint

The temporal bone (see Fig. 2.15) is located behind and in front of the ear. It is also part of the skull base. All sutures are difficult to palpate precisely. In the squamous suture, the temporal bone overlies the parietal bone. In the petrosquamous suture the mastoid process of the temporal bone touches the petrous bone. The petrous bone is generally seen as a part of the temporal bone. In the sphenosquamous suture it connects with the sphenoid bone. The sutures are difficult to locate exactly in the adult, whereas their preceding fontanelles are easy to palpate in the neonate.

The temporal bone contains the pore and external auditory meatus, the opening of the ear. The styloid process can be found mediocaudal to this opening. Many muscles are attached to this bony rod, which makes it hard to palpate. Relatively easy to palpate, however, is the stylomandibular ligament, which is attached to the dorsal side of the angle of the mandible.

The cheek bone is found immediately in front of the ear. The dorsal side of this zygomatic arc is part of the temporal bone and called the zygomatic process. It meets the zygomatic process of the zygomatic bone to build the temporozygomatic suture. The cheek bone is usually easy to palpate, although the suture is more probably estimated than palpated. The cranial side of the cheek bone is usually smooth; at the dorsocaudal side we find the articular eminence, part of the temporomandibular joint (TMJ).

The sternocleidomastoid muscle inserts at the mastoid process and continues ventrally over the temporal bone, thus producing a horizontal ridge, the supramastoid crista, that can be palpated immediately behind the auricula. The TMJ is to be found close to the ear opening, at the caudal side of the dorsal part of the cheek bone. Moving the jaw helps to confirm the exact location. With the jaw open wide, the mandibular fossa can be palpated immediately in front of the ear. Closing the mouth brings the mandibular head under the palpating finger. The palpation should be gentle, because it is easy to provoke pain in this position.

The TMJ has a relatively loose capsule, allowing rotational movements in the posterior part of the joint when opening the mouth a little as in normal conversation and permitting translational movements towards the ventral part of the joint (the articular tubercle) when swallowing (bilateral) or chewing (more unilateral). With protrusion or opening the mandible widely, the caput mandibulae slides ventrally and caudally to the top of the articular tubercle and might even dislocate to the ventral side of the tubercle. This movement is guided by the temporomandibular ligament which has an oblique course with the mandible at rest, and a more vertical position with a wide open jaw. The stylomandibular and sphenomandibular ligaments, both at the medial side of the joint, are slightly thickened parts of muscle fascia.

The articular disc of the TMJ consists of two parts. The ventral part has fibrous cartilage tissue and is well connected to the lateral pterygoid muscle. This muscle plays a role in protrusion and laterotrusion of the joint, thus shifting the disc ventrally along with the caput mandibulae. The fibrous dorsal part is functionally split into two layers: the upper part of loose fibrous tissue is connected to the dorsal side of the TMJ, the lower part of dense fibrous tissue is connected to the mandibular neck along with the capsule.

With the mouth closed, the caput mandibulae rests in a dorsal position close to the pars tympanica of the temporal bone, which is in itself a part of the auditory canal. The tissue in between the jaw and the ear canal has many elastic fibres, fat cells and blood vessels.

The functional movements of the TMJ can be compared with the shoulder joint. The shape of the bony parts and the looseness of the capsule make it an unstable joint. Therefore it is not surprising that minor craniomandibular dysfunction is present in 50–80% of the population, although therapy is needed in only 5%.

The parietal bones

The parietal bones (see Fig. 2.15) form a large part of the dome of the skull and part of the side of the head. The two parietal bones contact at the sagittal suture. It is possible to locate this suture, like most other sutures, by palpating a slight groove. Palpating the actual suture is difficult, however, as it is covered by skin and hair, and the aponeurotic galea, an aponeurosis within the epicranial muscle (occipitofrontal muscle) with the use of which most people raise their brows, and some people can shift their scalp.

In the coronal suture the parietal bones are connected with the frontal bone. In some people the frontal bone is considerably 'higher' than the parietal bone.

The lambdoid suture binds the parietal bones to the squama of the occipital bone and continues in the parietomastoid suture with the petrous bone. The squamous suture has already been described in the temporal bone section. It continues in the sphenoparietal suture at the ventrolateral side.

The parietal tubercle is the most convex part of the parietal bone. It is located craniodorsally to the ear and is best palpated with the palm of the hand.

Above the ear two lines can be found: the superior temporal line and the inferior temporal line. These lines are part of the parietal bone, not, as their names might suggest, of the temporal bone. Both lines have a functional relationship with the temporal muscle. At the superior line the fascia is inserted; at the inferior line the muscle fibres themselves are inserted. The inferior line is difficult to palpate. Palpating while the patient makes chewing movements tells you where the muscles are attached. The superior line is best found by starting at the dorsal side of the lateral border of the orbit. There might be a marginal tubercle located near the frontozygomatic suture. From there one can palpate the superior temporal line: first cranially, then dorsally and finally caudally, where it terminates in the supramastoid crista of the temporal bone. The line actually starts at the frontal bone.

The frontal bone

The frontal bone (Figs 2.15 and 2.16) has sutures with the following:

- Parietal bones – coronal suture
- Sphenoidal bone – sphenofrontal suture
- Zygomatic bone – frontozygomatic suture
- Maxilla – frontomaxillary suture
- Nasal bones – frontonasal suture.

The frontal bone is the result of two fused bones, and two diffuse frontal tubercles can be palpated a few centimetres above the eyebrow. Below the eyebrow is the supraorbital margin, most easily palpable by pressing cranially. When following this ridge from medial to lateral, you will feel the supraorbital incisure about 3 cm lateral to the nose, with the supraorbital nerve and artery leaving the orbit. The incisure is sometimes not palpable, i.e. when it is developed as a foramen. Especially in the male, the superciliary arch is developed as a bony ridge at the craniomedial side of the orbit. In between these ridges in the midline, a smooth horizontal ridge – a glabella – can sometimes be found; this often contains the remnants of the former frontal sinus.

The frontomaxillary suture can be palpated as a horizontal groove, along with the frontonasal suture at the deepest part of the bridge of the nose.

The sphenoid bone

The sphenoid bone (see Figs 2.15 and 2.16) is an important part of the skull base. Its greater

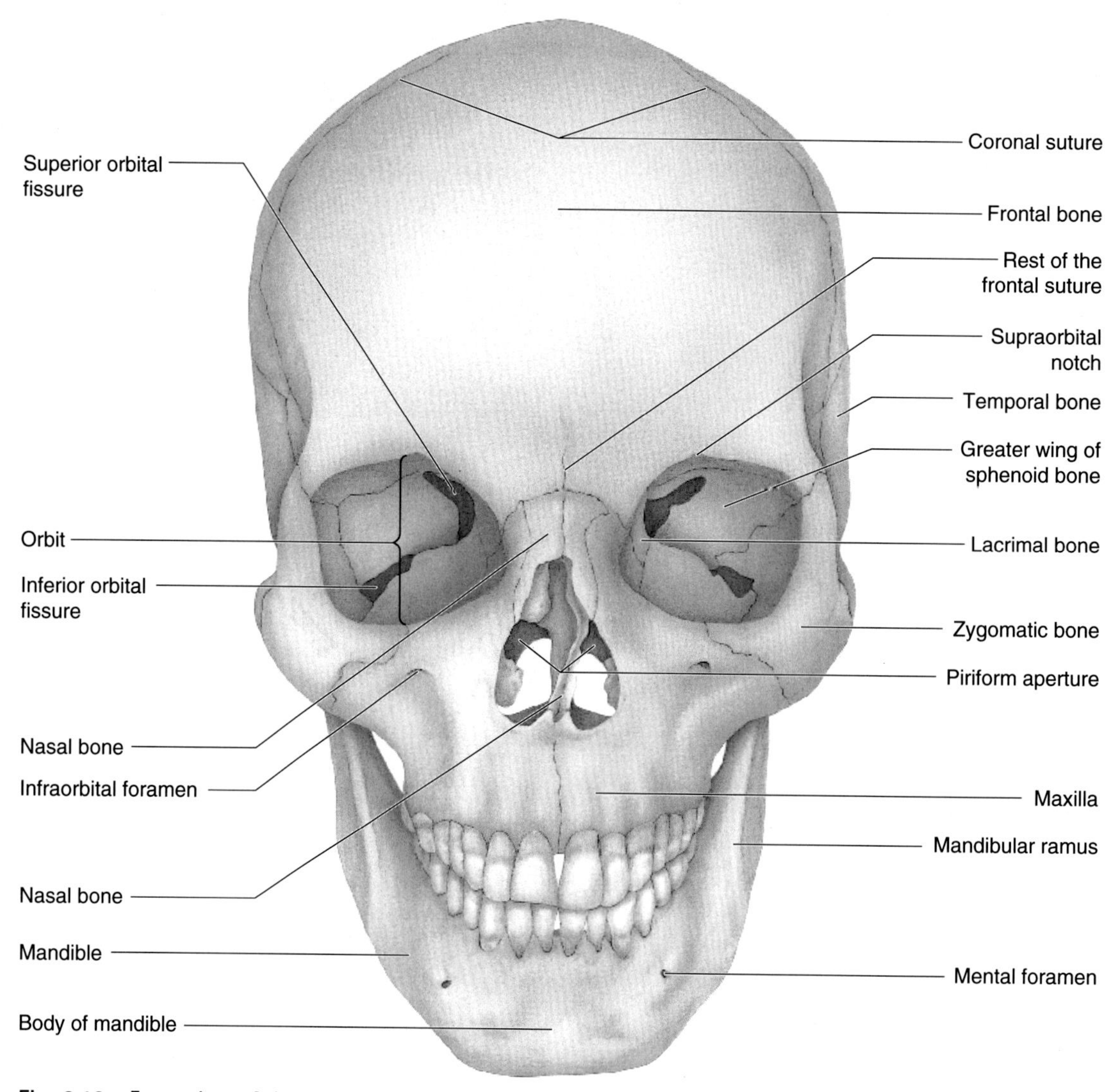

Fig. 2.16 Front view of the skull.

wing, the ala major, takes part in the calvaria, and is located in between the temporal, parietal, frontal and zygomatic bones. The respective sutures are all discussed at sections on the other bones.

In the part of the sphenoid bone forming the skull base we can palpate the pterygoid hamulus. You have to feel inside the mouth at the dorsal side of the hard palate, behind the last molars of the maxilla.

THE VISCEROCRANIUM (THE FACE)

Cues for palpation of the viscerocranium

- The sutures of the viscerocranium are mostly squamous or smooth. They are narrower, so are more difficult to feel than those of the neurocranium.
- They are more sensitive than the sutures of the neurocranium, so that when a dysfunc-

tioning suture is palpated the patient can experience a fierce, sharp pain.

- To palpate more precisely, greater flexion of the distal interphalangeal joint (about 110°) is advised, so that palpation is carried out with the tip of the finger to achieve better contact with the viscerocranial sutures (and their surroundings).

The nasal bone

The base of the nose is formed by both nasal bones and both frontal processes of the left and right maxilla (see Fig. 2.16). With the nose held with thumb and index finger one can easily feel that the point of the nose is more flexible because of the elastic cartilage.

The connection between both nasal bones – the internasal suture – is easy to palpate as a vertical groove. To palpate the horizontal groove of the nasofrontal suture, use the nail of your index finger at the deepest point of the bridge of the nose. The nasomaxillary suture is less easy to palpate.

The lacrimal bone

The lacrimal bone is situated at the dorsal side of the medial border of the orbit. When pressing softly, medially in the corner of the eye, a slight elevation can be felt.

The vomer

The vomer is the dorsocaudal part of the nasal septum. It can be palpated by entering the cavity of the nose and palpating along the chondral part of this septum until reaching the bony vomer. The possibility of palpating this bone will of course depend upon the dimensions of your finger and the patient's nose.

The zygomatic bone

This bone builds the lateral side and part of the caudal side of the orbit and builds the ventral side of the cheek bone. It is often one of the prominent features of the face.

The entire infraorbital margin is easy to palpate. In the lateral margin of the orbit, the frontal process of the zygomatic bone forms a frontozygomatic suture with the zygomatic process of the frontal bone. This suture can be relatively easily palpated in a groove.

The temporal process of the zygomatic bone is part of the cheek bone and is discussed with the temporal bone.

The maxilla

The maxilla is an important bone for the shape of the face above the mouth.

The maxilla articulates with the nasal bone (nasomaxillary suture) and with the frontal bone (frontomaxillary suture), both of which are discussed with the nasal and frontal bones, respectively.

The infraorbital margin is formed by the frontal process of the maxilla, which in fact forms part of the bottom of the orbit.

The infraorbital foramen can be palpated as a slight decline, slightly caudal to the middle of the infraorbital margin. The infraorbital foramen contains the infraorbital nerve and artery.

In between the nose and the mouth, both maxillae form the intermaxillary suture. The best way to palpate this vertical groove is under the upper lip. The anterior nasal spine can be felt by palpating under the nose cranially.

The roots of the teeth and molars are in the alveolar processes. Most of them are easy to palpate under the upper lip, as well as through the skin.

The anterior part of the roof of the mouth is built by the palatine process of the maxilla. The medial palatine suture can be found in the midline as a ridge.

The palatine bone

The most dorsal and smallest part of the roof of the mouth is formed by the paired palatine bones (Fig. 2.17). The transverse palatine suture can be found in between the dorsal and ventral part of the roof of the mouth. Further dorsally, in the midline, the dorsal nasal spine is palpable.

Although both maxillae are facial bones, they form part of the roof of the mouth, which in itself is considered part of the skull base.

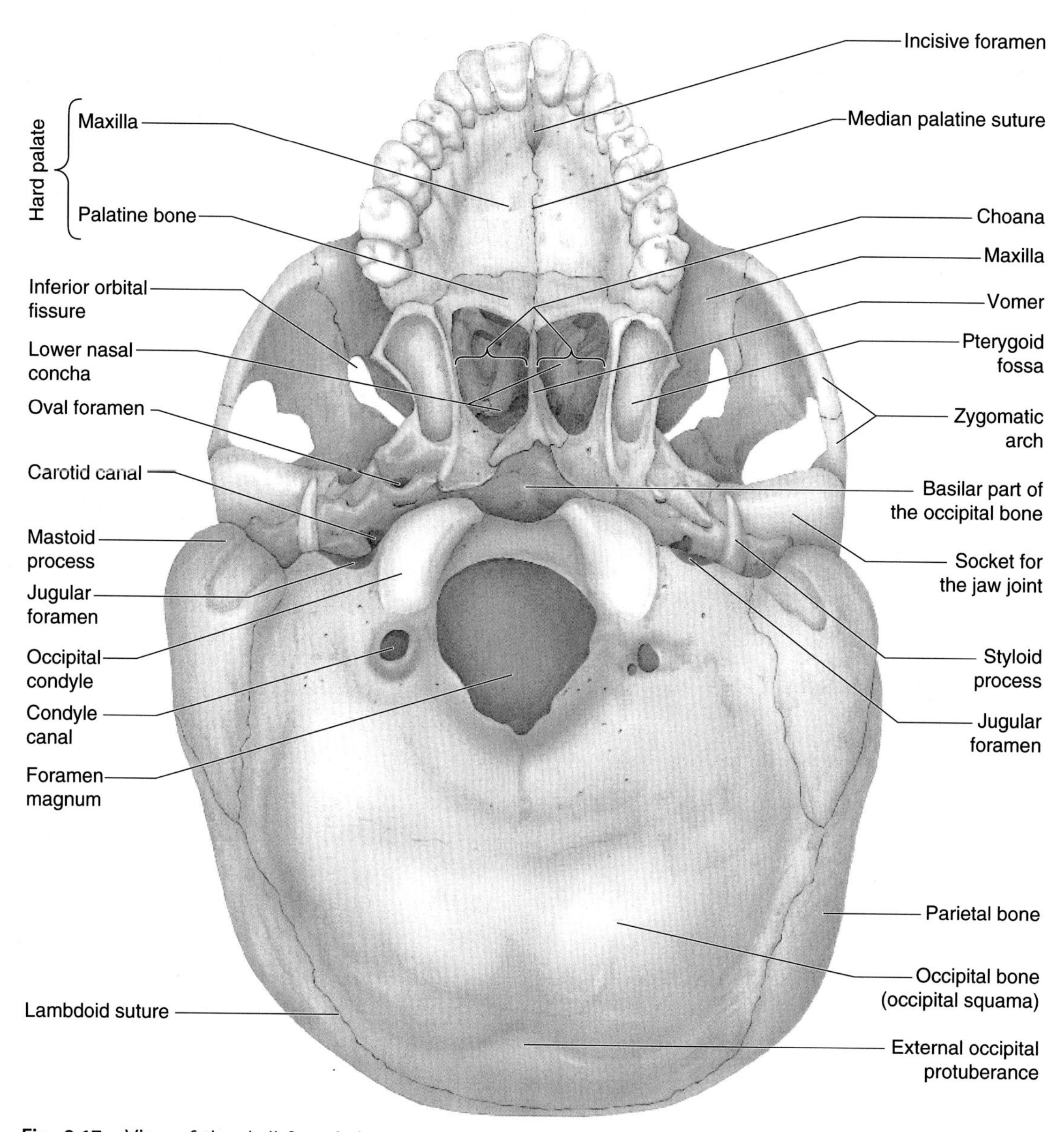

Fig. 2.17 View of the skull from below.

The mandible

The mandible (Fig. 2.18) is usually described with a horizontal part, the mandibular body, and a vertical part, the mandibular ramus. At the point where the horizontal body changes into the vertical ramus, we find the mandibular angle, easy to palpate and often used as a reference point. As in the maxilla, the roots of the teeth are held in the alveolar processes, and again, these can be palpated through the skin as well as under the lower lip. In the midfrontal line, an easily palpable ridge (the original suture) terminates in

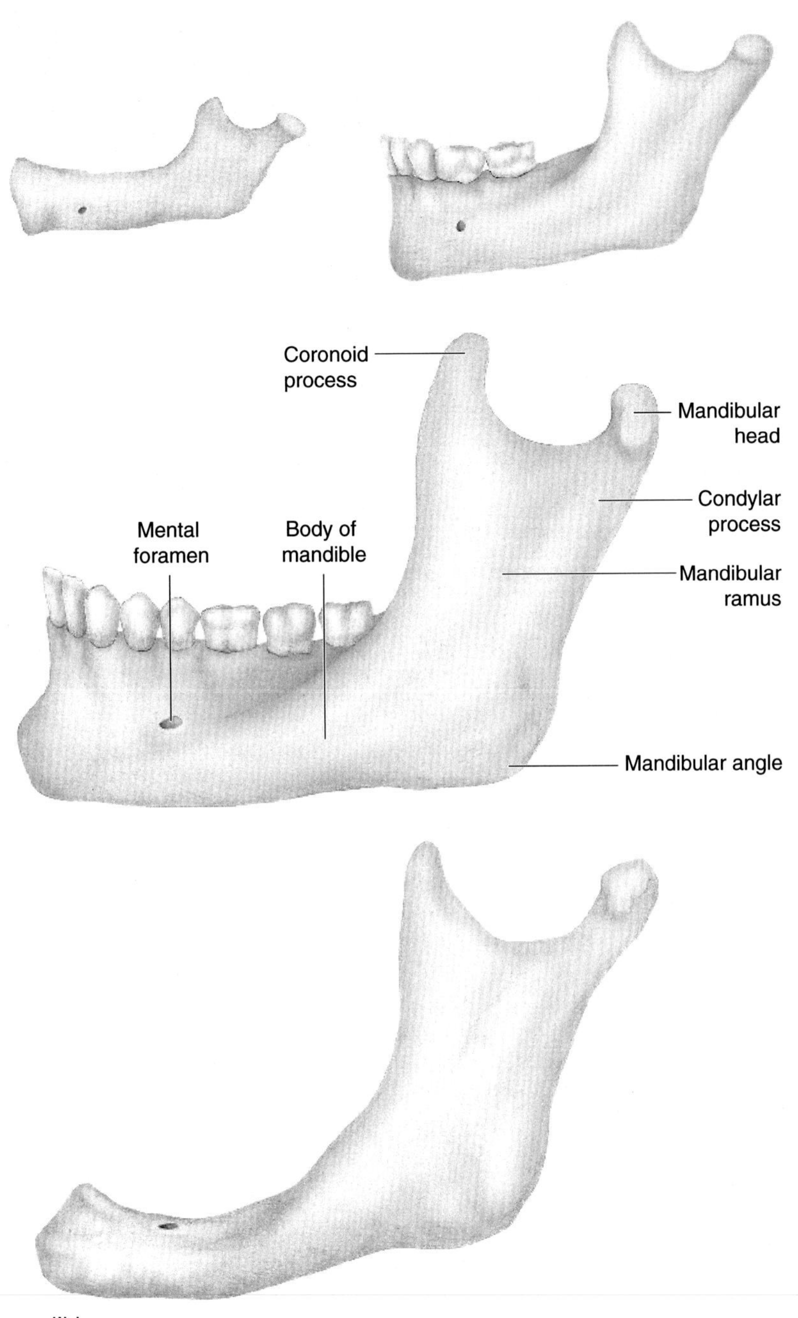

Fig. 2.18 The mandible.

the mental process, the chin. The mental foramen is palpable under the last premolar, in between the alveolar process and the body of the mandible. A shallow ridge – beginning dorsal to the mental foramen and gradually curving cranially – is the oblique line that terminates in the coronoid process, the insertion of the masticatory temporalis muscle. On palpation it is necessary to press quite firmly to feel 'through' the masseter muscle. The palpating finger can be placed just caudal to the zygomatic arch. The condylar process, the dorsal part of the mandibular ramus, is easy to palpate; it terminates in the mandibular head (Figs 4.6–4.10) in the temporomandibular joint. The mandibular head can be palpated immediately in front of the ear opening. It is helpful if the patient opens their mouth.

SUMMARY

- The main goal of this chapter is to provide the clinician with useful functional anatomy for palpation of the craniofacial tissue.
- The information gathered by palpation has to be combined with information from other manual techniques, such as passive movements. This may contribute to decision-making.
- The information from palpation should be interpreted utilizing knowledge of the nature of the sutures, their variations and their respective mobility. One should take account of changes that occur with age, and be aware of the wide scope of individual variations that have no effect on the health of the individual.

References

Enlow D H 1986 The human face. Harper and Row, New York

Kahle W, Leonhardt H, Platzer W 1975 Taschenatlas der Anatomie für Studium und Praxis. Thieme, Stuttgart

Oudhof H A J 2001 Skull growth in relation to mechanical stimulation. In: von Piekartz H, Bryden L (eds) Craniofacial dysfunction and pain. Butterworth-Heinemann, Oxford, p 1–21

Pernkopf E 1980 Atlas of topographical and applied human anatomy. Vol. I, Head and neck. Urban and Schwarzenberg, Baltimore

Spermon-Marijnen H E M, Spermon J R 2001 Manual therapy movements of the craniofacial region as a therapeutic approach to children with long-term ear disease. In: von Piekartz H, Bryden L (eds) Craniofacial dysfunction and pain. Butterworth-Heinemann, Oxford, p 63–100

van Cranenburg B 1993 Inleiding in de toegepaste neurowetenschappen, deel 3 pijn. Lemm BV, p 68–74

von Piekartz H J M 2001 Features of cranial tissue as a basis for clinical pattern recognition, examination and treatment. In: von Piekartz H, Bryden L (eds) Craniofacial dysfunction and pain. Butterworth-Heinemann, Oxford, p 22–45

Chapter 3

Guidelines for assessment of the craniomandibular and craniofacial region

Harry von Piekartz

CHAPTER CONTENTS

HISTORY

INTRODUCTION

This chapter will describe guidelines for collecting information by subjective examination, focusing on the craniomandibular and craniofacial regions and the cranial nervous system.

Methods of collecting information vary between clinical settings, especially when therapists are comparing different specialties (e.g. orofacial, knee, or low back pain).

One therapist may employ a hypothesis-oriented strategy of enquiry (Higgs & Jones 1995), another may prefer classification according to a particular protocol (Aufdemkampe 2001), and yet another may collect physical data before the subjective enquiry. Some combine all these strategies. Hypothesis-oriented strategies of enquiry entail collection of data by interview related to the patient's complaint and prior history (Maitland 1986). The aim of collecting such data is to recognize clinical patterns and to verify these later through physical testing (clinical evidence) (McNeill 1993, Jones et al 1995).

Data collection by a written questionnaire (protocol taking) is a screening evaluation by standardized written questionnaire or protocol for the assessment of complex signs and symptoms in the head region in order to detect contributory factors such as bruxism or head trauma.

One thing that all therapists have in common is that they search for clues, both diagnostic (i.e. source and cause of the patient's impairment) and non-diagnostic (e.g. physiological, social and cultural aspects of the patient's problem) in order to arrive at management decisions that holistically relate to all relevant aspects of individual health (Maitland 1986, Jones et al 1995).

It has not yet been proven which of these strategies of inquiry is the best. It is for the therapist to use whichever strategy is most adequate for a patient in a given situation.

The most important differences in these two main strategies of inquiry are summarized in Table 3.1.

Some circumstances in which one strategy is preferred over the other are suggested below:

- Type of care provider: Dentists, orthodontists and neurologists are probably more interested in the diagnosis. Physiotherapists, manual therapists, osteopaths and chiropractors on the other hand seem to be more interested in dysfunction, pain mechanisms and the most relevant physical signs which they can use for examination, treatment and further management.
- Type of patient: If an oral interview is impossible or difficult (e.g. because of aphasia or confabulation), a written questionnaire can be helpful, and the best available questionnaire should be selected (Butler 2000).
- Therapist's training level: When the therapist wishes to identify new clinical patterns (forward reasoning), written questionnaires do not stimulate the active thinking process which is needed to link signs and symptoms related to pathology and thereby recognize patterns (Jones et al 1995, Jones & Rivett 2004).
- Purpose of the examination: If the intention is research or classification of the disorder, a different method of enquiry is necessary. For example, a question which could be asked in a population with chronic temporomandibular dysfunction is whether or not the cervical spine influences their symptoms (de Wijer 1995). A written questionnaire would probably be more effective, in conjunction with an oral interview.

SUBJECTIVE EXAMINATION OF THE DIFFERENT REGIONS

The purpose of the subjective examination is to get a general impression of:

- The type and localization of the symptoms
- Involved pain mechanisms
- Activity and participation level of the patient
- Precautions and possible contraindications
- The examination plan.

Table 3.1 Advantages and disadvantages of hypothesis- and protocol-oriented assessment

Strategy	Advantages	Disadvantages
Hypothesis oriented	Facilitates active thinking, creativity Stimulates pattern recognition and discovery of new patterns Phenomenological approach	May miss relevant information Non-specific interview routines Time factor
Protocol oriented	Standardized Useful for classification and research Clinical patterns already described Diagnosis oriented Not time intensive	Inhibits lateral thinking Does not promote recognition of new clinical patterns Not always congruent with the patient's concerns

The proposed assessment and management of the patient with complicated head/neck and face pain by a specialized therapist can be divided into four categories:

- Patient history and profile
- Localization and description of the symptoms
- Behaviour of the symptoms
- Special questions.

Patient history and profile

The patient profile refers to personal information such as gender, family history, personal status (marital status, children, etc.), age, employment situation, free-time activities, etc.

This information immediately gives the therapist some clues as to which clinical patterns can be suspected on the basis of epidemiological studies. For example:

- The incidence of a migraine type of headache is higher in females than in males (Seidel et al 1993, Boissonault 1995).
- Atypical facial pain is seen more often in women older than 50 years and there appears to be a positive correlation with physical passivity (Zakrzewska & Hamlyn 1999).

Localization, quality and intensity of symptoms

An overview of the localization, quality and intensity of the patient's symptoms can be described on a body chart – see, for example, Figure 3.1. Symptoms from elsewhere can be noted on the same body chart. Patients diagnosed with fibromyalgia frequently have other systemic diseases alongside craniomandibular and facial symptoms. In these cases it is wise to note in detail the patient's main problem (head, neck and/or face pain). If there is sufficient time, questions about the clinical pattern of the rest of the body might be possible.

Pain intensity can be measured using a visual analogue scale (VAS). This is a line, 10 cm long, which starts with a zero point, representing no pain or symptoms, and a score of 10 for maximal conceivable pain. The VAS can be applied to many symptoms besides pain, such as vertigo, disturbance of concentration or olfactory hypoaesthesia. The VAS appears to be a reliable test for the loss of smell and is often used because there are no good diagnostic tests for such disorders (Spillane 1996). More details about the VAS are given in Chapter 19.

Body Chart

Name of the patient:........................ Profession:..................
Date of birth:.................................. Hobby:.........................
Diagnosis:..
GP:..
Date of first assessment:...
Physiotherapist:..

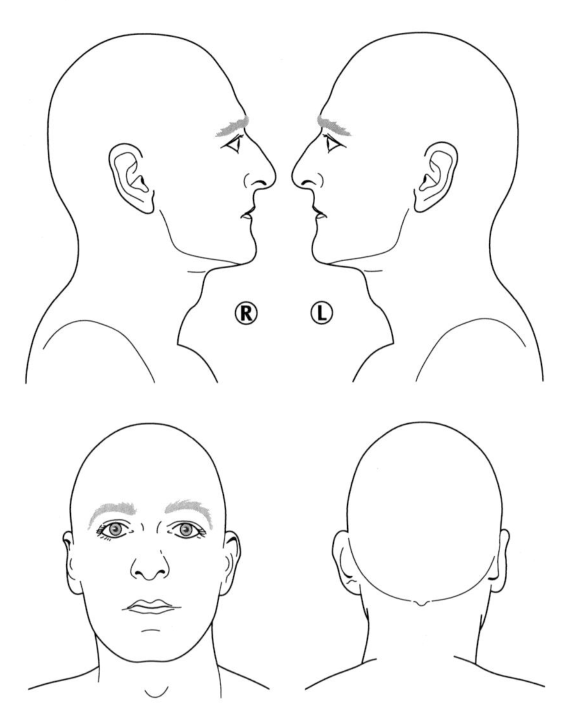

Fig. 3.1 Example of a body chart which is useful during the first interview to get an impression of the localization and quality of the symptoms.

Special questions

Special questions may point towards so-called 'red flags' (AHCPR 1994). These are a useful new concept, standing for precautions and contraindications. For example, in the case of a patient with longstanding head, neck and facial symptoms without a clear medical diagnosis, the therapist should bear in mind possible causes outwith the neuromusculoskeletal system (Okeson 1995). Patients may present with one of the following examples of facial pain without neuromusculoskeletal involvement:

- Headache as the first symptom caused by compression of central nervous tissue by slowly developing tumours at the cerebellopontine angle, most commonly found in middle-aged males (Lang 1995).
- A persistently numb chin with no change in the area or intensity of numbness due to a tumour of the skull base (Masset et al 1981).
- Persistent pain in the temporal region may be due to a mandibular osteosarcoma (Bar-Ziv & Asalsky 1997, Gavilán et al 2002, Schwenzer & Ehrenfeld 2002).

Screening questions that could motivate you to send the patient to another specialist for detailed medical examination are:

- Weight loss without reason
- Spontaneous increase of symptoms during the night which is not influenced, or only minimally influenced, by posture or movement
- Tiredness without a known reason.

For further information on this subject in the craniomandibular and facial region, see Boissonault (1995), Pertes & Gross (1995) and Okeson (1996). Boissonault's overview shows that, when required, special questions used in screening tests can be useful.

It is not known how frequently red flags are identified in patients who consult a medical specialist for head, neck or facial pain and are referred for physiotherapy. The therapist should always be alert for noteworthy symptoms or inexplicable clinical patterns (Maitland et al 2001, Lavigne et al 2005). This accelerates the decision to refer the patient to a specialist for further clarification (Jones 1994, Boissonault 1995) (Fig. 3.2).

THE CRANIOMANDIBULAR REGION

LOCALIZATION AND NATURE OF THE PAIN

Pain is often localized, severe and mainly limited to the temporomandibular joint (TMJ) and surrounding areas. In distal regions such as the temporal region, ear and mandible pain is more typically diffuse (Naeije & Van Loon 1988, Okeson 1995). When muscles are dominantly involved, pain is less localized and diffuse in the muscles of the area. This pain can also be sharp, especially during wide mouth opening, such as when yawning or chewing. In these zones ischaemic changes in the chewing muscles are often present; these are known as tender or trigger points (Friction et al 1985). Pressure on the exact location of one of these areas causes referred pain (see Chapter 8). Dysfunction of the masticatory musculature often results in stiff or 'heavy' jaws (Palla 1998).

There is some indication that the craniomandibular region has a contributory role in referred pain in the craniocervical region (de Wijer 1995, Okeson 1995). On a VAS, the score of the neck pain in most cases is lower than in the craniomandibular region, where there is a clear pattern of craniomandibular dysfunction (von Piekartz 2001).

Noises during mouth activity

Joint noises can often be experienced by the patient and can vary from a minimal popping sound through crepitations up to a loud snapping sound. Noises during movement are mostly directly related to intra-articular craniomandibular dysfunctions (Pertes & Gross 1995, Buhmann & Lotsman 2000). Arthrogenic dysfunctions of the craniomandibular region are described in detail in Chapter 9. An important question is whether or not the crepitus and/or clicking sounds are painful and how the patient controls these phenomena during daily activity. There is evidence that there is no direct correlation between this intra-articular phenomenon and the craniomandibular symptoms (Schiffmann et al 1992, Wabeke & Spruijt 1994).

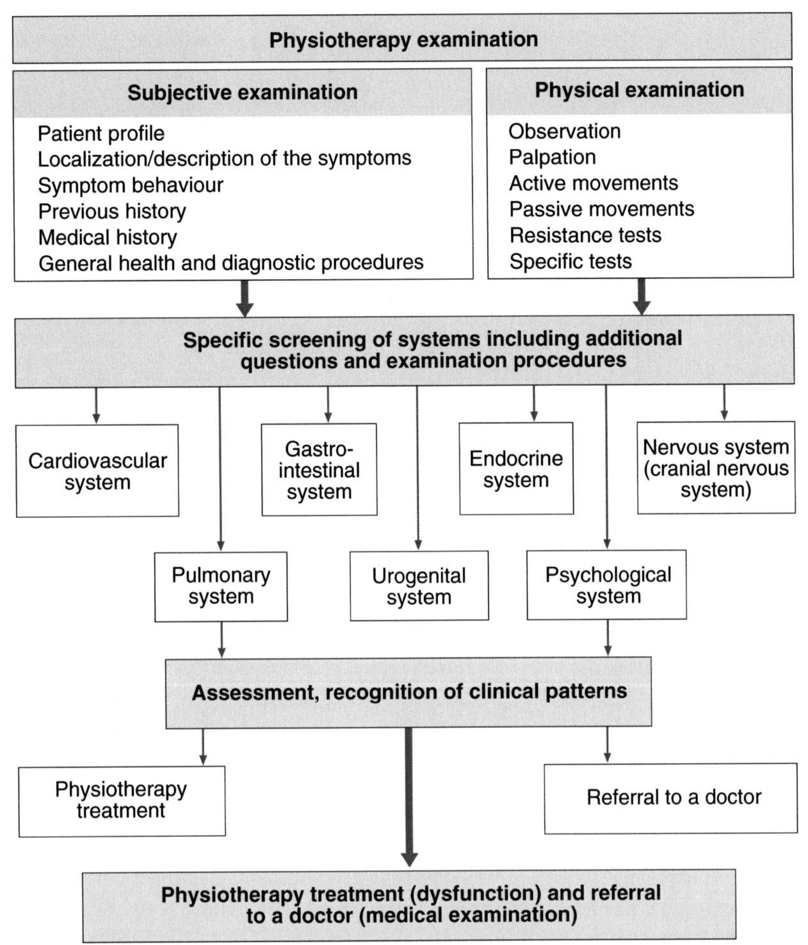

Fig. 3.2 Components of physiotherapeutic examination for gathering subjective data, physical examination and a possible trial treatment. This can be used to decide whether the patient needs to be referred back to a doctor. The neuromuscular system is not named as this is always the physiotherapist's first choice.

Limitation of physiological movements of the jaw

Movement of the TMJ can cause extreme limitation of orofacial movement during, for example, chewing, yawning, singing, biting and kissing (de Leeuw 1993, Wabeke & Spruijt 1994). Special questions about individual oral facial activity are therefore helpful.

Associated symptoms

In the literature it is noted that craniomandibular dysfunction often has associated symptoms where the patient and the therapist do not necessarily consider the craniomandibular region as a direct primary source (Kraus 1994). For a classic overview, see Figure 3.3 (after Pinkham 1986) in which the associated symptoms are summarized.

BEHAVIOUR OF SYMPTOMS

Variability of symptoms

Talking, chewing, yawning, brushing the teeth, washing the face, singing and kissing are essential activities which must be considered in relation to the patient's problems (Okeson 1995). In my experience, patients without joint noise and without limited

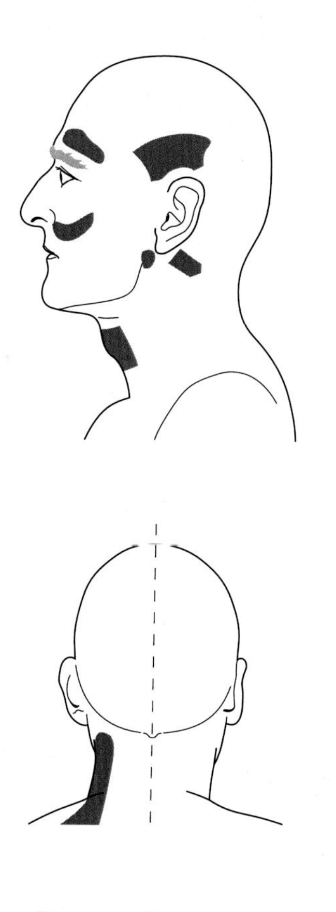

Location	Symptoms
Head	* Frontal head * Temporal area - Hemicranial pain, migraine * Frontal sinus pain - Stabbing headache - Sensitivity of the hair roots
Jaw	* Clicking - Crepitation - Muscle ache * Uncontrolled jaw movements - Derangement
Ear	* Ringing, buzzing in the ears (tinnitus) - Loss of hearing * Earache without inflammation - Dizziness - 'Clicking' in the ear
Mouth	* Limited opening - Coordination dysfunction on opening * Deviation on opening and closing * Locking on opening and closing

Location	Symptoms
Spine	- Stiffness * Cervical pain - Muscle ache * Shoulder pain * Scoliosis - Numbness of arms and fingers
Teeth	* Abrasion * Parafunctions - Malocclusion - Toothache
Eyes	* Pain behind the eye(s) * Sensitivity to light - Redness of the eye(s)
Throat	- Swallowing dysfunction - Throat pain without inflammation - Laryngitis - Throat feels swollen

*Most common symptoms

Fig. 3.3 The most important symptoms of craniomandibular dysfunction.

movement are seldom aware that use of the mouth may influence their symptoms.

Diurnal behaviour

In classic craniomandibular dysfunction discomfort or pain often slowly increases and/or decreases during the day. The patient is often not conscious of these factors and therefore has no influence on activities that may increase symptoms. For example, after talking for longer than an hour, a patient may feel temporal pain together with eye pain on the same side, limiting the patient's activity. The patient recognizes this pain but does not know where it comes from. They accept the diagnosis of 'migraine' and take their medicine.

In this example you may also think about the influence of abnormal oral habits (parafunctions) which the patient has not noticed until now (Naeije & Van Loon 1998). In such cases the patient should be advised to complete a 24-hour pain diary in order to record the intensity and behaviour of the pain (Fig. 3.4). Pain can then be correlated with activities performed before, during and after episodes of pain.

History

The history is an important part of the subjective examination in patients with head, neck and face pain. Patients often give descriptions in non-medical terms with an emotional component. This can give not only vital information about the aetiology of their complaints (Okeson 2005) but also additional information about pain mechanisms, contributory factors and prognosis (Jones & Rivett 2004).

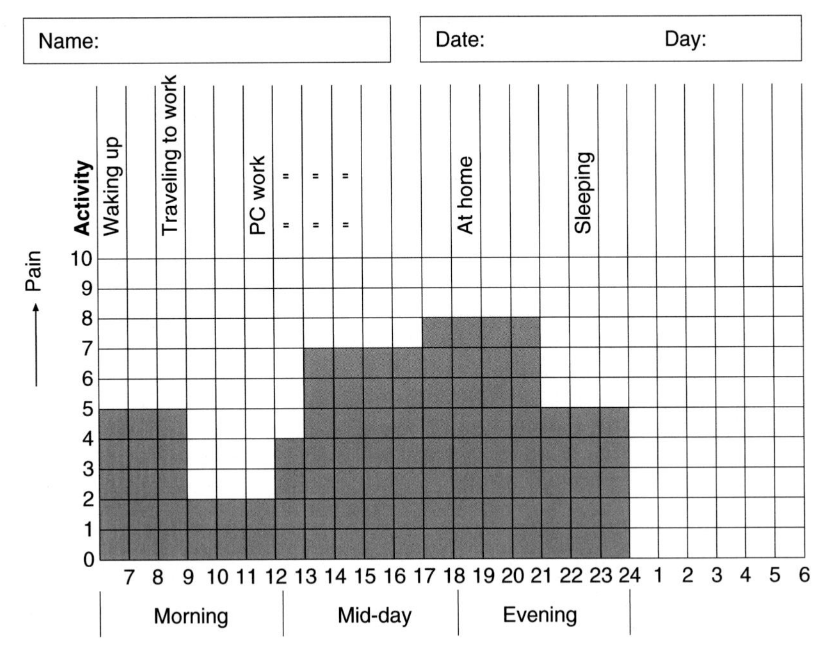

Fig. 3.4 An example of a symptom table of a patient with bruxism and unilateral face pain. Up until now the patient saw no correlation between the increasing symptoms in the afternoon and activity at the computer. The patient became aware of the connection because the table clarified the relationship between increasing pain and working patterns.

Onset

Minimal or severe trauma is often seen in the aetiology of craniomandibular symptoms (Freesmeyer 1993, Okeson 1995). The symptoms will not always appear directly after the trauma, but can be latent, manifesting even quite a long time after the initial trauma.

Trauma may be direct, such as a jaw fracture, or indirect, as in craniocervical trauma. A patient with a whiplash-associated disorder (WAD), for example, has a greater chance of developing craniomandibular dysfunction than a person who has not (Braun et al 1992, Stutzenegger et al 1994, Garcia & Arrington 1996). Minor sports injuries (e.g. a ball or a hand in the face) and extended mouth opening during dental treatment are often contributory factors in (long-term) craniofacial pain (Kraus 1994).

As already discussed, the history can gives clues as to contributory factors and so-called yellow flags which can influence long-term cranial facial dysfunction and pain (Baile & Myers 1986). The most important contributory factors are described in the next section.

CONTRIBUTORY FACTORS

'Contributory factors' is one of the hypothesis categories which should give the therapist subtle information regarding the patient or factors directly linked to the problem itself. For example:

- Trauma or overuse of the craniomandibular region while biting into a large apple or during tooth extraction
- Prone sleepers have more chance of problems in the craniocervical and craniomandibular regions than non-prone sleepers, possibly due to the increased long-term stress on these regions in this position (Kraus 1994)
- Facial asymmetry and dysgnathia predispose to craniomandibular dysfunction (Slavicek 2000)

- Stress and parafunctions can be seen as a maintaining influence.

In the last decade there has been increasing evidence of the importance of the psychosocial factors that influence long-term craniofacial pain (Naeije & Van Loon 1998, Lund et al 2000, Turp 2000). Thus a brief overview is essential for the therapist. Some of these factors will be discussed, along with other contributory factors related to head, neck and face pain. An overview of the various influences of relevant factors on craniofacial pain is shown in Box 3.1.

CRANIOCERVICAL TRAUMA AND CRANIOMANDIBULAR DYSFUNCTION

In the literature there is controversy about the incidence and onset of craniomandibular dysfunction following WADs (Garcia & Arrington 1996, Bergman et al 1998). For the therapist it is important to ask detailed questions about the possible craniomandibular complaints and their behaviour before and after the neck trauma. If you recognize overlap in the aetiology of the sources in a patient, then a craniomandibular assessment must be included alongside the craniocervical assessment (see Chapter 5) (Naeije & Van Loon 1998).

SPECIAL QUESTIONS

Parafunctions

Parafunctions refer to abnormal oral behaviour such as bruxism (chewing or biting the teeth), bracing, lip and tongue biting, unilateral chewing and other oral habits. Often patients are not aware of the relationship between their complaints and their daily oral activities. Some of these parafunctions have a tendency to increase during the course of the day (Okeson 1995). The patient can keep track of their symptoms in relation to oral habits using a simple table which enables the formation of hypotheses. Examples are shown in Box 3.1.

Medicines

Information on current use of medicines is required – type, dosage and the prescribing physician. Experience is frequently that a patient is taking a range of medications, some prescribed by the general practitioner and some purchased 'over the counter'. Regular assessment and fine tuning of medication is needed in most cases of chronic craniofacial pain (Okeson 2005). If a therapist thinks that the use of medication is unclear or doubtful, they should contact the prescribing physician.

Juvenile rheumatoid arthritis

Patients with juvenile rheumatoid arthritis have a higher incidence of degeneration of the discus articularis when older. As a result, dysfunction and pain may increase with time (Pertes & Gross 1995, Palla 1998).

Sleep disturbances

Sleep disturbances can be of considerable importance in a variety of craniofacial pain syndromes (Moldolfsky et al 1986, Molony et al 1986). Therefore it is important to analyse the quality of sleep and the symptoms of the patient. Box 3.1 is also relevant here.

Psychosocial factors, living situation, etc.

Emotional stress, living and family situations, and the patient's job situation have a clear influence and can result in idiopathic orofacial pain (Woda & Pionchon 2000). For further information, see 'Contributory factors' above.

The Clinical Dysfunction Index (after Helkimo 1974) is a frequently used questionnaire. Over the years it has proven to be a reliable standardized measure for estimating the prevalence of craniomandibular dysfunction. Classic symptoms of craniomandibular dysfunction can be recognized and easily classified with the help of this questionnaire.

The Helkimo questionnaire, assessment and its grades of classification of dysfunction are described in Table 3.2.

Box 3.1 Influence of relevant factors on craniofacial pain*

History

- A history of physical and sexual abuse is significantly related to greater pain severity, depression and psychological distress among CFP patients (Curran et al 1995, Riley et al 1998)
- Traumatic events during childhood (physical and sexual abuse, hospitalization) are significantly related to chronic pain. More than 50% of CFP sufferers are in this group (Goldberg et al 1999)
- A long history of illness without diagnosis has a poor prognosis, more so for women than for men (Pfaffenrath et al 1992)
- After an operation or injury to the face patients will take longer to recover and have a higher prevalence of AFP (Pfaffenrath et al 1992)
- More than a quarter (27%) of children with head injuries develop chronic headache, mainly tension type headache (Lemka 1999)

Moods, emotions

- AFP is increased and is maintained longer when anxiety, catastrophizing and depression are present (Madland et al 2000)
- Higher levels of anxiety and depression are strongly correlated with AFP (Lascelles 1966, Riley et al 1998)

Personality

- Some types of CFP and CMD seem to correlate with the presence of accompanying symptoms and with changes in personality (Mongini et al 2000)
- Chronic CMD patients present personality characteristics similar to those of other chronic pain patients (Michelotti et al 1998)
- AFP patients have an increased somatic preoccupation and are less likely to accept professional reassurance and psychological reasons for their pain (Speculand et al 1981)
- AFP patients show a tendency toward neurosis, psychosis and personality disturbances (Mongini et al 2000)

Behaviour

- The diagnosis of the primary help provider has a strong effect on the prognosis and further management (Turp et al 1998)
- Sleep disturbances and bruxism are common clinical characteristics of chronic facial pain patients (Bailey 1990)
- Poor sleep is a bad prognostic indicator of psychological distress related to chronic facial pain (Harness et al 1992)
- Bruxism is not associated with psychological disturbance in chronic facial pain (Harness et al 1990)
- Parafunctions such as bruxism, nail biting and thumb sucking in children are significant risk factors for oral/facial pain (Widmalm et al 1995).

Neurochemistry

- A diet high in carbohydrate and low in fat and protein with the addition of 3 g tryptophan per day resulted in decreased AFP and greater tolerance of pain but had no effect on anxiety and depression (Seltzer et al 1982)
- Lower levels of monoamine in the brain cerebrospinal fluid increased AFP, probably by a dysfunction of dopamine and serotonin (Bouckoms et al 1993)

* The literature is not always clear about terminology and definitions. Craniomandibular dysfunction (CMD), atypical facial pain (AFP) and craniofacial pain (CFP) are often used without a clear definition.

Table 3.2 The modified Helkimo Index and its interpretation

Criterion	Symptoms	Points
Restricted mobility	Normal ROM	0
	Restricted vertical ROM (mouth opening <40 mm)	1
	Additional horizontal restriction (right, left, laterotrusion and protrusion <6 mm)	2
	Restricted vertical ROM (mouth opening <30 mm) and horizontal ROM (<3 mm)	3
Pressure sensitivity of muscles	No sensitivity of masticatory muscles	0
	Sensitivity at 1–3 locations	1
	Sensitivity at 4–6 locations	2
	Sensitivity at >6 locations	3
Impaired jaw function	Smooth movement, no crepitation, no sensitivity (deviation <2 mm)	0
	Crepitation on one or both sides	1
	Additional deviation >2 mm and/or impaired resistance or pressure sensitivity in one or both TMJs	2
	Locking or luxation of the TMJs	3
Occlusion dysfunction	No occlusion dysfunction	0
	Early contact without centric position	1
	Early contact with centric and/or balance deficiencies	2
	Early contact and balance deficiencies or loss of the vertical support zone	3
Pain on mandibular movements	Pain-free movements	0
	Pain in one movement direction	1
	Pain in more than one movement direction	2
The sum of all points from the five categories allows the differentiation of dysfunction indices:		
0 points	Clinically symptom free	(Di 0)
1–3 points	Slight dysfunction	(Di I)
4–6 points	Moderate dysfunction	(Di II)
7 points	Severe dysfunction	(Di III)

ROM, range of movement; TMJ, temporomandibular joint.

THE CRANIOFACIAL REGION

SUBJECTIVE EXAMINATION

This section describes questions that are specific for signs and symptoms originating in the craniofacial region, and are suggested for the subjective examination.

These questions are based, firstly, on experience with patients using retrospective re-assessment and, secondly, relevant literature. These can be applied to both strategies of enquiry.

NATURE AND LOCALIZATION

Symptoms can vary from pain, stiffness and instability to motor deficit in the head region. Some typical examples are:

- Pain, often described as sharp, superficial and well localized. It is found more commonly in the region of a suture, for example in the nasofrontal, petro-occipital or frontozygomatic region. Onset is often after trauma and/or through changes in stress transducer forces in the skull, for example the application of an orthodontal brace.

- A deep pressure on the head, which can be divided into general and localized pressure. The general pressure is commonly felt relatively deep compared to the localized pressure and is often associated with sympathetic symptoms such as sweating, dizziness and temperature changes.
- Localized deep pressure in the ear(s), eye(s) and teeth, especially the maxilla.
- Symptoms such as a general feeling of stiffness in the head and/or neck independent of neck movements; fluctuating concentration disturbances, often associated with autonomic responses such as pressure on the throat, sweating, respiratory disturbances and tiredness may all indicate cranial dysfunction.

The presence of sympathetic symptoms, for example, could be explained by the anatomical position of the hypothalamus in the sella turcica of the sphenoid bone, the innervated sutures and the rich innervation of the internal part of the cranial dura (Wagemans et al 1988).

Behaviour of symptoms

During questioning it is essential to differentiate the behaviour of the various symptoms. Aggravation and easing of the symptoms may be associated with typical patterns of movement, or postures that are specific for the individual sutures which are the possible sources of symptoms. Cranial dysfunction appears to have specific classic patterns of symptom variability:

- Symptoms often accumulate during the day and without a direct stimulus–response reaction.
- Latent hyperpathic reactions are often felt during or after oral functions such as swallowing, eating, talking or parafunction, or after long-term pressure on the head in a lying position when sleeping.
- Wearing a crash helmet can alter symptoms, as can tooth extraction or using an electric toothbrush.
- Localized dull pressures in the facial palate and zygomatic and occipitoparietal regions may indicate strength imbalance of stress transducer system forces in the cranium.
- Patients may not always recognize the relationship between severe headaches and these factors because the pain often manifests itself after some time delay.
- Pain can be reduced by spontaneous indication of change of pressure in the craniofacial region. For example, pressure on the nasofrontal region with thumb and index finger, bilateral pressure with the palm of the hand on the occiput, unilateral pressure on the pars lateralis of the sphenoid bone. In children, pressure on the palatinum by the use of a dummy or thumb sucking can ameliorate pain.

History

Taking the patient's history is one of the most important parts of the examination process and requires a considerable amount of skill on the part of the therapist (Jones et al 1995). The history should be viewed as a continuous account which is subject to the therapist's influence (de Wijer 1995). It contains general information about onset, the cause of the problem, stability and progression of the pathology (Boissonault 1995, Jones et al 1995).

During the history taking it is always relevant to ask about the patient's delivery (birth). Trauma during delivery (e.g. suboccipital subluxation) can have consequences for cranial formation and spinal development, among other repercussions. Minor dysfunctions such as prolonged traction of the upper cervical spine and skull can result in morphological changes expressed in syndromes such as crying baby's torticollis, dyslexia and postural changes (van Duin 1991). Sustained pressure on the cranial bones during delivery can result in an abnormal 'moulding' behaviour during and after the delivery. Predisposing factors for later signs and symptoms can be minor and major traumas in youth such as contusion, concussion or whiplash, as well as skull and facial surgery in adolescence, when the skull and neurodynamics of cranial nerves have the potential to adapt maximally to such forces. A history of disease such as encephalitis or meningitis could have disturbed the development of the skull and can stimulate minor craniosynostosis (Johman 1994).

Protracted dural inflammation alters the inner balance between the cranium, neck and trunk and produces abnormal forces on the skull by changes in the tone of the neck muscles and masticator system (Hu et al 1995). When there is a long history of orthodontic intervention by brace therapy it is important to ask whether symptoms increased, decreased or developed during or after the therapy. The answer can vary from patient to patient. In literature reviews there is no correlation between asymmetry of the cranium and symptoms (Dibbets et al 1985).

SPECIAL QUESTIONS

This section covers questions which give more detailed information on the possible development of signs and symptoms from the cranium. Conditions for which passive techniques may be dangerous are noteworthy, such as weight loss, non-mechanical (spontaneous) pain, night pain, neurological or other 'bizarre' accompanying symptoms, and particular medical diagnoses (Higgs & Jones 1995).

The following section discusses relevant aspects of special questions for which so-called 'hands on' therapy is indicated.

Cranial synostosis

From the literature it is known that clear or minor cranial synostosis (premature closure of the cranial sutures) predisposes the individual to abnormal forces not only in childhood but also in adulthood (Proffit 1993). Relative growth differences between the cranial bones can take two forms:

- Two or more cranial bones can grow at different rates
- Two or more cranial bones grow for different durations.

For example, the frontal bones are paired at birth by a metopic suture that usually fuses during the second year. The coronal suture separates the frontal bone from the parietal bones in adulthood. Assuming similar growth rates at these sutures, relatively more growth must occur at the coronal suture by the time of adulthood simply because of the longer time interval.

Trigonocephaly (synostosis of the coronal suture or part thereof) gives an extreme shape to the cranium and predisposes to cranial pain or other cranial dysfunctions. If the patient is not aware of this phenomenon, inspection of the cranium can provide evidence. Cranial synostosis of various sutures is shown in Figure 3.5.

Extreme cranial synostosis is usually detected at birth. Patients with minor abnormalities who have not been diagnosed as having cranial synostosis often present with complaints of symptoms in the head and cranial region. These minor dysfunctions can be a predisposing factor and are related to the presenting symptoms (van Duin 1991); in most cases they react well to manual therapy for the craniofacial region (Case study 3.1).

Chronic sinusitis

Chronic sinusitis and inflammatory conditions of paranasal sinuses are generally misunderstood. Inflammatory conditions of the nasal mucosa cause primary pain. It is often the autonomic and sensory disturbances induced by the primary pain that cause the dull facial pain.

Waltner (1955) reported that, in his experience, no more than 20% of patients treated for sinusitis had any disease at all! The conclusion of van Duin (1991) during a major echoscope study was that acute sinus maxillaries occurred less often than suspected (see also Chapter 16). Frontal sinusitis was rare, just like chronic sinusitis, but symptoms mimicking chronic sinusitis were frequent. This study showed that there was no clear borderline between true sinusitis and symptoms imitating sinusitis.

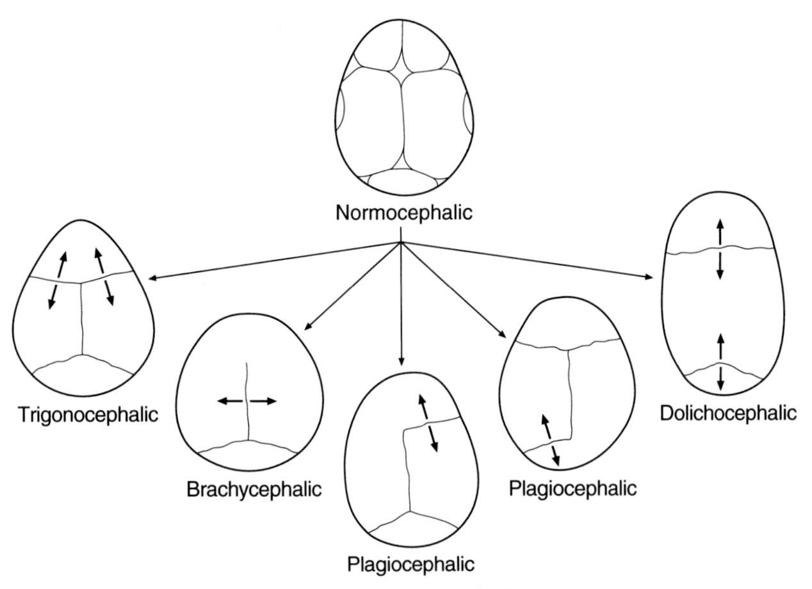

Fig. 3.5 Types of craniosynostosis (premature closing of sutures):

- Trigonocephaly: malformation characterized by triangular configuration of the cranium, mostly in the frontal region.
- Brachycephaly: premature closure of the sutures between both parietal bones (sagittal sutures).
- Plagiocephaly: an asymmetric craniostenosis due to premature closure of the lambdoid and coronal sutures on one side.

Case study 3.1

An 8-year-old boy with a paediatric diagnosis of 'myogenic torticollis' of 2 years' duration complains about a dull headache, dominantly in the vertex region. This occurs two or three times a week for several hours, especially in the evening. He has difficulties with concentration and the school teacher noted dyslexic behaviour. He has no intellectual deficit.

During inspection and palpation a small right orbit, a small but not prominent right zygomatic bone and a prominent left frontal bone were recorded (Fig. 3.6). He had antalgic head posture to the right and increased muscle tone in the right cervical spine region (trapezium I semispinalis and levator scapula muscles all with pain on local pressure). Extreme protraction of both scapulae was also visible. Palpation of the right coronal suture was, in comparison to the left, not possible. The suture felt hard and caused local pain on pressure. The hypothesis was that a minor frontal right plagiocephaly was probably relevant for these symptoms.

After six treatments over 5 months, focusing on craniofacial tissue and minor upper cervical spine mobilization together with muscle balancing exercise, his facial asymmetry decreased (see Fig. 3.6b). There was a visibly more active posture with less antalgic head posture and the increased muscle tone and palpation pain was gone. His parents and teacher agreed he had improved results at school.

Pain from the maxillary sinus often refers to the nose, jaw and specifically to the maxillary teeth (Wolff 1963). Dental sepsis seen during dental examination and radiographically often has an autonomic component (Proffit 1993).

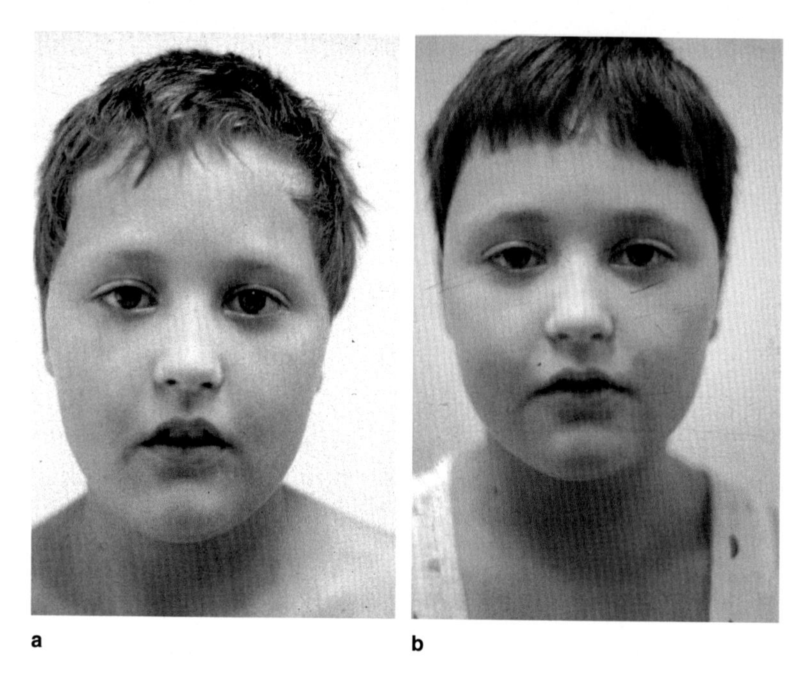

Fig. 3.6
a Patient with a diagnosis of myogeneic torticollis with a stable history. Note the contours of the right sternocleidomastoid muscle and the prominent orbits.
b The same patient after 5 months of craniofacial treatment (six times) and sensomotor integration once a week by a paediatric physiotherapist.

Solow and Sierbaek-Nielsen (1992) and Idema and Damsté (1994) described a correlation between airflow and craniofacial morphology. Long-term airflow occlusion, especially in childhood, can cause retarded development of the craniofacial region and the head (Hellsing et al 1987, Mahan & Alling 1991). Folweiler and Lynch (1995) emphasized, in a literature review, that cranial motion and passive movement of cranial bones in chronic sinusitis can change nasal and sinus airflow and has an influence on the pain pattern. Passive investigation of the skull bones is indicated for patients who have had dull facial pain for a long time, sinus x-rays are negative, antibiotics do not help and there is no fever, allergy or rhinitis, and where no abnormalities are found by the dentist or otolaryngologist.

Headache

Chronic headaches due to cranial dysfunction are often not recognized and the patients are often labelled with another diagnosis such as tension headache, (cervical) migraine, craniomandibular dysfunction, vasomotor headache, atypical facial pain, etc.

From the literature in this field we know that it is difficult to differentiate between the several types of headache because there is considerable overlap (see Chapter 20). Different researchers believe, for example, that migraine and tension-type headache are two different presentations of the same pathophysiological mechanisms (Proffit 1993, Nelson 1994). The same could be said for migraine and cervical headache (Buzzi & Moskowitz 1992).

It is known that long-term migraine influences cranial blood flow and the circulation to the cranial nerves, which could indicate that the neurodynamics of cranial nerves can be changed by migraine (Heisey & Adams 1993, Proffit 1993). Although cranial dysfunction can trigger other types of headache, a clear correlation between cranial dysfunction and prevalence of headache has not yet been found in relevant literature (Nelson 1994).

Surgery

Surgery to the eyes (diplopia, ptosis), nose (septum correction), ears, TMJ and cervical spine can influence the stress transducer components of the cranium (Enlow 1982). The onset of symptoms related to the surgical intervention is relevant, for example if symptoms changed after a septum correction of the nose; if not, they were possibly not originating from the nasofrontal region but somewhere else in the cranium.

If the dominant symptoms do start after the septum correction, a possible hypothesis is that the forces in the skull were responsible for the problem. For more postsurgery data related to clinical management of these patients, see the comments in the chapters on examination and treatment of cranial tissue (Chapters 15 and 16).

Associated symptoms

The five D's of Coman (diplopia, dysarthria, dizziness, dysphagia and drop attacks) (Coman 1995), as well as questions about behaviour, such as lack of concentration, sleep disturbances and personality changes, are all relevant. This is because chronic pressure on brain tissue may give clues leading to caution in the treatment with passive movements on the cranium (Coman 1995). Detailed questioning has to follow. For example, the five D's of Coman can also indicate a dysfunction of the cranial nervous tissues, such as the abducens, facial, vestibular and hypoglossal nerves.

Treatment by braces changes the form of the skull and is predisposed to change signs and symptoms (Koskinen 1977, Solow & Sierbaek-Nielsen 1992, De Bruin 1993, Palla 1998). It should be remembered that the main problem of children who have orthodontic care is dysfunction of the TMJ or asymmetry of the cranium rather than pain (Palla 1998). The current literature does not indicate any correlation between changes in subjective symptoms and correction of skull morphology (Herring et al 1979, Proffit 1993). In addition, the role and the precise mechanism of occlusion in craniomandibular and cranium dysfunction are not yet clear. Because of these unpredictable factors it is important to ask when, why and how long this treatment continued and when symptoms started and/or changed in relation to orthodontic treatment. The therapist should not forget to ask if the symptoms improved or worsened after orthodontic treatment.

CRANIAL NERVOUS TISSUE

Classic questions and described patterns are dominantly related with peripheral neurogenic pain mechanisms. For an excellent review of pain mechanisms, see Butler (2000). More specialized in the craniofacial region are the publications of Okeson (1995). Pain patterns not directly caused by the musculoskeletal system (e.g. aneurysms or brain tumours and other neoplasms) are considered only briefly with 'special questions'.

WHAT IS PERIPHERAL NEUROGENIC PAIN?

Peripheral neurogenic pain is defined as a nociceptive stimulus that comes from the nervous system, and which is regenerated (or generated) outside the dorsal horn or brainstem (Merskey & Bogduk 1994). In an anatomical sense this will include not only those nerves of the lower and upper extremity but also those from the (cranial) dura and the cranial nerves (Lunborg 1988).

Abnormal impulses, also called abnormal impulse generating sites (AIGS), develop by demyelinization. Neuronal cross-excitation can provoke peripheral neurogenic pain (Devor & Seltzer 1999). Cranial ganglia and dorsal root ganglia can also result in AIGS (Kulisch et al 1991, Devor 1994). The cranial ganglions are more mechano- and adrenaline sensitive in comparison to the dorsal root ganglia (Sugawara et al 1996, Chen et al 1997). Clinically this means that a mechanical load or increased stress influence quickly alters the behaviour of AIGS. For example, it is known that specialized intracranial surgery can

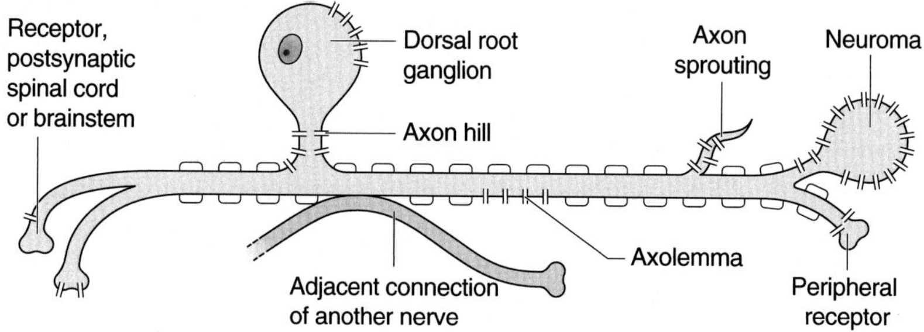

Fig. 3.7 Branches of the trigeminal nerve (modified from Butler 2000).

damage the trigeminal ganglion. Movement of the head and stress can lead to severe facial pain in the area of the trigeminal branches (Fig. 3.7) (Zakrzewska 1995).

INTRACRANIAL NEUROGENIC PAIN

The cranial dura and nerves, which are enormously pain-sensitive structures, are richly supplied by connective tissue (Kumar et al 1995, Shankland 1995). Mechanical, chemical and electrical stimulation of cranial nerves may alter neurodynamics (Breig 1978). Minimal movements of the large sinus, compression of the cerebellopontine angle, cavernous sinus and dilatation of cranial arteries can all provoke a clear peripheral neurogenic pain pattern (Schwenzer & Ehrenfeld 2002). Typical features are described below.

Nature and localization

The pain is often described in the direction of the nerve trunk towards the trigeminal ganglion. Patients often describe this as a 'line' of pain, for example an acute neuropathy of the mandibular nerve after a tooth extraction (LeResche 2000). Spot pain is also a classic description in the face, for example in front of the ear behind the head of the mandible (auriculotemporal nerve), between the ear and mastoid process (facial nerve) or on the infraorbital foramen (maxillary nerve). A diffuse, dull or 'heavy' feeling over a wider area is also classic but is seldom recognized as a cranial neuropathy. Entrapment of the lingual nerve in the medial pterygoideus is often related to a 'heavy' jaw (von Piekartz & Bryden 2001, Gavilán et al 2002). Burning, paraesthesia or a sharp shooting pain in the craniofacial region is classic (Lippton et al 1993). Different qualities in different locations are not always easy to identify as cranial neuropathic problems.

Behaviour

The severity of cranial neuropathic pain can be very variable. It is seldom that neuropathic pain in the face scores higher on a VAS than a non-neuropathic pain (Zakrzewska 1995). Okeson (1995) divided the behaviour of craniofacial neuropathic pain into two types: episodic pain and constant neuropathic pain. The main difference is their qualities and their behaviour, which will be discussed below.

EPISODIC NEUROPATHIC PAIN

There are often relatively short or sometimes long (weeks, months) pain-free periods. Mechanical and thermal stimuli are often triggers but stress situations for the patient can also be a factor (Okeson 1996).

Within the group two different clinical patterns are seen: vascular and neurogenic. Table 3.3 gives an overview of the differences.

CONTINUOUS NEUROPATHIC PAIN

Anatomical changes or disturbances are directly related to the pain. Examples are neuromas, demyelinization or cross-excitation

Table 3.3 Differences between neurovascular and neurogenic pain

	Neurovascular pain	Neurogenic pain
Mechanism	Imbalance of the autonomic nervous system	Abnormal impulses along the nerve, often without clear aetiology
Pain quality	Throbbing, pulsating	Electrical, shooting pains, spontaneous
Behaviour	Starts slowly	Mechanical stress, stress, latency after repetitive activities
Diagnosis	Migraine, cluster headache, vasomotor headache	Paroxysmal, trigeminal and glossopharyngeal neuralgia

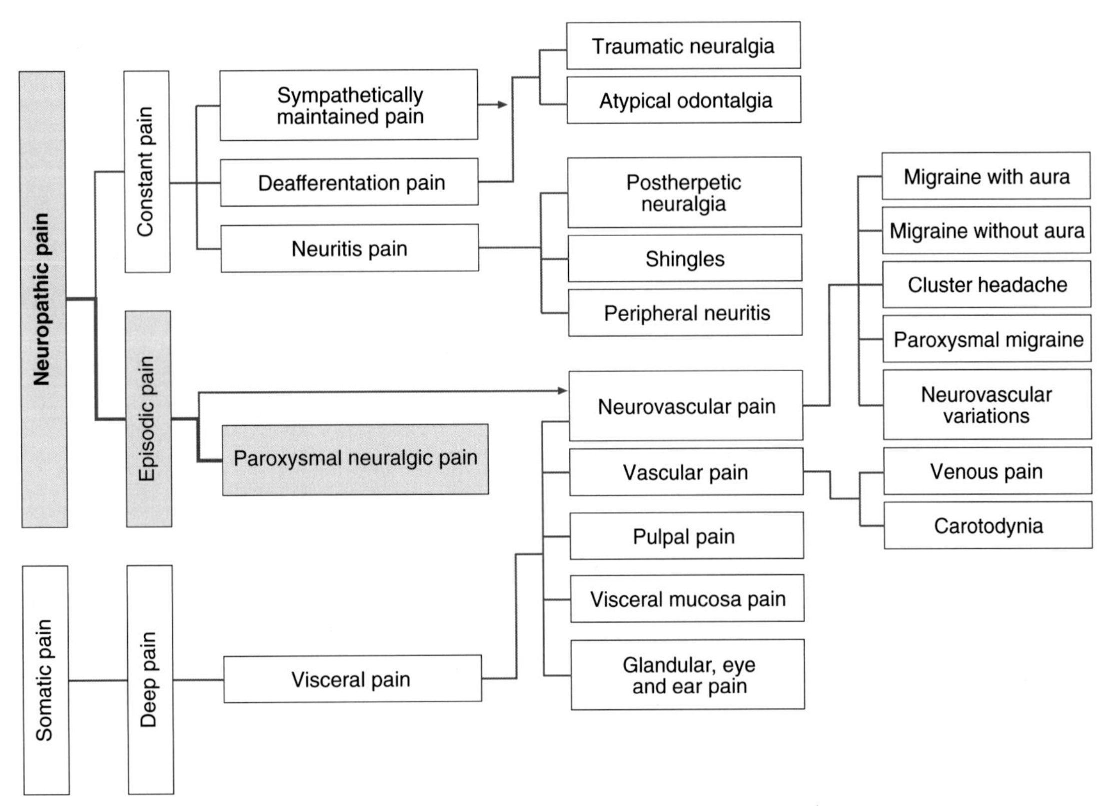

Fig. 3.8 Classification of neuropathic pain (Axis I) (modified from Okeson 2005).

which result from abnormal and sometimes spontaneous stimuli of the nerve due to AIGS:

- Pain intensity is variable
- The patient is rarely pain free
- In many cases there has been some talk of central sensitization, whereby the pain is independent of a clear external stimulus (Ejlersen et al 1992).

Diagnoses such as postherpetic pain or an atypical facial neuralgia are the most common (Fig. 3.8).

DOUBLE CRUSH

The 'double crush' hypothesis proposed by Upton and McComas (1973) is that local pathobiological changes in a nerve predispose to the development of other neuropathic changes elsewhere in the same nerve. Classically the changes start proximally and move distally. There are also so-called reversed crush and multiple crush syndromes (Butler 2000).

Classic questions which cover double crush include:

- Have any other regions in your head, face or body ever been symptomatic?
- If yes, when were these symptoms reduced or absent?
- Was there in the past a (possibly painless) traumatic event such as tooth extraction, septum correction, minor sports injury, long-term inflammation of your mouth or sinusitis?

Patients frequently do not notice the correlation between late arising symptoms and a previous minimal trauma. Here you have to consider mechanisms such as AIGS which often develops days or weeks after trauma rather than immediately (Devor & Seltzer 1999). Neurogenic inflammation may also be influenced by changes in neurotransmitter functionality or in the neuroendocrine system (Dickerson et al 1998, Watkins & Maier 2000). Useful questions relating to such a situation include (Box 3.2, Table 3.4):

- How was the period following your trauma? Did you have any problems?
- If yes, were the facial symptoms the same as they are now?

Box 3.2 Key questions to recognize minor craniofacial neuropathy

Localization

- A sharp local pain, mostly 'burning' and 'pulling'
- 'Line' of pain along the nerve?
- Not well localized pain area in the face or head?

Quality

- Is the pain 'burning', 'tickling', 'sharp' or 'shooting'?
- Is the pain (severely) 'pulling' or 'tearing'?
- Does a part of your head feel 'heavy'?

Target tissue function/contributory factors

- Does your face feel the same on both the right and the left side?
- If it is different, is it stronger (hyperaesthesia or -algesia) or weaker (hypoaesthesia) on the affected side?
- Do you have problems with short- or long-term functions of your head and/or face, e.g. chewing, talking, singing, swallowing, eating, observing, etc.?
- Are your head and face complaints dependent on your posture or activity?
- Are there other symptoms such as double or blurred vision, sensory phenomena such as an asymmetric feeling of the head and/or changed orientation of the head or the trunk?
- Do distress, rest and/or weather changes influence your complaints?
- Do you wake up because of your complaints, and if so, what do you do about it?

History

- Have you suffered trauma or had surgery on the head/face area or anywhere else in the body (double crush)?
- Was there a sudden onset or did the problem start after a time (weeks, months)?
- Do/did the complaints increase after a period of stress?

Special questions

- Do you suffer from fibromyalgia, diabetes, multiple sclerosis or HIV?
- Have you ever had any disease of your mouth, throat, eyes, ears or sinuses in the past?
- Do these kind of complaints run in your family?

Table 3.4 Short target tissue questions for cranial nerves

Question	Cranial nerve(s) involved
Any loss of smell?	I
Any loss of taste?	VII, IX
Any loss of vision or visual acuity?	II
Double vision?	III, IV, VI
Numbness of face or frontal scalp?	V
Hypersensitivity to sound?	VIII
Any loss of hearing or ringing in the ears?	VIII
Difficulty with swallowing?	IX, X
Chronic cough, loss of voice?	X

- Following the pain-free period, did your symptoms start up again without a cause?
- Did you experience extreme stress or anxiety at the time of the trauma?
- If yes, do you still suffer from these same feelings?
- How is your health? Are you often ill?
- Do you often have colds or do you tire quickly?
- Do you have minor inflammations in your body?
- Do you suffer from fibromyalgia, diabetes, multiple sclerosis or HIV?

What to do before the physical examination

After consideration of the information from the subjective examination, a decision must be made as to which structures to examine at the first consultation, i.e. craniocervical, cranio-mandibular, the craniofacial region or the cranial nervous tissue. At the same time, the following questions need to be addressed:

- May I or may I not produce pain during examination?
- Do I need to abort passive tests before first encountering resistance or can I go through the resistance?
- How many tests can I carry out without causing a deterioration in the patient?

Answering these questions should permit a general impression of the type of pain and probable pathobiological mechanism.

SUMMARY

- During gathering of subjective data about head, neck and face pain, the therapist can choose between an open interview, a systematic questionnaire or a combination of both. Each form has advantages and disadvantages and the choice is dependent on several criteria established by the therapist.
- The subjective data can be categorized into patient profiles, quality and behaviour of symptoms, special questions and history.
- The most important questions for the three sources of symptoms (craniomandibular, facial region and cranial nervous tissue) are discussed.
- This information will help to gain a general overview of the hypotheses categories such as pathobiological mechanisms, sources, contributory factors (yellow flags), contraindications (red flags), prognosis and further management.

References

AHCPR 1994 Acute low back problems in adults. Clinical Practice Guideline Number 14. Agency for Health Care Problems and Research. US Department of Health and Human Services, Rockville, MD

Aufdemkampe G 2001 Clinimetrics for the therapist: the use of some indices applicable in the craniocervical and craniofacial regions. In: von Piekartz H, Bryden L (eds) Craniofacial dysfunction and pain: manual therapy, assessment and management. Butterworth-Heinemann, Oxford

Baile W F, Myers D 1986 Psychological and behavioural dynamics in chronic atypical facial pain. Anesthesia Progress 33(5):252–257

Bailey D 1990 Tension headache and bruxism in the sleep disordered patient. Cranio 8(2):174–182

Bar-Ziv J, Asalsky B 1997 Imaging of mental neuropathy; the numb chin syndrome. American Journal of Roentgenology 168:371

Bergman H, Andersson F, Isberg A 1998 Incidence of temporomandibular joint changes after whiplash trauma: a prospective study using MR imaging. American Journal of Roentgenology 171(5):1237–1243

Boissonault W 1995 Examination in physical therapy practice. Screening for medical diseases, 2nd edn. Churchill Livingstone, Philadelphia

Bouckoms A, Sweet W, Poletti C 1993 Monoamines in the brain cerebrospinal fluid in facial pain patients. Anesthesia Progress 39:201

Braun L, DiGiovanna A, Bonnema J, Friction J 1992 Cross-section study of temporomandibular joint dysfunction in post-cervical trauma patients. Journal of Craniomandibular Disorders: Facial and Oral Pain 6:24

Breig A 1978 Adverse mechanical tension in the central nervous system 1: relief by functional neurosurgery. Alqvist and Wiksel International, Stockholm; Wiley, Chichester

Buhmann A, Lotzman U 2000 Funktiondiagnostik und Therapieprinzipen. Band 12. Thieme, Stuttgart

Butler D 2000 The sensitive nervous system. NOI Group Publications, Adelaide

Buzzi M, Moskowitz M 1992 The trigeminovascular system and migraine. Pathologie-biologie 40:313

Chen C, Cavanaugh J, Ozaktay A C et al 1997 Effects of phospholipase A2 on lumbar nerve root structure and function. Spine 22(10):1057–1064

Coman W 1995 Dizziness related to ENT conditions. In: Grieve G (ed.) Modern manual therapy of the vertebral column. Churchill Livingstone, Edinburgh, p 303

Curran S, Sherman J, Cunningham L et al 1995 Physical and sexual abuse among orofacial pain patients: linkages with pain and psychological distress. Journal of Orofacial Pain 9:340

De Bruin R 1993 A mathematical model applied to craniofacial growth. Thesis, University of Groningen, The Netherlands

de Leeuw J 1993 Psychosocial aspects and symptom characteristics of craniomandibular dysfunction. Thesis, University of Utrecht, The Netherlands

de Wijer A 1995 Temporomandibular and cervical spine disorders. Thesis, Elinkwijk BV

Devor M 1994 The pathophysiology of damaged peripheral nerves. In: Wall P, Melzack R (eds) Textbook of pain. Churchill Livingstone, Edinburgh, p 79

Devor M, Seltzer Z 1999 Pathophysiology of damaged nerves in relation to chronic pain. In: Wall P, Melzack R (eds) Textbook of pain, 4th edn. Churchill Livingstone, Edinburgh

Dibbets J, Weele van der L, Uildriks A 1985 Symptoms of TMJ dysfunction: indicators of growth patterns. Journal of Pedodontics 9:265

Dickerson C, Undem B, Bullock B et al 1998 Neuropeptide regulation of proinflammatory cytokine responses. Journal of Leukocyte Biology 63:602

Ejlersen E, Anderson H B, Eliasen K et al 1992 A comparison between preincisional and postincisional lidocaine infiltration and postoperative pain. Anesthesia and Analgesia 74:495

Enlow D 1982 Handbook of facial growth. W B Saunders, Philadelphia

Folweiler D S, Lynch O T 1995 Nasal specific technique as part of a chiropractic approach to chronic sinusitis and sinus headaches. Journal of Manipulative and Physiological Therapeutics 18(1):38–41

Freesmeyer W 1993 Zahärztliche Funktionstherapie. Hanser, Munich

Friction J, Kroening R, Haley D, Siegert R 1985 Myofascial pain syndrome of the head and neck: a review of clinical characteristics of 164 patients. Oral Surgery, Oral Medicine and Oral Pathology 60:615

Garcia R, Arrington J A 1996 The relationship between cervical whiplash and temporomandibular joint injuries: an MRI study. Cranio 14(3):233–239

Gavilán J, Herranz J, DeSanto L, Gavilán C 2002 Functional and selective neck dissection: frequently asked questions. Thieme, New York, p 139

Goldberg R, Pachas W, Keith D 1999 Relationship between traumatic events in childhood and chronic pain. Disability and Rehabilitation 21:23–30

Harness D, Donlon W, Eversole L 1990 Comparison of clinical characteristics in myogenic TMJ internal derangement and atypical facial pain patients. Clinical Journal of Pain 8:174
Harness D, Peltier B 1992 Comparison of MMPI scores with self report of sleep disturbance and bruxism in the facial pain population. Cranio 10(1):70–74
Heisey S, Adams T 1993 Role of cranial bone mobility in cranial compliance. Neurosurgery 33:869
Helkimo M 1974 Studies on function and dysfunction of the masticatory system. II. Index for anamnestic and clinical dysfunction and occlusal state. Swedish Dental Journal 67(2):101–121
Hellsing E, McWilliam J, Reigo T, Spangfort E 1987 The relationship between craniofacial morphology, head posture and spinal curvature in 8, 11 and 15 year old children. European Journal of Orthodontics 9:254
Herring S, Rowlatt U, Pruzansky S 1979 Anatomical abnormalities in mandibulofacial dysostosis. American Journal of Medical Genetics 3:225
Higgs J, Jones M 1995 Clinical reasoning in the health profession. Butterworth-Heinemann, Oxford
Hu J, Vernon H, Tatourion I 1995 Changes in neck electromyography associated with meningeal noxious stimulation. Journal of Manipulative and Physiological Therapeutics 18:577
Idema N, Damsté P 1994 Habitueel mondademen. Een terreinver-kenning. Bohn Stafleu Van Loghum, Houten
Johman J 1994 Perspectives of craniofacial growth. Clinics in Plastic Surgery 21:489
Jones M 1994 Clinical reasoning process in manipulative therapy. In: Boyling J, Palastanga N (eds) Grieve's modern manual therapy, 2nd edn. Churchill Livingstone, Edinburgh, S. 577
Jones M, Rivett D (eds) 2004 Introduction to clinical reasoning. In: Clinical reasoning for the manual therapist. Butterworth-Heinemann, Oxford, p 3
Jones M, Jensen G, Rothstein J 1995 Clinical reasoning in physiotherapy. In: Higgs J, Jones M (eds) Clinical reasoning in the health profession. Butterworth-Heinemann, Oxford, p 72
Koskinen L 1977 Adaptive sutures. Thesis. Proceedings of the Finish Dental Society 73(Suppl 10–11):3–80
Kraus S 1994 Temporomandibular disorders, 2nd edn. Churchill Livingstone, New York
Kumar R, Berger R J, Dunsker S B, Keller J T 1995 Innervation of the spinal dura; myth or reality? Spine 21:18–26
Kuslich S, Ulstrom C, Micheal C 1991 The tissue origin of low back and sciatica. Orthopedic Clinics of North America 22:181–187
Lang J 1995 Skull base and related structures. Atlas of clinical anatomy. Schattauer, Stuttgart
Lascelles R 1966 Atypical facial pain and depression. British Journal of Psychiatry 112:651–659
Lavigne G, Woda A, Truelove E, Ship J A, Dao T, Goulet J P 2005 Mechanisms associated with unusual orofacial pain. Journal of Orofacial Pain 19(1):9–21
Leeuw de R 1993 Psychosocial aspect and symptom characteristics of craniomandibular dysfunction. Thesis, University of Utrecht, The Netherlands
Lemka M 1999 Headache as the consequence of brain concussion and contusion in closed head injuries in children. Neurologia i Neurochirurgia Polska 33:37
LeResche L 2000 Epidemiology of orofacial pain. In: Lund J, Lavigne G, Dubner R, Sessle B (eds) Orofacial pain: from basic science to clinical management. Quintessence, Chicago, p 15
Lippton J, Ship J A, Larach-Robinson D 1993 Estimated prevalence and distribution of reported orofacial pain in the United States. Journal of the American Dental Association 124:115–121
Lund J, Lavigne G, Dubner R, Sessle B 2000 Orofacial pain: from basic science to clinical management. Quintessence, Chicago
Lundborg G 1988 Nerve injury and repair. Churchill Livingstone, Edinburgh
Madland G, Feinmann C, Newman S 2000 Factors associated with anxiety and depression in facial arthromyalgia. Pain 84:225
Mahan P, Alling C 1991 Facial pain. 3rd edn. Lea and Febiger, Philadelphia, p 311
Maitland G 1986 Vertebral manipulation, 5th edn. Butterworth-Heinemann, Oxford
Maitland G, Hengeveld E, Banks K, English K 2001 Maitland's vertebral manipulation, 6th edn. Butterworth Heinemann, Oxford
Masset E, Moore J, Schold S 1981 Mental neuropathy from systemic cancer. Neurology 31:1277
McNeill C 1993 Temporomandibular disorders: guidelines for classification, assessment and management. American Academy of Orofacial Pain. Quintessence, Chicago
Merskey H, Bogduk N 1994 Classification of chronic pain: descriptions of chronic pain syndromes and definitions of pain terms. IASP Press, Seattle
Michelotti A, Martina R, Russo M, Romeo R 1998 Personality characteristics of temporomandibular joint disorder patients using MMPI. Journal of Craniomandibular Practice 16:119
Moldofsky H, Tullis C, Lue F A 1986 Sleep related myoclonus in rheumatic pain modulation disorder (fibrosis syndrome). Rheumatology 13:614–617
Molony R, MacPeck D, Schiffman P et al 1986 Sleep, sleep apnea, and the fibromyalgia syndrome. Journal of Rheumatology 13:797
Mongini F, Ciccone G, Iberts F, Negro C 2000 Personality characteristics and accompanying symptoms in temporomandibular joint

dysfunction, headache and facial pain. Journal of Orofacial Pain 14:52

Naeije M, Van Loon L A J 1998 Craniomandibulaire functie en disfunctie. Bohn Stafleu Van Loghum, Houten/Diegem

Nelson G 1994 The tension headache–migraine headache continuum: a hypothesis. Journal of Manipulative and Physiological Therapeutics 17:156

Okeson J 1995 Bell's orofacial pains, 5th edn. Quintessence, Chicago

Okeson J 1996 Orofacial pain. Guidelines for assessment, diagnosis, and management: the biopsychosocial model of disease. Quintessence, Chicago

Okeson J 2005 Bell's orofacial pains, 6th edn. Quintessence, Chicago

Palla S 1998 Myoartropathien des kausystems und orofaziale Schmerzen. Fotoplast, Zurich

Pertes R A, Gross S G 1995 Clinical management of temporomandibular disorders and orofacial pain. Quintessence, Chicago, p 69

Pfaffenrath V, Rath M, Keeser W, Pollmann W 1992 Atypical facial pain – quality of IHS (International Headache Society) criteria and psychometric data. Nervenarzt 63:595

Pinkham I 1986 The dental treatment of migrainous and tension headaches. In: Grieve G P (ed.) Modern manual therapy of the vertebral column. Churchill Livingstone, Edinburgh, p 283

Proffit W R 1993 Fixed and removable appliances in contemporary orthodontics, 2nd edn. Mosby, St Louis, p 318

Riley J, Robinson M, Kvaal S, Gremillion H 1998 Effects of physical and sexual abuse in facial pain: direct or mediated? Cranio 16:259

Schiffmann E, Anderson G, Fricton J et al 1992 The relationship between level of mandibular pain and dysfunction and stage of temporomandibular joint internal derangement. Journal of Dental Research 71:1812

Schwenzer N, Ehrenfeld M (eds) 2002 Tumoren im Mund-Kiefer-Gesichts-Bereich. In: Spezielle Chirurgie. Thieme, Stuttgart, p 116

Seidel H, Ball J, Dains J, Benedict G 1993 Mosby's guide to physical examination. Saunders, Philadelphia

Seltzer S, Dewart D, Pollack R, Jackson E 1982 The effects of dietary tryptophan on chronic maxillofacial pain and experimental tolerance. Journal of Psychiatric Research 17:181

Shankland W 1995 Craniofacial pain syndromes that mimic temporomandibular joint disorders. Annals of the Academy of Medicine, Singapore 24:83

Slavicek R 2000 Das Kauorgan – Funktionen und Dysfunktionen: Gamma, Klosterneuburg, p 219

Solow B, Sierbaek-Nielsen S 1992 Cervical and craniocervical posture as predictors of craniofacial growth. American Journal of Orthodontics and Dentofacial Orthopedics 101:449

Speculand B, Gross A, Spence N, Pilowsky I 1981 Intractable facial pain and illness behaviour. Pain 11:213

Spillane J 1996 Bickerstaff's neurological examination in clinical practice, 6th edn. Blackwell, Oxford

Sturzenegger M, DiStefano G, Radanov B P, Schnidrig A 1994 Presenting symptoms and signs after whiplash: the influence of accident mechanisms. Neurology 44(4):688–693

Sugawara O, Atsuta Y, Iwahara T et al 1996 The effects of mechanical compression and hypoxia on nerve roots and dorsal ganglia. Spine 21:2089

Turp J 2000 Temporomandibular pain. Clinical presentation and impact. Quintessence, Berlin

Turp J, Kowalski C, Stohler C 1998 Treatment-seeking patterns of facial pain patients: many possibilities, limited satisfaction. Journal of Orofacial Pain 12:61

Upton A R M, McComas A J 1973 The double crush in nerve entrapment syndromes. Lancet 2:359–362

van Duin N 1991 Sinusitis maxillaris' symptomen verloop en diagnostiek. Thesis, Meditext

von Piekartz H 2001 Neurodynamik des kranialen Nervensystems (Kranioneurodynamik). In: Piekartz von H, Bryden L (eds) Kraniofaziale Dysfunktion und Schmerzen, Untersuchung, Beurteilung und Management. Thieme, Stuttgart, S. 115

von Piekartz H, Bryden L 2001 Craniofacial dysfunction and pain, assessment, manual therapy and management. Butterworth-Heinemann, Oxford

Wabeke K, Spruijt R 1994 On the temporomandibular sounds, dental and psychological studies. Thesis, Academisch Centrum Tandheelkunde Amsterdam (ACTA)

Wagemans P, Van de Velde J, Kuipers-Jagtman A 1988 Sutures and forces: a review. American Journal of Orthodontics and Dentofacial Orthopedics 94:129

Waltner J 1955 Otolaryngeal sources of pain. Journal of the American Dental Association 51:417

Watkins L R, Maier S F 2000 The pain of being sick: implications of immune-to-brain communication for understanding pain. Annual Review of Psychology 51:29–57

Widmalm S, Christiansen R, Gunn S 1995 Oral parafunctions as temporomandibular disorder risk factors in children. Journal of Craniomandibular Practice 13:242

Woda A, Pionchon P 2000 Unified concept of idiopathic orofacial pain: pathophysiological features. Journal of Orofacial Pain 14:196–212
Wolff H 1963 Headache and other head pain, 2nd edn. Oxford University Press, New York, 3:28
Zakrzewska J 1995 Trigeminal neuralgia: surgery at the level of the Gasserian ganglion. Saunders, London, p 125
Zakrzewska J, Hamlyn P 1999 Facial pain. In: Crombie I K (ed.) Epidemiology of pain. IASP Press, Seattle

Chapter 4

Therapeutic communication during management of craniofacial pain

Anke Handrock

CHAPTER CONTENTS

INTRODUCTION

Pain, in particular chronic pain, represents one of the greatest health problems in the industrial world (Schors & Ahrens 2002). Many types of pain, in particular chronic pain conditions, can be positively influenced with the help of psychological methods (Basler et al 1990). Obviously, this also applies to pain in the head area. It is therefore useful to have a brief oversight of communication techniques which may help or hinder pain management. Some basic mechanisms for the psychological treatment of pain and for guidance of patients are dealt with here.

Prerequisites for good communication contact with patients include:

- Treatment agreement
- The concept of secondary gains arising from the condition
- Definition of aims
- Hidden goals of therapist and patient
- Psychological aspects of the development of pain and the perception of pain
- Some simple therapeutic interventions
- An overview of further therapeutic options.

Patients with craniofacial pain syndromes have often already been suffering for a considerable period of time. Whether pain is considered more organic or psychosomatic will depend on the overall experience – a stronger psychosomatic component strengthens the indication for ancillary psychotherapeutic care, while it is precisely these patients who reject the possibility of a psychological contribution to their illness (Schors & Ahrens 2002). Some pointers are shown in Table 4.1.

In practice, specific psychological reactions should be considered in almost all chronic craniofacial pain patients. These patients have often seen several therapists and had many frustrating experiences. They generally have very high expectations of the therapist while, to a certain extent, expecting treatment failure (in the sense of a self-fulfilling prophecy). Sternbach (1968) mentioned patients' so-called 'pain games' in this context. Some broadly defined typical reactions the therapist should be aware of in order to select an appropriate communication strategy from the outset are listed here.

- The *tormented* person who requires immediate help – Example: 'You can see how much I am suffering. The pain is agonizing, do something now.'
- The *martyr* who patiently bears his suffering – Example: 'You can see how patiently I am coping with this whole situation. I am worthy of admiration.'
- The *accuser,* who arouses feelings of guilt – Example: 'Look what you have done to me. You are responsible for my suffering.'
- The *understater* who (even in the face of obvious suffering) plays down their symptoms – Example: It's not so bad really, hardly worth talking about, I'm still OK.'
- The *brave, experienced sufferer* – Example: 'You can do what you like with me, I'll cope.'
- The *authority killer* who first sees the therapist as a saviour and then pronounces them in the worst case to be a charlatan and even in some cases sues – Example: 'Please help me, I'm in constant pain. You are the only one who can help me.'

Table 4.1 Features of pain

Feature	Mainly organic	Mainly functional (non-organic)
Localization of pain	Exact localization, clearly described	Vague, unclear, shifting
Emotions/feelings expressed by patient	Fit the pain described	Not suitable, inappropriate
Duration of pain	Phases of pain and lessening or absence of pain	Pain is continual and of approximately the same intensity
Dependent on voluntary movement	Present	Barely present or totally absent
Reactions to pain killers	Pharmacologically appropriate	Unclear
Pain and human relationships	Independent of one another	Linked
Visual description of pain	Picture described fits	Picture described is unsuitable, partly theatrical
Cause of illness as given by patient	Stresses psychological causes	Stresses organic causes
Patient's speech	Simple, clear, matter-of-fact	Irritated, angry, bored, impatient
Therapist's feelings while listening	Calm, attentive, understanding	Anger, fury, boredom, impatience, helplessness, confusion

Modified from Adler (1996).

When such reactions are found in patients, this means that the therapist cannot assume that the patient is able to realistically judge the success of therapy. The patient's expectations are either unrealistically high or extremely low – 'nobody can help me anyway'. In either case, the patient will not recognize successful treatment, particularly if the effect is small. Successful treatment outcomes lag far behind those achieved with patients with a realistic understanding of their treatment. As this is a well-known situation, Keeser and Bullinger (1990) suggest questioning two typical medical assumptions when dealing with chronic pain patients:

- Firstly that the patient really (i.e. consciously and subconsciously) wants to be cured
- As a result of the above, such a cure can be effected with the appropriate means and methods available.

Under favourable conditions of communication it is possible to structure contact with these patients, who are mainly described as 'difficult', in such a way that the chances of successful therapy are substantially increased. To this end, a certain communicative attitude based on the following assumptions has been found to be helpful.

ASSUMPTIONS FOR FAVOURABLE COMMUNICATION CONDITIONS

These assumptions are creations of thought which are neither true nor false. They have been found useful for communication with patients because numerous treatment options arise from the resultant therapeutic disposition, allowing considerable therapeutic flexibility. These prerequisites promote therapeutic communication within the framework of an existing treatment agreement.

These communication basics are, of course, not new, and for this reason historical notes have been added in certain places. These come either from philosophers or from monks, the great orators of the past.

People act from their own personal viewpoint (individual reality), irrespective of actual reality. Understanding someone therefore means meeting them in their reality.

Each type of behaviour has a positive intention for the person concerned. Each person does the best they can do at the time in each situation. This also means that a negative or inappropriate type of behaviour will only be abandoned when a better form of behaviour is available. ('A wrong passion is not removed by quashing it but by driving it out with a real passion' – Bernhard of Clairvaux, co-founder of the Cistercian Order 1090–1153.)

The speaker (transmitter) is responsible for communication: 'It is not what I say, but what is understood that counts.' The importance of communication lies in the result it achieves. ('Because you were angry and corrected him with more candour than was your right, you did not improve him, but only angered him; in future pay attention not only to the truth of what you say, but also whether he to whom you speak can bear the truth' – Seneca, Roman philosopher ca. 0–65.)

Resistance is the result of a lack of flexibility in the speaker (in particular with regard to structuring contact, preparation of the message and timing of the communication). As a rule, more time is used in dealing with resistance after the fact than in correct preparation of messages; thus avoid resistance as far as possible.

In communication there are no mistakes, only new information. If you receive the information that a counselling technique has not functioned as you had hoped, then try something else. Do not, however, repeat the first technique – and certainly not without sufficient further preparation. One reason for this is that you have already encountered a reaction of resistance and this resistance would only increase.

Behaviour and thinking are guided by the direction of the attention given. The questioner steers attention and in so doing guides the conversation in the direction required. The person who orientates the conversation toward goals and resources (e.g. exceptions in the course of the illness) gives the patient the possibility of dealing with their problems in a new way. For potentially curable illnesses one can even say that each human being already has what they need to achieve their goals.

Behind every complaint there is a wish. Those who understand this wish and refer to it meets the patient in their world and the patient feels understood. Dealing with wishes is also far more pleasant than dealing with complaints and 'moaning'.

The above assumptions result in an involved, interested questioning attitude on the part of the therapist. Protracted lecturing of the patient should be the exception, not the rule. The patient is listened to and experiences understanding and goodwill from the therapist. This enables an open conversation in which a patient will divulge far more information than in a 'normal' consultation.

CONTACT

A prerequisite for such communication is that contact with the patient is built up in an appropriate manner. A basic rule is that, in communication, people react far more strongly to *how* something is said rather than to *what* is said.

Good communicative contact is often described as *rapport*. When people have a rapport with one another you can see this from a distance. Their behaviour patterns resemble each other. Use can be made of observable patterns of behaviour by consciously adapting to the patient. This 'virtual mirroring' is also referred to as pacing. With pacing, adaptation of behaviour occurs in the following areas.

The therapist adapts their attitude – at least in certain areas – to that of the patient. Where there is good contact this happens spontaneously (as seen with couples or business partners negotiating in a restaurant). What this means in practice is that the conversation partners, as far as possible:

- Meet at the same eye level
- Adapt to one another's hand, foot and head movements.

Patterns of behaviour are mirrored, which means that the conversation partners have:

- A similar tempo in movement and speech
- A similar style of language (number of foreign words, length and complexity of sentences, emotionality, etc.).

Very often, spontaneous adaptation of breathing patterns then results.

If good professional contact is to be established with the patient it is necessary to accompany the person until rapport has been recognizably established. Good conversational contact can be recognized by the following indications: the patient begins to slightly nod his head in agreement, body language becomes more open, when the therapist smiles the patient smiles back, if the therapist moves soon after the patient will also move, eye contact increases. At the point where good conversational contact has been established it is advised to move from accompanying the patient to leading the conversation. Unpleasant or difficult topics can now be dealt with. Should rapport diminish during the conversation, return immediately to pacing.

For therapeutic counselling there is usually an *implicit treatment agreement*. As a rule there are two conditions for such an agreement:

- The patient really wants to get better and is prepared to do everything necessary to achieve this. The patient will therefore keep to the agreements (shows high compliance).
- The therapist has ways and means to alleviate the symptoms and, if possible, to cure the illness.

This relatively simple model usually functions extremely well with many acute treatments such as therapy for acute inflammation. For this reason it is often generalized and applied to chronic conditions. Here, however, various special points should be noted.

PAIN-INFLUENCING FACTORS

The sensation of pain (in particular chronic pain) consists of several components (Fig. 4.1).

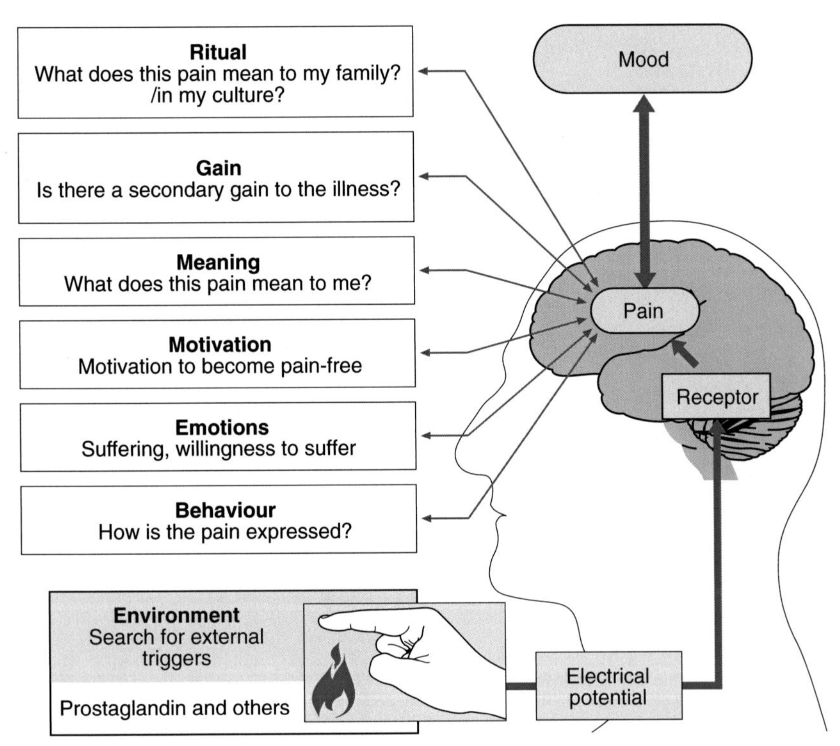

Fig. 4.1 Factors influencing pain.

Stimuli in the wider sense are responsible for the basis of the sensation of pain, be they mechanical, chemical, caused by temperature, inflammatory or similar. Different patients react very differently to stimuli of comparable intensity. Here, among other things, the following psychologically influenced factors play a part:

- Mood: Patients with negative mood (e.g. depressive patients) have a low tolerance of pain (Flor 1990) (see Case study 4.1). For this reason some clinics are starting to employ clowns to improve the mood of seriously ill cancer patients and so reduce the use of analgesic drugs (in addition to stimulating the immune system).
- Attitude to pain: Many patients tend to adopt extreme, partly cramped postures or work methods which actually increase pain. Ergonomic training, relaxation and breathing techniques and behavioural therapy approaches can effect positive changes.
- Emotions: The amount the patient is prepared to suffer and the intensity of suffering varies greatly between patients. The more intensively the patient concentrates their emotions on the pain, the greater will be the sensation of pain.
- Motivation: The will to cope as best as possible with the pain and the illness varies greatly. Sensation of pain is reduced with increasing motivation to cope with the pain and more realistic expectations of therapeutic outcomes. The more realistically the patient views their being cured and the higher the motivation to cope with the pain, the lower the sensation of pain.
- Meaning: The sensation of pain varies with the meaning that is attached to the pain (Müller-Busch 1990). When an injury during a competition is regarded as unimportant compared with the chance of victory, the real extent of the injury will only be realized after achieving the goal. If, on the other hand, a mild pain means the growth of a

tumour, then this pain, when it occurs, will be felt much more strongly.

- Gain: People always live in relationships and systems. These systems react to the pain of a patient. In this way, for instance, a migraine patient will receive special attention during a migraine attack (e.g. not having to carry out their duties). When the migraine

Case study 4.1

Not all factors are always of equal relevance for an episode of pain. A 75-year-old patient who has been widowed for 4 months (a pensioner, former metal-worker) goes to the surgery of a young colleague again and again because of painful tender spots following his receiving new dentures (the new dentures had been absolutely necessary). They know that the patient does not want morning appointments. Over a course of several weeks the patient comes to afternoon surgery with the same subjective complaints. He has no appointment and puts up with long waiting times.

The tender spots cannot be seen on examination of the mouth, although according to the patient the dentures have been worn continuously. The dentures are in a hygienic condition. An allergy test carried out by the man's general practitioner after some appointments shows no indication of allergic reaction. As the dentures sit perfectly, treatment consists of two components: placing the dentures in an ultrasound bath (this apparatus lies in another room, cannot be seen by the patient but heard) and treatment of the mouth with a mild diluted camomile solution. The dentures are not altered because there are no obvious tender spots and the dentures sit as they should.

During the treatment the patient seems to want to talk a lot and complains about his present situation in life. When the dentures again start to press, he cannot eat properly and also not speak properly. Not speaking wasn't so bad, he had no-one to talk to anyway, but not eating was a problem. On being advised to go to his GP because of his difficult situation, he brusquely rejects this advice and blames the apparently functional pains on his dentures. Each treatment is followed by about 5 days of subjective freedom from pain. Although the patient continues rinsing his mouth at home, the symptoms reappear in another place after about 5 days.

The treatment which led to freedom from pain in three sittings consisted of changing the pattern of treatment. Every 3 days the patient was given an appointment at 7.45 a.m. before the start of morning surgery for 'systematic oral treatment' with a mild, dilute camomile solution. Treatment was the same as before, except it was carried out by an older, resolute dental assistant. The dentist only briefly checked the result of treatment and then sent the patient home. After three sittings there was subjective freedom from pain. The patient cancelled the fourth appointment and only returned 6 months later for the agreed check-up.

The patient's reactionary depressive basic mood led to reduced tolerance of pain. Normal adjustment procedures when fitting the dentures are subjectively experienced as acute pain. Because of his grief, the patient at present experiences great willingness to suffer. The gain resulting from this pain situation is quite high. The patient regulates his need for contact and his need for conversation via the dentures. Minimizing the illness gain then also leads to a reduction of the symptoms. The unwillingness to go to his GP for talks is a result of the purely dental treatment agreement. In order to successfully suggest such treatment, a preparatory conversation about the possibilities of a psychological component in the illness would have been necessary. It seemed a good idea to minimize the illness gain by achieving freedom from the symptoms in order to prevent a chronic situation in the sense of habitual incompatibility with the dentures.

is over, the so-called illness gain is also lost. For this reason some psychosomatic clinics wait to see if the patient's request to retire will be granted (where medically possible) before they admit the patient.

- Ritual: In various ethnic groups and also within families there are rituals regarding illnesses and pain (Müller-Busch 1990). In this way a family tendency to 'keep a stiff upper lip – no complaining' can lead to serious delays in the diagnostic measures necessary. At the other end of the scale the presumption that 'a boy who is not brought forth in pain will become a weakling' can lead to an enhanced subjective sensation of pain during childbirth despite an effective epidural.

When one considers all these pain-influencing factors, it is easy to understand that the above-mentioned implicit treatment agreement is not always enough for treating chronic pain patients. An explicit treatment agreement clarifies the conditions of treatment and the intentions of patient and therapist.

Efficient methods of communication are very effective. When these methods are openly applied in the medical context within the framework of the existing treatment agreement they serve to achieve the predetermined aim of treatment in the fastest way possible. This procedure, if an open one, is acknowledged and respected by the patient. Where there is no such treatment agreement the following risks arise:

- The therapist intervenes in order to pursue their own personal (legitimate) interests (e.g. tries to achieve success in treatment by a certain method). The patient feels that this procedure is manipulative and reacts with resistance.
- The therapist intervenes in order to use secret 'areas' of the patient for treatment purposes (e.g. asks personal questions about possible psychological causes of illness without first clarifying the framework of treatment and the treatment agreement). The patient senses the intrusion and feels embarrassed. The patient either resists or breaks off treatment.
- The patient desires (due to personal factors, e.g. illness gain) that success of treatment be limited. For inexplicable reasons a difficult and limited process of healing results.

In order to avoid these obvious difficulties it is important to ensure that there is always a clear treatment agreement before these methods are applied.

> **!** In personal relationships there are no treatment agreements. Here all such intervention using professional communication techniques are to be absolutely avoided!

TREATMENT AGREEMENT

Within the framework of the treatment agreement a clear definition of aims is compiled with the patient. Following this the exact framework of the course of treatment is agreed. In doing this the patient receives security, the relationship with the therapist is intensified and compliance increased. When determining the aim of treatment the following aspects are considered:

- What exactly do you want to achieve/have? (the aim must be positively formulated): Only a positive description allows an exact idea of the state required such that one can exactly and clearly imagine an idea of the desired goal. In goal definition, therefore, there can be no negation and no comparison. A negation firstly produces an image of the problem and then the accompanying negation of the aim. A goal which contains comparisons produces two ideas of goal: one positive and desired, and another that reflects the undesired problem. Both negations and comparisons lead to failure.

- The patient is encouraged to describe the goal concretely with his senses: This is a pattern of speech from the area of hypnosis. The patient is requested to give an exact goal description using his senses (what will you see, hear, feel and smell when you have reached this goal?) In doing this the aim of treatment will become even more real for the patient. The more exact the description, the more exact the picture. The more exact the picture, the more attractive the goal and the greater the compliance!

> **!** The desired goal attitude must lie within the patient's reach. Several small, successful and successive treatment agreements are more effective than one that is too ambitious.

Patients often want something to happen passively to them (e.g. massages) which leads to recovery without their own active participation. Within the framework of goal definition of the treatment agreement, the part which the patient themselves must play is precisely defined. In doing so it is important to check whether the demands made on each patient lie within the area of their *subjective* possibilities.

- Cost–benefit analysis – examining the greater framework of the aim: What are the consequences which arise from achieving this goal? How does one's life change in achieving this goal?

Failure to consider the impact of a patient reaching their goal on the other people in the patient's life can have disastrous consequences. The questions used to examine the greater framework are unusual. Therefore, it is often necessary to first explain the advantages of an exact cost–benefit analysis to the patient (Table 4.2).

- How does the patient know that he has reached his goal? This question sounds strange, but it is very helpful when the patient knows exactly how to recognize that a particular stage of treatment was successful.

Table 4.2 Cost–benefit analysis

	The problem remains, the goal is not achieved?	The problem is solved – the goal is reached?
What do you gain when . . .	What is the good side of the problem?	What is good about the goal?
	What is good about the current situation?	**What can you do when you have reached your goal?**
What do you lose when . . .	What is the worst thing that can happen if the problem remains?	What is the disadvantage of the goal? What do you lose when you have reached your goal?
	What is the good in this?	**What do you have to do in order to achieve your goal? What do you have to do when you have reached your goal?**
What do other people gain when . . .	Who profits when you do not reach your goal?	Who else profits when you do reach your goal?
What do other people lose when . . .	Who else loses something when you do not reach your goal?	Who else loses something when you do reach your goal?

When checking success, there are two different situations. For the interim steps, brief feedback is important (feedback curve), i.e. when the patient notices success immediately after the treatment step, this motivates the patient to take the next step. When the final treatment goal has been reached it is necessary to note this in order to adjust behaviour to the state achieved (e.g. resuming normal fitness training).

Example 1

Diets often fail because, while people know how to lose weight, when they have reached their ideal weight they do not know how to recognize that they are full.

If treatment aims, treatment steps, the criteria by which the patient can recognize their progress and any conditions under which the treatment agreement must be altered are included in the treatment agreement, it is possible to use communication techniques to influence conditions of pain. If such methods are to be employed they must be expressly agreed within the framework of the treatment agreement.

Example 2

For years a patient has had recurring chronic nocturnal grinding of teeth. When during goal definition the question arose as to what he would lose if he lost this symptom he burst out: 'Then I could no longer grit my teeth when my wife starts yelling. Then I don't know how I would react!' In this way he recognizes that grinding his teeth allows him to tolerate a difficult marital situation with an extremely jealous wife. As a result he decides to undergo psychotherapy (indicated for several reasons) as advised, something he has rejected up to now.

VERBAL METHODS OF INTERVENTION

Patients with chronic pain frequently have indications for more general psychotherapeutic treatment (e.g. of concomitant depression). In such cases treatment by a psychotherapist may also be necessary. However, there is a whole spectrum of specific communication techniques to influence pain conditions that can be used by any trained doctor. To what extent the therapist themselves can and wish to apply these techniques depends on their particular qualifications. This spectrum ranges from classic relaxation methods (Jacobson training, autogenic training, self-hypnosis) via hypnotic guidance of speech during general treatment to psychotherapeutic intervention.

Hypnosis, in particular self-hypnosis, as a relaxation method has a similarly wide range as, for instance, the self-hypnosis of autogenic training. It can be used as a supportive form of therapy in the whole area of psychosomatics and to stimulate learning and creativity. Here it is important to pay careful attention to positive expression of the often unspecific suggestions. The transition to hypnotherapy is flexible.

Trance experiences are routinely used in many societies for healing, reflection or in order to deepen experiences. In Western Europe, however, the expression 'trance' belongs mainly to the area of hypnotherapy. In our everyday life we are expected to be fully oriented and conscious. Day-dreaming, for instance, is strictly forbidden to schoolchildren, whereby this is nothing more than a (good) daily trance. Trance experiences are completely normal; they are practised by every healthy person daily. According to Rossi (Schors & Ahrens 2002), one's day is composed of so-called ultradianous 90-minute rhythms. Following a phase of activity of 90 minutes a roughly 10-minute rest phase – a light trance phase – is inserted. In jobs requiring high concentration one can observe this in an increased number of mistakes. These phases of day-dreams which help one to recover are helpful in influencing pain conditions.

Therapeutic communication makes use of these trance conditions. They are partly applied within the framework of imagination techniques, partly within the framework of formal hypnosis. Hypnosis in the treatment of acute pain conditions has been particularly successful and for this reason use has begun in many dental practices. Hypnosis is also becoming more important in midwifery and anaesthetics.

Imaginative approaches lead to considerable improvement in eating problems, smoking and alcohol abuse. They are also being applied more and more to treat cancers. Here the aim is to reduce the side effects of chemotherapy, to strengthen the immune system, reduce pain, increase life expectancy and improve the quality of life.

The following types of intervention are especially suitable for influencing pain conditions.

IMAGINATIVE IMAGES LEAD, THROUGH INTENSIVE 'DAY-DREAMS' TO SPONTANEOUS TRANCE CONDITIONS

Metaphoric patterns and imagination

With the help of metaphors and stories it is often possible to achieve considerable changes in conditions of pain. Professional usage of such stories produces spontaneous trance conditions. With these methods one also speaks of indirect hypnotic intervention. As one works with images a (light) trance spontaneously develops.

- The patient is asked to imagine a control desk to regulate undesired symptoms and to adjust the values accordingly.
- The patient imagines the pain as a symbol, following which the symbol is altered or a different symbol chosen.
- Images are developed by inner helpers. These inner helpers give the patient suggestions as to how the pain can be changed. Religious patients often encounter their guardian angels in such images.
- Images of ritual healing ceremonies can be used, e.g. bathing in a healing spring.
- A concept is explained to the patient in which one can imagine the work of the subconscious in such a way that various parts take on different duties. When one part is impeded in its work it starts to send signals. If one fails to hear the quiet signals, then loud signals are sent – the symptoms. Imaginative images are then developed as to what the part sending the symptom might look like. Following this, questions are asked about this 'part': What would it like to say? What is its true function? Why is it sending out a signal? This results in the development of a metaphoric insight into the illness.
- Shifting of modalities: we receive all our perceptions via our sensory channels – one refers to sensory modalities (e.g. visual – seeing). These perceptions are again divisible into smaller subunits (e.g. with sight, considering the colour, the size of the image, picture or film, etc.). These subunits are called submodalities. When one alters a submodality, the sensation of pain changes.

Other techniques

- Finding and acknowledging exceptions: It is especially important that chronic pain patients take note of even small improvements and value these. It is, therefore, critical to ensure that all exceptions to the experience of chronic pain are acknowledged. It is then essential to find out exactly what led to this exception and how this state can again be reached. When patients realize their own potential to influence the situation, this stabilizes their self-confidence.
- Activating all resources: Many patients have the tendency to 'root around' in negative memories. In doing so their general mood worsens and their pain threshold is lowered. If, on the other hand, one trains the patient to independently and regularly relive positive memories and situations (resources) within the framework of relaxation exercises, their mood stabilizes and the pain threshold is increased.
- Reinterpretation (reframing of context and meaning): When pain occurs, a catastrophic

meaning is frequently ascribed to it (e.g. 'It's got to be cancer'). In such cases it can be very helpful to assign a different meaning to the pain. Fear is then reduced and the pain threshold increased (Case study 4.2).

Case study 4.2

A 45-year-old male teacher, married with two children, had great tension in his masticator muscles. On noting his medical history it was found that this tension and pain had arisen suddenly. Following this a connection was sought to his present situation in life and it turned out that the tension had arisen at the time of his father's death.

On further questioning the following additional connections were revealed. The patient's father had always expressed a wish to die at home. Due to a serious illness he had been admitted to hospital. His condition continued to worsen and he had asked his son to take him home. The doctors had, however, strongly advised the son against this because they expected his condition to improve with treatment. The son had therefore persuaded his father to remain in hospital where the father then died following a sudden deterioration in his condition. Shortly before his death the father had complained that his last wish, to die at home, had not been granted. Since then the son had suffered from feelings of guilt and extreme nocturnal grinding of teeth. On being asked what would have actually happened if the son had taken his father home and he had then died there, although the doctors had assumed that his father's condition would improve within a few days, the son's face brightened at once and he replied: 'Then I would have actually been partly responsible for my father's death.'

When questioned about how he now viewed the situation, he replied: 'In the particular circumstances my behaviour would seem to have been right.' In a check-up 2 weeks later it was found that the muscle pains had disappeared and the patient could not recall grinding his teeth in the meantime.

The situation described in Case study 4.2 is a classic case of reinterpretation of meaning. The patient's behaviour at having left his father in the hospital is no longer seen by him as not having carried out his father's last wishes but as having behaved responsibly with respect to his father's health.

FORMAL HYPNOSIS: USEFUL IN CERTAIN CIRCUMSTANCES

Direct suggestions are often used as 'gut feelings'. They are not usually particularly effective without proper hypnosis; however, when a patient is already in a trance they can be very helpful.

- Direct address: The pain is, for instance, linked to another bodily function. 'The unpleasant feeling decreases with each breath.'
- Changing the signalling system: 'Pay attention to another signal rather than the pain.'
- Altering area and intensity: 'Perceive the pain in a lower intensity over a larger area.'

Shifting the pain

In these procedures replacement ideas instead of the pain are offered. Such images are so effective in hypnotic trances that they are used to carry out operations under hypnoanaesthesia.

- Glove anaesthesia: A glove is suggested which causes the patient not to feel the pain. This numbness is then applied to other areas of the body (Schmierer 1997).
- Analgesics: Feeling the pain differently is suggested to the patient (e.g. as numbness, cold, etc.).
- Paradoxical intervention: 'This is pain and it does not hurt you.' (This pattern matches physiological discoveries in the brain regarding fighting pain with hypnosis. The pain is transmitted to the brain but is not felt as pain.)

- Disorientation: Pains can also be shifted whereby the pain is directed to a different part of the body.

> **!** This procedure can lead to shifting of symptoms, especially when the patient forgets the shifting of pain (amnesia).

Distraction techniques

By focusing attention on other activities or ideas the sensation of pain can be greatly reduced.

- Focusing attention (disassociation): The attention of the patient is concentrated on a different emotionally intensive situation (e.g. imagining playing sport intensively just at this moment).
- Disorientation – out-of-body experience: The patient is asked to leave his body behind and at the same time to be in another place (e.g. his favourite place).

Time gaps

Through the use of imagination the patient is 'sent' into a pain-free time or is trained to experience some periods of time as longer and others as shorter.

- Time without pain: Going into the past or future
- Distortion of time: The way one experiences time is changed, e.g.:
  - *Fast time* – time goes faster – in a contraction during labour
  - *Slow time* – time goes slower – in the break between contractions.

Amnesia suggestions

One can directly or indirectly (e.g. using pictures of drifting snow covering everything) request a patient to consciously not remember certain things (e.g. unpleasant and painful interventions).

Contraindications

Trance conditions work with images. At best, these images were once real but are not, however, real at the present time. As a rule psychotic people have great difficulty in recognizing hallucinations for what they are and differentiating them from images. For this reason one must proceed very carefully with all imagination techniques, as well as autogenic training. This also applies to all symptoms where the relationship between patient and therapist is not clearly stable and good. Most personality disorders, in particular borderline disturbance, are included in this category. Aggressive patients should not be placed in a trance: in lowering the inhibition threshold they could become more aggressive.

PATTERN OF ADJUSTMENT FOR PAIN CONDITIONS

Finally, a procedure will be described which very often leads to a swift reduction of symptoms in both acute and chronic pain. A prerequisite for employing this procedure is that the cause of the pain has been physiologically completely determined. (Altering unclear, not fully diagnosed pain is regarded as medical malpractice, as an important diagnostic criterion would be missing.)

The aim of this procedure is to change the pain sensation with features of the patient's experience (submodalities) (Handrock 1999).

First of all it is necessary to create the conditions which apply to every therapeutic communication intervention:

- Establish good contact with the patient and maintain this.
- Extend the treatment agreement in such a way that the patient is prepared to work with visual images.
- Carry out a cost–benefit analysis (see Table 4.2).

The patient is then asked to describe the pain precisely. As a support measure one can, for instance, use the question system outlined in Table 4.3, which can be extended at will. In

Table 4.3 Scheme of questions for pain conditions

Area of perception	Appropriate type of question
Bodily feeling	How large is the area that hurts? Where are the borders? How would you describe this sensation (e.g. stabbing, dragging, pressing)? When is the pain stronger – when does it lessen somewhat? How bad is the pain now on a scale of 1 to 10? If you concentrate totally on the pain can you then intensify it? (This is a so-called 'convincing question' because if the patient can increase the pain it means that they can alter the pain!) If you were to touch the area in your imagination would it tend to be hard or soft, rough or smooth, warm or cool?
Visual imagination	If the pain had a colour, what colour would this be? Are there colour variations in this area? Where is it lighter or darker? Is it matt or glossy? What do the contours look like – do they tend to be sharp or blurred with no clear border?
Aural imagination	If the pain had a tone how would it sound? Would it tend to be loud or quiet? Is the sound continual or does it rise and fall, rhythmic or non- rhythmic?

order to answer these questions the patient must be prepared to use their imagination. (Should the patient directly resist and say they cannot imagine all this, it is not a good idea to work against their feelings, and other intervention techniques can be applied.)

When the painful area is described in this way the patient is instructed to describe the surrounding healthy area with the same intensity and detail. The question system can again be used for this.

One now builds a further framework for change by asking the patient what would happen if the colour or the tone was slightly altered (e.g. from red to pale red). Which would be better? It may be helpful to ask the patient to imagine a control desk or a remote control with which all suggested changes can be directed (or, if necessary, be reversed). As the patient has by this point already experienced some inner pictures it is usually quite easy for them to imagine such a thing.

Following this the patient is instructed to effect change in the individual submodalities of the unpleasant area and to try to reach the submodalities of the 'normal condition' in the visual and auditory areas as precisely as possible. The area of kinetics is not involved at this point.

The patient must be carefully observed after each suggestion of change. Only pleasant changes are retained – otherwise the change is immediately reversed.

When the colour and tone characteristics of the painful area have been adjusted as far as possible to those of the healthy area, one first talks for a few minutes about a neutral subject (so that the change can stabilize). The patient is then asked about how they feel in general (and not specifically about the pain).

Within the framework of a text like this it is only possible to give brief consideration to the use of the techniques described and to demonstrate these with examples (Case study 4.3). However, the use of these methods broadens the rather somatic-oriented procedure considerably.

Case study 4.3

A 52-year-old female patient with bilateral disc inflammation and a background of rheumatoid arthritis was taught to use this procedure in a form of self-hypnosis when she noticed that her daily maximum dose of pain killers is inadequate. She needed approximately 20 minutes each time for this procedure. She described the painful temporal areas in her imagination as being taut, thick, hot, smooth, shiny, hard, red with orange patches in the middle surrounded by a clear border. The tone was felt to be a high buzzing, like a swarm of bees.

She described the surrounding healthy area in her imagination as smooth, soft, dull, green, like a meadow with many flowers on it.

The patient was then asked to watch how the red colour became very slightly paler. She experienced this as very pleasant. She was then asked to note at the same time how the meadow very slowly grew in from the sides into this paling area. She then spontaneously described how the noise of the 'swarm of bees' calmed down.

At the same time the redness of the inflamed areas substantially decreased. This resulted in a considerable reduction of pain which lasted between 1 and 3 hours on each occasion.

SUMMARY

- **The use of verbal therapeutic methods to influence pain (and in this particular instance craniofacial pain) clearly widens the range of available treatment options.**
- **Verbal support is particularly helpful for patients with chronic pain.**
- **Due to a change in the subjective experience of pain a clear improvement in the general situation of the patient can often be observed, even when the somatic conditions have not changed or have even worsened.**

References

Adler R 1996 Schmerz. In: von Uexküll T et al (eds) Psychosomatische Medizin, 5th edn. Urban and Schwarzenberg, Munich

Basler H-D et al (eds) 1990 Psychologische Schmerztherapie. Springer, Berlin

Flor H 1990 Verhaltensmedizinische Grundlagen chronischer Schmerzen. In: Basler H-D et al (eds) Psychologische Schmerztherapie. Springer, Berlin

Handrock A 1999 Sprache und Verständlichkeit. Quintessenz, Berlin

Keeser W, Bullinger M 1990 Psychologische Verfahren bei der Behandlung von Schmerzen. In: Pongratz W (ed.) Therapie chronischer Schmerzzustände. Springer, Berlin

Müller-Busch H C 1990 Kulturgeschichtliche Bedeutung des Schmerzes. In: Basler H-D et al (eds) Psychologische Schmerztherapie. Springer, Berlin

Rehfisch H P, Basler H D 1990 Entspannung und Imagination. In: Basler H-D et al (eds) Psychologische Schmerztherapie. Springer, Berlin

Schmierer A 1997 Einführung in die zahnärztliche Hypnose, 2nd edn. Quintessenz, Berlin

Schors R, Ahrens S 2002 Schmerzsyndrome. In: Ahrens S, Schneider W (eds) Lehrbuch der Psychotherapie und der Psychosomatischen Medizin, 2nd edn. Schattauer, Stuttgart

Sternbach R A 1968 Pain: a psychophysiological analysis. Academic Press, New York

Chapter 5

Reciprocal connection between the craniocervical and the craniomandibular region: a hypothetical model

Harry von Piekartz

CHAPTER CONTENTS

INTRODUCTION

Most clinicians and researchers regard the reciprocal connection between the craniocervical and the craniomandibular region as poorly understood (Kraus 1994). One of the first publications on the topic is from 1926 and was extremely advanced for that time. The Austrian dentist Martin Schwarz concluded from his observations that the mandibular resting position is not fixed but depends on the position of the head. He emphasized the importance of a vertical mid-position of the head to achieve a mandibular resting position when assessing occlusion (Schwarz 1926).

This chapter will discuss the various ideas and studies regarding a connection of two regions which is of great importance for the therapeutic decision-making process. Finally, some recommendations for research and management are presented.

Studies may be grouped into two categories: those which investigate the influence of the craniocervical region on the craniomandibular region and vice versa. Aetiological studies outline four major explanatory models:

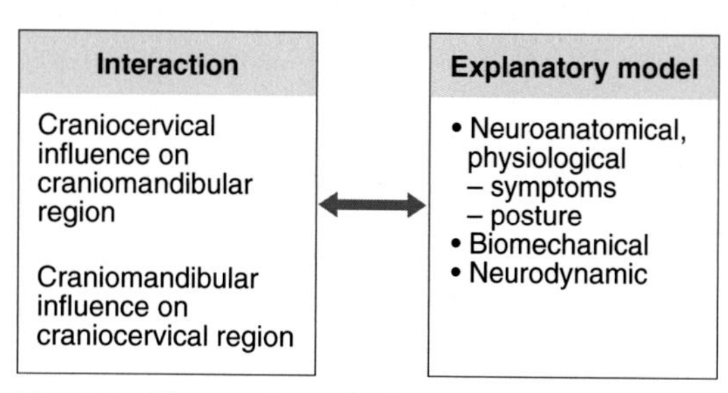

Fig. 5.1 The craniocervical region interacts with the craniomandibular region.

- Neuroanatomical/physiological model, based upon pain and posture
- Biomechanical
- Neurodynamic
- Clinical/functional.

As some overlap occurs naturally between those groups, this is not an absolute classification.

Figure 5.1 gives an overview. Examples of the explanatory models are described in the following sections.

NEUROANATOMY

Pain

Nociceptive input from craniocervical tissue is sent to the trigeminocervical nucleus, which is also the receptor for input from the trigeminal nerve. The trigeminal nucleus consists of neurones responsible for the transmission of afferent information to the cortex where pain is perceived. As the synapses of the trigeminal neurones and the neurones of the brainstem are in close proximity and influence each other, pain may be referred into the facial, head or jaw region (Kerr 1961a,b, 1963, Bogduk 1986a, Okeson 1995).

As a result of secondary hyperalgesia (caused by the craniocervical region), tests for the craniomandibular region may show false-positive results (Fig. 5.2).

Mandibular position

The mandibular resting position is the ideal position of the mandible in relationship to the cranium, allowing for all physiological mandibular movements (Kazis & Kazis 1956, Preiskel 1965). The ideal mandibular resting position is mandatory for an optimum occlusal relationship and an optimum muscle balance of the masticatory muscles (Murphy 1967, Kraus 1994). A number of studies showed that different positions of the head strongly influence the mandibular resting position (Preiskel 1965, Makofsky 1989, Gonzalis 1996, Miralles et al 2001). Sometimes the term 'upright postural position of the mandible (UPPM)' is used. One should also look out for the functional influences of head, neck and hyoid (Rugh & Drago 1981), since an ideal head position alone does not automatically guarantee an ideal mandibular position (Michelotti et al 2000). Sometimes the correction of head and neck position may result in an increase of masticatory muscle tone (EMG activity) (Kawamura & Fujimoto 1957, Wessberg et al 1983). Classic experimental studies showed an increase of EMG activity of the temporal muscle, the masseter and the digastricus anterior with cervical extension followed by a slight retrusion of the mandible, therefore influencing occlusion (Funakoshi et al 1976, Forsberg et al 1985, Kraus 1994). Increased activity of the digastricus anterior and the masseter muscle increased cervical extension which then reduced the EMG activity of these muscles (Funakoshi & Amano 1973).

Experimental studies on healthy volunteers using different head positions confirmed that the position of the head influences the movement and therefore the function of mandibular closing. Positions evaluated were: natural position (NP), anteroposition (forward head posture, FHP), maximal anteroposition (maximal forward head posture, MFHP) and military position (MP). Each position is associated with different muscle activity patterns and different occlusion types (Goldstein et al 1984). The craniomandibular muscles are also influenced by neurological reflex systems such as the tonic neck reflex (TNR) (Bratzlavsky & van der Eecken 1977). Cervical afferent information enters the subnucleus caudalis via the dorsal horn and

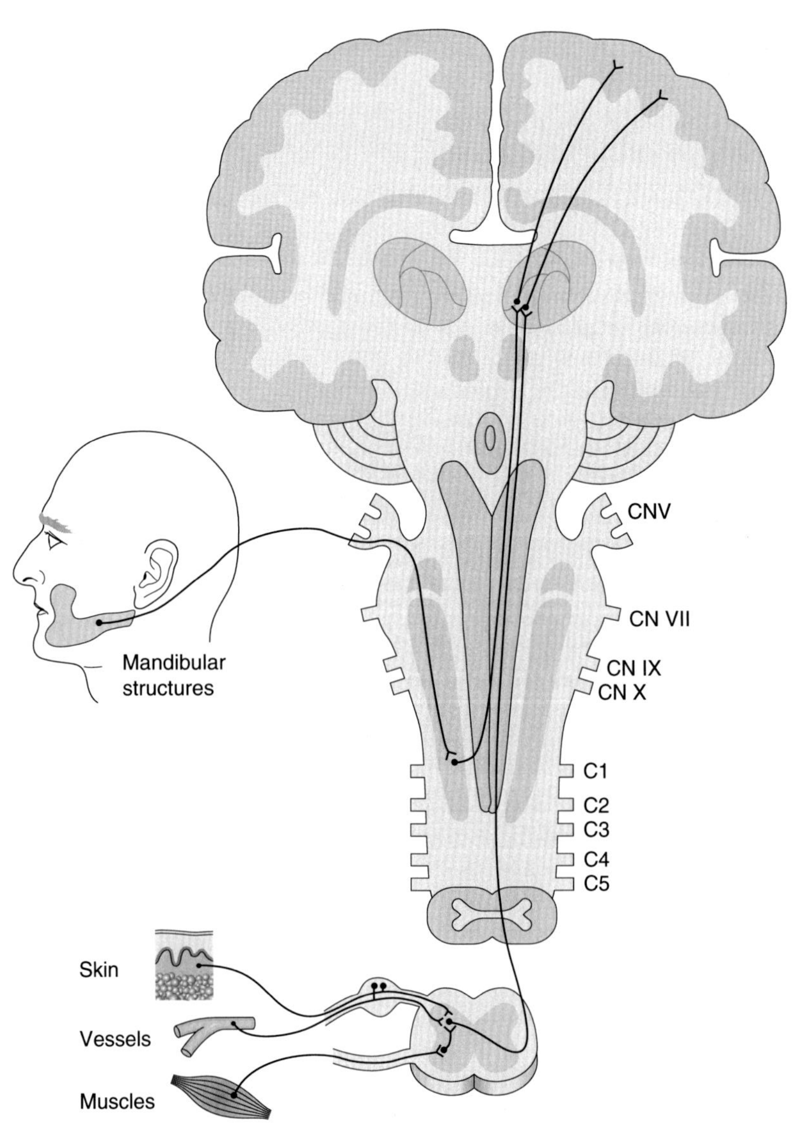

Fig. 5.2 Schematic overview of the afferent input from muscles, joints, and blood vessels from the craniocervical junction (primary afferent neurone = 1st neurone). These end in synaptic junctions to the 2nd neurone in the trigeminocervical nucleus, where the afferent craniomandibular neurones may also interfere (2nd neurone). Afferent information is passed on via the spinothalamic tract to the thalamus. The 3rd neurone projects the information to the somatosensory cortex (modified from Okeson 1995).

triggers neck reflexes by stimulating the trigeminocervical nucleus which stimulates the motor neurones of the masticatory muscles (Funakoshi & Amano 1973, Sumino et al 1981). Hu et al (1993) observed that prolonged nociceptive (inflammatory) stimuli from the paraspinal muscles not only increased the activity of the superficial and deep neck muscles but also those of the masticatory system. This may explain the clinical observations of facial pain and of parafunctions after whiplash injury.

BIOMECHANICS

Cephalometric measurements show a clear reciprocal influence of the craniocervical region, the mandibular position and the hyoid. Rocabado (1983) made the following statements:

- The angle between the two cephalometric lines MGP (McGregor's plane) and OP (odontoid plane) is 96° in *normal cervical lordosis*. The vertical hyoid position is below the C3 line and the outermost inferoposterior part of the mandible (retrognathion, RGN). There is a triangle between the C3 line, RGN and hyoid (Fig. 5.3a).
- A *flat cervical spine* (loss of physiological lordosis) shows an MGP–OP angle of less than 96° and the hyoid lies on the C3–RGN line.
- Kyphotic cervical spines show a MGP–OP angle that is either normal or less than 96°. The hyoid is above the C3–RGN line with a negative triangle between C3, RGN and hyoid (Fig. 5.3b).

Following whiplash-associated disorders (WAD), clinical and radiological cervical kyphosis is diagnosed frequently (Deltoff 2001). This is also true for adolescents with a history of craniocervical birth trauma, for example kinematic imbalance due to suboccipital strain (KISS) (Fig. 5.3c).

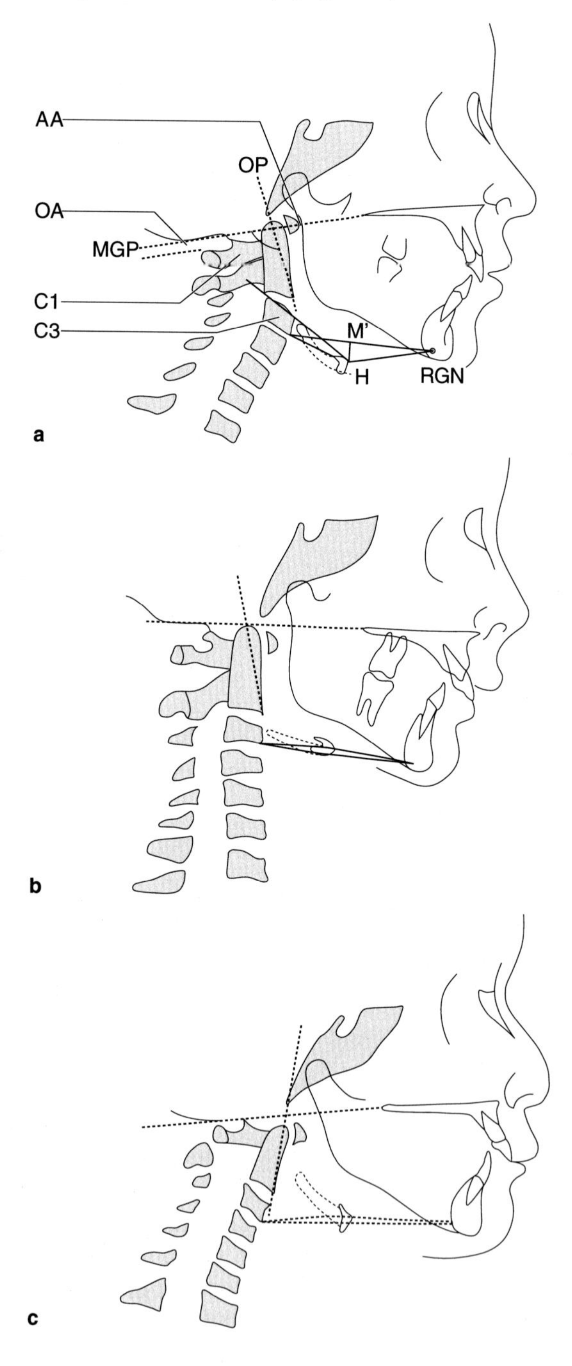

Fig. 5.3

a Cephalometric picture of a healthy volunteer. AA, atlas anterior; H, hyoid; MGP, McGregor's plane (a line that connects the base of the occiput with the side of the nose); RGN, retrognation (the part of the hyoid bone that lies the most superior and anterior).
The MGP–OP angle is 101° on average
The distance between occiput and atlas (OA) is between 4 and 9 mm on average
The hyoid is positioned underneath the C3–RGN line.

b Cephalometric picture of a patient with a craniocervical kyphosis. Note the differences from the healthy volunteer:
MGP–OP angle is greater than 96°
OA distance is greater than 9 mm
Hyoid is above the C3–RGN line and the RGN–H–C3 triangle is smaller.

c Comparison with a person in craniocervical extension. Note that:
MGP–OP angle is less than 96°
OA distance is less than 4 mm
Hyoid is on the RGN–C3 line and RGN–H–C3 triangle is smaller compared to the healthy volunteer. The C3–RGN line becomes longer.

On the basis of these biomechanical effects it is easy to see how the activity of the cervical muscles and of the infra- and suprahyoid muscles influence each other as well as the position of the tongue and the mandible.

The examples described all refer to postural correlations. Winnberg et al (1988) showed how differences in head position may not only influence range and quality of movement regarding hyoid and mandible but also change EMG activity of the masseter and suprahyoid muscles. Clinical observations as well as cephalometric measurements demonstrated that maximum mouth opening moves the hyoid downwards and causes an upper cervical extension of the occiput in relationship to the atlas (Muto & Kanazawa 1994).

If the head is held in permanent extension, the atlas morphology will influence the direction of growth and the size of the mandible. Huggare and Cooke (1994) showed in several studies how the mandible tends to grow anteriorly towards a prognathic position in such cases. This will also have an effect on dental occlusion (McClean et al 1973, Rocabado et al 1983, Chapman et al 1991, Urbanowicz 1991, Kraus 1994, Makofsky & Sexton 1994, Salonen et al 1994). Makofsky found that the initial occlusal pattern (IOCP) was significantly changed in forward head posture (FHP), and that there were individual differences but no age dependency (Makofsky 2000) (Fig. 5.4).

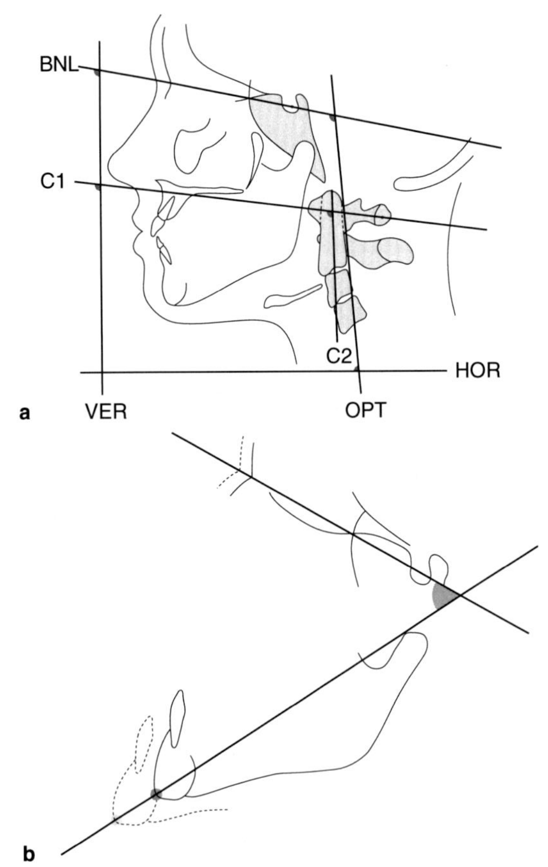

Fig. 5.4 Relation between the range of craniocervical extension and the expected prognathic mandibular growth.
a The craniocervical position and the relevant cephalometric lines and angles according to Huggare and Cooke (1994).
BNL = bridge of the nose line
HOR = horizontal line
OPT = orthodontal process tangential line (line between the dens and the vertebral body of C2)
VER = vertical line.
b The relation between BNL and the line through retrognation (RGN) and the junction of the BNL–OPT lines (see Fig.5.4a).
The smaller the BNL–OPT angle, the more likely is the mandible to develop prognathically.

NEURODYNAMICS

A number of studies emphasize the connection between the craniocervical and the craniomandibular nervous systems. Some examples are mentioned here.

Cervical movement

Cervical movements influence brain structures and cranial nerves because the nervous system is an anatomic continuum (Lang 1995). When the head is moved from flexion into extension, the spinomedullary angle increases, the brainstem gets longer and the load on the inner and outer layers of the dura increases (Breig et al 1966, Doursounian et al 1989). The load on the cranial nerves is particularly high near the critical zones, for example the cerebellopontine angle (CPA), the sinus cavernosus (SC) and the foramina (Profitt 1993, Smirniotopoulos et al 1993, Schick et al 1996). The most important cranial nerve for the craniomandibular region is the trigeminal nerve. It innervates the craniomandibular region, divides into branches there and is (co-)responsible for facial pain (Zakrzewska 1995, Zakrzewska & Hamlyn 1999). The nerve originates from the dorsolateral part of the brainstem and runs within the cerebellopontine angle (CPA; runs through the sinus cavernosus). The maxillary and mandibular branches run through the foramina of the sphenoid bone towards maxilla and mandible. The CPA, SC, foramina and tissues – including muscle, fascia and the mandible – are critical zones (parts of the body that demand the most adaptation to movement) and may restrict neurodynamic function significantly (Butler 2000). In the author's opinion, this knowledge is not applied sufficiently for the recognition of typical patterns that commonly indicate cranioneural dysfunctions. Examples are:

- Antalgic head position, typically upper cervical extension and lateroflexion away from the painful side
- Active and/or passive craniocervical flexion and lateroflexion towards the painful side, frequently leading to brief motor output reactions of the facial, masticatory and swallowing muscles. Sensory reactions such as facial pain are also commonly observed.

For more about other aspects of nervous system testing, see Chapters 16 and 17 (Fig. 5.5).

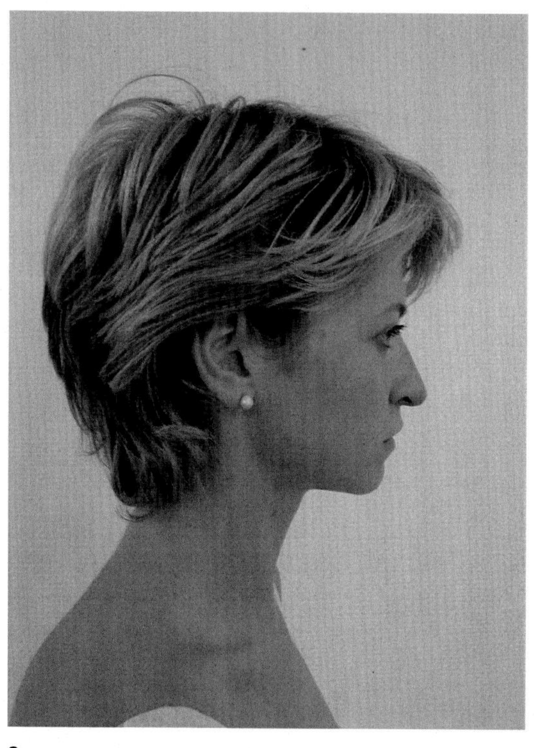

a

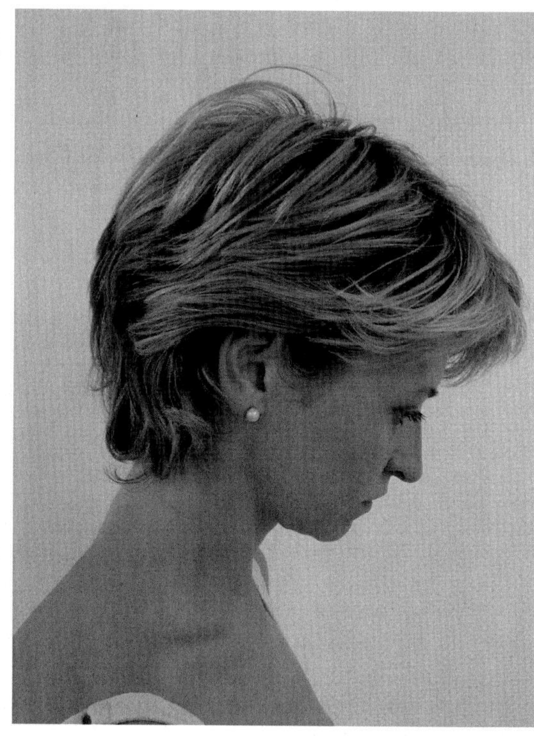

b

Fig. 5.5

a The classic posture of a patient with pathodynamic changes of the craniocervical and facial regions. Note the head forward position, the increased midcervical lordosis and the flat upper thoracic spine.

b Even in flexion the upper cervical extension is maintained and active cervical flexion is restricted. Reactions and restriction of flexion are commonly enhanced by a neurodynamic sensitizing manoeuvre of the legs (e.g. knee extension).

Neurophysiology

It has only recently been recognized that the craniocervical and cranial dura itself has a large number of nociceptors and plays an important role in the pathogenesis of vascular headaches (Moskowitz 1984, Andres et al 1987, Kumar 1995 (in Kumar et al 1996)). Hu et al (1995) found in experimental animal studies that irritation of dural vascular tissue in rats with mustard oil caused an irreversible activation of the masticatory and neck muscles. This may be an explanation for the clinical observation of hypertonic muscles, trigger points, bruxism and teeth clenching in patients with cervical symptoms.

CLINICAL/FUNCTIONAL

Maitland (1991) observed that accessory movements of the atlas and the axis led to reactions in the facial region and to pain or reflex muscle contractions of the masticatory and facial muscles in healthy subjects as well as in neck pain patients. Within the patient group the pain was regularly perceived as more severe and the resistance during accessory movements clearly changed whenever the mandibular position was shifted (Fig. 5.6).

In 1994 both Kraus and Mohl independently observed a change in mandibular movement quality with different neck positions. With

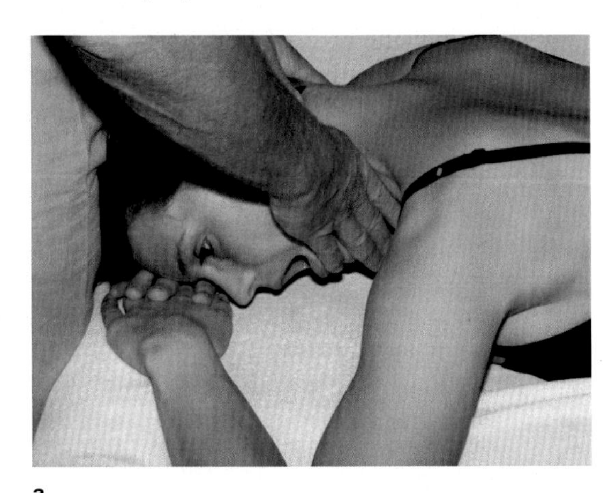

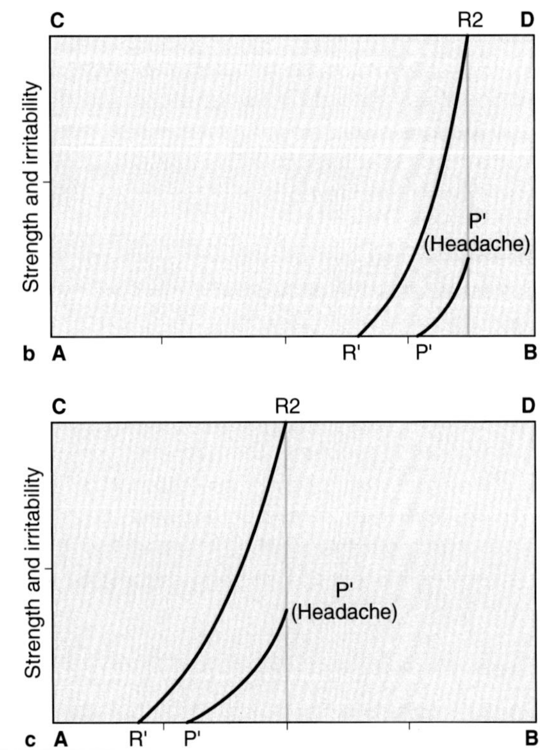

a

Fig. 5.6

a The patient lies prone. Both thumbs are in contact with the right lamina of the axis (C2). Both index and middle fingers hold the mandible to prevent mandibular movement. The position also allows variation of the mouth opening angle during the test procedure.

b Unilateral posterior–anterior movement on the C2 lamina without mouth opening. The movement is slightly restricted with resistance being the limiting factor. The patient perceives a slight dorsal sensitivity to pressure.

c Unilateral posterior–anterior movement on the C2 lamina with mouth opening. Note that the movement is restricted by 50% and limited by resistance (R1–R2) and that the patient's headache symptoms are clearly reproduced (P). In this case the mandibular position changes the quality of movement and the patient's reaction to the posterior-anterior C2 movement.

extension, a significant retrusive movement was noted whereas in upper cervical flexion the tendency was towards a protrusive mandibular shift. The mandibular resting position was changed as well as habitual occlusion patterns (Kraus 1994, Mohl 1994).

In a study on 230 participants, Wright (2000) showed that pressure on cervical trigger points (trapezius, splenus capitis and sternocleidomastoid muscles) led to referred pain into the head and face, more so than trigger points of the masticatory muscles were referred into the neck.

Visscher et al (2000) demonstrated that there is a great variability of posture and curvature among healthy subjects without headaches, facial or neck pain. The same applies for patients with craniocervical and craniofacial symptoms. This observation led to the conclusion that posture is an unlikely cause or risk factor for craniomandibular and cervical dysfunction and pain.

In a study that included 111 cervical patients and 103 craniomandibular patients, de Wijer and Steenks (1995) showed, based upon an anamnestic self-administered questionnaire and active/passive orthopaedic physical tests, that:

- Patients with craniocervical dysfunction do not show a greater prevalence of craniomandibular problems than others.
- The active and passive assessment of the neck and the shoulder showed no significant patterns that differentiated between craniocervical and craniomandibular patients.

De Wijer concluded that signs and symptoms in the craniomandibular region do not necessarily derive from craniocervical structures. He also stated that mouth opening and retrusion of the mandible was significantly restricted in the craniomandibular group compared to the craniocervical group. He recommended the inclusion of the craniomandibular region in assessment of craniocervical patients and vice versa.

An unpublished randomized pilot study investigated 100 participants diagnosed with cervical complaints for a craniomandibular component (von Piekartz 2005). Inclusion criteria were:

- More than 3 months of physiotherapy or manual therapy without any notable result
- No dental treatment or craniomandibular physiotherapy during these 3 months.

The measurement tool was the Conti Anamnestic Questionnaire that is validated in the Dutch language (Box 5.1). Based on the Helkimo Index, this questionnaire showed a reliable detection rate of craniomandibular dysfunction (Conti et al 1996) (Fig. 5.7). The investigation showed that 78% had a moderate to severe

Box 5.1 Conti Anamnestic Questionnaire

- Do you find it difficult to open your mouth?
- Do you find it difficult to move your jaw?
- Are your jaw muscles sensitive?
- Do you have muscular pain when chewing?
- Do you have headaches?
- Do you have neck or shoulder pain?
- Do you have pain in or around the ear?
- Do you notice noises in your temporomandibular joints?
- Do you feel that your bite is normal?
- Do you only use one side of your mouth when chewing?
- Do you have facial pain in the morning?

Reproduced with permission from Conti (1996).

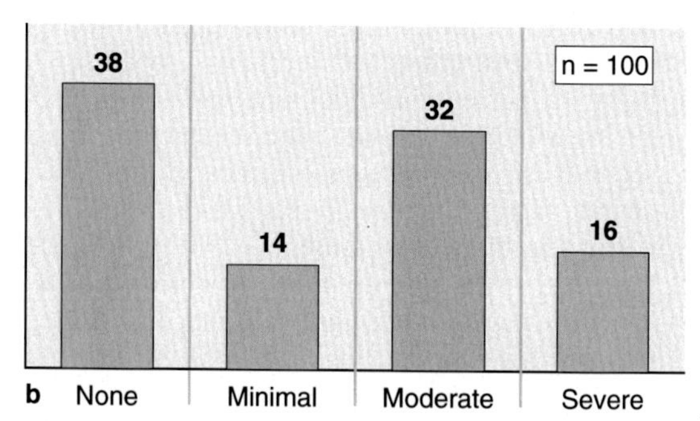

Fig. 5.7 The results of the Conti Anamnestic Questionnaire (AQ) of patients diagnosed as 'cervical syndrome' sufferers who did not or only slightly improved after 3 months of physiotherapy. The score is expressed as a percentage.

craniomandibular component. This is 20% higher than the estimated average prevalence of craniomandibular dysfunction in the Western world (Dao et al 1994). Therefore it seems that the prevalence increases in a patient sample with persistent unspecific craniocervical pain and no firm diagnosis. Obviously no conclusions can be made as to whether the craniomandibular component is responsible for the persistence of the craniocervical complaints. Further studies are needed to show an influence of craniomandibular dysfunction on prolonged cervical symptoms.

As the reader may have realized, the von Piekartz (2005) study does not offer any particular clarity. The therapist should still depend on the clinical presentation of the individual patient. Possibly some interesting aspects are gained by studying cervical trauma such as WAD for influences on the craniomandibular region. Here are some postulates.

WHIPLASH-ASSOCIATED DISORDERS AND THEIR INFLUENCE ON THE CRANIOMANDIBULAR REGION

In daily practice with patients who suffer from whiplash injuries and associated disorders, it is frequently observed that facial and neck pain may be provoked by manual craniomandibular tests. When treating craniomandibular dysfunction in subacute or chronic WAD patients, the reactions to conservative approaches such as physiotherapy or manual therapy are often unpredictable. Sometimes improvements may be impressive; at other times nothing is gained. The question is whether results may simply be due to chance or whether there is a clear connection. The literature does not provide any answers. Within the different disciplines there are some contradictory models and theories about the connection between cervical whiplash injuries and craniomandibular disorders. Some arguments that support or contradict the hypotheses are discussed below. They are categorized as:

- Neurophysiological/histological
- Anatomical/biomechanical
- Articular dysfunction
- Muscular dysfunction
- Mental distress and culture
- Clinical.

Neurophysiological/histological

Studies have showed significant neurophysiological changes after neck injury, for example:

- The *inhibitory reflex* of the temporal muscles was affected without any neurological or arthrogenic injuries of the cervical spine (Keidel et al 1994). This may influence the muscle tone regulation of the masticatory system (Dao et al 1994).
- *Nociceptive neurogenic convergence* occurs after whiplash injury; 50% of all nociceptive facial afferent neurones of the cervical spine converge and may cause pain to project into the deeper layers of the craniofacial tissues (Radanov et al 1993).
- *Dysfunction of the trigeminovascular system,* the site of the cranial autonomic nervous system. The result is a dysfunction of cerebral vascularization and an increase of the intercranial cerebrospinal fluid pressure (Lindvall et al 1978, Mathew et al 1996). This imbalance of output mechanisms in the sympathetic and the neuroendocrine systems may increase symptoms in the head, face or neck (Pillemer et al 1997).
- After whiplash injuries with indirect vascular trauma to the brainstem and the trigeminal nerve, fewer neurotransmitter substances such as 5-HT (serotonin) are produced. The immediate result may be emotional imbalance and impaired pain reduction (in the craniomandibular region among others) (Westerhuis 2001, Kasch et al 2002).

Anatomical/biomechanical

Anatomical and biomechanical explanations arise from the acceleration–deceleration model for the mandible and the cervical structures (Fig. 5.8a). The temporomandibular joint is a synovial joint, therefore symptoms in the craniomandibular region may occur due to overstretching of the ligaments, capsule, muscles, nervous tissue and other soft tissues (Bogduk 1986b). Some hypotheses about

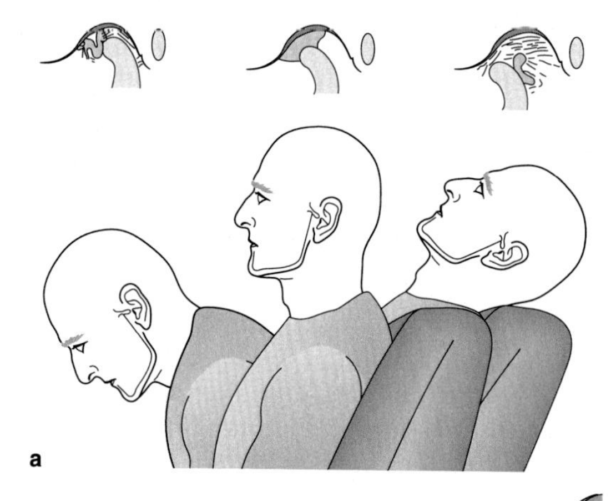

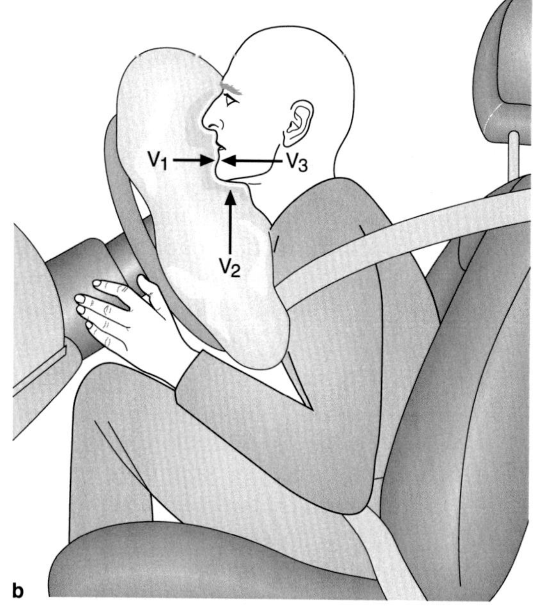

Fig. 5.8
a The mandible-whiplash model. (Is the anatomical–biomechanical model a realistic expression of what really happens? Opinions regarding anatomical, clinical and epidemiological results vary widely.)
b Diagram of influencing forces of an airbag deployment. The velocity forces of the head (V1) are enhanced by the velocity of the airbag and the compression (V2, V3) (reproduced with permission from Levy et al 1998).

which structures are injured during which phase of the impact were also investigated (Mannheimer et al 1989, O'Shaughnessy 1994).

In a literature review about the anatomy and pathophysiology of whiplash injuries, Bogduk (1986b) emphasizes that radiological and surgical findings frequently confirm destruction of the temporomandibular joint and the disc capsule with retrodiscal tears. Moreover, various structures of the cervical spine may be pathological (discs, zygapophyseal joints, muscles), so that it is suggested that multiple structures may be responsible for the patient's symptoms in the craniomandibular region and elsewhere (Frankel 1972).

Several case studies warn of the effect of airbags on the craniomandibular region. Garcia and Arrington (1996) reported a 20-year-old motorist who suffered from muscle spasm and restricted mouth opening after airbag deployment. MRI of his temporomandibular joints showed bilateral inflammation and disc displacement with reduction. Craniomandibular trauma seems more complex after airbag deployment than after blunt mandibular injury (Levy et al 1998). According to Levy, three forces interact resulting in a very large force on the TMJ:

- Vector 1: anterior movement of the mandible during the impact
- Vector 2: the cranial force that is loading the airbag
- Vector 3: the posterior movement of the airbag during the impact (Fig. 5.8b).

Knowing that airbags can cause bone fractures in the cervical and thoracic spine, as well as cardiac trauma (Lancaster et al 1993), helps us to understand the enormous force that loads the mandible during such accidents. On the other hand, some authors state that craniomandibular dysfunction after whiplash injuries is overdiagnosed. Clark et al (1993) stated that only 3–5% of the population with signs and symptoms really require treatment and that includes the whiplash patients. Ferrari and Leonard (1998) and Ferrari et al (1999) take the hypothesis one step further and say that anatomical changes of the temporomandibular joints are not significant compared to a control group and that the complaints are due to psychological profiles and cultural influences.

Various publications show that after whiplash injuries there are indeed neurological dysfunctions that include injuries of the brainstem and the cranial nerves (Hohl 1974, Balla 1980, Deans et al 1987, Maimaris et al 1988, Barry 1992). Sturzenegger et al (1994) showed in a cohort study on 137 whiplash patients that 33% (45 patients) showed symptoms due to pathology of the brainstem and the cranial nerves. The incidence of cervical nerve root and cervical spinal cord injury was significantly lower at 10% (14 patients) and 4% (5 patients), respectively.

Articular dysfunction

Various MRI studies confirmed the frequent occurrence of articular dysfunction such as disc displacement, joint inflammation and oedema in the retrodiscal space. The incidence of articular disc-related problems is around 80–97% (Kirkos et al 1987, Shellock et al 1990, Pressmann et al 1992, Garcia & Arrington 1996). The most common dysfunction is disc displacement with reduction. Garcia states that the prevalence is about 72% (Garcia & Arrington 1996). These authors are convinced that whiplash-related disorders such as headaches, facial pain, neck pain, earache, tinnitus and swallowing problems may be maintained by mandibular dysfunction.

Bergman et al (1998) conclude from a prospective MRI study that there is no increase of disc dysfunction, joint effusion or other craniomandibular trauma after cervical whiplash injury. They criticize previous investigations and claim that subjects were selected from those who already suffered from craniomandibular dysfunction.

It is clear that the authors are attempting to establish whether articular dysfunction shows an unambiguous positive correlation with the patients' signs and symptoms.

It should be added that it still remains uncertain whether MRI is the gold standard for the assessment of articular dysfunction (Chen et al 2002) and not every craniomandibular articular dysfunction causes symptoms.

Muscular dysfunction

A number of studies confirmed the increase of masticatory muscle tone and a lowered pain threshold after cervical whiplash injury (Deans 1980 (in Deans et al 1987), Kasch et al 2002). Various authors do not accept the theory that the increased muscle tone after whiplash injury is due to an acceleration–deceleration injury to the mandible (Mohl 1974, Kraus 1994). This may be because there is sufficient clinical evidence that muscle-related craniomandibular complaints such as bruxism, teeth clenching and muscle ache can be reduced by neuromuscular braces that 'deprogramme' muscle activity arising from occlusal irregularities (Nielsen et al 1990, Naeije & Hansson 1991, Wilkinson et al 1992, Losert-Bruggner 1998). These authors are convinced that muscular pain after whiplash injury is a reaction to the cervical pain. It was also shown that the jaw opening reflex in whiplash patients is significantly reduced similar to the clinical presentation of migraine or tension headache patients. This phenomenon might be explained by a dysfunction in the reflex chain at the brainstem level that regulates the opening reflex (Keidel et al 1994, Christensen & McKay 1997). The loss of this reflex may increase the activity of the mandibular elevator muscles followed by local trophic changes within the muscles and pain (Boismare et al 1985, Bottin et al 1989). In a similar study by Christensen and McKay (1997), no significant change of jaw opening reflex could be shown in whiplash patients, and the diagnosis of mandibular acceleration–deceleration trauma was dismissed.

It is common for cervical trauma patients to show a change in neck muscle EMG activity followed by a change of head position (Lader 1983, Sterling et al 2001). Therefore the neck muscles need to adapt to a new situation. This may influence occlusion, the position of the temporomandibular joint and the hyoid (Boyd et al 1987). A useful working model based upon the current literature was suggested by Rocabado (1981) (Fig. 5.9).

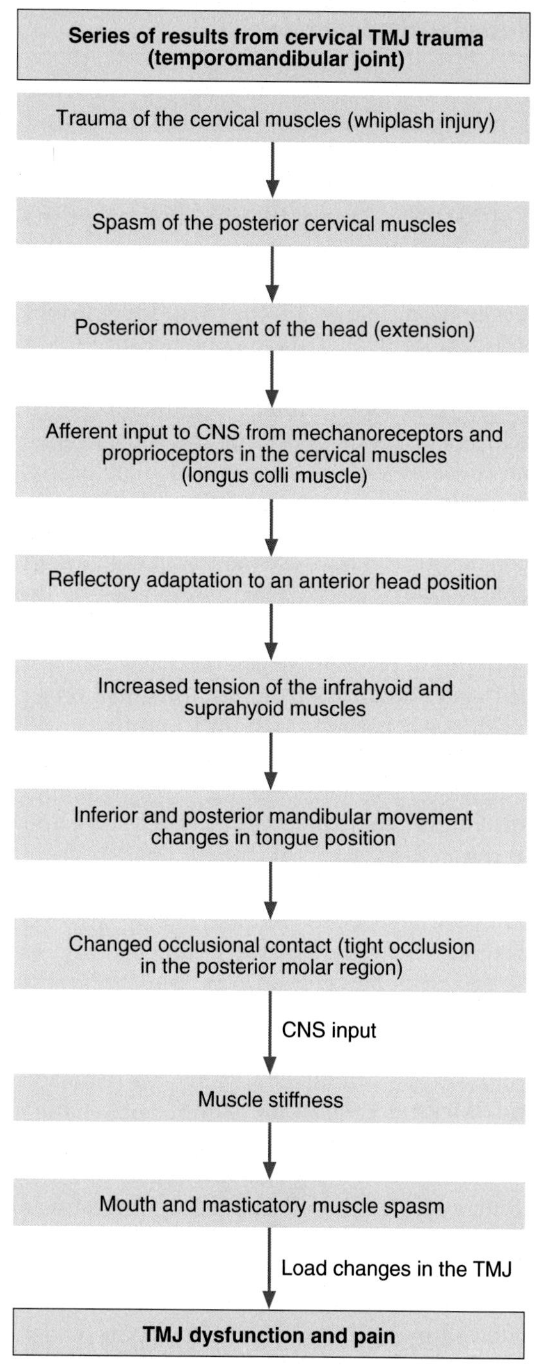

Fig. 5.9 Predominantly muscular dysfunction model of the craniomandibular region due to craniocervical trauma (modified from Rocabado 1981).

Mental distress and culture

Neuropsychological studies show that whiplash-related craniomandibular disorder patients show a significantly greater incidence of obsessions, somatization, depression and rage (Goldberg et al 1996). There is also a greater chance for symptoms to spread to the head, neck and shoulders within the group of whiplash patients (Burgess 1991, Braun et al 1992, Krogstad et al 1998). In a comparison of treatment efficacy for whiplash patients and patients with idiopathic temporomandibular dysfunction, Krogstad et al (1998) showed that the whiplash injury patients obtained only a minimal decrease in the proportion of tender muscles on standard palpation following treatment. The incidence and the visual analogue scale (VAS) values for intensity of headache remained unchanged, unlike in the idiopathic group. It has been known for some time that cervical whiplash injury may influence emotional and cognitive functions and lead to personality changes, depression and non-specific physical symptoms (Sternbach et al 1980, Balla 1982, Drottning et al 1995). Patients who suffer from prolonged whiplash symptoms (symptoms for more than 6 months post-injury) apparently show secondary hyperalgesia in the head and face regions. The therapist will therefore frequently have to consider false-positive results when assessing the craniomandibular region and should be aware of cognitive and behavioural aspects.

Ferrari and Leonard caused great turmoil in the late 1990s when they stated that there was no convincing proof for mandibular acceleration–deceleration trauma. Their epidemiological observations and meta-analyses concluded that craniomandibular symptoms in late whiplash injury patients were not caused by the injury itself but by psychological distress (Ferrari & Leonard 1998). They added that the quality and duration of the symptoms were strongly influenced by the cultural background of the individual patient. They investigated the symptoms of 165 Lithuanian whiplash patients in a controlled cohort study 14–27 months post-injury for craniomandibular dysfunction.

The signs and symptoms included were clicking noises on jaw movements, pain in and around the ear, mouth opening deficits, craniofacial pain and tinnitus. The results showed that only 2.4% of patients (4 out of 165) had such symptoms for a day or more. A healthy Lithuanian control group showed an incidence of 3.3% (6 out of 180). The result was that these numbers do not bear any resemblance to the prevalence in the rest of the Western world. This varies between 34 and 82%, depending on the study (Ferrari et al 1999).

Clinical

The site of the symptoms, the quality of the symptoms and the clinical tests regarding quality and range of movement as well as palpation of the masticatory muscles may indicate, retrospectively, whether the craniomandibular region was affected by a whiplash injury. To gain some insight, the following is a summary of the literature:

- Braun et al (1992) showed that whiplash patients referred for physiotherapy had a higher incidence of craniomandibular dysfunction and pain (between 2 days and 10 weeks). Compared with a group of volunteers, pain was rated higher, mouth opening was restricted and intracapsular craniomandibular dysfunctions were detected. These authors postulated that assessment and, if required, treatment of the craniomandibular region should be mandatory for effective management of post-traumatic cervical patients.
- Kronn (1993) compared a group of whiplash patients (n = 40) with a control group of idiopathic craniomandibular dysfunction patients (n = 40). He investigated mouth opening, shift, palpation of the masticatory muscles and clicking on jaw movements. The two groups were found to differ only with respect to mouth opening and sensitivity of the masticatory muscles. Kronn concluded that the combination of relatively authoritative clinical tests such as the ones mentioned above cannot provide sufficient information about the involvement of the craniomandibular region in the patient's symptoms. Routine investigation and treatment of the craniomandibular region of whiplash patients was strongly recommended.
- Intensity of craniofacial pain determined by algometry and sensomotor function in terms of mouth opening after whiplash injury does not significantly differ from the state after an ankle injury. This was the result of a prospective study by Kasch et al (2002). They did not find any significant changes 4 weeks and 6 months post-injury in 19 whiplash patients compared with 19 ankle trauma patients, and concluded that cervical trauma is not a clear risk factor for the development of craniomandibular symptoms.

Conclusions and state of the art clinical reasoning strategies in WAD patients and craniomandibular dysfunctions

Scientific and clinical opinions on the development and occurrence of craniomandibular dysfunction and pain due to whiplash associated disorders vary between disciplines. This implies that the therapist needs to carefully consider craniomandibular symptoms in WAD patients. The therapist should always investigate the quality of the symptoms and include special tests such as muscle palpation, the mouth opening test and passive assessment of the craniomandibular region. A detected dysfunction should be treated initially on a trial basis; subjective symptoms and physical signs from the craniocervical and craniomandibular regions should be continuously evaluated during treatment sessions. Whether a craniomandibular dysfunction is relevant for the individual complaints can only be shown retrospectively when signs and symptoms change after an appropriate technique.

INFLUENCE OF THE CRANIOMANDIBULAR REGION ON THE CERVICAL SPINE

For unknown reasons, the influence of the craniomandibular region on the cervical spine has not been investigated as thoroughly as the opposite influence described in the section above. Nevertheless, some important studies and ideas relating to this complex but interesting field can be cited.

Neurophysiology

PAIN PROJECTION

The somatosensory projections of craniomandibular structures project mainly on secondary trigeminal neurones in the trigeminal nucleus of the brainstem. Here, synaptic connections with neurones of other cranial nerves and the cervical spine may occur (Hu et al 1992, Yu et al 1995, Hu 1999). Hence, pain projection from the craniofacial on the craniocervical region is theoretically possible (Hu 2001).

Clinical studies showed that the pain projection from the craniomandibular region to the neck is more diffuse and less severe than the pain projection from the cervical spine to the face.

POSTURE

The muscle tone of the craniocervical region may change in reaction to nociceptive input from the craniomandibular region. This may also influence the positioning of the head. Noxious craniofacial stimulation of the deeper tissues (e.g. bone, capsule, ligaments and disc) triggers the output system. Autonomic reactions such as changes in blood pressure and breathing and also an increase in muscle activity within the craniomandibular region and the neck may be the result (Cairns et al 1998).

Biomechanics

Chinapi and Getzoff (1994) postulated that the reduction of radiographically measured cervical lordosis may be the result of a unilateral craniomandibular dysfunction. Cranialization of the hyoid may be another indicator and possibly correlates directly with the compensatory changes in cervical lordosis. Moreover, EMG measurements of the supra- and infrahyoid muscles showed an increase in activity.

Knutson and Jacob (1999) showed in two case studies that the craniomandibular region can have a strong influence on the biomechanical function of the upper cervical spine in patients with multiple craniocervical dysfunctions such as dizziness, migraine, acute locked neck and pain. The craniomandibular region was treated with muscle and joint techniques. After the intervention the symptoms were reduced significantly. After 30 days both patients' radiological investigation showed a normal cervical lordosis.

In a similar study on 16 young volunteers with craniomandibular dysfunction, Huggare and Raustia (1992) found similar effects. They assessed the craniocervical region radiologically and observed significantly increased cervical extension compared with an age-matched control group. They also found that the patient group showed a narrower atlas, the base of the cranium was flatter and the posterior–anterior relationship of the facial height was reduced. Treatment consisted of braces as well as active and passive muscle exercises. The post-treatment x-rays showed that 13 out of the 16 patients now had a normal cervical lordosis. Huggare concluded that the masticatory muscles directly influence the stabilizing cervical muscles. He further hypothesized that dysfunctions of both regions may change craniofacial morphology (Huggare 1991, Huggare & Raustia 1992).

Neurodynamics

Little is known about the influence of neurodynamic changes in the cranial nervous system on the craniofacial region. Responsible for the innervation of the region are the trigeminal and the facial nerves which are embedded in the craniofacial tissues. Like most of the cranial nerves they are connected to the brainstem which in turn has a close connection to the craniocervical region (von Piekartz et al 2001).

It is known that the mandibular nerve is 8 mm longer on mouth opening than in the resting position (Segter et al 1993). Hypothetically, due to the continuity of the nervous system, this may influence (dural) nervous structures such as the brainstem, CPA and dura mater. This again may change the arthrokinematics of the craniocervical junction that is closely connected to dural tissue (Breig et al 1966, Lang 1995). Clinically this is observed frequently as shown in the two examples that follow.

- A patient experiences peripheral neurogenic pain whenever she bends her neck with maximum mouth opening. Commonly upper cervical flexion is impossible but flexion occurs in the mid- and lower cervical spine (Fig. 5.10).
- When stimulating activity of the mimic muscles in patients with facial paresis one may observe compensatory upper cervical extension and ipsilateral lateroflexion. On correction of the head position the patient complains of a 'pulling' or 'tearing' sensation and the contraction of the mimic muscles becomes more difficult to perform (Fig. 5.11). For further information, see Chapters 17 and 18.

Clinical/functional

In a descriptive study on 13 healthy volunteers, Daly et al (1982) observed that an experimental brace (8 mm) increased neck extension by 2.9°. An hour after removal of the brace, head extension was back to normal. The same observation was made by Vig et al (1980). A potential explanation is that, since the eyes are moved into the horizontal plane by the oculomotor reflex for balance reasons, the head adapts to the position of the eyes (Kraus 1994) (Fig. 5.12).

According to Kraus, two types of adaptation may occur: an axial head–neck position with the head being moved into extension, or an anteriorly directed caudal adaptation that

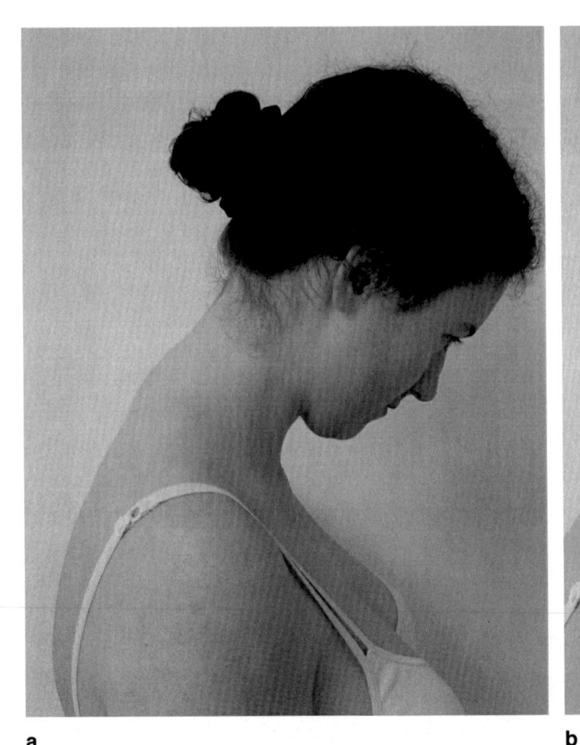

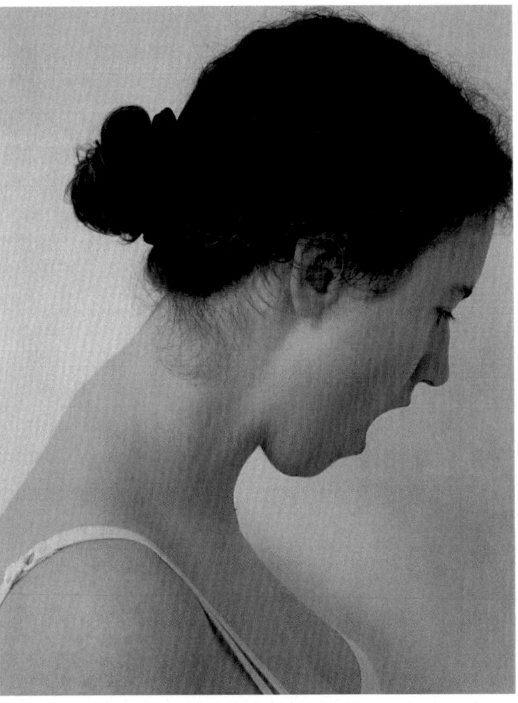

a b

Fig. 5.10
a Patient suffering from a minimal neurodynamic dysfunction of the right mandibular nerve. Flexion without mouth opening.
b Flexion with mouth opening of 40 mm and slight laterotrusion to the left. The patient perceives a severe pulling sensation in the left mandibular region. Note the quality of movement in the craniocervical region.

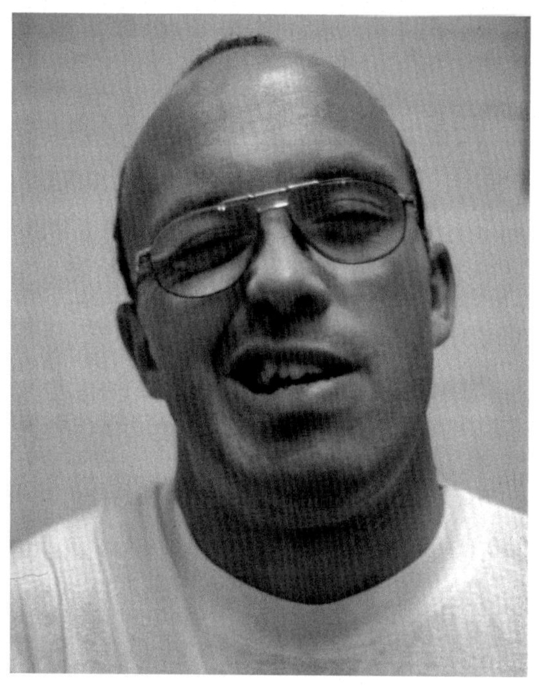

Fig. 5.11 A patient with peripheral facial nerve paresis on the right. The mimic muscles on the affected side are stimulated to contract. Note the compensatory craniocervical extension and ipsilateral lateroflexion that the patient performs to achieve a better muscle contraction.

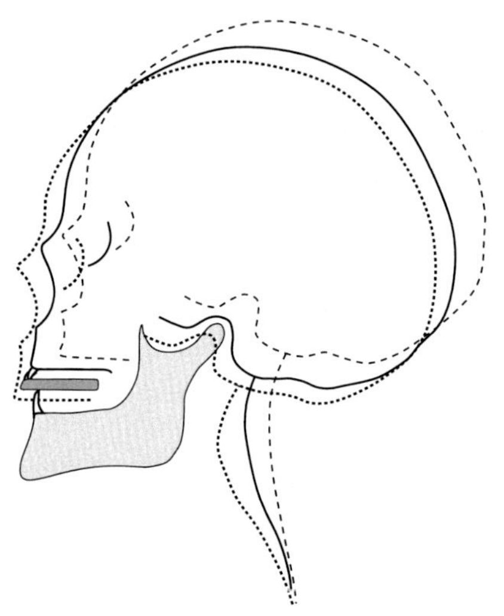

Fig. 5.12 Adaptation of the craniocervical region due to changes in the vertical dimension, e.g. after intraoral orthodontic intervention.
Dotted line: Axial adaptation of the head–neck position. The cranium tilts posterior on the atlas to keep the eyes horizontal.
Line: Adaptation of the cranium towards anterior and flexion to maintain the eye position on a horizontal line (modified from Kraus 1994).

changes muscle activity and arthrokinematics of the upper cervical spine (Kraus 1994).

To what extent craniocervical adaptive posture changes morphology in adolescents, while the viscerocranium is not fully developed, remains unknown. Some high-quality studies have been published in the past about neck extension as a compensation for nasal obstruction and mouth breathing and about the developmental capacities of the facial bones (Rickets 1968, Solow & Tallgren 1976, 1977).

Hülse et al (2001) described in various case studies that post-cervical trauma patients with diffuse and diagnostically challenging symptoms such as vertigo, tinnitus and swallowing difficulties improved significantly when supplied with neuromuscular braces. Retrospectively, the authors believe that upper cervical dysfunction may cause craniofacial symptoms and vice versa. They explain that the connection between the neck, masticatory and hyoid muscles is normalized by the brace.

As mentioned by Hülse et al (2001) the symptoms commonly occur as diffuse sensations that are difficult to diagnose and whose sources are hard to detect. Sometimes it is not clear whether they derive from the craniocervical or the craniomandibular region. Descriptive clinical studies show that:

- These diffuse symptoms as well as shoulder–arm pain may be caused by both regions and may overlap considerably (de Wijer 1995).
- Muscular craniomandibular dysfunctions are known to cause pain in the neck (Lobbezoo-Scholte 1993, de Wijer et al 1996).
- Craniocervical dysfunctions do not project as strongly to the craniomandibular region as the other way round (de Wijer 1995).

These findings frequently lead therapists to believe that the neck can be excluded if the diagnosis is a craniomandibular dysfunction. However, in the author's experience, the craniomandibular region is too often neglected in patients with longstanding neck pain. Possibly therapists are misguided by the location of the pain, especially if the symptoms are localized dominantly in the neck and not in the face. For further information, read Chapter 3.

De Wijer et al (1996) therefore recommend:

- Assessing the craniomandibular region in patients with longstanding neck pain and treating potential dysfunctions.
- Assessing the neck region orthopaedically if, during a course of craniomandibular treatment, improvement of dysfunction and symptoms is not satisfactory. If craniocervical dysfunction is found, the dentist should be informed and cervical dysfunction should be treated.
- Using a standardized anamnestic screening list to evaluate the dominant region. This is an important clinical instrument and may assist the therapist in the clinical decision-making process.

A QUESTION OF COMPLETENESS

This text does not claim to be exhaustive. For example, the influence of peripheral control mechanisms such as the vestibular and oculomotor systems on head and mandibular position has not been discussed (Ganong 1978, Kraus 1988). In addition, the influence of craniofacial growth during posture changes of the mandible and the craniocervical region deserves more attention (Oudhof 2000). Unfortunately more in-depth literature does not exist at present.

SUMMARY

- The craniocervical and the craniomandibular regions and their reciprocal influence have been discussed in their various aspects.
- The result is that there is no definite conclusion although a number of authors are convinced of a direct connection.
- Therapists should remember to examine the craniomandibular region whenever they are confronted with longstanding craniocervical symptoms; potential dysfunctions need to be evaluated for their relevance to the problem.
- Probationary treatment of craniomandibular structures followed by a reassessment of the craniocervical and craniomandibular regions constitutes clinical proof of the relevance of craniomandibular dysfunction. This implies that the problem is of a dominantly nociceptive nature.

References

Andres K H, Düring von M, Muszynski K, Schmidt R F 1987 Nerve fibres and their terminals of the dura mater encephali of the rat. Anatomy and Embryology 175:289–301

Balla J I 1980 The late whiplash syndrome. Australian and New Zealand Journal of Surgery 50:610–614

Balla J I 1982 The late whiplash syndrome: a study of an illness in Australia and Singapore. Culture, Medicine and Psychiatry 6:191–210

Barry M 1992 Whiplash injuries. British Journal of Rheumatology 31:579–581

Bergman H, Andersson F, Isberg A 1998 Incidence of temporomandibular joint changes after whiplash trauma: a prospective study using MR imaging. American Journal of Roentgenology 171:1237–1243

Bogduk N 1986a Cervical causes of headache and dizziness. In: Grieve G (ed.) Modern manual therapy. Churchill Livingstone, Edinburgh, p 289

Bogduk N 1986b The anatomy and pathophysiology of whiplash. Clinical Biomechanics 1:92–101

Boismare F, Boquet J, Moore N, Chretien P, Saligaut C, Daoust M 1985 Hemodynamic behavioural and biochemical disturbances induced by experimental craniocervical injury (whiplash) in rats. Journal of the Autonomic Nervous System 13:137–147

Bottin D, Sulon J, Schoenen J 1989 The second silent period of temporalis muscles is reduced during menstruation, but not at mid-cycle, in women reporting menstrual headaches. Cephalalgia 9:115–116

Boyd C H, Slagle W F, Boyd C M, Bryant R W, Wiygul J P 1987 The effect of head position on electromyographic evaluations of representative mandibular positioning muscle groups. Cranio 5:50–54

Bratzlavsky M, van der Eecken H 1977 Postural reflexes in cranial muscles in man. Acta Neurologica Belgica 77:5

Braun B L, DiGiovanna A, Schiffman E, Bonnema J, Fricton J 1992 A cross-sectional study of temporomandibular joint dysfunction in post-cervical trauma patients. Journal of Craniomandibular Disorders: Facial Oral Pain 6:24–31

Breig A, Turnbull I, Hassler O 1966 Effects of mechanical stresses on the spinal cord in cervical spondylosis: a study on fresh cadaver material. Journal of Neurosurgery 25:45–56

Burgess J 1991 Symptom characteristics in TMD patients reporting blunt trauma and/or whiplash injury. Journal of Craniomandibular Disorders: Facial and Oral Pain 5:251–257

Butler D 2000 The sensitive nervous system. NOI Press, Adelaide

Cairns B E, Sessle B J, Hu J W 1998 Evidence that excitatory amino acid receptors within the temporomandibular joint region are involved in the reflex activation of the jaw muscles. Journal of Neuroscience 16:8052–8060

Chapman R J, Maness W L, Osorio J 1991 Occlusal contact variation with changes in head position. International Journal of Prosthodontics 4:377–381

Chen Y, Gallo L, Palla S 2002 The mediolateral temporomandibular joint disc position: an in vivo quantitative study. Journal of Orofacial Pain 16:29

Chinappi A S, Gertzoff H 1994 A new management model for treating structural based disorders: dental, orthopedic and chiropractic co-treatment. Journal of Manipulative and Physiological Therapeutics 17:614–619

Christensen L V, McKay D C 1997 Reflex jaw motions and jaw stiffness pertaining to whiplash injury of the neck. Journal of Craniomandibular Practice 15(3):247–264

Clark G T, Delcanho R E, Goulet J P 1993 The utility and validity of current diagnostic procedures for defining temporomandibular disorder patients. Advances in Dental Research 7:97–112

Conti P C, Ferreira P M, Pegoraro L F, Conti J V, Salvador M C 1996 A cross-sectional study of prevalence and etiology of signs and symptoms of temporomandibular disorders in high school and university students. Journal of Orofacial Pain 10:254–262

Daly P, Preston C B, Evans W G 1982 Postural response of the head to bite opening in adult males. Department of Orthodontics, School of Dentistry, University of Witwatersrand, p 157–160

Dao T T, Lavigne G J, Charbonneau A, Feine J S, Lund J P 1994 The efficacy of oral splints in the treatment of myofascial pain of the jaw muscles: a controlled clinical trial. Pain 56:85–94

Deans G T, Magalliard J N, Kerr M, Rutherford W H 1987 Neck sprain – a major cause of disability following car accidents. Injury 18:10–12

Deltoff M N 2001 Diagnostic imaging of the cranio-cervical region. In: Vernon H (ed.) The cranio-cervical syndrome, mechanisms, assessment and treatment. Butterworth-Heinemann, Oxford, p 49–88

de Wijer A 1995 Temporomandibular and cervical spine disorders. PhD dissertation, Utrecht University, The Netherlands

de Wijer A, Steenks M H 1995 Cervical spine evaluation for the TMD patient. In: Fricton J, Dubner R (eds) Advances in orofacial pain and temporomandibular disorders. Raven Press, New York, p 351–361

de Wijer A, Rob J, Leeuw de J, Steenks M H, Bosmans F 1996 Temporomandibular and cervical spine disorders. Self-reported signs and symptoms. Spine 21:1638–1646

Doursounian L, Alfonso J M, Iba-Zizen M T et al 1989 Dynamics of the junction between the medulla and the cervical spinal cord: an in vivo study in the sagittal plane by magnetic resonance imaging. Surgical and Radiologic Anatomy 11:313–322

Drottning M, Staff P H, Levin L, Malt U F R 1995 Acute emotional response to common whiplash predicts subsequent pain complaints. Nordic Journal of Psychiatry 49:293–299

Ferrari R, Leonard M S 1998 Whiplash and temporomandibular disorders: a critical review. Journal of the American Dental Association 129:1739–1745

Ferrari R, Schrader H, Obelieniene D 1999 Prevalence of temporomandibular disorders associated with whiplash injury in Lithuania. Oral Surgery, Oral Medicine, Oral Pathology, Oral Radiology and Endodontics 87:653–657

Forsberg C, Hellsing E, Linder-Aronson S, Sheikholeslam A 1985 EMG activity in neck and masticatory muscles in relation to extension and flexion of the head. European Journal of Orthodontics 7:177–184

Frankel V H 1972 Whiplash injuries to the neck. In: Hirsch C, Zotterman Y (eds) Cervical pain. Pergammon, Oxford, p 97–112

Funakoshi M, Amano N 1973 Effects of the tonic neck reflex on the jaw muscles of the rat. Journal of Dental Research 52:668

Funakoshi M, Fujita N, Takehana S 1976 Relation between occlusal interference and jaw muscle activities in response to changes in head position. Journal of Dental Research 55:684
Ganong W F 1978 Manual de Fisiologia Medica. El Manual Moderno SA, Mexico
Garcia R, Arrington J A 1996 The relationship between cervical whiplash and temporomandibular joint injuries: an MRI study. Journal of Craniomandibular Practice 14(3):233–239
Goldberg M B, Mock D, Ichise M et al 1996 Neuropsychologic deficits and clinical features of posttraumatic temporomandibular disorders. Journal of Orofacial Pain 10:126–139
Goldstein D F, Kraus S L, Williams W B, Glasheen-Wray M G 1984 Influence of cervical posture on mandibular movement. Journal of Prosthetic Dentistry 52:421–426
Gonzalez H E, Manns A 1996 Forward head posture: its structural and functional influence on the stomatognathic system: a conceptual study. Journal of Craniomandibular Practice 14(1):71–80
Hohl M 1974 Soft tissue injuries of the neck in automobile accidents. Journal of Bone and Joint Surgery 56A:1675–1682
Hu J W 1999 Neurophysiological mechanisms of head, face and neck pain. In: Vernon H (ed) The cranio-cervical syndrome, mechanisms, assessment and treatment. Butterworth-Heinemann, Oxford, p 31–48
Hu J 2001 Neurophysiological mechanisms of head, face and neck pain. In: Vernon H (ed.) The craniocervical syndrome. Butterworth-Heinemann, Oxford, p 31
Hu J W, Sessle B J, Raboisson P et al 1992 Stimulation of craniofacial muscle afferents induces prolonged facilitatory effects in trigeminal nociceptive brainstem neurones. Pain 48:53–60
Hu J W, Yu X-M, Vernon H, Sessle B J 1993 Excitatory effects on neck and jaw muscle activity of inflammatory irritant injections into cervical paraspinal tissues. Pain 55:243–350
Hu J W, Vernon H, Tatourian I 1995 Changes in neck electromyography associated with meningeal noxious stimulation. Journal of Manipulative and Physiological Therapeutics 18:577–587
Huggare J A 1991 Association between morphology of the first cervical vertebra, head posture and craniofacial structures. European Journal of Orthodontics 13:435–440
Huggare J A, Cooke M S 1994 Head posture and cervicovertebral anatomy as mandibular growth predictors. European Journal of Orthodontics 16:175–180
Huggare J A, Raustia A M 1992 Head posture and cervicovertebral and craniofacial morphology in patients with craniomandibular dysfunction. Journal of Craniomandibular Practice 10(3):173–177
Hülse M, Losert-Bruggner B, Kuksen J 2001 Schwindel und Kiefergelenkprobleme nach HWS – Trauama. Manual Medizin und Osteopathic Medizin 39:20–24
Kasch H, Hjorth T, Svensson P, Nyhuus L, Jensen T S 2002 Temporomandibular disorders after whiplash injury: a controlled, prospective study. Journal of Orofacial Pain 16:118–128
Kawamura Y, Fujimoto J 1957 Some physiologic considerations on measuring rest position of the mandible. Medical Journal of Osaka University 8:247
Kazis H, Kazis A J 1956 Complete mouth rehabilitation. Kimpton, London
Keidel M, Rieschke P, Juptner M, Diener H C 1994 Pathological jaw opening reflex after whiplash injury. Nervenarzt 65:241–249
Kerr F 1961a A mechanism to account for frontal headache in cases of posterior fossa tumors. Journal of Neurosurgery 18:605
Kerr F 1961b Structural relation of the trigeminal spinal tract to upper cervical roots and the solitary nucleus in the cat. Experimental Neurology 4:134
Kerr F 1963 Mechanism, diagnosis and management of some cranial and facial pain syndromes. Surgical Clinics of North America 43:951
Kirkos L T, Ortendahl D A, Mark A S, Arakawa M 1987 Magnetic resonance imaging of the TMJ in asymptomatic volunteers. Journal of Oral and Maxillofacial Surgery 45:852–854
Knutson G A, Jacob M 1999 Possible manifestation of temporomandibular joint dysfunction on chiropractic cervical X-ray studies. Journal of Manipulative and Physiological Therapeutics 22:32–37
Kraus S L (ed.) 1988 Cervical spine influence on the craniomandibular region. In: Temporomandibular disorders: management of the craniomandibular complex. Churchill Livingstone, New York
Kraus S L (ed.) 1994 Cervical spine influences on the management of TMD. In: Temporomandibular disorders, 2nd edn. Churchill Livingstone, New York, p 348–353
Krogstad B S, Jokstad A, Dahl B L, Soboleva U 1998 Somatic complaints, psychologic distress, and treatment outcome in two groups of TMD patients, one previously subjected to whiplash injury. Journal of Orofacial Pain 12:136–144
Kronn E 1993 The incidence of TMJ dysfunction on patients who have suffered a cervical whiplash injury following a traffic accident. Journal of Orofacial Pain 7:209–213
Kumar R, Berger R J, Dunsker S B, Keller J T 1996 Innervation of the spinal dura: myth or reality? Spine 21:18–26

Lader E 1983 Cervical trauma as a factor in the development of TMJ dysfunction and facial pain. Journal of Craniomandibular Practice 1:85–90
Lancaster G I, DeFrance J, Borruso J 1993 Air-bag associated rupture of the right atrium [letter] New England Journal of Medicine 4:358
Lang J 1995 Skull base and related structures: atlas of clinical anatomy. Foreword by Samii M. Schattauer, Stuttgart
Levy Y, Hasson O, Zeltser R, Nahlieli O 1998 Temporomandibular joint derangement after air bag deployment: report of two cases. Journal of Oral and Maxillofacial Surgery 56:1000–1003
Lindvall M, Edvinsson L, Owman C 1978 Sympathetic nervous control of cerebrospinal fluid production from the choroid plexus. Science 201:176–178
Lobbezoo-Scholte A M 1993. Diagnostic subgroups of craniomandibular disorders. PhD dissertation, Utrecht University, The Netherlands
Losert-Bruggner B 1998 Myofunktionelle Untersuchungen bei Schmerzen im Kieferbereich. Manuelle Medizin. Springer, Heidelberg, p 213–217
Maimaris C, Barnes M R, Aleen M J 1988 'Whiplash injuries' of the neck: a retrospective study. Injury 19:393–396
Maitland G D 1991 Peripheral manipulation, 3rd edn. Butterworth-Heinemann, London
Makovsky H W 1989 The effect of head posture on muscle contact position: the sliding cranium theory. Journal of Craniomandibular Practice 7:286–292
Makofsky H W 2000 The influence of forward head posture on dental occlusion. Journal of Craniomandibular Practice 18(1):30–39.
Makofsky H W, Sexton T R 1994 The effect of craniovertebral fusion on occlusion. Journal of Craniomandibular Practice 12:38–45
Mannheimer J, Attanasio R, Cinotti W R, Pertes R 1989 Cervical strain and mandibular whiplash: effects upon the craniomandibular apparatus. Clinical Preventive Dentistry 11:31
Mathew N T, Ravishankar K, Sanin L C 1996 Coexistence of migraine and idiopathic intracranial hypertension without papilledema. Neurology 46:1226–1230
McClean L F, Brenman H S, Friedman M G 1973 Effects of changing body position on dental occlusion. Journal of Dental Research 52:1041–1045
Michelotti A, Farella M, Tedesco A, Cimino R, Martina R 2000 Changes in pressure–pain thresholds of the jaw muscles during a natural stressful condition in a group of symptom-free subjects. Journal of Orofacial Pain 14:279–285
Miralles R, Dodds C, Palazzi C et al 2001 Vertical dimension. Part 1: Comparison of clinical freeway space. Journal of Craniomandibular Practice 19(4):230–6
Mohl D M 1994 The role of head posture in mandibular function. In: Solberg W K, Clark G T (eds) Abnormal jaw mechanics: diagnosis and treatment. Quintessence, Chicago, p 97
Moskowitz M A 1984 The neurobiology of vascular head pain. Annals of Neurology 16:167–168
Murphy W M 1967 Rest position of the mandible. Journal of Prosthetic Dentistry 17:329
Muto T, Kanazawa M 1994 Positional change of the hyoid bone at maximal mouth opening. The first department of oral surgery. Mosby-Year Book, p 451–455
Naeije M, Hansson T 1991 Short-term effect of stabilization appliance on masticatory activity in myogenous craniomandibular disorder patients. Journal of Craniomandibular Disorders: Facial and Oral Pain 5:245
Nielsen I, McNeill C, Danzig W et al 1990 Adaptation of craniofacial muscles in subjects with craniomandibular disorders. American Journal of Orthodontics and Dentofacial Orthopedics 97:20
O'Shaughnessy T 1994 Craniomandibular/temporomandibular/cervical implications of a forced hyper-extension/hyper-flexion episode (i.e. whiplash). Functional Orthodontist 11(2):5–10, 12
Okeson J P 1995 Neuropathic pains; behavior of neuropathic pains. In: Bell's orofacial pains, 5th edn. Quintessence, Chicago.
Oudhof H A J 2000 Skull growth in relation to mechanical stimulation. In: Piekartz von H J M, Bryden L (eds) Craniofacial dysfunction and pain: manual therapy, assessment and management. Butterworth-Heinemann, Oxford, p 1–22
Pillemer S R, Bradley L A, Crofford L J, Moldofsky H, Chrousos G P 1997 The neuroscience and endocrinology of fibromyalgia. Arthritis and Rheumatism 40:1928–1939
Preiskel H W 1965 Some observations on the postural position of the mandible. Journal of Prosthetic Dentistry 15:625
Pressman B D, Shellock F, Schames J, Schames M 1992 MR imaging of temporomandibular joint abnormalities associated with cervical hyperextension/hyperflexion (whiplash) injuries. Journal of Magnetic Resonance Imaging 2:569–574
Profitt W R 1993 Concepts of growth and development. In: Profitt WR, Fields HW (eds) Contemporary orthodontics. Mosby-Year Book, p 18–55
Radanov B P, Sturzenegger M, DiStephano G, Schnidrig A, Aljinovic M 1993 Factors influencing recovery from headache after common whiplash. British Medical Journal 307:652–655
Rickets R M 1968 Respiratory obstruction syndrome. American Journal of Orthodontics 54:495–503

Rocabado M 1981 Selected papers. Rocabado Institute, Tacoma, Washington
Rocabado M 1983 Biomechanical relationship of the cranial, cervical, and hyoid regions. Journal of Craniomandibular Practice 1:62–63
Rocabado M, Johnson B E, Blakney M G 1983 Physical therapy and dentistry: an overview. Journal of Craniomandibular Practice 1:47–49
Rugh J D, Drago C J 1981 Vertical dimension. A study of clinical rest position and jaw muscle activity. Journal of Prosthetic Dentistry 45:670
Salonen M A M, Raustia A M, Huggare J A 1994 Changes in head and cervical-spine postures and EMG activities of masticatory muscles following treatment with complete upper and partial lower denture. Journal of Craniomandibular Practice 12(4):222–226
Schick B, Weber R, Mosler P et al 1996 Duraplasty in the area of the sphenoid sinus. Laryngorhinootologie 75:275–279
Schwarz M 1926 Kopfhaltung und Kiefer. Zeitschrift für Stomatologie: Organ für wissenschaftliche und praktische Zahnheilkunde
Segter R G M, Arzouman M J et al 1993 Observation of the anterior loop of the inferior alveolar canal. International Journal of Oral and Maxillofacial Implants 8:295–300
Shellock F, Pressman B D et al 1990 MR imaging evaluation of the temporomandibular joint following cervical extension–flexion injury (whiplash). Radiological Society of North America Meeting, Chicago
Smirniotopoulos J G, Yue N C, Rushing E J 1993 Cerebellopontine angle masses: radiologic–pathologic correlation. Radiography 13:1131–1147
Solow B, Tallgren A 1976 Head posture and craniofacial morphology. American Journal of Physical Anthropology 44:417–436
Solow B, Tallgren A 1977 Dento-alveolar morphology in relation to craniocervical posture. Angle Orthodontist 47:157–163
Sterling M, Jull G, Wright A 2001 The effect of musculoskeletal pain on motor activity and control. Journal of Pain 2:135
Sternbach R A, Dallessio D J, Kunzel M 1980 MMPI patterns in common headache disorders. Headache 20:311–315
Sturzenegger M, DiStefano G, Radanov B P, Schnidrig A 1994 Presenting symptoms and signs after whiplash injury: the influence of accident mechanisms. Neurology 44:688–693
Sumino R, Nozaki S, Katoh M 1981 Trigemino-neck reflex. In: Kawamura Y, Dubner R (eds) Orofacial sensory and motor functions. Quintessence, Tokyo, p 81
Urbanowicz M 1991 Alteration of vertical dimension and its effect on head and neck posture. Journal of Craniomandibular Practice 9:174–179
Vig P S, Showfety K, Phillips C 1980 Experimental manipulation of head posture. American Journal of Orthodontics 77:258–268
Visscher C M, Huddleston Slater J J, Lobbezoo F, Naelie M 2000 Kinematics of the human mandible for different head postures. Journal of Oral Rehabilitation 27(4):299–305
von Piekartz H 2005 Intern clinic study. (In press)
von Piekartz H, Coppieters M, De Weerdt W 2001 Vorschlag für einen neurodynamischen Test des N. Mandibularis. Reliabilität und Referenzwerte. Manuelle Therapie 5:56
Wessberg G A, Epker B N, Elliot A C 1983 Comparison of mandibular rest positions induced by phonetics, transcutaneous electrical stimulation, and masticatory electromyography. Journal of Prosthetic Dentistry 48:100
Westerhuis P 2001 Zervigogener Kopfschmerzen: Perspektive eines Kliniker. In: von Piekartz H (ed.) Kraniofaziale Dysfunktionen und Schmerzen. Untersuchung, Beurteilung und Management. Thieme, Stuttgart, p 83–95
Wilkinson T, Hansson T, McNeil C et al 1992 A comparison of the success of 24-hour occlusal splint therapy versus nocturnal occlusal splint therapy in reducing craniomandibular disorders. Journal of Craniomandibular Disorders: Facial and Oral Pain 6:64
Winnberg A, Pancherz H, Westesson P 1988 Head posture and hyo-mandibular function in man: a synchronized electromyographic and videofluorographic study of the open–close–clench cycle. American Journal of Orthodontics and Dentofacial Orthopedics 94:393–404
Wright E F 2000 Referred craniofacial pain patterns in patients with temporomandibular disorder. Journal of the American Dental Association 131:1307–1315
Yu X-M, Hu J W, Sessle B J 1995 Effects of inflammatory irritant application to the rat temporomandibular joint on jaw and neck muscle activity. Pain 60:143–149
Zakrzewska J M 1995 Trigeminal neuralgia: major problems in neurology. Saunders, London
Zakrzewska J, Hamlyn P 1999 Facial pain. In: Crombie I K (ed.) Epidemiology of pain. IASP Press, Seattle

Chapter 6

Cervical instability

Pieter Westerhuis

CHAPTER CONTENTS

INTRODUCTION AND DEFINITIONS

A variety of different aspects related to the concept of cervical instability can be differentiated. Depending on the individual focus, clinicians have defined spinal instability in various ways (Adams 1999). Panjabi (1992a) divides the spinal stabilizing system into three subsystems (Fig. 6.1):

- The passive subsystem (joints, capsule, ligaments, etc.)
- The active subsystem (muscles, strength, endurance, etc.)
- The regulating or controlling subsystem (coordination, control, proprioception).

THE PASSIVE SUBSYSTEM

The stability of the passive subsystem is influenced by several factors, including orientation of the zygapophyseal joints, the integrity of the joint capsule and ligaments and the integrity of the discs. Damage of these structures potentially causes structural instability (Zhu et al 1999, Wilmink & Patijn 2001, Lomoschitz et al 2002).

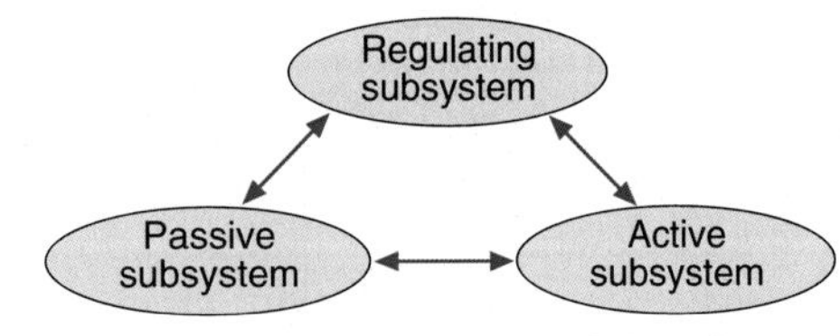

Fig. 6.1 The stabilizing system of the spine.

Some biomechanical aspects are particularly relevant. If one performs an instability test on a peripheral joint (e.g. the anterior drawer test to examine the anterior cruciate ligament of the knee) the examiner is evaluating the integrity of the passive subsystem. The examiner seeks the following information:

- The available range of motion before any resistance is felt (neutral zone, NZ) (Panjabi 1992b)
- The behaviour of resistance once the movement is continued into resistance. This is to assess 'stiffness' within the 'elastic zone' (EZ) (Pope & Panjabi 1985)
- The overall range of motion (ROM)
- Perceived pain
- Protective muscle spasm.

From a biomechanical point of view the following definitions can be made.

> **Definitions**
>
> A structural *instability* is an excessive range of motion of an accessory movement that shows an abnormal behaviour of resistance with an increased neutral zone and a loss of stiffness (adapted from Panjabi et al 1994 and Maitland et al 2001).
>
> *Hypermobility:* This is defined as above-average mobility in a physiological direction with normal resistance (R_1–R_2) behaviour. Hypermobility may also occur at one or more intervertebral joints, in which case these joints are excessively mobile with respect to neighbouring joints. A hypermobile joint is not necessarily unstable. Instability refers to a joint with loose supporting ligaments, which allows the joint to move more than normal (see page 121).

According to Panjabi (1992b), changes in the neutral zone are more significantly correlated with the occurrence of instability than changes in range of motion. This was confirmed in recent studies.

On clinical examination evaluation of range of motion is sometimes difficult due to protective muscle spasm. An important clue in the assessment of instability is a delayed onset of resistance when accessory movements are examined (Maitland et al 2001).

All traditional segmental instability tests will primarily assess structural rather than functional instability (among others, Aspinall 1990, Pettman 1994).

According to Sanchez Martin (1992) the most common causes of structural instability are:

- Trauma:
  - Massive external forces, e.g. whiplash injuries
  - Repetitive microtrauma
- Congenital, for example:
  - Occipitalization of C1
  - Down syndrome
- Metastases
- Diseases such as:
  - Rheumatoid arthritis
  - Ehlers–Danlos syndrome
  - Ankylosing spondylitis.

The greatest difficulty is that structural instability is not correlated with any specific symptoms (Cattrysse et al 1997, Pitkanen et al 1997, Eisenstein 1999).

THE ACTIVE AND REGULATING SUBSYSTEM

The stability of the active subsystem depends on the capacity of the muscle units to develop force and to maintain it over a prolonged period of time. Therefore the combination of force and endurance is relevant.

The regulating subsystem coordinates the timing and intensity of individual muscle contractions. It depends on sensory input provided by the joints (McLain 1994), discs (Mendel et al 1992) and muscles (Heikkiläa & Astrom 1996). The regulating system processes all inputs to coordinate an adequate muscular reaction.

Dysfunctions of the regulating subsystem can affect either input (afference/proprioception) or output (efference/coordination).

Panjabi proposed in 1992 that dysfunctions of one of the three subsystems can be compensated by the two other subsystems (Panjabi

1992a). Kettler et al (2002) demonstrated that mechanically stimulated muscle forces have the capacity to stabilize an unstable segment.

Studies on patients with lumbar spine instability show that specific muscle rehabilitation significantly relieves symptoms (O'Sullivan et al 1997). Hence therapists examining potential instability patients will need to evaluate the function of each subsystem separately.

CLINICAL/FUNCTIONAL INSTABILITY

If the three subsystems fail to stabilize the spinal segment adequately, this results in clinical/functional instability.

> **Definition**
> Clinical instability of the spine is defined as the loss of the ability to maintain the orientation between vertebrae under physiological loads in such a way that there is neither initial nor subsequent damage to the spinal cord and there is no development of incapacitating deformity or severe pain (White et al 1999).

According to this definition, stability is assessed functionally, in terms of the spine's ability to control the orientation of individual segments with respect to each other without neurological problems, symptoms or deformity arising.

This implies that patients with structural instabilities (e.g. whiplash) do not always become functionally unstable as long as they can still control the positioning of the vertebrae. From the opposite perspective, however, this also means that patients may exhibit functional instability in the absence of structural instability.

> **!** A structural instability is not, by definition, necessarily a functional instability.

One test for functional instability includes the observation of cervical control on bilateral arm elevation. With this movement upper trapezius and levator scapulae will show activity. Both muscles originate at the cervical spine and both muscles are neck extensors. The counterbalance of neck extension requires activity of deep cervical neck flexors (Mayoux-Benhamou et al 1995). Dysfunction of those stabilizing muscles leads to excessive neck extension on normal movements and may cause symptoms.

CLINICAL PRESENTATION OF CERVICAL INSTABILITY

BODY CHART

During the subjective examination, location of the symptoms and type of symptoms are recorded on a body chart. Pettman (1994) pointed out the importance of so-called 'cardinal symptoms'. These are symptoms indicative of obvious structural instability and therefore warning signs for a negative prognosis. Cardinal symptoms for structural instability include spinal cord signs and vertebrobasilar insufficiency.

SPINAL CORD SIGNS

Authors as early as Fielding et al (1974) have shown that instability of C1–C2 negatively influences spinal cord integrity. Patients with an atlantodental interval (Fig. 6.2) larger than 7 mm commonly show neurological signs and symptoms.

These might be (Wiesel & Rothman 1979, Delphini et al 1999):

- Instability on walking
- Stumbling
- Ataxia
- Extrasegmental sensitivity dysfunctions (arms/legs)
- Loss of bladder/bowel control
- Hyperreflexia
- Pathological reflexes (e.g. Babinski, clonus)
- Muscle spasms.

Physiotherapists in private practice will rarely come across such patients since they are usually

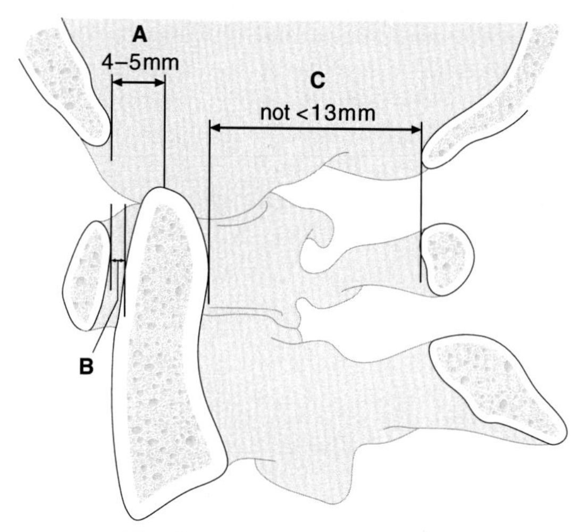

Fig. 6.2 The distance between the dorsal margin of the anterior atlas arch and the anterior side of the dens is called the atlantodental interval (ADI = B). The ADI should be <3 mm in adults (after White & Panjabi 1990).

referred to surgery. However, they should keep an eye out for subtle spinal cord signs, since they may indicate a definite worsening of the situation and will need adequate management immediately.

VERTEBROBASILAR INSUFFICIENCY

Abnormal translation in the midcervical segments and/or excessive rotation in the upper cervical spine may cause impaired blood flow in the vertebrobasilar system (McDermaid 2001). One of the main symptoms is dizziness. Coman (1986) states that dizziness may have a great variety of causes. If the dizziness is caused by impaired blood flow in the vertebral artery, other parts of the brain will also suffer a lack of blood flow. This may present as:

- Dysphagia
- Diplopia
- Dizziness
- Dysarthria
- Drop attacks (the patient experiences sudden loss of muscle control without losing consciousness, or falls on certain activities or movements).

According to Coman, these five D's are indicative for vertebral artery dysfunction (compare also Endo et al 2000).

PAIN

Instability causes abnormal segmental movement patterns. Joints and discs compensate abnormal mobility by bearing an increased load and may respond with pain (Bogduk 2001). Additionally, nerves may also react due to abnormal compression and/or stretch, leading to nerve impingement and pain (Bogduk 1981, Rydevik & Olmarker 1999).

Lance and Anthony (1980) describe the so-called 'neck–tongue' syndrome in which patients report unilateral occipital/suboccipital pain and paraesthesia of the tongue. Symptoms are exacerbated by sudden movements of the head. These symptoms are viewed as indicative for a segmental C1–C2 instability. Bogduk (1981) mentions the following neuroanatomical explanation: the hypoglossal nerve is responsible for motor innervation of the tongue. The ansa hypoglossi makes a connection between the hypoglossal nerve and the cervical plexus (Fig. 6.3). Afferent fibres of the hypoglossal nerve run parallel to the second spinal nerve. If the patient performs a sudden cervical movement this might irritate the C2 nerve and its dorsal root ganglion. As fibres of the hypoglossal nerve would also be irritated, tongue symptoms will be produced along with cervical symptoms.

DIZZINESS

Proprioceptive input of the upper cervical spine has a great influence on the balance system. Consequently any changes of this input may cause dizziness (Karlberg et al 1996).

Clinical features of cervical arthrogenic dizziness include the following:

- Patients rarely complain of true vertigo; rather they perceive their symptoms as modest instability on walking.

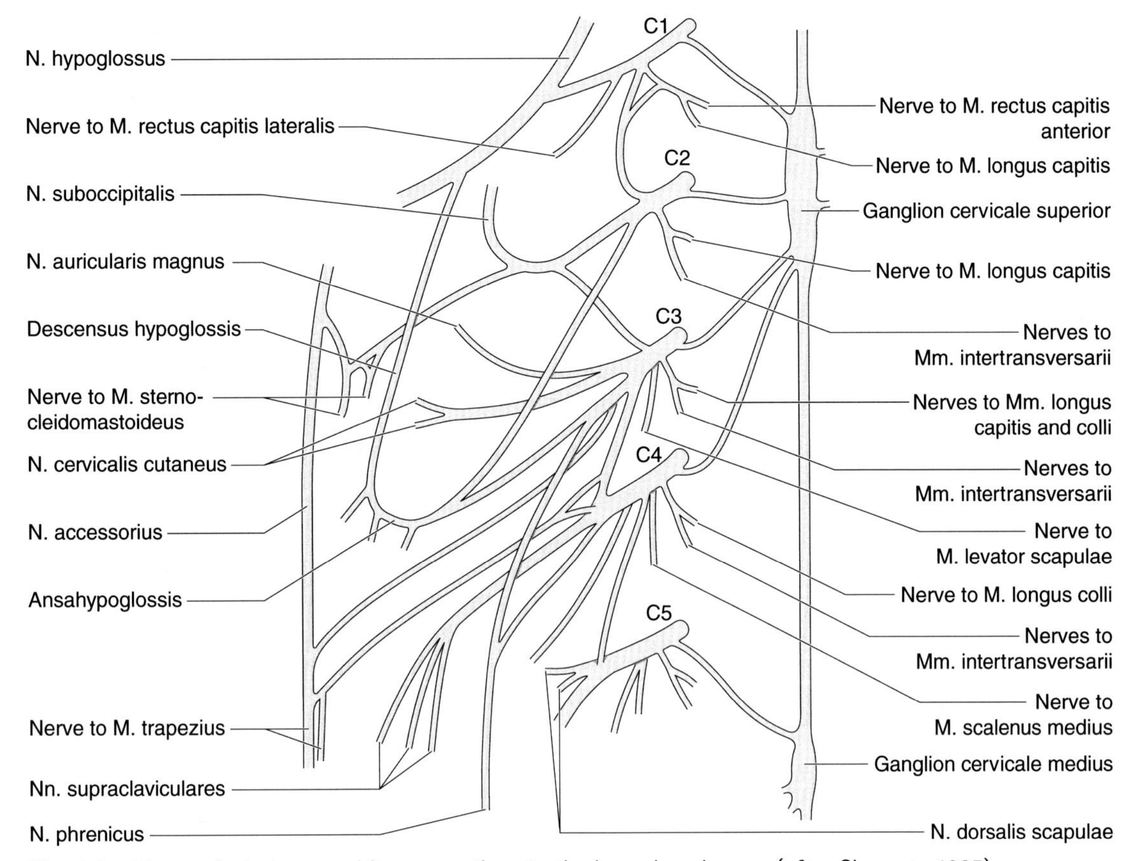

Fig. 6.3 The cervical plexus and its connections to the hypoglossal nerve (after Clemente 1985).

- Although associated symptoms are quite common, Coman's five D's do not occur.
- The dizziness can be clearly provoked by neck movements (clear on/off effect).
- Dizziness immediately follows a provoking movement (no latency).
- If a provoking position is held for any length of time, dizziness usually decreases with time.
- The history often indicates that the initial episode of dizziness is correlated with cervical trauma or cervical symptoms.
- The physical examination of the cervical spine will detect signs and symptoms (ROM limitations, instability, pain, etc.).
- The hypothesis of cervical dizziness is confirmed if treatment of the neck clearly influences the symptoms.

OTHER SYMPTOMS

- Movement limitations: It seems counterintuitive to hear patients with instability problems complain of stiffness in the neck. A possible explanation is the occurrence of protective muscle spasm.
- Locking: Patients frequently state that certain movements cause their neck to lock. Biomechanically, insufficient control of zygapophyseal joints due to lack of muscle control might cause an imbalance of rolling and gliding components in the joints.
- Crepitation: Patients notice noises in their neck such as clicking or cracking on certain movements.
- Insufficient muscle control: Indicators for muscle deficits are statements such as: 'I

have to hold my head with my hands', 'My head feels too heavy for my neck', 'My neck gets very tired', 'My neck feels as if it's made of glass and will break any minute', 'I can hardly hold my head up when I am shaving'.

- 'Something feels stuck in my throat'/'I have problems swallowing': Besides neural causes for problems with swallowing (e.g. vertebral artery dysfunction) a marked anterior glide of C1 in relation to C2, as is common in rheumatoid arthritis, can mechanically obstruct the oesophagus.
- Associated symptoms, for example:
  - Vomiting
  - Tinnitus
  - Seeing spots in front of the eyes (Wenngren et al 1998).

BEHAVIOUR OF SYMPTOMS

The dominant feature of symptom behaviour in cervical instability is the apparent inconsistency of the symptoms. Patients may be able to perform physically exhausting tasks without any problems, but then complain of symptoms on some very light activities. Some patients can, for example, play volleyball quite easily but suffer on sudden head movements during daily life. This seemingly contradictive phenomenon can be explained by muscle control deficits.

Hogdes et al (1996) and Moseley et al (2002) showed that primary stabilizing muscles of the lower back have a delayed reaction to sudden movements in patients with low back pain compared to pain-free controls. If the person is involved in an activity like playing volleyball the stabilizing muscles are constantly active; however, if the person is relaxed the stabilizing muscles are not activated. Sudden movements may now cause symptoms since the stabilizing muscles cannot control joint movement (Laurén et al 1997).

Patients frequently state that they experience symptoms when they are passengers in a car. This can be explained by hypothesizing that the driver knows his moves (acceleration, slowing down, changing gear) in advance so the muscles in the neck anticipate any changes whereas the passenger needs to react.

Instability patients commonly feel better in the morning than in the evening since the muscles were rested during the night. During the course of the day the symptoms usually increase.

Some patients describe a painful arc on particular movements. A lack of muscle control within the neutral zone might be the explanation here.

HISTORY

Again the dominant feature is inconsistency. Commonly patients have had their symptoms for a long time or have experienced recurrent episodes of symptoms. Duration and intensity of painful episodes may vary greatly. Patients may report that they could hardly move their head 2 days ago whereas yesterday their range of movement was almost back to normal.

Triggering activities frequently do not correlate with the intensity of the symptoms. It is quite possible that a patient cannot move their head for a whole week, suffering from great pain, while the triggering movement was merely a sudden turn of the head when reversing the car.

It is important to ask for a previous history of trauma. Studies have shown that whiplash injuries may cause instabilities (Barnsley et al 1993, Spitzer et al 1995, Siegmund et al 2001). Even if the x-ray taken directly after the traumatic event is clear, instabilities may still be present. Many x-rays are 'false negatives' (Jonsson et al 1991, Taylor & Twomey 1993).

Furthermore, authors like Foreman and Croft (1995) and Delphini et al (1999) point out the possibility of 'delayed instability' – defined as instabilities that become symptomatic 20 or more days after a trauma. Patients do not show any lesion on the initial x-rays (Herkowitz & Rothman 1984).

Taylor and Twomey (1993) demonstrated that whiplash injuries may cause so-called 'rim lesions'. These are fine tears that run horizontally at the anterior side of the disc with the disc being torn off the deck plate. Rim lesions cannot be detected by ordinary x-ray but may increase the degenerative process of the segment. The mobile segment loses height and hence causes ligament laxity (Twomey & Taylor 1991).

Consequently, clinicians will need to examine the segmental stability of any patient who reports previous trauma. However, instability is not always the result of severe trauma. Seemingly light activities may trigger instability symptoms. Examples are dental treatment or a visit to the hairdresser. End of range positions that had to be maintained over a stretch of time are commonly reported events to trigger first episodes of neck pain. A combination of muscle fatigue and creep effect lead to malpositioning of the vertebrae. If this is followed by a relatively small impact like the fitting of a tooth crown, instability may occur. Patients who have previously suffered a whiplash injury or other trauma, or who are generally hypermobile, are especially at risk.

The clinician should also ask about throat infections just before the first onset of neck pain. Grisel described how bacteria might use the lymphatic system to reach C1–C2 and cause deficits of ligament integrity there (Aspinall 1990).

PHYSICAL EXAMINATION

INTRODUCTION

If the results of the subjective examination point towards cervical instability, the following guidelines apply:

- Even if active movements do not produce any pain one should refrain from adding overpressure since this might massively worsen the situation.
- Instability patients tend to react negatively when structures are stressed at the end of a range of movement too frequently. If the hypothesis is cervical instability, as little testing as necessary should be performed.
- If the examiner feels an increased neutral zone and/or a loss of stiffness on passive testing, the movement should not be continued to the end of range. It is contraindicated in this situation to assess for end-feel. For an extensive description of the manual therapy examination of the cervical spine, see Maitland et al (2001).

The following examination procedure focuses on the particular aspects of the assessment of unstable cervical segments. The individual results of one test alone do not confirm instability. Only if a number of tests are positive can the presence of an instability be hypothesized.

Each patient needs a thorough cervical spine examination. The clinical pattern evolves from the overall impression gained throughout the examination. To confirm or deny the diagnosis of cervical instability, the following aspects of the physical examination are particularly relevant:

- Inspection
- Active movements
- Passive physiological intervertebral movements (PPIVMs)
- Linear movements including specific tests for ligament integrity
- Passive accessory intervertebral movements (PAIVMs)
- Muscle control tests.

INSPECTION

Many patients, and particularly female patients, may have a relatively thin neck ('swan neck'). Some patients seem to move their neck constantly during the subjective examination ('patients talk with their necks').

Another common feature is an increased kyphosis of the upper thoracic spine accompanied by a lordotic bend at C5–C6 with visible creasing of the skin. These patients typically show instability on neck extension.

ACTIVE MOVEMENTS

One of the most important features that needs to be evaluated is the quality of movements.

- Which part of the cervical spine shows hypermobility and which part shows hypomobility?
- Does the cervical spine show an even segmental opening?
- Is there a visible translation of one vertebra or is there any visible hinging in one segment?
- Is there a painful arc? (This could point towards control deficits within the neutral zone.)
- Shaky muscle activity?
- Protective muscle spasm?
- Does the patient show apprehension? (This indicates fear of movement and is frequently found on cervical extension.)

When analysing a passive movement (see Fig. 6.4), the behaviour of various factors can be depicted graphically in a movement diagram. The A–B line indicates the extent of the movement, with B defined as the normal average limit of movement. L stands for the limit and indicates the limit of mobility for the individual patient. On a normal movement diagram, L and B are the same. The A–C line indicates the intensity of the individual factors. R stands for resistance (of the passive structures), P for pain, and S for spasm. C indicates the maximum intensity that the therapist is prepared to exert. The shape of the resistance curve indicates stiffness through the range of movement.

In this example of cervical rotation towards the right, the normal range of movement is approximately 85°. The therapist notices the onset of resistance at about 30°. Resistance increases slowly at first, and then increases exponentially after 60°. There is pain without protective spasm. Figure 6.4a shows a normal movement diagram.

The movement diagram in Figure 6.4b indicates that right rotation is restricted by about 20°, the onset of resistance is observed at 15° and the onset of pain occurs at 45°. At the end of the movement this pain has an intensity of about 6 on a 10-point visual analogue scale (VAS).

The movement diagram in Figure 6.4c shows an onset of resistance at 45°, i.e. the neutral

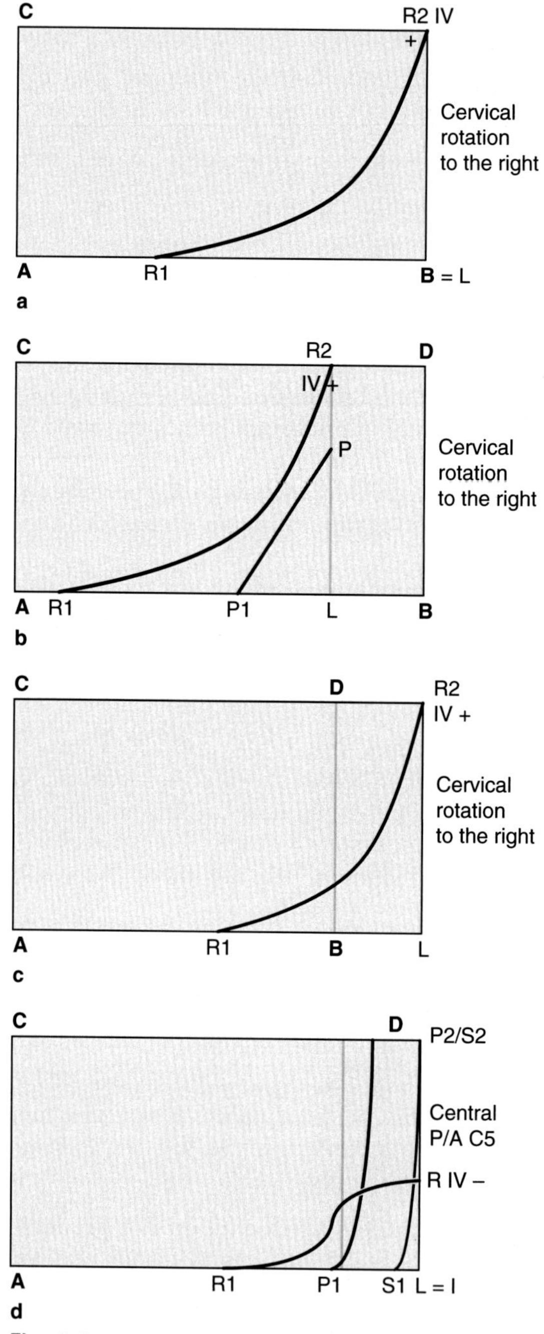

Fig. 6.4
a Movement diagram of normal cervical rotation to the right.
b Movement diagram of hypomobile painful cervical rotation to the right.
c Movement diagram of hypermobile cervical rotation to the right.
d Movement diagram of cervical instability.

zone is increased in size. This patient also shows above average right rotation, with the limit of range of movement exceeding the B value. The limit of movement is about 100°. This is therefore not a case of instability, but rather of hypermobility. The basis for this is that, firstly the exponential resistance curve is normal and there is no loss of stiffness, and secondly the movement diagram is showing a physiological movement, not an accessory movement.

The movement diagram in Figure 6.4d shows a central posteroanterior movement on C5, i.e. an accessory movement. Normally the A–B line is just 15 mm and the onset of resistance is rather early. However, in this case, the onset of resistance is delayed and the neutral zone is enlarged. Furthermore, resistance does not increase exponentially, with the movement showing loss of stiffness. Often these cases show limitation at the end of the range of movement by a protective spasm or symptoms which the investigator is not able to resolve, indicating that this is an example of structural instability.

It is also important to assess these aspects during return from end of range positions. For example, a cranial to caudal movement should be initiated as a return movement from end of range extension (Hino et 1999). The deep cervical flexors are mainly responsible for segmental control during this activity. With some pathologies these muscles are inhibited (Jull 2000). This leads to an excessive activity of superficial muscles such as sternocleidomastoid producing shear forces (Winters & Peles 1990). Clinically these patients initiate return from extension by moving the midcervical segments first while increasing upper cervical extension. The neck moves with a protracted chin until at the very end of the movement the head is repositioned to neutral alignment. Similarly inadequate muscle control has been observed on return from end of range flexion. If the deep-lying stabilizing muscles (deep neck flexors, multifidi and semispinalis) are inhibited, the more superficial extensors such as the splenius capitis and the upper trapezius first pull the head in extension on the neck until this movement is complete. Only then is the head moved backwards. This abnormal action will also increase shear forces in the midcervical spine.

During the examination of active movements the relative restriction of ranges of motion should be evaluated. During flexion and extension, the head's centre of gravity moves away from the perpendicular. These movements are therefore more difficult than rotation and lateroflexion, and extension is often much more restricted than rotation by instability.

Example

A patient shows extension limited at 45° with unilateral symptoms on the left-hand side. If this restriction is caused by cervical instability of a zygapophyseal joint on the left side, rotation towards the left is usually relatively normal. If the restriction is due to a hypomobile zygapophyseal joint, rotation to the left will also usually be limited at about 45°.

PASSIVE PHYSIOLOGICAL INTERVERTEBRAL MOVEMENTS (PPIVMS)

PPIVMs examine the intersegmental range of motion in a physiological direction. For a detailed description of these tests, see Maitland et al (2001).

LINEAR MOVEMENTS AND SPECIFIC TESTS FOR LIGAMENT INTEGRITY

The so-called 'linear stress' tests consist of translational movements without any physiological movement. The test results are negative if no distinct movement is possible. The end-feel should be hard–elastic. The reproduction of symptoms should also be evaluated.

Pettman (1994) hypothesizes that linear tests might cause translational stress on the vertebral artery and the nervous system in patients with cervical instability.

Linear stress tests assess the passive subsystem as a whole for structural integrity. A positive result implies a possible segmental instability but does not point towards any specific structural deficit.

There are additional, more specific tests for the upper cervical spine (occiput–C2) that can be used to selectively examine ligament integrity. The examiner evaluates the same aspects as with PPIVM testing. The validity of these tests has not been researched in large scale studies of trauma patients to date.

Alar ligament

The anatomy, biomechanics and pathology of the alar ligament have been studied extensively by Dvorak and Panjabi (1987). The alar ligament usually consists of two portions: an occipital and an occasionally missing atlantal portion (Fig. 6.5).

The occipital portion originates at the dens and inserts at the occipital condyles. Depending on the size of the dens, its fibres run craniocaudally, horizontally or caudocranially. In the transverse plane the left and the right occipital ligament form an angle of 150–180°: the smaller the angle, the more tension on the ligament on upper cervical flexion due to the dorsal glide of the occiput (Penning 1998). Therefore stability testing should be performed in extension as well as in flexion (Willauschus et al 1995).

The atlantal portion originates at the dens and inserts at the massa lateralis of C1. The alar ligaments limit rotatory movements of the occiput–atlas–axis complex. According to Dvorak and Panjabi (1987) rotation towards the right loads the left alar ligament while the right alar ligament is relaxed (Fig. 6.6).

Lateroflexion to the right loads the left occipito-alar ligament, limiting the extent of movement. It also produces tension of the right atlanto-alar ligament. This produces rotation of C2 to the right. The spinous process of C2 moves to the left (Fig. 6.7).

Lateroflexion to the right therefore causes a relative left rotation of the C1–C2 segment (lateroflexion to the right is coupled with left rotation of the C1–C2 segment).

Dvorak and Panjabi (1987) described how flexion combined with rotation causes maximum loading of the ligament. Clinically, patients with whiplash injury are often seen after rear impact motor accidents. If the patient's head was in a flexed position and turned to the right at the time of the impact (e.g. while waiting

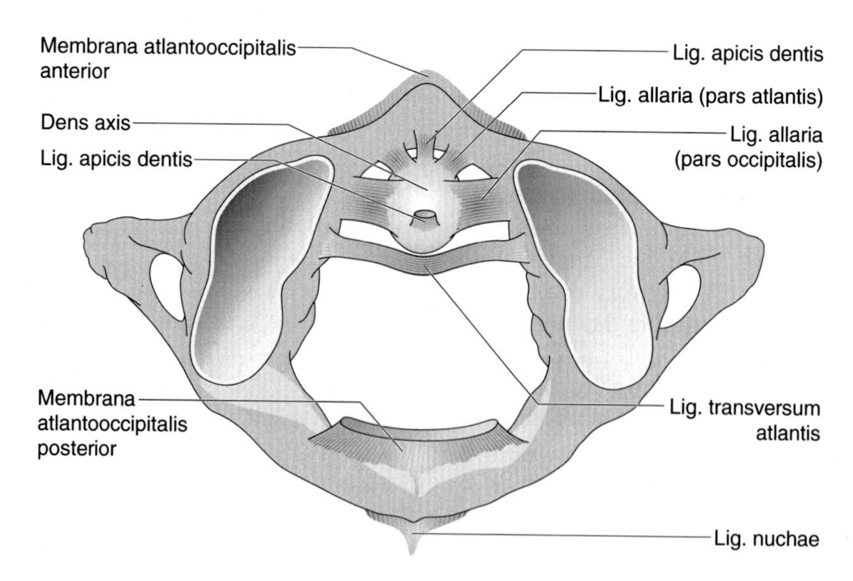

Fig. 6.5 Alar ligaments and transverse ligament in the horizontal plane (reproduced with permission from Dvorak & Panjabi 1987)

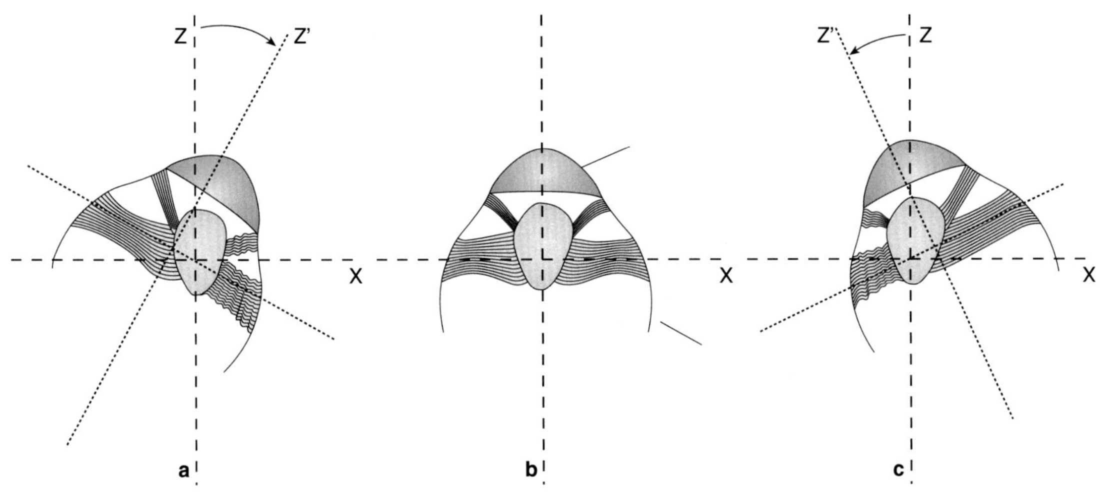

Fig. 6.6 Dorsal view onto the alar ligaments. On rotation to the right the left alar ligament and on rotation to the left, the right alar ligament are tensed (see text) (reproduced with permission from Dvorak & Panjabi 1987).

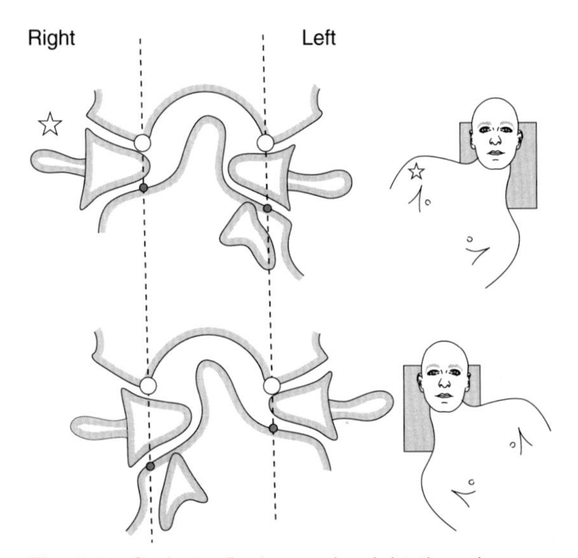

Fig. 6.7 On lateroflexion to the right the atlas shifts to the right and the axis rotates to the right. This means that the spinous process of C2 moves to the left (after Penning 1998).

at traffic lights and opening the glove compartment), the patient is at specific risk of having injured the left alar ligament.

Besides the C1–C2 rotation, Penning (1998) has studied atlas translation on lateroflexion. He describes how lateroflexion to the right causes the atlas to move to the right relative to the occiput. This is due to the wedge-shaped massa lateralis of C1. This atlas movement additionally stresses the atlantal portion of the alar ligament.

Based on the knowledge of anatomy and biomechanics it is hypothesized that clinicians will find the following test results in patients with left alar ligament insufficiency:

- Increased right rotation of occiput–C1 (rotation PPIVM occiput–C1).
- Increased lateroflexion of occiput–C1 with reduced glide of C1 towards the right compared to the left (lateroflexion PPIVM occiput–C1). Panjabi et al (1991a,b) demonstrated that not the overall range of motion but mainly the neutral zone increases in this case (see also Brodeur 2001).
- Increased right rotation of occiput–C2 (rotation PPIVM occiput–C2).
- Lack of movement of the C2 spinous process to the left on lateroflexion to the right (specific alar ligament test).
- Fixation of the C2 spinous process allows lateroflexion of the occiput to the right (specific alar ligament test).
- Increased translation to the right of occiput and C1 towards C2 on linear side force (specific alar ligament test).

Lateroflexion of occiput–C2 to the right in sitting

This test evaluates the integrity of the left alar ligament (Fig. 6.8).

Starting position

- The patient is sitting, with the neck relaxed.
- The neck is in a mid-position of cervical flexion and extension.

Position of the examiner

- The therapist stands on the patient's right.
- The therapist holds the patient's head with the right hand.
- The left thumb and index finger hold the spinous process of C2.

Fixation

- There is no fixation.

Method

- The right hand of the therapist moves the head towards right lateroflexion.
- It is important to avoid rotatory movements.

Interpretation

- An intact left alar ligament will produce an immediate rotation of C2.
- The therapist should therefore feel an immediate rotation of the C2 spinous process.

Lateroflexion of occiput–C2 to the right in supine

This test evaluates the integrity of the left alar ligament (Fig. 6.9).

Starting position

- The patient is lying supine.
- The patient's head is positioned in the right hand and is supported against the stomach of the therapist.
- This test is performed in upper cervical flexion, extension and neutral position.

Position of the examiner

- The therapist is sitting or standing behind the patient.

Fixation

- The left index finger holds the spinous process of C2 from the left side.

a

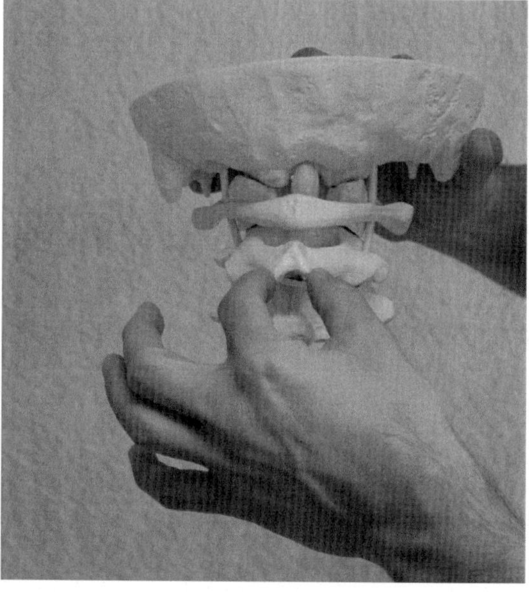

b

Fig. 6.8 Alar ligament test in sitting (see text).

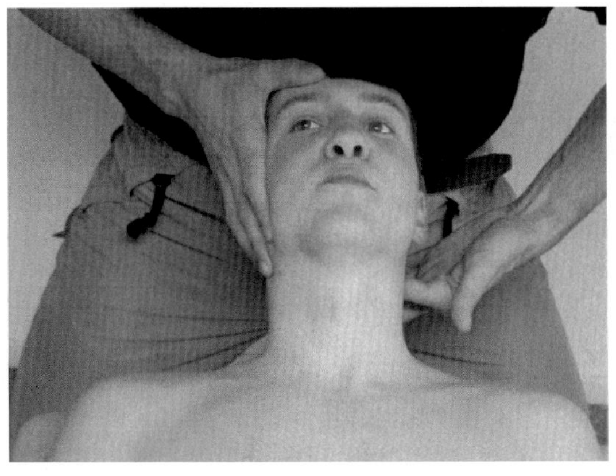

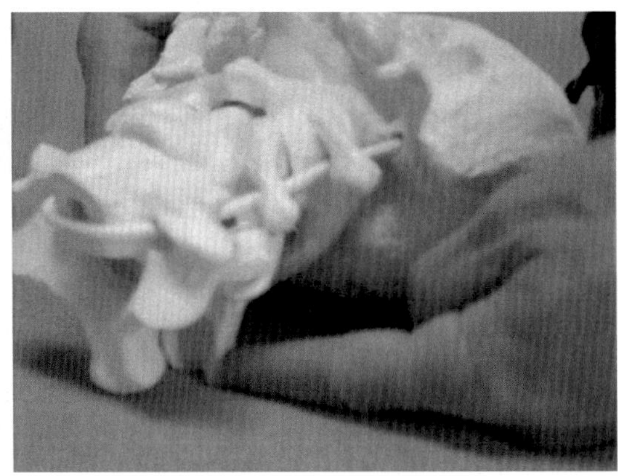

Fig. 6.9 Alar ligament test in supine (see text).

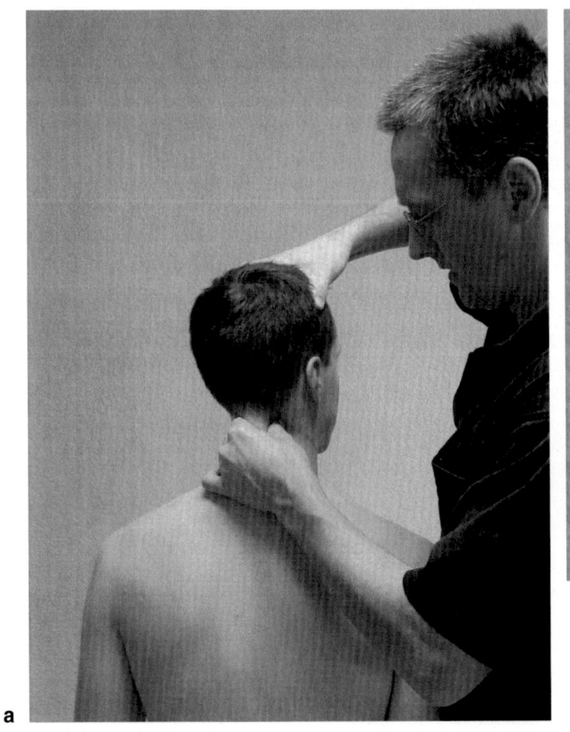

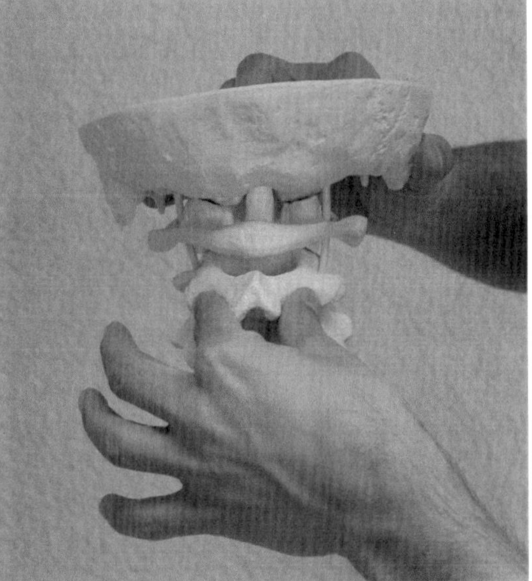

Fig. 6.10 Rotationary stress to the right in sitting (occiput–C2) (see text). Note that the fixating hand at the spinous process of C2 is positioned flatter and with more contact than in the previous test.

- The index finger should be positioned as far dorsal as possible.

Method

- The therapist attempts to perform an upper cervical lateroflexion to the right using the body and right hand.

Interpretation

- An intact alar ligament should not allow for any movement if the C2 spinous process is fixed.

Rotatory stress to the right: occiput–C2 test in sitting

This test evaluates the integrity of the left alar ligament (Fig. 6.10).

Starting position

- The patient is sitting with the neck relaxed.

Position of the examiner

- The therapist is standing on the patient's right.

- The therapist holds the patient's head from cranial with the right hand.

Fixation

- With the left thumb and index finger the lamina is held from dorsal.

Method

- The right hand rotates the head towards the right.

Interpretation

- An intact left alar ligament should limit rotation to the right at 30–35°.
- The discrepancy between right and left rotation should be no more than 8°.

Transverse stress test to the left: occiput–C2 in supine

This test evaluates the integrity of the left alar ligament (Fig. 6.11).

Starting position

- The patient is lying supine.

Position of the examiner

- The therapist is sitting or standing behind the patient.
- The patient's head is positioned in the right hand and is supported against the stomach of the therapist.
- The radial side of the metacarpophalangeal joint of the therapist's right index finger is positioned laterally against the C1 transverse process.

Fixation

- The radial side of the metacarpophalangeal joint of the therapist's left index finger is positioned laterally against C2 transverse process.

Method

- With the right hand the therapist attempts to shift the occiput and C1 to the left, relative to C2.
- It is important to take up the soft tissue slack first to avoid false-positive results.

Interpretation

- Normally, no movement should be possible.

Transverse ligament

The transverse ligament is the primary stabilizer for C1–C2 flexion. It originates at the massa lateralis of C1 on one side and inserts at the massa lateralis on the other. It runs posterior to the dens and prevents ventral glide of C1 during flexion (or dorsal movement of the dens which would impair the spinal medulla).

The following tests are designed to assess the integrity of the transverse ligament:

- Sharp–Purser test (Sharp & Purser 1961, Uitvlugt & Indenbaum 1988)
- Anterior shear test (Aspinall 1990)
- Posterior–anterior movement of C2, with the neck positioned in upper cervical flexion.

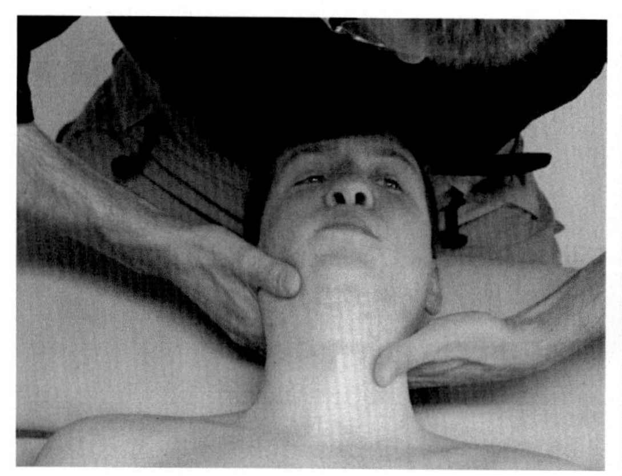
a

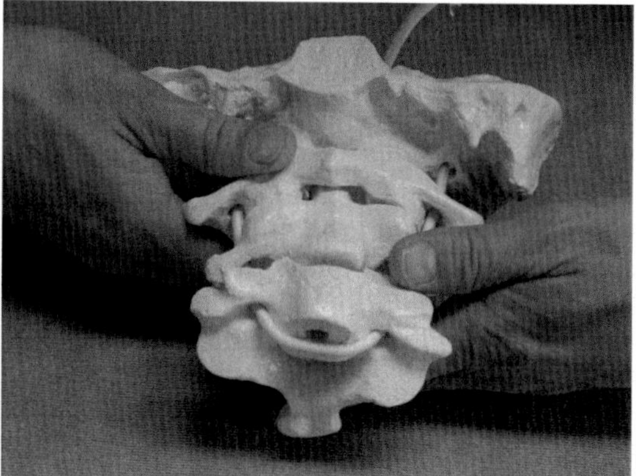
b

Fig. 6.11 Transverse stress occiput–C2 to the left in supine.

Sharp–Purser test (Fig. 6.12)

Starting position

- Sitting.
- Head is relaxed.
- Neck in slight flexion (possibly move until onset of symptoms).

Position of the examiner

- Standing next to the patient.
- Cradles the head of the patient with the left forearm and biceps.

Fixation

- With the right hand (thumb and index finger) the spinous process and both laminae of C2 are held from dorsal.

Method

- The left hand attempts to move the head, and therewith the occiput and C1 dorsally, relative to C2.

Interpretation

- An insufficient transverse ligament allows C1 to translate ventrally on C2 on cervical flexion. In that case the examiner will find the following results:
  - Dorsal movement of occiput and C1
  - Possibly a palpable 'click'
  - Reduced symptoms
  - A stable segment should not allow any movement and should show a hard–elastic end-feel.

Anterior shear test (Fig. 6.13)

Starting position

- Supine with head on bench.

Position of the examiner

- Sitting or standing behind the patient with both index fingers positioned on the atlas and fingers 3–5 against the occiput.

Fixation

- Both thumbs fixate the C2 transverse processes bilaterally from ventral.

Method

- The therapist attempts to move the atlas and occiput ventrally against C2.

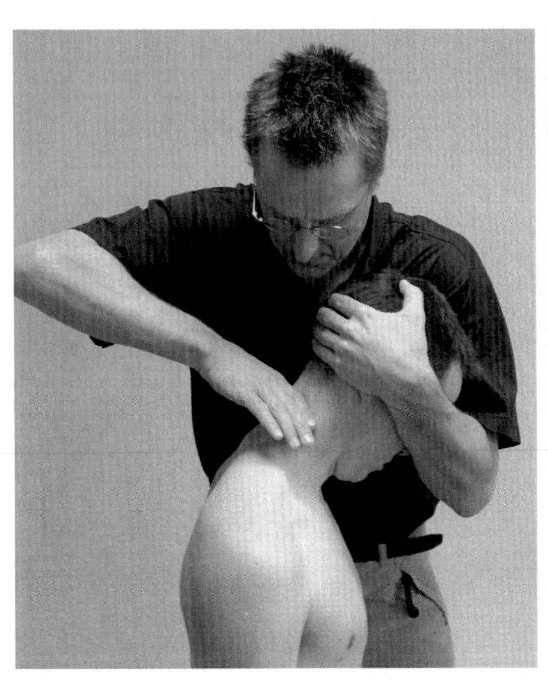

a

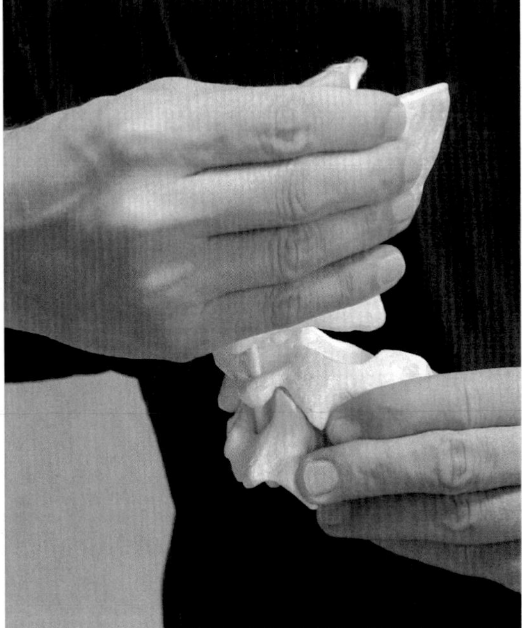

b

Fig. 6.12 Sharp–Purser test.

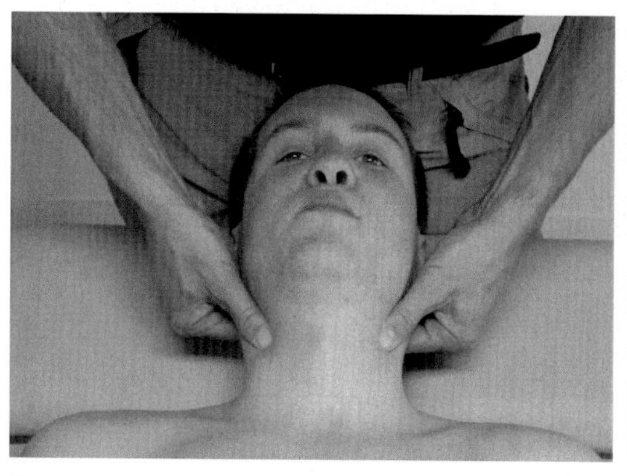

a

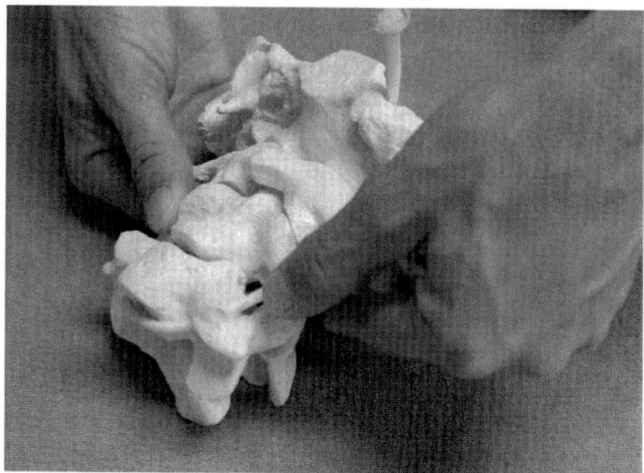

b

Fig. 6.13 Anterior shear test.

Interpretation

- Normally there should be no movement.

Posterior–anterior relative to C2 in upper cervical flexion

The posterior–anterior test on C2 is an adaptation of the Sharp–Purser test in supine.

Starting position

- Supine.
- The head is positioned in upper cervical flexion in the position of onset of symptoms.

Position of the examiner

- The examiner is sitting or standing behind the patient.

Fixation

- Both thenar eminences hold the head on either side.

Method

- Both middle fingers attempt to move C2 ventrally, relative to C1.

Interpretation

- In the case of an instability, this test will reduce subluxation (analogous to the Sharp–Purser test). This leads to the following findings:
  - Ventral movement
  - Possibly a palpable 'click'
  - Reduction of symptoms.

In the case of a hypomobility dysfunction the therapist will find:

- No noticeable movement
- No 'click'
- Possibly an increase of symptoms, since the occiput should perform a dorsal glide on upper cervical flexion.

Tectorial membrane

The tectorial membrane is an extension of the posterior longitudinal ligament. It is a large and strong ligament. It originates from the posterior vertebral body of C2, runs posterior to the dens and inserts at the ventral foramen magnum (Fig. 6.14) (Oda et al 1992, Harris et al 1993).

According to Pettman (1994), it is the primary stabilizer for distraction of the head on the neck. Furthermore, it assists the transverse ligament to stabilize C1–C2 flexion (Oda et al 1992, Harris et al 1993). Harris et al (1993) dissected the tectorial membrane and found instability on flexion but not extension. The study did not assess behaviour on head distraction.

Since the occiput moves ventrally on C1 during extension, Pettman (1994) hypothesized that the ligament is loaded in extension. Therefore the instability tests should be performed in end of range flexion, extension and in mid-position.

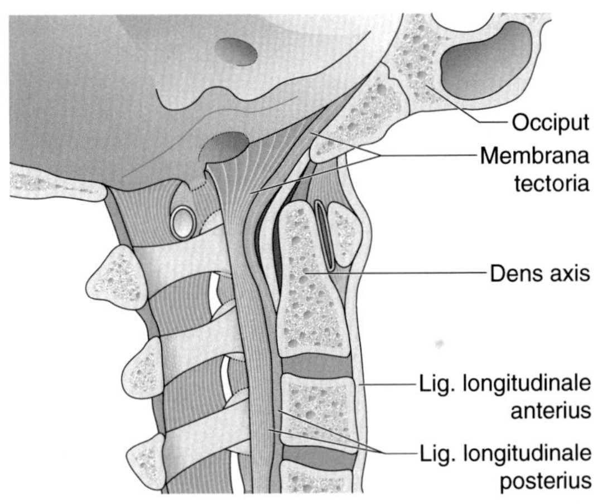

Fig. 6.14 Tectorial membrane (after Oda et al 1992).

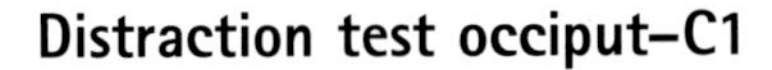

Distraction test occiput–C1

This test evaluates the integrity of the tectorial membrane (Fig. 6.15).

Starting position

- Supine.
- The head is rested on the hands of the examiner on the bench.
- Occiput–C1 is positioned in either end of range extension, end of range flexion or mid-position.

Position of the examiner

- The therapist is sitting or standing behind the patient.
- Both hands hold the head of the patient. Fingers 3–5 hold the occiput while the bases of the thumbs hold the head on either side.
- The tips of the thumbs palpate the space between the mastoid process and the transverse process of C1.

Fixation

- The bodyweight of the patient is sufficient for fixation.

Method

- By leaning backwards the examiner applies traction to the neck.

Interpretation

- The separation of mastoid process and transverse process C1 should be no more than 1 mm.

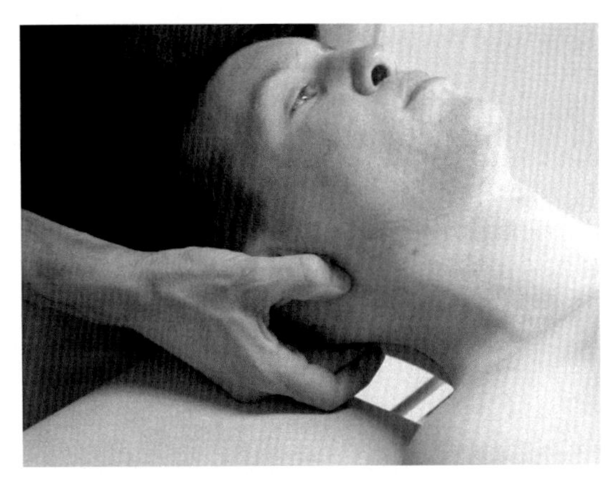

a

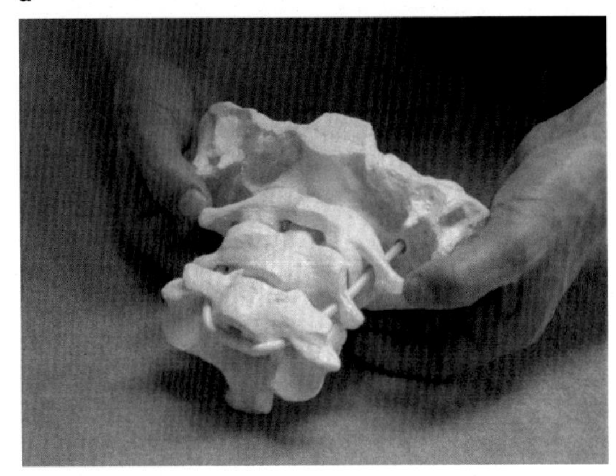

b

Fig. 6.15 Distraction test occiput–C1.

- In flexion as well as in extension the movement should feel 'tight'.

Linear stress occiput–C1 towards anterior (Fig. 6.16)

Starting position

- Supine with head on the bench.

Position of the examiner

- Standing or sitting behind the patient.
- Fingers 3–5 hold the occiput from dorsal.

Fixation

- Both thumbs carefully hold the C1 transverse processes from ventral.

Method

- Fingers 3–5 attempt to move the occiput ventrally.

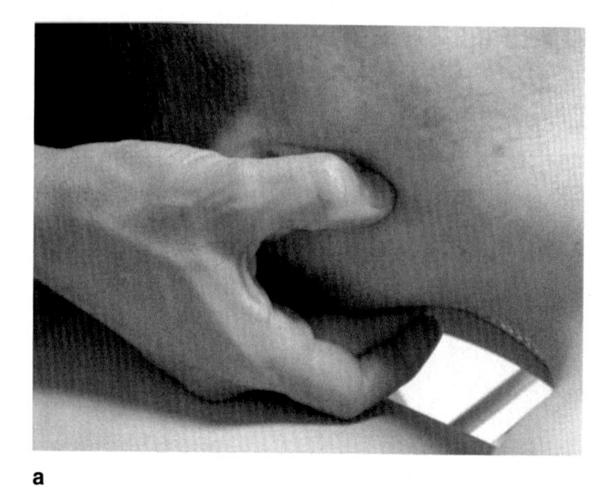

a

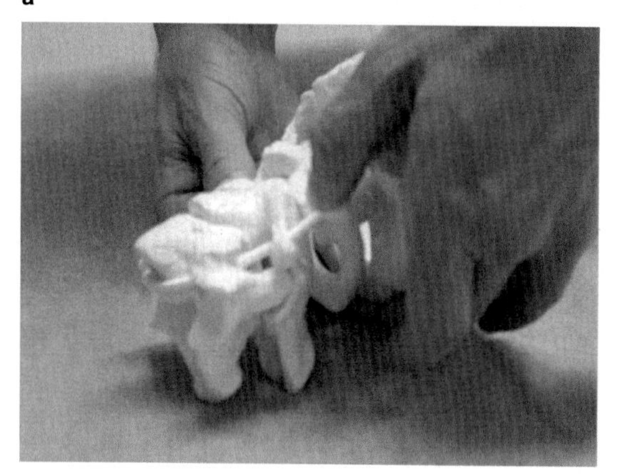

b

Fig. 6.16 Linear stress occiput–C1 towards anterior.

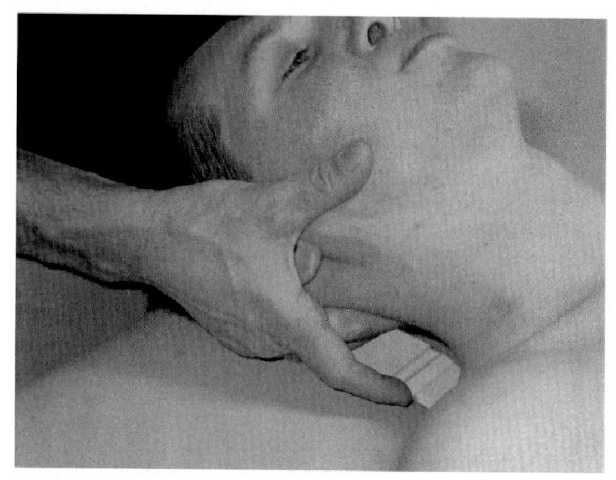

a

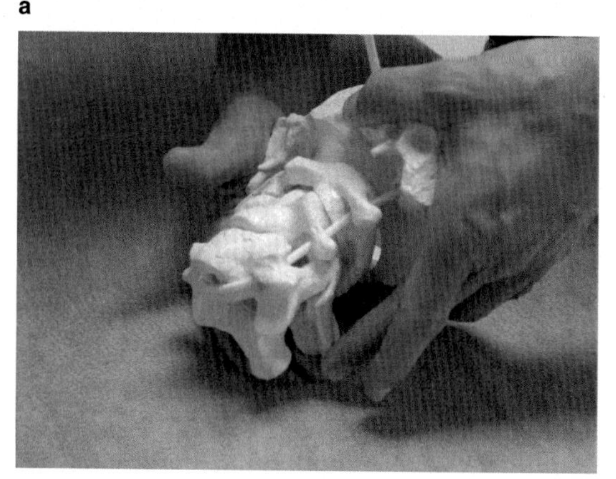

b

Fig. 6.17 Linear stress occiput–C2 towards anterior.

Interpretation

- Normally, no movement should be felt.

Linear stress occiput–C2 towards anterior (Fig. 6.17)

Starting position

- Supine with head on the bench.

Position of the examiner

- Standing or sitting behind the patient.
- Both middle fingers held against the spinous process of C2 from dorsal.

Fixation

- Both thenar eminences hold the head from either side.

Method

- Both middle fingers attempt to move C2 ventrally.

Interpretation

- Normally there should be no movement.
- It can be difficult to find a direct bony contact to C1 since it is covered by the suboccipital muscles. If the therapist attempts to palpate through the soft tissue this might feel like a movement and cause false-positive results.
- If both dens and transverse ligament are intact, the dens of C1 will move to anterior relative to the occiput during a posterior–anterior movement against C2.
- If there should be palpable movement the examination should be continued with atlantoaxial instability tests to evaluate whether the problem is caused by an occiput–C1 or by a C1–C2 instability.

Linear stress C2–C3 towards anterior (Fig. 6.18)

Starting position

- Supine with head on the bench.

Position of the therapist

- Standing or sitting behind the patient.

Fixation

- Both thumbs carefully fixate the C3 transverse processes from ventral.

Method

- With both middle fingers against the laminae, C2 is moved ventrally.

Interpretation

- Normally, there should be no movement.

The same principles apply for instability testing of C3–C7.

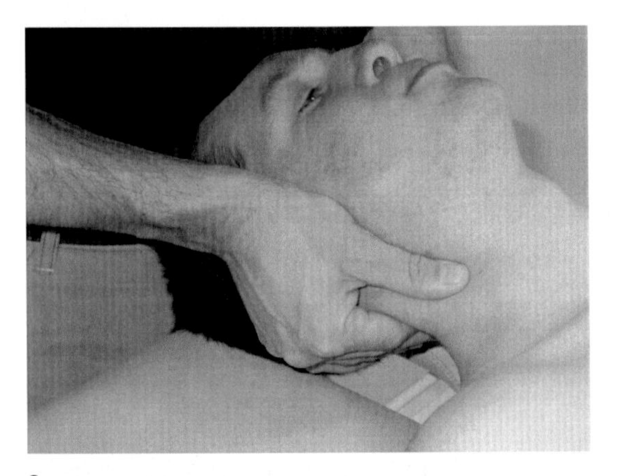

a

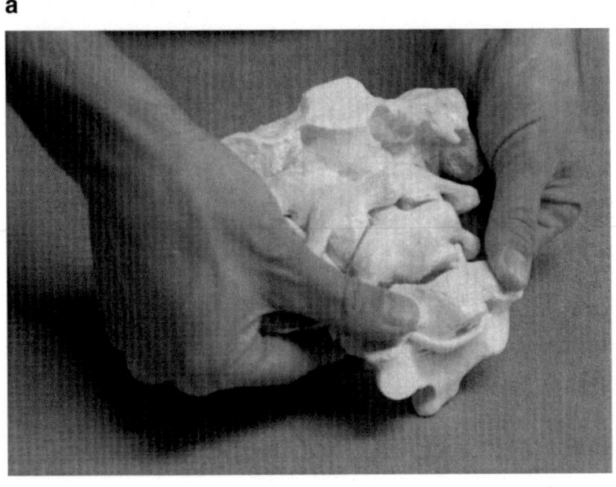

b

Fig. 6.18 Linear stress C2–C3 towards anterior.

Linear stress C3–C2 towards anterior (Fig. 6.19)

Starting position

- Supine with head on the bench.

Position of the examiner

- Standing or sitting behind the patient.

Fixation

- Both thumbs carefully hold the C2 transverse processes from ventral.

Method

- With the middle fingers against the C3 laminae, C3 is moved ventrally.

Interpretation

- Normally, there should be no movement.
- Clinically one will frequently reproduce symptoms with this test in patients with a dorsal extension instability.

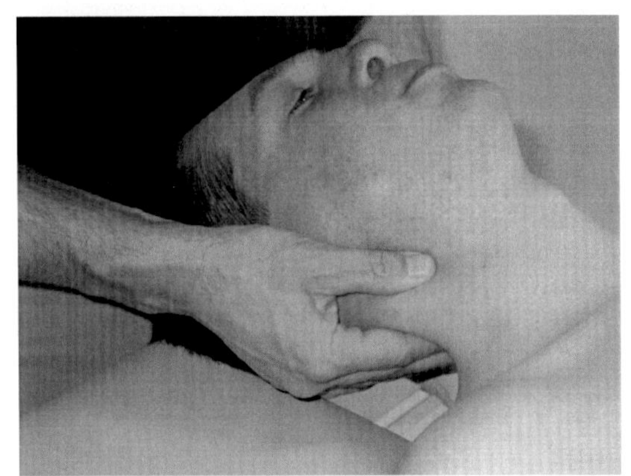

a

b

Fig. 6.19 Linear stress C3–C2 towards anterior.

The same principles apply for instability testing of C3–C7.

Transverse stress test to the left for C2–C7

The principle of the transverse stress test for C2–C7 is the same as for transverse stress test of occiput–C1 (Fig. 6.20). The cranial hand of the examiner attempts to move the occiput and the cranial segment that needs to be examined (e.g. C2) against the caudal segment (in this case C3) to the left.

PASSIVE ACCESSORY INTERVERTEBRAL MOVEMENTS (PAIVMS)

PAIVMs examine segmental mobility during accessory movements. For a detailed description of the techniques, see Maitland et al (2001).

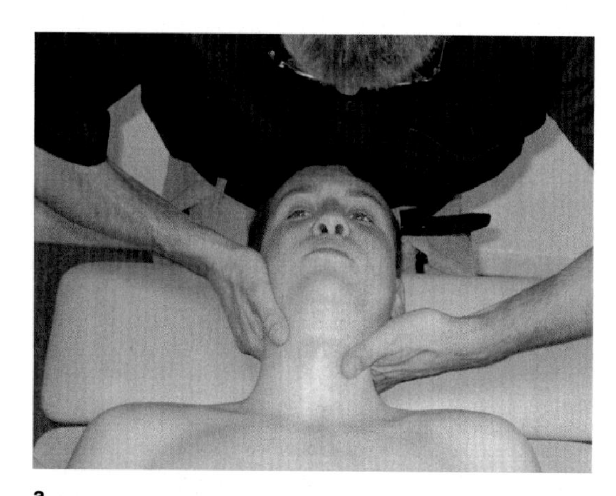

a

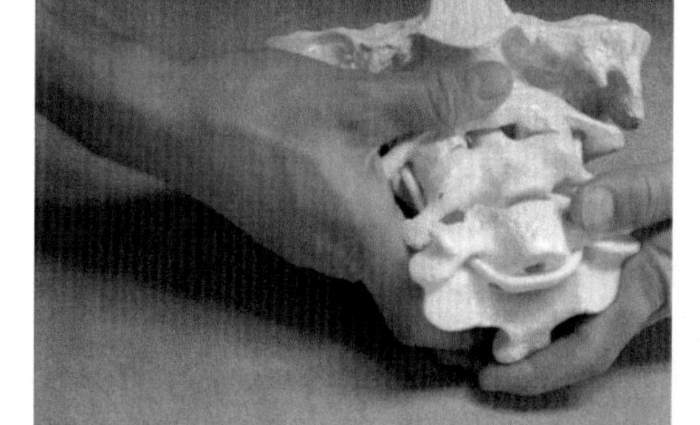

b

Fig. 6.20 Transverse stress test to the left, C2–C3.

A number of studies have confirmed the validity of manual assessment of intersegmental mobility. PPIVM and PAIVM techniques have been compared with discography, facet joint injection and ultrasound (Jull et al 1988, 1994, 1997, Hides et al 1994, Lord et al 1994, Philips & Twomey 1996).

Since most of these studies investigated validity of manual testing on hypomobile joints one cannot assume that the same applies for the examination of hypermobile/unstable joints.

MUSCLE CONTROL

Introduction

All muscles of the neck and shoulder girdle contribute to stability and control of the cervical spine. However, there is one group of muscles that functions mainly as stabilizers whereas other muscles dominantly produce movement (mobilizers) (Bergmark 1989, Conley et al 1995, Jull 2000, Sahrmann 2002).

Features of muscles which primarily serve for stabilization:

- They are monoarticular and are positioned near the joint in the deep muscle layers. Bergmark (1989) calls these muscles the 'local system'.
- Their fibres frequently insert into joint capsules and function as capsule tighteners (Taylor & Twomey 1986).
- Origin and insertion of the muscles are in close proximity to the joint. The resultant short leverage prevents muscle activity from producing major joint movement. Muscle contraction compresses the joint, thereby enhancing joint stability.
- According to Conley et al (1995), these muscles show a tonic activity essential for postural support.
- Mayoux-Benhamou et al (1995) demonstrated that, for example, the longus colli muscle functions as a stabilizer for the cervical lordosis.

The primary stabilizers of the neck are:

- Rectus capitis anterior and lateralis
- Longus colli

- Longus capitis
- Semispinalis cervicis
- Multifidus.

The first three muscles are called the 'deep cervical flexors'.

Features of the mobilizer muscles are:

- They are polyarticular and are therefore called 'global system' (Bergmark 1989). Since these muscles pass more than one segment they do not have the capacity to stabilize an individual segment.
- They are more superficially positioned. This enhances the force they can produce and therefore gives them the capacity to produce joint movement.
- According to Conley et al (1995), they normally do not show tonic activity.

The primary mobilizers of the neck are:

- Sternocleidomastoid (SCM)
- Scaleni
- Semispinalis capitis
- Splenius capitis.

For adequate stability during functional loading the primary stabilizers and the primary mobilizers will need to function in a state of balance (Sahrmann 2002). Studies have demonstrated that pathologies principally tend to affect the function of the local stabilizers (Hallgren et al 1994, Treleaven et al 1994, Watson 1994, McPartland et al 1997, Jull et al 1999, Jull 2000, Sterling et al 2001, Falla 2004, Falla et al 2004a, 2004b).

Uhlig et al (1995) stated that dysfunctions are not specific for any particular pathology and hypothesize that pain inhibition might be the cause of muscle insufficiency. Clinically, inhibition of flexor stabilizers seems more common than inhibition of extensors (Vernon 1992, Jull 1998). Inhibition of deep cervical flexor muscles produces anterior translation of the head. Watson and Trott (1993) found that headache patients show significantly greater head forward posture than control subjects. Muscles are therefore continuously forced into a stretched position and cannot generate sufficient force when repositioned to normal length. The muscle is actively insufficient (Sahrmann 2002).

To compensate for dysfunction of the deep cervical flexors, uninhibited superficial muscles (e.g. sternocleidomastoid) are activated and react with hyperactivity and muscle shortening. Jull et al (1999) therefore developed the 'graded craniocervical flexion test' which specifically assesses function of the deep cervical flexors.

Graded craniocervical flexion test (Fig. 6.21)

Starting position

- Supine with head on the bench.
- Cervical spine neutral.
- Teeth are slightly apart and the tongue is placed at the roof of the mouth and relaxed. This is to avoid hyperactivity of infra- and suprahyoid muscles.
- A 'pressure biofeedback unit' (PBU) is placed under the cervical lordosis.
- The PBU is adjusted to 20 mmHg.

Method

- To avoid hyperactivity of upper trapezius and levator scapulae muscles the patient is first asked to move the shoulder blades slightly backwards and downwards.
- The patient is instructed to perform an upper cervical flexion, a movement similar to the nodding of the head when saying 'yes'.
- This position is maintained for 10 seconds.
- It is important to perform the activity without any visible muscle force.
- The examiner carefully observes for compensation strategies (see below).

Interpretation

- If the deep cervical flexors are activated correctly the cervical lordosis will decrease and therefore increase the pressure on the PBU.
- For the graded craniocervical flexor test the pressure should first increase by just 2 mmHg to 22 mmHg. If this is achieved without superficial muscle substitution a further 2 mmHg is attempted. The test is continued until the patient is able to hold

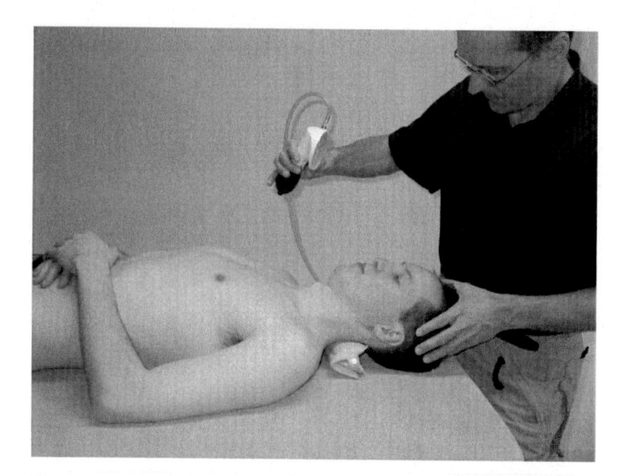

a

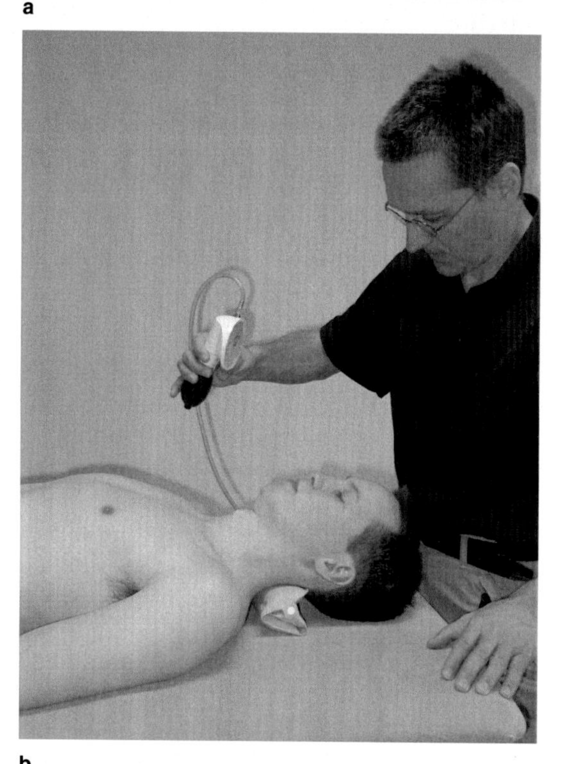

b

Fig. 6.21 Graded craniocervical flexion test with PBU.

30 mmHg without substitution 10 times for 10 seconds.

Variation

- Instead of a PBU the examiner may place a hand under the patient's head.
- The examiner's right hand is placed underneath the occiput; the fingers of the left hand support the cervical lordosis. The left thumb palpates for SCM activity (Fig. 6.22).
- If the patient performs the task correctly the pressure on the left hand will increase while the pressure on the right hand will not change.

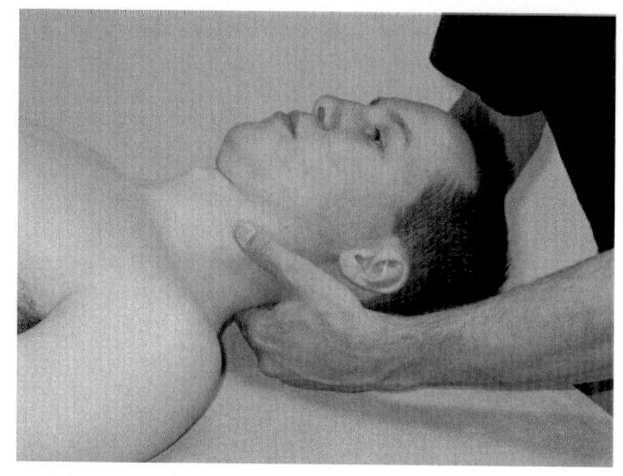

Fig. 6.22 Graded craniocervical flexion test with manual control.

How to control substitution strategies:

- Hyperactivity of SCM:
  - Ideally surface electrodes check for activity of SCM.
  - There should be no visible or palpable contraction of SCM.
  - The pressure of the occiput on the hand/bench should not decrease.
- Retraction of the head:
  - Some patients attempt to increase the pressure on the PBU by activating their extensor muscles. The pressure of the occiput should not increase.
- Hyperactivity of infra-/suprahyoid muscles:
  - The jaw should be relaxed.
  - The patient must be able to maintain pressure on the PBU while opening and closing the mouth.

Jull (2000) demonstrated that patients who suffered from neck pain after whiplash injury (minimum of 3 months after the accident) showed:

- Increased activity of SCM
- Greater difficulty in controlling deep cervical flexor activity.

Scapulothoracic muscles

As well as dysfunction of the deep cervical flexors, clinicians frequently observe dysfunction of the lower trapezius muscle (Jull 1998, Sahrmann 2002). Again substitution strategies apply. In this case it is principally the upper trapezius that becomes hyperactive. Nederhand et al (2000) examined the activity of upper trapezius in patients with chronic (>6 months) pain after whiplash injury. Compared to a control group they found:

- Increased activity on light arm usage
- Difficulties in relaxing the upper trapezius after arm activity.

Functional testing of the trapezius muscle pars ascendens (Fig. 6.23)

Starting position

- Lying prone with arms in 30° abduction.
- The physiotherapist positions the patient's scapula in a position of retraction, depression and slight upward rotation. The patient is asked to maintain this position.
- The other scapula is placed into the same position.

Method

- The therapist attempts to move the scapulae anterior/cranial/lateral with minimal pressure on the spinal scapulae while the patient tries to resist this pressure.

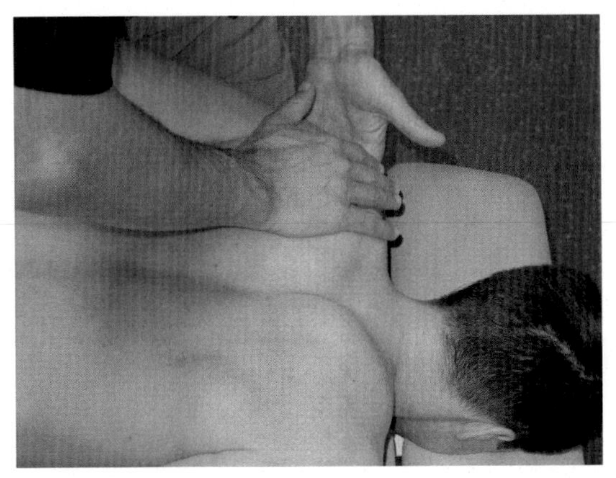

Fig. 6.23 Functional test for the trapezius muscle pars ascendens.

Interpretation and substitution strategies

- If the lower trapezius is weak the patient will not be able to maintain the starting position and will try to substitute lower trapezius by activating latissimus dorsi or the rhomboid muscles.
- Hyperactivity of the latissimus dorsi will adduct the arms and/or move them backwards. Overactivity of the rhomboids will move the inferior angle of the scapula medial and dorsal (medial rotation of the scapula).

Assessment of functional stability

As well as the specific muscle tests described above, the examiner will need to evaluate muscle control on active movements. The examiner may also decide to assess the stability of the cervical spine on functional loading. The patient is asked to perform activities of daily living while the examiner observes the capacity of the stabilizing muscles to maintain control of the neck. The following dysfunctions may be clinically relevant:

- Opening of the jaw is accompanied by cervical extension (Fig. 6.24).
- Arm elevation is accompanied by neck extension (Fig. 6.25).
- Bending forward while standing produces a hingeing of the lower cervical spine.

CASE REPORT

History

A 28-year-old female complains of burning pain at the radial side of her left forearm (Fig. 6.26). Furthermore, she has a slight numbness of the left thumb and a dull ache in the neck. During the subjective examination she confirms a loss of muscle strength (she finds it difficult to carry her breakfast plate) which supports the hypothesis of nerve root dysfunction.

The arm symptoms are continuously present, and increase with computer work (30 minutes) and during the night. Extension of the neck (her hobby is climbing which involves

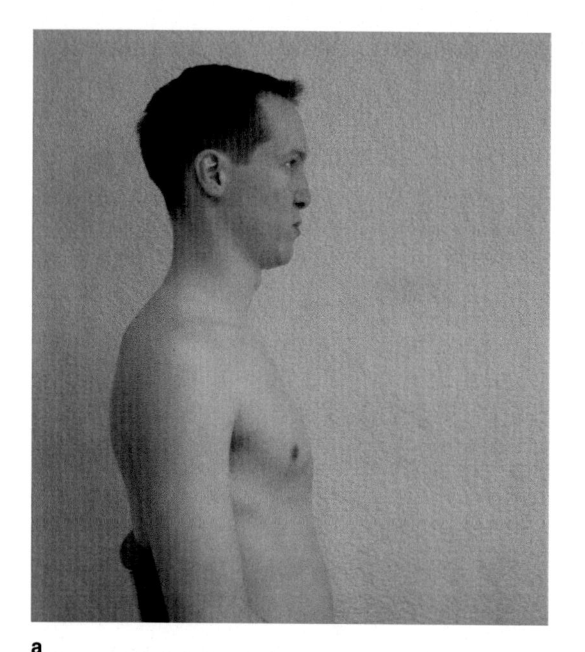

a

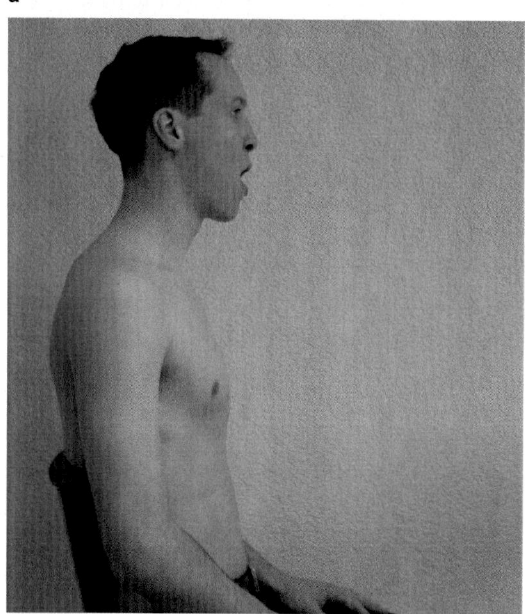

b

Fig. 6.24 Functional instability on mouth opening.

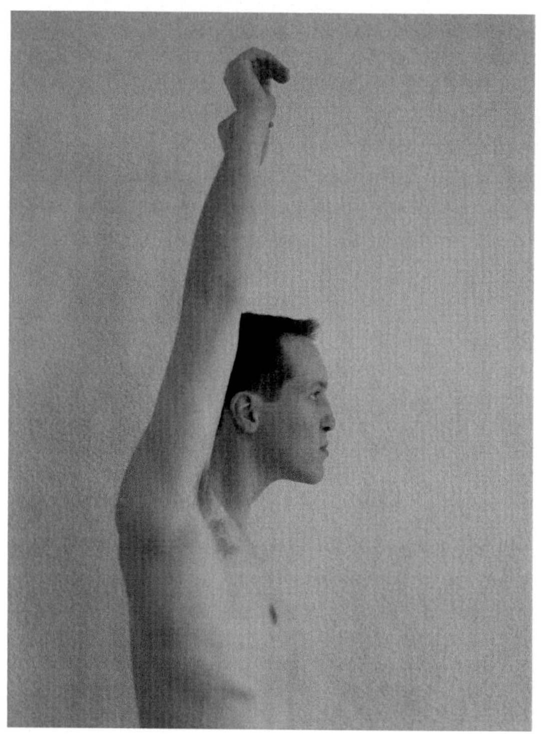

Fig. 6.25 Functional instability on elevation of the arms.

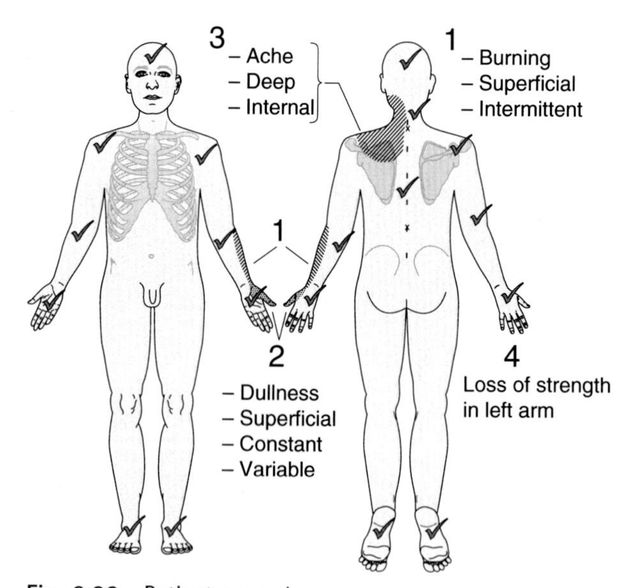

Fig. 6.26 Patient example.

protracted neck extension) increases the symptoms in her neck. The more she provokes neck symptoms the more intense she will feel her arm symptoms within the next few hours.

Generally she suffers more in the evenings. Her neck feels very tired at night and she needs to lie down to support the neck. Six days ago she slipped three times while walking downhill and fell on her bottom. This caused a strong impact on her neck. That night she woke at 4 a.m. with a tingling sensation and a burning pain in her arm.

Previous history shows that she had experienced four episodes of a stiff neck within the past 5 years which had been treated successfully by a chiropractor (>20 manipulations). The patient works full time in administration. Her hobbies are jogging, mountain biking and climbing (6 hours/week). As a child she did gymnastics and has always been very flexible.

No x-rays have been taken and the patient does not use any medications.

Hypothesis and plan for physical examination

The following facts support the hypothesis of cervical instability:

- General hypermobility
- Torticollis
- More than 20 manipulations
- Tiredness of the neck in the evenings
- A relatively small event causes radicular symptoms.

The physical examination will be performed without the use of overpressure. A radicular inflammation is assumed because of:

- Symptoms at the C6 dermatome
- Loss of muscle strength
- Increase of symptoms during the night.

A neurological examination is therefore compulsory.

Since the nerve root C6 leaves the spinal canal between the segments of C5 and C6 these segments will need special attention during the examination.

Physical examination

Present pain

- Burning of the forearm with VAS intensity of 2/10.

Inspection

- Mild flattened cervical lordosis.

Active movements

- Extension limited at 40°, pronounced 'hingeing' at the lower cervical spine.
- On return from extension the chin is pushed forwards and she describes a 'jamming' of the neck.
- Rotation to the left is 90°.
- Rotation to the right is 80° with a slight pulling sensation in the neck.
- Side bending is normal.
- At the end of the active movements she feels a slight increase of her symptoms (2.5/10 VAS).

Neurological examination

- Sensitivity of the left thumb is reduced.
- Strength of biceps and extensor carpi radialis muscles are 4/5.
- Biceps reflex is weak.

Neurodynamic examination

- ULNT 1 (upper limb neurodynamic test) of the right arm is limited at 5° elbow extension and the patient feels a pulling at the medial elbow. This is reduced by cervical lateroflexion to the right (a normal reaction).
- ULNT 1 of the left arm is limited at –10° elbow extension and the patient complains of tingling of her thumb. Lateroflexion to the left improves the tingling.

Passive physiological intervertebral movements

- Hypermobility of C4–C5 and C5–C6 extension.
- No stiffness of the neighbouring joints.

Linear movements

- Posteroanterior movement of C6 against C5 shows segmental instability.
- The patient complains of a local stabbing pain during that movement.

- Transverse linear movement of C5 to the left is also positive.

Passive accessory movements

- C5–C6 shows an increased neutral zone.
- The general range of motion is increased.
- At reassessment cervical extension and ULNT 1 left are unchanged. Resting pain is increased to 3/10 VAS.

Analysis of the results and treatment plan

- The neurological examination confirms a C6 radicular syndrome.
- Neurodynamic tests are only slightly affected, therefore disc contribution to the nerve root pain is not likely.
- The results of active movements and passive testing support the hypothesis that C5–C6 instability causes the radicular symptoms.
- Since no hypomobilities were found, end of range mobilization is not indicated.
- The focus of the physiotherapy treatment should be on cervical stabilization exercises.
- To prepare the segments for the stabilization, light mobilizations (grade II = large amplitude before onset of resistance) of the unstable segments can be helpful.

References

Adams M A 1999 Biomechanics of the intervertebral disc, vertebra, and ligaments. In: Szpalski M, Gunzburg R, Pope M H (eds) Lumbar segmental instability. Lippincott, Williams and Wilkins, Philadelphia, p 3–13

Aspinall W 1990 Clinical testing for craniovertebral hypermobility syndrome. Journal of Orthopaedic and Sports Physical Therapy 12:47–54

Barnsley L, Lord S, Bogduk N 1993 Whiplash injury. Pain 58:283–307

Bergmark A 1989 Stability of the lumbar spine. A study in mechanical engineering. Acta Orthopaedica Scandinavica 230(Suppl):20–24

Bogduk N 1981 An anatomical basis for the neck–tongue syndrome. Journal of Neurology, Neurosurgery and Psychiatry 44:202–208

Bogduk N 2001 Mechanisms and pain patterns of the upper cervical spine. In: Vernon H (ed.) The cranio-cervical syndrome. Butterworth-Heinemann, Oxford, p 110–116

Brodeur R R 2001 Biomechanics of the upper cervical spine. In: Vernon H (ed.) The cranio-cervical syndrome. Butterworth-Heinemann, Oxford, p 88–109

Cattrysse E, Swinkels R A H M, Oostendorp R A B et al 1997 Upper cervical instability: are clinical tests reliable? Manual Therapy 2:91–97

Clemente C D 1985 Gray's anatomy, 13th American edition. Lea and Febiger, Philadelphia

Coman W B 1986 Dizziness related to ENT conditions. In: Grieve G P (ed.) Modern manual therapy of the vertebral column. Churchill Livingstone, Edinburgh, p 28

Conley M S, Meyer R A, Bloomberg J J, Feeback D L, Dudley G A 1995 Noninvasive analysis of human neck muscle function. Spine 23:2505–2512

Delphini R, Dorizzi A, Facchinetti G et al 1999 Delayed post-traumatic cervical instability. Surgical Neurology 51:588–595

Dvorak J, Panjabi M 1987 Functional anatomy of the alar ligaments. Spine 2:183–189

Eisenstein S M 1999 'Instability' and low back pain: a way out of the semantic maze. In: Szpalski M, Gunzburg R, Pope M H (eds) Lumbar segmental instability. Lippincott, Williams and Wilkins, Philadelphia, p 39–51

Endo K, Ichimaru K, Shimura H et al 2000 Cervical vertigo after hair shampoo treatment at a hairdressing salon. Spine 25:632–634

Falla D 2004 Unravelling the complexity of muscle impairment in chronic neck pain. Manual Therapy 9:125–133

Falla D, Bilekij G, Jull G 2004a Patients with chronic neck pain demonstrate altered patterns of muscle activation during performance of a functional upper limb task. Spine 29(13):1436–1440

Falla D, Jull G, Hodges P 2004b Patients with neck pain demonstrate reduced electromyographic activity of the deep cervical flexor muscles during performance of the craniocervical flexion test. Spine 29(19):2108–2114

Fielding J, Cochran G, Lawsing J, Hohl M 1974 Tears of the transverse ligament of the atlas: a clinical and biomechanical study. Journal of Bone and Joint Surgery 56:1683–1691

Foreman S M, Croft A C 1995 Whiplash injuries. The cervical acceleration/deceleration syndrome, 2nd edn. Williams and Wilkins, Baltimore
Hallgren R C, Greenman P E, Rechtien J J 1994 Atrophy of suboccipital muscles in patients with chronic pain: a pilot study. Journal of the American Osteopathic Association 94:1032–1038
Harris M, Duval M, Davis J et al 1993 Anatomical and roentgenographic features of atlanto-occipital instability. Journal of Spinal Disorders 6:5–10
Heikkiläa H V, Astrom P G 1996 Cervicocephalic kinesthetic sensibility in patients with whiplash injury. Scandinavian Journal of Rehabilitation Medicine 28:133–138
Herkowitz H, Rothman R H 1984 Subacute instability of the cervical spine. Spine 9:348–357
Hides J A, Stokes M J, Saide M, Jull G A, Cooper D H 1994 Evidence of lumbar multifidus wasting ipsilateral to symptoms in patients with acute/subacute low back pain. Spine 19:165–172
Hino H, Abumi K, Kanayama M, Kaneda K 1999 Dynamic motion analysis of normal and unstable cervical spines using cineradiography Spine 24:163–168
Hodges P W, Richardson C A, Jull G A 1996 Inefficient stabilisation of the lumbar spine associated with low back pain: a motor evaluation of transverse abdominus. Spine 21:2640–2650
Jonsson H, Bring G, Rauschning W, Sahlstedt B 1991 Hidden cervical spine injuries in traffic accident victims with skull fractures Journal of Spinal Disorders 4:251–263
Jull G A 1997 Management of cervical headache. Manual Therapy 2:182–190
Jull G A 1998 Physiotherapy management of neck pain of mechanical origin. In: Giles L G F, Singer K P (eds) Clinical anatomy and management of the cervical spine. Butterworth-Heinemann, Oxford, p 168–191
Jull G A 2000 Deep cervical flexor muscle dysfunction in whiplash. Journal of Musculoskeletal Pain 8:143–154
Jull G, Bogduk N, Marsland A 1988 The accuracy of manual diagnosis for cervical zygapophyseal joint pain syndromes. Medical Journal of Australia 148:233–236
Jull G, Treleaven J, Versace G 1994 Manual examination: is pain provocation a major cue for spinal dysfunction? Australian Physiotherapy 40:159–165
Jull G, Zito G, Trott P, Potter H, Shirley D, Richardson C 1997 Inter-examiner reliability to detect painful upper cervical joint dysfunction. Australian Physiotherapy 43:125–129
Jull G A, Barrett C, Magee R, Ho P 1999 Further clinical clarification of the muscle dysfunction in cervical headache. Cephalalgia 19:179–185
Karlberg M, Magnusson M, Malström E-M et al 1996 Postural and symptomatic improvement after physiotherapy in patients with dizziness of suspected cervical origin. Archives of Physical and Medical Rehabilitation 77:874–882
Kettler A, Hartwig E, Schultheiss M et al 2002 Mechanically simulated muscle forces strongly stabilize intact and injured upper cervical spine specimens. Journal of Biomechanics 35:339–346
Lance J W, Anthony M 1980 Neck–tongue syndrome on sudden turning of the head. Journal of Neurology, Neurosurgery and Psychiatry 43:97–101
Laurén H, Luoto S, Alaranta H et al 1997 Arm motion speed and risk of neck pain. Spine 22:2094–2099
Lomoschitz F M, Blackmore C C, Mirza S K, Mann F A 2002 Cervical spine injuries in patients 65 years old and older: epidemiologic analysis regarding the effects of age and injury mechanism on distribution, type, and stability of injuries. American Journal of Roentgenology 178:573–577
Lord S M, Barnsley L, Wallis B J, Bogduk N 1994 Third occipital nerve headache: a prevalence study. Journal of Neurology, Neurosurgery and Psychiatry 57:1187–1190
Maitland G D, Hengeveld E, Banks K, English K 2001 Maitland's vertebral manipulation, 6th edn. Butterworth-Heinemann, Oxford
Mayoux-Benhamou M A, Revel M, Vallee C et al 1995 Longus colli has a postural function on cervical curvature. Surgical and Radiologic Anatomy 16:367–371
McDermaid C 2001 Vertebrobasilar incidents and spinal manipulative therapy of the cervical spine. In: Vernon H (ed.) The cranio-cervical syndrome. Butterworth-Heinemann, Oxford, p 244–253
McLain R F 1994 Mechanoreceptor endings in human cervical facet joints. Spine 19:495–501
McPartland J, Brodeur R R, Hallgreen R C 1997 Chronic neck pain, standing balance, and suboccipital muscle atrophy – a pilot study. Journal of Manipulative and Physiological Therapeutics 20:24–29
Mendel T, Wink C S, Zimny M L 1992 Neural elements in human cervical intervertebral discs. Spine 17:132–135
Moseley G L, Hodges P W, Gandevia S C 2002 Deep and superficial fibers of the lumbar multifidus muscle are differentially active during voluntary arm movements. Spine 27:E29–E36
Nederhand M, Ijzerman M, Hermens H et al 2000 Cervical muscle dysfunction in the chronic whiplash associated disorder, Grade II. Spine 25:1938–1943
O'Sullivan P B, Twomey L, Allison G 1997 Evaluation of specific stabilising exercise in the treatment of chronic low back pain with radiological diagnosis

of spondylosis or spondylolisthesis. Spine 22:2959–2967

Oda T, Panjabi M M, Crisco J J et al 1992 Role of the tectorial membrane in the stability of the upper cervical spine. Clinical Biomechanics 7:201–207

Panjabi M M 1992a The stabilising system of the spine. Part I: Function, dysfunction, adaption, and enhancement. Journal of Spinal Disorders 5:383–389

Panjabi M M 1992b The stabilizing system of the spine. Part II: Neutral zone and instability hypothesis. Journal of Spinal Disorders 5:390–397

Panjabi M M, Dvorak J, Crisco J et al 1991a Flexion, extension, and lateral bending of the upper cervical spine in response to alar ligament transactions. Journal of Spinal Disorders 4:157–167

Panjabi M M, Dvorak J, Crisco J et al 1991b Effect of alar ligament transaction on upper cervical spine rotation. Journal of Orthopedic Research 9:584–593

Panjabi M M, Lydon C, Vasavada A, Grob D, Crisco J J, Dvorak J 1994 On the understanding of clinical instability. Spine 19:2642–2650

Penning L 1998 Normal kinematics of the cervical spine. In: Giles L G F, Singer K P (eds) Clinical anatomy and management of the cervical spine. Butterworth-Heinemann, Oxford, p 53–70

Pettman E 1994 Stress tests of the craniovertebral joints. In: Boyling J D, Palastanga N (eds) Grieve's modern manual therapy. The vertebral column, 2nd edn. Churchill Livingstone, Edinburgh, p 529–537

Philips D R, Twomey L T 1996 A comparison of manual diagnosis with a diagnosis established by a uni-level lumbar spinal block procedure. Manual Therapy 2:82–87

Pitkanen M, Manninen H I, Lindgrer K A et al 1997 Limited usefulness of traction–compression films in the radiographic diagnosis of lumbar v spinal instability: comparison with flexion–extension films. Spine 22:193–197

Pope M H, Panjabi M M 1985 Diagnosing instability. Clinical Orthopaedics 279:60–67

Rydevik B L, Olmarker K 1999 Instability and sciatica. In: Szpalski M, Gunzburg R, Pope M H (eds) Lumbar segmental instability. Lippincott, Williams and Wilkins, Philadelphia, p 75–84

Sahrmann S A 2002 Diagnosis and treatment of movement impairment syndromes. Mosby, St Louis

Sanchez Martin M M 1992 Occipital–cervical instability. Clinical Orthopaedics and Related Research 283:63–73

Sharp J, Purser D W 1961 Spontaneous atlanto-axial dislocation in ankylosing spondylitis and rheumatoid arthritis. Annals of the Rheumatic Diseases 20:47–77

Siegmund G P, Myers B S, Davis M B 2001 Mechanical evidence of cervical facet capsule injury during whiplash. Spine 26:2095–2101

Spitzer W O, Skovron M L, Salmi L R et al 1995 Scientific monograph of the Quebec Taskforce on whiplash-associated disorders: redefining 'whiplash' and its management. Spine 20:10S–68S

Sterling M, Jull G, Wright A 2001 The effect of musculoskeletal pain on motor activity and control. Journal of Pain 2:135–145

Taylor J R, Twomey L T 1986 Lumbar multifidus: 'rotator cuff' muscles of the zygapophyseal joints. Journal of Anatomy 149:266–267

Taylor J R, Twomey L T 1993 Acute injuries to cervical joints. Spine 18:1115–1122

Treleaven J, Jull, G A, Atkinson L 1994 Cervical musculoskeletal dysfunction in post-concussional headache. Cephalalgia 14:273–279

Twomey L T, Taylor J R 1991 Age related changes of the lumbar spine and spinal rehabilitation. Physical and Rehabilitation Medicine 2:153–169

Uhlig Y, Weber B R, Grob D 1995 Fiber composition and fiber transformations in neck muscles of patients with dysfunction of the cervical spine. Journal of Orthopedic Research 13:240–249

Uitvlugt G, Indenbaum S 1988 Clinical assessment of atlantoaxial instability using the Sharp–Purser test. Arthritis and Rheumatism 31(7):918–922

Vernon H T, Aker P, Aramenko M et al 1992 Evaluation of neck muscle strength with a modified sphygmomanometer dynamometer: reliability and validity. Journal of Manipulative and Physiological Therapeutics 15:343–349

Watson D A 1994 Cervical headache: an investigation of natural head posture and upper cervical flexor muscle performance. In: Boyling J D, Palastanga N (eds) Grieve's modern manual therapy. The vertebral column, 2nd edn. Churchill Livingstone, Edinburgh, p 349–359

Watson D A, Trott P 1993 Cervical headache: an investigation of natural head posture and upper cervical flexor muscle performance. Cephalalgia 13:272–284

Wenngren B I, Toolanen G, Hildingsson C 1998 Oculomotor dysfunction in rheumatoid patients with upper cervical dislocation. Acta Otolaryngologica 118:609–612

White A A, Panjabi M M 1990 Clinical biomechanics of the spine, 2nd edn. Lippincott, Philadelphia

White A A, Bernhardt M, Panjabi M M 1999 Clinical biomechanics and lumbar spinal instability. In: Szpalski M, Gunzburg R, Pope M H (eds) Lumbar segmental instability. Lippincott, Williams and Wilkins, Philadelphia, p 15–25

Wiesel S, Rothman R 1979 Occipitoatlantal hypermobility. Spine 4:187–191

Willauschus W, Kladny B, Beyer W et al 1995 Lesions of the alar ligaments. Spine 20:2493–2498

Wilmink J T, Patijn J 2001 MR imaging of alar ligament in whiplash-associated disorders: an observer study. Neuroradiology 43: 859–863

Winters J M, Peles J D 1990 Neck muscle activity and 3D kinematics during quasistatic and dynamic tracking movements. In: Winters J M, Woolsley H (eds) Multiple muscle systems: biomechanics and movement organisation. Springer, New York, p 461–480

Zhu Q, Ouyang J, Lu W et al 1999 Traumatic instabilities of the cervical spine caused by high-speed axial compression in a human model. Spine 24:440–444

Chapter 7

Treatment and management of cervical instability

Pieter Westerhuis

CHAPTER CONTENTS

INTRODUCTION

When planning treatment the therapist will need to analyse and prioritize individual findings. During this process the therapist will need to consider particular hypotheses categories (Butler 1998, Gifford 2000).

This chapter will focus principally on peripheral nociceptive pain mechanisms. Peripheral nociceptive symptoms are consistently dependent on activities, positions and loading (Gifford 2002a). The primary sources of the symptoms are found in the craniocervical region and healing has reached the stage of consolidation and reorganization (from day 21) (van den Berg 1999). The treatment examples will focus on structures and function of the neck.

For further information on aspects of treatment of patients with predominantly central pain mechanisms or with problems predominantly at the level of participation, see Gifford (2002a, 2002b).

TREATING NEUROMUSCULOSKELETAL DYSFUNCTION

Dysfunction of the neuromusculoskeletal system causes abnormal movements and may lead to symptoms. Symptoms may again cause abnormal muscle activity (Svensson & Graven-Nielsen 2001). Sterling et al (2001a) described the following musculoskeletal pains in their literature review:

- Increased activity of superficial muscles, e.g. sternocleidomastoid
- Decreased activity of the deep stabilizing muscles, e.g. longus colli
- Changes of the neural control of muscles
- Proprioceptive deficits.

These changes may persist even after the acute symptoms have subsided (Hides et al 1996). This may be a contributory factor for the persistence of symptoms or for relapses (Hides et al 2001). The result is a *vicious circle*: dysfunction – symptoms – abnormal muscle activity – dysfunction.

The treatment will therefore need to address the various neuromusculoskeletal aspects of the syndrome. Since pain of the motor segments inhibits physiological muscle function, the joints should be approached before muscular control exercises are attempted (Stokes & Young 1984).

Sterling et al (2001b) demonstrated how mobilization of the lower cervical spine in patients with unilateral cervical pain decreases sternocleidomastoid activity in the graded craniocervical flexor test. Management of an instability problem should therefore include the following components:

- Treatment of the joints
- Treatment of the muscles
- Treatment of neurodynamics
- Contributory factors.

TREATING JOINT DYSFUNCTION

For a detailed description of joint mobilization techniques, see Maitland et al (2001). Functional cervical instabilities are commonly found in combination with the following joint dysfunctions:

- Hypomobile painful joints
- Hypomobile adjacent joints
- Unstable painful joints.

Hypomobile painful joints

Figure 7.1 shows the movement diagram of lateroflexion occiput–C1 to the right. Applicable

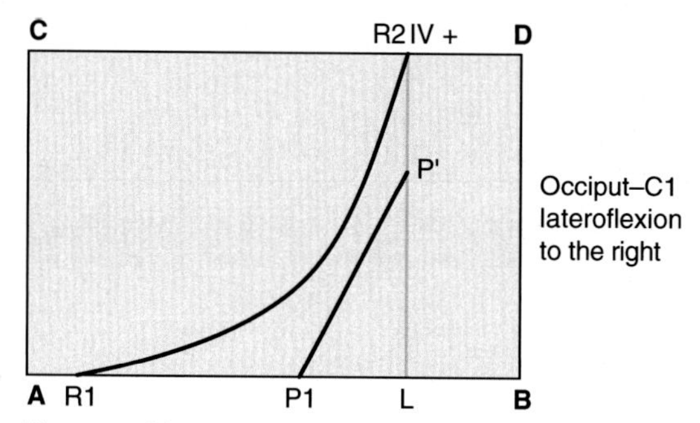

Fig. 7.1 Movement diagram showing a restricted range of lateroflexion to the right. Pain at the end of range is 6/10 VAS.

treatment techniques are grade IV mobilizations, a small amplitude oscillation at the limit of range of movement (Maitland et al 2001). The initial techniques should not provoke any symptoms. If the reassessment does not show any improvement, mobilization can be progressed until pain is produced. It is important that the pain comes and goes in rhythm with the oscillation and that its intensity does not increase.

Passive accessory intervertebral movements (PAIVMs) are techniques worth considering, for example left unilateral posterior–anterior mobilization of C1. Sterling et al (2001b) demonstrated that unilateral posterior–anterior mobilization of the lower cervical segments decreased local pain perception and also decreased symptoms on end of range rotation. If local hypersensitivity does not allow for direct techniques, indirect techniques such as lateral flexion to avoid manual contact with the painful segments can be considered.

If the patient has been assessed for contraindications, manipulations such as unilateral posterior–anterior thrust occiput–C1 might also prove beneficial (Fig. 7.2).

Hypomobile adjacent joints

Hypomobility of adjacent joints causes an increased load and hypermobility of the neighbouring segments. To reduce the load, hypomobility should be treated by manual therapy, being careful not to accidentally load the adjacent hypermobile joints.

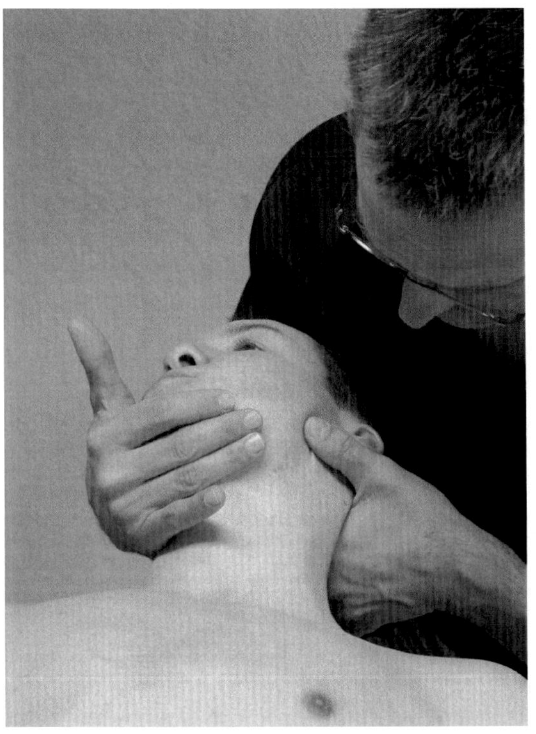

Fig. 7.2 Unilateral posterior–anterior mobilization of C1 on the left.

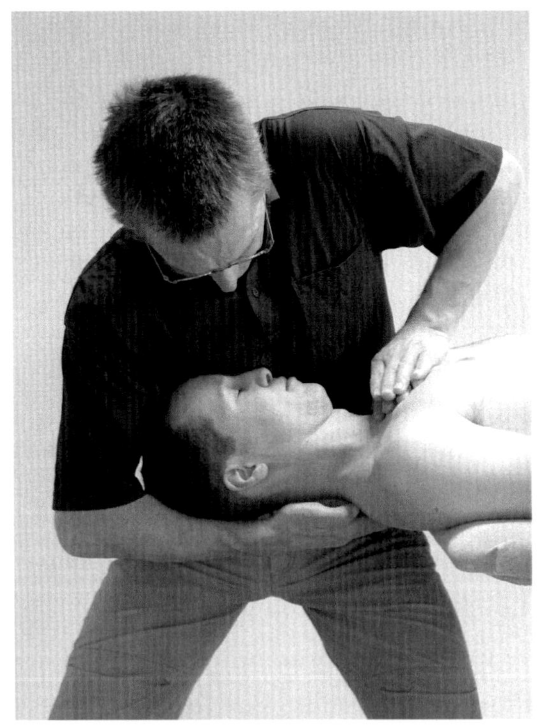

Fig. 7.3 Anterior–posterior mobilization T4–T5 via the sternum.

Example 1

Patient A has hypomobility of the cervicothoracic junction on extension and rotation to the right and instability/hypermobility in the upper craniocervical segments.

The following techniques might be beneficial:

- Anterior–posterior mobilization through the sternum (Fig. 7.3).
- Localized rotation to the right. The right hand holds the seventh cervical segment and is primarily responsible for the rotation/mobilization.
- Automobilization of the craniothoracic junction: The patient sits on a chair with the fourth to sixth thoracic segments against the backrest of the chair, folding their hands behind their neck and the craniocervical area. The patient then draws in the stomach to avoid compensatory movements of the lumbar spine and mobilizes the thoracic spine into extension.

Example 2

Patient B has hypomobility of the upper two cervical segments on rotation to the left. The patient also shows compensatory hypermobility of the lower cervical segments on extension and rotation to the left. Since rotation to the left is coupled with lateroflexion to the right, the therapist may decide to mobilize the upper segments by lateroflexion to the right (see also Chapter 6). This would lead to an increase in upper cervical rotation to the left without overstressing the lower segments.

For the automobilization technique the patient will need a large towel. The patient sits on a chair with the towel behind the neck. The patient's hands are crossed in such a manner that the right hand holds the left end of the towel and is positioned underneath the left hand which holds the right end of the towel. The edge of the towel is placed on the left side of the dorsal articular process of C3 and on the right onto the articular processes of C1 or C2. The patient's right hand pulls on the towel to fix C3 while they attempt to turn the head to the left supported by the left hand which also pulls on the end of the towel.

Unstable painful joints

For patients with structural instabilities passive mobilization of the unstable joints is not the first choice. Priorities are rather mobilization of adjacent hypomobile joints and muscle control.

From a clinical point of view, grade II mobilizations might still be an option to reduce sensitivity of the hypermobile segments (Maitland et al 2001). The Maitland Concept defines grade II mobilizations as oscillating movements with a large amplitude without resistance. These mobilizations do not aim to increase the passive range of motion but rather to positively influence pain perception by offering non-nociceptive joint input (Melzack 1996).

Thus, for example, a patient with midcranio-cervical instability could be treated in the supine position by unilateral posterior–anterior mobilization (Fig. 7.4).

TREATING NEURAL STRUCTURES

Introduction

Instability of a mobile segment might cause nerve root irritations (Rydevik & Olmarker 1999). In this case dysfunction of neurodynamics is a secondary problem. Clinically, one will often find that neurodynamic signs will improve automatically with increased stability of the unstable segment. Therefore it is not surprising that ULNT 1 (upper limb neurodynamic test) will show increased elbow extension after activation of the deep cervical flexor muscles.

Detailed instructions, techniques and management of neural mobilization are described in Hall and Elvey (1999) and in Butler (2000).

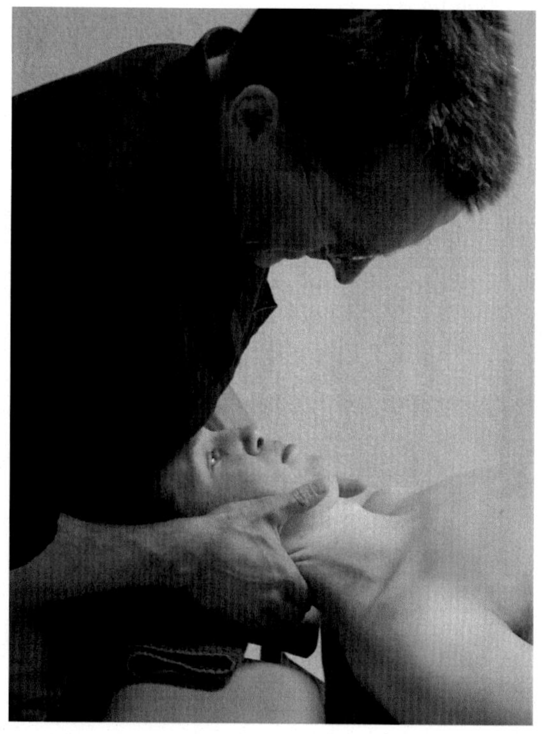

Fig. 7.4 Unilateral posterior–anterior mobilization on the right side.

A commonly applied technique to improve sensitivity and mobility of the nervous system is the sideglide technique.

Sideglide to the left

Starting position

- The patient is supine with the head positioned just beyond the edge of the bed.

Position of the examiner

- The therapist is standing behind the patient.
- The patient's head is positioned in the left hand and is supported against the stomach of the therapist (Fig. 7.5).
- The patient's hands rest on their stomach.

Fixation

- The therapist's left hand holds C4 from dorsal and the left index finger is placed on the right side of the patient's neck.

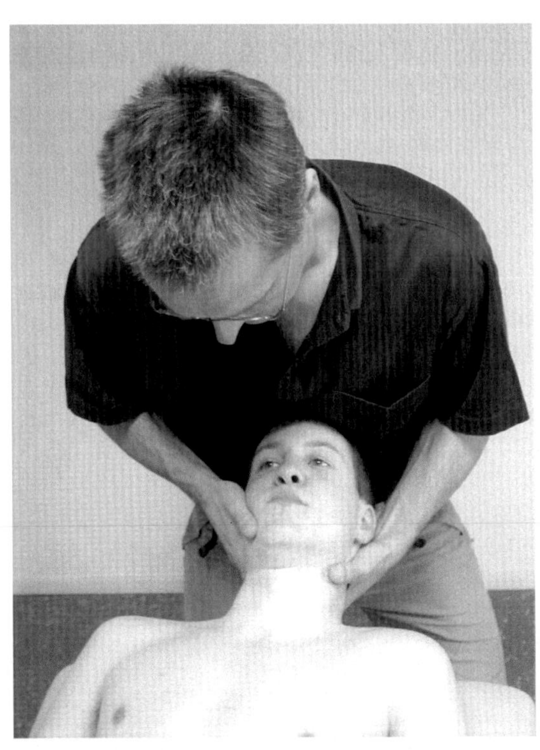

Fig. 7.5 Lateral glides to the left for the midcervical spine.

- The right hand is at the side of the neck as far down as C4, taking care not to apply pressure on the spinal nerves.

Method

- By transferring weight to the left leg, the therapist moves the upper body, and with it the patient's head sideways to the left.
- This transverse movement should be performed slowly with a large amplitude.

Interpretation

- Initially the movement should stop before any resistance is felt.
- To increase the intensity one might then decide to move into resistance. To control the elevation of the right shoulder of the patient, the therapist can put their right hand onto the patient's acromion.
- A further increase in intensity can be achieved by positioning the patient's right arm in elbow extension and slight abduction of the shoulder (Fig. 7.6).

Validity of the therapeutic approaches

Vicenzino et al (1996) demonstrated how this technique decreased local sensitivity at the lateral epicondyle and increased grip strength in patients with lateral epicondylitis. No changes in temperature sensitivity were observed. Since the technique also changed

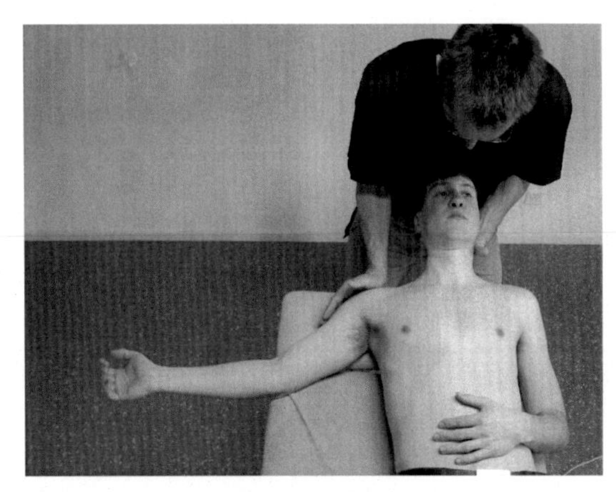

Fig. 7.6 Lateral glides to the left with the right arm in slight neurodynamic tension.

sympathetic activity, the authors hypothesized that the sideglide technique activates the dorsal periaqueductal grey, thereby causing hypoalgesia.

Hall et al (1997) and Cowell and Phillips (2002) observed an effect of neural mobilization on cervicobrachial pain syndromes. They also used cervical sideglide techniques.

IMPROVING MUSCULAR STABILITY

Basic exercise

Exercises for muscle stability are based on the graded cervical flexion test. All exercises are designed to focus on deep cervical flexor activity and should be performed with low intensity muscle force. To gain control over muscle coordination the exercises should be performed two or three times a day, 10 repetitions of 10 seconds holding time.

The exercise is performed in exactly the same way as the test for the deep cervical flexors. Additionally, an exercise in the sitting position should be performed (Fig. 7.7). Initially it will be easier for the patient to perform the exercise with the back leaning against a wall or a door, as far back against the wall as possible. The patient's hands rest on their lap and the back of the head leans gently against the wall. Patients with a thoracic kyphosis who cannot adopt this position are allowed to move their buttocks slightly away from the wall.

The stomach is drawn in, and the shoulder blades are positioned in slight retraction and gentle elevation or depression depending on the habitual position of the individual patient. If the nervous system is highly mechanosensitive, shoulder depression should not be performed since this might cause an additional irritation of the nervous system. The final movement that is added is a gentle nod of the head. It is important that the head maintains contact with the wall and slides upwards against the wall. The advantages of performing the exercise in this position are:

- The patient can perform the exercise throughout the day wherever they are.
- It is a functional position.

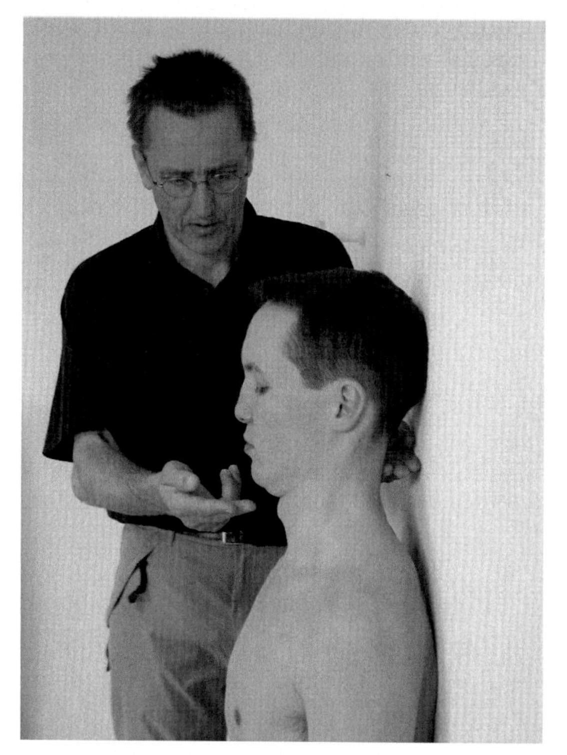

Fig. 7.7 Reactivation of the deep cervical flexors in sitting.

- Sliding against the wall provides sensory feedback.
- The wall prevents retraction.

Once comfortable with the wall exercise, the patient should learn to continue the activity without the feedback of the wall. He should imagine 'growing tall' while doing the exercise.

The patient is then asked to correct their posture throughout the day whenever it comes to mind. Reminders could be red traffic lights or the sound of the telephone ringing; on seeing or hearing the cue, the patient should perform a single 10-second hold of the exercise. The progression of this exercise depends on the normal activities of daily living of the patient and the treatment goals. For example, a young footballer who has problems when heading the ball will need an exercise progression for the deep cervical flexors that is designed to withstand the load of a ball on the head. Alternatively, a mountain biker with problems on downhilling might need strength and endurance of the neck extensors. Those patients who do not put any specific load on their necks in their day-to-day lives should focus on functional muscle stability.

The following exercise examples do not require specific equipment to allow the patient to exercise where and whenever it comes to mind. Naturally, the therapist is free to adapt the exercises for their own purposes and supplement them with any equipment felt to be required (e.g. elastic exercise bands, pulleys, etc.).

Focus on deep cervical flexors

Initially the patient performs the basic exercise in supine, then attempts to decrease the pressure of the occiput on the bed while the pressure of the cervical lordosis is maintained. The back of the head should then be gradually raised about 0.5 cm. Since this exercise is very difficult in supine one might first try to perform the movement in half-sitting or with a tilted headrest. At home the patient might try to sit on the floor by the bed. For an inclined position the patient may want to try an ironing board.

To lift the head off the bed, activity of the superficial flexor muscles (e.g. sternocleidomastoid) is needed. It is essential that the therapist constantly checks whether the patient continues to have control over the cervical lordosis (the patient is not allowed to push their chin forward).

Progression of the exercise requires performance on a flat surface or to move the chin towards the sternum. It is also important to change the starting position more towards extension. This is achieved by placing a small pillow underneath the thoracic spine and thereby positioning the craniocervical region into slight extension. The patient is now asked to perform an upper cervical flexion ('head on neck') before lifting the head off the bed.

The final stage of the exercise programme could be to perform the movement in a supine position with the head hanging over the end of the bed. Only those patients who need to perform high load activities in their daily life will need to train at this level.

The football player mentioned above was also asked to do a specific ball exercise. For this, he was positioned standing 1 metre from a wall, facing the wall, and held a football against the wall with his forehead. Progression of this exercise included decreased base (standing on one leg) or fast movements with hand weights.

Focus on extensor muscles

After the patient has learned the basic exercise they are now positioned prone. The patient draws in the stomach, positions the shoulder blades in retraction and slight depression and lifts the forehead off the bed with the chin tucked in. Since the muscles in the back of the neck are much stronger than the ventral muscles this exercise can usually be performed in a flat position straight away.

To increase the intensity of this exercise, a light weight (e.g. 1 kg) may be placed on the back of the head. Otherwise the patient should be standing, not only lifting the forehead but also extending the neck. It is very important to carefully observe maintenance of deep cervical extension and cervical lordosis. For example, no bending should occur. A further progression can be to ask the patient to support themselves on their elbows with the chin towards the sternum. Starting from this flexed position the patient now performs a controlled extension.

Exercises in standing that involve arm movements have also shown good results. The patient stands with the trunk bent to 60° by hip flexion, holding 1-kg weights in both hands. First of all the patient needs to position the head correctly before starting to quickly move the arms into flexion and/or abduction while trying not to loose the position of the neck. Again exercises with a ball against a wall might be indicated.

Focus on functional stability

The exercise routine depends on the test position in which the patient failed to maintain the position of the head and neck. The test that was failed is turned into the exercise (Sahrmann 2002). Two cases will explain this procedure.

Example 3

Patient C shows a hingeing of cervical segments to extension on bilateral arm elevation. This patient should begin his training by performing the exercise against the wall. He positions his fingers in his cervical lordosis to feel and control the pressure he builds up on correct performance of the exercise. The other arm is moved into elevation. Increased speed of the arm movement or hand weights will progress this exercise. Once this exercise is learned the training can be continued in a freestanding position.

Example 4

Patient D is a physiotherapist who suffered a whiplash injury 3 years ago with continuing cervical symptoms ('My neck gets very tired and feels like snapping'). The symptoms increase during the course of the day so that she commonly needs a brace in the afternoons around 3 p.m. Her symptoms depend on her work posture: the more manual therapy she does (in a position of slight forward bending), the worse her symptoms become.

The physical examination shows a hingeing in the cervical spine on lumbar forward bending. If she pretends to perform a manual therapy mobilization her head moves into protraction in the rhythm of her movements.

This patient was supplied with exercises focusing on extensor muscles. Additionally, lumbar flexion was performed in sitting and standing with control of craniocervical stability. The patient was also asked to do controlled cervical flexion and extension while sitting with her elbows positioned on a bed. Finally, she practised posterior–anterior mobilization techniques on a ball while maintaining craniocervical stability.

CONTRIBUTORY FACTORS

Following the treatment of neuromusculoskeletal dysfunction, potential contributory factors should also be addressed. These include biopsychosocial aspects (Gifford 2002a, 2002b) and ergonomic factors as well as an analysis of activities of daily living.

Repetitive activities in a non-physiological position or compensatory movement patterns might maintain symptoms or lead to further episodes of symptoms.

Some examples will underline these thoughts:

- The first patient shows a slight instability of the C4–C5 segment on extension. Additionally, his cervicothoracic junction is hypomobile. Although he religiously performed his stabilization and mobilization exercises he was never symptom-free and suffered frequent relapses. An analysis of his daily activities showed that his symptoms occurred whenever he rode his mountain bike. He generally preferred flat surfaces but the low position of the handlebar and the hypomobility of his cervicothoracic junction forced his hypermobile cervical segments into extension. He was advised to change the height of the handlebar to achieve a more upright posture.
- The second patient is a woman with mild insufficiency of the right alar ligaments whose hair was parted on the right side so her hair covered her left eye. She thus had a tendency to hold her head in slight lateroflexion to the right and habitually performed quick left rotations of her head to reposition her hair. This frequently caused new episodes of symptoms. After the third painful episode in a year she accepted that she needed to change her hairstyle.
- The third patient suffered from a hypermobility of the C2–C3 segment on rotation to the left and extension. Additionally, his neck was stiff on rotation and lateroflexion to the right. He is an architect who spends a number of hours a day on the telephone which he habitually held between his left shoulder and his left ear to keep his hands

free to write. This caused frequent lateroflexion to the left and an increased activity of the left levator scapulae muscle. Muscle shortening will cause movement restriction on rotation and lateroflexion to the right. The patient was informed of the biomechanical background of his symptoms and he bought a headset for his phone. He has never had a relapse since.

Finally, it is important to assess the posture and activities at the workplace. Good ergonomic advice might be even more beneficial than mobilization and stabilization treatment in some computer users.

SUMMARY

- Successful management of cervical instability problems includes consideration of all biopsychosocial aspects (Gifford 2002a, 2002b).
- During neuromusculoskeletal treatment any signs and symptoms need to be evaluated for priority and relevance.
- To avoid relapses it is of enormous importance to include a workplace and daily life activity intervention.

References

Butler D S 1998 Integrating pain awareness into physiotherapy – wise action for the future. In: Gifford L S (ed.) Topical issues in pain 1. Whiplash – science and management. CNS Press, Falmouth, p 1–23

Butler D S 2000 The sensitive nervous system. NOI Group Publications, Adelaide

Cowell I M, Phillips D R 2002 Effectiveness of manipulative physiotherapy for the treatment of a neurogenic cervicobrachial pain syndrome: a single case study – experimental design. Manual Therapy 7:31–38

Gifford L S 2000 Schmerzphysiologie. In: Van den Berg F (ed.) Angewandte Physiologie Teil 2: Organsysteme verstehen und beeinflussen. Thieme, Stuttgart, p 467–518

Gifford L S 2002a Perspektiven zum biopsychosozialen Modell. Teil 1: Müssen einige Aspekte vielleicht doch akzeptiert werden? Manuelle Therapie 6:139–145

Gifford L S 2002b Perspektiven zum biopsychosozialen Modell. Teil 2: Einkaufskorb-Ansatz Manuelle Therapie 6:197–206

Hall T M, Elvey R L 1999 Nerve trunk pain: physical diagnosis and treatment. Manual Therapy 4:63–73

Hall T M, Elvey R L, Davies N, Dutton L, Moog M 1997 Efficacy of manipulative physiotherapy for the treatment of cervicobrachial pain. In: Tenth Biennial Conference of the MPAA. Manipulative Physiotherapists Association of Australia, Melbourne

Hides J A, Richardson C A, Jull G A 1996 Multifidus muscle recovery is not automatic after resolution of acute first episode low back pain. Spine 21:2763–2769

Hides J A, Jull G A, Richardson C A 2001 Long-term effects of specific stabilising exercises for first episode low back pain. Spine 26: E243–E248

Maitland G D, Hengeveld E, Banks K, English K 2001 Maitland's vertebral manipulation, 6th edn. Butterworth-Heinemann, Oxford

Melzack R 1996 Gate control theory. On the evolution of pain concepts. Pain Forum 5:128–138

Rydevik B L, Olmarker K 1999 Instability and sciatica. In: Szpalski M, Gunzburg R, Pope M H (eds) Lumbar segmental instability. Lippincott, Williams and Wilkins, Philadelphia, p 75–84

Sahrmann S A 2002 Diagnosis and treatment of movement impairment syndromes. Mosby, St Louis

Sterling M, Jull G, Wright A 2001a The effect of musculoskeletal pain on motor activity and control. Journal of Pain 2:135–145

Sterling M, Jull G, Wright A 2001b Cervical mobilisation: concurrent effects on pain, sympathetic nervous system activity and motor activity. Manual Therapy 6:72–81

Stokes M, Young A 1984 The contribution of reflex inhibition to arthrogenous muscle weakness. Clinical Science 67:7–14

Svensson P, Graven-Nielsen T 2001 Craniofacial muscle pain: review of mechanisms and clinical manifestations. Journal of Orofacial Pain 15:117–145

van den Berg F 1999 Angewandte Physiologie Teil 1: Das Bindegewebe des Bewegungsapparates verstehen und beeinflussen. Thieme, Stuttgart

Vicenzino B, Collins D, Wright A 1996 The initial effects of a cervical spine manipulative physiotherapy treatment on the pain and dysfunction of lateral epicondylalgia. Pain 68:69–74

Chapter 8

Physical examination of dysfunctions in the craniomandibular region

Harry von Piekartz

CHAPTER CONTENTS

INTRODUCTION

In this chapter the most common examination techniques will be described and their clinical benefits discussed. Knowledge from evidence-based medicine (EBM) will be outlined. The techniques are described from a physiotherapy and manual therapy perspective. In this case, the principal aim is not to find a diagnosis but rather to analyse the craniomandibular dysfunctions and their functional connection to other regions such as the craniofacial region and the cranial nervous system.

Unilateral techniques will always be described for the *right* craniomandibular region. These tests will be introduced in the following:

- Observation and craniomandibular and craniofacial measurements
- Differentiation of the craniomandibular region and other regions
- Active movements:
  - In sitting
  - In supine with overpressure
- Muscle tests:
  - Static (isometric) tests
  - Dynamic tests
  - Prolonged sustained tests (endurance or repeated movements)
  - Muscle control and (dynamic) muscle endurance

  - Functional coordination
- Palpation:
  - Craniomandibular joint
  - Salivary glands and lymph nodes
  - Muscles
  - Cranial nervous tissue.

This list is not meant to be ticked off from top to bottom by the therapist. Depending on the type and the intensity of the symptoms, as well as the symptomatic region, only a selection of these techniques will be required.

OBSERVATION AND CRANIOMANDIBULAR AND FACIAL MEASUREMENTS

Introduction

During the subjective assessment the therapist will already have an idea of the hypotheses (pathobiological mechanisms, cause of the symptoms, dysfunctions, contributing factors, precautions, prognosis and treatment) which were discussed in Chapter 1. To perform a physical examination in the symptomatic region is still necessary. Although we know that the majority of the clinical decisions are already made during the subjective examination (Butler 2000) (Box 8.1), a number of reasons still justify the need for a physical assessment. It is also known that the combination of an adequate subjective examination and tests that are not gold standard tests (the most widely accepted and most valid known tests) may result in the same orofacial diagnosis as, for example, imaging procedures (Mohl 1991). The most essential questions are often: 'Which region needs to be examined first?' and 'In which functional position should the patient be examined?' This is followed by the decision as to whether or not other regions are also associated with the problem (Fig. 8.1).

There are some clear indicators from the subjective assessment, as discussed in Chapter 3, that point towards the region which needs to be examined first. Observation and optometry may strongly influence clinical decision-making during the initial physical examination. Some important, and often easy, observational principles and measurements that apply before the beginning of the physical examination are discussed below. Examination and treatment techniques of the craniofacial region and the cranial nervous system are described in detail in Chapters 9, 16, 17 and 18 (Fig. 8.2).

General impression

A head forward position influences the function of the cervical spine as well as the craniomandibular region (Rocabado 1985, Kraus 1994). Some clinical measurements that may assist the assessment of posture are given below.

Box 8.1 Reasons for performing a physical examination

- Movement includes the patient
- Hypotheses may be confirmed or dismissed quickly
- Documentation of an activity level that cannot be assessed with psychosocial measurement tools
- Exclusion or confirmation of contraindications
- Foundation for treatment techniques

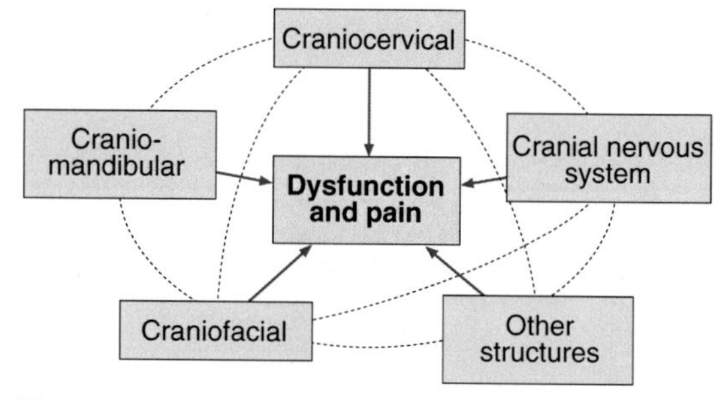

Fig. 8.1 Regions which may influence craniofacial dysfunction and pain and their interrelationships.

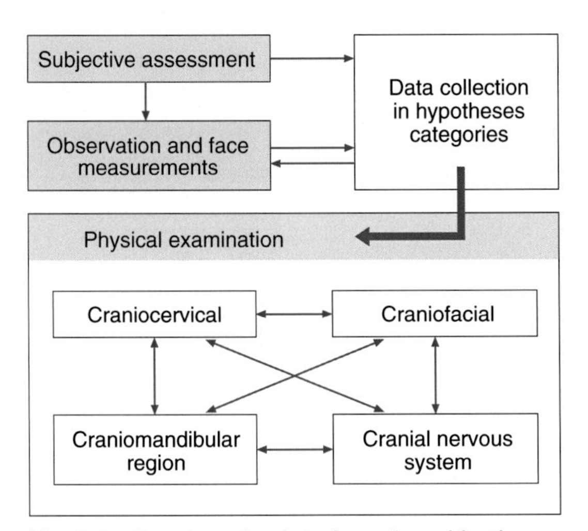

Fig. 8.2 Based on the data from the subjective examination, inspection and face measurements, the therapist may establish a priority list and decide which structures need to be assessed first. This will also provide indications for potential relationships to other regions.

Assessment of the craniocervical region

A normal posture can be identified by drawing a vertical line from the thoracic curve to the apex of the occiput. The average distance of this fictitious plumb line towards the deepest point of the cervical lordosis is 6 cm (Rocabado 1985). A global impression is often gained by placing the patient against a wall to observe the relation of thoracic spine, head region and mandibular joints.

A fictitious line from the most prominent part of the zygomatic bone to the clavicle may also give a good indication of posture. On average, this line will end at the anterior part of the clavicle. If the distance is more than 2 cm, this points towards a bad orthostatic posture (Rocabado & Iglash 1991). Unfortunately there are no reference data for these measurements.

Assessment of the craniomandibular region

The fictitious line from the dorsal edge of the nostrils to the *retrognathion* must be vertical. For a detailed description of the analysis of the face profile, see the classification according to Angle in Chapter 10.

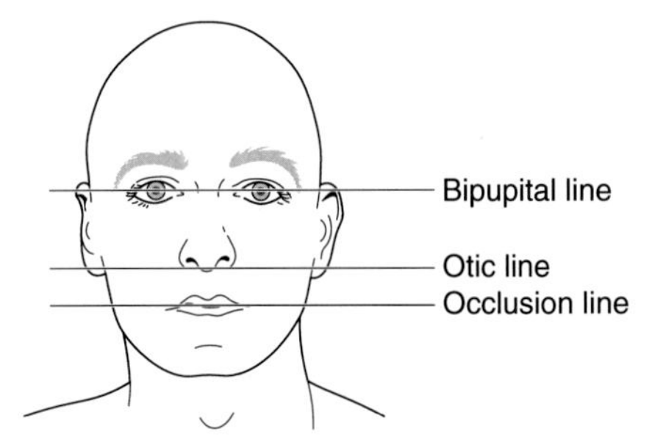

Fig. 8.3 Measurements of the bipupital line, the otic line and the occlusion line will provide reliable information about facial asymmetry.

By palpating the orientation of the hyoid this impression may be confirmed. Normally the hyoid is situated at the level of the third cervical segment. The hyoid may be palpated with the index finger and thumb while the other hand locates C3. If the hyoid is significantly further cranial than C3 this may confirm the previously identified data.

Frontal extraoral observation and measurements

(MACROSCOPIC) FACIAL ASYMMETRY (THE BIPUPITAL, OTIC AND OCCLUSION LINES)

Check whether the bipupital, otic and occlusion lines run parallel. The bipupital line is determined by standing in front of the patient holding a ruler of 15 cm length from the corner of one eye to the other. For the otic line it is easiest to palpate the most dorsal points of the left and right zygomatic bones and to mark these on the skin with a washable pen. The occlusion line is measured from the right to the left corner of the mouth. In a study by Schokker et al (1990), 110 patients with chronically recurrent headaches and facial pain showed, compared to a control group, significant asymmetry of the size and shape of the face and the mandibles. It is the author's experience that a great number of patients with intra-articular dysfunction show a convergence of these lines at the symptomatic side, combined with a smaller mandibular ramus (for mandibular measurements, see below) (Fig. 8.3).

Masticatory muscles

In the case of a clear craniomandibular dysfunction increased unilateral muscle tone is usually found (Friction & Dubner 1994, Palla et al 1998). The muscle relief of the masseter and the temporal muscles have been compared in detail. An increased muscle tone of the masseter is dominantly visible cranially to the mandibular ramus. Relief changes of the temples point towards an increased tone of the temporal muscle. Swelling around the medial pterygoid muscle is shown near the middle of the mandibular angle. A quick comparison can be made by asking the patient to slightly tilt the head backwards. A brief palpation of the most sensitive areas of muscles and ligament, comparing sides and assessing pain and resistance (muscle tone), often confirms the dysfunction (Clark et al 1989). The muscles of the neck should not be left out during the palpation. The sternocleidomastoid and the suprahyoid muscles, such as the digastric muscle, are particularly known for their high levels of excitation associated with orofacial dysfunction and pain (Tsai et al 2002) (Fig. 8.4).

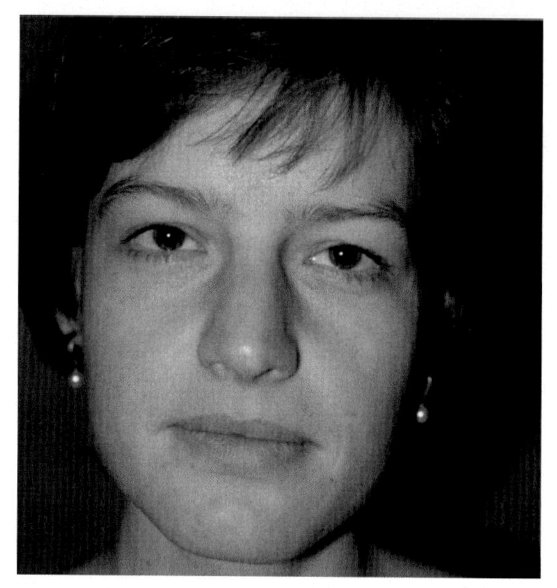

Fig. 8.4 Patient with clear craniofacial dysfunction. Note the masseter muscle relief and compare right and left side. The facial asymmetry (drawn from bipupital line, otic line and occlusion line) indicates that the dysfunction was probably already present during adolescence.

Upper lip and prominent incisors

The shape and the size of the upper lip and the incisor teeth are determined, like the shape of the face, substantially by ethnic origin (Proffit & Ackerman 1993). A relatively short and tight upper lip may be due to:

- Bimaxillary protrusion: The maxillary front teeth are prominent but the upper lip is small.
- Compensatory mechanisms due to bad posture: A head forward position increases the muscle tone of the masticatory and facial muscles (Hu 2001). Clinically either increased or decreased tension of the upper lip is noted.
- Parafunctional behaviour: Aesthetically the upper lip may function to cover large front teeth. This will increase the tension of the whole orofacial region (Subtelny 2000, Biates & Cleese 2001).

ASSESSMENT

- Excessive separation of the lips in a relaxed position: Ask the patient to relax the lips. This procedure may be more standardized by initially pressing the lips together followed by a more maximal relaxation. The general guideline is that the lips should be no further than 4 mm apart (Proffit & Ackerman 1993).
- Putting the lips together: In the case of dysfunction, this is difficult for the patient to do and is associated with activity of the facial and masticatory muscles.
- Assessment of the face profile: A clearly seen bilateral protrusion is commonly associated with bilabial protrusion. A short upper lip is often observed in dysfunctions of the craniocervical and craniomandibular regions.

Dysfunction of the cranial nervous tissue and inspection

On inspection the therapist may already gain an impression of the function of the cranial nerves that is subtly mirrored by dysfunction of the target tissue (Okeson 1995, Butler 2000). Some potential indicators for cranial nerve dysfunctions are listed below:

- Asymmetry of the relief, fasciculation or trismus of the facial and masticatory muscles may point towards a dysfunction of the facial nerve (VII) or the trigeminal nerve (V).
- Upper cervical extension (nose pointing upwards and forwards) may indicate an olfactory dysfunction (olfactory nerve), but may also point towards increased muscle tone of the neck and throat muscles (glossopharyngeal nerve, vagus nerve and hypoglossal nerve) (Spillane 1996).
- If the head is turned with the ear pointing towards the therapist, this may indicate a hearing disorder or a dysfunction of the visual field (acoustic nerve or optic nerve). If this is associated with asymmetry of sternocleidomastoid or trapezoid muscle tone, this may indicate a dysfunction of the accessory nerve (XII).
- The eye often shows the function of various cranial nerves. Notable changes are:
  - A difference in eye position (divergence, diplopia) which points towards dysfunction of the motor nerves (oculomotor nerve, trochlear nerve, abducens nerve).
  - Asymmetry of the pupil size, indicating a parafunction of either the oculomotor nerve or the vagus nerve (Okeson 1995).
- Intraorbital swelling caused by malfunction of lacrimation and salivation can result in a diffuse pressure at the medial side of the eye. This indicates dysfunction of the facial nerve (VII), the glossopharyngeal nerve (IX) and the vagus nerve (X) (Fig. 8.5).
- Colour changes of the skin often indicate malfunction of the autonomous nervous system, with various cranial nerves being affected, e.g. trigeminal nerve (V), facial nerve (VII), trochlear nerve (IV), glossopharyngeal nerve (IX) and vagus nerve (X) (Wilson-Pauwels et al 1998). The influence of the cervical spine should not be ignored in this context (Hu 2001).

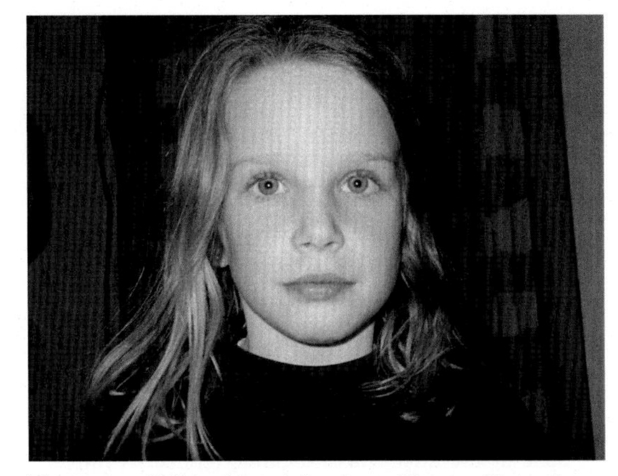

Fig. 8.5 Child with minimal strabismus. Note the eye asymmetry (slight deviation of the right eye), which may be caused by a dysfunction of the abducens and trochlear nerves (see Chapter 17).

For further information regarding target tissue tests for the cranial nerves, see Chapter 18.

GENERAL VERTICAL FACE PROPORTIONS (FRONTAL VIEW)

Asymmetrical facial soft tissue (e.g. skin and mimic muscles) proportions may easily lead to wrong conclusions regarding general facial symmetry. The normal proportions are:

- The vertical height of the facial middle line from the suborbital upper edge and the wrinkles to the base of the nose (*upper face*) is the same as the height of the *lower face* (Fig. 8.6a).
- In the *lower face* the mouth should be positioned about one-third of the way from the base of the nose to the tip of the chin (Fig. 8.6b) (Proffit & Ackerman 1993).

In the clinical assessment the measuring points are marked and measured with a ruler. The ruler needs to be pressed hard against the soft tissue towards the underlying bone. If this should be difficult – for whatever reason – the following method might be easier to perform.

MEASURING THE VERTICAL FACE DIMENSIONS

A quick overview of the vertical face dimensions can be performed using Trott's method.

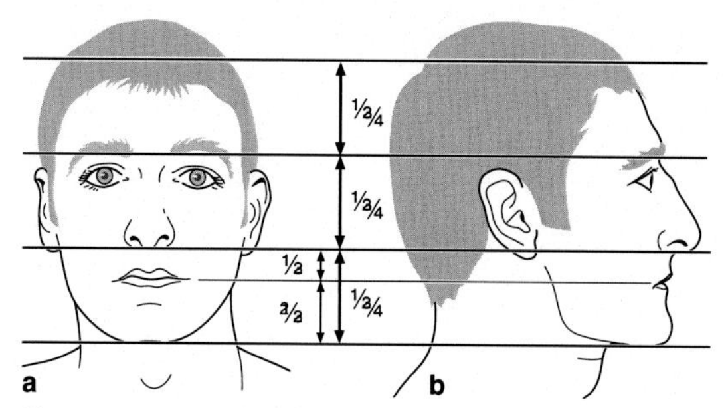

Fig. 8.6 Normal facial proportions. Vertical face proportions in the frontal plane. The vertical height of the midface (from the supraorbital prominence to the base of the nose) has the same length as the height of the lower face (lower third of the face). In the lower face the mouth is positioned in the first third between the base of the nose and the chin.

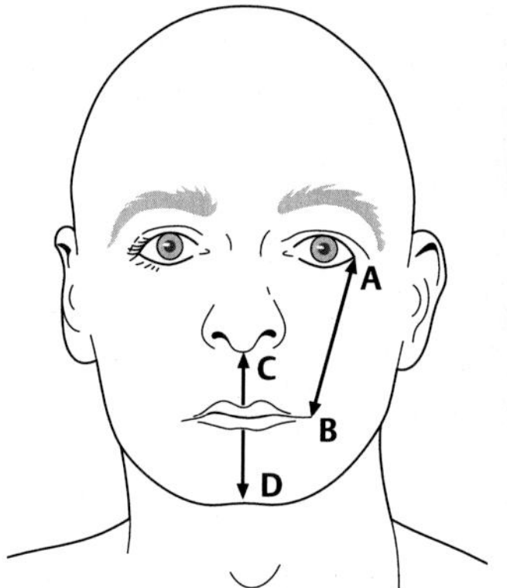

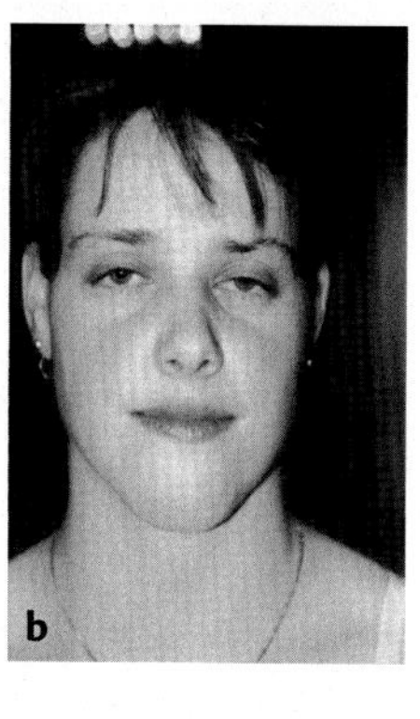

Fig. 8.7 Facial measurement, Trott's method.
a The relationship between the AB line (from the lateral corner of the eye to the ipsilateral corner of the mouth) and the CD line (below the tip of the nose to the tip of the chin) is calculated. If the CD line is more than 10 mm shorter than the AB line this is a clear contributing factor for symptoms in the craniomandibular region.
b Patient with increased CD line after inappropriate orthodontic treatment.

With a 15 cm long ruler, the distance between the lateral corner of the eye and the corner of the mouth (same side) is measured (AB line). Afterwards the distance between the anterior nasal spine and the retrognathion (tip of the chin) is measured (CD line). If the CD line is 10 mm or more shorter than the AB line, this indicates an overbite, crossbite or loss of one or more teeth (Graber 1969, Trott 1985). While measuring, the ruler should have as much contact with the hard tissue as possible along its entire length (Fig. 8.7).

Inspection and measurement of the mandible

Visual position of the tip of the chin (protuberantia mentalis): Is the chin centred or deviated? If an obvious deviation is observed the therapist should also note whether:

- There are relief changes of the masticatory muscles. Often a clear unilateral hypertonus is found (muscle imbalance).
- The position of the incisors is not parallel, indicating a dysfunction.
- Observed from cranially with the patient supine any changes of mandibular position, zygoma relief and forehead are found. If the mandibular deviation is as clearly seen as in the vertical position, structural changes are likely. If the deviation seems less, gravity seems to play a role, so that an output mechanism is hypothesized (motor system). If the deviation remains, the following tests apply.

Identifying the resting position of the mandibular head

EXTRAOTAL

A general impression of the position of the heads of the mandible is gained by placing both middle fingers symmetrically behind the mandibular head and in front of the ears. The index fingers are placed ventrally of the mandibular heads. The therapist can now estimate the distance between the dorsal mandibular head and the auricular articular eminence, the height of the mandibular joint processes and potentially of the mandibular translation in the frontal plane. It is useful to ask the patient whether the palpation provokes any of their symptoms.

INTRAOTAL

If the mandibular joint heads are positioned too far dorsocranially, one may try to place

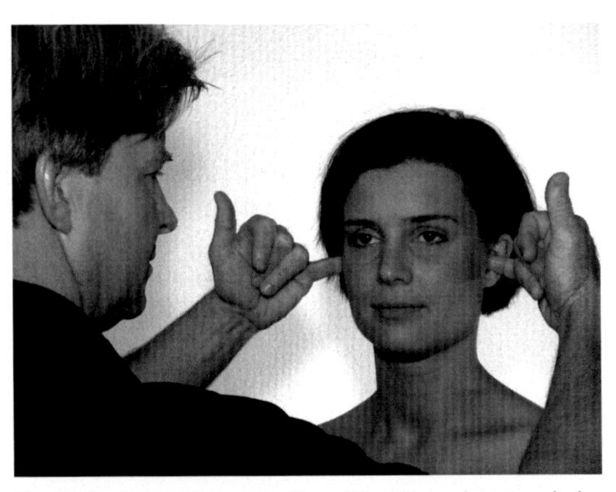

Fig. 8.8 Intraotal palpation. The therapist stands in front of the patient with the arms supinated, and places the little fingers or ring fingers into the outer ear canal. The position of the mandibular head and the retrodiscal space is compared with the non-symptomatic side.

both little fingers into the external ear canal with the lower arms supinated (Fig. 8.8). The dorsal part of the mandibular joint processes and the retrodiscal space are easily palpated. If pain is provoked this is compared with the non-symptomatic opposite side. A small mouth opening activity may further provoke symptoms, indicating a craniomandibular dysfunction rather than otitis media (Berghaus et al 1996).

MANDIBULAR RESTING POSITION

With a ruler, the distance between the upper lip and the tip of the chin may be measured in a resting position. The patient is asked to make minimal teeth contact and then return to habitual occlusion. The difference is calculated. In a normal resting position the distance between the upper and lower molar teeth due to gravity is 2–3 mm at habitual occlusion (Harzer 1999). This interocclusal distance changes with muscle imbalance, orthostatic posture changes, dysgnathia or parafunctions.

MANDIBULAR MEASUREMENTS

Length measured from the mandibular head to the tip of the chin: Mandibular asymmetry is a predisposing factor for craniomandibular dysfunction, headaches and facial pain (Schokker et al 1990, Palla et al 1998). First the measuring points are marked (tip of the mandibular head and tip of the chin). The distances are then measured with a ruler and compared. An unpublished study showed significant differences in length and symmetry between patients with craniomandibular dysfunctions and healthy volunteers.

Another unpublished pilot study (von Piekartz 2004) that included 120 Dutch volunteers (68 male/52 female) aged over 18 years (average age 28.6 years) without headaches, neck or face pain, showed an average distance of 14.3 cm on the left and 14.6 cm on the right side (standard deviation 0.2 and 0.3 cm). The average ratio of the left/right distances was 0.98.

The second group included patients ($n = 86$) who suffered from headaches, neck or face pain for more than 3 months and who were classified as Helkimo III or IV. The average age was 32.8 years. The average distance was 13.6 cm on the left and 13.2 cm on the right side. The standard deviation was 0.4 cm and 0.5 cm, respectively. The average ratio of left/right was 1.12.

It can therefore be tentatively concluded that the difference in left to right side mandibular length differs significantly between the dysfunction and control groups. The average difference was 1.12 cm comparing the left side with the right side (Table 8.1).

Mandibular plane angle and profile

The inclination of the mandibular plane, which is the horizontal plane, needs to be observed. This is important because:

- A steep mandibular plane angle with a prolonged anterior vertical face dimension correlates with an anterior open bite malocclusion.
- A shallow mandibular plane angle correlates with a short face height and overbite malocclusion (Proffit & Ackerman 1993).

This line may be visualized clinically by placing a ruler or any other measuring tool

Table 8.1 Average mandibular length

	Healthy volunteers (n = 120)		CMD patients (n = 86)	
	Left	Right	Left	Right
Mandibular length (cm)	14.3 (0.2)	14.6 (0.3)	13.6 (0.4)	13.2 (0.5)
Ratio	0.98		1.12	

CMD, craniomandibular disorders.

(e.g. a goniometer) along the mandibular edge. The angle towards the fictitious horizontal line is measured and should be approximately 45–50°. Naturally both sides are compared (Fig. 8.9).

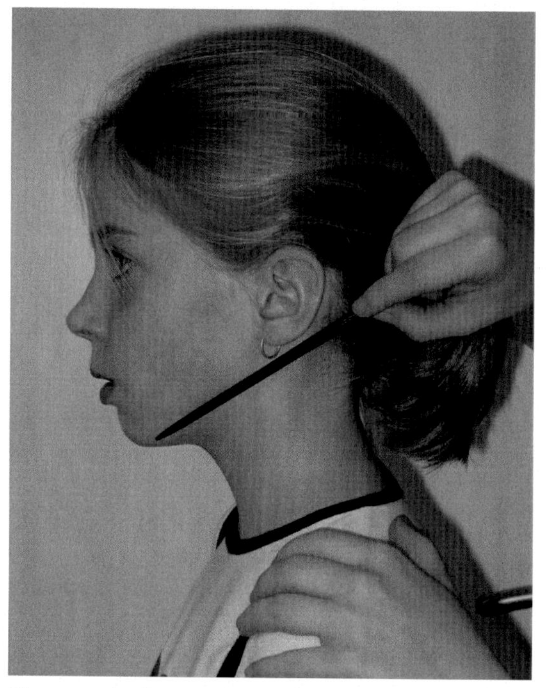

Fig. 8.9 Inclination of the mandibular angle. Placing a ruler or a pen along the mandible will help to visualize the mandibular angle. The inclination is estimated and compared with the other side. This 10-year-old girl appears to have similar mandibular angles that fit to the development of the face (see text).

ANTHROPOMETRIC FACE MEASUREMENT

In some cases it is advisable to measure the proportions of the facial bones and to compare the results with reference data from cephalometry. The measurements show a good intratester and intertester reliability, are easy and inexpensive. The disadvantage of cephalometry is that only the bony structures and not the soft tissue are assessed (Proffit & Ackerman 1993). A clinical evaluation, as described below, will also integrate the soft tissue. The therapist therefore gains:

- An overview of any (ab)normal development of the face and the consequences of the stress transducer phenomenon of the craniofacial region (see Chapters 15 and 16)
- A confirmation of the recognized patterns of abnormal face development
- A reliable measuring method for reassessment after the course of treatments.

A confirmation of the recognized patterns of abnormal face development may, for example, be a patient with an anterior open bite and an increased size of the lower face.

The vertical measurements (height) need to be proportional, with a certain value, which is called face width. Unilateral craniomandibular dysfunction arising during facial growth shows proportional values that clearly differ from average values (Farkas & Munro 1987).

Take, for example, a patient with long-term facial pain, who suffered from protracted sinusitis in the past. Anthropometric measurements showed an increased facial height (n–gn), increased zygomatic width (zy–zy) and an increased height of the lower face (sn–gn).

The midface proportions are therefore abnormal, indicating that the therapist should consider a potential dysfunction in this area. The measurements may be performed with a hard 15 cm (metal) ruler or a slide calliper. The calliper and the ruler need to show the millimetres clearly and be of at least 15 cm length. A reliable measuring tool is the electronic digital calliper (Pro-fit 2520 150 D, Mitutayo Ned. B.V. Veenendaal, Netherlands) that measures with a precision of 0.03 mm (von Piekartz 2001). The most important measurements and their reference data are shown in Tables 8.2 and 8.3.

The measurements are divided into:

- Transverse measurements
- Vertical measurements
- Profile measurements.

Transverse measurements

ZYGOMATIC WIDTH (ZY–ZY)

The therapist identifies the most prominent lateral part of the zygomatic bone. In adults this is found 3–4 cm cranial to the auricular articular eminence. The highest point is marked with a washable pen and the distance between the points on the right and the left sides is measured.

MANDIBULAR WIDTH (GONION WIDTH, GO–GO)

An imaginary line is drawn through the upper lip. It ends at the mandibular angles on the right and on the left. A small mark is placed at the most lateral point of the mandibles, the distances measured and the difference between the marked points on each side is compared.

NASOFRONTAL REGION (INTERCANTHAL DISTANCE)

An imaginary line is drawn between the corners of the right and left eyes. The distance between the medial corners of the right and left eyes is then measured. Be careful with the sharp callipers around the eyes. It is easiest to place one indicator at, for example, the medial corner of the right eye and to then carefully

Table 8.2 Anthropometric face measurements in young adults

Parameter	Male	Female
1. Zygomatic width (zy–zy) (mm)	137 (4.3)	130 (5.3)
2. Gonion width (go–go) (mm)	97 (5.8)	91 (5.9)
3. Intercanthal distance (mm)	33 (2.7)	32 (2.4)
4. Pupil–midface distance (mm)	33 (2.0)	31 (1.8)
5. Base of the nose width (mm)	35 (2.6)	31 (1.9)
6. Mouth opening (mm)	53 (3.3)	50 (3.2)
7. Face height (n–gn) (mm)	121 (6.8)	112 (5.2)
8. Lower face height (subnasal–gn) (mm)	72 (6.0)	66 (4.5)
9. Upper lip vermilion (mm)	8.9 (1.5)	8.4 (1.3)
10. Lower lip vermilion (mm)	10.4 (1.9)	9.7 (1.6)
11. Nasolabial angle (°)	99 (8.0)	9.7 (1.6)
12. Nasofrontal angle (°)	131 (8.1)	134 (1.8)

As stated by Farkas & Munro (1987). The measurements are presented in Proffit & Ackerman (1993).
Standard deviation in parentheses.

Table 8.3 Facial indices in young adults

Index	Parameter	Male	Female
Facial	n–gn/zy–zy	88.5 (5.1)	86.2 (4.6)
Mandibular width/face width	go–go/zy–zy	70.8 (3.8)	70.1 (4.2)
Upper face	n–sto/zy–zy	54.0 (3.1)	52.4 (3.1)
Mandibular width/face height	go–go/n–gn	80.3 (6.8)	81.7 (6.0)
Mandible	sto–gn/go–go	51.8 (6.2)	49.8 (4.8)
Mouth/face width	ch–ch × 100/zy–zy	38.9 (2.5)	38.4 (2.5)
Lower face/face height	sn–gn/n–gn	59.2 (2.7)	58.6 (2.9)
Mandible/face height	sto–gn/n–gn	41.2 (2.3)	40.4 (2.1)
Mandible/upper face	sto–ng/n–sto	67.7 (5.3)	66.5 (4.5)
Mandible/lower face	sto–ng/sn–gn	69.6 (2.7)	69.1 (2.8)
Chin/face height	sl–gn × 100/sn–gn	25.0 (2.4)	25.4 (1.9)

From Farkas & Munro (1987).
Standard deviation in parentheses.

move the other indicator, so that it can be placed without much pressure and without shifting into the medial corner of the left eye.

DISTANCE TO CENTRE OF THE FACE (PUPIL–MIDFACE DISTANCE)

An imaginary line is drawn from the lower eyelid to the centre of the nose (internasal suture). A mark is placed onto the centre of the nose and the lowest part of the eyelid with a washable pen. The distance between the two points is measured and compared with the opposite side.

WIDTH OF THE BASE OF THE NOSE

The distance between the right and the left nose wing fold is measured. These are usually easily recognized and do not need to be marked.

WIDTH OF THE MOUTH

In a relaxed position the distance between both corners of the mouth is measured. To achieve maximum standardization the patient is asked to initially open the mouth wide and thereby stretch the lips. The measurement is taken on return to the relaxed position.

Vertical measurements

FACE HEIGHT (N–GN)

The distance from the internasal suture at the level of the medial corner to the tip of the chin (mental protuberance) is measured.

LOWER FACE HEIGHT (SUBNASAL–GN)

The distance from the base of the nose (anterior nasal spine) to the tip of the chin (mental protuberance) is measured.

DISTANCE UPPER LIP–LOWER LIP (UPPER LIP VERMILION)

The distance from the highest point of the upper lip to the highest point of the lower lip is measured (= width of the upper lip). The jaw needs to be completely relaxed. For a better standardization it is helpful to ask the patient to open the mouth wide and to then return into a relaxed position before measuring.

WIDTH OF THE LOWER LIP (LOWER LIP VERMILION)

The distance between the lowest point of the upper lip and the lowest point of the lower lip is measured.

Profile measurements

The profile measurements require a goniometer or a protractor to achieve good standardized results. As the goniometer is easier to use in the face region and shows better reliability (Proffit & Ackerman 1993), it is the preferred tool for the following two measurements. It is fixed onto a square piece of plexiglas that can be turned easily. The resulting data are noted in degrees and not in millimetres.

FRONTONASAL ANGLE (BETWEEN FOREHEAD AND NOSE)

One side of the plexiglas with the goniometer is held firmly against the forehead with the bottom corner at the very top of the nose (frontomaxillary suture). The goniometer is calibrated to 0°. The plexiglas is then turned so that the opposite side now touches the nose line. The angle is indicated on the goniometer (Fig. 8.10).

NASOLABIAL ANGLE (BETWEEN NOSE AND LIP)

One side of the plexiglas is held at the lower edge of the nose with the corner of the plexiglas resting against the anterior nasal spine.

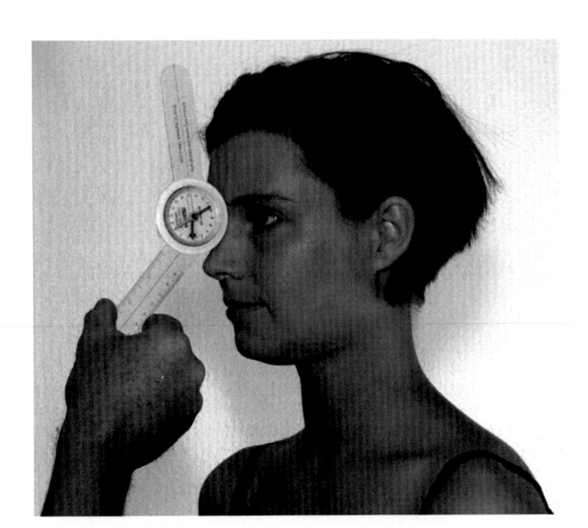

Fig. 8.10 This important anthropometric measurement calculates the angle between forehead and nose in the profile.

The goniometer is calibrated to 0°. The opposite side is then placed against the mandible and the maxilla and the degrees are read from the goniometer.

PROFILE ASSESSMENT ACCORDING TO ANGLE

Once the anthropometric measurements are performed the clinician should have a better idea as to whether the patient shows a retrognathia or a prognathia, and may form a hypothesis according to the classification system by Angle (1900) which distinguishes three categories of malocclusion:

- Neutral bite
- Distal bite (two variations)
- Mesial bite.

Clinical experience shows that patients with different types of malocclusion frequently show a predisposition for typical craniofacial and craniocervical dysfunctions (see also Chapter 10).

INTRAORBITAL INSPECTION

The assessment of occlusion and the condition of the orofacial region is partly the job of dentists (see Chapter 10); however, a therapist who assesses the neuromusculoskeletal system also needs to perform intraoral inspection for the following reasons:

- To detect potential pathologies such as parodontitis, gingivitis and inflammation of the salivary glands
- To then refer the patient to a specialist (Schwenzer et al 2002).

Occlusion mainly reflects the growth of the craniofacial region (Okeson 1995). This may clarify or confirm hypothesized dysfunctions of the cranium or the craniomandibular region. For example, a crossbite and a unilaterally increased muscle tone of the masseter could prove to be related to parafunctional behaviour (Jäger 1997).

The following components are important to assess.

Teeth

Occlusion

Note the position of the upper and lower incisors and the maximum 'multiple point contact' (maximum intercuspidation) as well as malocclusion in the sagittal and frontal plane (for detailed information, see Chapter 10).

Abrasion

Abrasion and wear and tear of teeth, especially the incisors, may give an indication of potential parafunctional behaviour. Incisors and canines are the most commonly affected (Okeson 1995) (Fig. 8.11).

Tooth contact

A quick test, frequently performed during the inspection, is the quick repetitive contact of the teeth elements. If the resulting noise is consistently light and short, the static contact would appear to be normal. If the noise decreases with the repetitions, changes its quality or becomes non-rhythmical, the dynamic occlusion is dysfunctional and potentially associated with muscle imbalance (Naeije & Van Loon 1998).

Colour of the gums

Colour changes (bluish and shiny) of the gums may reflect general parafunctions (Freesmeyer 1993, Jäger 1997). Prolonged abnormal pressure on the teeth joints (gomphoses) causes trophic dysfunction of the dental region and may cause periodontal pain (Okeson 1995).

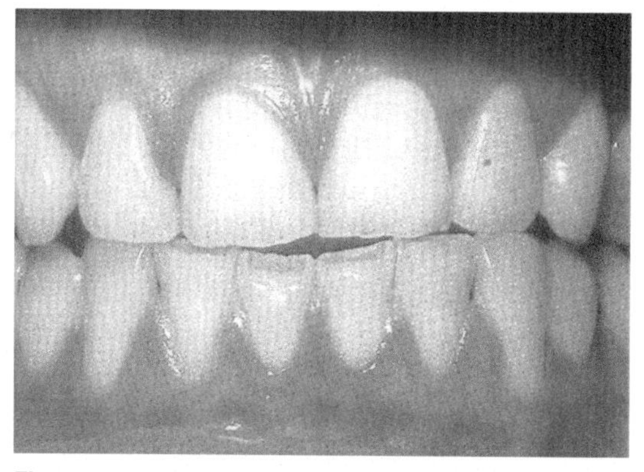

Fig. 8.11 Abrasions of the incisor teeth in a patient with bruxism.

Tongue

Tongue impressions, especially at the lateral sides, may indicate an increased tongue protrusion, a small oral cavity or parafunctions like gritting of the teeth. The patient is asked to open the mouth and to put out the tongue. Many patients show an increased muscle tone of the tongue which is shown by a pointed tongue or by a cranial movement of the tip of the tongue when it leaves the oral cavity.

Sometimes a pressure line (hyperkeratotic mucosal fold) is seen inside the cheek at the occlusal level.

DIFFERENTIATION OF THE CRANIOMANDIBULAR REGION FROM OTHER REGIONS

Features of structural differentiation

The patient may mention daily activities or positions that trigger the symptoms during subjective assessment. If the symptoms occur locally and do not show hyperpathic and latent qualities, a structural differentiation may be possible.

The pain pattern needs to show a clear on/off behaviour and the pain needs to be primarily hyperalgesic. In this case the differentiation may identify the dominant structural sources of the symptoms.

The principle of a differentiation test is that the therapist attempts to form a hypothesis about the responsible structures by assessing resistance and symptoms.

Not only the dominantly suspected structure but also other potential contributing structures are tested. The pain pattern should show a clear peripheral nociceptive input.

Principle of functional differentiation

THE FIRST DIFFERENTIATION TESTS

After the inspection it makes sense to form a hypothesis about the patient's structure and the pain mechanisms. If the pain classification points towards an input mechanism (nociceptive or peripheral neurogenic), further differentiation tests apply. These tests may confirm or dismiss the hypothesis. Another great advantage is that the tests reflect the activity level of the patient. Frequently exactly these activities or postures are the ones that need to be improved. These tests give evidence for a later new assessment or re-assessment (Maitland et al 2001, von Piekartz 2001). Naturally this is not always possible. If the following conditions apply, there is a good chance that the tests will be useful and will not worsen the patient's condition:

- The patient needs to be able to indicate clearly which activities provoke which symptoms.
- The pain quality shows an on/off behaviour. The pain is quite intense and occurs locally.
- The pain does not accumulate and does not show hyperpathic or latent behaviour.

TEST PRINCIPLES

The patient demonstrates the pain-provoking position and is then placed in a manner that no pain is suffered or is just at the point of the onset of pain. One structure is then physiologically changed and the patient is asked whether the symptoms increase or decrease with the change. The therapist's hypothesis is either confirmed or dismissed. A second structure is then changed without moving the initial structure. Again the changes in symptoms will influence the hypothesis.

TEST VALIDITY

Obviously, as with many manual tests, there is inadequate sensitivity and specificity in the identification of structures that are responsible for the symptoms (Gross et al 1996). However, this is not the main intention of the tests: they simply assess functional disorders and the range of dysfunction in the various regions. The subjective examination indicates the movements that need to be tested to confirm or dismiss the therapist's hypotheses (Schon 1983, Jones 1994). Some frequently performed differentiation manoeuvres are described below.

Regions and differentiations discussed in this chapter

- Differentiation of craniomandibular vs craniocervical region:
  - Cervical physiological occlusion differentiation (spatula technique)
  - Physiological cervical movements
  - Cervical rotation differentiation
  - Cervical accessory movements in various mandibular positions
  - Mandibular movements in various cervical positions
- Differentiation of craniomandibular vs craniofacial: temporal–craniomandibular differentiation
- Differentiation of craniofacial vs craniocervical: differentiation in physiological cervical positions (rotation and flexion)
- Differentiation of cranial nervous system vs craniocervical: cervical flexion and slump position
- Differentiation of cranial nervous system vs craniomandibular: mandibular laterotrusion in various cervical positions
- Differentiation of cranial nervous system vs craniofacial: cranial accessory movements in slump position.

DIFFERENTIATION OF CRANIOMANDIBULAR VERSUS CRANIOCERVICAL

Cervical physiological occlusion differentiation (spatula technique)

SPATULA TECHNIQUE

If the temporomandibular joint (TMJ) is suspected as contributing to the signs and symptoms that occur on active cervical movements, the spatula technique – among other tests performed during the functional demonstra-

Example 1

A young female patient shows a flexion deficit of 30°. She is given a normal spatula to hold between her teeth and is asked not to tighten her masticatory muscles more than necessary. She is then asked to repeat the cervical flexion. Any change in pain quality, range of motion and other responses compared to the test without the spatula will point towards a contribution of the craniomandibular region.

tion – may serve to confirm or dismiss the hypothesis.

This technique applies not only for cervical flexion but for any other movement (extension, lateroflexion, rotation). If a lateroflexion movement was spontaneously performed by dominantly moving the upper cervical spine, the spatula between the molar teeth may change this into a more harmonic movement, performed by all cervical segments. The spatula may also change symptoms. If, for example, a patient complains of symptoms on cervical extension that diminish with the spatula technique, a craniomandibular component is hypothesized. The position of the spatula may be important here (molar teeth or incisor teeth) and influence the result of the test.

How does it work?

The spatula technique changes pain quality and reactions significantly in patients with cervical and craniomandibular dysfunctions. This may be explained by various mechanisms.

Mechanical explanation

A slight contact of the teeth keeps the mandibular head in the same place in the fossa during physiological cervical movements. Normally the mandibular head shifts during cervical activities. It has been stated that the mandibular head shifts by 1 mm in an anterior–posterior direction for every 8° of cervical movement (Rocabado & Iglash 1991). Presumably this will change the afferent sensory input and the cervical muscles are no longer facilitated (Omae et al 1989).

Neurophysiological explanation

The neurophysiological chain of afferent input from the masticatory system (teeth and TMJ) is altered and the associated motor engram in the sensomotor cortex is no longer facilitated (Manni et al 1975, Palzzi et al 1996). Motor output can therefore be changed and this will influence aspects of the movement of the cervical spine (Omae et al 1989).

Where do I place the spatula?

If the intraoral inspection reveals abrasions and changes in teeth contact, this will indicate areas of relatively increased pressure during occlusion (Hannson et al 1987, Freesmeyer 1993). It makes sense to choose these areas to place the spatula. The therapist may also try to identify the area at which the teeth first make contact and place the spatula there.

Differentiation during physiological cervical movements

Assessing the cervical spine and applying overpressure will also influence the craniomandibular region.

To examine cervical flexion, one hand is placed onto the mandible and the other hand onto the occiput. Cervical flexion is then performed. During this manoeuvre the craniomandibular region is put under significant stress and will influence the patient's reaction. To differentiate between the two regions the movement is repeated. This time the hand is supinated and placed onto the maxilla and not on the mandible. If the symptoms change significantly, the symptoms on cervical flexion derive from a craniomandibular component.

During cervical extension one hand is placed on the mandible to support the movement. Clinically, a compression occurs in the temporomandibular joints. For the differentiation this hand is supinated and placed onto the occiput when guiding the neck into extension.

Rotation differentiation of the craniocervical region versus the craniomandibular region in sitting position

On cervical end of range rotation to the left, the mandible moves into a laterotrusion to the left. Therefore the mandibular position changes during tooth contact and with it the occlusion (Chapman et al 1991). If the patient complains of unilateral pain in the temple region, this may indicate upper cervical or craniomandibular dysfunction as a nociceptive input. In the following example the TMJ is responsible for the symptoms.

Starting position

- The patient sits on the short side of the plinth.

Position of the examiner

- The therapist stands behind the patient on the right side.

Fixation

- If able to tolerate the pain, the patient is asked to turn the head to the left until the onset of pain is felt.
- The therapist holds the patient's forehead with the left hand with the fingers placed above the patient's right eye.
- The right thumb is placed onto the right half of the mandible, the right index finger in front of and the middle finger behind the patient's chin.

Method

- The therapist reduces the lateroflexion to the left with the right hand. The cervical spine remains unchanged, fixed by the left hand. The pain is reduced.
- In a similar way cervical rotation is decreased by releasing the left hand slightly. This will reduce the cervical stress but increase the craniomandibular stress. Pain remains the same or increases slightly.
- After the joints have been de-rotated separately, the rotation may now be selectively increased. The right hand may increase the left laterotrusion. If the pain is aggravated, the 'craniomandibular region' hypothesis is confirmed.
- With the left hand the rotation of the patient's head may be increased. The craniomandibular joint will be simultaneously relaxed, so that in our example the pain should remain unchanged or decrease slightly.
- The fifth test is an isolated laterotrusion to the left in a neutral cervical position, performed with the therapist's right hand. The pain will return if the 'craniomandibular region' hypothesis is correct.
- The last test is an isolated cervical rotation. The therapist now stands on the left in front of the patient and places the hands on either side of the patient's head. The thumbs hold the mandibles bilaterally. The TMJ is not allowed to move into laterotrusion. If the therapist moves the hands as one, a pain-free cervical rotation occurs (Fig. 8.12).

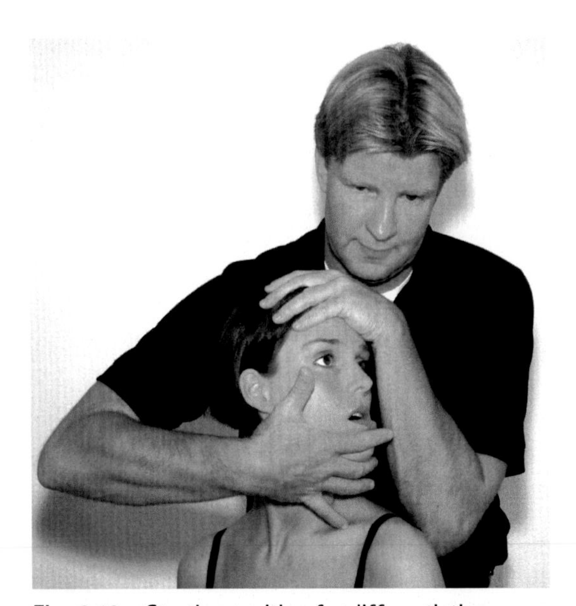

Fig. 8.12 Starting position for differentiation between the craniocervical and craniomandibular regions. This example shows rotation to the left. It is important that the left hand holds the head firmly in the rotation position. The right index finger and middle finger lie on the mandible. To allow a physiological laterotrusion, the forearm needs to be held horizontally.

Rotational differentiation of the craniocervical region versus the craniomandibular region in prone position

Since a number of patients complain of jaw symptoms when lying prone, it is sometimes useful to perform the tests in a prone position.

Starting position

- The patient lies prone with the head turned to the left.

Position of the examiner

- The therapist stands on the right side of the plinth.

Fixation

- The therapist places the right hand onto the frontal bone and the left index and middle fingers on the patient's chin.
- The patient's head is turned to the point of the onset of symptoms. In this example the TMJ is again responsible for the symptoms.

Method

- With the left hand the therapist slightly reduces the laterotrusion to the left; this will relieve the TMJ and the pain decreases.
- Back in the starting position the therapist's right hand now minimally reduces the cervical rotation. This will decrease the cervical tension but increase the craniomandibular stress. The pain does not change or might even increase slightly.
- The third test is an increase of the laterotrusion to the left, performed with the therapist's left hand. If the TMJ is the source of pain, the symptoms will increase significantly with this test.

Interpretation

- Increasing the cervical rotation with the therapist's right hand will reduce the tension on the TMJ and thereby reduce the symptoms.

Since there is no 'gold standard' for craniomandibular dysfunction in manual therapy, more than one test is required to support our clinical reasoning in the search for the source of the symptoms. If the pain is due to input mechanisms, the rotation differentiation may be a valuable contribution for the identification of the dysfunctional structure.

Cervical accessory movements in various mandibular positions

As already mentioned, there is a clear neurophysiological, biomechanical, neurodynamic and functional connection between the craniocervical and the craniomandibular regions (see Chapter 5). Various accessory movements such as passive intervertebral movements (PAIVMs) (Maitland et al 2001) may be evaluated in different mandibular positions. These results are shown as the parameters of resistance, pain and spasm during the assessment of PAIVMs. The EMG activity will also change in healthy volunteers but are more significant in patients with craniocervical and craniomandibular dysfunctions. Clinically the therapist can expect clear alterations when performing PAIVMs (Maitland et al 2001). Some examples follow.

UNILATERAL POSTERIOR–ANTERIOR MOVEMENT OF C2 IN VARIOUS MANDIBULAR POSITIONS

Example 2

A middle-aged man with symptoms suspected to arise mainly from the upper cervical spine complains of symptoms when eating an apple or visiting the dentist.

These activities may point towards an influence of a submaximal mandibular depression. The patient lies prone with his hands underneath his forehead. The therapist assesses the upper cervical spine by performing PAIVMs and identifies an abnormality of C2 on unilateral posterior–anterior movement on the right-hand side. Based on the data from the subjective examination, the therapist

Example 2—cont'd

hypothesizes that the patient's neck symptoms are related to craniomandibular activities.

The therapist now holds the mandible with both middle and index fingers and positions it in, for example, submaximal depression. In this position the intensity of resistance, pain and/or spasm is assessed and compared to the signs when the submaximal depression is released.

TRANSVERSE MOVEMENT OF C1 IN VARIOUS MANDIBULAR POSITIONS

Example 3

A female student complains of perceived water in her ear. Additionally she has slight tinnitus. She can reproduce her symptoms by end of range mandibular movements, especially in cervical lateroflexion. The tinnitus increases on cervical lateroflexion with additional gentle pressure onto her ear.

In this case the patient is positioned lying on the right side, with her neck supported on a small pillow. The therapist stands at the short end of the plinth and holds the head with the thenar and hypothenar eminences of both hands. Both thumbs rest beside each other on the transverse process of C1 while the left middle and index fingers are positioned on the left side of the mandible. In this position a gentle transverse movement of C1 may be performed. This is repeated in mandibular depression and in laterotrusion. The reactions and the alterations in resistance are noted and compared.

The therapist takes care to perform the transverse movements slowly and gently since the periosteum of C1 is extremely sensitive and various branches of the cranial nerves run along the C1 transverse process (Fig. 8.13).

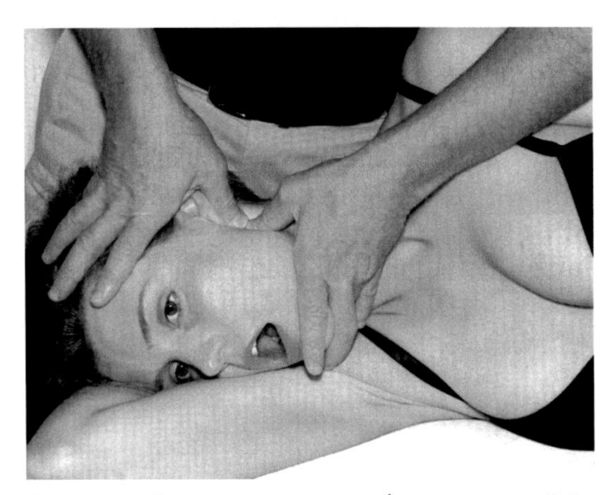

Fig. 8.13 Accessory movement (transverse medial of C1) in various mandibular positions. This example shows laterotrusion to the right and slight depression. The plinth needs to be low to allow the therapist to position the sternum above the craniocervical region.

Mandibular movements in cervical positions

The same principle applies when the therapist hypothesizes that a cervical component is contributing to a predominantly craniomandibular dysfunction. Various upper cervical positions will result in different reactions when testing the physiological and accessory movements of the mandible, the two most common examples being depression (mouth opening) and transverse mandibular movements.

DEPRESSION (MOUTH OPENING) IN VARIOUS CERVICAL FLEXION AND EXTENSION POSITIONS

If the flexion or extension position of the upper cervical spine is altered, this will influence the quality and range of mandibular movements (Rocabado & Iglash 1991, Higbie et al 1999). Opening the mouth is the most functional craniomandibular movement.

The following example supports this: A patient potentially suffers from an anterior–posterior disc displacement without reposition and performs an extension before maximally opening the mouth. This is an indication to assess this patient in supine for quality, resistance and symptoms on mandibular movements in a neutral cervical position and in flexion.

TRANSVERSE MANDIBULAR MOVEMENTS

Transverse mandibular movements towards medial in a slight lateroflexion to the left reproduce ear pain and temporal pain on the right hand side, whenever the patient lies on a pillow for more than 10 minutes. In this case, the patient is assessed in lying on the left with a slight upper cervical lateroflexion and the therapist performs transverse movements medially on the right neck of the mandible. The signs and symptoms are compared to the reactions when the same movement is performed in a neutral position.

DIFFERENTIATION OF CRANIOMANDIBULAR VERSUS CRANIOFACIAL

Temporal–craniomandibular differentiation

The quality of the active mandibular movements may be assessed by slightly changing pressure on the cranium aspects as described in 'General techniques for the neurocranium' in Chapter 14.

> **Example 4**
>
> A 35-year-old accountant presents with complaints of noises in his jaw and a feeling of pressure in the right ear. Active mouth opening produces a clicking and shows a deviation to the right. Maximum opening is 42 mm.
>
> On bilateral temporal rotation the clicking disappears, the shift is reduced and the range of motion increases to 49 mm. The pressure in the ear has also diminished. This points towards a craniofacial contribution to a craniomandibular dysfunction.
>
> This principle may be repeated with any generalized cranium technique, and combined with any physiological mandibular movement.

DIFFERENTIATION OF CRANIOFACIAL VERSUS CRANIOCERVICAL

Generally a standard occiput technique is applied in exactly the position in which the patient has symptoms. For example, if the patient complains of neck pain when working at the PC for 5 minutes, the therapist will choose to stand while the patient sits in a position similar to the work posture until the pain or discomfort sets in.

The therapist stands in front of the patient, holding the occiput with both hands. From this position, compression and rotations around various axes may be performed (see Chapter 14). If the symptoms change with changing pressure on the occiput, the cranium may contribute to the problem. Temporal and sphenoid techniques are also possible, but with the occiput neighbouring directly to the atlas, occiput techniques are the most relevant.

DIFFERENTIATION OF CRANIAL NERVOUS SYSTEM VERSUS CRANIOCERVICAL REGION

If the symptoms occur dominantly on upper cervical flexion and lateroflexion, and the subjective examination points towards a neurodynamic component, the therapist may apply sensitizing manoeuvres in the symptomatic position (Butler 2000). Let us return to the patient above, who suffers from pain on upper cervical flexion during PC work.

Now the hypothesis 'nervous system' needs to be assessed as a source of the symptoms.

Differentiation of cervical flexion and slump position

The patient sits at the short end of the plinth with the therapist standing in front towards one side.

If the status is irritable, the head is now bent to the first onset of symptoms or discomfort. The therapist then places the left hand on the patient's neck with the left thumb in contact with the occiput. The left little finger touches the spine. The therapist asks the patient to bend the thoracic spine. During this movement, which is sensitizing for the nervous system, the head should not move into extension or flexion. The therapist watches the distance between the occiput and the thoracic spine, which should not change throughout the movement. If the symptoms change (better or worse) this points towards a neurodynamic contribution (Fig. 8.14a). If the therapist feels that one or more cranial nerves are contributing to the problem, contralateral upper cervical lateroflexion can be carried out. More information on neurodynamic tests and treatment techniques are found in Chapters 16–18.

If the symptoms are not clearly irritable, the manoeuvre should be performed with fixation of the head. The therapist now places the right hand in supination onto the patient's maxilla. The left hand holds the occiput in this position (Fig. 8.14b). This way, the head should easily move into resistance of upper cervical flexion and can be held here while lateroflexion is added (to the right).

If the therapist believes that one or more cranial nerves are contributing to the problem, lateroflexion to the opposite side can be added.

For more detailed information on cranial neurodynamics, see Chapters 16 and 17.

DIFFERENTIATION OF CRANIAL NERVOUS SYSTEM VERSUS CRANIOMANDIBULAR REGION

If no other structure becomes relevant during functional differentiation, it seems logical to continue by collecting clinical data from the craniomandibular region. It is almost impossible to perform all of the tests that are described in the following paragraphs, so the therapist will have to decide, according to the results from the subjective examination, which of the available tests are likely to be most productive in the time available (Mohl 1991).

Clinically and scientifically supported evidence shows that mandibular movements have altered functions during neurodynamically altered positions of the cervical spine (Isberg et al 1987, von Piekartz 2000). One example is mandibular laterotrusion in a position of cervical lateroflexion.

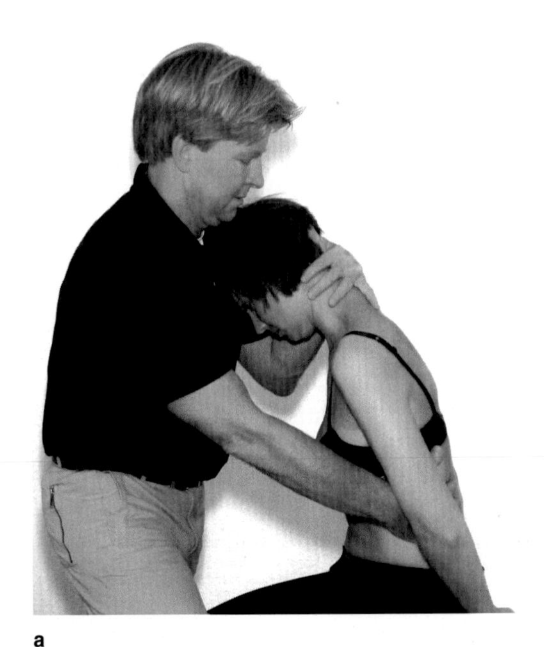

a

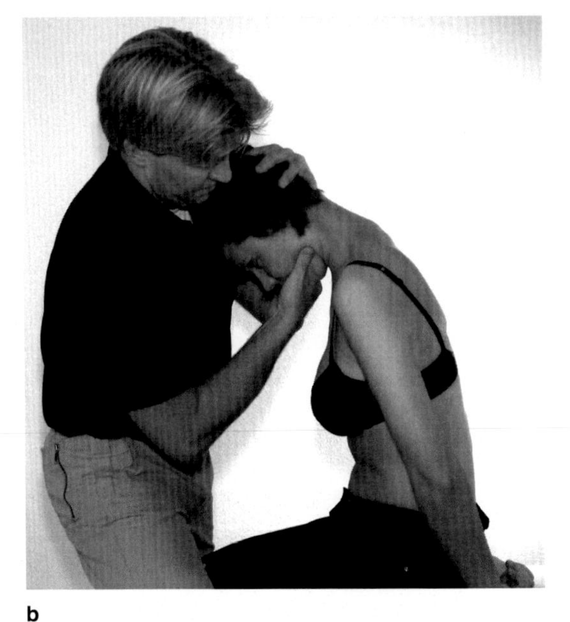

b

Fig. 8.14
a Cervical slump test in an irritable situation.
b Cervical slump test in a non-irritable situation. Note the different position of the right hand.

Mandibular laterotrusion in upper cervical flexion and lateroflexion

A patient complains of lower right molar toothache. Mandibular laterotrusion to the right is performed. The toothache is slightly reproduced. The therapist now reasons that the mandibular nerve may contribute neuropathically to the problem. The patient is then positioned in upper cervical flexion and lateroflexion to the left, putting the structures into further neurodynamic tension (Breig 1978, Doursonian et al 1989). The laterotrusion is repeated actively in this position. Active laterotrusion to the right is now limited, more clearly reproduces the toothache and a protective spasm of the masseter muscle occurs. This clinical pattern may point towards (neuropathic) involvement of the mandibular nerve. The standard neurodynamic tests for the mandibular nerve now need to be evaluated (von Piekartz 2000).

DIFFERENTIATION OF CRANIAL NERVOUS SYSTEM VERSUS CRANIOFACIAL

Anatomical and clinical signs show a direct correlation of the symptoms that may be produced by these structures. The dura, for example, is attached to the cranium, plays an important role in cranial growth (Wagemans et al 1988) and is a mechanosensitive structure (Kumar et al 1996). It is quite common for patients with dominantly neurogenic pain to react to spontaneous pressure changes within the cranium (pain may increase or decrease). If this pattern is apparent on subjective examination, the therapist may add various general cranium techniques in a craniocervical position of gentle neurodynamic tension.

Occiput techniques in slump position

The therapist asks the patient to perform thoracic and lumbar flexion. During this manoeuvre, which is sensitizing for the nervous system, the head should not change its flexion–extension position. The therapist monitors the distance between occiput and thoracic spine so that this does not change during the movement. If the symptoms change, this may indicate a neurodynamic component. In this position the therapist performs some standard neurocranium techniques of the occipital, temporal, sphenoid, frontal and parietal regions depending on the hypothesized sources of the symptoms. In this case the hands gently hold the occiput to perform rotation about various axes.

ACTIVE MOVEMENTS

ACTIVE MOVEMENTS IN SITTING

The standard active movements are:

- Depression: mouth opening
- Protrusion: forward movement of the mandible
- Retrusion: dorsal movement of the mandible
- Laterotrusion: sideways movement of the mandible.

Starting position, methods and some clinical tips are described in the following.

Mouth opening (depression)

STARTING POSITION AND METHOD

The patient sits in a standardized position on the plinth. Commonly this is an upright position. The therapist stands directly in front of the patient and palpates for both mandibular heads. To assess the right TMJ, the therapist places the index finger in front of and the middle finger behind the mandibular head. The right hand does the same on the left mandibular head. The patient is now asked to open their mouth. The therapist assesses the symmetrical rolling movement of the mandibular head and the ventrocaudal glide.

If the patient simultaneously performs cervical extension, or any other cervical movement, the therapist attempts to standardize the head position by starting with the opening of the mouth. This is essential since neck position strongly influences the mandibular range of motion. While the patient opens the mouth, the therapist reminds the patient that an isolated mandibular movement is required. If the patient cannot control this by themselves, the therapist stabilizes the patient's head by placing a hand on the occiput. The lower arm of the stabilizing hand is held parallel to the spine, so that the patient cannot move into more thoracic flexion (Higbie et al 1999). On inspection of the depression movement from lateral, an arched curve of the chin towards caudal and dorsal is observed; this is considered as normal.

INDICATIONS FOR DYSFUNCTIONS

If a deviation or shift is observed on mouth opening, this is corrected by gentle thumb pressure on the chin. If signs occur (clicking, resistance) or symptoms are provoked, the changes in movement patterns are potentially due to protective deformities (Maitland et al 2001). A continued deviation, with the lower jaw shifting laterally on initiation of depression, that corrects back to the mid-position at the end of range, may be an indicator for an intra-articular problem. If the deviation varies, this points more towards a muscular imbalance (Hochstedler et al 1996). If opening is accompanied by a constant lateral shift, this may indicate a homolateral (intra-articular) problem.

MOUTH OPENING

A number of studies proved that the inter- and intrareliability of measurements for mouth opening with a ruler is moderate to good (Lund et al 1995, Walker et al 2000, Leher et al 2005). A calliper or goniometer may also be used clinically and both achieve similar results (Graff-Rafford 1985).

The following measurements should be performed with a hard ruler of 15 cm length so that all important mandibular ranges of motion may be measured quickly and easily (Fig. 8.15).

The patient opens the mouth and the ruler is placed between the upper edge of the lower incisors and the lower edge of the upper incisors.

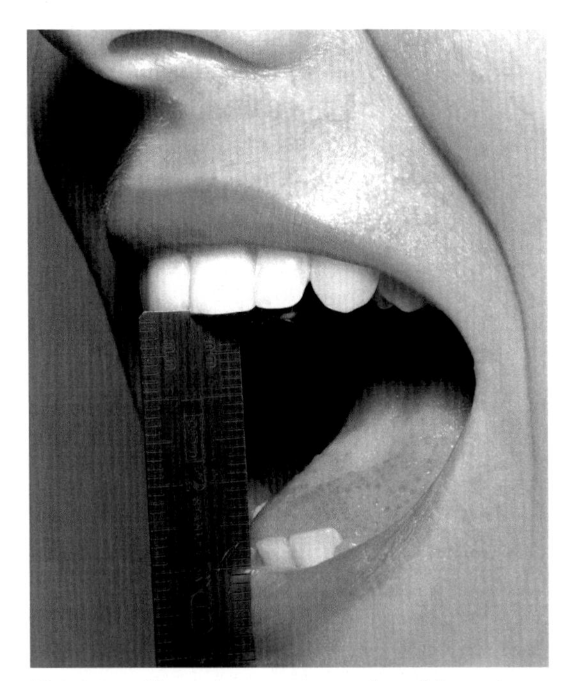

Fig. 8.15 Measuring mouth opening with a ruler. The distance between the upper edge of the lower incisors and the lower edge of the upper incisors is measured.

> **!** To test the reliability of the use of a ruler between experienced and inexperienced examiners, Lehrer et al (2005) used 27 patients with craniomandibular dysfunction who were rated blindly and in random sequence by two experienced and two inexperienced examiners. An excellent reliability was found for vertical dimension motions and there were no significant differences in the measurement results between the experienced and inexperienced examiners. The conclusion is that examiner calibration is a more important factor than professional experience for vertical dimension motion measurement with a ruler.

OVERBITE

Overbite indicates to what extent the upper incisor teeth cover the lower incisor teeth (Harzer 1999). The therapist draws a horizontal line onto the lower incisors where the upper incisors stop at maximum intercuspidation. The patient is then asked to half open the mouth to allow the therapist to measure the vertical distance between the line and the upper edge of the lower incisors. The average distance for patients without craniomandibular dysfunction is 3.0 mm (Walker et al 2000) (Fig. 8.16).

Overjet is the horizontal distance between the upper and lower incisor teeth when the mouth is closed. The ruler is placed perpendicularly onto the upper incisors until it reaches the lower incisors and the distance is noted in millimetres. The average distance for patients without craniomandibular problems is 3.2 mm (Walker et al 2000).

VROM SCALE (VISUAL RANGE OF MOTION SCALE)/REGISTRATION OF THE QUANTITATIVE AND QUALITATIVE MOUTH OPENING DATA

It is of enormous importance not only to record the range of motion but also to describe the quality of the lower jaw movements which provoke or ameliorate symptoms. It is important to know whether a clicking occurs before, during or at the end of a shift or where during the range of motion the shift is most dominant. These data may be analysed in combination with a *visual range of motion scale.*

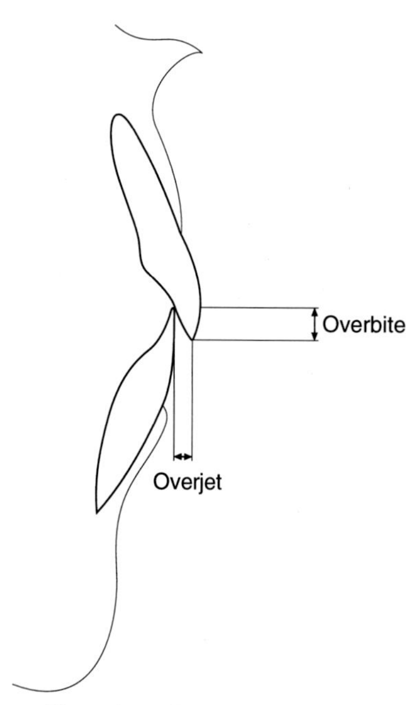

Fig. 8.16 Normal overjet and overbite. These are easily assessed with a ruler (see text).

VROM in the frontal plane

An example for a VROM scale in the frontal plane is shown in Figure 8.17a. The vertical line represents mouth opening from the beginning (A) to the average limit (B). The horizontal line represents laterotrusion, for which 10 mm to the left (L) and 10 mm to the right (R) were chosen. In Figure 8.17b the example described above is shown graphically. The shift to the right sets in at 8 mm, reaches its climax at 21 mm opening with 8 mm shift and disappears at 39 mm opening. The clicking occurs at 14 mm opening. The maximum depression is 45 mm. Even if the therapist does not always need all these data, the most important for each individual case can be chosen. The advantages of the VROM scale are:

- Information: It offers a lot of information in very little time. This helps to identify clinical patterns such as intra-articular dysfunctions, limitations and muscle imbalances.
- Straightforward: It is easy to integrate into the daily clinical routine, easy to draw and for most clinicians easy to visualize.
- Reassessment: It does take a little practice and time to draw the scale. Since it has shown good intrarater reliability, it is a valuable reassessment tool (Shellhas 1989).
- Uniformity: This scale is frequently used in dental practices as well as in orthodontic clinics and protocols, and is therefore a useful communication tool (Sheppard & Sheppard 1965, Rosenbaum 1975, Curl 1992).

VROM in the sagittal plane

In some cases it may be important to draw a VROM scale of depression in the sagittal plane. The movement should normally show an arched line towards caudal and dorsal. The tip of the chin should stay behind an imaginary line that originates from the nose wings.

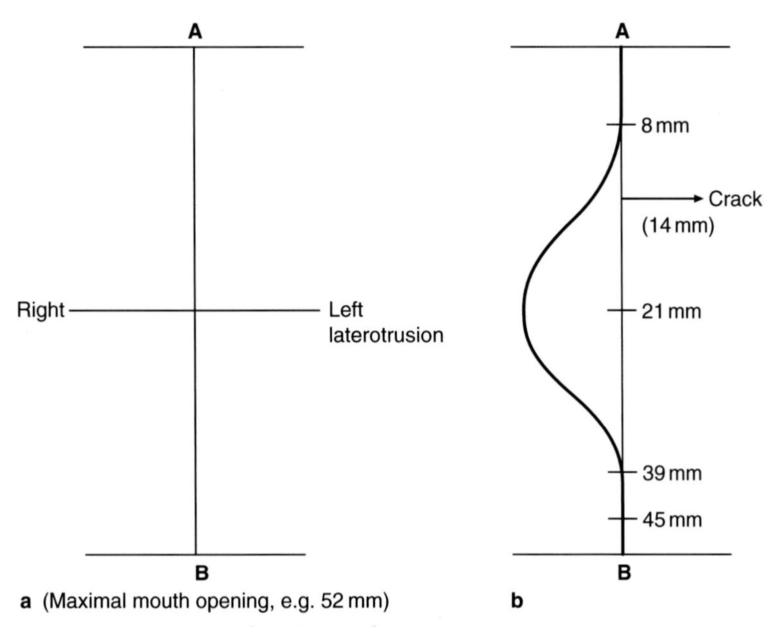

Fig. 8.17 Visual range of motion scale (VROM scale) in the frontal plane.
a Example of a VROM scale in the frontal plane (see text).
b VROM scale in the frontal plane on mouth opening with mandibular shift to the right.

Abnormal movements towards protrusion and retrusion are easy to register and combine with other symptoms with the aid of the VROM scale.

Protrusion

STARTING POSITION AND METHOD

The therapist stands to the side of the seated patient and asks them to move the lower jaw forwards. Normal movement shows an arch like the lower jaw itself: initially towards caudal and ventral, then towards cranial and ventral. The tip of the chin moves forward on the frontal plane.

INDICATIONS FOR DYSFUNCTIONS

During the movement the patient should not perform any additional compensatory cervical activities. If this is the case, the therapist corrects these activities gently and asks the patient to repeat the movement.

A shift to the right or to the left, with or without pain, may also occur. The mandible deviates to one side, visible by a movement of the chin. Potential causes are intra-articular dysfunction or muscle imbalance (Okeson 1995, Palla et al 1998, Bryden & Fitzgerald 2001). Again the chin position may be corrected during the movement. The range of motion, the reactions, the clicking, the muscle spasm and the symptoms can be compared to the movement without the correction.

DISTANCE MEASUREMENT

To assess protrusion, the distance between the upper and lower incisors is measured in the transverse plane with a ruler or calliper and this value is added to the distance between the incisors in a resting position (overbite distance) (Fig. 8.18).

The average value is 6–11 mm in men and 6–12 mm in women (Burch 1983, Clark et al 1989).

Retrusion

STARTING POSITION AND METHOD

The starting position is the same as for protrusion. The patient is asked to move the jaw backwards. If the patient has difficulties with this activity, the therapist may add a gentle tactile stimulus with the fingers on the patient's chin.

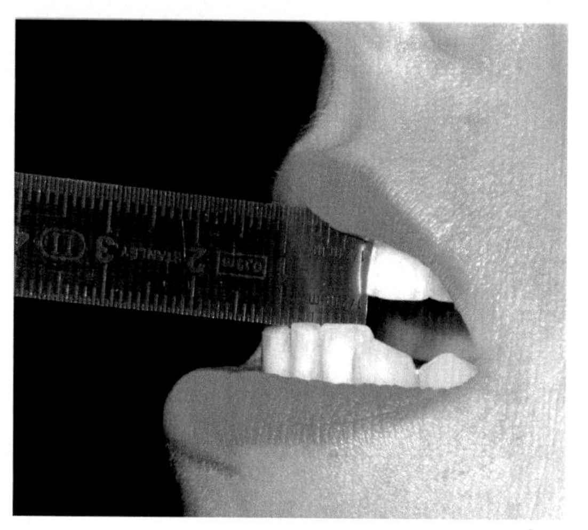

Fig. 8.18 Measuring protrusion with a ruler. It is important that the craniocervical region remains in the same position.

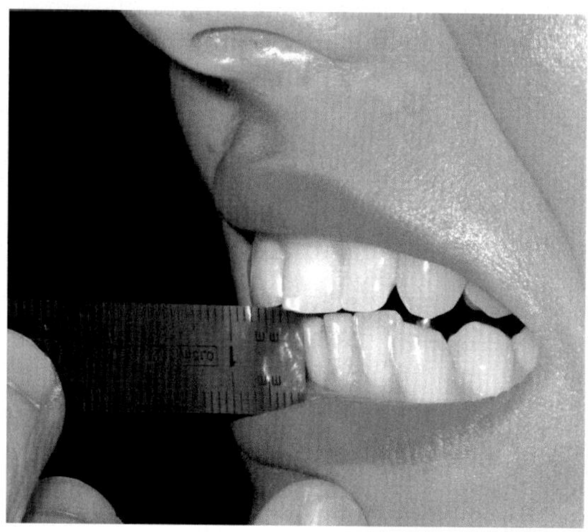

Fig. 8.19 Measuring retropulsion with a ruler (same technique as overjet measurement).

INDICATIONS FOR DYSFUNCTIONS

This movement is difficult to perform for many patients with craniomandibular dysfunction. It is only saved in the motor cortex in a reduced version (Ramachandran & Blakeslee 1998, Kaas 2000). Retrusion is commonly associated with increased muscle activity of the masticatory and suprahyoid muscles and pressure of the tongue. If the therapist repeats the movement passively or assists the patient with the movement, the patient then generally finds it easier to do it by themselves. If this is the case the therapist gains important information and remembers to integrate coordination exercises into overall patient management.

DISTANCE MEASUREMENT

The distance between the incisor teeth may again be measured with a ruler or a calliper in the transverse plane (Fig. 8.19). The resting distance of the incisor teeth now needs to be subtracted from the measured value. The average value is 4 mm (Graber 1969) and is significantly lower in healthy volunteers than in patients with protrusion.

Laterotrusion

STARTING POSITION AND METHOD

As for depression, the therapist stands directly in front of the seated patient. The patient is asked to relax the jaw and to shift the lower jaw to the left with the mouth slightly opened. The movement is compared to the lateral shift to the right.

INDICATIONS FOR DYSFUNCTION

The reaction of patients with craniomandibular dysfunction to laterotrusion may be different from the reactions to the previous active movements. This is because laterotrusion is a horizontal movement which implies different effects on the joints and the neuromuscular system (Herring 2001, Murray et al 2001). If a clear difference of more than 5 mm is noted between sides, this indicates an intra-articular dysfunction on the side where the movement is limited (Graber 1969, Bell 1982).

DISTANCE MEASUREMENT

The distance between the central upper and lower incisor teeth is measured in the end of range positions. If the lower jaw is already shifted to the left in a resting position, this shift needs to be subtracted from the overall measured value of laterotrusion to the left, or added to the laterotrusion to the right; 12 mm to each side is the average range of motion. If the difference between left and right laterotrusion is greater than 5 mm, this may indicate an intra-articular problem on the side with restricted movement. The average value varies in different studies between 8.6 mm and 12 mm (Graber 1969, Curl 1992, Walker et al 2000). A difference between sides of up to 3 mm is considered normal (Burch 1983, Curl 1992) (Fig. 8.20).

Reference data for the mandibular range of motion

Mandibular range of motion measurements are considered to be valid and reliable clinical indicators for dysfunction (Hannam 1991, Karlsson et al 1991). Reference data, average values from populations of healthy volunteers (Agterberg 1987), may be used to compare and analyse patient data. Unfortunately not all studies indicate the same values. Potential causes are the different numbers of volunteers (*n*), the starting position for the measurement and the type of measurement tool. There follow some examples of studies where the measurements have been performed with a ruler and that the author considers sufficiently straightforward for the clinician to interpret.

MOUTH OPENING

Measuring the opening capacity is usually the most important measurement. This value not only informs about the situation of the joints and the masticatory muscles but is also the most useful reassessment parameter (Palla et al 1998). Carlsson and Magnusson (1999) emphasize the importance of the classic study by Agterberg (1987), who evaluated the average range of mouth opening in a large population. The advantage of his data is that the age and sex of the volunteers were also recorded and evaluated. Although the minimum and maximum values are clearly indicated, unfortunately the standard deviation was not mentioned in the article. The study describes active opening without passive overpressure (Table 8.4).

MEASURING OPENING IN VARIOUS CERVICAL POSITIONS

It is usually sensible to measure in a functional cervical position, especially if the patient has described functional positions in which the

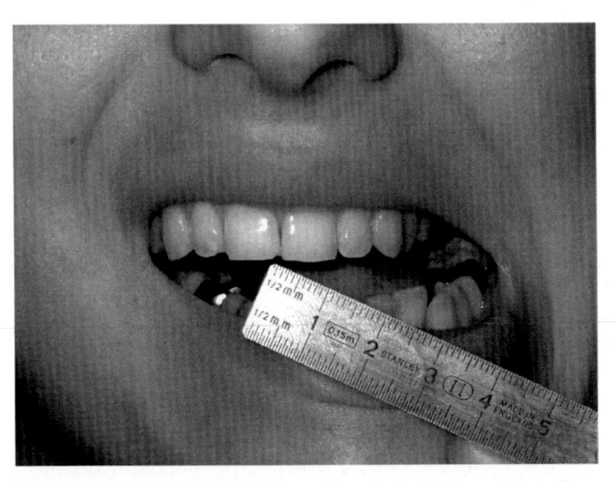

Fig. 8.20 Measuring laterotrusion with a ruler. At the end of range, the distance between the central incisor teeth of the upper and lower jaw are calculated.

Table 8.4 Average maximum mouth opening in dependence of age and sex

	Main results (mm)		
Age (years)	Male	Female	Range (mm)
1.5	38.6	38.1	32–44
6	44.3	45.2	33–60
13	53.4	54.4	41–73
16	57.0	55.0	39–82
20	58.6	53.3	42–77
70	52.7	49.3	38–65

From Carlsson & Magnusson (1999).

symptoms are provoked. Higbie et al (1999) have calculated the average values for maximum opening in neutral position, upper cervical extension and upper cervical flexion. The disadvantage of this study is the small number of volunteers ($n = 19$).

To summarize, the maximum opening in most individuals is more than 40 mm (average value minus 2 mm standard deviation) (Dworkin & LeResche 1992, Salaorni & Palla 1994) (Table 8.5).

PROTRUSION AND LATEROTRUSION

Various studies state a large range of motion with a relatively small average value. Although women show a larger amplitude of opening than men, protrusion and laterotrusion seem fairly equal (Dworkin & LeResche 1992, Salaorni & Palla 1994). Table 8.6 shows an overview of the range, the minimum values and the average values of protrusion and laterotrusion in females and in males in a population of more than 100 volunteers (Clark et al 1989, Curl 1992).

Interpretation of the maximum mandibular ranges of motion

RELATIVITY OF MAXIMUM OPENING

Limited mouth opening is usually a clear indicator for a craniomandibular dysfunction. According to the frequently used Helkimo Index, an opening capacity of 30–39 mm indicates a slight disability and less than 30 mm a severe disability (Helkimo 1974). It is important to mention in this context since a number of different variables determine the range of mouth opening. As shown in Table 8.4, the opening capacity depends, among other factors, on age and sex (Agterberg 1987). Facial height and mandibular length also influence the range of motion (Carlsson & Magnusson 1999). This explains the large physiological range and the meaning of reference data should not be overestimated. One recorded patient showed a range of 45 mm before treatment and 52 mm after treatment – the therapy therefore resulted in a definite improvement! Retrospectively, this patient showed an opening limitation (Palla et al 1998).

Table 8.5 Mouth opening measurements in various cervical positions

Cervical position	Mean value (mm)	Standard deviation (mm)	Range (mm)
Head bent forwards	44.5	5.3	32.0–55.3
Neutral head position	41.5	4.8	31.7–50.7
Head bent backwards	36.2	4.5	26.3–46.3

Table 8.6 Overview of the range of motion of depression, protrusion and laterotrusion

	Maximum depression	Protrusion	Laterotrusion
Male	45–60 mm Minimum 40 mm Mean value 55 mm	6–11 mm Minimum 4 mm Mean value 2.0 mm	Range of motion (roughly 3 mm) from side to side in both sexes Minimum 4 mm Mean value 2.4 mm
Female	40–55 mm Minimum 40 mm Mean value 50 mm	6–12 mm Minimum 4 mm Mean value 2.0 mm	Range of motion (roughly 3 mm) from side to side in both sexes Minimum 4 mm Mean value 2.4 mm

Only differences of more than 4 mm, or for laterotrusion of more than 2 mm, are clinically significant (Agterberg 1987).

ACTIVE VERSUS PASSIVE MOUTH OPENING

The range of motion may be smaller on active opening without deviation than on passive overpressure. If the difference is greater than 4 mm, the soft tissue may be responsible for the restriction (Carlsson & Magnusson 1999). Palpation of the soft tissue and the dynamic and static tests for the masticatory muscles may confirm this hypothesis.

If active *and* passive mouth opening is restricted (less than 30 mm), the end-feel is hard and the patient complains of a sharp pain localized around the joint, the source of the symptoms is probably an intra-articular dysfunction (Kraus 1994, Palla et al 1998, Bumann & Lotzmann 2000).

LATEROTRUSION DURING MOUTH OPENING

If a deviation occurs on opening and laterotrusion is restricted more than 5 mm compared with the opposite side, this may indicate an intra-articular dysfunction on the restricted side (Graber 1969).

INFLUENCE OF VARIOUS CERVICAL POSITIONS ON MAXIMUM OPENING, LATEROTRUSION AND PROTRUSION

Various test results may indicate whether the nociceptive input is dominantly arthrogenic, muscular or neurogenic. Some clinical patterns are discussed below.

- A dominantly muscular mouth opening problem shows no changes of protrusion and laterotrusion since the elevator muscles are usually not involved (Cacchiotti et al 1991).
- If mouth opening is not or only slightly affected, the protrusion is restricted and unilaterally painful, and the same reaction is found on contralateral laterotrusion, the potential source may be the pterygoid muscles.
- With mouth opening restricted and unilateral laterotrusion affected, and possibly painful, the hypothesis of an intra-articular problem is confirmed if the lower jaw deviates to the ipsilateral side on protrusion (Palla et al 1998).
- If active opening is restricted but the jaw moves freely but painfully on passive overpressure, and laterotrusion to both sides is not affected, it is most likely to be a muscular problem.
- If retrusion is severely restricted and the end-feel is hard, and protrusion and laterotrusion are not affected, this may indicate a dorsal intra-articular dysfunction (Bumann & Lotzmann 2000) or a strong muscular protective mechanism that frequently occurs in patients with dysgnathia III as classified by Angle (Proffit & Ackerman 1993) (see also Chapter 9).
- If laterotrusion and protrusion are restricted and produce a deep unilateral, sometimes burning pain behind or directly inside the joint or along the mandible, this may point towards a (minimal) neuropathy of the mandibular nerve. The hypothesis is confirmed if the pain increases on a static test in protrusion. The potential explanation for this provocation is an impingement of the buccal or the lingual nerves (branch of the mandibular nerve) in the superior aspect of the lateral pterygoid muscle (Dupont & Matthews 2000).

INTERPRETATION OF THE MANDIBULAR MOVEMENT DATA

The cervical spine may change the central position of the mandible and may therefore influence the quality of movement (Rocabado & Iglash 1991) and potentially also the neurodynamics (von Piekartz 2001). For example:

- If an opening click with or without pain accompanies an asymmetrically changed laterotrusion and a restricted protrusion with pain around the ear, a disc displacement towards the anterior may be the source of the symptoms. This hypothesis is confirmed if active as well as passive protrusion

in sustained upper cervical flexion deviates, produces pain or shows a restriction.
- If active as well as passive laterotrusion is restricted and painful heterolaterally, and a pulling, burning pain along the mandible (which increases with cervical flexion) occurs, a contribution of the mandibular nerve is likely (von Piekartz 2000, 2001).

ACTIVE MOVEMENTS WITH OVERPRESSURE IN SUPINE

The same movements may also be performed with overpressure. Overpressure is defined as a gently passive continuation of the physiological movement at the end of active range of motion (Cyriax 1982, Maitland et al 2001). The therapist assesses the following aspects:

- Does it provoke symptoms more clearly if they could not be reproduced convincingly? (This may guide clinical decision-making.)
- Behaviour of the range of motion when comparing active movement with passive overpressure: In a normal situation the range of motion is larger on overpressure due to the non-contractile structures and does not provoke symptoms (Silman et al 1986, Hesse & Hansson 1988).
- End-feel: The therapist may differentiate between qualities such as 'hard', 'elastic' and 'tight'.

Interpretation of the end-feel

Various studies show that the type of end-feel is independent from the specific structure (Hesse 1990, Hesse et al 1996). This implies that tests can only register dysfunctions, act as reassessment parameters and point only retrospectively towards potential structures, depending on the response to the treatment technique.

ACTIVE TESTS WITH OVERPRESSURE

The following tests are all performed with the patient lying supine. The advantage of this position is that the patient's head can be placed in a standardized manner. It is also a helpful position if the therapist decides to apply one of the assessment techniques as a treatment technique. Depending on the therapist and the patient, the techniques may also be performed in sitting. Overpressure means that the therapist continues the physiological movement passively from the end of the active range. Usually this requires between two and four small amplitude oscillating movements. The advantage is that the behaviour of resistance and symptoms is noted instantly and the therapist can stop the movement immediately if severe symptoms occur (Jones 1994, Maitland et al 2001).

Mouth opening (depression)

STARTING POSITION AND METHOD

The patient is lying supine with a small pillow, if required (Fig. 8.21). The therapist is standing on the left side of the plinth near the patient's shoulder girdle and holds the patient's head with the right forearm. With the arm resting on the plinth, the right hand is free to palpate the right mandibular head with the index and middle fingers.

The patient is asked to open the mouth maximally. The therapist places the left index and middle fingers onto the floor of the patient's mouth and the thumb underneath the patient's chin. The therapist now performs gently oscillating movements towards depression as an

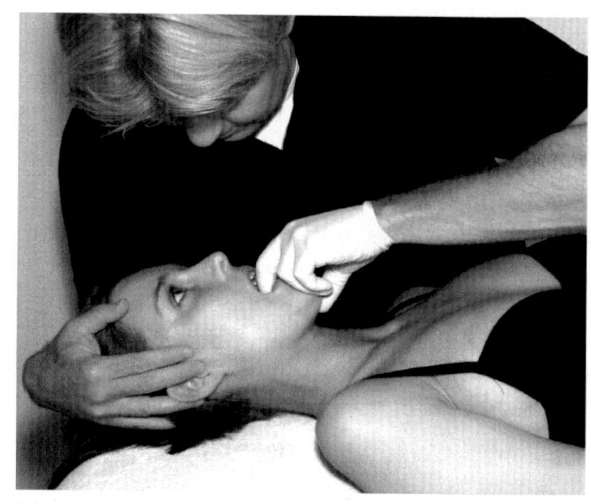

Fig. 8.21 Depression (mouth opening) in supine with intraoral overpressure.

overpressure. It is important not to let the hand perform the activity but to move the shoulder and the trunk. This will make the movement less painful for the patient and the therapist will find it easier to evaluate resistance. To control his own movement the therapist needs to be careful that the tip of his elbow (olecranon) moves in an arch towards the patient's trunk.

Protrusion

STARTING POSITION AND METHOD

Again the therapist stands on the left next to the supine patient at shoulder level. For protrusion it is especially important to hold the head steady to avoid cervical movements. The therapist holds the patient's head with the distal part of the right forearm and the right hand. The therapist's elbow is supported on the plinth. The therapist palpates for the right mandibular head with the right middle and index fingers (Fig. 8.22).

With the mouth slightly open the patient moves the jaw as far forward as possible. The therapist places the left thumb on the floor of the patient's mouth and holds the chin by positioning the left middle and index fingers underneath and behind the chin. The left elbow points towards the ceiling so that the forearm is vertical. By moving the trunk the therapist produces small oscillating movements towards a protrusion overpressure. It is important not to perform a linear movement, but to move along a ventrocranial arch, continuing the physiological motion. With the right middle and index finger the movement can be palpated.

Overpressure on protrusion causes stress on the intra-articular structures and the lateral pterygoid muscle (Naeije & van Loon 1998, Bumann & Lotzmann 2000).

Retrusion

STARTING POSITION AND METHOD

The patient is lying relaxed in supine and the therapist, positioned on the patient's left, holds the patient's head with the right forearm and hand. The right forearm is supported on the plinth and the right middle and index fingers palpate for the right mandibular head (Fig. 8.23). The left hand is placed on the chin, so that the thumb is on the left and the index finger on the right side of the mandibular body. The left forearm is almost vertical. In a dorsocranial arch the overpressure is now applied with oscillating movements. It is important not to produce the activity with the wrist but by moving the trunk. The therapist watches for resistance, stiffness and the subjective response of the patient. In most cases the patient will

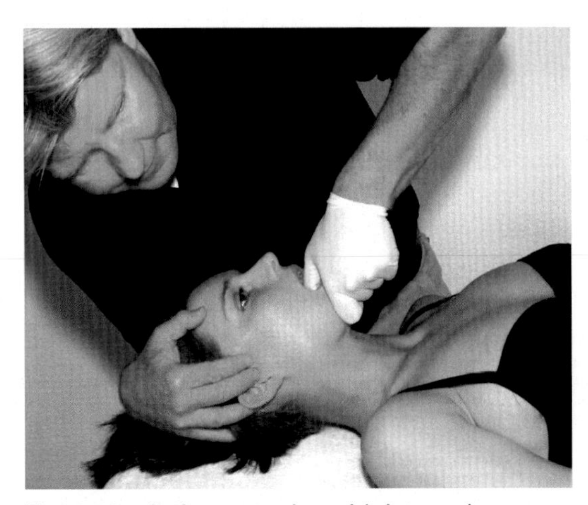

Fig. 8.22 Active protrusion with intraoral overpressure.

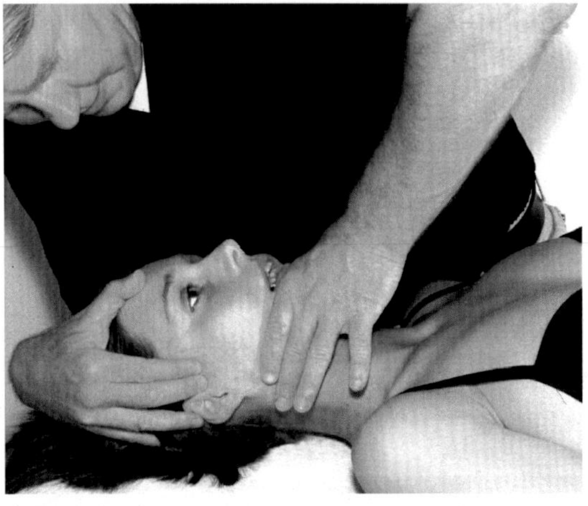

Fig. 8.23 Active retropulsion with overpressure in supine.

perceive an increase of pressure ventral to the ear. This pressure may become relevant if there is a clear difference in intensity or the patient's pain is reproduced.

> **!** *Hint for difficulties during active retrusion:* Many patients find it difficult to actively perform retrusion. It can be helpful to introduce the movement by briefly placing the tip of the tongue against the hard palate. On relaxation after that activity a retrusion automatically occurs and the patient only needs to enhance this automatic reaction. If the therapist supports the activity or performs it passively, most patients are then able to actively move the jaw into retrusion

Laterotrusion

Laterotrusion is a movement to the right or to the left. This chapter describes laterotrusion to the right.

STARTING POSITION AND METHOD

For laterotrusion to the right, the therapist stands on the left side of the plinth. The patient's head is turned 30–35° to the right for easier handling. The therapist's right hand stabilizes the patient's head by embracing it from cranially (Fig. 8.24). (If the therapist is absolutely certain that no neurodynamic contribution may alter the test result, the patient may also support their own head with the right hand.) The therapist's forearm is supported by the plinth and the middle and index fingers palpate for the right mandibular head. The middle and index fingers of the left hand are placed on the mandible and the thumb lies lateral to the mandibular angle. The patient now performs an active laterotrusion to the right and the therapist continues the movement passively by applying oscillating overpressure. Again the movement is produced by moving the trunk and not the arm joints. The movement does not represent transverse accessory movements but a physiological arched motion.

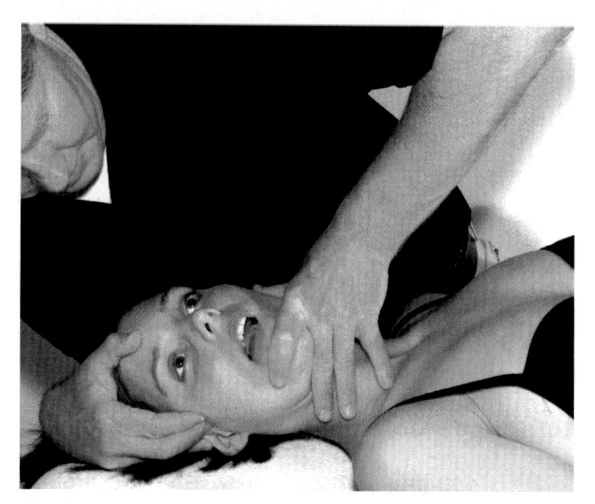

Fig. 8.24 Active laterotrusion with overpressure in supine.

EXAMPLE OF A CLINICAL EVALUATION OF THE TEST

If the test is applied towards the right hand side, it compromises structures of the right craniomandibular region. In particular, the TMJ and the left side experience less stress. This applies, for example, when laterotrusion provokes the patient's symptoms on the right side and the movement is restricted. If the patient's history points towards intra-articular dysfunction (e.g. trauma of the TMJ, disc displacement without reduction), mouth opening is clearly restricted and the mandible is shifted to the right, the hypothesis of an intra-articular dysfunction is supported. Accessory movements to the right TMJ are then expected to provoke signs and possibly symptoms. If this is the case, the altered directions of movement can be treated by manual therapy techniques. The retrospective assessment will decide whether the hypothesis is confirmed or dismissed.

MUSCLE TESTS

To gain an impression of the status of the masticatory muscles, various muscle tests apply:

- Static (isometric) tests
- Dynamic tests

- Length tests
- Muscle control: endurance and functional coordination
- Palpation
- General tests
- Trigger points.

Depending on experience, the therapist may be able to recognize certain clinical patterns and to decide according to the collected clinical data which tests should be applied first (Jones & von Piekartz 2001). Commonly the first choice tests are the isometric and muscle control tests, similar to other regions of the body. Palpation is usually performed at the end of the physical examination. The following paragraphs will introduce the various testing procedures, including their indications.

STATIC (ISOMETRIC TESTS)

Static or isometric tests are defined as techniques where the therapist applies a certain force in one direction against the resistance of the mandible (Cyriax 1982, Maitland et al 2001). The patient reacts by holding against this force with the same force in the opposite direction. The resultant movement should be zero. This means that a static action without any movement occurs. Muscle physiology states that in this case an isometric muscle contraction occurs (Mense 1998).

In the craniomandibular region the following parameters can be easily assessed:

- Force
- Pain
- Coordination
- Willingness to move.

Force

The therapist gains an impression of the potential muscle force. If muscle force appears reduced it does not automatically imply that the muscular system is dysfunctional. The static mandibular tests have been evaluated for validity (as a muscle test) and reliability (Lobbezoo-Scholte et al 1993). A number of studies of the neuromuscular system have shown that a nociceptive input from a certain region may function as an inhibition to the contractile structures, thereby protecting the tissue. This is called *pain inhibition* or *disorder inhibition* (Stokes 1984, Hurley 1997, Sterling et al 2001). Such phenomena have also been found in patients with TMJ capsulitis with swelling (Kraus 1994).

A loss of force towards one direction should therefore not only be interpreted as a morphological alteration of the neuromuscular system but also as a physiological reaction.

CLINICAL INTERPRETATION

If passive mobilization (e.g. accessory movements) significantly improves the force of isometric laterotrusion, the loss of muscle force was not due to morphological changes such as muscle atrophy, but results from neurophysiological inhibition mechanisms.

Pain

If pain is provoked by isometric tests, this may indicate dysfunctions of the contractile structures (Cyriax 1982). The therapist should also be aware that the increased muscle tension during isometric tests will result in increased intra-articular compression in synovial joints (Kaltenborn 1992, Maitland et al 2001). It is known that isometric tests, for example at the elbow, increase the intra-articular compression of the glenohumeral joint (Ellenberker 1996).

This also applies for the TMJ. A slight static contact increases the intra-articular compression (De Laat et al 1993). Therefore an isometric craniomandibular test may be false-positive if the clinician hypothesizes that the contractile structures alone are the source responsible for the reproduction of pain. Experience has shown that muscle inhibition is the common reason for a reduced force on isometric testing if the test is accompanied by pain.

Coordination

Static craniomandibular tests are often an ideal method to gain an impression of the patient's capacity to perform isolated mandibular movements. It is known that if a movement has not been performed for a prolonged period of time the somatotopy of the primary somatosensory cortex (homunculus) is reduced (Penfield & Boldrey 1937). The result is a disturbed sensomotor feedback, presented as coordination difficulties (Held 1965). The craniomandibular region, together with the hand, shows the largest projection area on the homunculus (Ramachandran & Blakeslee 1998) with a great plasticity (see Chapter 1).

The area of projection becomes smaller when the structures are not (or only very little) used. On isometric testing of the craniomandibular region, features of coordination deficiencies as outlined in Box 8.2 may be found.

Willingness to move

Patients with craniomandibular dysfunction often fear orofacial movements (Kino et al 2001), especially after trauma or surgery (Morris et al 1997). Isometric testing will show the therapist whether the patient is willing to forcefully perform a movement. The results, for example significant fear of performing laterotrusion to the right because it may produce a clicking, need to be considered for pain management strategies at a later stage (Butler 2000).

Box 8.2 Coordination deficiencies

- Associated cervical movements (mainly towards extension)
- Increased pressure of the tongue against the palate, registered as an upward shift of the hyoid and contour changes of the suprahyoid muscles
- Parafunctions such as 'bracing', 'tongue pressure' or 'biting the lips' are not uncommon
- Associated, generally unilateral activities of the mimic muscles
- Loss of force or inability to initiate the required mandibular movement
- If one or more indicators is found, the therapist needs to introduce static and later on dynamic coordinative exercises into the patient management programme at an early stage.

GENERAL STARTING POSITION AND METHOD

The therapist stands or sits behind the patient, who is positioned in supine. Supine is the first choice position since overpressure tests may be followed immediately by isometric tests. It also helps the patient to perform the movements easily and the therapist will find the activities simple to control (in the case of deviations). Laterotrusion to the right can be directly compared with laterotrusion to the left. The only disadvantage is that the upright position would be more functional. If symptoms cannot be provoked in lying, or the therapist decides to use the test as an exercise, sitting upright is also an option.

During the test, muscle tension is increased gently, held for a moment and slowly released.

The patient should be able to increase force steadily and to hold it constant without an actual movement of the mandible.

Elevation

STARTING POSITION AND METHOD

The therapist places the index finger underneath and the thumb on the patient's chin, so that the fingertips almost touch. With the patient's mouth slightly open, the thumb will now increase its pressure towards depression. The patient attempts to prevent any mandibular movement.

Depression

STARTING POSITION AND METHOD

Index finger and thumb are positioned as described above for elevation. The therapist applies pressure with the index finger towards elevation and the patient uses their depressor muscles to prevent any movement.

Laterotrusion to the left

STARTING POSITION AND METHOD

For isometric laterotrusion to the left, the therapist places the left thumb ventrolaterally on the left mandibular head and the left index finger around the tip of the patient's chin. With the mouth slightly open, the jaw is pushed gently towards laterotrusion to the right while the patient is asked to hold the jaw steady.

Protrusion

STARTING POSITION AND METHOD

The therapist places the thumb and index finger as described for elevation around the patient's chin. The tips of the fingers may touch. The tip of the chin is pushed dorsocranially. By controlled muscle activity, the patient prevents any movement of the jaw.

Retrusion

STARTING POSITION AND METHOD

Both therapist's forearms are positioned in supination with the middle and ring fingers behind the mandibular angle so the jaw may be moved forwards (Fig. 8.25).

If this causes pain, alternatively the web spaces between thumbs and index fingers may be positioned at the same place. The therapist needs to pronate the forearms for this technique. The patient is asked to prevent protrusion by muscle force. As this may be a difficult task for some patients, it sometimes helps to repeat the movement from the same starting position several times. If the patient is then able to perform the activity symmetrically, it may be hypothesized that coordination problems are contributing to the dysfunction.

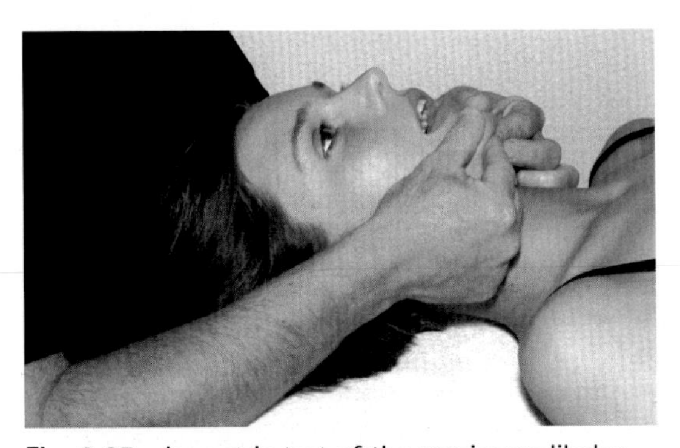

Fig. 8.25 Isometric test of the craniomandibular region. Both thumbs and index fingers are positioned symmetrically on the mandible to allow movement in all directions. In this position the patient is unable to guess which movement the therapist will initiate.

SUMMARY: ISOMETRIC TESTS

- Standard position is supine. The head is always in the same position.
- The therapist stands behind the patient. Thumb and index finger produce equal pressure on the right and the left side of the chin.
- During the test the tension is increased slowly and the therapist observes associated facial and cervical activities.
- The parameters *pain*, *force* and *coordination* and their relationship to each other are assessed.

DYNAMIC TESTS

Dynamic tests are defined as physiological mandibular movements that are performed against gentle pressure of the therapist's hands. The starting position may be the same as for the isometric tests.

Interpretation

These movements are normally pain-free and not accompanied by any noises in the joint. The dynamic tests clearly stress the intra-articular structures and are not dominantly dependent on muscle function (Kaplan 1991, Kaltenborn 1992). Both static and dynamic tests may point towards an articular pathogenesis, although opinions differ (de Wijer et al 1995). The tests are generally good reassessment parameters to evaluate the effect of a manual mobilization retrospectively and to answer the question as to whether the dysfunctions are arthrogenic or non-arthrogenic.

If the therapist needs further information about articular status, accessory movements with compression or other specific static and dynamic tests may be used. The advantage of these tests is that they are easy to perform and may be converted into coordinative home exercises. One situation where this test may be relevant for assessment and further management is the whiplash-associated disorder (WAD) group. This is also pointed out by Haggman-Henrikson et al (2004) who observed significantly faster fatigue during oral activities such as chewing and talking in a WAD group (n = 50) than in a healthy subject group (n = 50).

Specific static/dynamic tests

These tests place an accumulating load onto the TMJs by increasing static and dynamic resistance. Although these tests cannot be performed with all patients since they put severe stress onto the structures, they do give a clear impression of the intra-articular status.

There are three types of load test: static, dynamic and dynamic in the superior region.

STATIC LOAD TEST

Starting position and method

Patient and therapist are seated at the same level, facing each other. The therapist's thumbs (radial sides) are placed in pronation on the patient's chin. The patient's neck is supported by the rest of the hands, preventing compensatory movements. In a position of mouth opening that is most likely to provoke symptoms, the therapist applies an increasing pressure against the patient's chin in the direction of opening. The patient is asked to hold against the pressure so that no movement occurs.

DYNAMIC LOAD TEST

Starting position and method

The starting position is the same as for the static test. The patient is asked to apply more force so that a controlled mouth closure occurs.

DYNAMIC LOAD TEST IN THE SUPERIOR REGION

The starting position remains the same. The patient's mouth is maximally opened. The therapist's thumbs apply gentle pressure to the mandible in the (dorso)cranial direction, so that the mandibular head is positioned high in the articular fossa. The patient is now asked to close the mouth while the therapist resists the movement by maintaining the dorsocranial pressure on the mandible.

Interpretation of these tests

The tests are referred to as 'if necessary' tests. They may be applied whenever the physiological movements have not shown clear results regarding the articular contribution that seemed likely after the subjective examination. They should not be applied if the patient has severe or irritable symptoms. A conspicuous test may be used as a reassessment parameter, which is especially useful when insufficient signs are found (Maitland et al 2001).

LENGTH TESTS

Craniomandibular muscles, like any other muscle, can be tested for stiffness and physiological responses (pain). On any active and passive mandibular movement in different cervical positions the fibres of the masticatory muscles are loaded and lengthened in various ways (Keller 2001). The following descriptions of length tests for the masticatory muscles follow anatomic classification.

The therapist must be aware of other craniomandibular structures that are also loaded on these tests, since signs and symptoms provoked by these combinations of physiological and accessory movements may also be caused by other structures. For example, lengthening of the right masseter muscle and a resulting disc derangement in the right TMJ may lead to a severely restricted laterotrusion to the right. Pain and resistance are caused by other structures and the left masseter is not lengthened. In the following, the length tests for the four masticatory muscles are described.

Masseter muscle

The fibres of the masseter muscle run from the zygomatic arch caudodorsally to the mandibular angle. The main activities are mouth closure, retrusion and ipsilateral laterotrusion (Nakzawa & Kamimaru 1991, Bumann & Lotzmann 2000). A direct or an indirect technique may be chosen to influence the length of the masseter muscle.

DIRECT LENGTH TEST (INTRAORAL)

Starting position and method

The patient lies supine with the mouth half opened. The head is rotated 20–30° to the left. The therapist puts on examination gloves and places the right thumb intraorally on the right side medial to the masseter muscle. The middle and index fingers gently touch the masseter from lateral. The right forearm is supported by the plinth and stabilizes the right lateral side of the patient's head. If the therapist has difficulties in locating the muscle the patient may be asked to press their teeth together slightly. The therapist will feel the thumb being pushed medially by the masseter muscle and should now find it easier to localize the muscle belly and can place the thumb into the middle of it. With the forearm positioned vertically onto the lateral part of the joint the therapist can perform controlled transverse movements perpendicularly on the muscle belly towards lateral. Throughout the technique the patient's mouth stays slightly open (Fig. 8.26).

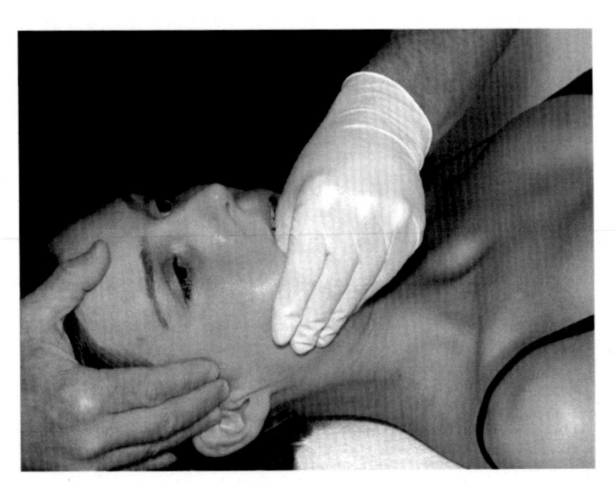

Fig. 8.26 M. masseter. Intraoral (direct) length and stretch test. The movement is towards lateral.

> **!** Movement should come from the therapist's trunk and not the thumb. This will make the technique more comfortable for the patient.

INDIRECT TEST (INTRAORAL)

Starting position and method

The patient is supine with the head in midposition. The mouth is opened about 2 cm, so that the therapist can place the left thumb onto the molar teeth of the right mandible and to facilitate the greatest possible amplitude of laterotrusion (Sheppard & Sheppard 1965). The other fingers lie extraorally on the right mandibular angle. The therapist is supported on the plinth with the right forearm and holds the right side of the patient's head. The movement which can thus be performed is a combination of posterior–anterior and a laterotrusion to the left. This may be repeated in various positions of depression. Again the therapist remembers to move the trunk and not the thumb.

> **!** During the movement the therapist communicates verbally and non-verbally with the patient to assess resistance and pain. If there are clear differences in the range of motion of depression the most conspicuous position may be the starting position at which the masseter muscle best lengthens.

Temporal muscle

The temporal muscle originates from the linea temporalis on the lateral side of the head, converges towards distal and inserts at the coronoid process. It consists of an anterior part with fibres that run directly caudally and a posterior part with fibres that run in a posterior–anterior direction. The main movements are elevation, retrusion and ipsilateral laterotrusion of the mandible (Bumann & Lotzmann 2000).

STARTING POSITION AND METHOD

The patient lies supine with the head in a relaxed mid-position. The therapist's left thumb is placed on the right mandibular molar teeth while the other fingers lie extraorally on the right mandibular angle, as described in the starting position for the indirect masseter technique. The right forearm is positioned comfortably on the plinth and holds the patient's head from the right side. The movement depends on which part of the temporal muscle the therapist intends to focus. For all parts of the muscle, the dominant movement is laterotrusion of the mandible to the contralateral side. For the anterior part, it is laterotrusion with an anterior–posterior movement, for the middle part it is laterotrusion alone, and for the posterior part it is laterotrusion combined with a posterior–anterior movement. Again the movement is initiated by the therapist's trunk (Fig. 8.27).

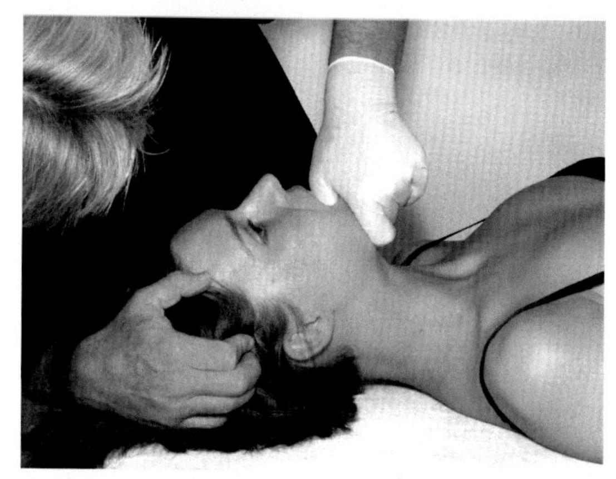

Fig. 8.27 M. temporalis. Intraoral length test. This way, depression and laterotrusion to the other side can be tested easily. Moreover, modifications of the caudal movement may be used to emphasize specific components of the muscle (posterior, middle and anterior part) (see text).

> **!** Muscle pain caused by the posterior part of the temporal muscle often goes unnoticed by clinicians (Bumann & Lotzmann 2000). The test for the posterior muscle part is often positive in patients with dorsal headache. The neck is then usually the suspected source of the symptoms. The therapist needs to make sure that the patient's head is kept upright during the test and that no cervical movements occur. The temporal muscle length tests can be combined nicely with the trigger point palpation. If the trigger points of the temporal muscle provoke pain on lengthening, this further supports the hypothesis (see Chapter 9).

Medial pterygoid muscle

The medial pterygoid muscle originates at the sphenoid bone and runs ventrolaterally to the medial aspect of the ascending mandibular ramus. The most important activities of this muscle are elevation, retrusion and laterotrusion of the mandible towards the contralateral side (Ide et al 1991, Bumann & Lotzmann 2000).

STARTING POSITION AND METHOD

The patient lies supine with the head in mid-position and the mouth 2–3 cm opened. The therapist sits or stands behind the patient, the right forearm resting on the plinth and touching the right side of the patient's head. The right arm is supinated and the index and middle fingers palpate the medial pterygoid muscle at the mandibular ramus. The left index and middle fingers lie on the left side of the chin and the left forearm is placed vertically onto the mandibular ramus. Laterotrusion to the right may now be performed, since most muscle fibres are loaded in this position (Bumann & Lotzmann 2000) (Fig. 8.28).

> **!** This starting position is ideal to treat local trigger points in general lengthening, since skin and supraspinal muscles are relaxed on the right side due to ipsilateral laterotrusion.

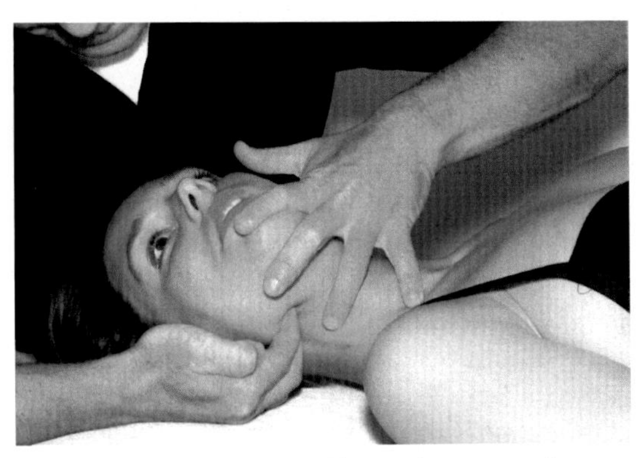

Fig. 8.28 Medial pterygoid muscle, extraoral lengthening technique. The therapist's ipsilateral hand is free for trigger point techniques, if necessary.

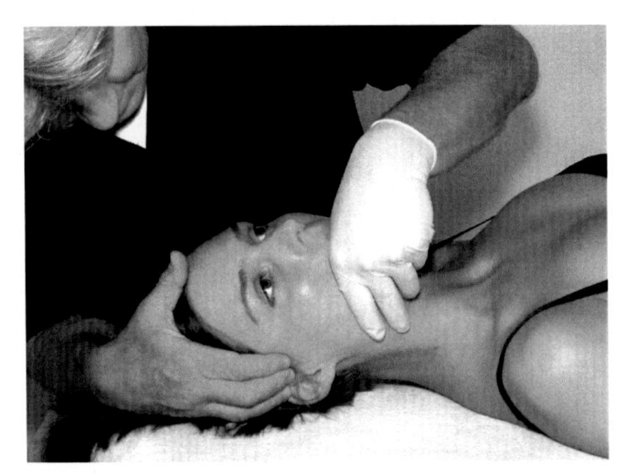

Fig. 8.29 Lateral pterygoid muscle. Starting position and method are the same as for the standard accessory movement towards lateral with an additional anterior movement.

Lateral pterygoid muscle

This muscle originates, like the medial pterygoid muscle, at the sphenoid bone and consists of an inferior and a superior part. The superior part originates at the disc and the inferior at the mandibular neck. It is the only muscle to produce the important protrusion movement and can pull the disc ventromedially (Bumann & Lotzmann 2000).

STARTING POSITION AND METHOD

The plinth is adjusted to hip level and the patient's head is held by the therapist's right forearm and the right hand. The therapist stands on the left side of the patient. The right index and middle fingers palpate the mandibular head on the right side. The therapist places the left thumb intraorally lateral of the upper molar teeth, if possible directly below the mandibular head at the mandibular neck. The other fingers of the left hand hold the patient's right jaw from lateral (Fig. 8.29).

By slowly increasing the pressure the therapist may now move the mandible lateroventrally (transverse movement). This is the direction that lengthens the fibres of the lateral pterygoid muscle. It is important that the left forearm moves as one unit, and that the movement is initiated by the trunk, to make the technique more comfortable for the patient.

> **!** This technique looks similar to the standard accessory movement towards lateral. The major difference is that the plinth is adjusted at a higher level and that the movement is directed more ventrally. If the movement is performed too quickly or initiated by the left thumb instead of the trunk, this technique will often be uncomfortable for the patient. Alternatively, the left thumb may be positioned on the medial side of the mandibular angle. If the therapist finds that the ventral component of the technique in particular cannot be performed well, the plinth may be adjusted a little higher.

MUSCLE PALPATION

Muscle palpation is described at the end of this chapter.

ASSESSMENT OF THE NERVOUS SYSTEM

The sensitivity, mechanics and general health of the nervous system in the craniofacial region may be assessed by three types of test (Butler 2000):

- Manual nerve conduction tests:
  - Cervical region
  - Facial region (cranial nerves): Most therapists will know the neurological tests for the cervical region. Excellent reviews have been published by Spillane (1996), Butler (2000), and Petty and Moore (2001). Specific tests for the relevant target tissue and the conductivity of the cranial nerves are discussed in the Chapters 16 and 17.
- Palpation of the cranial nerves (see Chapter 18): This may also be integrated into the general palpation (see below).
- Active and passive neurodynamic tests for the cranial nervous system: These tests and their indications are discussed in detail in Chapters 16 and 17.

None of these tests alone shows a high validity or reliability in isolation. Therefore the therapist needs the results from various tests. The relevance increases when the therapist chooses appropriate tests for nerve conditions based on clinical experience (Matheson 2000). An experienced therapist will always perform more than one test on a structure before deciding whether the structure contributes to the problem (Jones 1994).

PALPATION OF THE CRANIOMANDIBULAR REGION

Palpation is a manual technique that is not only part of the physical examination but is also a treatment technique (see Chapter 19). It frequently helps to confirm the hypothesis about the source of the symptoms. Palpation may also give an impression of the underlying pain mechanisms.

Example 5

Patient A shows a locally inflamed and swollen retrodiscal space with primary hyperalgesic reactions and a local on/off pain on pressure. Patient B, who has had facial pain for years, perceives pain on palpation of the skin, the muscles and the joint. In this case, as there is

Example 5—cont'd

no specific tender structure but a secondary hyperalgesia, it is suspected that the pain is not dominantly nociceptive (Coderre & Katz 1997). For patient A, a 'high-tech-examination' – i.e. a targeted, structure palpation – will be of great value (Butler 2000); this is less so for patient B. However, the therapist now has a strong case to explain central maladaptive pain (Gifford 2000).

Quantification and qualification of the responses to palpation

If the localization, intensity of pressure and responses are well defined, craniomandibular palpation shows a moderate to high inter- and intratester reliability (Chung et al 1992, Gracely & Reid 1994, Turp 2000).

One method to measure sensitivity to touch in correlation with the pain response is algometry, which will be explained later. The best option to document pain is the use of the visual analogue scale (VAS). In the author's experience a 5-point scale is the ideal tool for reassessment although it may sometimes not be clinically practical for the palpation of some regions. Alternatively, a 4-point ordinal scale may be used:

- 0 no pain and no sensitivity
- 1 mild to minimal pain response
- 2 moderate pain and/or motor facial reaction
- 3 severe pain reaction with an avoidance manoeuvre.

Motor responses are slight contractions of the facial or masticatory muscles during palpation. An avoidance reaction is a pulling away of the head while the therapist attempts to palpate certain areas. This differentiation is therapist- and patient-friendly and time efficient (Pertes & Gross 1995).

The therapist should note the following components:

- Temperature of the area
- Local sweating
- Swelling and oedema
- Constitution of the superficial tissue
- Constitution of the ligaments, capsule and muscles
- Position of the mandible
- Pain provocation and pain reduction.

Some of the main clinical findings of the craniomandibular region are now presented.

TEMPERATURE AND SWEATING OF THE CRANIOFACIAL REGION

With the back of the hands the therapist may feel for temperature changes and local sweating in the affected region, compared with other areas. Local temperature changes may indicate local inflammation. Examples are retrodiscal, salivary gland or lymph node inflammation. To be able to compare temperature and sweating, the therapist should always use the same hand for the palpation (Maitland et al 2001). If the surface is very small, only a part of the back of the hand may be used.

Changes in the autonomic nervous system may influence sweating (Jänig 1996). Local sweating can be easily assessed by gently stroking the skin and noticing the resistance. Wet skin will usually produce a greater resistance (Petty & Moore 2000, Maitland et al 2001). Sweating often occurs in regions of increased temperature (Vicenzino et al 1998).

SWELLING AND OEDEMA

Typical locations for swelling are the mandibular head, the salivary glands, the lymph nodes at the neck and the orbital region.

The region around the mandibular head

The patient lies supine and the therapist sits behind the patient. The index fingers are placed ventrally of the mandibular head and the middle fingers dorsally, approximately 3–5 mm in front of the outer auditory canal. With gentle pressure the therapist may assess the localization of swelling and oedema, sensitivity to touch and the position of the mandibular head.

If in doubt, the therapist may ask the patient to open the mouth a maximum of 10 mm, so that swellings (especially in the retrodiscal space) become easier to palpate and symptoms occur more clearly. This can make it easier to differentiate between capsulitis and retrodiscitis. Sometimes it is also helpful to palpate ventrocranially of the mandibular head, where the disc is in contact with the articular eminence. In (anterior) medial disc derangements, the disc is loaded more in this area and may produce swelling and pain (Dolwick & Dimitroulis 1996). Palpation with the middle finger may be an easy option to differentiate the localization (Pertes & Gross 1995).

Salivary glands

There are three subgroups of salivary glands: the *parotid, submandibular* and *sublingual* glands.

The parotid is the largest salivary gland. It is positioned in front of the ear at the masseter muscle. It can be palpated with the index and middle fingers 1 cm caudally of the mandibular head. The pressure is superficial and swellings are often found over an extended region (larger than 1–2 cm).

If the masseter muscle is hypertrophic, superficial sensitivity to touch and tightness of the muscle occur.

The submandibular gland is found between the jaw and the two digastric muscle bellies (Fig. 8.30). It is palpated superficially ventromedial of the mandibular angle. The therapist's forearms are supinated, so that palpation may be performed with the tips of the index and middle fingers.

The sublingual gland is located at the floor of the mouth on the mylohyoid muscle and outlets with the mandibular gland. The therapist stands or sits in front of the patient. In this case the right index finger is placed intraorally underneath the tongue onto the floor of the mouth. The left forearm is pronated and supports the floor of the mouth extraorally. By applying gentle pressure with both hands, the consistency, size, mobility and sensitivity can be assessed (Berghaus et al 1996).

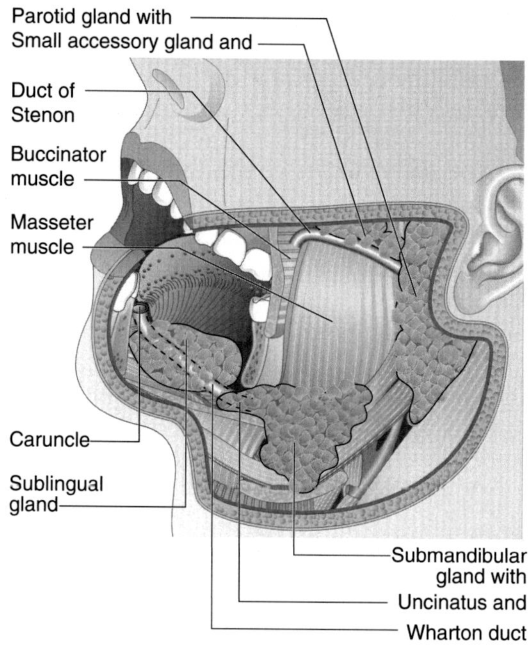

Fig. 8.30 Topography of the salivary glands.

> **!** If the patient's symptoms have not yet been clearly diagnosed by an ENT specialist or any other doctor, and the therapist detects abnormal swelling or well-localized hard areas in the salivary glands and the lymph nodes, but the findings do not correlate with the clinical patterns of the neuromusculoskeletal system in the craniomandibular and craniofacial regions, the patient should be sent back to the doctor for further investigation.

Lymph nodes

Asymmetries are fairly common in the craniofacial and craniomandibular regions. Affected lymphatic tissue may cause facial asymmetries, masking, for example, craniomandibular dysfunction. Enlarged lymph nodes may have three causes:

- Specific and non-specific inflammation
- Metastases of tumour cells from the surrounding tissue
- Tumours of the lymphatic system (Schwenzer et al 2002).

If no clear indicators for craniomandibular and/or craniofacial dysfunction have been found on subjective examination, but a clear soft tissue asymmetry is seen and the complaints have not been investigated by a medical specialist, the therapist may perform a global palpation of the lymph nodes. The therapist feels for size, sensitivity, mobility and consistency of the abnormalities.

The following quick examination, as suggested by Berghaus et al (1996), is usually sufficient to detect abnormalities and to potentially refer the patient back to the specialist.

The therapist sits behind the patient, who sits in an upright position (with 20–30° cervical flexion). The palpation is performed with both hands in comparison with the other side. It saves time to assess the submental region initially and then to move on to the mandibular angle, rather than anterocranially to the sternocleidomastoid muscle, the subclavicular space and along the edge of the trapezius muscle (pars descendens) towards the occiput (Fig. 8.31).

Muscles

A generally accepted method to assess changes in muscle tone and muscle pain is manual palpation (Mahan & Alling 1991, Okeson 1995). Manual palpation has been investigated for reliability and, in the craniomandibular region, shows acceptable inter- and intratester reliability (Dworkin et al 1988). It depends significantly on the standardization of the applied technique, on the quantification of sensitivity, the facial responses and the conduction and interpretation by the therapist (Bendtsen et al 1994, Jensen 1986).

Types of palpation

Muscle palpation includes:

- General palpation of the muscle regions: The intention is to gain a general impression of muscle tone and sensitivity to touch. Once various regions have been palpated, the therapist may decide whether central sensitization or dysregulation of pain-inhibiting mechanisms contribute to the problem (Palla et al 1998, Butler 2000).

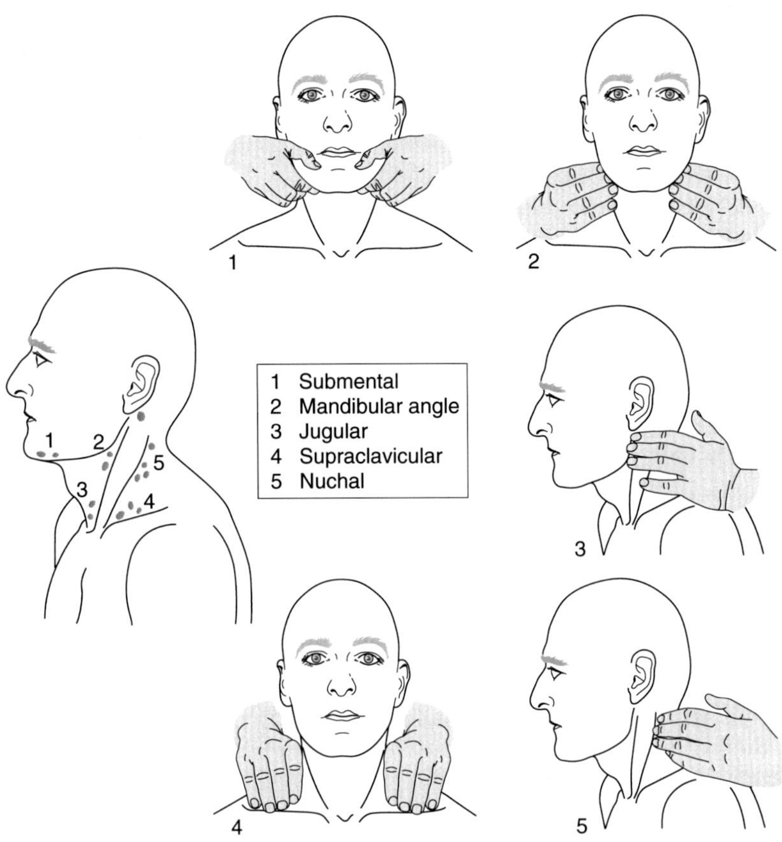

Fig. 8.31 Assessment of the cervical and neck lymph nodes by palpation from dorsal. The following nodes are palpable: (1) submental, (2) at the mandibular angle, (3) jugular, (4), supraclavicular and (5) nuchal (after Berghaus et al 1996).

- Specific local (standardized) pain areas: These pain areas (e.g. trigger points) are assessed for local pain, referred pain and the patient's motor reaction (Widmer et al 1992). In this chapter the general techniques are first described; trigger points are discussed in depth in Chapter 9.

METHOD AND EVALUATION

Even if starting position, localization and method are well defined, various therapists may not always achieve the same responses. Other parameters, such as intensity of pressure, speed and duration, may influence pain and facial responses. The conclusion from various studies is that the quality of the palpatory pressure in the craniofacial region varies strongly between testers but not for a single tester (Bendtsen et al 1994). The consequence is that inexperienced clinicians will achieve an insufficient intertester reliability and a moderate intratester reliability (Dworkin et al 1988). Measurement faults may be improved by algometry, which will be discussed in the next section.

Interpretation of the responses may also vary. Experienced clinicians will recognize clinical patterns more quickly and more accurately than novices. They will assess the responses more accurately in relation to their clinical relevance (Jones & von Piekartz 2001).

> **!** Increased sensitivity to touch is a clinical sign that will only indicate a clinical pattern if combined with other clinical signs and symptoms. The quality of clinical decision-making will always depend on the therapist's experience.

Algometry (dolometry)

Various authors have investigated the reliability of pressure algometry – measurement of pressure on a body in kiloPascals (kPa) – in patients with masticatory muscle pain (Palla et al 1998). In most studies the pain threshold of certain trigger points was assessed. The results show that the inter- and intratester reliability is good to excellent (Reeves et al 1986, Schiffman et al 1988, Vernon et al 1990, Sung-Chang et al 1992, Gracely & Reid 1994). Pressure measurements are an easy tool for therapists to compare individual results with the average data of healthy volunteers and for retrospective reassessment. For a discussion on the algometry of painful trigger points, see Chapter 9.

The algometer may be used not only at painful points but also in areas of increased muscle tone. In the author's experience the pain threshold is higher at these points. This implies that the therapist may use more force, if allowed by the patient's clinical pattern. Again, algometry may be useful for reassessment.

General palpation of the most important craniomandibular and craniofacial muscles

Muscle tone, pain quality and quantity, autonomic and motor responses may be evaluated by the criteria suggested by Tanaka (1984):

- In the resting position, lengthened and shortened status
- In the muscle belly and the area of insertion
- Bilaterally, if possible (side differences)
- Vertically and parallel to the muscle belly and the insertion.

It is impossible to assess all the above criteria in daily practice. Only in very localized problems, for example of the masseter muscle, can most of the above qualities be evaluated. If the examination is performed in more generalized problems (e.g. craniofacial pain in fibromyalgia patients, one criterion should be evaluated for various muscles.

The masticatory muscles are discussed here together with the most important cervical muscles and the supra- and infrahyoid muscles. Detailed anatomical information is found in Chapters 2 and 9.

Starting position

In this case the starting position is horizontal or half sitting (angle of 45°). The patient's head rests on the plinth; the therapist sits or stands behind the patient. In this position the craniocervical and craniomandibular muscles are in maximum relaxation and the therapist can easily compare right and left side (Pertes & Gross 1995). During palpation the patient's teeth should not be in contact since this might influence the results (Hagberg 1991).

THE MASTICATORY SYSTEM

Temporal muscle

The therapist palpates with the tips of the middle and index fingers for the anterior region superior of the zygomatic arch, 1.5 cm in front of the TMJ. The medial region is found 1 cm above the TMJ and superior to the zygomatic arch. The muscle fibres run horizontal on the lateral part of the temporal bone. The posterior part runs horizontally and is easy to palpate, 1.5 cm dorsocranially of the ear.

Masseter muscle

This muscle may be palpated intra- or extraorally. The inferior and the superior insertions of the muscle belly can be palpated.

Intraoral palpation

The little finger of the right hand (forearm in supination) palpates the muscle insertion intraorally at the zygomatic ramus. The index and middle fingers of the left hand simultaneously investigate the same region extraorally. The same may be repeated at the inferior region of the mandibular ramus (Fig. 8.32).

If there is any difficulty in locating the masseter muscle, the therapist may ask the patient to gently put the teeth together. The therapist will then immediately feel the masseter muscle push against the little finger.

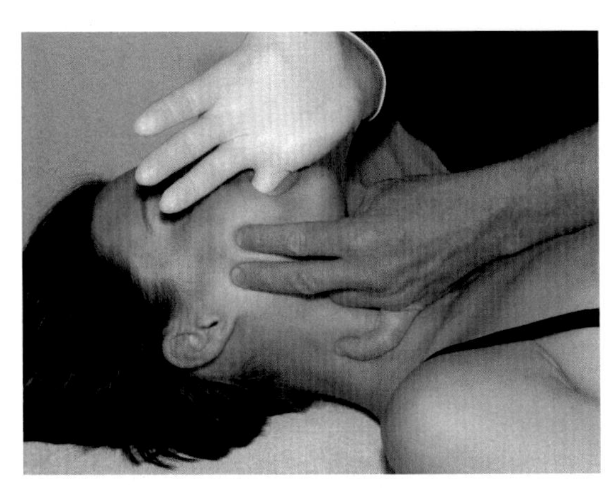

Fig. 8.32 Intraoral palpation of the masseter muscle.

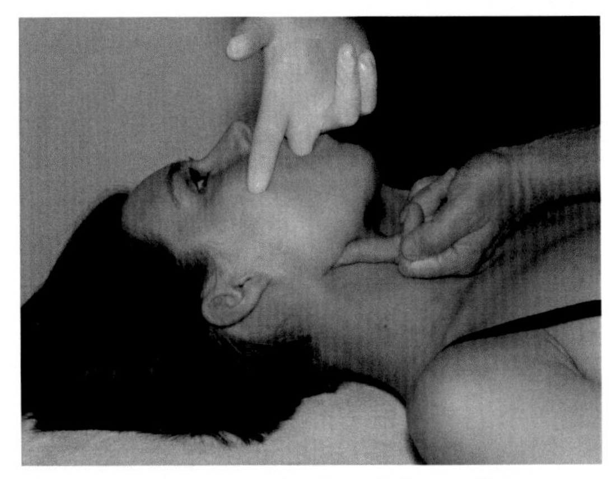

Fig. 8.33 Intraoral palpation of the medial pterygoid muscle.

Extraoral palpation

The same region is now palpated bilaterally. It is usually easier to assess the muscle belly extraorally.

Medial pterygoid muscle

Extraoral palpation

The patient's mouth is held relaxed and without teeth contact. The therapist positions the hands in supination ventral of the mandibular ramus. The index and middle fingers are moved towards medial so that the soft tissue medial of the mandibular ramus becomes palpable. From here, the therapist moves the fingers simultaneously towards dorsal and compares function and responses.

If the tissue on the neck is very sensitive or tensed, passive ipsilateral laterotrusion may relax the neck.

Intraoral palpation

Occasionally the direct contact on extraoral palpation of the pterygoid muscle may be very pain sensitive, for example after radiotherapy for cancer of the floor of the mouth. One may attempt to palpate intraorally by placing the ipsilateral index finger and possibly also the middle finger on the mandibular ramus. From this position the therapist may execute a small caudolateral movement to the belly of the medial pterygoid muscle. The other hand supports the patient's neck or the mandible to ease unnecessary tension (Fig. 8.33).

Lateral pterygoid muscle

A number of studies mention the lateral pterygoid muscle as the most pressure-sensitive muscle. For anatomical reasons it is not possible to palpate the lateral pterygoid muscle (Johnstone & Templeton 1980). It is more likely that the sensitive structure is the tendon of the temporal muscle. If it is not the temporal muscle and a clear side difference is found, it may be the lateral pterygoid muscle (Palla et al 1998). The patient's mouth needs to be open wide and the therapist places the little finger medial of the mandibular head. The right hand is placed into supination and the little finger is positioned medially of the mandibular head intraorally. The left index and middle fingers help to find the right location extraorally. During this test, non-verbal communication with the patient is extremely important, since it may potentially cause a retching reflex.

CERVICAL MUSCLES

Sternocleidomastoid

The sternocleidomastoid muscle (SCM) does not directly move the mandible, but frequently becomes important in craniomandibular dysfunction. This muscle is easy to palpate (Clark et al 1993). With the tips of the thumb and index finger, the therapist palpates bilaterally inferior of the mastoid processes. To differentiate whether it is more the anterior or the posterior part that shows responses, the therapist may either increase the thumb (anterior part) or the index finger (posterior part) pressure. The therapist slowly follows the SCM inferiorly down to the clavicle.

Frequently, clinical changes become obvious when the SCM is lengthened (contralateral lateroflexion and ipsilateral rotation). This may provoke referred pain into the face and motor responses of the masticatory muscles. In the lengthened position it is also easier to locate trigger points (Fig. 8.34).

Splenius capitis muscle

The splenius capitis muscle and the semispinal capitis muscle react frequently with muscle tone changes in craniomandibular dysfunction (Travell & Simons 1983, Friction et al 1988). The insertion of the splenius capitis muscle is found at the cranium, posterior of the SCM insertion. The muscle is very superficial here, and it is also frequently the site of dysfunction. The therapist palpates with the middle and index fingers in supination 2–3 cm further inferior. Here the muscle converges with the other neck muscles (Williams et al 1989) (Fig. 8.35).

Semispinal capitis muscle

The muscle insertion is located at the edge of the occiput and is connected to the nuchal ligament. The therapist positions both hands in supination lateral of the spinous processes of the upper cervical spine. The therapist then palpates the splenius capitis muscle with the index and middle fingers from the edge of the occiput medial to approximately 5 cm caudal. It sometimes helps to ask the patient to perform a parafunction, such as bracing or biting a pen. In patients with craniomandibular dysfunction this may provoke muscle tone changes and pain responses.

Trapezius muscle (pars descendens)

Various studies show that the trapezius muscle typically changes its tone significantly in patients with malocclusion and craniomandibular dysfunction (Zufiga et al 1995). This large muscle has a great influence on cervical and shoulder girdle function (Sahrmann 2001). The edge of the muscle can be palpated bilaterally from the midcervical spine laterally towards inferior. Again the therapist may want

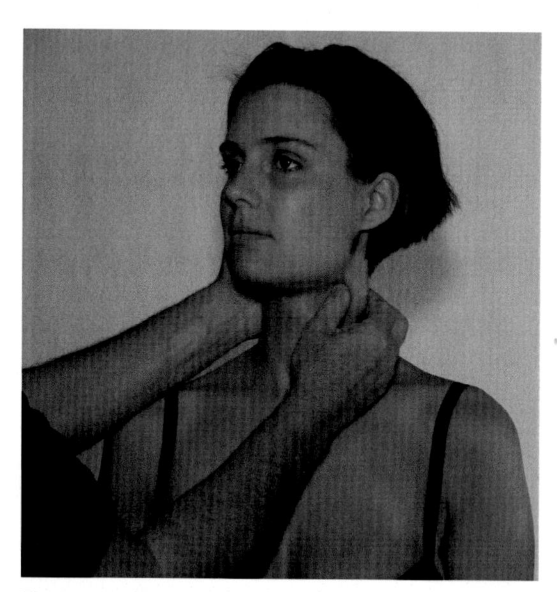

Fig. 8.34 Palpation of the sternocleidomastoid muscle.

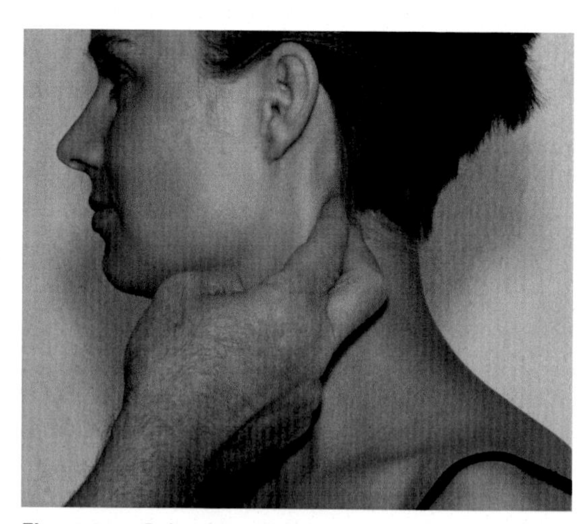

Fig. 8.35 Palpation of the splenius capitis muscle with index and middle fingers.

to place the head in various positions of lateroflexion to lengthen the trapezius muscle and provoke different responses.

INFRA- AND SUPRAHYOID MUSCLES

Digastric muscle

The muscle has both an anterior and a posterior muscle belly that inserts with a thick tendon at the anterior side of the hyoid. The insertion of the anterior part is located below the tip of the mandible (fossa digastricus); the posterior insertion can be palpated dorsal of the mastoid (incisura mastoidea). The muscle is active on swallowing, speaking and tongue positions and movements. The main function is hyoid elevation (Moller 1966, Munro 1974, Ide et al 1991). A number of studies proved that muscle tone varies significantly with changes of tongue position that frequently accompany craniomandibular dysfunction (Rocabado & Iglash 1991, Zufiga et al 1995) (Fig. 8.36).

Anterior part

The anterior muscle belly is best palpated superficially with the tips of the index and middle fingers bilaterally medial of the mandibular ramus. The emphasis here is on 'superficial' palpation. In the author's experience, responses are most easily provoked on transverse palpation of the muscle belly 1.5 cm posterior to the tip of the chin.

Posterior part

This is located on a line from the posterior mastoid to the hyoid. With both hands in supination the therapist follows the soft tissue to 2 cm anterior of the mastoid. This is where the muscle belly is palpated. When the patient swallows, the muscle tightens and the muscle belly is palpated in transverse direction. The various responses are evaluated (see also Chapter 13) (Fig. 8.37).

Mylohyoid muscle

This muscle runs cranial of the digastric muscle and forms the floor of the mouth. It originates at the medial part of the mandible and is attached in the middle to connective tissue. It is active on minimal opening and supports swallowing and excessive tongue protrusion (Munro 1974, Kraus 1994).

In this case the therapist stands in front of the patient and places the right index finger intraorally on the right part of the floor of the mouth. The left index finger palpates extraorally at the same level and compares the right and left sides.

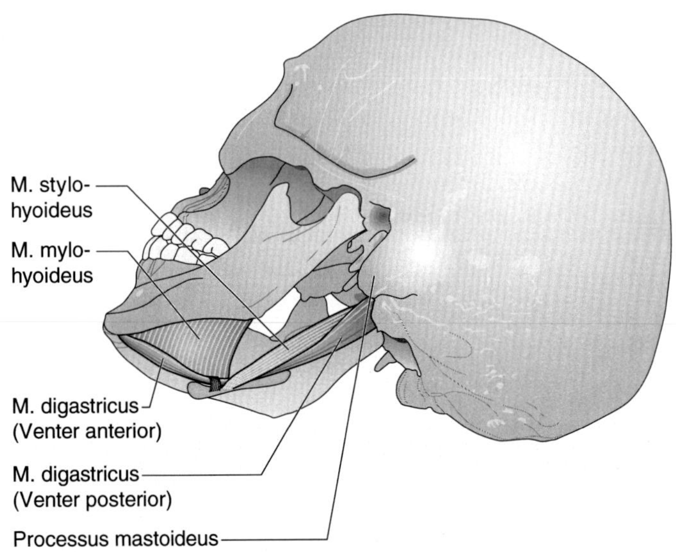

Fig. 8.36 Localization of the digastric muscle. The anterior part of the muscle runs transverse to the mylohyoid muscle, the posterior part inserts dorsal of the mastoid.

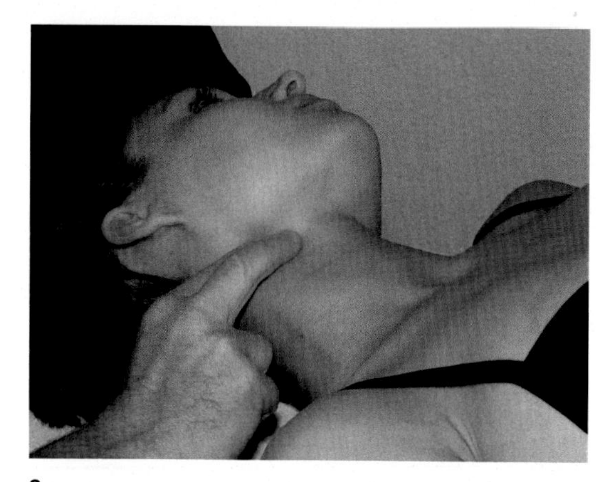

a

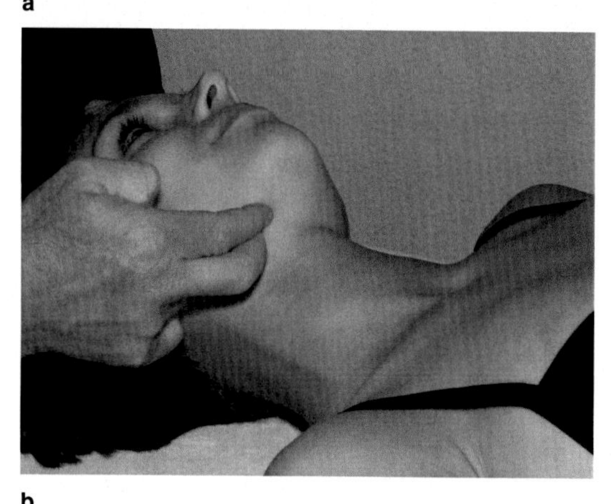

b

Fig. 8.37 Palpation of the digastric muscle.
a Anterior part. Superficial palpation with the tips of the index and middle fingers.
b Posterior part. Index and middle fingers are slightly bent and palpate superficially.

Omohyoid muscle

The omohyoid muscle has a superior and an inferior part, connected by an intermediate tendon. The inferior part originates at the superior margin of the scapula. The superior part runs along the cricothyroid cartilage and inserts at the caudolateral edge of the hyoid. It is active on swallowing and tongue movements (Okeson 1995). The inferior part may be visible on the neck of slim female patients on swallowing (Wong & Li 2000). A permanent band is commonly visible in the case of a dysfunction, often combined with a protracted elevated shoulder. Palpation is indicated to support the hypothesis.

Superior part

Index and middle fingers palpate bilaterally in a lateral direction along the muscle near the cricothyroid cartilage. If it is difficult to locate the muscle, the therapist may elevate the hyoid with the right index and middle fingers to lengthen the right infrahyoid muscle. Superficial transverse movements may provoke severe responses.

Inferior part

The muscle belly is easy to palpate with index and middle fingers in the supraclavicular space. If the clavicle is used as a reference point and the therapist palpates 1–2 cm cranial of this point, it is likely that the fingers are touching the muscle belly of the omohyoid muscle, inferior part. To clarify one may ask the patient to swallow a few times and/or to move the shoulders into retraction and depression. Palpation should now be easier.

Nerve palpation

If the clinical pattern points towards a (minimal) cranial neuropathy, or the therapist wants to confirm the hypothesis that the nervous system does not dominantly provoke the symptoms, palpation of the most important superficial cranial nerves is indicated. Detailed information is found in Chapters 17 and 18.

ACCESSORY MOVEMENTS

Accessory movements are movements that cannot be performed actively by the patient but are initiated by the therapist (Maitland et al 2001). They are usually assessed at the end of the physical examination, since they may strongly influence the local tissue of the craniofacial region. Accessory movements are also commonly used as treatment techniques.

Why are accessory movements tested at the end of the physical examination?

In the assessment of a patient with chronic neck, head and face pain, mainly cervical and craniomandibular dysfunctions are detected. Based on the previous history and the revealed signs, the therapist suspects that the craniomandibular dysfunctions influence the cervical as well as the craniomandibular symptoms. At the end of the initial appointment there is only limited time to confirm this hypothesis. The therapist found that accessory movements, for example transverse lateral movement of the mandibular head on the symptomatic side, were significant. The dominant pain mechanism appears to be input related (peripheral nociceptive) without any signs of irritability.

The therapist decides to perform a manual trial technique of 1 minute's duration, bearing in mind the patient's pain. Afterwards a reassessment of the most important cervical signs and craniomandibular movements is performed. In this example the therapist finds that three of the four cervical signs have significantly changed with regard to range of movement and intensity of the symptoms. All three of the craniomandibular signs had also improved slightly. The therapist reasons that the dysfunctions on the symptomatic side may be influenced by transverse movements and that this is relevant for the cervical as well as the craniomandibular symptoms. The accessory movement may be the basis for further treatment and management of the problem, although the therapist does not yet know which structure was dominantly affected by this technique.

The following standard techniques will be described in this section:

- Longitudinal caudal movement
- Bilateral movement
- Unilateral movement
- Transverse lateral movement
- Transverse medial movement
- Anterior–posterior movement
- Posterior–anterior movement.

To achieve optimum relaxation and for better standardization, all tests are performed in supine.

Longitudinal caudal, bilateral

STARTING POSITION AND METHOD

For this extraoral technique, the therapist sits behind the patient's head. The therapist places his hands gently on the lateral part of the cranium with the palms placed on the temporal and parietal regions. The ring, middle and index fingers are positioned bilaterally behind and lateral of the mandibular ramus. With the patient's mouth slightly open, the therapist initiates a caudal movement by extending the interphalangeal joints of the fingers of both hands (Fig. 8.38).

The movement is very small and should be performed gently and slowly to avoid pain (initially 2 seconds per movement cycle).

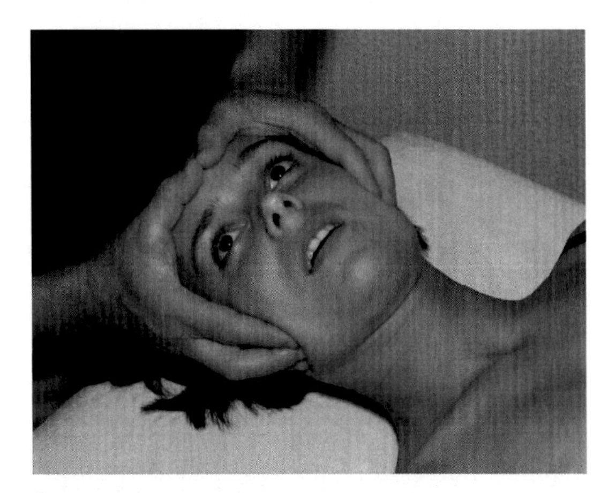

a

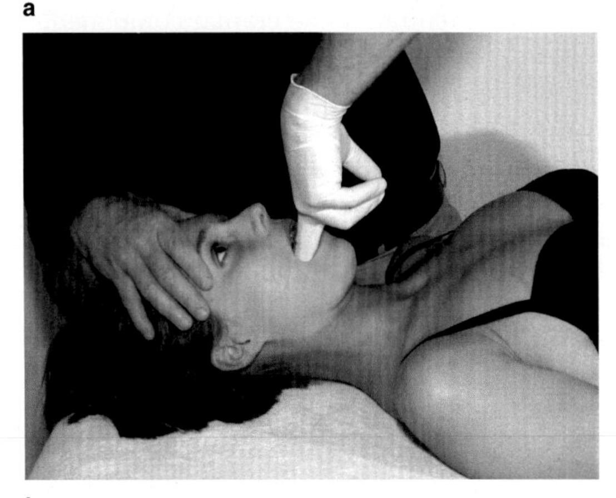

b

Fig. 8.38 Accessory movements.
a Bilateral longitudinal movement towards caudal (distraction).
b Alternative bilateral longitudinal movement towards caudal with index and middle fingers on the lower molar teeth on the right and on the left.

INDICATIONS

The technique is particularly useful after surgery at the TMJ, after active disc displacement with strong swelling and pain or embedded in a programme to manage pain for patients with strong fears and bad experiences with orofacial stimuli (Woda 2000).

Longitudinal caudal, unilateral

STARTING POSITION AND METHOD

The therapist stands on the right side of the patient, close to the patient's head. The therapist's right forearm is resting on the plinth and holds the patient's head. With the index and middle fingers the therapist palpates for the right mandibular head. The left thumb is placed intraorally on the right molar teeth, the other fingers hold the right mandible extraorally. The left forearm is parallel to the patient's sternum. By rotating the trunk to the left, the therapist performs a controlled longitudinal movement of the right TMJ. During the technique, the movement behaviour of the mandibular head is assessed. If symptoms are provoked, palpation with the right index and middle fingers may provide information as to whether the symptoms are caused by the dorsal, the ventral or the cranial components of the mandibular head (Kraus 1994). Unwanted muscle contractions or cervical movements are reduced by slow performance of the technique (Fig. 8.39).

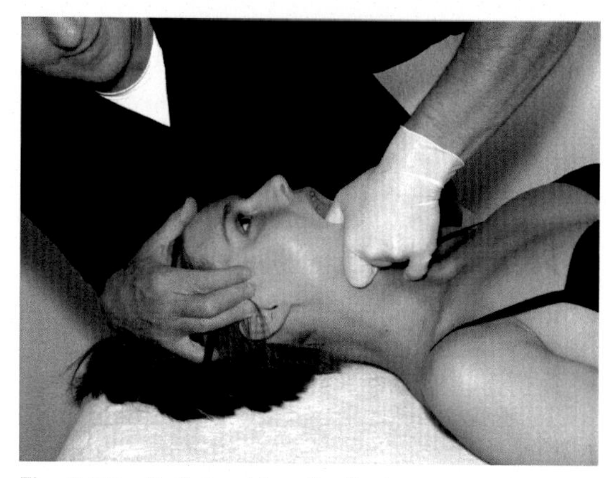

Fig. 8.39 Unilateral longitudinal movement towards caudal (distraction). The thumb of the active hand is placed tightly onto the lower molar teeth, the index finger holds the mandibular angle.

INDICATION

This technique and its variations are described and applied by various authors and clinicians from different disciplines. It is often recommended for articular disc problems as well as for disc displacement, with or without reposition (Kraus 1994, Palla et al 1998, Bumann & Lotzmann 2000). Even extra-articular dysfunctions such as fibrosis or craniomandibular capsulitis (Kraus 1994, Pertes & Gross 1995) and neurodynamic dysfunctions of the mandibular or the auriculotemporal nerve may respond to this technique (Schwenzer et al 2002).

TEST RELIABILITY

Like the mouth opening test, this test has been investigated thoroughly for reliability and construct validity. Assessment variables such as end-feel, clicking and range of motion are usually evaluated. The result of most of these studies is that the test alone does not show great reliability, with intrarater reliability higher than interrater reliability (Lobbezoo-Scholte et al 1993, Vermeiren et al 1995). Based on this test alone no statement on a specific structure can be made (Rugh 1991, Lund et al 1995, Hesse et al 1996). Unfortunately most of the aforementioned studies show methodological weaknesses, such as small populations, insufficiently described designs or manipulation of systematic or incidental faults (Portney & Watkins 1993). The question arises, therefore, whether this test should be included at all.

Those therapists who analyse the patient's problem individually, and who combine the results from the subjective examination with some clinically relevant physical tests, have achieved results comparable to the gold standard (e.g. computed tomography) (Mohl 1991).

Transverse lateral, to the right

STARTING POSITION AND METHOD

The patient's head is held with the right forearm and the right hand of the therapist who is standing left of the patient. The right index and middle fingers palpate the right mandibular head. The therapist's left thumb is placed intraorally lateral of the upper molar teeth, directly below the mandibular head on the neck of the mandible. All other fingers of the left hand hold the right jaw extraorally from lateral.

By slowly increasing the pressure the therapist now produces a transverse lateral movement of the right jaw. The therapist must be careful that the left arm moves as one unit and the movement is initiated by the trunk to make this technique comfortable for the patient. (If the patient feels uncomfortable or experiences a retching reflex, an alternative technique should be chosen.) The therapist then moves the thumb slowly towards caudal and feels with the medial side for the arcus mandibularis. The left index and middle fingers continue to hold the lateral part of the mandible and the movement is repeated. In this way, retching reflexes occur very rarely and local pain is usually not provoked. The disadvantage is that the resulting movement is not purely transverse lateral but incorporates a slight rotation around a sagittal axis (Fig. 8.40).

INDICATION

In the author's experience, this technique provokes signs or symptoms in various types of craniomandibular dysfunction. It can be significantly restricted compared to the non-symptomatic side and the movement may provoke a deep dull pain around the ear. A brief transverse lateral mobilization may dramatically change signs and symptoms. Typical signs are:

- Improved mouth opening
- Improved mobility with pain reduction on laterotrusion (horizontal plane)
- Changed intensity of opening click and the clicking occurs at a different point in the range (usually towards the beginning of mouth opening)
- Decreased muscle tension of the masseter on mouth opening.

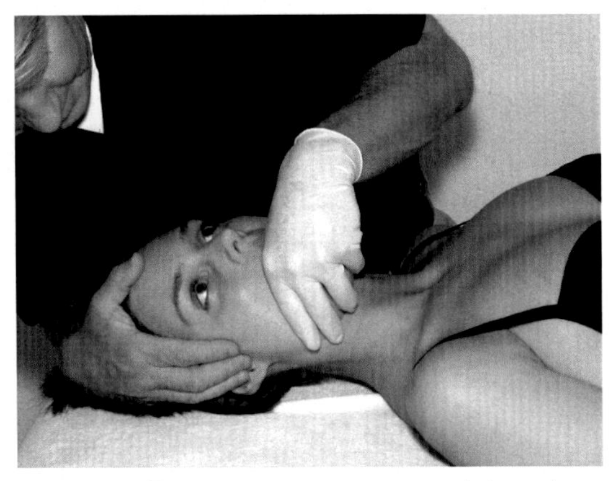

Fig. 8.40 Transverse movement towards lateral (intraoral technique). If a retching reflex is provoked, the therapist moves the thumb 1–2 cm towards caudal, medial to the mandibular angle.

Some explanations as to why this movement may be clinically effective include:

- Stretching of the lateral pterygoid muscle: This muscle runs intracranially, lateroventrally (see Chapter 2) and shows an increased muscle tone and morphological changes in craniomandibular dysfunctions (Murray et al 2001). Transverse lateral movements may strongly influence the muscle tone of the lateral pterygoid.
- Influence on the (ventro) medialization of the articular disc: Computed tomography may show that physiological medial movement of the disc is possible. This movement is limited in craniomandibular dysfunction (Chen et al 2002). Transverse movements may change the disc dynamics and therefore also the classic signs of disc displacement.
- Influencing the mandibular nerve neurodynamics: Once the mandibular nerve has split up into its branches – lingual nerve, alveolar nerve and auriculotemporal nerve

– a great variety of abnormalities occur. These are frequently found in the lingual nerve that runs through the pterygoid muscle. Increased muscle tone may influence potential neuropathies (Isberg et al 1987). The neural mechanical interface of the nerve may be influenced by transverse TMJ movements (von Piekartz 2000).

Transverse medial, to the left

STARTING POSITION AND METHOD

For this technique, the therapist stands on the left of the patient. The patient's head is slightly rotated to the right and the mouth is not quite shut. The therapist's right hand is placed on the temporal bone and the frontal bone, the left on the patient's chin. The thumbs lie close together on the neck of mandible directly below the mandibular head (Fig. 8.41).

By bending and extending the trunk the therapist can now perform a very controlled transverse movement on the left side of the patient's chin. The movement will influence both the left and right TMJs. *Be careful*: if the thumbs are placed on top of each other, rather than beside each other, the movement may become very painful for the patient.

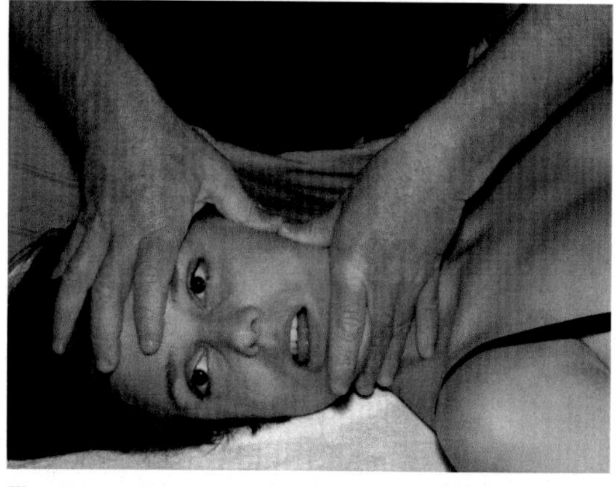

Fig. 8.41 Transverse movement towards medial (extraoral). The therapist needs to stabilize the patient's head with the right hand. If this is not sufficient stabilization, the patient supports their own neck with their right hand.

Should the technique be accompanied by large cervical movements, the patient may be asked to stabilize the neck with their right arm.

Anterior–posterior movement

Generally this movement is performed extraorally; however, an intraoral technique may be chosen.

EXTRAORAL

Starting position and method

The therapist stands at the head end of the plinth, supported by the left knee next to the patient's head. This will allow the therapist to position the sternum directly above the patient's right TMJ, resulting in a more economical performance of the movement. The therapist's right hand stabilizes the patient's neck from dorsal and the right thumb is placed on the right mandibular angle. The left hand holds the patient's chin, and the index and middle finger may rest on the left pectoralis major muscle and the left clavicle. The left thumb lies next to the right thumb on the mandibular angle.

By moving the body, the anterior–posterior movement is initiated principally through the therapist's left hand/thumb. The right hand functions as a stabilizer, but is also involved in the movement. This technique is particularly useful for disc problems and muscle tension.

INTRAORAL

Starting position and method

The patient's head is held and stabilized by the therapist's right forearm and right hand. The index and middle fingers of the same hand palpate for the right mandibular head. The left thumb is placed intraorally on the right molar teeth; the left index finger is placed parallel on the body of the mandible. This way, the right mandibular side is clasped. The therapist's left elbow points towards the ceiling. It is now possible to produce an anterior–posterior movement by moving the trunk (Fig. 8.42).

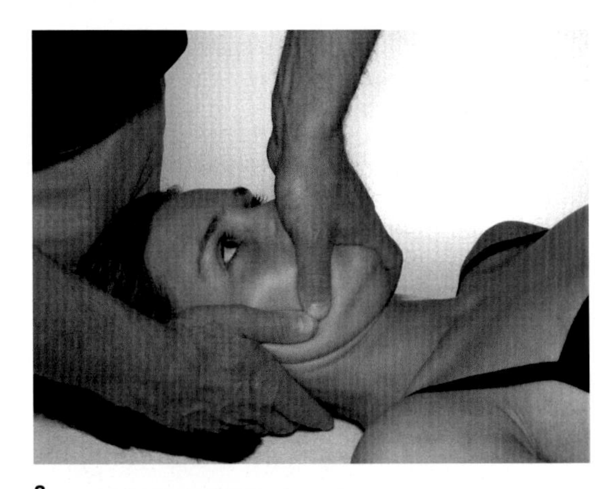

a

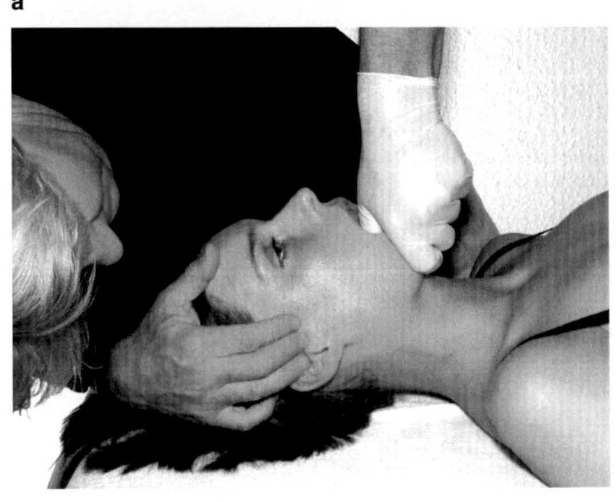

b

Fig. 8.42 Anterior–posterior movement.
a Extraoral. The plinth is relatively low so that the therapist is positioned directly over the patient's head.
b Intraoral. The starting position is the same as for the unilateral longitudinal movement towards caudal, but the direction is different.

Posterior–anterior movement

EXTRAORAL

Starting position and method

The patient's head is slightly rotated to the left. The patient supports this position by stabilizing the neck with the left hand. The therapist stands on the right side and puts the hands onto the patient's forehead and chin. The therapist's thumbs are placed directly underneath the mandibular head onto the mandibular neck, if possible. As many sensitive structures run through this region, it may be more comfortable to move the thumb slightly caudal towards the mandibular angle. A trunk movement will allow a posterior–anterior movement, mainly through the right hand since the left serves more to stabilize the cranium.

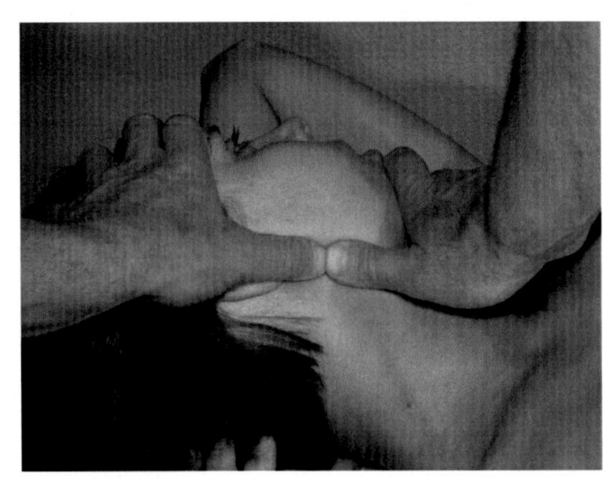

Fig. 8.43 Posterior–anterior movement.

Indication

This technique is often used for disc derangements towards anterior or anterior/medial but may also be indicated in other morphological tissue changes around the TMJ.

INTRAORAL

Starting position and method

Starting position and hand placement are similar to the intraoral anterior–posterior movement. Only the movement direction is different. The mandible is moved towards anterior (Fig. 8.43).

Interpretation of accessory movements

Accessory movements are not primarily tissue-specific tests but rather tests to analyse movements. The behaviour of stiffness, pain and muscle spasm is assessed (Maher 1995, Maitland et al 2001). Based on this information, clinical patterns that point towards certain structures can be recognized (Jones 1994). For example:

- Accessory movements provide information as to whether the nociceptive source of the symptoms is located in the anterior or the posterior part of the articular disc. If the anterior–posterior and longitudinal–caudal accessory movements produce more signs and symptoms with an on/off bias than the posterior–anterior and longitudinal accessory movements, the retrodiscal structures are the potential source of the symptoms (Bumann & Lotzmann 2000).

- The longitudinal–caudal movement causes a sudden tension in the masseter muscle that depends on the speed of the technique. On contralateral laterotrusion in longitudinal position a limited range of motion is found. The tentative hypothesis is that a local muscle problem causes the symptoms (Visser 2000).
- The transverse lateral movement compared to the other side is limited and causes a dull, sometimes burning pain on the ipsilateral side of the jaw. Signs and symptoms change clearly on upper cervical flexion, lateroflexion and/or positioning the homolateral arm in neurodynamic tension. In this case, a peripheral neurogenic problem of the mandibular nerve is likely, caused by a local craniomandibular problem (Butler 2000, von Piekartz 2001).

SUMMARY

- Targeted physical examination of the craniomandibular neuromusculoskeletal system with tests, although not the gold standard, are necessary to confirm the hypothesis about the sources of the symptoms gained from the subjective examination (Mohl 1991, Greene 2001).
- The test results and the types of the reaction provide an impression of the patient's dominant pain mechanisms.
- Most tests or components of the active and passive tests that reproduce a (potentially) relevant dysfunction may also be used as treatment techniques.

References

Agterberg G 1987 Longitudinal variation of mandibular mobility: an intra-individual study. Journal of Prosthetic Dentistry 58:370

Angle E 1900 Treatment of malocclusion of the teeth and fractures of the maxilla, Angle system. SS White Dental Manufacturing Co., Philadelphia

Bell W 1982 Clinical management of temporomandibular disorders. Year Book Medical Publishers, Chicago

Bendtsen L, Jensen R, Jensen N et al 1994 Muscle palpation with controlled finger pressure: new equipment for the study of tender myofascial tissues. Pain 59:235

Berghaus A, Rettinger G, Böhme G 1996 Speicheldrüsen. Hals-Nasen-Ohren-Heilkunde. Hippocrates, Stuttgart, p 456

Biates B, Cleese Journal of 2001 The human face. BBC Worldwide, London

Breig A 1978 Adverse mechanical tension in the central nervous system 1. Relief by functional neurosurgery. Alqvist and Wiksel, Stockholm; Wiley, Chichester

Bryden L, Fitzgerald D 2001 Einfluss von Haltung und Funktionsänderung auf die kraniozervikale und kraniofaziale Region. In: von Piekartz H (ed.) Kraniofaziale Dysfunktionen und Schmerzen. Thieme, Stuttgart, p 163

Bumann A, Lotzmann U (eds) 2000 Manuelle Funktionsanalyse. In: Funktiondiagnostik und Therapieprinzipen. Thieme, Stuttgart, p 53

Burch Journal of 1983 History and clinical examination. In: Laskin D, Greenfield W, Gale E, Rugh J, Ayer I V A (eds) The president's conference on the examination, diagnosis and management of temporomandibular disorders. American Dental Association, Chicago, 51:6

Butler D 2000 The sensitive nervous system. Noigroup Publications, Adelaide

Cacchiotti D, Plesh O, Bianchi P et al 1991 Signs and symptoms in samples with and without temporomandibular disorders. Journal of Craniomandibular Disorders 5:167

Carlsson G, Magnusson T 1999 Symptoms associated with TMD in management of temporomandibular disorders in the general dental practice. 51

Chapman R, Maness W, Osorio J 1991 Occlusal contact variation with changes in head position. International Journal of Prosthodontology 4:377

Chen Y, Gallo L, Palla S 2002 The mediolateral temporomandibular joint disc position: an in vivo quantitative study. Journal of Orofacial Pain 16:29–38

Chung S, Um B, Kim H 1992 Evaluation of pressure pain threshold in head and neck muscles by

electronic algometry: intrarater and interrater reliability. Journal of Craniomandibular Practice 10:28–34
Clark G, Seligman D, Solberg W, Pullinger A 1989 Guidelines for the examination and diagnosis of temporomandibular disorders. Journal of Craniomandibular Disorders 3:7
Clark G, Browne P, Nakano M et al 1993 Co-activation of sternocleidomastoideus muscles during maximal clenching. Journal of Dental Research 72:1499
Coderre T, Katz J 1997 Peripheral and central hyperexcitability. Behavioral and Brain Sciences 20:404
Curl D 1992 The visual range of motion scale: analysis of mandibular gait in a chiropractic setting. Journal of Manipulative and Physiological Therapeutics 15(2):115–122
Cyriax J 1982 Textbook of orthopaedic medicine: diagnosis of soft tissue lesions, 8th edn. Baillière Tindall, London
De Laat A, Horvath M, Bossuyt M, Fossini E, Baert A 1993 Myogenous or arthrogenous limitation of mouth opening: correlation between clinical findings, MR and clinical outcome. Journal of Orofacial Pain 7:150
de Wijer A, Lobbezoo-Scholte A, Steenks M et al 1995 Reliability of clinical findings in temporomandibular disorders. Journal of Orofacial Pain 9(2):181–191
Dolwick M, Dimitroulis G 1996 A re-evaluation of the importance of disc position in temporomandibular disorders. Australian Dental Journal 41:184
Doursonian L, Alfonso J, Iba-Zizen M et al 1989 Dynamics of the junction between the medulla and the cervical spinal cord: an in vivo study in the sagittal plane by magnetic resonance imaging. Surgical and Radiological Anatomy 11:313
Dupont J, Matthews E 2000 Orofacial sensory changes and temporomandibular dysfunction. Journal of Craniomandibular Practice 18:174
Dworkin S, LeResche L 1992 Research diagnosis criteria for temporomandibular disorders: review, criteria, examinations and specifications, critique. Journal of Craniomandibular Disorders 6:301–355
Dworkin S, LeResche L, DeRouen T 1988 Reliability of clinical measurement in temporomandibular disorders. Clinical Journal of Pain 4:59
Ellenberker E 1996 Muscular strength relationship between normal grade manual muscle testing and isokinetic measurements of the shoulder internal and external rotators. Isokinetics and Exercise Science 6:51
Farkas L, Munro I 1987 Anthropometry of the head and face in medicine. Elsevier Science, New York
Freesmeyer W 1993 Zahnärztliche Funktionstherapie. Hanser, Munich, p 25
Friction J, Dubner R 1994 Orofacial pain and temporomandibular disorders. Advances in pain, research and therapy, Vol 21. Raven Press, New York
Friction J, Kroening R, Hathaway K 1988 TMJ and craniofacial pain: diagnosis and management. Ishiyaku Euro-America, St Louis
Gifford L (ed.) 2000 The patient in front of us: from genes to environment. In: Topical issues of pain 2: biopsychosocial assessment and management. Relationships and pain. CNS Press, San Francisco
Graber T 1969 Overbite. 'The dentist' challenge. American Dental Association Journal 79:1135
Gracely R, Reid K 1994 Orofacial measurement in orofacial pain and temporomandibular disorders. In: Friction J, Dubner R (eds) Advances in pain research and therapy. Raven Press, New York, p 114
Graff-Radford S 1985 Objective measurement of jaw movement: a comparison. Two measuring instruments. Journal of Craniomandibular Practice 3:240
Greene C S 2001 Etiology of temporomandibular disorders. Implications for treatment. Journal of Orofacial Pain 15:93
Gross A, Haines, Thomson M, Goldsmidt C, McIntosh J 1996 Diagnostic tests for temporomandibular disorders: an assessment of the methodologic quality of research reviews. Manual Therapy 1:250
Hagberg C 1991 General musculoskeletal complaints in a group of patients with craniomandibular disorders (CMD). A case control study. Swedish Dental Journal 15:179
Haggman-Henrikson B, Osterlund C, Eriksson P O 2004 Endurance during chewing in whiplash-associated disorders and TMD. Journal of Dental Research 83(12):946–950
Hannam A 1991 The measurement of jaw motion. In: McNeill C (ed.) Current controversies in temporomandibular disorders. Proceedings of the Craniomandibular Institute's 10th Annual Squaw Valley Winter Seminar. Quintessence, Chicago, p 130
Hansson T, Honee W, Hesse J 1987 Funktionsstörungen im Kausystem. Hüthig, Heidelberg
Harzer W 1999 Diagnostik in Lehrbuch der Kieferorthopädie. Hanser, Munich, p 126
Held R 1965 Plasticity in sensory-motor systems. Scientific American 213:84
Helkimo M 1974 Studies of function and dysfunction and occlusal state. Swedish Dental Journal 76:101
Herring S 2001 Clinical commentary: the role of the human lateral pterygoid muscle in the control of horizontal jaw movements. Journal of Orofacial Pain 15:292

Hesse R 1990 Craniomandibular stiffness toward maximum mouth opening in healthy subjects: a clinical and experimental investigation. Journal of Craniomandibular Disorders 4:257

Hesse J, Hansson T 1988 Factors influencing joint mobility in general and in particular respect of the craniomandibular articulation: a literature review. Journal of Craniomandibular Disorders 2:19–28

Hesse J, Naeije M, Hansson T 1996 Craniomandibular stiffness in myogenous and arthrogenous CMD patients and control subjects: a clinical and experimental investigation. Journal of Oral Rehabilitation 23:379

Higbie E, Seidel-Cobb D, Taylor L, Cummings G 1999 Effect of head position on vertical mandibular opening. Journal of Orthopaedic and Sports Physical Therapy 29:127

Hochstedler J, James D, Allen J, Follmar M 1996 Temporomandibular joint range of motion: a ratio of interincisal opening to excursive movement in a healthy population. Journal of Craniomandibular Practice 14:296

Hu J 2001 Neurophysiological mechanisms of head, face and neck pain. In: Vernon H (ed.) The craniocervical syndrome. Butterworth-Heinemann, Oxford, p 31

Hurley M 1997 The effects of joint damage on muscle function, proprioception and rehabilitation. Manual Therapy 2:11

Ide Y, Nakazawa K, Kamimura K 1991 Anatomical atlas of the temporomandibular joint. Quintessence, Tokyo

Isberg A, Isaacson G, Williams W, Loughner B 1987 Lingual numbness and speech articulation deviation associated with the temporomandibular joint disc displacement. Oral Surgery, Oral Medicine, Oral Pathology 64:12

Jäger K 1997 Stressbedingte Kaufunktionsstörungen, Konsequenzen für den zahnärztlichen Praxisalltag. Quintessenz, Berlin, p 51

Jänig W 1996 The puzzle of 'reflex sympathetic dystrophy'. In: Jänig W, Stanton-Hicks M (eds) Mechanisms, hypotheses, open questions in reflex sympathetic dystrophy: a reappraisal. Progress in Pain Research and Management. IASP Press, Seattle, 6:1

Jensen K 1986 Qualification of changes in myofascial trigger point sensitivity with the pressure algometer following passive stretch. Pain 27:20

Johnstone D, Templeton M 1980 The feasibility of palpating the lateral pterygoid muscle. Journal of Prosthetic Dentistry 44:318–323

Jones M, von Piekartz H 2001 Clinical reasoning – Grundlage für die Untersuchung und Behandlung in der kranialen Region. In: von Piekartz H (ed.) Kraniofaziale Dysfunktionen und Schmerzen. Thieme, Stuttgart, p 187

Jones M 1994 Clinical reasoning process in manipulative therapy. In: Boyling J, Palastanga N (eds) Grieve's modern manual therapy, 2nd edn. Churchill Livingstone, New York, p 577

Kaas J 2000 The reorganisation of sensory and motor maps after injury in adult mammals. In: Gazzaniga M (ed.) The new cognitive neurosciences, 2nd edn. MIT Press, Cambridge

Kaltenborn F 1992 Manuelle Mobilisation der Extremitätengelenke, 9th edn. Olaf Noris, Oslo

Kaplan A 1991 Examination and diagnosis. In: Kaplan A, Assael L (eds) Temporomandibular disorders: diagnosis and treatment. Saunders, Philadelphia, p 284

Karlsson S, Persson M, Carlsson G 1991 Mandibular movement and velocity in relation to state of dentition and age. Journal of Oral Rehabilitation 18:1

Keller D C 2001 Diagnostic orthotics to establish the functional mandibular–maxillary relationship for orthodontic corrections. Journal of General Orthodontics 12(1):21

Kino K, Sugisaki M, Ishikawa T, Shibuya T, Amagasa T 2001 Preliminary psychologic survey of orofacial outpatients. Part I: predictors of anxiety or depression. Journal of Orofacial Pain 15:235

Kraus S 1994 Cervical influences on management of temporomandibular disorders, 2nd edn. Churchill Livingstone, New York, p 325

Kumar R, Berger R J, Dunsker S B, Keller J T 1996 Innervation of the spinal dura. Myth or reality? Spine 21(1):18

Leher A, Graf K, PhoDuc J M, Rammelsberg P 2005 Is there a difference in the reliable measurement of temporomandibular disorder signs between experienced and inexperienced examiners? Journal of Orofacial Pain 19(1):58–64

Lobbezoo-Scholte A, Steenks M, Faber J et al 1993 Diagnostic value of orthopedic tests in patients with temporomandibular disorders. Journal of Dental Research 72:1443

Lund J, Widmer C, Feine J 1995 Validity of diagnostic and monitoring tests used for temporomandibular disorders. Journal of Dental Research 74:1133

Mahan P, Alling C 1991 Facial pain, 3rd edn. Lea and Febiger, Malvern, PA, p 145

Maher C 1995 Perception of stiffness in manipulative physiotherapy. Physiotherapy Practice 11:35

Maitland G, Hengeveld E, Banks K, English K 2001 Maitland's vertebral manipulation. Butterworth-Heinemann, Oxford

Manni E, Palmier G, Marini R et al 1975 Trigeminal influences and extensor muscles of the neck. Experimental Neurology 47:330

Matheson J 2000 Research in neurodynamics; is neurodynamics worthy of scientific merit? In: Butler D (ed.) The sensitive nervous system. Noigroup Publications, Adelaide, p 342

Mense S 1998 Pathophysiologische Grundlagen der Muskelschmerz-Syndrome in Myoarthropathien des Kausystems und orofaziale Schmerzen. Fotoplast, Zürich, p 17

Mohl N 1991 Temporomandibular disorders: the role of occlusion, TMJ imaging and electronic devices. A diagnostic update. Journal of the American College of Dentists 58:4

Moller E 1966 The chewing apparatus: an electromyographic study of the action of the muscles of mastication and its correlation to facial morphology. Acta Physiologica Scandinavica 69:1

Morris S, Benjamin S, Gray R, Bennett D 1997 Physical, psychiatric and social characteristics of the temporomandibular disorder pain dysfunction syndrome: the relationship of mental disorders to presentation. British Dental Journal 182:25

Munro R 1974 Activity of the digastric muscle in swallowing and chewing. Journal of Dental Research 53:530

Murray G, Phanachet I, Uchida S, Whittle T 2001 The role of the human lateral pterygoid muscle in the control of horizontal jaw movements. Journal of Orofacial Pain 15:279

Naeije M, van Loon L (eds) 1998 Diagnostiek van craniomandibulaire dysfunctie. In: Craniomandibulaire functie en dysfunctie. Bohn Stafleu van Loghum, Houten, p 139

Nakzawa K, Kamimaru K 1991 Anatomical atlas of the temporomandibular joint. Quintessence, Tokyo

Okeson J 1995 Bell's orofacial pains, 5th edn. Quintessence, Chicago, p 147

Omae T, Inoue S, Saito O et al 1989 Electromyographic study on the effects of head position to head and neck muscles. Nippon Otetsu Shika Gakkai Zasshi 33:352

Palla S, Koller M, Airoldi R 1998 Befunderhebung und Diagnose bei Myoarthropathien. In: Palla S (ed.) Myoarthropathien des Kausystems und orofaziale Schmerzen. Fotoplast, Zürich, p 73

Palzzi C, Miralles R, Soto M, Santander H, Zuniga C, Moyda H 1996 Body position effects on EMG activity of sternocleidomastoideus and masseter muscles in patients with myogenic cranio-cervical-mandibular dysfunction. Journal of Craniomandibular Practice 14:200

Penfield W, Boldrey E 1937 Somatic motor and sensory representation in the cerebral cortex of man as studied by electrical stimulation. Brain 60:389

Pertes R, Gross S 1995 Clinical management of temporomandibular disorders and orofacial pain. Quintessence, Chicago, p 146

Petty N, Moore A (eds) 2001 Examination of the temporomandibular joint. In: A handbook for therapists: neuromusculoskeletal examination and assessment. Churchill Livingstone, Oxford, p 113

Portney L, Watkins M 1993 Foundations of clinical research. Application to practice. Appleton and Lange, Norwalk, CT

Proffit W, Ackerman J 1993 Orthodontic diagnosis: the development of a problem list. In: Proffit W, Fields H W (eds) Contemporary orthodontics. Mosby, Philadelphia, p 139

Ramachandran V, Blakeslee S 1998 Phantoms in the brain. William Morrow, New York

Reeves J, Jaeger B, Graff-Radford S 1986 Reliability of the pressure algometer as a measure of myofascial trigger point sensitivity. Pain 24(3):313–321

Rocabado M 1985 Diagnose und Behandlung einer abnormalen kraniozervikalen und kraniomandibulären Mechanik. In: Solberb W, Clark G (eds) Kieferfunktionen, Diagnostik und Therapie. Quintessenz, Berlin, p 145

Rocabado M, Iglash Z 1991 Musculoskeletal approach to maxillofacial pain. Lippincott, Philadelphia

Rosenbaum M 1975 The feasibility of a screening procedure regarding temporomandibular joint dysfunction. Oral Surgery, Oral Medicine, Oral Pathology 39:382

Rugh J 1991 TMJ diagnostic test in current controversies in temporomandibular disorders. Quintessence, New York

Sahrmann S 2001 Diagnosis and treatment of movement impairment syndromes. Mosby, St Louis, p 193

Salaorni C, Palla S 1994 Condylar rotation and anterior translation in healthy human temporomandibular joints. Schweizer Monatsschrift für Zahnmedizin 104:415

Schiffman E, Fricton J, Haley D, Tylka D 1988 A pressure algometer and the myofascial pain syndrome: reliability and validity testing. In: Dubner R, Gebhart G, Bonds M (eds) Proceedings of the Vth World Congress on Pain. Elsevier, Amsterdam, p 407

Schokker R, Hansson T, Ansink B, Habets L 1990 Craniomandibular asymmetry in headache patients. Journal of Craniomandibular Disorders 4(3):205–209

Schon D 1983 The reflective clinician. Basic Books, New York

Schwenzer M, Ehrenfeld M (eds) 2002 Zahn-Mund-Kiefer-Heilkunde. In: Spezielle Chirurgie, Band 2. Thieme, Stuttgart

Shellhas K 1989 Diagnostic criteria for intra-articular TMJ disorders. Community Dentistry and Oral Epidemiology 17:252

Sheppard I, Sheppard S 1965 Maximum incisal opening: a diagnostic approach index? Journal of Dental Medicine 20:13

Silman A, Haskard D, Day S 1986 Distribution of joint mobility in a normal population: results of the normal population: results of the use of fixed torque measure devices. Annals of the Rheumatic Diseases 45:27

Spillane J (ed.) 1996 The cranial nerves. In: Bickerstaff's neurological examination in clinical practice, 6th edn. Blackwell Science, Oxford, p 35

Sterling M, Jull G, Wright A 2001 The effect of musculoskeletal pain on motor activity and control. Journal of Pain 2:135

Stokes M, Young A 1984 The contribution of reflex inhibition to arthrogenous muscle weakness. Clinical Science 67:7–14

Subtelny J (ed.) 2000 Maxillary skeletal retrusion malocclusions. In: Early orthodontic treatment. Quintessence, Chicago, p 3

Sung-Chang C, Bo-Yong U, Hyung-Suk K 1992 Evaluation of pressure pain threshold in head and neck muscles by electronic algometer: intrarater and interrater reliability. Journal of Craniomandibular Practice 10:28–34

Tanaka T 1984 Recognition of the pain formula for head, neck and TMJ disorders: the general physical examination. Journal of the California Dental Association 12(5):43–49

Travell J, Simons D 1983 Myofascial pain and dysfunction. The trigger point manual. Williams and Wilkins, Baltimore

Trott P 1985 Examination of the temporomandibular joint. In: Grieve G P (ed.) Modern manual therapy of the vertebral column. Churchill Livingstone, Edinburgh, p 521

Tsai C M, Chou S L, Galke E N, Mccall W D Jr 2002 Human masticatory muscle activity and jaw position under experimental stress. Journal of Oral Rehabilitation 29:44

Turp J 2000 Temporomandibular pain, clinical presentation and Impact. Quintessenz, Berlin

Vermeiren J, Heyrman A, Oostendorp R, Bos J, Duquet W, de Cock J 1995 Het joint-play onderzoek van het temporomandibulaire gewricht. Een experimenteel onderzoek naar de intra- en interbeoordelaarsbetrouwbaarheid. Nederlands Tijdschrift voor Manuele Therapie 14:32

Vernon H, Aker P, Burns P, Viljakaanen S, Short L 1990 Pressure pain threshold evaluation of the effect of spinal manipulation in the treatment of chronic neck pain: a pilot study. Journal of Manipulative and Physiological Therapeutics 13:13

Vicenzino B, Collins D, Benson H, Wright A 1998 An investigation of the interrelationship between manipulative therapy-induced hyperalgesia and sympatho-excitation. Journal of Manipulative and Physiological Therapeutics 21:448

Visser C M 2000 Cervical spinal pain in chronic craniomandibular pain patients, recognition, prevalence, and indicators. Thesis, ACTA Amsterdam

von Piekartz H 2000 Neurodynamik des kranialen Nervensystems (Kranioneurodynamik). In: von Piekartz H (ed.) Kraniofaziale Dysfunktionen und Schmerzen: Untersuchung, Beurteilung und Management. Thieme, Stuttgart, p 115

von Piekartz H 2001 Vorschlag für einen neurodynamischen Test des N. mandibularis. Reliabilität und Referenzwerte. Manuelle Therapie 56

von Piekartz H 2004 A comparative study of left to right side mandibular length in patients with headaches, neck or face pain and a healthy control group (unpublished pilot study)

Wagemans P, Van de Velde J, Kuipers-Jagtman A 1988 Sutures and forces: a review. American Journal of Orthodontics and Dentofacial Orthopedics 94:129

Walker N, Bohannon R, Caeron D 2000 Discriminant validity of temporomandibular joint range of motion measurements obtained with a ruler. Journal of Orthopaedics and Sports Physical Therapy 30:484

Widmer C, Huggins K, Friction J 1992 History questionnaire, specifications for TMD examination forms. Journal of Craniomandibular Disorders 6:335

Williams P, Warwick R, Dyson M, Bannister L 1989 Gray's anatomy, 37th edn. Churchill Livingstone, Edinburgh

Wilson-Pauwels L, Akesson E, Stewart P 1988 Cranial nerves, anatomy and clinical comments. Decker, Toronto

Woda A 2000 Mechanisms of neuropathic pain in orofacial pain. In: Lund J, Lavigne G, Dubner R, Sessle B (eds) From basic science to clinical management. Quintessence, Chicago, p 67

Wong D, Li J 2000 The omohyoid sling syndrome. American Journal of Otolaryngology 21:318

Zufiga G, Mirales R, Moran B, Santander H, Moya H 1995 Influences of variation in jaw posture on sternocleidomastoid and trapezius electromyographic activity. Journal of Craniomandibular Practice 13:157

Chapter 9

Craniomandibular region: clinical patterns and management

Harry von Piekartz

CHAPTER CONTENTS

INTRODUCTION

The aetiology of craniomandibular complaints is unknown (Greene 2001). Symptoms in this region are often associated with multistructural changes. The medical diagnosis is therefore usually only a secondary consideration during (conservative) treatment. Nevertheless, the therapist needs to be able to recognize clinical patterns of, for example, disc displacement or myogenic dysfunction with associated parafunctions in order to decide on further tests, treatment and future strategies. The therapist should also be able to evaluate the contribution of the various structures to enable a structure-specific treatment approach.

In this chapter, common syndromes with their associated clinical patterns are presented and their relationship to anatomical structures is discussed. Based on clinical evidence, guidelines and treatment ideas are introduced. This list of ideas makes no attempt to be complete and additions may be made.

Craniomandibular dysfunctions are often multistructural. It is the task of the therapist to find out which structures influence each other and which structures behave indifferently. The results will guide the choice of therapy and management.

Consider for example a patient with unilateral facial pain in the right mandibular region,

32 mm mouth opening and a mandibular displacement towards the right. Palpation of the masseter muscle is painful and three trigger points increase symptoms. History points towards a predominantly intra-articular dysfunction, possibly disc displacement without reduction. During the first treatment session the therapist chooses techniques that predominantly influence intra-articular structures. Following treatment, mouth opening has increased to 40 mm. At the beginning of the second session it is 38 mm. The unilateral facial pain has decreased, the masseter muscle is less inflamed and the trigger points are diminished. Retrospectively, it can be assumed that the muscular dysfunction is secondary to the intra-articular dysfunction, and that a more intra-articular strategy is the most appropriate.

Clinical patterns may generally be divided into three subgroups:

- Craniomandibular joint dysfunctions
- Neuromuscular dysfunctions
- (Cranio)neurodynamic dysfunctions.

The most common patterns of articular and neuromuscular dysfunctions are discussed in the following sections. For more information on cranioneurodynamic dysfunction, see Chapters 17 and 18.

CRANIOMANDIBULAR JOINT DYSFUNCTIONS

For a better understanding of the various clinical patterns, the commonest dysfunctions of mouth opening and their differential interpretation are presented here.

MANDIBULAR MOVEMENTS AND ARTICULAR STRUCTURES

Hypomobility

Hypomobility is defined as a restriction of functional mandibular movements (Kraus 1994). This may be due to various mechanisms, for example aplasia, hypoplasia, hyperplasia, dysplasia, neoplasia and fractures (McNeil 1993). Restriction may also be caused by dysfunctions of the masticatory muscles such as myofacial pain, trismus and contractures (McNeil 1993). Recent investigations show that patients with craniomandibular dysfunctions due to a co-contraction of the elevator muscles (m. masseter and the anterior part of the m. temporalis) commonly show mouth opening restrictions (Yamaguchi et al 2002). Dominantly arthrogenic dysfunctions such as ankylosis, arthritis, periarticular stiffness and specific intra-articular problems (disc displacement and inflammatory processes such as joint effusion) often show the classic features of hypomobility (Bays 1994).

Neurodynamic dysfunction is a frequently ignored influence. Several EMG studies incorporating neurodynamic tests have shown that there is a clear correlation between EMG activities during performance of the neurodynamic tests in both the control and dysfunction patient groups: EMG activity of neighbouring muscles increases with increased burdening of the mobility of the nervous system.

Apparently the body possesses a protection mechanism for sensitive nerves. In patients with neuropathy the EMG activity is clearly higher (Hu et al 1995, Zusman 1998). Clinical experience shows that this is a common phenomenon, especially in patients with mandibular nerve neuropathy (after tooth extraction, tooth implantation and mandibular trauma). To the author's knowledge, no studies have been conducted to date that show the EMG activity of the masticatory muscles in patients with mandibular nerve neuropathy in various neurodynamic positions. For more information on neuropathy and hypomobility, see Chapters 17 and 18.

If patients fear to move the mandible because they are scared of a clicking noise, (sub)luxation and pain, this may lead to guarding or a so-called *protective splint* (Asmundson et al 1999). This central mechanism is often connected with an unpleasant memory of symptomatic craniomandibular movements in the past (Flor et al 1992). In this case the hypomobility is not a constant phenomenon but depends on movement direction and situation. Passive movements might be more difficult to perform with mouth opening of less than 30 mm, while yawning at home may achieve 50 mm.

Hypermobility

Hypermobility may be caused by anatomical (position and movement of the head of the mandible in the fossa articularis) and functional (range of movement) features. These may occur independently of each other.

Anatomically, hypermobility is defined as an increased joint play of the condyle between the articular arch and the articular tubercle (Kraus 1994). On maximum mouth opening this is easily detected radiologically (Palla et al 1998). The therapist may observe a greater range of mouth opening than average. A slightly prominent mandibular head may be palpated laterally on either side.

The aetiology of hypermobility is unknown. Skeletal abnormalities, muscle imbalance and psychiatric disorders may contribute to the problem (Keith 1988). Constitutional hyperlaxity of the whole body may also affect the craniomandibular region (Buckingham et al 1991). Hypermobility of the craniomandibular region is not a risk factor for disc displacement (Westling 1989, Westling & Mattiasson 1991, Dijkstra et al 1992).

Quality of movement

Functional mouth opening and the patient's reaction during this movement point towards specific clinical patterns. The following features and reactions may be observed and interpreted:

- Shift or *swinging opening* (for dentists: *deflection*)
- Clicking noises or *crepitation* on opening and closing
- Contraction of the superficial masticatory muscles
- Pain alone or in combination with one or more of the above features.

The pathogenesis of individual dysfunctions is briefly presented in the following section. This is followed by evidence-based treatment approaches and discussed according to the recent literature. How to achieve the most appropriate technique and dosage based on biomedical and clinical knowledge and experience of the individual therapist is explained by applying the clinical reasoning approach (Jones et al 2001).

Intra- or periarticular dysfunction

Periarticular structures are tissues that are located outside the joint (Wyke 1972). Based on functional–anatomical evidence, the outermost two-thirds of the joint capsule is counted as a periarticular structure; the remaining one-third is intra-articular, as is the subchondral bone. The intra-articular structures are responsible for the production of synovial fluids (Wyke 1972, Clark 1976).

The periarticular components are responsible for proprioception and stabilization. Monoarticular muscles, nervous tissue, blood vessels and lymphatic tissue may functionally be counted as periarticular structures (Wyke 1972, Clark 1976, Bogduk et al 1995).

In the following section the most common intra- and periarticular dysfunctions and their clinical patterns are described and treatment suggestions are added.

INTRA-ARTICULAR DYSFUNCTIONS

Disc disease

Disc disease of the craniomandibular joint is defined as a morphological change due to a shift in disc position. The most common shift is towards anterior, anterior-laterally or anterior-medially; very rarely the disc moves posteriorly or laterally (Palla et al 1998, Chen et al 2002). This may cause degenerative changes of the joint (Wyke 1972, Clark 1976).

Generally it is possible to differentiate between disc displacement with or without reduction/reposition (Rocabado 1991, Erikson et al 1992, Okeson 1995, Perthes & Gross 1995).

DISC DISEASE WITH REDUCTION

One classic feature of disc displacement is a reciprocal clicking noise. Various explanations are found for the occurrence of the click. The following simplified model is the most common and is accepted by most authors (Gelb 1985,

Rocabado & Iglash 1991, Palla et al 1998, Bumann & Lutzmann 2000). It is easily applied for treatment.

- The disc is moved anteriorly or medially in relation to the condyle articularis on maximum intercuspidation (Fig. 9.1a).
- On mouth opening the disc is shifted forwards and/or medially, so that the condyle lies inferior and dorsal of the posterior band of the disc for a brief moment (Fig. 9.1b).
- On further opening the condyle accelerates forwards and the superior–anterior part of the condyle moves underneath the midzone of the disc. This quick movement may be accompanied by a 'click', the so-called opening click (Fig. 9.1c).
- Further mouth opening is possible to the physiological end of range due to a normal disc–condyle relationship (Fig. 9.1d).
- Just before maximum intercuspidation the condyle may again move briefly behind the posterior band, this time towards posterior. A clicking noise may be heard that is less obvious than the opening click; this is called the closing click (Fig. 9.3e–h).

Clinical features of disc displacement with reduction/reposition

- Reciprocal opening or closing 'click', with the opening noise louder than the closing noise (Westesson et al 1985).
- Usually swinging mouth opening or shift (displacement) and occasionally clear restriction of depression (mouth opening).

Restricted depression may also be caused by secondary phenomena, as described in 'Hypomobility', p. 216.

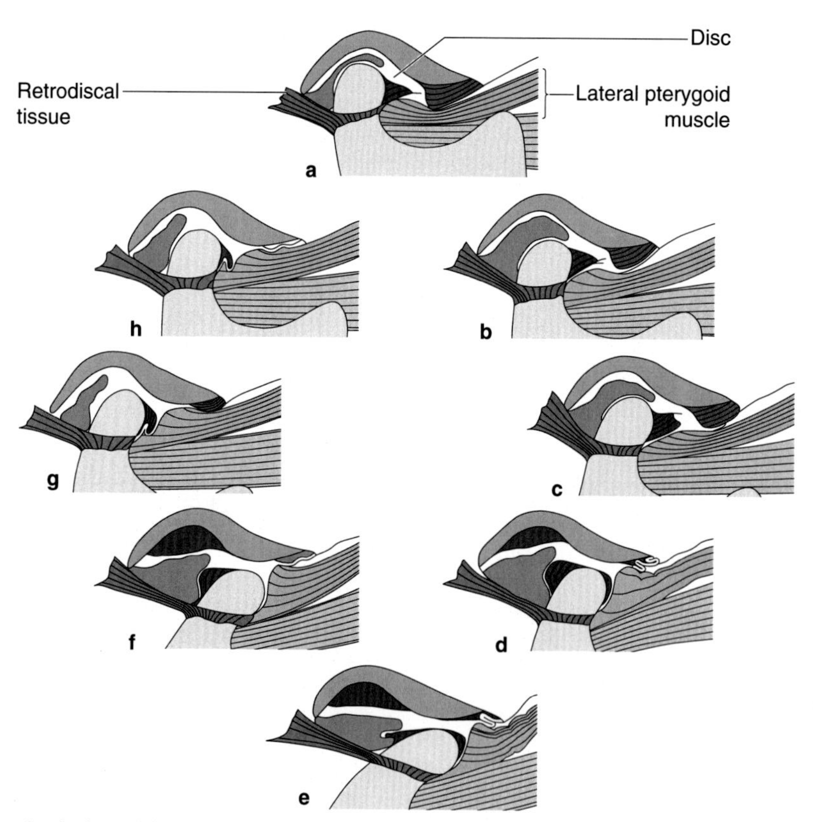

Fig. 9.1 Hypothetical model of a disc displacement with reduction and associated opening and closing click (b and h) (see text) (after Okeson 1995).

Does the 'click' always indicate disc displacement? If the answer is 'no', other explanations for joint crepitation are:

- Habitual (sub)luxation: If the caput articularis moves forward too quickly in the articular fossa, this may produce a clicking noise. It occurs towards the end of range of mouth opening and sounds dull. The therapist should see/palpate the prominent caput articularis laterally (Okeson 1995).
- Snapping of soft tissue such as ligaments, adhesions within the masticatory muscles along the articular condyle: There are a number of anatomical variations that may cause a clicking noise, e.g. the insertion of the lateral pterygoid muscle, the sphenomandibular and stylomandibular ligaments or the lateral (external) capsule (Zaki et al 1996). The quality of the noise may range from dull to sharp and short; it is generally reduced on repeated (more than 10 repetitions) mouth opening. Immediately after probationary manual therapy treatment of the peripheral tissue the clicking is commonly reduced significantly. With disc displacement, there will not be such an immediate symptom reduction.
- Intra-articular adhesion or loose bodies in the joint: Fibres of connective tissue may come off the articular disc, the joint surface and/or the temporal bone. Minimal adhesions may also cause a clicking and are usually associated with hypomobility. In most cases joint distraction will reduce the symptoms and increase the range of motion. Loose bodies in the joint (former adhesions, disc particles) may cause non-permanent joint locking. An arthroscopy or sometimes even an MRI may confirm the hypothesis of a loose body (Erikson & Westesson 1983, Rao 1995, Chen et al 2000).

Clicking due to disc displacement can be diagnosed by modern MRI (Farrar & Mcarthy 1982, Rasmussen 1983) and electronic axiography (Bumann & Groot Landeweert 1991). An easier option is the stethoscope. The clicking is a reproducible, reliable symptom for the recognition of disc displacement (Gallo et al 2000) (Table 9.1).

Treatment

Manual therapy

- Accessory movements: Generally longitudinal caudal, transverse movements and anterior–posterior movements will show some clinical signs. It is also possible that posterior–anterior movement will reproduce the clicking. If the same movement is performed with added distraction the symptoms become more bearable. The best results are commonly expected if accessory movements are applied in a position just before or during the click. This is also the position

Table 9.1 Joint sounds of the craniomandibular joint, the main features and their interpretation

Tissue hypothesis	Features
Hypermobility (subluxation)	Dull click at the end of range of mouth opening Head of the mandible moves laterally
Periarticular structures around the caput articularis	May range from dull to sharp click With or without pain Changes quickly with repeated movement (active/passive)
Intra-articular adhesions, free bodies	Severe click with or without pain Click and limited range of motion commonly occur simultaneously Quick and significant changes of noise and restriction after joint distraction techniques

that shows the most relevant clinical signs and symptoms (pain, increased resistance). Reassessment of mouth opening shows which techniques influence the problem best. If clicking is reduced and occurs earlier in the range this indicates a positive prognosis (De Naaije & van Loon 1998). Possibly the disc has increased space and the articular head may move underneath the disc more easily.

- Passive physiological movements/depression evaluation: If the clicking changes without a change in mandibular shift, large range depression and elevation movements may result in a more physiological shift-free quality of movement. The technique is identical to the longitudinal caudal movement. The advantage is that during the depression/elevation a slight distraction occurs which avoids clicking and other symptoms. Hence there is a double effect: first, stimulation of the somatosensory cortex (homunculus) by movements that were not registered for a long time (Allard et al 1991, Ramachandran & Blakesee 1998) and second, re-education of mandibular movements is initiated (discussed later in this chapter).

Dental treatment

Braces (see Chapters 10 and 11).

Home management

Exercises may be integrated into daily life, for example:

- Coordinated mouth opening
- Static stabilization in different positions of opening
- 'Snake' movements
- 'Touch-and-bite' exercise (see below).

It is most important for the treatment of disc displacement with reduction that clicking does not occur (or occurs only minimally) when exercising. The exercises are listed in an order from easy to difficult. If the clicking occurs during the 'snake' or the 'touch-and-bite', this indicates that those exercises are too difficult and the patient should stick with the first one or two exercises until the symptoms have improved.

DISC DISPLACEMENT WITHOUT REDUCTION

In the literature the models for disc displacement without reduction are more unidimensional than for disc displacement with reduction (Palla et al 1998, Bumann & Lotzmann 2000). The disc–condyle relation is affected and the disc is positioned further anterior (medial) of the articular head (Fig. 9.2a):

- On mouth opening the disc is stuck in front of the condyle and shows a tendency to shift anteriorly (Fig. 9.2b,c).
- Therefore, the retrodiscal space and the collateral ligaments are loaded. End of range movements will produce pain (Bumann & Lotzmann 2000) (Fig. 9.2d–h).

Clinical features

- In the past the patient has often experienced a phase of clicking, although the symptoms have now disappeared. The patient is left with a restriction in mouth opening.
- Opening restrictions are between 25 and 35 mm (Kraus 1994, Hesse 1996, Palla et al 1998).
- On mouth opening the neck is often moved into upper cervical extension. Correction of the neck position reduces mouth opening and/or provokes pain (Fig. 9.3).
- Moving the mandible to the right and left alternately leads to a short-term reduction of the opening restriction.
- Generally, there is no mandibular shift. If laterotrusion is present it occurs at the end of range and commonly the shift is towards the asymptomatic side; protrusions have also been observed with unilateral dysfunctions.
- Laterotrusion away from the symptomatic side and transverse medial and lateral movements, as well as posterior–anterior movements, are often restricted by rapidly increasing resistance, with or without pain.

Treatment

Manual therapy

- In maximum mouth opening, perform the most restricted accessory movement into

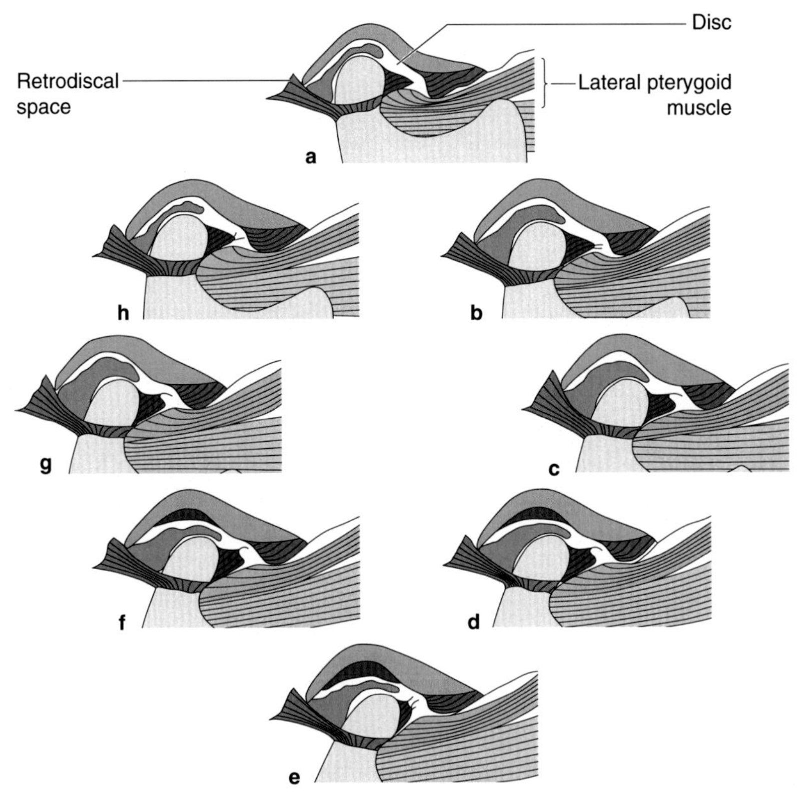

Fig. 9.2 Hypothetical model for an anterior disc displacement without reduction (see text).

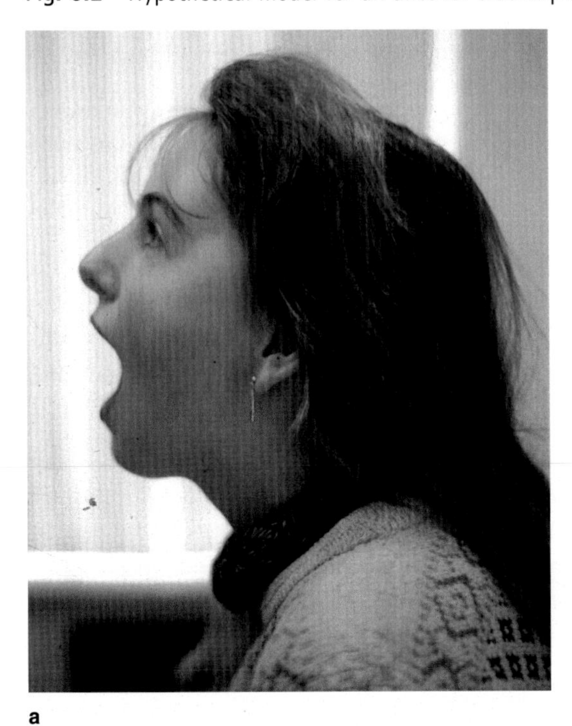

Fig. 9.3 Examples of disc displacement on mouth opening.

a Female patient (19 years) with an anterior disc displacement on active mouth opening. Note the upper cervical extension that serves as a compensatory activity to increase the range of opening.

b Movement diagram of passive opening (patient with disc displacement without reduction). Note the severe restriction of motion (range of opening 24 mm), the rapid increase of tension, in this case the masseter (S1–S') and the increase in pain (P1–P') associated with the increase in resistance (R1–R2).

resistance. These are often transverse movements.

- If mouth opening improves, emphasize the increased range of motion by adding a physiological depression combined with longitudinal (caudal) distraction.
- Progress the intensity by positioning the head more into flexion. Clinical experience shows that restricted mandibular (accessory) movements respond well to manual mobilization.
- When applying the 'Trott' (1986) method, take care that the spatula is well positioned on the molar teeth, so that a distraction is achieved and not a modified depression that would shift the disc even further towards ventral.

Dental treatment

Usually a distraction or relaxation brace is prescribed (see also Chapter 10).

Home management

- Accessory movements of the articular condyle that have been shown to be beneficial are taught as an automobilization routine, for example transverse medial mobilization.
- Active depression exercise with bilateral distraction. The patient's hands are pronated so that the thumbs point caudally and touch the mandibular angles. The tongue is kept at the roof of the mouth while the mouth is opened slowly. On opening the patient performs an interphalangeal extension of both thumbs, achieving a slight distraction.
- Exercises as described for disc displacement with reduction. Once mouth opening has improved towards end of range and protrusion does not provoke any symptoms, the 'snake' exercise should be added.
- If instructed well by the therapist, the patient may also perform the 'Trott' method at home.

LATERAL AND MEDIAL DISC DISPLACEMENT

Unilateral disc displacements towards medial or lateral without any anterior shift are extremely rare. Depending on the method of assessment the incidence varies between 16% (post-mortem) and 11–26% (imaging techniques) (Katzberg & Westesson 1983, Duvoisin et al 1990). Medial displacement is more common than lateral displacement (Duvoisin et al 1990, Dittmer & Ewers 1991). Correct disc behaviour can only be shown by modern CT imaging (Chen et al 2000).

In the author's opinion, transverse movements are the most noticeable. They often react more quickly with improved movement and reduced pain than classic anterior (medial) displacement.

DORSAL DISC DISPLACEMENT

The disc has shifted to dorsal and the syndrome may easily be misdiagnosed as a condyle luxation. This is the most uncommon type of disc displacement (Katzberg et al 1983). Young hypermobile females are particularly prone to this dysfunction (Westesson et al 1985). Prolonged maximum mouth opening or sudden uncontrolled mouth opening may be the triggering stimulus.

Clinical features

- Mouth closure is restricted and may be painful unilaterally.
- Mouth opening is often slightly reduced and sometimes associated with a mandibular shift away from the symptomatic side.
- On palpation the retrodiscal space feels swollen and is sensitive to touch.

Treatment

Most patients with dorsal disc displacement have already been seen by a dentist and/or orthodontist and have been provided with an 'emergency brace' and medication.

If the situation is acute and painful the therapist should opt for pain-reducing manual therapy techniques and exercises that will also achieve an improvement in function.

Manual therapy

- Pain-free longitudinal caudal mobilization (distraction) is recommended in an asymptomatic position of mouth opening, generally around mid-range. Bilateral distraction

is commonly the most beneficial technique if mouth opening or closing provokes severe pain.
- Anterior–posterior movements, possibly combined with slight traction, may improve closure and reduce pain.

Dental treatment

Usually the patient is provided with an 'emergency brace' that reduces the discal pressure and gently shifts the disc towards anterior.

Non-steroidal anti-inflammatory drugs (NSAIDs) may be prescribed to reduce swelling and local temperature increases due to inflammatory processes in the craniomandibular joint.

Home management

- In an acute phase the patient is advised to apply cool packs frequently for a short period of time.
- If able to perform pain-free opening and closing in mid-range (1.5–3.5 cm), the patient is advised to perform these as a home exercise. Clinical experience shows that the pain-free range of motion increases within a few days so that the exercise will need to be adapted.

DEGENERATION

Primary degeneration occurs after trauma of the discal cartilage whereas secondary degeneration is associated with synovitis and bone structure changes such as osteosclerosis of the eminentia articularis (De Bont et al 1986). Longitudinal studies have shown that disc displacement patients are significantly more likely to develop degenerative changes in the craniomandibular joints. At this point it has to be mentioned that degeneration of the craniomandibular joints is not directly correlated with the occurrence of pain (Schiffman et al 1992, Murakami et al 1996). Any variation up to severe arthritis and perforation may also occur at the craniomandibular joints. Severe arthrotic changes, usually associated with disc perforation, will show the classic clinical pattern for osteoarthrosis. A multidisciplinary approach is recommended, as described in the following sections.

Clinical features

- Obvious crepitation with or without pain on movement.
- Premature protrusion on mouth opening and restricted range of movement.
- Compression during mouth opening significantly increases or decreases the symptoms.
- Distraction during mouth opening usually causes minimal crepitation or pain.
- Radiological indicators are sclerosis, changes of joint shape and narrowing of the joint space (Gynther et al 1996, Hansson et al 1996).

Benefits of compression for manual therapy assessment and treatment

Compression has been shown to be clinically effective in the treatment of synovial joint degeneration. It was also confirmed that the joint itself benefits from compression techniques (Salter & Field 1960, van Wingerden 1990, 1997). The craniomandibular joint undergoes compressive forces regularly in daily activities such as chewing, swallowing and speaking. Research on other synovial joints such as the knee and foot has shown that gentle compression produces a growth stimulus in the cartilage of joints affected by slight degeneration and may even regenerate the cartilage to a certain degree (van Wingerden 1997). The pain becomes more bearable, range of movement increases and activities of daily living therefore become easier to perform (Maitland 1991). This may also be true for the craniomandibular joint. The following features and reactions point to a beneficial effect of compressive techniques:

- At first, minimal compression is executed during mouth opening and closing.
- On minimal compression during mouth opening and closing the pain and crepitation are slowly reduced (usually after 10–20 repetitions).
- On reassessment:
  - Pain has improved
  - Resistance on passive movement has decreased
  - Range of movement has increased (slightly).

If the above reactions are observed, it is likely that compressive techniques will be beneficial for the individual patient with degenerative joint complaints. If the most spectacular reactions do not occur, this might point towards a more advanced degenerative process. The cartilage is no longer capable of regenerating itself (van Wingerden 1990). It may also indicate that the disc tissue is destroyed (e.g. disc perforation) such that the head of the mandible and the temporal bone are in direct contact (Murakami et al 1996).

Treatment

Manual therapy

Stiffness is treated with accessory movements in end of physiological range positions. This is expected to improve craniomandibular movement towards a physiological intra-articular range of movement. Longitudinal caudal and transverse lateral accessory movements are often symptomatic.

A minimal longitudinal cranial movement (compression) is carried out during end of range mouth opening and closing (depression and elevation). The hand position is the same as for longitudinal caudal movements (see Chapter 8). The patient's pain responses direct the intensity of pressure for the longitudinal movement towards cranial. If the symptoms gradually decrease with this technique, the correct force is applied.

Dental treatment

Commonly a 'relaxation brace' is prescribed (see also Chapters 10 and 11).

Home management

- Accessory movements that have been beneficial in the treatment session may be effective if taught as a home exercise.
- Depression and elevation combined with axial compression onto the mandibular head. The hands are positioned as described for depression with distraction, but the thumbs now lie underneath the mandibular angle so that constant compression is applied throughout opening and closing (Fig. 9.4).

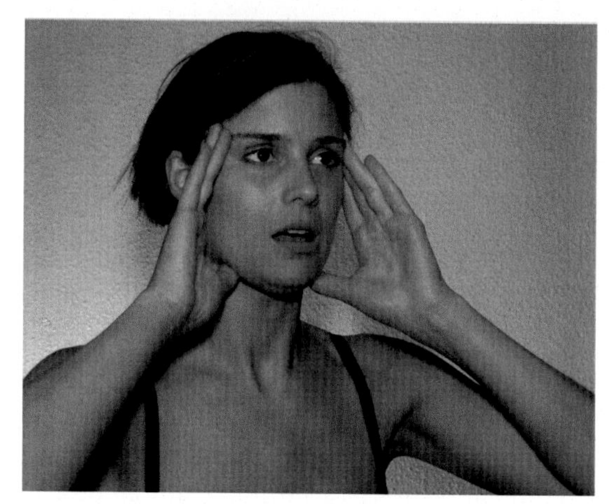

Fig. 9.4 A home exercise: with the tips of both thumbs in contact with the lower edge of the mandibular arch, the index, middle and ring fingers stabilize the head laterally.

Some facts on disc displacements are outlined in Box 9.1.

RETRODISCAL INFLAMMATION

Phylogeny shows how the development from the quadruped to *Homo erectus* etc. has an important influence on the position of the head of the mandible.

Once upright, the development of the human race occurred rather quickly in comparison to general evolution. This may be an explanation for the fact that the retrodiscal space of the human craniomandibular system is not ideally prepared to withstand constant compressive loading and tension forces (Slavicek 2000).

The retrodiscal space contains a number of sensitive and vascular structures that may react to compression and distraction overload by excessive inflammation (Westesson et al 1985, Bumann & Groot Landeweert 1997).

A disturbed disc–condyle relationship may cause retrodiscal inflammation due to an overstretched posterior joint capsule, stratum superior and stratum inferior on end of range movements such as singing, dental treatment or yawning (Freesmeyer 1993, Kraus 1994, Langendoen et al 1997, Bumann & Lotzmann 2000). Traumatic incidents may also cause dorsal compression, for example bicycle acci-

Box 9.1 Some facts about disc displacements

- The incidence of crepitation increases in the second decade of life (Magnusson 1986, Dibbets et al 1992).
- The clicking may spontaneously disappear with time (Magnusson et al 1994, Könönen et al 1996).
- Most anterior disc displacements also show a slight medial shift (Chen et al 2002). Distinct unidimensional shifts towards medial or lateral without anterior displacement are relatively uncommon. Post-mortem studies claim an incidence of 16% (Katzberg et al 1983) while imaging studies state 11–26% (Duvoisin et al 1990, Katzberg & Westesson 1993).
- The most uncommon disc displacement is the posterior variation.
- An ideal disc position as diagnosed by imaging techniques does not guarantee normal function of both temporomandibular joints (Westesson et al 1985, Davant et al 1993).
- There is no direct correlation between disc position and pain in the craniomandibular region (Schiffmann et al 1992).
- Disc displacements do lead to degeneration in the long term, but there is no direct correlation between degenerative changes and pain (Schiffmann et al 1992, Luder 1993, Carlsson & Magnusson 1999) (Table 9.2).

dents, motorbike accidents or being hit on the chin during ball games. In the acute stage, swelling and severe pain are present; in the long term, stiffness with or without anterior disc displacement occurs (Müller et al 1992, Okeson 1996, Bumann & Lotzmann 2000). Clinical practice shows that patients with craniomandibular hypermobility combined with parafunctions frequently show a slight constant swelling of the retrodiscal space, sometimes for years. This may result in diffuse short-term episodes of pain and sudden sharp pain on daily orofacial activities.

Clinical features

- Palpation: The retrodiscal space is sensitive to touch (and slightly swollen); frequently a slight anterior position of the head of the mandible in its fossa is palpated.
- Physiological end of range opening, as well as mid-range movements such as protrusion and laterotrusion, provoke pain. Sudden active physiological movements and/or parafunctions also provoke symptoms.
- Accessory movements such as anterior–posterior, posterior–anterior, longitudinal movements and combined movements strongly affect the retrodiscal structures (Bumann & Lotzmann 2000).

Functional assessment based upon the anatomical model and the clinical experience of, for example, Bumann and Groot Landeweert (1997) or Bumann and Lotzmann (2000) have led to the conclusion that specific movement directions load the tissue in the retrodiscal space:

- Stratum superior (tension): longitudinal combined with posterior–anterior movements
- Stratum inferior (compression): anterior–posterior movements
- Stratum posterior and stratum inferior (compression-)angulation of the anterior–posterior movement.

This requires a relaxed mandibular position (aperture) of 2 cm. The load changes with variations in mandibular position.

What makes the difference in the retrodiscal space?

Naturally, the above information will influence therapeutic decisions, but the therapist needs to be aware that accessory movements are not the gold standard for assessment of the retrodiscal space (Miller 1991, Palla et al 1998). There is a wide range of anatomical variation (Mahan 1980). From the manual therapy point of view the tests are useful to confirm the clinical pattern and may also contribute to the classification of pain mechanisms.

Table 9.2 Disc displacement: the most common disc displacements, clinical features and management suggestions

Displacement	Clinical features	Management guidelines
Anterior–medial with reduction	Reciprocal opening and/or closing click, commonly mid-range With or without opening limitation	Manual therapy: Accessory movements just before the click (longitudinal–caudal and transverse–lateral), anterior–posterior movements worsen the symptoms Carry out through-range depressions with slight longitudinal movement of the mandible towards caudal, active, without symptom reproduction Home exercises: Coordinated mouth opening Snake and touch-and-bite exercises Active stabilization without click Dental intervention: Distraction brace
Without reduction	Not always a shift on opening Mouth opening restriction <25 mm Usually no click End of range movements commonly painful Accessory movements restricted Compensatory neck movements	Manual therapy: Accessory movements: commonly caudal and transverse Mouth opening with longitudinal caudal movement Dental intervention: Joint distraction brace Home activities: Accessory movement on end of range active opening Active opening with longitudinal caudal movement Method according to Trott
Medial and lateral displacement	See: Disc displacement with reduction Signs and symptoms on transverse movements	See: Disc displacement with reduction Transverse movements frequently change signs and symptoms
Dorsal/posterior	Young female patients Hypermobile Sustained mouth opening Very painful Retrodiscal swelling and painful on palpation Elevation restricted and painful	Manual therapy: Longitudinal–caudal without pain Anterior–posterior in slight distraction Dental intervention: Emergency brace NSAIDs Home activities: Gentle cryotherapy Opening and closing in mid-range without pain

Table 9.2—cont'd

Displacement	Clinical features	Management guidelines
Degeneration/arthritis and perforation	Crepitation and clicking End of range restrictions With/without pain Compression techniques during mouth opening often influence the signs and symptoms	Manual therapy: Accessory movements in end of range opening Depression and elevation combined with longitudinal cranial movements (compression) Dental intervention: Relaxation brace Home activities: Accessory movements in end of range physiological positions Longitudinal cranial movements in elevation and depression

NSAIDs, non-steroidal anti-inflammatory drugs.

Treatment

Manual therapy

Use accessory movements as described above. In the acute stage techniques that do not directly affect the inflamed tissue and that do not hurt are preferable. A non-painful effective technique is frequently bilateral distraction as described in Chapter 8. For subacute and chronic cases dominated by stiffness, accessory movements which reproduce the stiffness are the first option. Reassessment of the main physiological movements and pain reaction remain the most important indicators for an effective technique.

Passive mouth opening and closure within a pain-free range of motion will not only stimulate proprioceptive joint information (Rocabado 1983) but may also positively influence trophism in the subacute and acute stage. The rhythmical movements may reduce swelling as it does in other peripheral joints by a pump mechanism to the genu vasculosum (which contains many arteriovenous anastomoses) (Westesson et al 1985). Moreover, this mobilization may be easily taught as an active exercise.

Dental treatment

Tooth restoration and brace therapy may reduce retrodiscal pressure and contribute to a reorganization of the posterior joint compartment. This can be confirmed by MRI (Müller et al 1992, 1993).

Medication

In the acute stage, anti-inflammatory medication may be beneficial (Okeson 1996).

Home management

- Active mouth opening and closing exercises in the mid-range of motion as described later in this chapter. The clinical decision depends on the effectiveness of the aforementioned passive mobilization techniques.
- Short-term cold pack applications, especially ventral of the ear (duration 10–20 minutes), are usually perceived as soothing and influence the inflammatory processes (Kraus 1994, De Naeije & van Loon 1998).
- Parafunctions need to be identified and given up.

CAPSULITIS

Capsulitis without additional pathologies is usually associated with parafunctions such as bruxism and other muscle hyperactivities (Yu et al 1992, Kraus 1993).

Clinical features

- Lateral temporomandibular joint palpation: swollen.

- Mouth opening: painful arc, end of range restriction due to hypertonic muscles.
- Muscles sensitive, especially on mouth closure.
- No findings on radiological assessment (Palla et al 1998).

Treatment

Manual therapy

Accessory and physiological movements as described for the treatment of the retrodiscal space are useful. The treatment should be painless with small amplitudes without resistance.

Dental treatment

If capsulitis persists for a long time or relapses occur frequently, a relaxation brace or tooth restoration may be indicated (see Chapter 10).

Home management

Exercises are as described for retrodiscal inflammation.

CAPSULE STIFFNESS

Aetiology

There may be various causes. Three broad categories can be defined:

- Intentional immobilization after surgical or orthodontic treatment, for examples orthognathic and temporomandibular surgery that requires maxillomandibular fixation for 6–8 weeks (Freesmeyer 1993, Proffit 1993). Immobility for more than 8 weeks may also be due to post-surgery muscle bracing and pain.
- Trauma. Macro- and microtrauma can be differentiated. *Macrotrauma* may be due to a thrust to the mandible, for example bicycle accidents, a child that jumps against the chin of father or mother from underneath, and surgery. Small adhesions develop between the joint surface and the articular disc causing end of range stiffness (Kraus 1994, De Naeije & van Loon 1998). *Microtrauma* may be the result of tooth corrections that influence the maxillomandibular relation in the long term. The joint position changes and induces capsular stress (Clark 1976, Krogh-Poulsen & Olsson 1996). If the head–neck position changes over a long period of time this may also result in a 'pseudoregulation occlusion' as described by Kraus (1988) and consequently lead to connective tissue changes in the craniomandibular joint. Small accidents that the patient might not even remember (e.g. a minor blow to the face during sports), a prone sleeping position and habits such as chewing gum may also count as microtrauma.
- Secondary consequences of degenerative processes, rheumatoid and infectious arthritis may also cause capsular stiffness (Okeson 1996).

Consequences of capsular stiffness

Capsular stiffness leads to arthrokinetic dysfunctions, affecting in particular maximal mouth opening. If the situation is maintained for a prolonged period of time (months, years) this may have consequences for the craniomandibular joint.

The blood supply may be insufficient for peri- and intra-articular structures, leading to hypoxia and insufficient nutrition of the cartilage and the disc. With a restricted range of physiological motion the synovial distribution in the joint is not sufficient. Waste products may accumulate leading to degeneration and dystrophy of the cartilage cells. The consequence may be craniomandibular arthritis (Glineburg et al 1982, De Bont et al 1986, Dijkgraaf et al 1989).

Another consequence is mechanoreceptor activity and projection to the sensomotor cortex. More than 40 years ago an excellent article on the innervation of the human craniomandibular joint was published, stating that the capsule is indeed richly innervated (Thilander 1961). Not only mechanoreceptors (Aα) but also nociceptors (Aδ and C-fibres), which are the basis of pain, are present. It is known that the craniomandibular region and the thumb show the largest sensomotor projection areas. This implies that the temporomandibular joint (TMJ) has a strong influence on the motor output system (Butler 2000). Clinical studies show that if the capsule has a nociceptive or an inhibiting effect, this will also influence the patient's balance. Disturbed balance occurs more frequently in whiplash patients with craniomandibular components than in patients without TMJ symptoms (Braun et al 1992, Chole & Parker 1992). If an anaesthetic is injected into the craniomandibular capsule of healthy individuals, they show impaired static balance (Danzig et al 1992, Shankland 1993). It would appear therefore that the TMJ has a greater influence on balance than expected. Some clinical observations confirm this; for example balance tests and dizziness (sometimes in combination with tinnitus) frequently improve after TMJ treatment techniques.

Clinical features

- Physiological movements: The active aperture is variable. Usually 20–25 mm is observed since the rolling component of the joint movement is not affected. On mouth opening an increased masticatory muscle tone (*muscle guarding*) can be observed. Frequently a compensatory cervical movement into extension and lateroflexion towards the symptomatic side occurs.
- Accessory movements are severely restricted. In particular, longitudinal (distraction) and transverse movements in various positions of mouth opening provoke symptoms. In addition, combinations of accessory movements may show an increased early resistance, pointing to a capsular contribution. Examples for combined movements are longitudinal plus posterior–anterior or transverse lateral movements. The resistance increases further when a slight laterotrusion towards the symptom-free side is added.
- Hypermobility of the opposite craniomandibular joint. With hypomobility on one side the opposite side may react with a compensatory hypermobility, especially in cases of mild cranial asymmetry (Proffit 1993). Its influence depends on the degree of cranial asymmetry and the occurrence of symptoms.
- Increased unilateral masticatory muscle tonus and muscle guarding as a reaction to capsular stiffness. Trigger points might also become increasingly sensitive.

Treatment

Manual therapy

Accessory techniques towards the direction of the greatest perceived resistance are indicated. Commonly these are the techniques described above. There follow some additional recommendations for the application of accessory movements:

- Knowing that the disc might already have experienced increased pressure (Westling et al 1990), adding a slight longitudinal caudal movement to the posterior–anterior glide is recommended. This will reduce intra-articular pressure and relieve the disc. It is recommended strongly whenever clicking occurs on manual mobilization.
- It might be helpful to palpate the area around the head of the mandible. The therapist gains information on the mobility and the relation to the surrounding tissues. If pain occurs, the therapist might consider the contributing structures.
- Assessment and treatment in various head positions. The head position also changes the position of the mandibular head and therefore has an influence on the loading of the soft tissue including the capsule (Kawamura & Fujimoto 1957, Murpy 1967, Rocabado & Iglash 1991). The positions might reflect the pain-provoking working posture of the patient (Nicolakis et al 2000). Sitting in front of the computer or electronic notebook might be an example of a position that provokes stiffness in the neck and pain unilaterally. The patient should consequently be examined and also treated in slight thoracic flexion and upper cervical extension, a position that has a unique influence on the joint capsule.
- Physiological movements. If the aperture is 25 mm or more and there is no hard end of range feel to it or stabbing pain (which may indicate disc displacement without reduction), passive physiological movements might be indicated. Depression and laterotrusion are commonly the most symptomatic movements. These patients may be treated by small amplitude movements at the end of

range to ameliorate capsular stiffness. Large amplitude through range movements to influence mechanoreceptors, improve trophism and initiate active movements may also be indicated (Wyke 1972, Newton 1982, Salter et al 1983, Maitland et al 2001).

- Muscle techniques. If the muscular signs and symptoms do not change on reassessment after joint techniques it may be helpful to approach the muscles directly, as discussed later in this chapter.
- Dynamic coordination exercises with passive overpressure on physiological mouth opening. Normal movement is relearned such that the mandibular head does not translate or subluxate on orofacial activities.

Home management

Passive mobilization stimulates a gentle inflammatory reaction that evokes neurobiological responses, promoting regeneration of the capsular connective tissue. Functional stimulation also seems to play an important role (van Wingerden 1997, van den Berg 1999). Therefore the achieved range of motion and function need to be maintained constantly by exercises during daily activities.

SUBLUXATION

Condyle subluxation occurs when the articular condyle translates excessively anterior on the eminentia. The disc–condyle relationship remains unaffected (Kraus 1994, Palla et al 1998).

Clinical features

- Hardly any pain apart from situations where capsulitis occurs due to overuse.
- The patient is conscious of the subluxation.
- Increased range of aperture: often more than 50 mm, sometimes combined with a mandibular shift.
- On inspection from lateral or ventral: the condyle is laterally more prominent on maximum mouth opening.
- May produce a painless dull 'click'.

Treatment

Manual therapy

Passive mobilization for stretching purposes is not indicated. Passive physiological movements may be beneficial to stimulate mechanoreceptors and thereby provide the homunculus with correct information on jaw movements (Ramachandran & Blakesee 1998, Butler 2000). Experience shows that this should be initiated before starting on coordinative exercises. The patient will re-learn the correct movements quicker and more efficiently after experiencing the correct movements passively.

Neuromuscular re-education exercises

Static stabilization exercises in various positions of mouth opening are particularly useful.

Home management

- Un-learn parafunctions. This may reduce the incidence of subluxation significantly.
- Neuromuscular re-education exercises as taught in the treatment sessions should be performed regularly.

In most cases the patient does not suffer too much from subluxation. Unfortunately this frequently leads to inadequate patient compliance.

(HABITUAL) LUXATION

On maximum aperture the head of the mandible translates forward beyond the articular tubercle. If the patient is unable to return the jaw to its normal position, this is called 'luxation'. If this occurs frequently, it is called 'habitual luxation' (Okeson 1995, De Naeije & van Loon 1998).

Clinical features

- Occurs commonly in young hypermobile individuals on sudden or prolonged mouth opening (e.g. yawning, singing, dental treatment).
- Fear of relapse.
- During luxation there is pain and spasm in the masticatory musculature.

Treatment

Manual therapy

- The condyle can be influenced by a manual longitudinal movement towards caudal (distraction), enabling the therapist to slide the condyle slowly back into the fossa with relative muscular hypotonia.
- If intra- or periarticular contusions or sprains occur, these should be treated in the following therapy session.

Neuromuscular re-education exercises

Dynamic and static stabilization exercises in maximum aperture are indicated. Watch for a neutral head position and prevent upper cervical extension.

Home management

- Repeat the described exercises regularly.
- Avoid maximum mouth opening by supporting the chin with the hand whenever wide opening is required (e.g. yawning or biting into an apple).

SUMMARY

- Craniomandibular joint dysfunctions may be grouped generally into extra- and intra-articular syndromes. They are differentiated by their clinical patterns.
- The literature and clinical experience show that monostructural diagnoses are usually impossible due to the anatomy of the joint and individual anatomic variations as well as complex pathogenesis.
- Clinical patterns and treatment suggestions are presented for the most common dysfunctions and syndromes (see Table 9.3).

CRANIOMANDIBULAR MYOGENIC DYSFUNCTIONS AND PAIN

To properly understand myogenic dysfunctions of the masticatory system this section will give a brief introduction to the current concepts of pathobiological mechanisms and the potential influence of the muscles on the craniomandibular region. Naturally, not every possible dysfunction can be mentioned and only the most common muscular reactions known to therapists in their daily practice are discussed.

PATHOBIOLOGICAL INPUT AND OUTPUT MECHANISMS

The motor system as a part of the output mechanism

The neural system is constantly active and evaluates every input. Some output effects are easily recognized – for example, sympathetic reactions (sweating, blushing) and motor reactions (spasms, learned and subconscious movements) (Butler 2000).

In the craniomandibular and craniofacial regions these reactions may be differentiated:

- Functional activities: These include chewing, swallowing, sucking, speaking, mimic expressions and eye movements.
- Parafunctions: (Abnormal) oral habits such as teeth clenching, chewing on the inner cheeks/lips/nails and thumb sucking. In certain circumstances, but by no means always, these may lead to symptoms in this region. Parafunctions are also present in individuals without craniofacial problems (Lobbezoo et al 1996).
- Abnormally increased or decreased activities: Increased or decreased motor reactions due to nociception and/or tissue destruction (Flor & Turk 1996, Ohrbach & McCall 1996). Examples are atonia after facial nerve paresis, trismus of the masticatory muscles after tooth extraction and strabismus after orbital fracture. Reactions may be adaptive or maladaptive.

Adaptive or maladaptive reactions

Changes in motor activity may be adaptive protection mechanisms, for example immediately after plastic surgery that included dissection of the temporal muscle (Schwenzer & Ehrenfeld 2002). Maladaptive or inadequate

Table 9.3 Diagnosis and therapy for other joint dysfunctions

Dysfunction	Clinical features	Management guidelines
Retrodiscal inflammation	Retrodiscally swollen and painful on palpation End of range opening, laterotrusion and protrusion are painful Accessory movements anterior–posterior, posterior–anterior and longitudinal provoke signs and symptoms	Manual therapy: Accessory movements without pain Passive physiological movements in mid-range Passive physiological movements without pain Dental intervention: Teeth restoration Distraction brace NSAIDs Home activities: Active physiological movements Gentle cold application Un-learn abnormal habits which provoke symptoms
Capsulitis	Lateral palpation painful Painful arc on opening Opening slightly restricted Muscles sensitive on closure Accessory movements change the symptoms Imaging procedures show changes	Manual therapy: Accessory and physiological movements without pain Dental intervention: Relaxation brace, if necessary teeth restoration Home activities: See: Retrodiscal inflammation
Capsule stiffness	Physiological and accessory movements Mandibular position changes level of stiffness Muscle signs on the ipsilateral side Contralaterally possibly hypomobile or subluxated	Manual therapy: Accessory and physiological movements into the stiff direction Muscle treatment Dynamic coordination
Hypermobility or subluxation of the condyles	Opening range more than 50 mm Unilateral glide of the head of the mandible Variable force on isometric testing	Manual therapy: Active movements and exercises Dynamic coordination (load test) Stabilization in ± 25–30 mm opening Slight cervical extension if luxation occurs too easily

NSAIDs, non-steroidal anti-inflammatory drugs.

muscle activity, mainly due to increasing or prolonged nociceptive inputs, is also included (Ohrbach & McCall 1996). Pain that is associated with stressful life situations regularly shows an increased motor response in the painful region (Flor et al 1991, 1992, 1995).

Some parafunctions such as bruxism and teeth clenching may result in symptoms if the person is additionally confronted with stressful life or emotional situations (Hathaway 1995). Other psychological influences, such as fear of movements that have previously produced symptoms, may also influence maladaptive motor responses (Vlaeyen & Crombez 1999). A classic example is the patient with restricted aperture due to a clicking noise who will hesitate if asked to spontaneously open the mouth. Other activities such as singing, yawning or eating a hamburger will not be restricted if the patient does not associate them with the clicking.

Recognizing and classifying clinical patterns of craniofacial motor dysfunctions correctly is therefore a challenge that may greatly contribute to appropriate patient management.

Physiological changes of the masticatory muscles resulting from abnormal output mechanisms

Abnormal output of the masticatory muscles or any other muscle in the human body results in changes of muscle tension (Bumann & Lotzmann 2000). Such changes in muscle tension and their underlying mechanisms are described in the following from a craniomandibular point of view.

Physiologically, muscle tension depends on two influences:

- The viscoelastic properties of the soft tissue
- The grade of activity in the contractile muscle system (Simons & Mense 1998).

The viscoelastic structures generally increase tension and thereby stiffness as soon as external forces are applied to the muscle. This may be viewed as the 'independence of the contractile structures' (Kimura & Watson 1989). The viscoelastic stiffness may be evaluated by an external passive force and consists of two components:

- Elastic stiffness: Structures that contain little water, e.g. the capsule and ligaments.
- Viscoelastic stiffness: Fluids in the muscle including contents such as proteins.

Contractile muscle activity consists of:

- Electrogenetic stiffness: Tension in a normal but not completely relaxed muscle, due to an electric muscle contraction, commonly called basic muscle tone.
- (Electrogenetic) spasm: Involuntary, posture dependent (EMG) activity (Simons & Mense 1998).
- Contracture: Endogenic shortening of the contractile system, independent of electric (EMG) activities (DiMauro & Tsujino 1994, Layzer 1994) (Fig. 9.5).

On the basis of this model, muscle tension may be defined as elastic and/or viscoelastic stiffness without contractile activity. Clinical masticatory phenomena can be explained in a simplified manner using this model:

- If the masseter shows morphological changes, early onset of resistance and general stiffness are felt on stretching tests due to an increase of viscoelastic muscle tone (Sharmann 2002).
- Patients with parafunctions commonly show an increased masticatory muscle

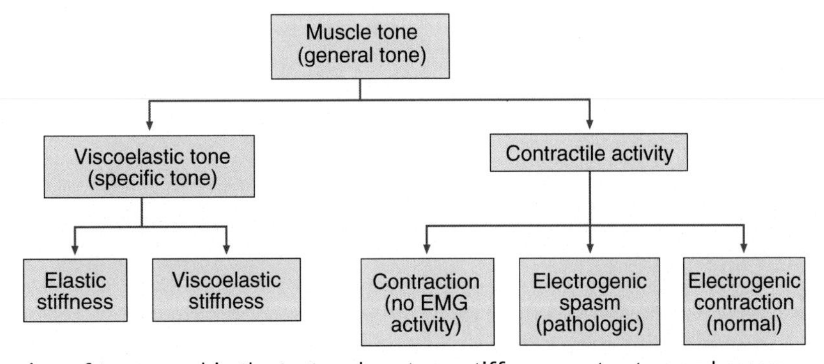

Fig. 9.5 Overview of terms used in the text such as tone, stiffness, contracture and spasm.

contraction, particularly of the masseter and temporal muscles, on testing of sudden passive craniomandibular movements that may even be visible to the therapist. The end of range feel is 'hard' or 'locked'. This might be due to an increase of contractile muscle activity.

- After treatment of trigger points the muscle strength will improve noticeably on reassessment of the static tests and fatigue will occur later on repetitive active testing. The restricted motion will also improve. It is known that muscle stiffness depends on the tension of the trigger point's taut band. The muscle stiffness is due to an endogenous muscle contracture and not to contraction (Simons & Mense 1998). A trigger point may also be responsible for decreased contractile muscle activity (Jaeger & Reeves 1986, Donaldson et al 1994).
- On physical examination after radiotherapy for cancer of the floor of the mouth a trismus occurs on mouth opening. The movement is severely restricted and passive testing shows a hard end-feel as well as trismus of both masseter muscles. It was shown in this case that the electrical activity (spasm) was pathologically increased, possibly due to an increase of viscoelastic stiffness caused by radiogenic fibrosis (Gonzalez et al 1992).

These natural occurrences are related to muscular dysfunction but they do not help us to understand the various mechanisms that are frequently based on complicated counteractions between peripheral and central nervous system mechanisms (Sterling et al 2001). The therapist has the task of finding out the underlying mechanisms based upon the behaviour of the symptoms. Excellent current reviews on this topic have been published by Sterling et al (2001) and Svensson (2001).

The influence of central mechanisms on the masticatory muscles

Several models have been developed over the last few decades in which the contribution of neuromusculoskeletal dysfunction and pain in the craniomandibular region is derived from central nervous system mechanisms.

INCREASED CONTRACTILE ACTIVITY

Prolonged nociceptive input by joint and muscles may result in an increased motor response (Gronroos & Pertovaara 1993, Andersen et al 2000). This is also true for the peripheral nervous system. It has been shown that during neurodynamic upper limb tests the excitation of the motor neurones in the arm flexors increases. Hu et al (1995) confirmed the same mechanism for the cranial peripheral nervous system. Nociceptive input of the cranial meningeal structures provoked by an irritating substance and an inflammation-stimulating chemical resulted in a significant increase of jaw and neck muscle EMG activity. This mechanism is believed to rely on the flexor withdrawal reflex that depends on central changes and sensitization of peripheral mechanisms (Cook et al 1986). In this case it is likely that inhibitory reflexes (e.g. the jaw reflex: mandibular elevators) are modulated and lead to a prolonged and increased motor response manifested as muscle spasm and morphological changes (Johansson & Sjolander 1993, Anderson et al 1998, Svensson et al 1998, Wang et al 1999). With time this may cause a vicious circle of muscle tension (combined with pain), changed masticatory muscle activity and more muscle tension (and pain) (Johansson & Sjolander 1993).

DECREASED CONTRACTILE ACTIVITY – A PAIN ADAPTATION MODEL

The statement that increased nociceptive input from craniomandibular muscles or joints will always result in increased muscular activity could not be confirmed in recent investigations. Stohler et al (1996) showed that increased masseter activity and pain significantly reduced the maximal voluntary contraction. Range of motion, coordination and endurance of the mandible on repetitive active movements was also reduced (Svensson et al 1995, 1998). This phenomenon is known as the pain adaptation model (interaction between muscular pain and coordination; Lund et al 1991).

Muscle inhibition may generally occur with or without pain (Shakespeare et al 1985). A number of studies on peripheral joints showed an inhibitory effect of articular pressure changes and aspiration techniques on the surrounding muscles without the presence of pain (Shakespeare et al 1985, Stokes & Cooper 1993). Clinical studies on animals and humans confirmed that craniofacial motor function may be either inhibited or increased by pain in the craniofacial muscles. Clinically this is observed as reduced velocity and fatigue on repetitive mandibular movements (Svensson 2001). Craniomandibular inflammation frequently reduces the static force and coordination of the muscles on the affected side without causing severe pain. Retrospectively, force and static and dynamic coordination improve significantly once nociceptive input has diminished.

The influence of stress on craniomandibular muscle dysfunction

Studies have shown that stress during daily life may influence the basic muscle tone of the masticatory system (Moss & Adams 1984, Rugh & Montgomery 1987, Kapel et al 1989). For example, patients with chronic craniomandibular dysfunction in stressful situations show a slightly increased EMG activity on the symptomatic side (Flor et al 1992). An increase of muscle tension is often associated with pain. This has led to the current discussion as to whether prolonged minimally increased muscle tension can really be responsible for prolonged pain. So far there is insufficient evidence (Svensson et al 1998).

The same applies for bruxism. Its aetiology remains unknown but it has been shown that external stress and the environment may influence the frequency of its occurrence (Yemm 1986, Lavigne et al 1995). Other studies have found that distress directly correlates with sleep disorders in chronic bruxism patients (Mulligan & Clark 1979, Harness & Peltier 1992). Another important aspect is the patient's personality, with emotions such as fear and depression leading to an increased prevalence of bruxism (Solberg et al 1972).

Trigger points also react differently under the influence of long-term stressors. During attacks of tension headache, for example, trigger points become electrically more active and more sensitive than in a relaxed situation (Travell & Simons 1992, McNulty et al 1994, Molina et al 1997).

In summary, it can be said that there are signs indicating that stress and the environment do indeed influence masticatory muscle tension, but an increase of tension does not necessarily explain pain.

Pain and motor output changes

As mentioned in the previous section, clinicians and scientists have long assumed that pain will always increase masticatory muscle activity and will therefore inevitably result in a vicious circle of pain and muscle tension.

It is known that:

- Nociceptors in muscles may provoke a brief pain reaction that may linger for a while if the contraction has been excessively strong (Arima et al 1999).
- Mechanically stimulated trigger points in the masseter muscle provoke a local electrical muscle activity that disappears with the stimulation (Simons & Hong 1995).
- Pain may be present in the masticatory muscles on minimally elevated EMG (Lund et al 1991, Sessle 1995, 2000).

Other experimental studies recorded increased EMG activity within chronic craniofacial pain regions only when the affected muscle works antagonistically (Lund et al 1991, Svensson et al 1995, 1997).

This phenomenon was interpreted as a functional reflex adaptation that prevents excessive force, excessive range of motion and excessive speed of mandibular movement to protect against further impairments and pain.

The underlying mechanism derives from inhibitory and excitatory changes in the premotor brain neurones and the central generators in the brainstem (Lund 1991, Svensson 2001). This might also potentially explain why the supra- and infrahyoid muscles are sensitive to palpation and why chronic craniomandibular patients sometimes complain of swallowing difficulties, pressure on the throat and the feeling as if something is stuck in the throat.

Painful masticatory muscles – which pain mechanisms are relevant?

While the aetiology and pathophysiology of deep craniofacial hyperalgesia remains unknown, muscular sources may be a possibility. The sensitivity of the masticatory muscles to pressure, for example, increases in patients with craniofacial muscular dysfunction. Pain may spread within the region (Wang et al 1999). It is hypothesized that prolonged afferent nociceptive input from the masticatory muscles is processed in the somatosensory cortex. Somatosensory reactions are manifested as referred pain and hyperalgesia of the superficial and deeper craniofacial structures (Vecchiet et al 1993, Okeson 1995).

A great number of craniofacial pain patients also complain of pain in other body parts (Türp et al 1997). Svensson (2001) suggested that somatosensory changes potentially spread to other brain regions. The intensity, duration and location of the sensitized peripheral nociceptors determine whether central mechanisms will also contribute to the problem.

- If local pressure causes a stabbing pain that is referred into the symptomatic area, this is called a trigger point (Travell & Simons 1992).
- In fibromyalgia patients (Henriksson 1999), deep facial (or other) hyperalgesia may be associated with a less effective endogenous pain inhibitory system (Maixner et al 1998) or a dysfunction of the excitatory and inhibitory cortical system (Møller et al 1984).

The therapist should therefore question if the pain is really due to direct local muscular changes connected to possible pain (primary hyperalgesia) or, if this is not the case, that false-positive results are caused by broad-based pain in the masticatory musculature arising from secondary hyperalgetic pain. This decision is important for subsequent treatment procedures. Some obvious differences that the therapist may observe are listed in Table 9.4. These are fairly extreme examples and clinically there is some overlap between peripheral nociceptive and central pain mechanisms (Wall 1995).

Table 9.4 Craniomandibular muscle pain: clinical differentiation based on pain mechanisms

Peripheral mechanism	Central mechanism
Pain quality: stabbing, superficial and/or deep	Pain quality: diffuse and deep, often associated with general autonomous symptoms such as sweating, abdominal sensitivity
Localization: local, potentially referred into the ipsilateral face	Localization: widely spread, referred to the rest of the body
Tissue changes on palpation, with/without pain	No tissue changes on palpation
Active tests restricted (restriction and pain), may fit to the hypothesized muscle	Active tests not always restricted Restrictions occur in all directions
On stretching, on/off mechanism of the symptoms	Pain independent of mandibular movement Stretching does not necessarily increase the symptoms
If muscle tone is increased, only a part of the muscle is affected, commonly near the palpated tissue; increases on stretching	Muscle tone increases in the whole muscle group Often triggered by slight mechanical impulse or verbal interaction

The influence of nervous system plasticity and craniofacial motor output

The plasticity of the brain has an influence on the output systems including the motor system (Woolf 1984). It is accepted that the somatotopic representation (homunculus) is not a specific region of the brain (Ramachandran & Blakesee 1998). The representation will change with every peripheral input (Buonomano & Merzenich 1998, Kaas 2000). If a patient is unable to use the lips and oral muscles for several weeks due to a mandibular fracture immobilized by external fixation, the representation of this area will shrink and it will be taken over by other regions (Ramachandran & Blakesee 1998). The opposite is also true: it was shown that musicians (e.g. guitarists and violinists) show a greater representation of the fingers than non-musicians (Recanzone 2000).

Changes in representation take place not only in the somatosensory cortex but also subcortically in the thalamus and the cerebellum (Dostrovsky 1999, Kaas 1999). This might explain why balance disorders occur more frequently in craniofacial or craniomandibular pain patients and it might also offer an explanation for the increase in muscle tension during emotional reactions such as anger or fear (Møller et al 1984, Kumai 1993, Stohler et al 1996).

Muscles also react to cognitive processes. The cortical activities associated with movement show the same patterns as the cortical reactions to imagined movements (Lotze et al 1999) – for example, an imagined mouth opening may enhance the real performance of mouth opening. Another phenomenon that influences the cognition of the motor system is pain due to 'stressful' situations.

Flor et al (1991, 1992, 1997) recorded EMG activity and observed that patients suffering from craniomandibular and other dysfunctions showed significantly increased activity and tension, both when experiencing pain and when confronted with personal stress situations. Compared with a healthy control group, the muscular reaction in the symptomatic craniomandibular region was significantly increased. The same EMG pattern emerged when the person was only thinking of a stressful situation. These results may potentially explain the following clinical patterns that are frequently observed in patients:

- Muscle tension generally depends on the environment and experienced stress as well as on cognitive processes related to the problem (Flor et al 1992).
- Coordination of mandibular movements is reduced. Isolated movements such as protrusion and laterotrusion cannot be performed if the problem is not arthrogenic or neurogenic, possibly due to decreased somatosensory presentation.
- Patients with muscular craniomandibular dysfunction show impaired balance functions that improve after treatment.

The following aspects should therefore be included in both the subjective and the objective examination:

- When do the symptoms occur (correlation with stressful events)? Does the patient actually have pain?
- Cognitive processes: What does the patient really think? Is the patient conscious of increased muscle tension and parafunctions?
- Do emotions influence the symptoms? Are such situations associated with abnormal motor outputs such as bruxism, bracing and other parafunctions?
- Physical examination of the motor system should not be restricted to the craniofacial region. Low-tech assessment of the head and neck as well as the balance system should be included.

Although not all patients are conscious of triggering situations, it is essential for future management to gain as much information as possible, especially if a reconditioning programme such as the tongue–teeth–breathing–swallowing (TTBS) exercise or the habitual reverse technique (HRT) is considered. A helpful tool is a pain diary that the patient is asked to keep over a number of weeks. The patient should record the pain intensity as well as the activity, time of day and quality of the symptoms (see also Chapter 3).

SUMMARY

- There is no direct link between pain and increased muscle tension.
- Even if masticatory muscle activity is increased over a prolonged period of time, this will not automatically provoke pain.
- Long-term muscle dysfunction influences the somatosensory qualities of the cortex. This will influence pain behaviour and pain referral into the facial region and may explain secondary hyperalgesia in other body parts.
- Long-term motor dysfunction and pain will change the somatosensory presentation in the large craniofacial area of the cortex (homunculus). This will influence local and general coordinative capacities.
- Motor output changes of the craniofacial region may be associated with pathophysiological, neuromuscular, biomechanical and cognitive–affective factors. These influences need to be evaluated for their contribution to the individual problem and integrated into the management approach.
- Craniofacial pain may influence the motor system although motor dysfunction does not automatically provoke pain. Pain management is therefore a priority before treating the motor dysfunction. This does not mean that restoration of motor function might not also influence the behaviour of the symptoms.

The next part of this chapter will present some dominantly motor clinical patterns and will discuss appropriate management guidelines. Included are:

- Bruxism/bruxomania
- Bracing
- Trismus
- Excessive mandibular protrusion
- Trigger points.

BRUXISM

Definition

Bruxism is viewed primarily as a parafunctional activity and is defined differently by various organizations. The American Academy of Orofacial Pain (AAOP) defines bruxism as 'a continued or rhythmic contraction of the masticatory muscles combined with tooth contact' (McNeill 1993, Hathaway 1995). This descriptive definition is considered inadequate by a number of clinicians since pathophysiological mechanisms are not mentioned and no specific criteria for pathological orofacial behaviour (e.g. during sleeping or swallowing) are stated.

The American Sleep Disorder Association (ASDA) defines bruxism as 'a movement disorder of the masticatory system characterized by bracing and grinding of the incisor and molar teeth'. This definition emphasizes nightly bracing and grinding. However, this may also occur during the day (Thorpy 1990, Lobbezoo & Naeije 1997). The behaviour is then called diurnal bruxism or bruxomania (Marbach et al 1990, Lobbezoo & Naeije 1997, Marie & Pietkiewicz 1997).

Of all patients assessed in sleep laboratories, 60% show rhythmic masticatory muscle activities without having craniomandibular symptoms (Lavigne et al 1995). Therefore the current consensus is that bruxism or bruxomania are normal behaviours that, under certain conditions, increase in a way that may be harmful to the masticatory system (Lobbezoo et al 1996).

Epidemiology

The prevalence of bruxism is estimated, according to studies on students (Glaros 1981, Gross et al 1988) and on the general population (Goulet et al 1993, Lavigne & Montplaisir 1994), as 6–20%. Of these, 10–20% are conscious of the bruxism (Carlsson & Magnusson 1999). The incidence decreases with age, especially beyond the age of 50 (Lavigne & Montplaisir 1995). There is a positive general correlation between parafunctional activities such as bruxism, lip/cheek/nail biting and craniofacial dysfunctions and pain (Magnusson et al 1991, Widmalm 1995). It is interesting to note that there is no direct correlation with bruxism, since only 17–20% of all bruxism patients suffer from dysfunctions and pain (Goulet et al 1993).

Aetiology

The literature on bruxism does not clarify its aetiology. Occlusal dysfunction and psychological stress seem to account for fewer of the symptoms than generally expected (Clark & Adler 1985, Okeson 1987, Goulet et al 1993). The only direct correlation is found with sleeping disorders. It appears that bruxism mainly occurs during phases of 'superficial sleep', predominantly when waking up or when sleep is disturbed (Lobbezoo et al 1996, Lavigne & Montplaisir 1995).

Stress is frequently mentioned as a dominant aetiological factor, but it is not clear whether it really is a cause of the symptoms. As described above, Flor et al (1991) found a correlation between masticatory muscle tension and individual experimental stressful situations. It is not recorded whether these parafunctions showed qualities of bruxomania.

In summary it should be said that there is no known direct cause for bruxism or bruxomania at this time. This implies that the therapist will need to assess a long list of potential contributing factors when examining and managing bruxism patients (Fig. 9.6). The following factors should be considered:

- Occlusal dysfunction: Further evaluation by the dentist is required (see also Chapter 10).
- Psychological and emotional influences: Is there a link to processing problems, extreme stress situations and/or fear, discontentment and frustration? By keeping a 24-hour diary that includes activities and symptoms, correlations between certain situations/environments/emotions and symptoms may be detected.
- Is the symptom related to a certain situation? Is the patient conscious of this? (This can be clarified in part from the symptoms diary.)
- Sleeping disorders: Poor superficial sleep and too little sleep may have an influence on the symptoms.

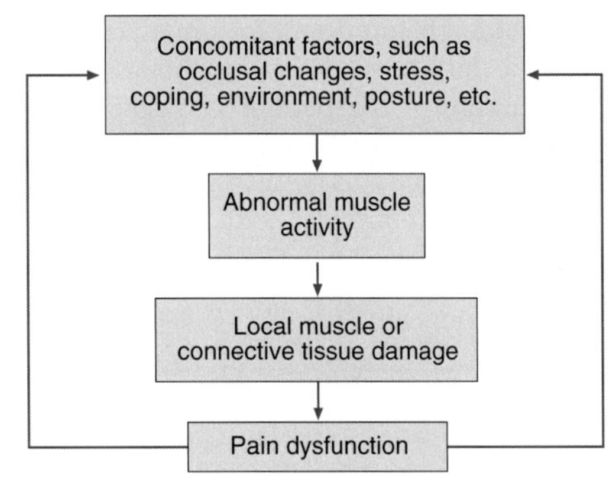

Fig. 9.6 Aetiology of bruxism. Potential contributing factors of parafunctions and bruxism in relation to morphological changes in the craniomandibular muscle system.

Correlation of bruxism and myofacial pain

It is not clear whether there is a causal correlation between bruxism and myofacial pain. First, there is no correlation of bruxism/bruxomania and increased masticatory muscle activity. Second, if masticatory muscle activity is increased due to parafunctions, there is still no proof that this dysfunction is relevant to the patient's symptoms. As discussed earlier, most authors doubt the hypothesis that increased muscle activity will automatically produce more pain (Lund et al 1991).

Lobbezoo et al (1996) hypothesized that the intensity and frequency of bruxism might have an influence on the development of symptoms. Genetic predisposition, intensity and frequency of parafunction determine whether dysfunctions and pain occur in the masticatory muscle system. This might also explain why craniomandibular dysfunction, bruxism and migraine type headaches frequently occur as a triad of symptoms (Molina et al 1997).

Therefore it is important for the therapist to gain an insight into the 24-hour behaviour of the symptoms if the patient is already conscious of intensity and frequency. The patient might also become more aware of symptom behaviour by preparing a logbook or table of the symptoms.

Characteristics of bruxism

The previous sections made it clear that bruxism is not a unidimensional phenomenon that is easy to identify. However, there is frequently a clinical pattern that points towards the parafunction. The following sections will present the most common clinical characteristics of bruxism.

Subjective examination

BEHAVIOUR

- The patient is conscious of teeth grinding and clenching during the day.
- The patient perceives the masticatory muscles as stiff and tensed.
- The patient and/or partner wake during the night because of tooth grinding.
- The masseter muscle feels 'tired' in the morning.
- Muscle tiredness during the day is associated with certain activities.
- The patient wakes with a locked jaw.
- The patient wakes with soreness of the masseter and temporal muscles.
- The patient experiences neck pain in the morning, usually combined with one or more of the above symptoms.
- The patient feels physically tired or has had disturbed sleep.
- The patient wakes with toothache or other unpleasant symptoms.

PREVIOUS HISTORY

- Recent history (previous 6 months) of grinding the teeth, usually observed by friends or partner.
- Recent history of craniomandibular dysfunction and/or dental treatment.

Physical examination

CLINICAL PATTERN OF GRINDING AND BRACING

Severe grinding and bracing might be observed by the therapist. This is important clinically since both parafunctions require slightly different management approaches. The following section describes the different features, some of which may naturally overlap.

GRINDING

- Tooth abrasions are visible.
- The parodontium shows changes.
- Unilateral hypertrophy of masseter or temporal muscles.
- Unilaterally increased tension of the sternocleidomastoid muscle.
- Trigger points often not obviously positive.
- Aperture restricted and frequently associated with laterotrusion towards the painful side.

BRACING/CLENCHING

- No sign of abrasions.
- Changes of the parodontium.
- Usually bilateral hypertrophy of the masseter and temporal muscles.
- Trigger points bilaterally positive.
- Aperture restricted without obvious asymmetry.

CHANGES OF THE PARODONTIUM

Abnormal pressure on the tooth surfaces and excessive mouth closure causes a deterioration in the condition of the parodontium. This is shown as changes in colour or bleeding and sometimes even by loosening of teeth (Freesmeyer 1993, Rosenbaum & Ayllon 1993, Okeson 1995).

TRIGGER POINTS

As mentioned previously, bruxism is not directly correlated with daytime motor reactions. Research in the author's clinic has shown that, of 28 bruxism patients, three showed a minimum of the expected reactions in the masseter and temporal muscles (right and left). The same reactions were found in 17 bracing patients ($n = 23$). The reactions were recorded by blinded examiners. Although this was an unofficial pilot study, it shows that bracing patients do have a greater number of bilateral trigger points than grinding patients.

FACTS ABOUT BRUXISM

- Bruxism is a parafunctional activity including grinding and bracing.
- A decade ago, occlusal dysfunction was considered the principal cause of the symptoms. Today we know that a number of factors may interfere with one another and result in such dysfunction.
- Nocturnal and diurnal bruxism are strictly differentiated.
- Nocturnal bruxism is considered to be a sleeping disorder, often associated with emotional situations. Diurnal bruxism is viewed as a subconscious muscle activity that depends on emotional and environmental factors. Bracing occurs mainly during the day (Lobbezoo et al 1996).

Treatment of bruxism

Since so little is known about the aetiology and so many factors may contribute to the problem, there is a great variety of therapy and management approaches.

The most common procedures are as follows.

OCCLUSAL TREATMENT

Various experimental studies have not confirmed a direct correlation between occlusal dysfunction and bruxism (Clark & Adler 1985). Influencing occlusion with night-time braces may have an effect on some patients but generally does not result in long-term improvement (Hathaway 1995, Okeson 1995). Evaluating the success of a treatment approach will always be empirical but is nevertheless obligatory.

PSYCHOLOGICAL INTERVENTION

Part of the aetiology is due to psychological stress. Modern stress management strategies and psychological interventions for general aggression among other disorders, including progressive muscle relaxation, hypnosis and biofeedback (Heller & Forgione 1975, Kardachi & Clarke 1977, Hathaway 1995), have shown short-term improvement of bruxism (Goulet et al 1993). Long term-effects have not been investigated.

BEHAVIOURAL TREATMENT

Behavioural intervention techniques have resulted in improvements of a number of maladaptive behaviours such as self-harming (e.g. banging the head), pathological hair pulling and weight loss (Hathaway 1995). The habitual reversal technique (HRT) described later in this chapter is one such technique that was analysed successfully by Ayer and Levin (1975) in a 1-year follow-up study. The results were positive but were not reproduced by later investigators.

PHYSIOTHERAPY

Modern pain management, treatment of tissue dysfunction, education and behavioural interventions such as the HRT and the TTBS exercise may help to reduce the symptoms and assist the patient to gain control over parafunctions (Kraus 1987). However, the effects can only be measured if the results are evaluated regularly.

HABITUAL REVERSE TECHNIQUE

The principles of the HRT were described by the psychologists Azin and Nunn (1973). The advantage of the technique is that the patient becomes more aware of the symptoms within the environment that triggers parafunctions. The patient is then taught to control the behaviour. Therefore, the technique is ideal for parafunctions such as bruxism. For the best results, the method should follow the steps outlined below:

- Response description: The type of dysfunction is described and awareness promoted; a mirror might be a helpful tool. Information about the consequences of the parafunctions such as asymmetrical atrophy and abrasion may also be of benefit.
- Early warning procedure: Early signs such as tension in the cheek muscles or pressure

in the throat need to be identified for the patient to react to and prevent bruxism activities.

- Situation awareness: In the author's opinion this is the most crucial step and depends entirely on the success of the previous steps. Together with the patient, triggering situations are identified. It sometimes takes days and weeks for the patient to identify these situations. If the previous steps were easy for the patient, this procedure will generally lead to good results. A logbook may assist the process.
- Habitual inconveniences: This is a description of the unpleasant emotions, thoughts and consequences experienced by the patient. If the patient cannot state these spontaneously the therapist should ask explicitly about these inconveniences. Imitation of the patient's behaviour may provoke them to talk about these experiences. It may also be helpful to analyse 24-hour behaviour according to the logbook or table of symptoms.
- Competing response: This describes the activity that the patient needs to perform whenever the onset of parafunctions is felt (early warning procedure). The activity or exercise has the following prerequisites:
  - Isometric activity that is opposed to the habitual movement
  - Performed until the signs of oncoming parafunctions wear off; generally this will take from a few seconds up to 1 minute
  - Should be easy to perform and fits in with normal daily activities.

The most common exercise is mouth opening against resistance. The exercise is important because the elevator muscles, especially in bruxism patients, clinically show increased tension.

If the observation during physical examination has shown a laterotrusional activity, laterotrusion to the opposite side is also an important exercise.

The most important feature of these exercises is that they are performed statically without associated movements of the neck or abnormal habitual postures.

Correction of posture is an important prerequisite for the success of the TTBS exercise. It is therefore recommended that some essential muscle balancing basics (as described in Chapter 12) are introduced.

INFLUENCING PARAFUNCTIONAL ACTIVITIES

The idea is to influence parafunctions by stimulating premotor neurones and the sensomotor cortex (Flor et al 1991). The following principles apply:

- Learning of static reverse actions.
- Once in a controlled position the patient needs to be made aware of the interference of the neck posture with the overall posture. Ask the patient to explain to you what they have understood.
- Guide the patient's attention towards their neck posture and ask them to perform the isolated static reverse activity. The patient should describe the difference perceived.
- If control is gained, the exercise is performed in the triggering situation (e.g. in a traffic jam while driving or working at the computer). How quickly this step is achieved depends on the patient's understanding of the situation, the complexity of the symptoms and the number of triggering situations.
- Symbolic rehearsal. After a number of treatment sessions, the exercise is reviewed regarding performance and effect. If a logbook was kept, the therapist and patient will evaluate the effects according to the logbook. Talking about progress promotes a collaborative relationship and problem analysis. Collaborative reasoning is a good basis for control of the symptoms (Jones et al 2001).

TTBS EXERCISE

Parafunctions may increase facial muscle activity. Tooth contact increases under maximum intercuspidation and oral activities such as swallowing, chewing and breathing may be affected. Muscle imbalance may influence the position and function of the tongue:

- The tongue may be protruded and presses against the upper incisor teeth.
- The tongue does not perform a rhythmic activity on breathing (inhaling: tongue against the palate; exhaling: contact eases).
- The tongue produces a constant pressure on the central palate.

These motor reactions of the tongue can be viewed as parafunctions. They will influence the contact time of the teeth and lead to increased tension of the masticatory and cervical muscles (Ekberg 1986).

Physiologically the contact time is around 3–10 minutes and occurs only on swallowing, around 1200 times a day. Increased maximum intercuspidation may result in increased masticatory muscle tension (Rocabado & Iglash 1991).

Characteristics of the TTBS

The TTBS exercise was initially described by Steven Kraus (1987). It is a neuromuscular reeducation training and includes the components 'tongue-up', 'teeth apart' and 'breathing and swallowing' to gain control over diurnal parafunctions. It is a method to make patients aware of parafunctions and aims to control muscle activity during resting times and mandibular movements (Kraus 1994).

This method, as well as the habitual reverse technique, can be easily integrated into the patient's daily routine.

The exercise should be performed in a maximum mandibular resting position where muscle activity is minimal (Rugh & Drago 1981). The position is determined by patient and therapist as the position that feels the most relaxed to the patient and provokes as little masticatory muscle tension as possible, as evaluated by the therapist. The evaluation may be assisted by reliable EMG tests, although this may be a little time consuming. The TTBS exercise will be described chronologically in the following section.

TTBS, tongue-up

The tongue consists of a number of intrinsic and extrinsic muscles, with the genioglossus muscle being the largest and the most important for the positioning of the tongue within the mouth. It is motor innervated by the hypoglossal nerve (Wilson-Pauwels et al 2002). The genioglossus muscle is responsible for elevation and protrusion of the tongue.

During the 'tongue-up' phase of the exercise, the middle of the tongue is in contact with the central palate while the tip of the tongue lies behind the middle upper incisor teeth without producing too much pressure. This position promotes nose breathing and relaxes the mandibular elevator muscles (Derkay & Schechter 1998).

The therapist controls the position in collaboration with the patient. Personal experience has shown that patients with craniofacial dysfunction and pain are often unable to control their tongue position. In this case, some therapeutic tongue coordination exercises are indicated before continuing the TTBS exercise. Another option is to use a wooden spatula to assess tongue position and to gently touch the palate. It is then easy to assess any increased tension of the region.

TTBS, teeth apart

As mentioned in the Introduction, tooth contact may generally increase masticatory muscle tension; no contact decreases masticatory activity (Kraus 1994). The initial contact occurs commonly at the canine and the molar teeth (Freesmeyer 1993).

The patient is asked whether the tongue is in dorsal contact with the teeth in a resting position. This may be confirmed with the aid of a spatula that is inserted, if possible, between the upper and lower molar teeth (Fig. 9.7). If there is clear contact without the patient being aware of it this is a good method to improve awareness.

TTBS, breathing

Nose breathing is an important component of human wellbeing. The nose filters dirt particles and warms the incoming air. Nose

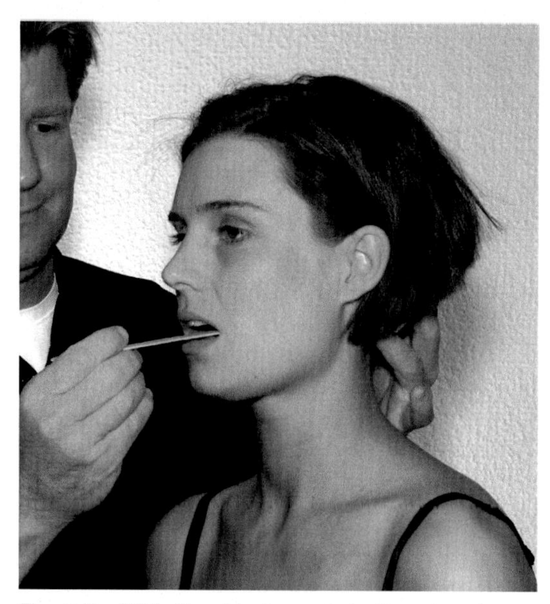

Fig. 9.7 With the aid of a spatula the relaxed position of the tongue on the floor of the mouth is examined. Furthermore, the spatula assesses whether there is contact between the maxillary and mandibular molar teeth.

breathing also promotes diaphragm activity and therefore has an influence on craniofacial morphology (Damste & Idema 1994; see also Chapter 22). Nose–diaphragm breathing stimulates the resting position of the tongue and inhibits the masticatory muscles (Lowe & Johnston 1979). In contrast, mouth breathing provokes upper cervical extension and facilitates accessory respiratory muscle activity such as sternocleidomastoid and scalenus activity (Sharp et al 1976). It also reduces diaphragm breathing (Sharp et al 1976, Ormeno et al 1999).

The therapist supports the patient by guiding them into a neutral thoracic position and by stimulating diaphragm breathing with a technique of the therapist's choice. While the patient inhales, the therapist makes sure that:

- The tongue pressure does not increase
- The diameter of the nose wings does not increase
- The neck is not moved into extension
- The masticatory muscle tension does not increase and the teeth do not touch.

TTBS, swallowing

Characteristics of swallowing

The purpose of swallowing is to transport food, fluids and mucus from the oral region towards the digestive system (oesophagus). The tongue is extremely active during this process and generally maximum intercuspidation occurs (Derkay & Schechter 1998). The adult swallows on average 1200 times a day (Gupta et al 1996). This takes about 6–10 minutes. In an abnormal situation (e.g. in neurology patients or children with an anterior bite) this causes hyperactivity of the genioglossus muscle (the most important muscle of the tongue) and of the infra- and suprahyoid muscles (Kelly et al 1973, Lawrence & Samson 1988). The activity of the genioglossus muscle also depends on the position of the neck (Milidonis et al 1993). For example, in extension it is more difficult to swallow since the teeth are closer together and the normal procedure of swallowing cannot be completed (Sauerland & Mitchell 1975, Bartolome et al 1999). It is therefore clinically important for the therapist to teach the patient a neutral neck position and to help the patient control the position throughout the exercise.

The physiological swallowing procedure, with the neck in mid-position between extension and flexion, occurs in the following order:

1. The tongue is positioned behind the upper incisor teeth.
2. Once food or fluids enter the mouth, the tongue moves to the floor of the mouth.
3. To initiate swallowing the tongue moves into the resting position but the pressure on the back of the incisor teeth increases.
4. Intermediate phase: The dorsal two-thirds of the tongue increase their tension while the activity of the tip of the tongue is reduced. The tongue performs a wave-like motion and the muscle activity occurs more dorsally. This takes place with or without contact with the (pre)molar teeth.
5. Final phase: The tongue moves back into the resting position and swallowing is completed (Derkay & Schechter 1998) (Fig. 9.8a).

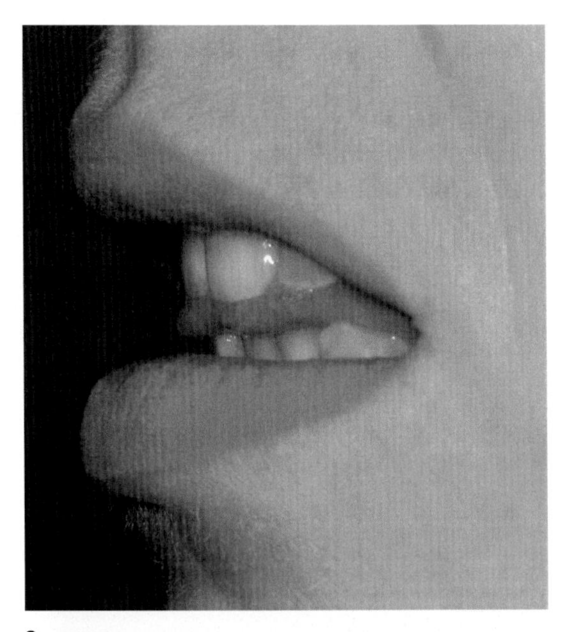

a

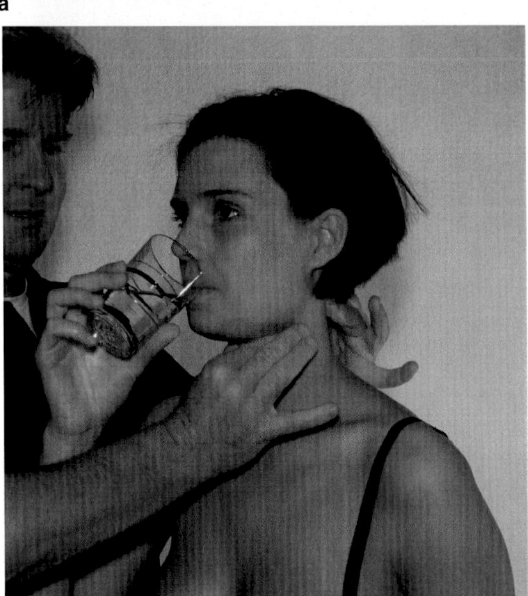

b

Fig. 9.8 Tongue–teeth–breathing–swallowing exercise: swallowing.

a Abnormal tongue position at the beginning and the end of swallowing (the tip of the tongue always has slight contact with the anterior palatinum).

b On normal swallowing an increase of the infra- and suprahyoid as well as the masseter and the temporal muscle tone is briefly visible and the upper cervical spine is in only minimal (or no) extension.

In summary, the following aspects are important for physiological swallowing:

- The head maintains a neutral position throughout the process.
- There is no dorsal tooth contact, thus decreasing the risk of excessive masticatory muscle activity.
- After the process is completed the tongue is returned to its position behind the incisors without pressure of the mid-tongue against the palate.

Performance of the exercise

The principles for this exercise were initially described by Baret and Hansson (1978) with the aim of understanding the position of the tongue during swallowing in children. If testing adults, the exercise needs to be slightly adapted.

A glass of water and optionally a mirror are required for this exercise. The therapist should be seated at the same height as the patient to optimally observe and correct muscle activity and compensatory movements.

The patient is asked to swallow a sip of water several times while the therapist observes the behaviour of the lips, the hyoid and the cervical spine. The therapist then places the thumb and index finger of one hand underneath the occiput onto the suboccipital muscles and the thumb and index finger of the other hand gently around the hyoid (Fig. 9.8b).

Indicators for dysfunctions are:

- Lips: During the tongue's resting phase the lips usually move slightly. They should then relax again. This is easily observed on the upper lip that slightly curls upwards. If the activity is increased this is observed consistently, and the upper lip curls slightly inwards.
- Hyoid: In the intermediate phase, swallowing can be palpated: the hyoid moves upwards and returns to the normal position. Indicators for dysfunctions are:
  - The hyoid is positioned higher than normal (above the C2–C3 line)
  - The range of motion is smaller than usual

  - On palpation the hyoid is positioned more cranially or tilted in the sagittal axis.

It is naturally difficult to assess normal hyoid range of motion. Generally the adult hyoid moves just beyond the palpating thumb and index finger and back in between the fingers on return. If the range of motion is restricted the hyoid stays in between the palpating fingers.

- Head: The head has to stay in mid-position without moving into upper cervical extension. The therapist palpates the suboccipital muscles with minimum pressure for an increase of tension.
- Awareness phase: If the patient has difficulty with components of the exercise, more time should be spent with this part of the movement. For example, if it is difficult for the patient to relax the lips, an additional lip exercise is indicated. The next treatment session should then repeat the complete TTBS exercise.

Examples for lip exercises include passive stretching of the upper lip, manually or with the aid of a small gauze plug. This may be combined with coordinative exercises and proprioceptive stimulation as known from mimic therapy in the treatment of facial nerve paresis, i.e. point the lips, spread the lips, suck lips into the mouth cavity, whistling, lip stretching by tongue movement, etc. (Fig. 9.9).

Clinical experience has shown that combining passive stretching alternately with coordination leads to surprisingly positive results.

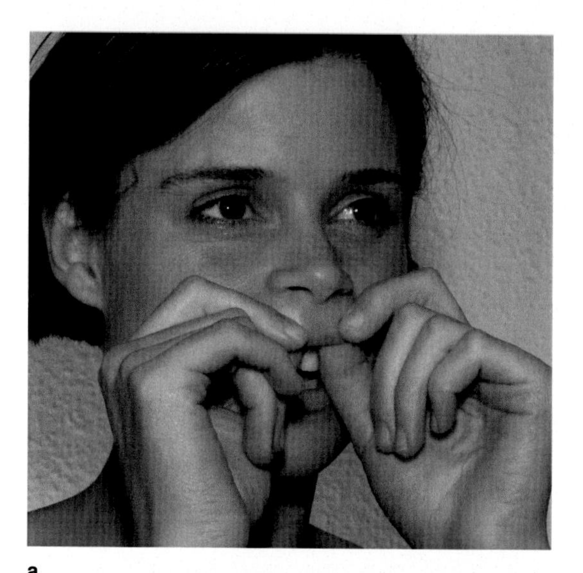

a

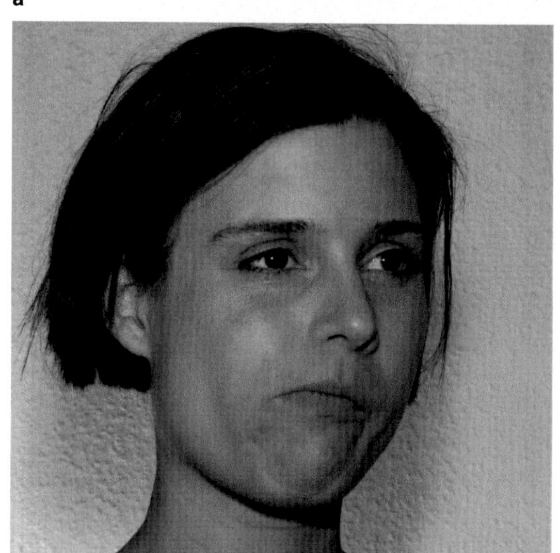

b

Fig. 9.9 Lip stretching.

a Passive lip stretching. Index fingers and thumbs hold the upper lip and move it towards ventral and caudal in an arc motion.

b If the tongue muscles work normally, a similar stretch may be performed by the tongue. The lips are kept together with the tip of the tongue attempting to stretch either the upper or the lower lip. The advantage of this version is the somatosensory input into the orofacial region.

BRACING

Bracing describes hyperactive masticatory muscles with tooth contact (Kraus 1988). Sensory craniomandibular input is answered directly by a motor response, shown as tension in the masticatory muscle system (agonists and antagonists). The therapist may assess bracing by applying a gentle resistance to the mandible and recording the reactive muscle tension. Often, this reaction is familiar to the patient, who immediately associates it with stressful life situations. This parafunctional activity is indicated by:

- Bilateral activity of the masticatory muscles on palpation
- Slightly restricted aperture, better on passive testing
- Passive movements and static testing trigger the motor reaction of the masticatory muscles. Resistance on passive testing is then clearly palpable in all directions and the muscle relief changes visibly.

Bracing and bruxism

As previously stated, the various parafunctions may occur simultaneously and influence each other (Lobbezoo & Naeije 1997). It is helpful to differentiate the clinical patterns of different parafunctions since the management may differ. This is also the case for bracing and bruxism. Some differences are listed in Table 9.5.

Proprioceptive stimulation to reduce bracing

The aim of this technique is to minimize the motor output reaction to normal sensory input by influencing the system with small oscillating painless passive or active movements. A prerequisite for the success of this technique is the ability of the patient to consciously relax the mandible.

BRACE–RELAX TECHNIQUE

The patient is informed about the aim of the exercise and is asked to concentrate on relaxation and 'letting go' of the jaw.

Starting position and method

The patient sits upright in a relaxed position on a chair. The patient is asked to gently press the tip of the tongue against the palate. The therapist holds the patient's head static with the right arm and puts the right hand on the patient's jaw without any pressure (Fig. 9.10).

In this position small amplitude oscillating movements are performed, initially only into laterotrusion to the right and left sides. The patient is asked to relax the jaw as much as possible. The following images may assist the patient in the relaxation of the mandible:

- The jaw is very heavy as if it weighs more than 10 kg.
- The bottom of the jaw is so big that it almost touches the floor.
- The jaw is so warm and heavy that it becomes impossible to shut the mouth.

Table 9.5 Differences between bruxism and bracing

Bruxism	Bracing
Cheeks feel stiff in the morning	No stiffness in the cheek area in the morning
Complaints improve during the day	Symptoms accumulate during the day
Tooth abrasions	No clear abrasions
Unilateral myogenic and arthrogenic dysfunctions	Mainly bilateral dysfunctions
Not aware of nocturnal parafunctions	No nocturnal parafunctions
Aware of diurnal bruxism and bracing	Aware of diurnal bracing
Awareness exercises for oral habits usually not successful	Awareness exercises successful
HRT and TTBS exercises indicated	Proprioceptive stimulating techniques and analysis of complaints indicated as well as 'wiggle' technique

HRT, habitual reverse technique; TTBS, tongue-teeth-breathing-swallowing.

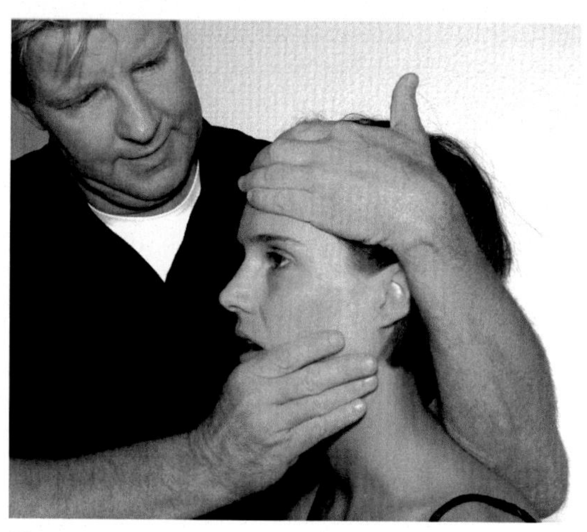

Fig. 9.10 The brace-relax technique. It is important that the patient has no tooth contact and that the tone of tongue musculature does not increase during the exercise.

Frequently the patient is initially able to relax but tension returns after a short period of time. The therapist should make the patient aware of this so that the patient can consciously influence the muscle tension. An increased awareness during the therapy sessions and during daily activities combined with exercises often results in very positive outcomes, with the duration and frequency of the muscle tension reducing significantly.

Variations

Once the basic exercise is mastered, variations may be introduced. For example:

- Speed: The speed of the oscillating movements may be increased to between four and eight times per second.
- Direction: Pro- and retrusion may be performed in the same position. If the result is satisfactory, combinations with laterotrusion may be introduced.
- Duration: The duration of a series may be extended. Even patients that progress well seem to experience some difficulties here. Sometimes the bracing recurs after 20–30 seconds of relaxation. In this case the exercise should be gradually extended.
- Position of the head: As the position of the head may influence masticatory motor output (see also Chapter 5), a range of positions may be used as a starting position. This increases or decreases the grade of difficulty for the individual patient. In most cases the therapist will aim for the position that usually triggers the symptoms.
- Mental exercise: Once the jaw is relaxed, the patient may be asked to think of a triggering situation. The therapist constantly assesses for motor reactions and gives feedback to the patient. The duration of this exercise depends on its result.
- *Combinations* of the above examples may increase the difficulty of the exercise even further.

Active exercises

WIGGLE TECHNIQUE

Once the feeling of a relaxed mandible has been experienced, the patient can now introduce exercises such as the wiggle technique into daily life activities.

Starting position and method

The patient sits in a relaxed position and moves the index fingers to within 2 mm of the skin surface of the mandible. The tongue is gently pressed against the palate such that no tooth contact occurs. The therapist then actively moves the mandible back and forward, until contact with the fingers is made. It is important that the patient does not experience any symptoms during the exercise and that no compensatory or associated movements occur.

RAPID OPENING AND CLOSING IN MID-POSITION

Starting position and method

The tongue is pressed gently against the palate so that the mouth cannot be opened more than 20–25 mm. Both index fingers are placed dorsally of the mandibular angle to add proprioceptive input. During the movement:

- Both index and middle fingers palpate the dorsal glide of the mandibular ramus

- No pain or neck activity should occur
- There should be no unpleasant feelings. The exercise is stopped at the earliest signs of tiredness.

If the movement is performed satisfactorily, some difficulty may be added by taking the fingers away.

TRISMUS

Trismus is defined as a significant restriction in aperture due to masticatory muscle spasm (Poulsen 1984, Magnusson et al 1994). This may severely impair (non-)verbal communication, eating, chewing and oral hygiene. The most common causes are trauma, inflammation or tumour (Goldstein et al 1999). Long-standing parafunctions with occlusal problems may also influence muscle and neurophysiological function in a manner that will ultimately result in trismus. Trismus is most commonly observed in the postoperative phase after tumour resection in the head or neck (Balm et al 1997). Postoperative muscle scarring may also cause trismus as may radiotherapy. Due to direct changes and long-term effects, fibrotic changes occur in the muscle (Engelmeier & King 1983, Dijkstra et al 1992b, 2001).

Characteristics of trismus

- Restricted aperture. There are no clear criteria for aperture restrictions due to trismus since various authors have defined them differently or not at all (Table 9.6) (Dijkstra et al 2001). If the mouth can only be opened 15 mm this will naturally impair mandibular function significantly and hinder the patient in daily life activities (Dijkstra et al 2001) (Fig. 9.11).
- Bilaterally increased muscle tone with or without pain on palpation. Generally the restricted motion is the main problem, not pain.
- Passive movement (e.g. aperture) shows a hard end of range resistance, possibly as a result of viscoelastic tissue stiffness and pathologically increased electrical muscle activity (spasm) (Gonzalez et al 1992).
- Compensation by craniocervical movements. The head is commonly held in slight extension. On mouth opening upper cervical extension increases. This may lead to further craniocervical dysfunction and pain.
- Associated symptoms such as lymphatic swelling after surgery and irritation of the mucosa can not only cause pain and a dry mouth but may also lead to a restricted range of motion (Steelman & Sokol 1986).

Treatment principles of trismus

The following principles apply:

- Mechanical influence: A gradually progressing external force (passive movement) not only influences (visco)elastic stiffness

Table 9.6 Trismus criteria

Authors	Criteria for trismus of less than:
Steelman & Sokol (1986), Nguyen et al (1988)	40 mm
Lund & Cohen (1993)	35 mm
Olmi et al (1990)	30 mm
Sakai et al (1988)	Severe trismus: <20 mm Moderate trismus: 20–30 mm
Thomas et al (1988)	Severe trismus: <15 mm Moderate trismus: ≤20 mm Slight trismus: ≤30 mm

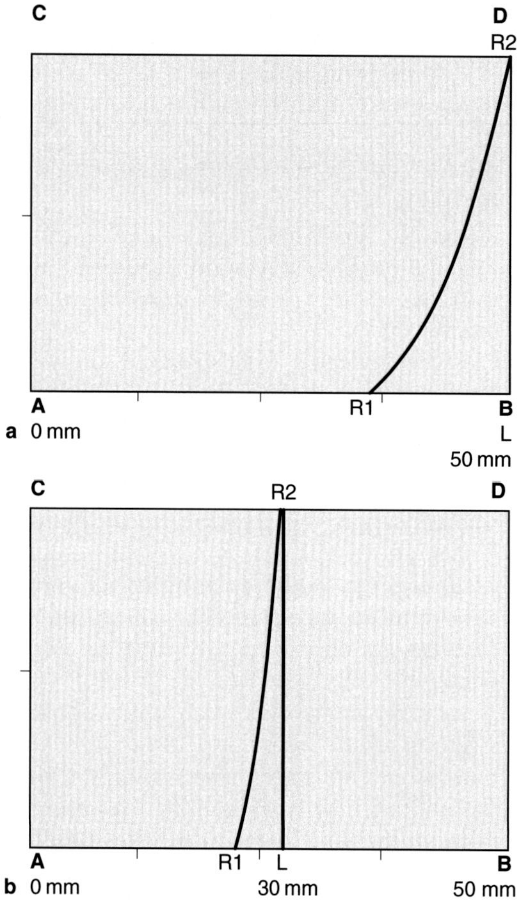

Fig. 9.11 Compared with the exponential increase of resistance on 'normal' passive mouth opening, the resistance in example **b** is severely limited and 'straight' as seen in the movement diagram. (AB, average range of motion; AC, quality and quantity of the movement; R1, first perceived onset of resistance; R2, maximum resistance; L, limit of the movement.)

a Exponential resistance, perceived by the therapist on passive mouth opening (control person without craniomandibular dysfunction).

b Severely limited mouth opening with a 'straight' line of resistance (patient with trismus).

but also changes mandibular elevator muscle spasm (Fonsesca 1969).

- Reciprocal inhibition: Facilitating the mandibular retractor muscles may inhibit the mouth closure muscles. Mouth closure is activated briefly to stimulate reactive opening. The expected effect of this phenomenon is usually not great since the elevator muscles are generally much stronger than the mandibular depressor muscles and because the central stimulation leading to trismus is more potent than the reflex inhibition (Lund & Cohen 1993).
- Changes in representation in the somatosensory cortex: As mentioned in the first section of this chapter, there are indications that the somatosensory representation is not limited to a certain area in the cortex but may change according to peripheral sensory stimulation (Ramachandran & Blakesee 1998). The orofacial sensory information is reduced and simplified once trismus occurs. Various stimulating inputs to the region may potentially inhibit the mandibular elevator muscles that are responsible for the trismus. For example:
    - Activities such as lip and tongue movements, preferably combined with affective facial expressions such as making an angry face, kissing, laughing, sticking the tongue out.
    - Tactile stimulation of this region, e.g. with a spatula or a wet towel.
    - Stimulating the taste buds by applying sweet, sour, bitter and salty ingredients (for further information, see Chapter 18).

Personal experience has shown that, after 6 months of orofacial stimulation, many trismus patients still show improvements (increased aperture) and that after even longer periods of time combinations with passive movements and active exercises will result in positive outcomes.

Treatment examples

PASSIVE MOBILIZATION

Any physiological and accessory movements as described in Chapter 8 may be applied. The choice of technique depends on the effect and the subjective response of the patient. Assessment of the type of movement and range of motion will also influence the decision. The method of Trott (1986) can easily be adapted to trismus patients.

MODIFIED SPATULA TECHNIQUE AFTER TROTT

Introduction

Trott described this method in her original publication for patients with severe, non-irritable but longstanding temporomandibular restrictions of mouth opening (Maitland 1991). Clinically this method is also useful for patients with disc reduction without displacement and for trismus patients.

The principle is that the elevator muscles are inhibited by contract–relax techniques including passive mobilization and maintained passive forces towards mouth opening. Short-term reduction of the contractile activity and increased external passive forces are meant to influence viscoelastic tension/stiffness (Simons & Mense 1998). The expected result is an increased aperture (Fig. 9.12).

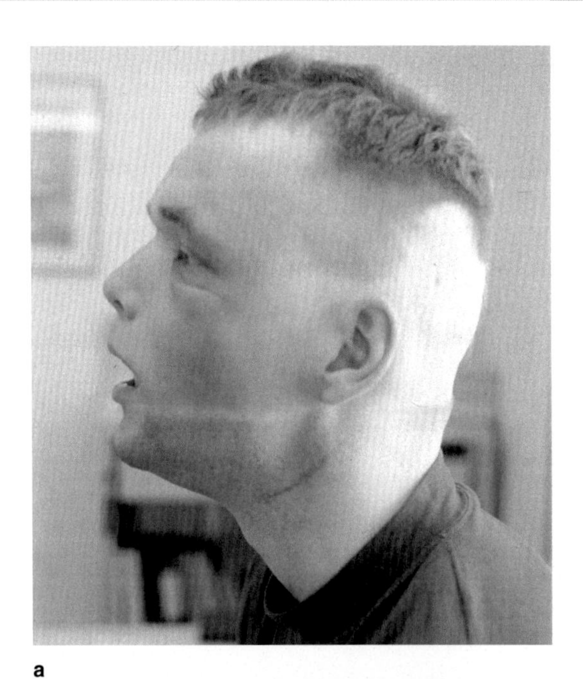

a

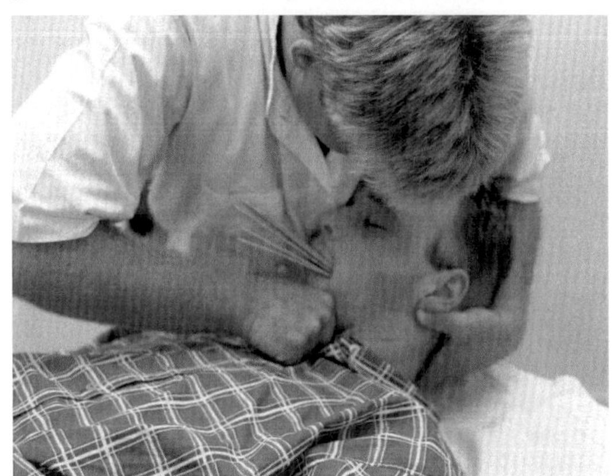

b

Fig. 9.12 A 23-year-old patient with trismus after radiotherapy following a carcinoma at the base of the skull.
a Maximum mouth opening of 1.7 cm, 4 weeks post-surgery.
b Spatula technique according to Trott; in this case the craniocervical flexion position marginally improves opening.

Starting position and method

The patient lies on a plinth with the head supported in a neutral position. The therapist explains the procedure step by step.

- The patient opens the mouth as far as possible. The therapist inserts as many spatulas as can be fitted between the upper and lower molar teeth. The patient will experience an increased tension in the masticatory muscles and the muscle relief becomes clearly visible.
- Extraoral accessory (glide) movements, which are generally restricted, are applied without pain (Fig. 9.13a).
- A contract–relax technique is applied. The patient is asked to gradually increase the closing force for a few seconds. For optimum recruitment of the motor units it is important to do this in a controlled manner (Sterling et al 2001).
- After asking the patient to open the mouth wider, the therapist attempts to insert another spatula between two others. The patient usually reports an increase of muscle tension that will decrease after a few seconds due to decreased activity in the contractile tissue (Fig. 9.13b).
- Afterwards, passive mobilization, contract–relax, mouth opening and inserting more spatulas is repeated (Trott 1986).

Please note:

- Since mouth opening occurs in the transverse axis of the head of the mandible,

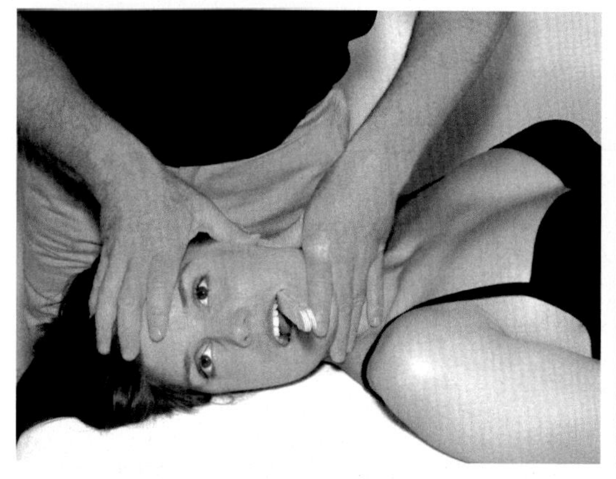
a

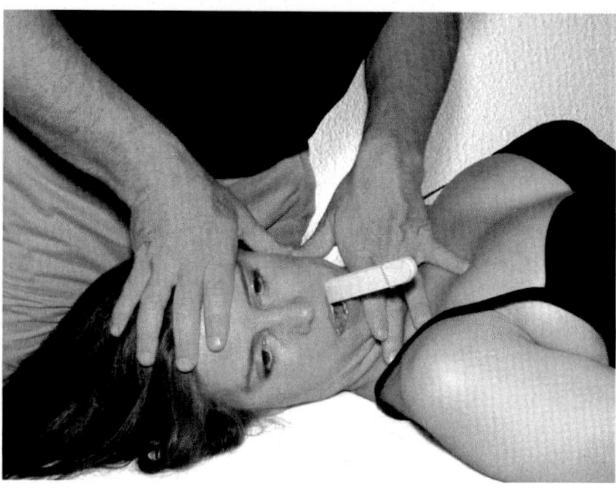
c

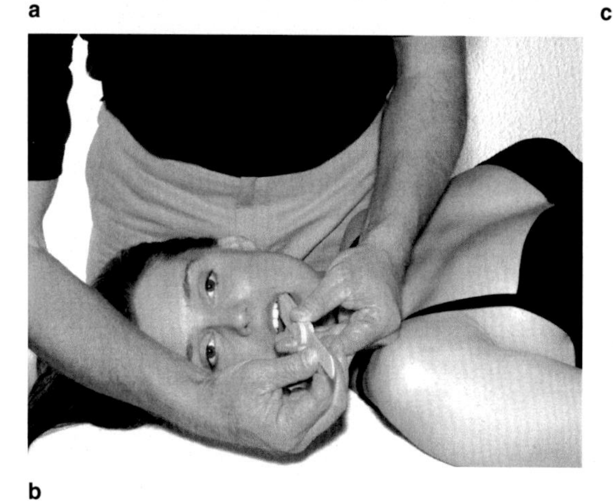
b

Fig. 9.13 Modified spatula technique according to Trott.
a Extraoral accessory movement in maximum active mouth opening supported by the spatula.
b After the hold–relax technique the patient attempts to carefully open the mouth further and the therapist tries to insert another spatula. The spatula *must* be inserted between the other spatulas and not adjacent to the teeth.
c The technique is performed in craniocervical flexion, often adding a few millimetres of opening.

the distance between the upper and lower molar teeth will always be smaller than between the incisors, where the range of motion is usually measured. Spatulas are around 2 mm wide, therefore only 3–7 spatulas are needed for an opening range of 20–30 mm.

- If more than 7–9 spatulas are used they frequently begin to slip and slide. It may be useful to tie them together with a rubber band.
- If more than 7–10 spatulas are inserted between the molar teeth, the mandible will shift slightly towards laterotrusion, usually away from the painful side. It may be useful to insert the same number of spatulas between the molar teeth of the opposite side. There will then be no laterotrusion and unnecessary tension and potential pain are reduced.
- Changes in neck position may influence the range of opening. In contrast to healthy subjects that generally show an increase of aperture on neck extension, the opposite may be the case in trismus patients. Accessory movements combined with the contract–relax technique performed in upper cervical flexion may improve the aperture by some millimetres if a plateau is reached in neutral neck position. No clinical or experimental data have been published regarding this phenomenon (Fig. 9.13c).

Recommended activities of daily living

EFFECT OF THE RECOMMENDED ACTIVITIES

Self-regulating activities performed at home, during sport or at work significantly influence craniofacial muscular pain in both the short and long term (Carlsson 2001). Performance of prescribed activities by trismus patients, either with or without appliances has also shown to result in positive outcomes (Buchbinder et al 1993). Clinical experience confirms that such activities lead to the best results when introduced at an early stage (Dijkstra et al 1992b). The therapist needs to control the quality of the performed exercises constantly and to reassess the effect in collaboration with the patient.

WHICH ACTIVITIES?

Any activity that improves the aperture may potentially be used. All three principles (mechanical influence, reflex inhibition and facilitation of the sensomotor cortex) apply. They may be performed with or without appliances.

WITH APPLIANCES

Cork and spatula exercise

With a cork cut to the appropriate size, exercises may be performed in end of range aperture. For example, performing rolling movements with the cork may have a positive influence on maximum aperture. Changes of neck position in flexion and extension may also lead to positive results. These movements may also be performed with a spatula instead of a cork as described for Trott's method.

WITHOUT APPLIANCES

All physiological movements that improve aperture are indicated.

Usually the best results are shown by exercises that include long-term stretching of the masticatory muscles in an end of range position. For example, the thumb depression technique is ideal. The advantage is that this exercise may be performed anywhere without appliances and with or without neck positioning or movements.

Thumb–chin–mouth opening technique

Starting position and method

The patient sits upright in front of a table with the elbows supported in pronation on the table. The thumbs palpate the ventral part of the lateral mandible while the middle or index fingers palpate the mandibular head. The patient actively attempts to open the mouth and symmetrically pronates the lower arms. The thumbs will automatically increase the aperture. The exercise may be performed in the following variations:

- Dynamic: The thumbs apply pressure to the chin throughout the movement.
- Static: Sustained pressure is applied at the end of range; however, the duration may vary.
- In various positions of neck flexion and extension: In trismus patients upper cervical flexion may increase the aperture by some millimetres in contrast to healthy subjects, whereas extension generally improves mouth opening (Higbie et al 1999). This may also apply to the static and dynamic variations of the exercise.
- During head movement in flexion and extension: This will integrate the interference of the proprioceptive input of the craniocervical and craniomandibular regions (Hu 2001). This may also be performed statically or dynamically.

The wiggle technique or sudden opening and closing of the mouth in mid-position as described for bracing patients may be added once the patient achieves an aperture of 20 mm or more.

EXCESSIVE MANDIBULAR PROTRUSION

If there is muscle imbalance in the craniomandibular region, increased activity of the lateral pterygoid muscle is regularly observed (Murray et al 2001, Phanachet et al 2001).

This phenomenon explains why craniomandibular pain patients frequently show excessive mandibular protrusion without any obvious joint signs.

> Definition
>
> Hansson et al (1992) defines protrusion as a regular but abnormal anterior shift of the mandible that is associated with the intercuspidal position, with or without contact of the upper and lower teeth. This definition, which depends on the occlusion and the mandibular

position, also includes other clinical features relevant for assessment and the treatment.

In summary, it can be said that excessive protrusion is mainly a muscular dysfunction that influences other structures such as the craniocervical and the thoracic region as well as the respiratory tract.

The most obvious clinical pattern is depicted in Figure 9.14.

Inspection

EXTRAORAL

- Nose–chin line: significant ventralization of the mandible.
- Increased extension in the craniocervical junction.
- Correction of the cervical extension does not change the symptoms, correction of the mandibular position does.
- Increased tension of the upper lip.

INTRAORAL

- Insufficient occlusal resting position; commonly not enough mesiobuccal contact.
- Tongue impressions visible due to increased tongue protrusion.
- Mouth breathing dominant over nasal breathing.

Physical examination

- Bilaterally increased tension and sensitivity to palpation of the masticatory muscles and of the sternocleidomastoid muscle.
- Retrodiscal space widened bilaterally.
- Active protrusion enhances the pattern described on inspection.
- Active retrusion difficult, commonly coordination problems.
- Passive retrusion and anterior–posterior movement is pain-free with a normal range of motion.
- On static testing patients tend to compensate protrusion by moving into lateral deviation. The force applied is often overly proportional.
- In many cases upper cervical extension or ventral shift is observed.

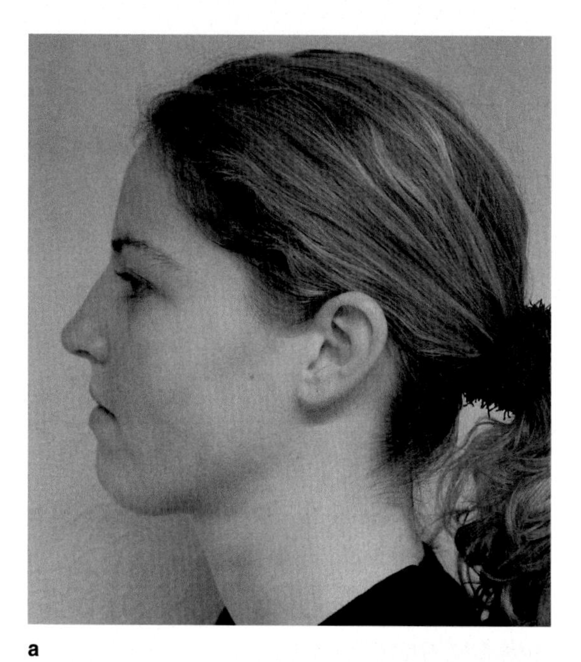

a

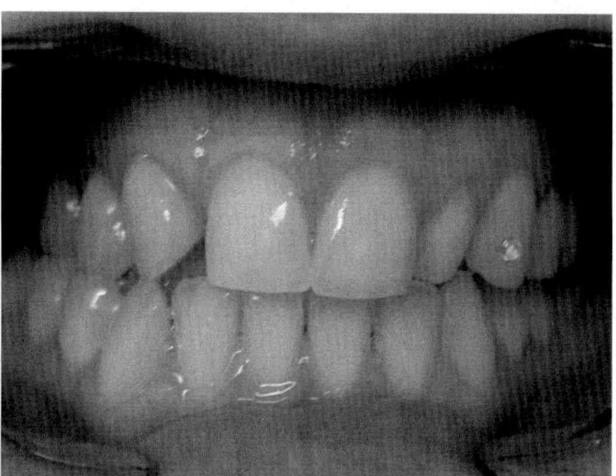

b

Fig. 9.14 A 29-year-old patient with excessive mandibular protrusion.
a Note the wing of the nose–chin line (retrognathion) and the excessive craniocervical extension.
b Occlusion of the same patient. Note the crossbite and the tongue position on the right.

Craniomandibular region

Coordination is in many cases significantly reduced. New orofacial–mandibular input may positively influence the muscle balance and the presentation on the somatosensory cortex. For example:

- Physiological position of the tongue combined with symmetrically isolated mouth opening.
- Static coordinative exercises in a position that is habitually associated with protrusion.
- Isolated protrusion and retrusion exercises.
- These movements are generally difficult for the patient to perform and may require proprioceptive assistance. The mandibular initiation manoeuvre and the touch-and-bite-exercise may be helpful to re-learn protrusion and retrusion movements.

Mandibular initiation manoeuvre

STARTING POSITION AND METHOD

The patient sits upright on a chair, if necessary with thoracic or lumbar support. The patient is asked to perform mandibular protrusion and retrusion and is corrected by the therapist.

- Compensatory thoracic or cervical movements are corrected.
- Protrusion and retrusion are initiated without additional lateral shift.
- The emphasis is put on the retrusion component of the exercise once the opposite direction can be performed in an isolated manner.
- Home exercise: The index finger gently presses against the chin while the patient actively performs retrusion guided by the pressure of the finger.

Touch-and-bite exercise

The principles of this exercise, performed to facilitate mechanoreceptors and thereby regain afferent input of mandibular positions and movements, were described by Kraus (1994). It is particularly useful for patients with extra-articular stiffness as a result of, for example, capsulitis. Coordinative deficiencies and a lack of proprioceptive feedback may be the cause of a restricted range of motion. The movements performed during this exercise are protrusion and laterotrusion.

The exercise is easy to learn, even for patients with excessive muscular mandibular protrusion since it focuses on an isolated movement and is performed actively. Retrusion is equally easy, because no articular restrictions apply. Another useful feature of this exercise is its association with biting, an essential daily life activity. This enables the patient to induce the activity using other cerebral neurocircuits. It may be that the craniomandibular symptoms have caused a strong motor reaction that is now memorized (Flor et al 1991). The result may be muscle imbalance with associated excessive protrusion. Automatic basic functions such as biting, licking and sucking may overcome these neurocircuits (Dougherty & Lenz 1994, Galea & Darian-Smith 1995). The major advantage of this exercise is that it is easy to integrate into the patient's daily routine.

STARTING POSITION AND METHOD

The patient sits upright. Thoracic and cervical positions are corrected if necessary.

Protrusion and retrusion

To prepare the patient for the active exercise the movements may initially be performed passively.

The therapist then places an index finger vertically onto the upper incisors and asks the patient to move the mandible forwards and to bite onto the finger. The therapist should ensure that the movement is not performed by changing neck position. The pressure of the incisors against the index finger should not increase. If the exercise is performed correctly, retrusion may be added. The patient is now asked to move the lower incisors away from the therapist's index finger. If this movement is associated with accompanying movements, the therapist may use the other index finger to rest on the jaw and guide the movement (Fig. 9.15a).

Laterotrusion

The therapist places an index finger vertically on the skin above the upper canines on the side which the patient needs to move the mandible towards. The patient is then asked to move the chin sideways to bite into the therapist's finger.

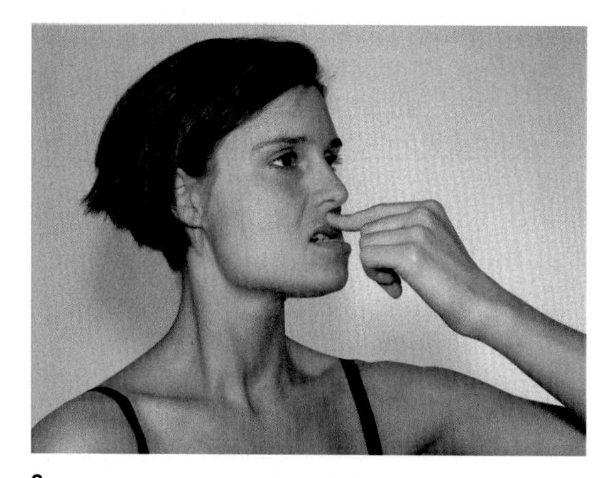

a

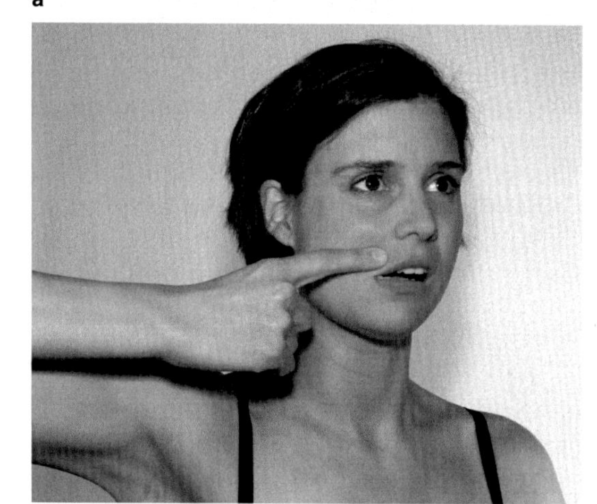

b

Fig. 9.15 Touch-and-bite-exercise.
a Initiated into protrusion.
b Initiated into laterotrusion. If possible, an isolated movement is facilitated without associated movements of the craniocervical and facial muscles.

This exercise cannot be carried out in the corrected direction but it does challenge the pterygoid muscle (Yang et al 2001) and provides proprioceptive information that in time leads to an improvement of protrusion and retrusion.

MYOFACIAL TRIGGER POINTS AND TENDER POINTS

Introduction

When working with craniofacial pain patients, therapists often note areas and spots that are sensitive to palpation. In a number of cases these are associated with autonomic reactions such as sweating or watering eyes.

Often symptoms such as toothache or eye watering in patients with no clear diagnosis (e.g. patients with frontal sinus complaints – although this is ultimately contradictory as the reader is immediately led to consider sinusitis, i.e. a 'clear' diagnosis) can be clearly reproduced by local pressure on a masticatory or craniomandibular muscle.

The therapist commonly notes that these spots feel hard and mobile. These might potentially be tender points or trigger points. This section provides an overview of current knowledge on trigger points:

- Definition
- Pathophysiological mechanisms
- Prevalence and aetiology
- Clinical features
- Treatment approaches
- Characteristics of most common craniomandibular and craniocervical trigger points.

Definitions

As is commonly accepted, it is often difficult to define medical and paramedical pathologies and dysfunctions. Various diagnostic terms are often used for one phenomenon (Mongini 1999). This is also true for the craniofacial and craniomandibular muscle system. The most common definitions as used in the current scientific literature are as follows:

Myofacial pain–dysfunction syndrome

Myofacial pain–dysfunction syndrome (or myofacial pain syndrome) is a synonym for craniomandibular dysfunctions. The clinical pattern includes periauricular pain and commonly unilateral muscular sensitivity combined with a qualitatively restricted range of motion. Additionally, unilateral clicking may occur, indicating disc dysfunction (Simons et al 1999).

Myofacial pain syndrome (MPS)

MPS is defined as muscular pain and/or dysfunctions that derive from referred pain and sympathetic reactions due to trigger points and myofacial structures (Friction et al 1986, Travell & Simons 1992). Frequently used synonyms are arthropathy, myofibrosis, fasciitis, myogelosis, myalgia and fibromyalgia.

Myofacial trigger points (TPs)

A local area of sensitive tissue, associated with a taut band of muscles, tendons and ligaments that refers pain into the symptomatic region potentially associated with autonomic reactions (Travell 1976, Friction 1985, Mense 1999). Specific criteria for trigger points were defined by Travell and Simons (1992, 1999) as follows:

- A taut band that includes a tender spot which is very sensitive to pressure.
- Sustained pressure on the spot produces a classic clinical pattern such as tingling, numbness or pain.
- Transverse movement on the band leads to local muscle tension (Travell & Simons 1983, Simons 1990, McNulty et al 1994).

Tender points

Tender points are defined as local tight or sensitive spots that do not necessarily occur in a taut band and do not produce referred pain. They should therefore be differentiated from trigger points (Mongini 1999). The term myogelosis is often used synonymously (Simons 1997).

Pathophysiological mechanisms of trigger points

The pathophysiological mechanisms that lead to the development of trigger points are not yet fully understood. At present there are only hypotheses (Mense 1997) as outlined in the following examples.

SECONDARY TO ZYGAPOPHYSEAL JOINT DYSFUNCTION

Some authors are convinced that trigger points are caused by increased nociception due to cervical zygapophyseal joint dysfunction (Aprill et al 1990, Dwyer et al 1990, Reitinger et al 1996). A study by Aprill and Bogduk (1992) concluded that 80% of post-traumatic pain (especially after whiplash-associated injuries) that can be reproduced by pressure on trigger points correlates with zygapophyseal joint impairments.

Trigger points are associated with muscular overuse in acute as well as in chronic situations (Simons 1988). Muscular overuse is very common in the craniocervical and craniomandibular regions. The neck muscles fulfil an important postural task by keeping the head balanced on the rest of the spine. The masticatory muscles show higher EMG activity in the case of parafunctions such as bruxism and grinding (Mongini 1999). This overuse is mainly due to eccentric contractions and may result in chronic muscle fatigue (Larsson et al 1990, Stauber et al 1990, Hendriksson et al 1993, Reitinger et al 1996). With time, muscle adhesions, tender points and trigger points develop (Christensen & Hutchings 1992).

THE ENDPLATE HYPOTHESIS

The hypothesis by Simons (1990, Mense 1997) of a disturbed endplate function is currently the most widely accepted (Fig. 9.16).

The hypothesis is based on the following assumptions:

- A lesion of the muscle tissue due to overuse or tension.
- Endplate dysfunction with excessive output of acetylcholine (ACh) into the synaptic junction of the neuromuscular endplate.
- Excessive ACh release causes a prolonged depolarization and the action potentials at the endplate are registered as spontaneous electrical activities. Calcium is released and results in sustained contraction of the actin and myosin filaments below the endplate.
- Other muscle fibre components are stretched by the prolonged contraction. These form a 'taut band'.
- The contracted muscle fibres compromise the surrounding capillary vessels resulting in local ischaemia.
- Increased energy consumption results in local hypoxia.

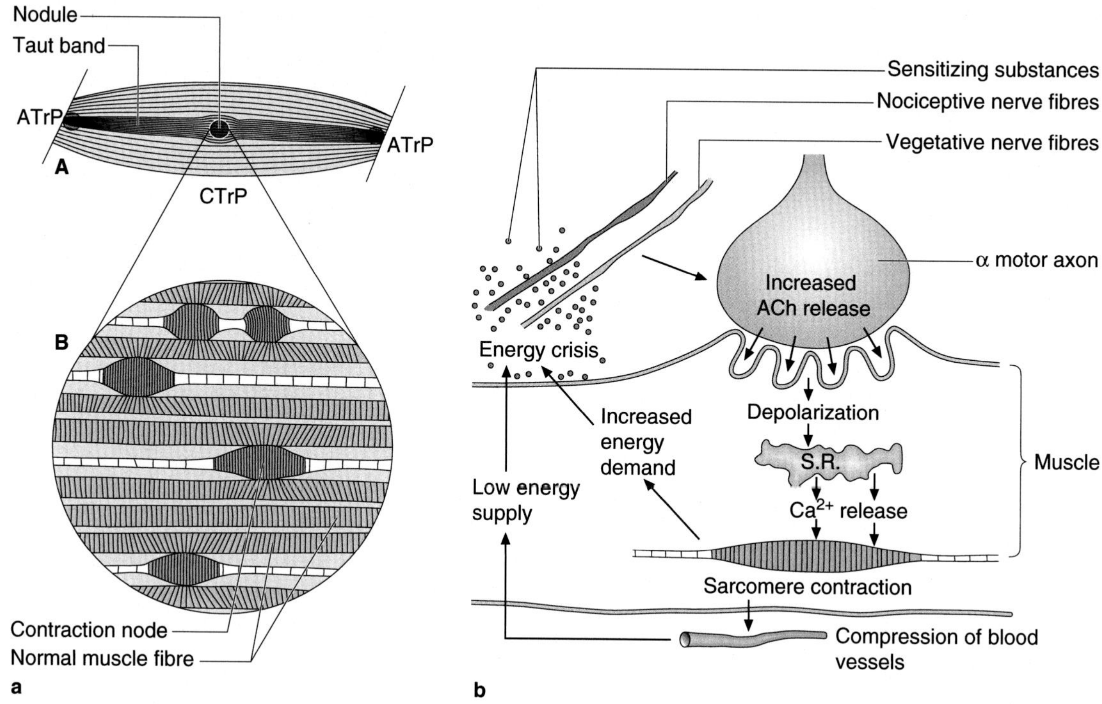

Fig. 9.16 Trigger point mechanisms.

a Structure of a trigger point. Commonly the trigger point is found in the end plate zone of a muscle (CTrP), roughly in the middle of a muscle fibre. Trigger points generally consist of a number of 'contraction knots' that may be palpated by the therapist. ATrP, insertion trigger point; CTrP, central trigger point.

b End plate hypothesis for the development of a trigger point. The process starts with a mechanical or chemical lesion of the presynaptic component of the end plate. This is characterized by concentrated changes in the local microstructure of the tissue (see text) (from Mense 1999).

- The energy crisis is due to ischaemia and increased energy consumption (activation of the actin–myosin system).
- Ischaemia is followed by a release of neurotransmitters such as bradykinin, prostaglandins, substance P, and CGRP (calcium gene-related peptide) and sensitizes the neurones in the dorsal horn (primary hyperalgesia).

CENTRAL SENSITIZATION

Devor (1991) defines trigger points as the result of impairments of the nerve endings, with the dorsal horn becoming more and more sensitized due to the transition from mechanical to chemical stimulation. The continuous barrage is due to a lack of normal regulation. This will increase cross-firing into the peripheral regions and cross-excitation in the central nervous system leading to referred pain (Devor 1991). Quinter and Cohen (1994) compared the clinical pattern of peripheral neuralgias with the clinical pattern of trigger points. They concluded that trigger points, based on their location and quality, should not be viewed as primary hyperalgesia but rather as a result of secondary hyperalgesia.

In summary, it can be said that the myofacial pain syndrome cannot always be explained by the model introduced by Travell and Simons. The topic of chronic pain is a modern clinical challenge because trigger point treatment in the craniomandibular region reduces symptoms, and processing and output mechanisms are clearly heavily involved.

Prevalence and aetiology of trigger points

Trigger points are equally common in males and in females. They can also be found in children (Bates & Grunwaldt 1958). Compared to other pathologies it is characteristic for fibromyalgia patients to show comparatively more of these sensitive muscular areas. The multiplication factor lies around 2.7–2.3 (Müller-Busch 1994). In a clinical study on 164 patients with dysfunction and pain in the head–neck region, Friction (1985) showed that a surprisingly high number of trigger points were present.

Box 9.2 provides an overview of the number and behaviour of trigger points.

The literature differentiates between three basic concepts regarding explanations for the development of trigger points:

- Muscle imbalance.
- Repetitive movements as they occur in parafunctions or abnormal behaviours may lead to pathological changes in the masticatory muscles and to the development of trigger points (Simons 1975, Weinberger 1977, Friction et al 1986, Amano et al 1988, Simons et al 1999). Muscle weakness and muscle inhibition are also viewed as predisposing factors for insufficient blood supply and the development of trigger points. This weakness may be due to a protracted mandible, disc displacements or dominantly unilateral chewing (Loiselle 1969, Kendall et al 1970, Molofsky et al 1975, Mongini 1999).
- Processing problems in the central nervous system due to prolonged stress, psychological problems or sleep disorders may also contribute to the development of trigger points (Friction et al 1986, Okeson 1995). Bendtsen et al (1996) found an increased mechanosensitivity of trigger points in the head–neck–facial region when patients were confronted with stress. They suggest that the mechanosensitivity results from the sensitization of the nervous system, especially the dorsal horn.

Box 9.2 Prevalence of trigger points in patients suffering from headaches, neck or facial pain for more than 6 months (n = 164)

Craniocervical region

- Trapezius: Insertion 67.7%, muscle 80.5%
- Splenius capitis: 85.9%

Craniomandibular region

- Posterior digastricus: 67.7%
- Lateral pterygoid: 92.7%
- Medial pterygoid: 81.7%
- Masseter, superficial: 76.8%
- Masseter, deep: 76.2%
- Temporalis, posterior: 20.0%
- Temporalis, deep: 68.8%
- Temporalis, anterior: 78.8%
- Temporalis, intermediate: 41.5%

From Friction (1985).

Clinical features of trigger points

Some general characteristics will be explained first, then special features of the craniomandibular region will be highlighted.

SUBJECTIVE EXAMINATION (GENERAL)

- The patient complains of localized stabbing pain or of an area of diffuse dull pain. Rest or activity may ease the symptoms.
- Perceived stiffness or limitation of the joint associated with a muscle that contains a symptomatic trigger point.

PHYSICAL EXAMINATION

To gain information on the site and features of a trigger point, the following methods apply:

- Palpation,
- Passive stretching
- Tests for muscular strength, endurance and coordination.

Palpation

Trigger points are found within a taut band of muscle fibres. In severe cases, a hard 'string' may be palpated in otherwise soft muscle tissue. Trigger points can be identified by their location and by the referred pain that occurs on pressure. Local twitching may sometimes be observed (Mense 1999).

Localization

Trigger points are localized in the neuromuscular endplate zone of a muscle (Simons 1975). The position of this zone varies with the shape of the muscle. The most common sites are in the muscle belly and in the mid-point between insertion and origin of the muscle. They are differentiated from tender points by their localization since tender points are typically found at the muscle–tendon junction (Mense 1999).

Referred muscle pain

Trigger points typically produce pain that is referred into peripheral areas. The source of the symptoms is the trigger point itself and not as sometimes assumed the muscle tissue.

The phenomenon of referred pain is due to central processing mechanisms of nociceptive input that lead to pain projection into other deep somatic structures (muscle, fascia, tendons, joints). The painful areas do not correlate with segmental innervation zones or innervation zones of peripheral nerves (Gröbli & Dommerholt 1997, Mense 1997).

Local muscle twitching

Local twitch responses (LTR) are visible reactions that occur on palpation of the taut band ('snapping palpation'). The cause is unknown but a possible explanation may be a spinal reflex arc (Hong 1994).

LTRs are often observed on dry needling of a trigger point. Results of this technique vary in the available literature (Cooper et al 1991, Gerwin et al 1997).

Autonomic reactions

This phenomenon is observed in the area of the trigger point but is not distributed segmentally (Mense 1999).

Reliability of the palpation of trigger points

Myofacial trigger points in the craniomandibular region have been researched thoroughly for their reliability by dentists. Moderate to high reliability has been shown for the exact manual location of trigger points (McMillan et al 1994, Reid 1994). The quantification of sensitivity is generally inaccurate (Travell & Simons 1983, Reeves et al 1986, McMillan & Blasberg 1994).

Intertester reliability of manual palpation and algometer measurements depends on experience and training (Gerwin et al 1997).

Therefore the validity of the study appears to depend on the assumption that the therapist applies the gold standard for the detection of trigger points.

Basic principles of manual palpation

The best position for palpation is when the muscle is in a state of two-thirds of its maximum length. The therapist uses the index and middle fingers to slide the skin over a muscle, searching for a taut band. The therapist then observes for muscle twitching and asks the patient about sensitivity and referred pain. The therapist may then choose from the following techniques:

- Index and middle fingers are positioned lateral of the taut band and roll the taut band back and forth between the fingers. The taut band is easiest to locate in large muscles such as the masseter or sternocleidomastoid. For the sternocleidomastoid muscle the 'rolling' technique described below is also a helpful method. For some muscles the rolling technique is impossible since they are too small or too flat for two fingers. Alternatively, one finger may be used for the palpation.
- Rolling movement of middle and index fingers: The therapist attempts to position the fingertips lateral of the taut band. The therapist then extends the interphalangeal joints so that the taut band rolls underneath the fingers. Muscles such as the medial pterygoid, temporal muscle, digastric muscle and facial muscles such as the orbicularis oculi and zygomaticus major may be easily palpated with this technique.

Passive stretching

Muscles that contain trigger points are often shortened and react with pain to end of range stretching (Mannheim & Lavett 1989, Gröbli & Dommerholt 1997). Craniofacial pain is mostly local and not referred as would be expected by trigger points. After a passive stretching technique the trigger point should be reassessed. A study by Jaeger and Reeves (1986) on 20 subjects with neck and facial pain showed that the sensitivity of trigger points was significantly reduced after passive stretching as measured by an algometer (Fig. 9.17).

Tests for strength, coordination and endurance

The strength of the masticatory muscles is often noticeably reduced. This may be associated with pain (Travell & Simons 1992).

If a certain mandibular movement is performed repetitively (depression, laterotrusion, protrusion) the therapist will observe that the quality of the movement deteriorates (Baker 1986, Palla et al 1998, Mongini 1999).

Clinical features of trigger points in the craniomandibular region

Clinicians will often detect trigger points in the face and head region. They are associated with combinations of the symptoms listed below.

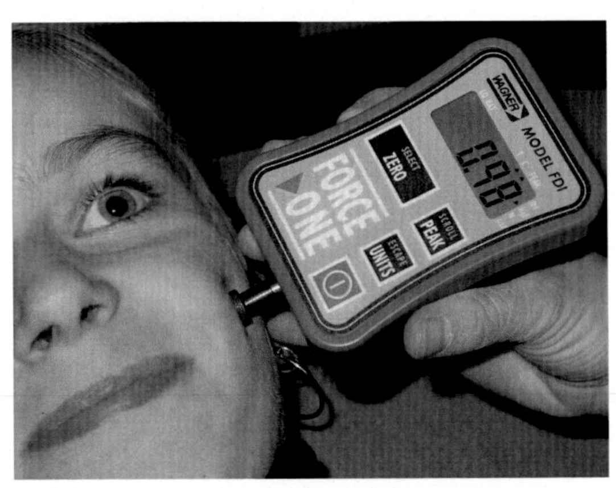

Fig. 9.17 Algometer. The pressure algometer or pain threshold indicator (a mechanical sensor that is connected to a calibrated pin with a 1 cm round rubber cap at the end) is considered a reliable instrument to measure the sensitivity of myofacial trigger points (Reeves et al 1986, Ohrbach & Gale 1989, Farella et al 2000).

Treatment of the trigger points will also reduce the symptoms, indicating a correlation between trigger points and symptoms (Travell 1976, Friction et al 1986, Jaeger & Reeves 1986).

SUBJECTIVE EXAMINATION

- Perceived craniomandibular stiffness
- Fatigue on mandibular movements
- (Spontaneous) stabbing or dull pain
- Deep diffuse non-segmental pain in the trigger point area
- Non-segmental thermic and mechanical hyperalgesia.

PHYSICAL EXAMINATION

- Stiffness reduces aperture
- Pain on active and passive physiological movements
- Reduced endurance
- Muscle weakness without atrophy on static and dynamic muscle testing
- Sympathetic reactions:
  - Pupil dilatation
  - Watering of the eyes
  - Sweating
  - Muscle spasms
  - Palpation: hypersensitivity apparent by the 'jump sign' (sudden motor reaction on palpation of a trigger point) and by the verbal reaction of the patient.

Treatment options for trigger points

Most of the evidence-based literature states reduction of input and thereby changes of the afferent input and central processing as the aim of treatment (Tschopp & Bachmann 1992, Gröbli & Dommerholt 1997, Mense 1999).

Treatment options include:

- Hands-on techniques
- Ice spray (ethyl chloride spray)
- Dry-needling acupuncture
- Muscle imbalance approach (see also Chapter 12)
- Combinations.

In this book, those hands-on techniques (direct local manual techniques) that have been shown to result in positive clinical outcomes are emphasized. The choice of technique depends not only on the therapist and their qualifications but also on the localization of the symptoms, the quality of the symptoms and the success of previously tried techniques as evaluated in the retrospective assessment. These manual therapy options are now described in detail.

HANDS-ON TECHNIQUES

These are categorized as *basic techniques* and *combined techniques* (Box 9.3).

Basic techniques

Active facilitation

It has been shown that active facilitation with post-isometric relaxation influences trigger points (Ingber 1989, Simons et al 1999).

The muscle is placed in a pain-free submaximal position; the patient is then required to hold against a minimal isometric resistance. If the technique is successful, muscle length, local sensitivity and referred pain are normalized (Lewit & Simons 1984).

Frictioning

For the treatment of trigger points, circular and transverse friction techniques are indicated. This is meant to improve trigger points and general muscular health (Simons 1999). On application of one of these techniques, local sensitivity levels need to be assessed continuously. The intensity should drop on sustained constant pressure. There is no scientific proof for the influence of friction techniques on trigger points but personal experience shows that circular friction in particular, combined with active facilitation, is beneficial for the treatment of myogenic craniofacial pain syndromes.

Box 9.3 Treatment options for trigger points: hands-on techniques

Basic techniques

- Active facilitation
- Frictioning
- Compression
- Transverse movements
- Percussions and vibrations

Combinations

- Transverse movements with or without muscle movement
- Combined with active restoration of the muscle balance (see later in this chapter)

(Ischaemic) compression

This technique consists of local pressure for 30–60 seconds. One finger or thumb applies vertical local pressure to the trigger point. It depends on the therapy concept as to exactly how much pressure should be applied. Most authors suggest pressure under 10 kg, in chronic cases even up to 50–60 kg (Tsujii 1993). The effect of sustained (ischaemic) compression is probably due to a release of opiates by the endogenous pain inhibition system (Gröbli & Dommerholt 1997). The disadvantage of the technique is that blood vessels may rupture under the great pressure and neuronal motor endplates may be damaged. This may even lead to the development of new trigger points (Mense 1999). For patients with craniofacial myogenic pain the pressure rarely needs to be higher than 5 kg since the pain is easily reproduced.

Transverse movements

The therapist attempts to locate the trigger point and positions the middle or index fingers transversely to the muscle fibres. The therapist then extends the interphalangeal joint of the palpating finger in a manner that applies a transverse 'stretch' to the muscle fibres. During this action the therapist may note a local muscle twitching, often accompanied by pain. This may influence the taut band (Mense 1999). The degree of transverse movement combined with muscle tension is very advantageous for adjustment of individual dosage (Fig. 9.18).

Percussions and vibrations

Light tapping or vibrating vertically onto the trigger point may be applied in 2–5 second intervals. The aim is to reduce pain intensity

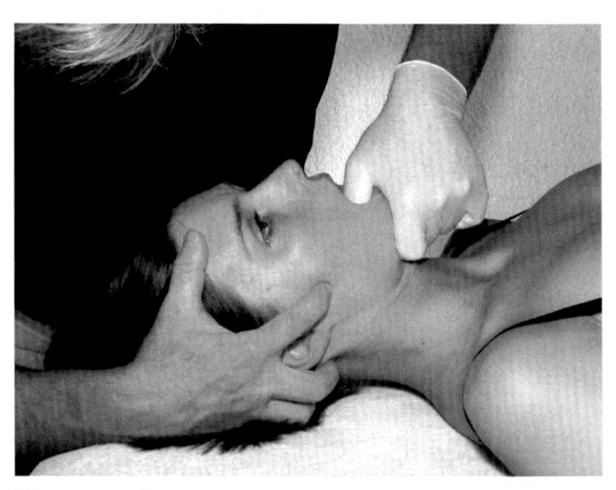

Fig. 9.18 Transverse movement of masseter muscle fibres. The muscle is positioned in slight muscle tension (depression and laterotrusion to the opposite side). It is important that only the tips of the fingers touch the muscle fibres containing suspected trigger points.

by counter-irritation and to thereby restore muscle function (Chaitow 1996, Gerwin et al 1997).

Combinations of techniques

Signs and symptoms are generally reduced clinically after the application of a certain technique. Once a plateau is reached those techniques that have been shown to improve the symptoms may be combined.

Experience has led to a number of particularly helpful combinations of hands-on techniques:

- Active facilitation combined with compression or transverse movements. Especially helpful for facial muscles such as the orbicularis oculi and zygomaticus major.
- Transverse movements combined with passive end of range muscle stretching. Particularly beneficial for trigger points in the masseter, temporal, medial pterygoid and trapezius (pars descendens) muscles.
- Transverse movements combined with vibrations. Particularly when transverse movements result in accumulating symptoms it is helpful to add one or two series of vibrations. Examples for muscles that benefit from this technique include m. sternocleidomastoideus pars sternalis and clavicularis, m. digastricus venter anterior and posterior.

Hands-on techniques combined with muscle balance exercises

Trigger points may have an inhibiting or abnormal facilitating influence on the function of stabilizing and mobilizing muscles (Comerford & Mottram 2001; see also Chapter 12). Friction found that patients with an abnormal posture (anteroposition of the head) and craniofacial dysfunction show significantly more trigger points than normal (Friction et al 1986, Nicolakis et al 2000).

The assessment of craniocervical and craniomandibular muscles, as suggested in Chapter 8, followed by treatment of the trigger points and muscle function reassessment will indicate whether trigger points directly influence muscle function and posture. If the procedure demonstrates that muscle balance exercises show a positive result, it is beneficial to include muscle balance exercises in the trigger point treatment.

SUMMARY

- **The aetiology of trigger points is unclear. Three models are discussed.**
- **Pathobiological explanations emphasize input mechanisms with sensitization of the central nervous system as an explanation for sustained symptoms (hyperalgesia).**
- **Manual therapy and other methods such as heat application or dry needling may have an effect on the function of various muscle groups.**
- **Hands-on techniques (manual techniques) are easily included in the treatment of craniofacial pain; the choice of technique depends on the reaction of the symptoms.**

Trigger points in the craniocervical and craniofacial regions

Based on the current literature and empirical knowledge, location, palpation, classic symptoms and predisposing factors are discussed.

Trigger points that are found in these regions but do not result in referred pain are not mentioned here.

MASTICATORY MUSCLES

M. masseter (superficialis)

TP1

Localization and palpation (Fig. 9.19a)

For palpation the patient opens the mouth to approximately 3 cm and the therapist's index finger is positioned 2–5 mm anterior of the mandibular angle.

Symptoms

- Pain above the eyebrows, in the temporal area and the zygomatic, mandibular and periauricular region. Symptoms are often associated with trismus.

Predisposing factors

- Bruxism, occlusal dysfunctions, orthopaedic instruments for cervical traction, overstretching, e.g. on dental treatments.
- Chronic inflammation of the periodontium or the pulp.
- This is commonly one of the first trigger points to occur with emotional stress.

TP2

Localization and palpation (Fig. 9.19b)

The mouth is opened 3 cm and the therapist's index finger is placed on the middle of the muscle belly, about 2 cm below the zygomatic bone. The therapist attempts to detect the trigger points transversely to the muscle fibres (that run craniodorsally).

Symptoms

- Pain in the mandibular area.
- Hyperalgesia at the molar, premolar and canine teeth.
- The canine teeth commonly react to pressure, heat and sweet or sour taste with pain.

Predisposing factors

- Bruxism, occlusal dysfunctions, orthopaedic devices for traction and stabilization of the cervical spine.
- Overstretching during, for example, dental procedures.
- Chronic inflammation of the periodontium or the pulp.

TP3

Localization and palpation (Fig. 9.19b)

The mouth is opened 3 cm and the therapist's fingers are placed 0.5 cm below the zygoma.

Symptoms

- Pain in the maxilla and the premolar and molar teeth.
- Hyperalgesia on pressure on the upper jaw, the premolar and molar teeth; also on temperature and sweet or sour food.
- Paraesthesia at the gingiva, the premolar and molar teeth as well as in the region of the canine teeth.
- Chronic inflammation of the periodontium or the pulp.
- Frequently this is one of the first trigger points to occur on emotional stress.

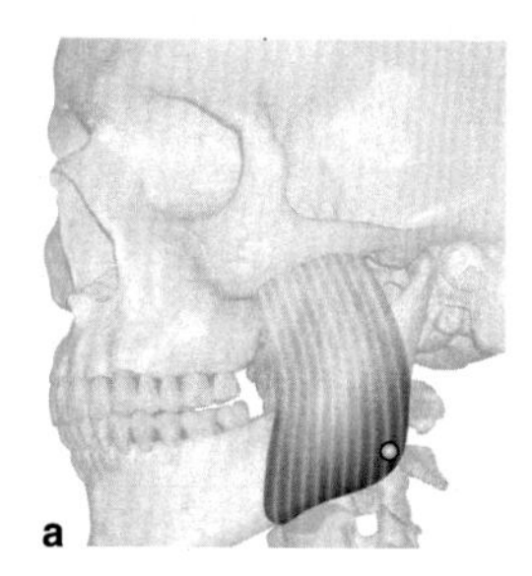

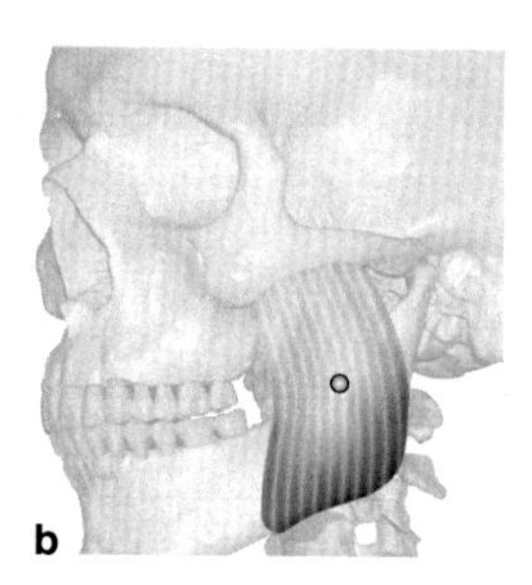

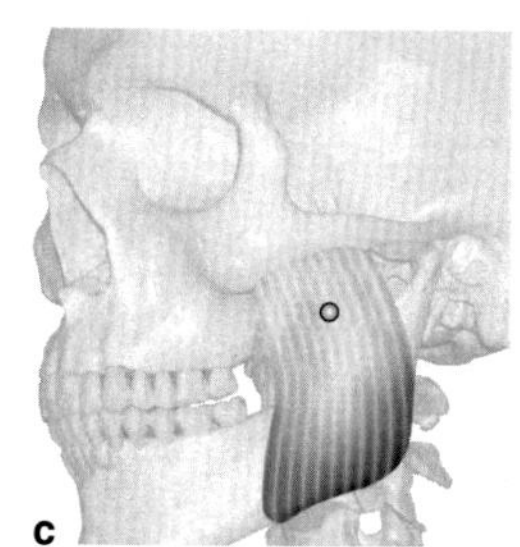

Fig. 9.19 Masseter (superficial) trigger points and referred pain: **a** TP1, **b** TP2, **c** TP3.

M. masseter (pars profunda)

TP1

Localization and palpation (Fig. 9.20a)
The patient's mouth is opened 3 cm and positioned into slight laterotrusion towards the opposite side. The therapist's finger palpates the muscle belly for a trigger point, which is usually found 2–3 cm distal of the zygoma.

Symptoms

- Diffuse retromolar pain in the cheek, possibly referred as far as the TMJ.
- Swelling below the eye due to a dysfunction of the lymphatic system.

Predisposing factors

- Bruxism, occlusal dysfunctions, orthopaedic devices for traction and stabilization of the cervical spine.
- Overstretching during dental procedures.
- Chronic inflammation of gingiva or pulp.
- Frequently this is one of the first trigger points to occur on emotional stress.

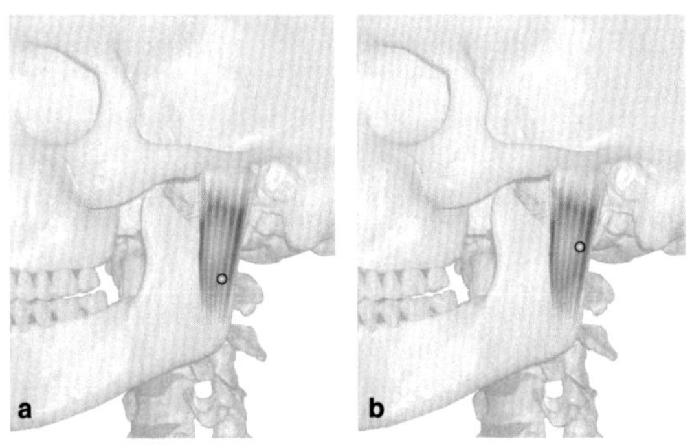

Fig. 9.20 Masseter pars profunda trigger points: a TP1, b TP2.

TP2

Localization and palpation (Fig. 9.20b)
The patient's mouth is opened with slight protrusion and the therapist's index finger is placed on the tendomuscular junction 0.5 cm below the zygomatic arch.

Symptoms

- Pain deep in the ear.
- Influences tinnitus, bilateral changes of the noise intensity.

Predisposing factors

- Bruxism, occlusal dysfunctions, orthopaedic devices for traction and stabilization of the cervical spine.
- Overstretching during dental procedures.
- Chronic inflammation of gingiva or pulp.
- Frequently this is one of the first trigger points to occur on emotional stress.

M. temporalis

TP1

Localization and palpation (Fig. 9.21a)
The patient's mouth is opened submaximally (around 4 cm). The therapist's index finger is placed 0.5 cm above the zygomatic bone at the extension of the coronoid process. The therapist palpates the tendon insertion.

Symptoms

- Pain in the maxilla, especially in the incisors.
- Hyperalgesia of the incisors on palpation and on contact with sweet or sour food.
- Paraesthesia of the gingiva.
- Pain in the cranial part of the orbita and around the zygomatic bone.

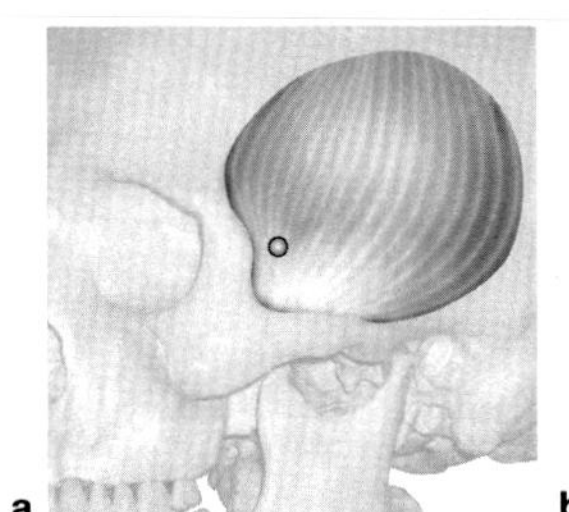

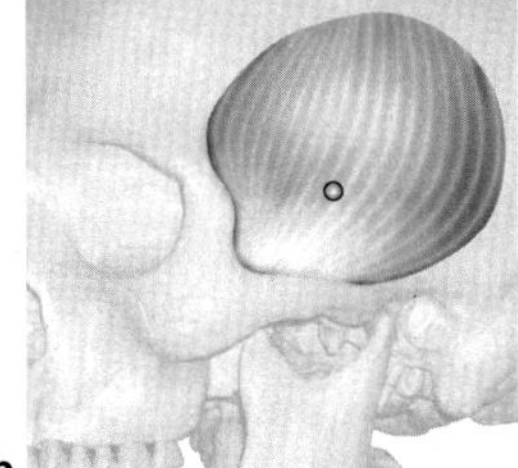

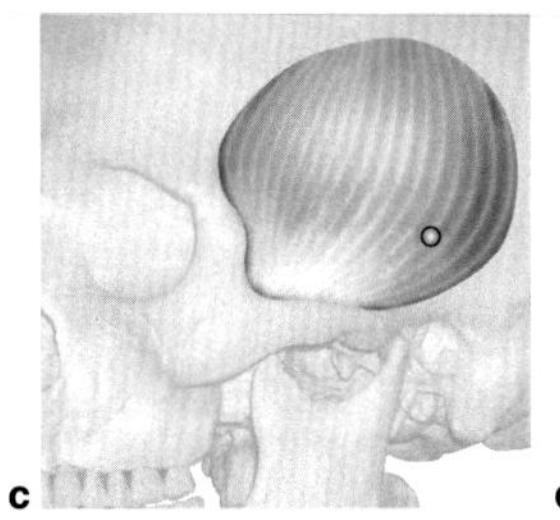

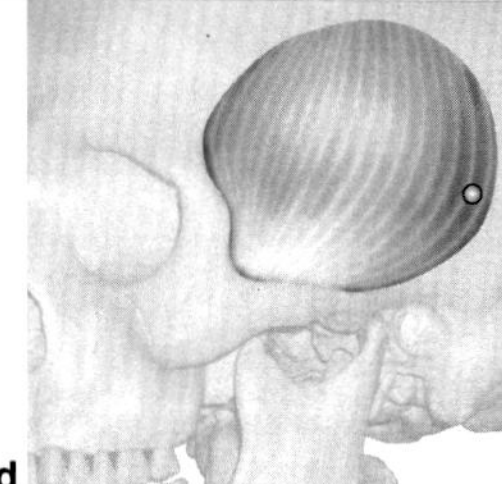

Fig. 9.21 Temporalis trigger points: a TP1, b TP2, c TP3, d TP4.

Predisposing factors

- Unilateral hypertrophia, usually dominantly on the prominent side, for example in plagiocephalia (see also masseter).

TP2

Localization and palpation (Fig. 9.21b)

The patient's mouth is opened submaximally (around 4 cm). The therapist's index finger is placed 1.5 cm ventral of the ear and 2 cm towards cranial in order to palpate the tendomuscular junction. The therapist finds the trigger point by palpating vertically to the muscle fibres.

Symptoms

- Pain at the canines and the upper premolar teeth.
- Hyperalgesia in the same area on palpation and on contact with sweet or sour food.
- Paraesthesia at the periodontium of the premolar and molar teeth.
- Pain in the temporal area.

Predisposing factors

See TP1.

TP3

Localization and palpation (Fig. 9.21c)

The patient's mouth is opened submaximally (around 4 cm) and the therapist places the index finger 1 cm above the head of the mandible and 1.5 cm ventral of the ear. The finger touches the muscle belly of the temporal muscle and feels for the trigger point.

Symptoms

- Pain in the canine teeth and the upper premolar teeth.
- Hyperalgesia in the same area on palpation and on contact with sweet or sour food.
- Paraesthesia at the gingiva of the premolar and molar teeth.
- Pain in the central temporal region.
- Occasionally sharp pain in the TMJ.
- Changes frequency of tinnitus.

Predisposing factors

See TP1

TP4

Localization and palpation (Fig. 9.21d)

The patient's mouth is opened 3 cm and actively placed into slight protrusion. The therapist palpates 0.5 cm craniodorsal of the tip of the ear helix for the trigger point.

Symptoms

- Pain in the dorsal parts of the temporal and the occipital areas, sometimes referred into the helix of the ear.
- Tinnitus frequency may change on palpation.

Predisposing factors

See TP1.

M. pterygoideus medialis

Localization and palpation (Fig. 9.22)

This trigger point is very common. The mouth is opened 2 cm with laterotrusion towards the symptomatic side. The tip of the therapist's middle finger is slightly flexed and palpates 1–2 cm medial of the mandibular angle.

Symptoms

- Diffuse pain in the tongue, the pharynx and the hard palate, behind the ear and dorsal of the craniomandibular joint.

Predisposing factors

- Trismus combined with swallowing difficulties, pain on maximum intercuspidation.
- Dysfunctions that affect the Eustachian tube (e.g. repetitive inflammation of the sinuses).

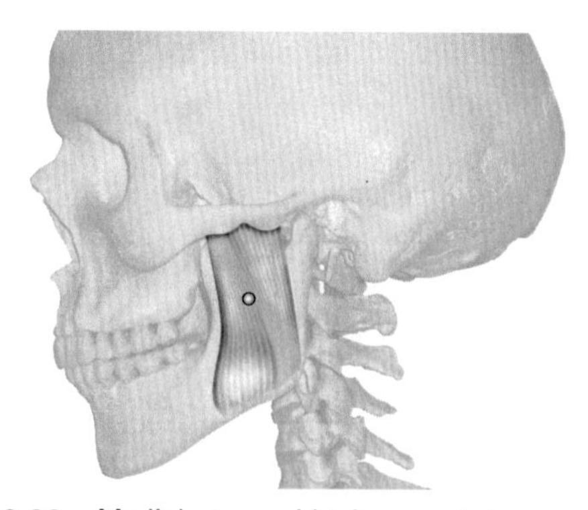

Fig. 9.22 Medial pterygoid trigger points.

M. pterygoideus lateralis (pars inferior)

Localization and palpation (Fig. 9.23a)

The trigger point is located in the muscle belly of the inferior part of the muscle but cannot be palpated. The patient relaxes the TMJ so that the teeth are not in contact. Local pressure of the therapist's index finger along the maxillary tubercle and medial onto the pterygoid process often reproduces some of the symptoms. Usually the local pressure pain increases when the patient performs slight protrusion against resistance.

Symptoms

- Pain in the TMJ and the maxilla (sinus region).

Predisposing factors

- Dynamic occlusion with early or missing teeth contact.
- Intra-articular dysfunction of the TMJ, e.g. on disc displacement.
- Minimal neuropathy of the mandibular nerve.
- Excessively protruded mandible, intensive wind instrument playing.

M. pterygoideus lateralis (pars superior)

Localization and palpation (Fig. 9.23b)

The trigger point is located in the muscle belly of the superior part of the muscle but cannot be palpated. Targeted pressure along the maxillary tubercle towards the pterygoid process reproduces the symptoms (partially). A clearer reproduction occurs commonly when the second and third molar teeth bite onto a wooden spatula.

Symptoms

- Pain in the TMJ or the maxilla (sinuses).

Predisposing factors

- Dynamic occlusion with missing or early teeth contact.
- Intra-articular dysfunction of the TMJ such as disc displacement.
- Minimal neuropathy of the mandibular nerve.
- Excessively protruded mandible.
- Intensive wind instrument playing.

SUPRAHYOID MUSCLES

M. digastricus venter anterior

Localization and palpation (Fig. 9.24a)

The patient sits or lies with the mouth slightly opened. The therapist's index finger is placed intraorally on the floor of the mouth 1–2 cm posterior of the mandibular tip. The index finger of the other hand is placed exactly opposite (extraorally). The therapist palpates for a rolling trigger point in between the fingers.

Symptoms

- Pain and hyperalgesia of the incisors, the affected alveolar bone and the gingiva.

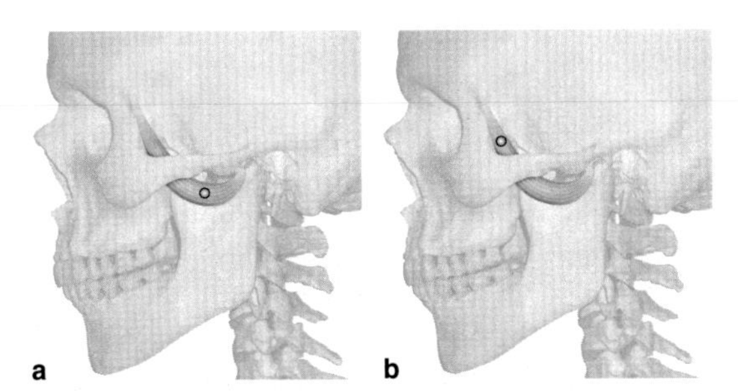

Fig. 9.23 Lateral pterygoid trigger points: **a** inferior part, **b** superior part.

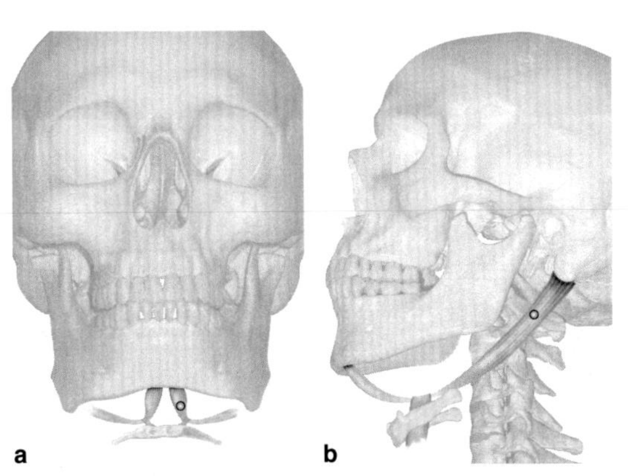

Fig. 9.24 Digastricus trigger points: **a** venter anterior, **b** venter posterior.

- Pressure on the throat, perceived cramping of the floor of the mouth.
- Swallowing difficulties.

Predisposing factors

- Surgery of the floor of the mouth, swallowing difficulties, muscle imbalance of the head and neck region.
- Mouth breathing, mandibular retrusion, bruxism, radiotherapy.

M. digastricus venter posterior

The m. stylohyoideus is positioned medially behind the m. digastricus and therefore cannot be palpated.

Localization and palpation (Fig. 9.24b)

The patient is in 10° of neck extension and the therapist gently moves the hyoid laterally towards the opposite side. The index finger of the other hand palpates for a trigger point in a taut band that is usually found 3 cm anterior of the mastoid process.

Symptoms

- Diffuse suprahyoid pain from the tip of the mandible up towards the ear.
- Perceived throat inflammation.
- Occasionally dysarthria on fatigue.
- Swallowing difficulties.

Predisposing factors

- Surgery to the floor of the mouth.
- Swallowing difficulties.
- Muscle imbalance of the head and neck region.

M. trapezius pars descendens

TP1

Localization and palpation (Fig. 9.25a)

The trigger point is found cranial of the suprascapular space, 5–8 cm anterior of the medial margin of the acromion. The patient performs a depression of the scapula. The therapist holds the shoulder in slight depression and places the index finger at the margin of the trapezius muscle. Thumb and index finger now palpate for the trigger point by performing rolling movements vertically to the muscle.

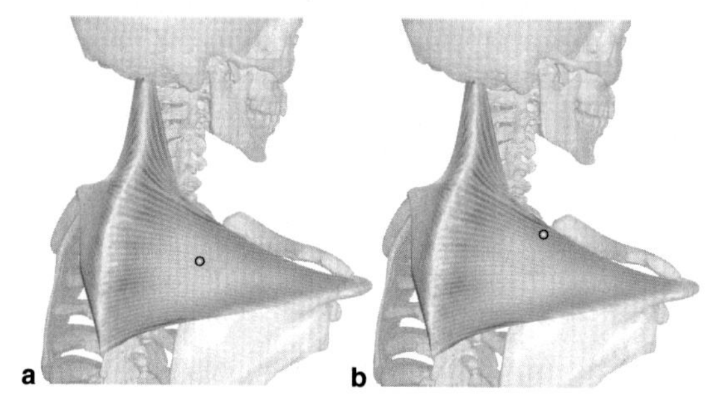

Fig. 9.25 Trapezius (pars descendens) trigger points: **a** TP1, **b** TP2.

Symptoms

- Pain in the posterolateral aspect of the neck up to the mastoid. Pain is not referred beyond the craniocervical junction.

Predisposing factors

- Postural dysfunction.
- Surgery in the neck region.
- Accessory nerve neuropathy.

TP2

Localization and palpation (Fig. 9.25b)

The trigger point is found in the anterior part of the muscle at the level of the fifth cervical vertebra. The patient performs a slight lateroflexion to the opposite side. The therapist places one hand on the lateral side of the head and performs a rolling movement with the other thumb and index finger to palpate for the trigger point.

Symptoms

- Pain posterolaterally of the neck up to the mastoid. Pain is referred beyond the craniocervical junction to the head.
- Pain in the cranial orbita and pain behind the eyes.
- Pain in the area of the mandibular angle.
- Diffuse, superficial earache, occasionally associated with vasomotor reactions ('red ears').

Predisposing factors

- Postural dysfunction.
- Surgery in the neck region.
- Accessory nerve neuropathy.

FACIAL MUSCLES

Trigger points also occur in the facial muscles. They are sometimes difficult to palpate, they produce a superficial pain and the area of referred symptoms is comparably small.

M. orbicularis oculi

Localization and palpation (Fig. 9.26)

With the patient's eyes maximally open, the therapist applies pressure to the cranial orbital edge just below the eyebrows with the tip of the index finger.

Symptoms

- Ipsilateral pain in the bridge of the nose and the cheek.
- Ptosis and watering of the eye.
- 'Jumpy-print syndrome'; when reading, the letters appear to move.

Predisposing factors

- Orbital trauma or surgery.
- Secondary to peripheral facial nerve paresis.

M. zygomaticus major

Localization and palpation (Fig. 9.27)

The patient opens the mouth and slightly widens the corners. The therapist positions one index finger in the mouth; the other index finger is placed extraorally 1–2 cm laterocranially of the corner of the mouth so that the tips of both index fingers face each other.

Symptoms

- Pain lateral of the nose towards the centre of the forehead.
- Difficulty in lifting the corner of the mouth.

Predisposing factors

- Craniomandibular dysfunction with mandibular shift.
- Secondary to facial nerve paresis.
- Secondary to salivary gland surgery.

M. buccinator

Localization and palpation (Fig. 9.28)

The patient parts the lips as if pronouncing the letter 'o'. The therapist palpates for the trigger point 1–1.5 cm lateral to the corner of the mouth.

Symptoms

- Hyperalgesia of the upper incisors.
- Diffuse pain in both cheeks.
- Deep pain in the ipsilateral TMJ.
- Dysphagia during prolonged or fast speech.

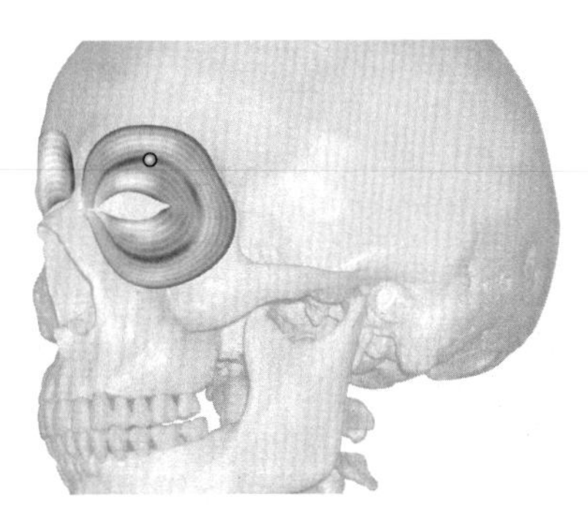

Fig. 9.26 Trigger point of the orbicularis oculi muscle and referred pain.

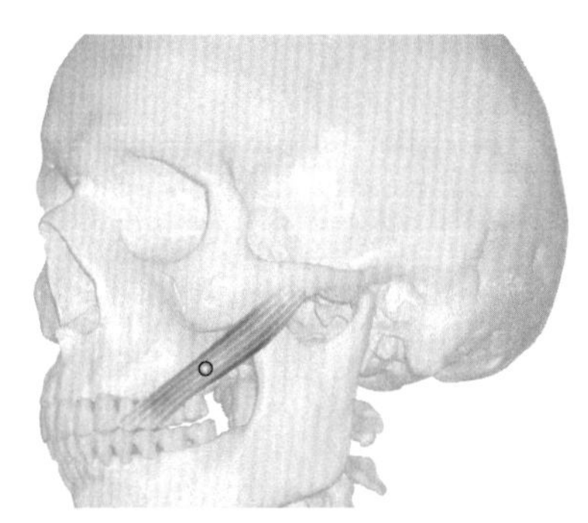

Fig. 9.27 Trigger points of the major zygomatic muscle.

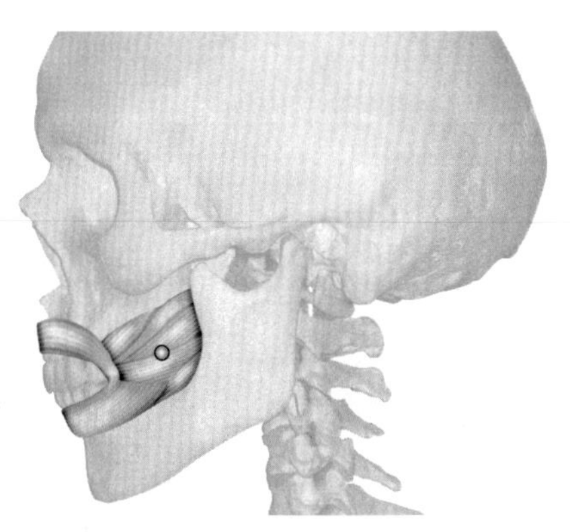

Fig. 9.28 Trigger points of the buccalis oris muscle.

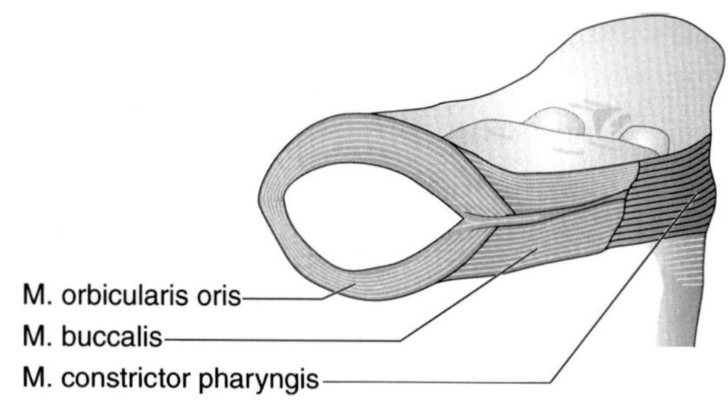

Fig. 9.29 Anatomical overview of the buccalis, orbicularis and constrictor pharyngis muscles.

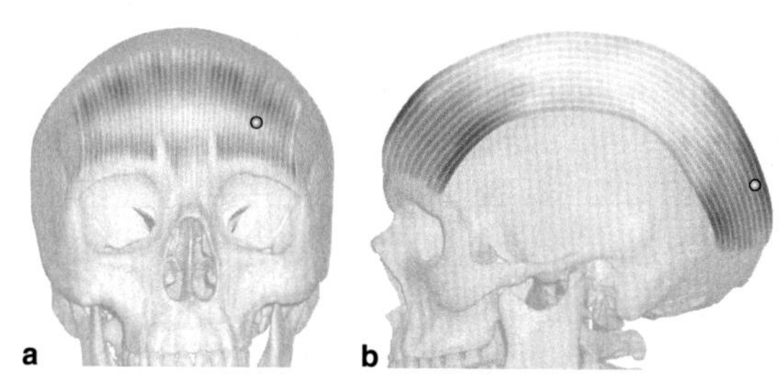

Fig. 9.30 Trigger points of the occipitofrontal muscle: **a** frontal part, **b** occipital part.

Predisposing factors

- Previous facial nerve paresis.
- Mouth floor surgery.
- Viscerocranial surgery.

How can the m. buccalis be responsible for swallowing dysfunctions?

The buccal muscles, orbicularis oris and constrictor pharyngis superior muscles form a continuous functional band (Williams et al 1989). This muscle group works like a sphincter muscle that moves the bolus towards the pharynx during the first phase of swallowing (Curl 1989) (Fig. 9.29).

M. occipitofrontalis pars frontalis

Localization and palpation (Fig. 9.30a)

With the patient's eyes slightly open, the therapist places the index finger 2–3 cm cranially of the centre of the orbita onto the muscle belly. Transverse movements on the muscle will detect the trigger point.

Symptoms

- Superficial unilateral pain in the forehead (sinus frontalis region), commonly slightly referred cranially. The pain does not increase with cervical flexion.

Predisposing factors

- Frequent frowning.
- Chronic sinusitis.
- Secondary to facial nerve paresis.

M. occipitofrontalis pars occipitalis

Localization and palpation (Fig. 9.30b)

The patient slightly bends the neck and the therapist palpates the muscle belly with the index finger 3–4 cm caudally of the lambdoid suture. The trigger point is detected by a transverse motion of the index finger.

Symptoms

- Diffuse, unilateral pain in the dorsolateral part of the head.
- Orbital pain.

Predisposing factors

- Scarring of the fascia occipitalis.
- N. occipitalis major neuropathy.
- Suboccipital surgery.

CRANIOCERVICAL MUSCLES

M. sternocleidomastoideus pars clavicularis

TP1

Localization and palpation (Fig. 9.31a)

The patient sits or lies supine. The patient's head is positioned in slight ipsilateral lateroflexion and rotation. The therapist's hand stabilizes the patient's head, with index finger and thumb palpating for the trigger point. The palpation starts underneath the mastoid process and continues caudally along the sternocleidomastoid muscle. The trigger point is located approximately 2 cm below the mastoid process. For palpation purposes it is rolled between index and middle finger.

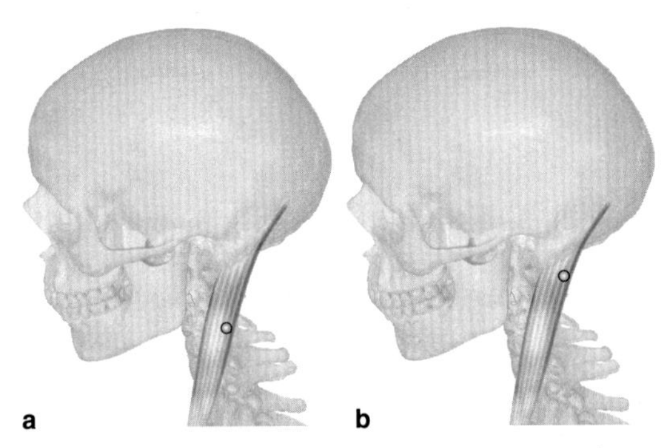

Fig. 9.31 Sternocleidomastoid (clavicular part) trigger points: a TP1, b TP2.

Symptoms

- Mainly unilateral pain in the forehead (sinus frontalis region).
- Changes of posture, especially movements of the head, trigger balance problems and dizziness.
- Vegetative reactions such as sweating and goose bumps are observed in the neck.

Predisposing factors

- Malocclusion (especially ipsilateral crossbite).
- Commonly associated with masseter muscle trigger points.
- Plagiocephalia.
- KISS (kinematic imbalance due to suboccipital strain) and KIDD (kinematically induced dysgnosia and dyspraxia) children with cranial dysfunctions.
- Unilateral cervical problems.

TP2

Localization and palpation (Fig. 9.31b)

The patient sits or lies supine. The head is slightly tilted to the heterolateral side and rotated to the homolateral side. The therapist stabilizes the patient's head with one hand and the index finger of the other hand palpates 2–3 cm below the mastoid process from dorsal.

Symptoms

- Pain inside or below the ear.
- Diffuse pain in the cheek.
- Referred pain into the molar teeth of the lower jaw and the gingiva.
- Spatial disorientation.
- Balance problems and dizziness on changes of the posture and the head position.
- Vegetative reactions such as sweating and goose bumps in the neck.

Predisposing factors

- Malocclusion.
- Commonly associated with trigger points of the masseter muscle.
- Plagiocephaly.
- KISS and KIDD children with cranial dysfunctions.
- Unilateral cervical problems.
- Post-surgery behind the ear, e.g. after surgery of the salivary glands or for acoustic neuroma.

M. sternocleidomastoideus pars sternalis

This part of the sternocleidomastoid muscle may host three important trigger points, all of which may be palpated in the same starting position.

All three trigger points show referred pain into the same regions, predisposing factors and dysfunctions.

TP1

Localization and palpation (Fig. 9.32a)

The patient's head is positioned into lateroflexion and rotation away from the symptoms. The therapist stabilizes the patient's head with one hand while the index finger and thumb of the other hand palpate for the trigger point. The palpation begins below the mastoid process and continues caudally along the sternocleidomastoid muscle. Approximately 4 cm above the clavicle the muscle belly is rolled between the index or middle finger and the thumb.

Symptoms

- The pain spreads from the cheek into the maxilla, zygoma and the supraorbital region, and usually also into the orbita.
- Pain in the outer ear canal.
- Vegetative reactions such as watering of the eyes and reddening of the conjunctiva.
- Ptosis.
- Perceived swelling of the nose and mouth mucosa.

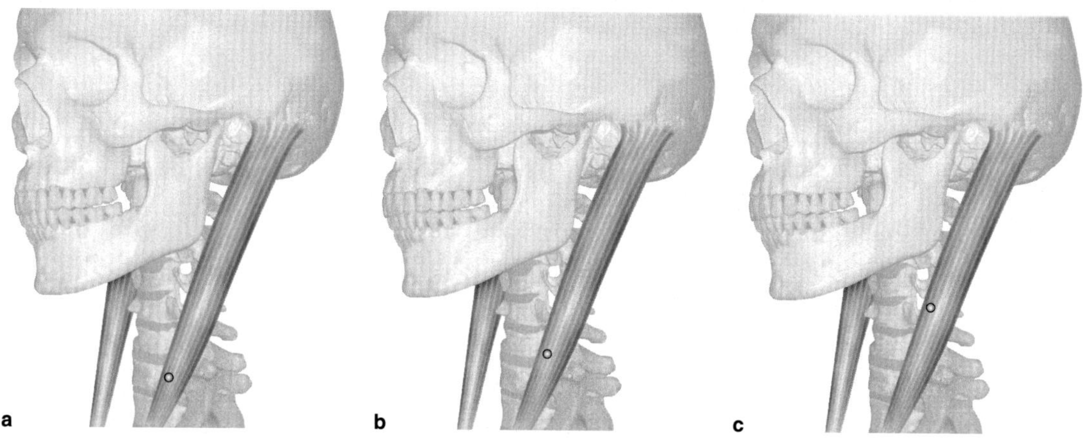

Fig. 9.32 Sternocleidomastoid (sternal part) trigger points: **a** TP1, **b** TP2, **c** TP3.

- Hearing dysfunctions and tinnitus due to activation of the tensor tympani muscle.
- Diplopia and accommodation dysfunctions.

Predisposing factors

- Malocclusion (especially ipsilateral crossbite).
- Commonly associated with trigger points of the masseter muscle.
- Plagiocephaly.
- KISS and KIDD children with cranial dysfunctions.
- Unilateral cervical problems.

TP2

Localization and palpation (Fig. 9.32b)

As TP1 but the trigger point is more towards the centre of the muscle, 7–8 cm cranial of the clavicle.

Symptoms

- See TP1.
- Pain is referred behind the ear and into the occipital region.

Predisposing factors

- See TP1.

TP3

Localization and palpation (Fig. 9.32c)

See TP1 but the trigger point is located less than 1 cm anterior and caudal of the mastoid.

Symptoms

- See TP2.

Predisposing factors

- See TP1.

M. semispinalis capitis

Localization and palpation (Fig. 9.33)

The patient performs upper cervical flexion (chin tuck) and the therapist palpates 1 cm under the nuchal line in the middle of the muscle belly with the index finger.

Symptoms

- Craniofacial pain referring to laterofrontal in the frontal region.

Predisposing factors

- Scarring of the occipital fascia.
- Neuropathy of the major occipital nerve.
- Suboccipital surgery.

M. semispinalis cervicis

Localization and palpation (Fig. 9.34)

The patient lies prone or sits at the short side of the plinth with the head supported. The head is positioned into midcervical flexion. The muscle fibres run 2–4 cm below the occiput. The therapist palpates with the index finger

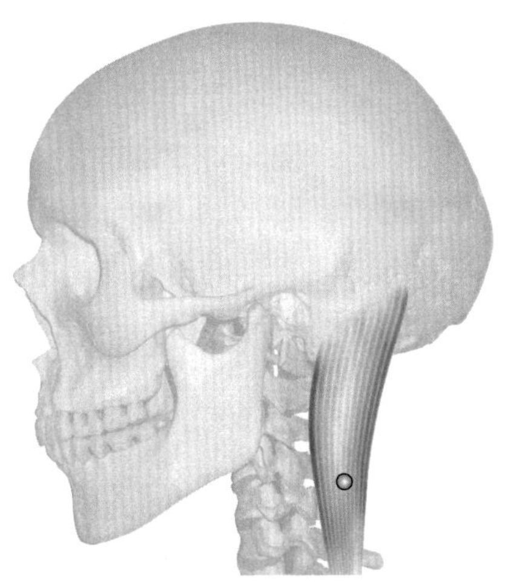

Fig. 9.33 Trigger points of the semispinal capitis muscle.

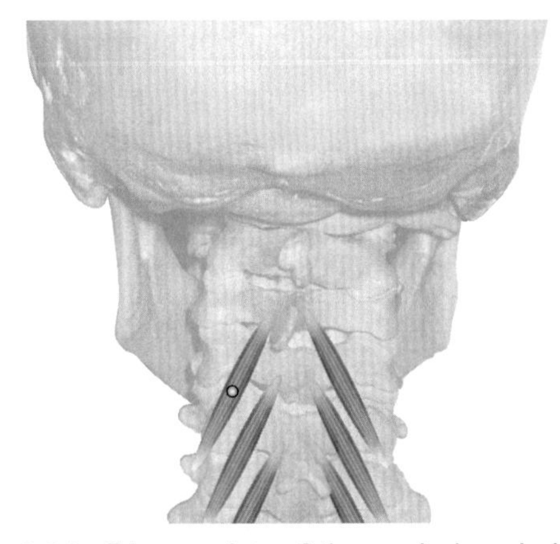

Fig. 9.34 Trigger points of the cervical semispinal muscle.

from laterocranially to mediocaudally 1–2 cm lateral of the spinous processes.

Symptoms

- Diffuse, superficial pain near the vertex.

Predisposing factors

- Arthrogenic dysfunctions of the zygapophyseal midcervical joints.
- Postural dysfunctions.

M. splenius capitis

Localization and palpation

The patient performs a slight upper cervical flexion and lateroflexion to the opposite side. The therapist follows the muscle fibres from the medial side of the mastoid to 1–2 cm mediocaudally of the mastoid. The index finger palpates with transverse movements for the trigger point.

Symptoms

- Pain below the crown of the head in the bregma region (connection between the coronal and sagittal sutures).

Predisposing factors

- Arthrogenic dysfunction of the zygapophyseal midcervical joints.
- Postural dysfunctions.

M. splenius cervicis

Localization and palpation

The patient's head is positioned into upper cervical flexion and rotation (30°) away from the therapist. The muscle is therefore in slight tension and it becomes possible to gently push aside the m. trapezius pars descendens (towards dorsal) and the m. levator scapulae (towards anterior). The therapist palpates the muscle belly of the splenius cervicis muscle from the laminae of the third cervical vertebra in between the trapezius and levator muscles.

Symptoms

- Unilateral, superficial temporal pain.
- Pain deep behind the eye.
- Unilateral disturbed vision on end of range eye movements.

Predisposing factors

- Arthrogenic dysfunction of the zygapophyseal midcervical joints.
- Postural dysfunctions with dominantly rotatory components, e.g. PC work with the monitor placed to the right or the left side, or working as a dentist or dental assistant.

Table 9.7 Overview of various areas of referred pain and the related trigger points based on the literature*

Symptomatic region	Muscle with trigger point
Vertex (2)	Cervical semispinal muscle, semispinalis capitis
Frontal region (3)	Orbicularis oris, zygomaticus major, occipitalis frontalis (processus frontalis),sternocleidomastoid TP1, sternocleidomastoid sternal part TP1, semispinalis capitis
Temporal region (5)	Temporalis TP3, TP4, semispinalis capitis
Zygoma region (6)	Masseter superior TP1, temporalis TP1, sternocleidomastoid sternal part TP1, TP2
Maxillary region (7)	Masseter superior TP3, temporalis TP1, lateral pterygoid (inferior), zygomaticus major, buccinator, sternocleidomastoid sternal part TP1
Mandibular region (8)	Masseter superior TP2, digastricus venter posterior, trapezius (pars descendens) TP2
Craniomandibular joint (9)	Temporalis TP3, medial pterygoid, lateral pterygoid (inferior, superior)
Intra-auricular region (10)	Temporalis profundus TP2
Periauricular region (11)	Masseter TP1, sternocleidomastoid TP2
Ear (12)	Temporalis TP4, trapezius (pars descendens) TP2, sternocleidomastoid TP2, sternocleidomastoid sternal part TP1, TP2, TP3
Intraoral region (13)	Medial pterygoid, digastricus venter posterior Soft tissue: paradontium, tongue
Intraoral region (2, 13) Maxillary teeth	Masseter TP1, TP2, TP3, masseter profundus TP1, sternocleidomastoid TP2, temporalis TP1, TP2, TP3
Intraoral region (3, 13) Mandibular teeth	Masseter TP1, TP2, TP3, digastricus venter anterior
Craniocervical region (14)	Trapezius (pars descendens) TP1, TP2, semispinalis capitis

* Friction (1985), Jankelson (1990), Travell & Simons (1992), Bogduk & Aprill (1993), Chaitow (1996), Mongini (1999); see also Figure 9.35 to which the numbers in parentheses refer.

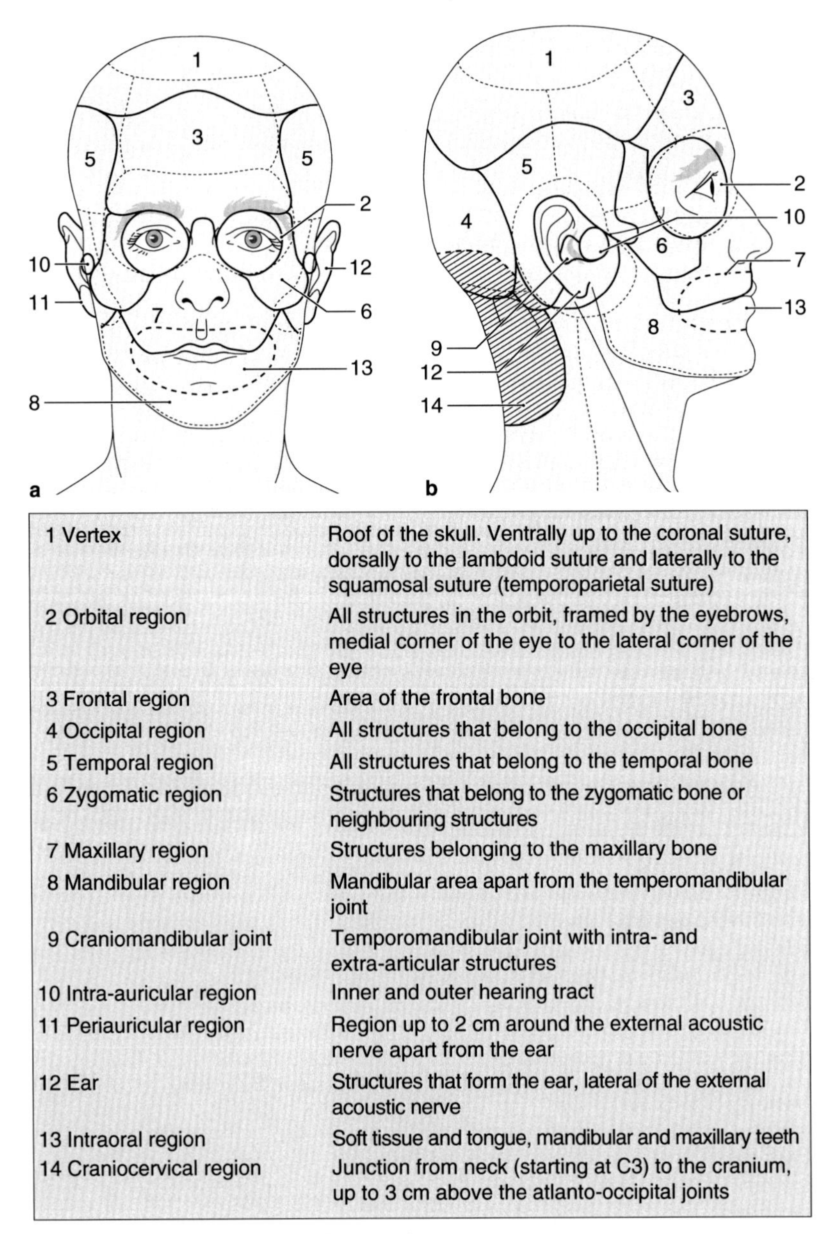

1 Vertex	Roof of the skull. Ventrally up to the coronal suture, dorsally to the lambdoid suture and laterally to the squamosal suture (temporoparietal suture)
2 Orbital region	All structures in the orbit, framed by the eyebrows, medial corner of the eye to the lateral corner of the eye
3 Frontal region	Area of the frontal bone
4 Occipital region	All structures that belong to the occipital bone
5 Temporal region	All structures that belong to the temporal bone
6 Zygomatic region	Structures that belong to the zygomatic bone or neighbouring structures
7 Maxillary region	Structures belonging to the maxillary bone
8 Mandibular region	Mandibular area apart from the temperomandibular joint
9 Craniomandibular joint	Temporomandibular joint with intra- and extra-articular structures
10 Intra-auricular region	Inner and outer hearing tract
11 Periauricular region	Region up to 2 cm around the external acoustic nerve apart from the ear
12 Ear	Structures that form the ear, lateral of the external acoustic nerve
13 Intraoral region	Soft tissue and tongue, mandibular and maxillary teeth
14 Craniocervical region	Junction from neck (starting at C3) to the cranium, up to 3 cm above the atlanto-occipital joints

Fig. 9.35 Overview of pain referred from trigger points.

References

Allard T, Clark S, Jenkins W 1991 Reorganisation of somatosensory area 3b representations in adult owl monkeys after digital syndactyly. Journal of Neurophysiology 66:1048

Amano M, Umeda G, Nakajima H, Yatsuki K 1988 Characteristics of work actions of shoe manufacturing assembly line workers and a cross sectional factor control study on occupational cervicobrachial disorders. Japanese Journal of Industrial Health 30:3

Anderson O, Svensson P, Ellrich J, Arendt-Nielsen L 1998 Conditioning of the masseter inhibitory reflex by homotopically applied painful heat in humans. Electroencephalography and Clinical Neurophysiology 109:508

Andersen O, Graven-Nielsen T, Matre D, Arendt-Nielsen L, Schömburg E 2000 Interaction between cutaneous and muscle afferent activity in polysynaptic reflex pathways: a human experimental study. Pain 84:29

Aprill C, Bogduk N 1992 The prevalence of cervical zygapophyseal joint pain: a first approximation. Spine 17:744

Aprill C, Dwyer A, Bogduk N 1990 Cervical zygapophyseal joint pain patterns: a clinical evaluation. Spine 15(6):458

Arima T, Svensson P, Arendt-Nielsen L 1999 Experimental grinding in healthy subjects: a model for postexercise jaw muscle soreness. Journal of Orofacial Pain 13:104

Asmundson G, Norton P, Nonon G 1999 Beyond pain: the role of fear and avoidance in chronicity. Clinical Psychology Review 19:97

Ayer W, Levin M 1975 Elimination of tooth grinding habits by massed practice therapy. Theoretical basis and application of massed practice exercise for the elimination of tooth grinding habits. Journal of Periodontology 46:306

Azin N, Nunn R 1973 Habit reversal: a method of eliminating nervous habits and tics. Behaviour Research and Therapy 11:619

Baker B 1986 The muscle trigger: evidence of overload injury. Journal of Neurology, Orthopedic Medicine and Surgery 7:35–43

Balm A, Plaat B, Hart A, Hilgers F, Keus R 1997 Nasopharyngeal carcinoma: epidemiology and treatment outcome. Nederlands Tijdschrift voor Geneeskunde 141:2346

Baret R, Hanson M 1978 Oral myofunctional disorders. Mosby, St Louis

Bartolome G, Buchholz D, Feussner H et al 1999 Schluckstörungen. Diagnostik und Rehabilitation, 2nd edn. Urban and Fischer, Munich

Bates T, Grunwaldt E 1958 Myofascial pain in childhood. Journal of Pediatrics 53:198

Bays A 1994 Arthrotomy and orthognathic surgery for TMD. In: Kraus S (ed.) Temporomandibular disorders. Churchill Livingstone, New York, p 237

Bendtsen L, Jensen R, Olesen J 1996 Qualitative nociception in chronic myofascial pain. Pain 65:259

Bogduk N, Aprill C 1993 On the nature of neck pain, discography and cervical zygapophyseal joint blocks. Pain 54:213

Bogduk N, Aprill C, Derby R 1995 Diagnostic blocks of synovial joints. In: White A (ed.) Spine care, Vol. 1: Diagnosis and conservative treatment. Mosby, St Louis, p 298

Braun B, DiGiovanna A, Schiffman E, Bonnema J, Friction J 1992 Cross-sectional study of temporomandibular joint dysfunction in post-cervical trauma patients. Journal of Craniomandibular Disorders, Facial and Oral Pain 6:24

Buchbinder D, Currivan R, Kaplan A, Urken M 1993 Mobilization regimens for the prevention of jaw hypomobility in the radiated patient: a comparison of three techniques. Journal of Oral and Maxillofacial Surgery 51:863

Buckingham R, Braun T, Harenstein D et al 1991 Temporomandibular joint dysfunction syndrome: a close association with systemic joint laxity (the hypermobile joint syndrome). Oral Surgery, Oral Medicine, Oral Pathology 7:514

Bumann A, Groot Landeweert G 1991 Reziproke Knackphänomene. Zuverlässigkeit der Axiographie. Wissenschaft und Praxis. Phillip Journal 6:377

Bumann A, Groot Landeweert G 1997 Manuelle Funktionsanalyse zur Diagnostik und Therapieplanung von Funktionsstörungen im Kausystem. Christian-Albrechts-Universitat, Kiel

Bumann A, Lotzmann U 2000 Manuelle Funktionsanalyse und Funktionsdiagnostik und Therapieprinzipien. Thieme, Stuttgart, p 53

Buonomano D, Merzenich M 1998 Cortical plasticity: from synapses to maps. Annual Review of Neuroscience 21:149

Butler D 2000 Pain mechanisms and peripheral sensitivity. In: The sensitive nervous system. Noigroup Publications, Adelaide, pp 46, 72

Carlsson G 2001 Physical self-regulation: training for the management of temporomandibular disorders. Journal of Orofacial Pain 15:47

Carlsson G, Magnusson T 1999 Management of temporomandibular disorders in general dental practice. Quintessence, Chicago

Chaitow L 1996 Modern neuromuscular techniques. Churchill Livingstone, New York

Chen Y, Gallo L, Meier D, Palla S 2000 Dynamic magnetic resonance imaging technique for the study of the temporomandibular joint. Journal of Orofacial Pain 14:65
Chen Y, Gallo L, Palla S 2002 The mediolateral temporomandibular joint disc position: an in vivo quantitative study. Journal of Orofacial Pain 16:29
Chole R, Parker W 1992 Tinnitus and vertigo in patients with temporomandibular disorder. Archives of Otolaryngology, Head and Neck Surgery 118:817
Christensen L, Hutchings M 1992 Methodological observations on positive and negative work (teeth grinding) by human jaw muscles. Journal of Oral Rehabilitation 19:399
Clark G, Adler R 1985 A critical evaluation of occlusal therapy: occlusal adjustment procedures. Journal of the American Dental Association 110:743
Clark R 1976 Neurology of the temporomandibular joints: an experimental study. Annals of the Royal College of Surgeons of England 58(1):43–51
Comerford M, Mottram S 2001 Movement and stability dysfunction – contemporary developments. Manual Therapy 6:31
Cook A, Woolf C, Wall P 1986 Prolonged C-fibre mediated facilitation of the flexion reflex in the rat is not due to changes in afferent terminals or motor neurone excitability. Neuroscience Letters 70:91
Cooper B, Cooper D, Lucente F 1991 Electromyography of masticatory muscles in craniomandibular disorders. Laryngoscope 101(2):150–157
Curl D 1989 Discovery of a myofascial trigger point in the buccinator muscle: a case report. Journal of Craniomandibular Practice 7:339
Damste P, Idema N 1994 Habitueel mondademen. Bohn Stafleu Van Loghum, Houten/Zaventem
Danzig W, May S, Macneil C, Miller A 1992 Effect of an anesthetic injection into the temporomandibular joint space. Journal of Craniomandibular Disorders 6:288
Davant T, Greene C, Perry H et al 1993 A quantitative computer-assisted analysis of disc displacement in patients with internal derangement using sagittal view magnetic resonance imaging. Journal of Oral and Maxillofacial Surgery 51:974
De Bont L, Boering G, Liem R et al 1986 Osteoarthritis and internal derangement of the temporomandibular joint: a light microscopic study. Journal of Oral and Maxillofacial Surgery 44:634
De Naeije M, Van Loon L 1998 Behandeling van craniomandibulaire Dysfunctie, Craniomandibulaire functie en dysfunctie. Bohn Stafleu Van Loghum, Houten/Diegem, p 188
Derkay C, Schechter G 1998 Anatomy and physiology of pediatric swallowing disorders, dysphagia in children. Otolaryngology Clinics of North America 31(3):397–404
Devor M 1991 Neuropathic pain and injured nerve: peripheral mechanisms. British Medical Bulletin 47:619
Dibbets J, van der Weele L 1992 The prevalence of joint noises as related to age and gender. Journal of Craniomandibular Disorders 6:157
Dijkgraaf L, de Bont L, Boering G, Liem R 1989 The structure, biochemistry and metabolism of osteoarthritic cartilage: a review of the literature. Journal of Oral and Maxillofacial Surgery 47:249
Dijkstra P, Lambert de Bont G, Stegenga B et al 1992a Temporomandibular joint osteoarthrosis and generalized joint hypermobility. Journal of Craniomandibular Practice 10:221
Dijkstra P, Kropmans T, Tamminga R 1992b Modified use of a dynamic bite opener-treatment and prevention of trismus in a child with head and neck cancer: a case report. Cranio 10:327
Dijkstra P, Wilgen v. C, Roodenburg J 2001 Trismus. NVG PT Bulletin. 19e jaargang
DiMauro S, Tsujino S 1994 Non-lysosomal glycogenoses. In: Engel A, Franzini-Armstrong C (eds) Myology, 2nd edn, Vol. 2. McGraw-Hill, Columbus, 59:1554
Dittmer D, Ewers R 1991 Die Verlagerung des Discus articularis im menschlichen Kiefergelenk. Deutsche Zahnärztliche Zeitschrift 46:476
Donaldson C, Skubiek D, Clasby R, Cram J 1994 The evaluation of trigger-points activity using dynamic EMG techniques. American Journal of Pain Management 4:118
Dostrovsky J 1999 Immediate and long-term plasticity in human somatosensory thalamus and its involvement in phantom limbs. Pain Supplement 6:37
Dougherty P, Lenz F 1994 Plasticity of the somatosensory system following neural injury. In: Boivie J, Hansson P, Lindblom U (eds) Touch, temperature, and pain in health and disease: mechanisms and assessments. IASP Press, Seattle, p 439
Duvoisin B, Klaus E, Schnyder P 1990 Coronal radiographs and videofluoroscopy improve the diagnostic quality of temporomandibular joint arthrography. AJR American Journal of Roentgenology 55:105
Dwyer A, April C, Bogduk N 1990 Cervical zygapophyseal joint patterns: a study in normal volunteers. Spine 15:453
Ekberg O 1986 The normal movements of the hyoid bone during swallowing. Investigative Radiology 21:408

Engelmeier R, King G 1983 Complications of head and neck radiation therapy and their management. Journal of Prosthetic Dentistry 49:514

Erikson L, Westesson P 1983 Clinical and radiological study of patients with anterior disc displacement of the temporomandibular joint. Swedish Dental Journal 7:55

Erikson L, Westesson P, Macher D, Hicks D, Tallents R 1992 Creation of disc displacement in human temporomandibular joints autopsy specimens. Journal of Oral and Maxillofacial Surgery 50:867

Farella M, Michelotti A, Steenks M, Romeo R, Cimino R, Bosman F 2000 The diagnostic value of pressure algometry in myofascial pain of the jaw muscles. Journal of Oral Rehabilitation 27:9

Farrar W, Mcarthy W 1982 A clinical outline of temporomandibular joint diagnosis and treatment. Normandie Publications, Montgomery

Flor H, Turk D 1996 Integrating central and peripheral mechanisms in chronic muscular pain. An initial step on a long road. Pain Forum 5:74

Flor H, Birbaumer N, Schulte W et al 1991 Stress-related EMG responses in patients with chronic temporomandibular pain. Pain 46:145

Flor H, Schugens M, Birbaumer N 1992a Discrimination of muscle tension in chronic pain patients and healthy controls. Biofeedback and Self-Regulation 17:165

Flor H, Birbaumer N, Schugens M, Lutzenberger W 1992b Symptom-specific psychophysiological responses in chronic pain patients. Department of Clinical and Physiological Psychology, Universität Tübingen 29:452

Flor H, Elbert T, Knecht C et al 1995 Phantom limb pain as a perceptual correlate of cortical reorganisation following arm amputation. Nature 375:482

Flor H, Braun C, Elbert T et al 1997 Extensive reorganisation of primary somatosensory cortex in chronic back pain patients. Neuroscience Letters 244:5

Fonsesca E 1969 Treatment of maxillomandibular constrictions. Journal of Prosthetic Dentistry 22:652

Freesmeyer W 1993 Zahnärztliche Funktionstherapie. Carl Hanser, Munich, p 301

Friction J 1985 Myofascial pain syndrome of the head and neck: a review of clinical characteristics of 164 patients. Oral Surgery, Oral Medicine, Oral Pathology 60:615

Friction, J, Kroening R, Haley D, Siegert R 1986 Myofascial pain syndrome of the head and neck: a review of clinical characteristics of 164 patients. Oral Surgery, Oral Medicine, Oral Pathology 60:615

Galea M, Darian-Smith I 1995 Voluntary movement and pain: focussing on action rather than perception. In: Shacklock M (ed.) Moving in on pain. Butterworth-Heinemann, Chatswood, p 40

Gallo L, Svoboda A, Palla S 2000 Reproducibility of temporomandibular clicking. Journal of Orofacial Pain 14:293

Gelb H 1985 Clinical management of head, neck and TMJ pain and dysfunction. Saunders, Los Angeles

Gerwin R, Shannon S, Hong C, Hubbard D, Gervitz R 1997 Interrater reliability in myofascial trigger point examination. Pain 69:65

Glaros A 1981 Incidence of diurnal and nocturnal bruxism. Journal of Prosthetic Dentistry 45:545

Glineburg R, Laskin D, Blaustein D 1982 The effects of immobilization on the primate temporomandibular joint: a histologic and histochemical study. Journal of Oral and Maxillofacial Surgery 40:3

Goldstein M, Maxym W, Cummings B, Wood R 1999 The effects of antitumor irradiation on mandibular opening and mobility: a prospective study of 58 patients. Oral Surgery, Oral Medicine, Oral Pathology, Oral Radiology and Endodontics 88:365

Gonzalez A, Sakamaki H, Hatori M, Nagumo M 1992 Evaluation of trismus after treatment of mandibular fractures. Journal of Oral and Maxillofacial Surgery 50:223

Goulet J, Lund J, Montplaisir J et al 1993 Daily clenching, nocturnal bruxism, and stress and their association with CMD symptoms. Journal of Orofacial Pain 7:120

Greene C 2001 The etiology of temporomandibular disorders: implications for treatment. Journal of Orofacial Pain 15:93

Gröbli C, Dommerholt J 1997 Myofaziale Triggerpunkte; Pathologie und Behandlungsmöglichkeiten. Manuelle Medizin 35:295

Gronroos M, Pertovaara A 1993 Capsaicin-induced central facilitation of a nociceptive flexion reflex in humans. Neuroscience Letters 159:215

Gross A, Rivera-Morales W, Gale E 1988 A prevalence study of symptoms associated with TM disorders. Journal of Craniomandibular Disorders, Facial and Oral Pain 2:191

Gupta V, Reddy N, Canilang E 1996 Surface EMG measurements at the throat during dry and wet swallowing. Dysphagia 11:173

Gynther G, Tronje G, Holmund A 1996 Radiographic changes in the temporomandibular joint in patients with generalized osteoarthritis and rheumatoid arthritis. Oral Surgery, Oral Medicine, Oral Pathology, Oral Radiology and Endodontics 81:613

Hansson T, Christensen Minor C, Wagnon Taylor D 1992 Physical therapy in craniomandibular disorders. Quintessence, Copenhagen, p 45

Hansson L, Westesson P, Erikson L 1996 Comparison of tomography and midfield magnetic resonance

imaging of the temporomandibular joint: comparison of imaging of the osseous changes of the temporomandibular joint. Oral Surgery, Oral Medicine, Oral Pathology, Oral Radiology and Endodontics 82:698
Harness D, Peltier B 1992 Comparison of MMPI scores with self-report of sleep disturbance and bruxism in the facial pain population. Cranio 10:70–74
Hathaway K 1995 Bruxism: definition, measurement and treatment. In: Fricton J, Dubner R (eds) Orofacial pain and temporomandibular disorders. Raven Press, New York, p 375
Heller R, Forgione A 1975 An evaluation of bruxism control: massed negative practice and automated relaxation training. Journal of Dental Research 54:1120
Henriksson K 1999 Muscle activity and chronic muscle pain. Journal of Musculoskeletal Pain 7:101
Henriksson K, Bengtsson A, Lindman R, Thornell L 1993 Morphological changes in muscle in fibromyalgia and chronic shoulder myalgia. In: Vaeröy H, Merskey H (eds) Progress in fibromyalgia and myofascial pain. Elsevier, Amsterdam, p 61
Hesse J 1996 Craniomandibular disorder characteristics and orofacial pain. Thesis, University of Amsterdam, ACTA
Higbie E, Seidel-Cobb D, Taylor L, Cummings G 1999 Effect of head position on vertical mandibular opening. Journal of Orthopaedic and Sports Physical Therapy 29:127
Hong C-Z 1994 Lidocaine injection versus dry needling to myofascial trigger points. American Journal of Physical and Medical Rehabilitation 73:256
Hu J 2001 Neurophysiological mechanisms of head, face and neck pain. In: Vernon H (ed.) The craniocervical syndrome. Butterworth-Heinemann, Oxford, p 31
Hu J, Vernon H, Tatourian I 1995 Changes in neck electromyography associated with meningeal noxious stimulation. Journal of Manipulative and Physiological Therapeutics 18:577
Ingber R 1989 Iliopsoas myofascial dysfunction: a treatable cause of 'failed' low back syndrome. Archives of Physical and Medical Rehabilitation 70:382
Jaeger B, Reeves J 1986 Quantification of changes in myofascial trigger point sensitivity with the pressure algometer following passive stretch. Pain 27:203
Jankelson R 1990 Neuromuscular dental diagnosis and treatment. Ishiyaku EuroAmerica, Tokyo
Johansson H, Sjolander P 1993 Neurophysiology of joints. In: Wright V, Radin E (eds) Mechanics of human joints. Dekker, New York, p 243
Jones M, Jensen G, Edwards I 2001 Clinical reasoning in physiotherapy. In: Higgs J, Jones M (eds) Clinical reasoning in the health professions, 2nd edn. Butterworth-Heinemann, Oxford
Kaas J 1999 Is most of the neural plasticity in the thalamus cortical? Proceedings of the National Academy of Sciences USA 96:7622
Kaas J 2000 The reorganisation of sensory and motor maps after injury in adult mammals. In: Gazzaniga M (ed.) The new cognitive neurosciences, 2nd edn. MIT Press, Cambridge
Kapel L, Giaros A, McGlynn F 1989 Psychophysiological responses to stress in patients with myofascial pain-dysfunction syndrome. Journal of Behavioral Medicine 12:397
Kardachi B, Clarke N 1977 The use of biofeedback to control bruxism. Journal of Periodontology 48:639
Katzberg R, Westesson P 1993 Diagnosis of the temporomandibular joint. Saunders, Philadelphia
Katzberg R, Keith D, Guralnick W et al 1983 Internal derangements and arthritis of the temporomandibular joint. Radiology 146:107
Kawamura Y, Fujimoto J 1957 Some physiologic considerations on measuring rest position of the mandible. Medical Journal of Osaka University 8:47
Keith D 1988 Surgery of the temporomandibular joint. Blackwell Scientific, Boston
Kelly J, Sanchez M, Van Kirk L 1973 An assessment of the occlusion of teeth of children. National Center for Health Statistics. US Public Health Service, Washington
Kendall H, Kendall F, Boynton D 1970 Posture and pain. Krieger Publishing, Huntington, New York
Kimura D, Watson N 1989 The relation between oral movement control and speech. Brain and Language 37(4):565
Könönen M, Waltimo A, Nystrom M 1996 Does clicking in adolescence lead to painful temporomandibular joint locking? Lancet 347:1080
Kraus S 1987 Tongue–teeth–breathing–swallowing: exercise pad. Stretching Charts, Tacoma, Washington
Kraus S 1988 Cervical spine influences on the craniomandibular region. Churchill Livingstone, New York, p 367
Kraus S 1993 Evaluation and management of temporomandibular disorders. In: Saunders H, Saunders R (eds) Evaluation, treatment and prevention of musculoskeletal disorders. Saunders, Minneapolis
Kraus S 1994 Cervical influences on management of temporomandibular disorders, 2nd edn. Churchill Livingstone, New York, p 325
Krogh-Poulsen W, Olsson A 1996 Occlusal disharmonies and dysfunction of the stomatognathic system. Dental Clinics of North America 10:627

Kumai T 1993 Difference in chewing patterns between involved and opposite sides in patients with unilateral temporomandibular joint and myofascial pain dysfunction. Archives of Oral Biology 38:467

Langendoen J, Muller J, Jull G 1997 The retrodiscal tissue of the temporomandibular joint. Clinical anatomy and its role in arthropathies. Manual Therapy 2(4):191–198

Larsson S, Bodegård L, Henriksson K, Öberg P 1990 Chronic trapezius myalgia. Morphology and blood flow studied in 17 patients. Acta Orthopaedica Scandinavica 61:394

Lavigne G, Montplaisir J 1994 Restless legs syndrome and sleep bruxism: prevalence and association among Canadians. Sleep 17:739

Lavigne G, Montplaisir J 1995 Bruxism: epidemiology, diagnosis, pathophysiology and pharmacology. Advances in Pain Research and Therapy 21:387

Lavigne G, Lobbezoo F, Montplaisir J 1995 The genesis of rhythmic masticatory muscle activity and bruxism during sleep. In: Morimoto T, Matsuya T, Takada K (eds) Brain and oral functions. Elsevier Science, Amsterdam, p 249

Lawrence E, Samson G 1988 Growth development influences on the craniomandibular region. In: Kraus S (ed.) TMJ disorders: management of the craniomandibular complex. Churchill Livingstone, New York

Layzer R 1994. Muscle pain, cramps and fatigue. In: Engel A, Franzini-Armstrong C (eds) Myology, 2nd edn. McGraw-Hill, New York, 67:1754

Lewit K, Simons D 1984 Myofascial pain: relief by post-isometric relaxation. Archives of Physical and Medical Rehabilitation 65:452

Lobbezoo F, Naeije M 1997 Bruxisme en myofasciale pijn van kauwspieren. De relatie kritisch bekeken. Nederlands Tijdschrift voor Fysiotherapie 107:70

Lobbezoo F, Montplaisir J, Lavigne G 1996 Bruxism: a factor associated with temporomandibular disorders and orofacial pain. Journal of Back and Musculoskeletal Rehabilitation 6:165

Loiselle R 1969 Relation of occlusion to temporomandibular joint dysfunction: the prosthodontic viewpoint. Journal of the American Dental Association 79:145

Lotze M, Montoya P, Erb M et al 1999 Activation of cortical and cerebellar motor areas during executed and imagined hand movements: an MRI study. Journal of Cognitive Neuroscience 11:491

Lowe A A, Johnston W D 1979 Tongue and jaw muscle activity in response to mandibular rotations in a sample of normal and anterior open-bite subjects. American Journal of Orthodontics 76(5):565–576

Luder H 1993 Articular degeneration and remodeling in human temporomandibular joints with normal and abnormal disc position. Journal of Orofacial Pain 7:391

Lund T, Cohen J 1993 Trismus appliances and indications for use. Quintessence International 24:275

Lund J, Donga R, Widmer C et al 1991 The pain-adaptation model: a discussion of the relationship between chronic musculoskeletal pain and motor activity. Canadian Journal of Physiology and Pharmacology 69:683

Magnusson T 1986 Five year longitudinal study of signs and symptoms of mandibular dysfunction in adolescents. Cranio 4:338

Magnusson T, Carlsson G, Egermark I 1991 An evaluation of the need and demand for treatment of craniomandibular disorders in a young Swedish population. Journal of Craniomandibular Disorders 5:57

Magnusson T, Carlsson G, Egermark I 1994 Changes in clinical signs of craniomandibular disorders from the age of 15 to 25 years. Journal of Orofacial Pain 8:207

Mahan P 1980 The temporomandibular joint in function and pathofunction. In: Solberg W, Clark W (eds) TMJ problems, biologic diagnosis and treatment. Quintessence, Chicago

Maitland G 1991 Peripheral manipulation. Butterworth-Heinemann, Oxford, p 290

Maitland G, Hengeveld E, Banks K, English K 2001 Vertebral manipulation, 6th edn. Butterworth-Heinemann, Oxford

Maixner W, Fillingim R, Sigurdsson A, Kincaid S, Silva S 1998 Sensitivity of patients with painful temporomandibular disorder to experimentally evoked pain: evidence for altered temporal summation of pain. Pain 76:71

Mannheim C, Lavett D 1989 The myofascial release manual. Slack, Thorofare, NJ

Marbach J, Raphael K, Dohrenwend B et al 1990 The validity of tooth grinding measures: etiology of pain dysfunction syndrome revisited. Journal of the American Dental Association 120:327

Marie H, Pietkiewicz K 1997 La bruxomanie: mémoires originaux. Revue de Stomatologie 14:107

McMillan A, Blasberg B 1994 Pain–pressure threshold in painful jaw muscles following trigger point injection. Journal of Orofacial Pain 8:384

McNeil C 1993 Temporomandibular disorders: guidelines for classification, assessment, and management. The American Academy of Orofacial Pain. Quintessence, Chicago

McNulty W, Gevirtz R, Hubbard D, Berkhoff G 1994 Needle electromyographic evaluation of trigger point response to a psychological stressor. Psychophysiology 31:313

Mense S 1997 Pathophysiologic basis of muscle pain; update in diagnosis and treatment, 8. Saunders, Philadelphia

Mense S 1999 Neue Entwicklungen im Verständnis von Triggerpunkten. Manuelle Medizin. Springer, Heidelberg, 37:115

Milidonis M, Kraus S, Segal R, Widmer C 1993 Genioglossi muscle activity in response to changes in anterior/neutral head posture. American Journal of Orthodontics and Dentofacial Orthopedics 103:39

Miller A 1991 The measurement of jaw motions in current controversies in temporomandibular disorders. Quintessence, Chicago, p 118

Molina O, Santos dos J, Nelson S, Grossman E 1997 Prevalence of modalities of headaches and bruxism among patients with craniomandibular disorder. Journal of Craniomandibular Practice 15:314–325

Møller E, Sheikholeslam A, Lous I 1984 Response of elevator activity during mastication to treatment of functional disorders. Scandinavian Journal of Dental Research 92:64

Molofsky H, Scarisbrick P, England R, Smythe H 1975 Musculoskeletal symptoms and non-REM sleep disturbance in patients with 'fibrositis syndrome' and healthy subjects. Psychosomatic Medicine 37:341

Mongini F 1999 Tender and trigger points. In: Headache and facial pain. Thieme, Stuttgart, p 42

Moss R, Adams H 1984 Physiological reactions to stress in subjects with and without myofascial pain dysfunction symptoms. Journal of Oral Rehabilitation 11:219

Müller J, Schmid C, Bruckner G, Vogl T 1992 Morphologisch nachweisbare Formen von intraartikulären Dysfunktionen der Kiefergelenke. Deutsche Zahnärztliche Zeitschrift 33:416

Müller J, Bruckner G, Nerlich A, Schmid C 1993 Articulating surfaces of the temporomandibular joint – a morphological study on autopsy specimens of all age categories. Part 1, upper joint compartment/Part 2, lower joint compartment. Journal of Prosthetic Dentistry 205

Müller-Busch C 1994 Klinik, Pathophysiologie und Therapie des Fibromyalgiesyndroms. Schmerz 8:133

Mulligan R, Clark G 1979 Effects of hypnosis on the treatment of bruxism. Journal of Dental Research 58:323

Murakami K, Nishida M, Beeho K et al 1996 MRI evidence of high signal intensity and temporomandibular arthralgia and relating pain. Does the high signal correlate with pain? British Journal of Oral and Maxillofacial Surgery 34:220

Murphy W 1967 Rest position of the mandible. Journal of Prosthetic Dentistry 17:329

Murray G, Phanachet I, Uchida S, Whittle T 2001 The role of the human lateral pterygoid muscle in control of horizontal jaw movements. Journal of Orofacial Pain 15:279

Newton R 1982 Joint receptor contributions to reflexive and kinesthetic responses. Physical Therapy 62:22

Nguyen T D, Panis X, Froissart D, Legros M, Coninx P, Loirette M 1988 Analysis of late complications after rapid hyperfractionated radiotherapy in advanced head and neck cancers. International Journal of Radiation Oncology, Biology, Physics 14(1):23

Nicolakis P, Nicolakis M, Piehslinger E et al 2000 Relationship between craniomandibular disorders and poor posture. Journal of Craniomandibular Practice 18:106

Ohrbach R, Gale E 1989 Pressure pain thresholds, clinical assessment and differential diagnosis: reliability and validity in patients with myogenic pain. Pain 39:157

Ohrbach R, McCall W 1996 The stress–hyperactivity pain theory of myogenic pain. Proposal for a revised theory. Pain Forum 5:51

Okeson J 1987 The effects of hard and soft occlusal splints on nocturnal bruxism. Journal of the American Dental Association 114:788

Okeson J 1995 Pains of muscular origin. In: Bell's orofacial pains, 5th edn. Quintessence, Chicago, p 259

Okeson J 1996 Orofacial pain: guidelines for assessment, diagnosis and management. The Academy of Orofacial Pain. Quintessence, Chicago, p 113

Olmi P, Cellai E, Chiavacci A, Fallai C 1990 Accelerated fractionation in advanced head and neck cancer: results and analysis of late sequelae. Radiotherapy and Oncology 17(3): 199

Ormeno G, Miralles R, Loyola R et al 1999 Body position effects on EMG activity of the temporal and suprahyoid muscles in healthy subjects and in patients with myogenic cranio-cervical-mandibular dysfunction. Journal of Craniomandibular Practice 17(2):132–142

Palla S, Koller M, Airoldi R 1998 Befunderhebung und Diagnose bei Myoarthropathien. In: Myoarthropathien des Kausystems und orofaziale Schmerzen. Fotoplast, Zürich, p 73

Perthes R, Gross S 1995 Disorders of the temporomandibular joint. In: Clinical management of the temporomandibular disorders and orofacial pain. Quintessence, Chicago, p 69

Phanachet I, Wanigaratne K, Whittle T, Uchida S, Peeceeyen S, Murray G 2001 A method for standardizing jaw displacements in the horizontal plane while recording single motor unit activity in the human lateral pterygoid muscle. Journal of Neuroscience Methods 105:201

Poulsen P 1984 Restricted mandibular opening (trismus). Journal of Laryngology and Otology 98:1111

Proffit W 1993 Fixed and removable appliances in contemporary orthodontics, 2nd edn. Mosby, St Louis, p 318

Quintner J, Cohen M 1994 Referred pain of peripheral nerve origin: an alternative to the 'myofascial pain' construct. Clinical Journal of Pain 10:243

Ramachandran V, Blakesee S 1998 Phantoms in the brain. William Morrow, New York

Rao V 1995 Imaging of the temporomandibular joint. Seminars in Ultrasound, CT and MR 16:513

Rasmussen O 1983 Temporomandibular arthropathy. Clinical, radiologic and therapeutic aspects with emphasis on diagnosis. International Journal of Oral Surgery 12:365

Recanzone G 2000 Cerebral cortical plasticity. In: Gazzaniga M (ed.) The new cognitive neurosciences, 2nd edn. MIT Press, Cambridge

Reeves J, Jaeger B, Graff-Radford S 1986 Reliability of the pressure algometer as a measure of myofascial trigger point sensitivity. Pain 24:313

Reid K, Gracely R, Dubner R 1994 The influence of time, facial side, and location on pain pressure thresholds in chronic myogenous temporomandibular disorder. Journal of Orofacial Pain 8:258

Reitinger A, Radner H, Tilscher H, Hanna M, Windisch A, Feigl W 1996 Morphologische Untersuchung und Triggerpunkte. Manuelle Medizin. Springer, Heidelberg, 34:256

Rocabado M 1983 Biomechanical relationships of the cranial, cervical and hyoid regions. Journal of Craniomandibular Practice 1:61

Rocabado M, Iglash Z 1991 Musculoskeletal approach to maxillofacial pain. J B Lippincott, Philadelphia

Rosenbaum M, Ayllon T 1993 Treating bruxism with the habit reversal technique. Behaviour Research and Therapy 19:87–96

Rugh J, Drago C 1981 Vertical dimension: a study of clinical rest position and jaw muscle activity. Journal of Prosthetic Dentistry 45:670

Rugh J, Montgomery G 1987 Physiological reactions of patients with TM disorders vs. symptom-free controls on a physical stress task. Journal of Craniomandibular Disorders, Facial and Oral Pain 1:243

Sakai S, Kubo T, Mori N et al 1988 A study of the late effects of radiotherapy and operation on patients with maxillary cancer. A survey more than 10 years after initial treatment. Cancer 62(10):2114

Salter R, Field P 1960 The effects of continuous compression on living articular cartilage. Journal of Bone and Joint Surgery 42A:31–49

Salter R, Hamilton H, Wedge J et al 1983 Clinical application of basic research on continuous passive motion for disorders and injuries of synovial joints: a preliminary report of a feasibility study. Journal of Orthopaedic Research 1:325

Sauerland E, Mitchell S 1975 Electromyographic activity of intrinsic and extrinsic muscles of the human tongue. Texas Reports on Biology and Medicine 33:258

Schiffman E, Anderson G, Fricton J et al 1992 The relationship between level of mandibular pain and dysfunction and stage of temporomandibular joint internal derangement. Journal of Dental Research 71:1812

Schwenzer N, Ehrenfeld M 2002 Spezielle Chirurgie. Thieme, Stuttgart

Selms van M K, Lobbezoo F, Wicks D J, Hamburger H L, Naeije M 2004 Craniomandibular pain, oral parafunctions, and psychological stress in a longitudinal case study. Journal of Oral Rehabilitation 31(8):738–745

Sessle B 1995 Masticatory muscle disorders: basic science perspectives. In: Sessle B, Bryant P, Dionne R (eds) Progress in pain research and management, Vol. 4. Temporomandibular disorders and related pain conditions. IASP Press, Seattle, p 47

Sessle B 2000 Acute and chronic craniofacial pain: brain stem mechanisms of nociceptive transmission and neuroplasticity, and their clinical correlates. Critical Reviews in Oral Biology and Medicine 11:57

Shakespeare D, Stokes M, Sherman K, Young A 1985 Reflex inhibition of the quadriceps after meniscectomy: lack of association with pain. Clinical Physiology 5:137

Shankland W 1993 Capsulitis of the temporomandibular joint. Journal of Craniomandibular Practice 11:75

Sharmann S 2002 Diagnosis and treatment of movement impairment syndromes. Mosby, St Louis, p 9

Sharp J, Druz W, Danon J et al 1976 Respiratory muscle function and the use of respiratory muscle electromyography in the evaluation of respiratory regulation. Chest 70(Suppl.):150

Simons D 1975 Muscle pain syndromes (Part I and II). American Journal of Physical Medicine 54:288, 55:288; 55:15

Simons D 1988 Myofascial pain syndrome due to trigger points. In: Goodgold J (ed.) Rehabilitation medicine. Taylor and Francis, St Louis, Chapter 45, p 686

Simons D 1990 Muscular pain syndromes. Advances in Pain Research and Therapy 17:1

Simons D 1997 Triggerpunkte und Myogelose. Manuelle Medizin. Springer, Heidelberg, 35:290

Simons D, Hong C 1995 Prevalence of spontaneous electrical activity at trigger spots and control sites in rabbit muscle. Journal of Musculoskeletal Pain 3:35

Simons D, Mense S 1998 Understanding and measurement of muscle tone as related to clinical muscle pain. Pain 75:1

Simons D, Travell J, Simons L 1999 Myofascial pain and dysfunction. The trigger point manual. Vol. 1

Upper half of the body, 2nd edn. Williams and Wilkins, Baltimore
Slavicek R 2000 Evolution. Das Kausystem. Med Wiss Fortbildungsgesellschaft, Klosterneuburg, p 17
Solberg W, Flint R, Brantner J 1972 Temporomandibular joint pain and dysfunction: a clinical study of emotional and occlusal components. Journal of Prosthetic Dentistry 28:412
Stauber W, Clarkson P, Fritz V, Evans W 1990 Extracellular matrix disruption and pain after eccentric muscle action. Journal of Applied Physiology 69:868
Steelman R, Sokol J 1986 Quantification of trismus following irradiation of the temporomandibular joint. Missouri Dental Journal 66:21
Sterling M, Juli G, Wright A 2001 The effect of musculoskeletal pain in motor activity and control. Journal of Pain 3:135
Stohler C, Zhang X, Lund J 1996 The effect of experimental jaw muscle pain on postural muscle activity. Pain 66:215
Stokes M, Cooper R 1993 Physiological factors influencing performance of skeletal muscle. In: Crosbie J, McConnell J (eds) Key issues in musculoskeletal physiotherapy. Butterworth-Heinemann, Oxford
Svensson P 2001 Craniofacial muscle pain: review of mechanisms and clinical manifestations. Journal of Orofacial Pain 15:117
Svensson P, Arendt-Nielsen L, Houe L 1995 Sensory–motor interactions of human experimental unilateral jaw muscle pain: a quantitative analysis. Pain 64:241
Svensson P, Houe L, Arendt-Nielsen L 1997 Bilateral experimental muscle pain changes electromyographic activity of human jaw-closing muscles during mastication. Experimental Brain Research 116:182
Svensson P, Arendt-Nielsen L, Houe L 1998a Muscle pain modulates mastication: an experimental study in humans. Journal of Orofacial Pain 12:7
Svensson P, Graven-Nielsen T, Arendt-Nielsen L 1998b Mechanical hyperesthesia of human facial skin induced by tonic painful stimulation of jaw-muscles. Pain 74:93
Svensson P, Graven-Nielsen T, Matre D, Arendt-Nielsen L 1998c Experimental muscle pain does not cause long-lasting increases in resting electromyographic activity. Muscle and Nerve 21:1382
Thilander B 1961 Innervation of the temporomandibular joint capsule in man. Transactions of the Royal Schools of Dentistry, Stockholm and Umeå 7:1
Thomas F, Ozanne F, Mamelle G, Wibault P, Eschwege F 1988 Radiotherapy alone for oropharyngeal carcinomas: the role of fraction size (2 Gy vs 2.5 Gy) on local control and early and late complications. International Journal of Radiation, Oncology and Biological Physics 15(5):1097
Thorpy M (ed.) 1990 Parasomnias. In: International classification of sleep disorders: diagnostic and coding manual. American Sleep Disorders Association. Allen Press, Rochester, MN, p 142
Travell J 1976 Myofascial trigger points: clinical view. In: Bonica J, Albe-Fessard D (eds) Advances in pain research and therapy, Vol. 1. Raven Press, New York, p 919
Travell J, Simons D 1983 Myofascial pain and dysfunction. In: The trigger point manual, Vol. 1. Williams and Wilkins, Baltimore, p 5
Travell J, Simons D 1992 Myofascial pain and dysfunction. In: The trigger point manual, Vol. 2. Williams and Wilkins, Baltimore
Travell J, Simons D 1999 Myofascial pain and dysfunction. In: The trigger point manual, Vol. 1. Upper half of body, 2nd edn. Williams and Wilkins, Baltimore
Trott P 1986 Examination of the temporomandibular joint. In: Grieve G (ed.) Modern manual therapy of the vertebral column. Churchill Livingstone, Edinburgh, 48:521
Tschopp K, Bachmann R 1992 Das temporomandibuläre Myoarthropathiesyndrom – eine häufige Ursache für Gesichtsschmerzen. Schweizerische Rundschau für Medizin Praxis 81:468
Tsujii Y 1993 Myotherapy: treatment of muscle hardening. Nagoya University College of Medical Technology, Nagoya
Türp J, Kowalski C, Stohler C 1997 Temporomandibular disorders: pain outside the head and face is rarely acknowledged in the chief complaint. Journal of Prosthetic Dentistry 78:592
van den Berg G 1999 Angewandte Physiologie. Das Bindegewebe des Bewegungsapparates verstehen und beeinflussen. Thieme, Stuttgart, p 271
van Wingerden B 1990 Compression and mobilisation in the evaluation of synovial joints. IAS Journal 4
van Wingerden B 1997 Connective tissue and rehabilitation. Scipro, Vaduz
Vecchiet L, Dragani L, Bigontina P, Obletter G, Giamberardino M 1993 Experimental referred pain and hyperalgesia from muscles in humans. In: Vecchiet L, Albe-Fessard D, Lindblom U (eds) Pain research and clinical management, Vol. 7. New trends in referred pain and hyperalgesia. Elsevier, Amsterdam, 114:390
Vlaeyen J, Crombez G 1999 Fear of movement/(re)injury, avoidance and pain disability in chronic low back pain patients. Manual Therapy 4:187
Wall P 1995 Independent mechanisms converge on pain. Nature Medicine 1:740

Wang K, Svensson P, Arendt-Nielsen L 1999 Modulation of exteroceptive suppression periods in human jaw-closing muscles by local and remote experimental muscle pain. Pain 82:253

Weinberger L 1977 Traumatic fibrositis: a critical review of an enigmatic concept. Western Journal of Medicine 127:99

Westesson P, Bronstein S, Liedberg J 1985 Internal derangement of the temporomandibular joint. Morphologic description with correlation to joint function. Oral Surgery, Oral Medicine, Oral Pathology 59:323

Westling L 1989 Craniomandibular disorders and general joint mobility. Acta Odontologica Scandinavica 47:293

Westling L, Mattiasson A 1991 General joint hypermobility and temporomandibular joint derangement in adolescents. Annals of the Rheumatic Diseases 51:87

Westling L, Carlson G, Hellkimo M 1990 Background factors in craniomandibular disorders with special reference to general joint hypermobility, parafunction and trauma. Journal of Craniomandibular Disorders, Facial and Oral Pain 4:89

Widmalm S, Christiansen R, Gunn S 1995 Oral parafunctions as temporomandibular disorder risk factors in children. Journal of Craniomandibular Practice 13:242

Williams P, Warwick R, Dyson M, Bannister L (eds) 1989 Gray's anatomy, 37th edn. Churchill Livingstone, Edinburgh, p 569

Wilson-Pauwels L, Akesson E, Stewart P, Spacey S 2002 Cranial nerves in health and disease. Decker, London, p 215

Woolf C 1984 Long term alteration in the excitability of the flexion reflex produced by peripheral tissue injury in the chronic decerebrate rat. Pain 18:325

Wyke B 1972 Articular neurology – a review. Physiotherapy 58:94

Yamaguchi T, Kaoru Satoh K, Komatsu K et al 2002 Electromyographic active jaw-closing muscles during jaw opening in patients with masseter muscle contracture. Journal of Craniomandibular Practice 20:1

Yang X, Pernu H, Pythinien J et al 2001 MRI findings concerning the lateral pterygoid muscle in patients with symptomatic TMJ hypermobility. Cranio 19:260–268

Yemm R 1986 A neurophysiological approach to the pathology and aetiology of temporomandibular dysfunction. Journal of Oral Rehabilitation 12:343

Yu X, Hu J, Vernon H, Sessle B 1992 Temporomandibular inflammatory irritant induces increased activity of jaw muscles. Journal of Dental Research 72:603

Zaki H, Greco C, Rudy Th, Kubinski J 1996 Elongated styloid process in a temporomandibular disorder sample: prevalence and treatment outcome. Journal of Prosthetic Dentistry 75:399

Zusman M 1998 Central nervous system contribution to mechanically produced motor and sensory responses. Australian Journal of Physiotherapy Monograph 3:75

Chapter 10

Craniomandibular dysgnathia: orthodontic classification, assessment and management

Antonia Werres

CHAPTER CONTENTS

INTRODUCTION

Despite the lack of scientific evidence, many years of empirical observation have shown that chronic pain syndromes – including non-specific facial pain, chronic headaches, craniocervical pain and even pelvic floor dysfunctions – can potentially be influenced by craniomandibular disorders (CMD). In some cases the craniomandibular disorder remains without symptoms whereas secondary problems caused by the CMD become relevant for the patient. Treating the symptoms rather than the causes will not result in long-lasting relief and an interdisciplinary search for the source of the dysfunction becomes necessary.

The temporomandibular joint (TMJ) is the only joint of the human body that is not only dominantly guided by muscular forces but is also influenced by the alignment of the teeth. As the position of the mandible and the posture of the trunk influence each other, changes of the occlusal relationships may lead to changes of the position and function of the mandible as well as postural changes (Kaufman 1980, Rocabado 1983, Makofsky et al 1989, Huggare & Raustia 1992, Esposito et al 1993, Kopp & Plato 1996, Plato & Kopp 1996, Fink et al 2003). The reverse is also true; craniocervical dysfunction may cause changes of the TMJ, the position of the mandible and the occlusion of the teeth (Balters 1964, Schöttl 1991, Capurso et al 1992, Kopp & Plato 1995, Slavicek 2000) (Fig. 10.1).

These interactions are controlled by the neuromuscular system which is responsible for the physiological function of muscular activities. These include the whole spectrum of the masticatory system functions, i.e. chewing, swallowing, speech (speaking), parafunctions such as clenching and grinding as well as the posture of the head, all of which are controlled by proprioceptive receptors of the craniomandibular system. Dysfunctional occlusion may be important in the development of craniomandibular dysfunction as the teeth may be responsible for functional interference of free movement of the lower jaw.

Besides genetic influences, functional influences play an important role for the development of dysgnathia. A complex interaction among multiple factors (genetic causes, external causes) results in malocclusion and it is usually impossible to describe a specific aetiologic factor.

Malocclusion may already be present in early childhood during development of the milk teeth, and might be carried on to permanent dentition. For example, incongruent dental arches in the primary dentition might cause a non-ideal occlusion such that the lower jaw frequently changes position to compensate. Functional influences such as prolonged use of pacifiers or thumb-sucking can also lead to malocclusion (Schopf 2000, Slavicek 2000).

During growth, malocclusion will be followed by functional and structural adaptation of the dentoalveolar and craniomandibular regions. When growth is complete the TMJs maintain a small but important range of adaptation capacity, so that throughout life a certain amount of remodelling and adaptation is performed (Bumann & Lotzmann 2000).

Since the capacity to adapt rapidly diminishes after growth is complete, the development of craniomandibular disorders becomes possible, usually presenting itself with incipient pain in the TMJ region. The occurrence of atypical facial pain, otalgia or tinnitus, tension headaches and craniocervical dysfunction often tends to become chronic and refractory to any orthopaedic therapy (Kopp & Plato 2001).

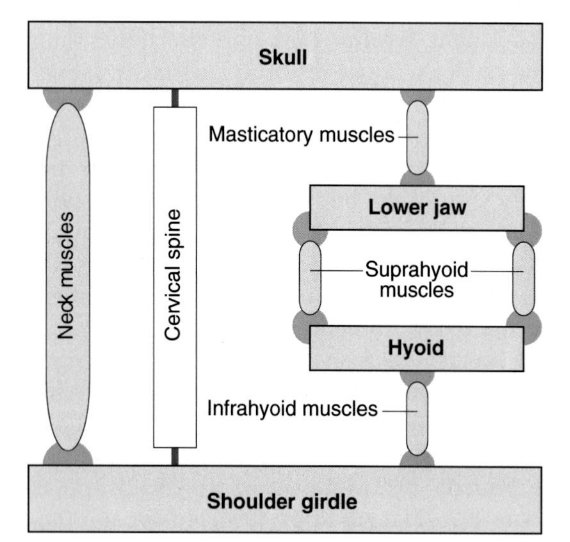

Fig. 10.1 The mandibular region as part of a functional chain including the craniocervical region, the hyoid, the cranium and the rest of the body.

CLASSIFICATION OF POSITIONAL ANOMALIES

The human permanent dentition consists of 32 teeth, following primary dentition with only 20 (milk) teeth.

The dentition is divided into four quadrants and each tooth is given a number from 1 (mesial incisor tooth) to 8 (wisdom tooth). Each quadrant (from mesial to distal) consists of two incisor teeth, one canine tooth, two premolar teeth and three molar teeth.

The dental arches can be formed in a variety of shapes. Generally the upper dental arch shows an ellipsoid form if viewed from above, whereas the lower dental arch is shaped parabolically.

For classification, the publication by Edward H. Angle at the beginning of the 20th century is usually used. Based on his postulate that the upper first molars were the key to occlusion he described three classes of malocclusion (Angle

1913). More detailed classifications, including causes and characteristics of the different types of dysgnathia, have been developed but have not become popular clinically.

For classification, generally the position of the canines and first molars on each side is used. Angle considered only the first molars in his definition. As he regarded this tooth as definitive, the position of a tooth's antagonists was defined in fractions of premolar width towards mesial, distal or neutral.

ANGLE CLASS I: NORMAL OCCLUSION

The upper and lower molars should be related so that the mesiobuccal cusp of the first upper molar occludes in the buccal groove of the first lower molar.

If the dental arches are congruent, there is a 1:2 relation of the teeth with the lower mesial incisor tooth and the distal molar only having one antagonist. The eugnath dentition shows a horizontal and vertical overbite of 2–2.5 mm.

The eugnath dentition is seen as the ideal constellation of teeth and is therefore used as a reference (Fig. 10.2).

ANGLE CLASS II/1: OVERBITE

The first lower molar is positioned distally relative to the first upper molar. The maxillary incisors are protruded, forming an increased overjet.

Increased overjet, usually in combination with a retruded mandible, is characteristic of this form of dysgnathia. Further principal symptoms commonly observed in Angle class II/1 disorders are protrusion of the incisors, narrow transverse dental arches, especially in the maxilla, caused by adaptation to the retruded mandible (Fig. 10.3) and an elongated mandibular front.

Patients classified as type II/1 frequently show a so-called 'double-bite' meaning that the TMJs are in a habitually protruded position, supported retrally by the bilaminal zone. This constellation can become symptomatic (Slavicek 2000).

Aetiology

Commonly, a combination of skeletal and dental causes is responsible for the development of malocclusion. It is difficult to differentiate between exogenous and endogenous factors. Skeletal abnormalities (e.g. a retrognathic or underdeveloped mandible, or prognathia of the maxilla) are more likely to be genetic if there is a family history, whereas dentoalveolar symptoms point towards exogenic influences. These can be habits such as biting the lips, sucking the lips or thumb-sucking over a prolonged period of time. Trauma in early childhood such as a condylar fracture, osteomyelitis, ankylosis and juvenile arthritis can also result in growth deficiencies of the jaw.

Clinical implications

In many respects, retrusion leads to both functional and aesthetic limitations.

Biting and chewing are restricted by the increased sagittal level and singular antagonism, and there is an increased risk of loss of

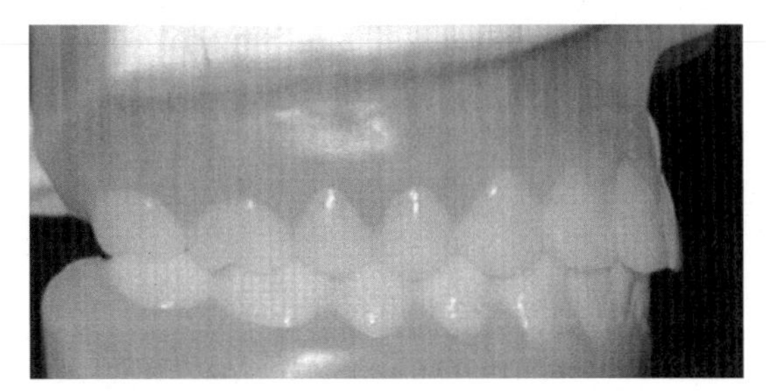

Fig. 10.2 Angle class I dentition.

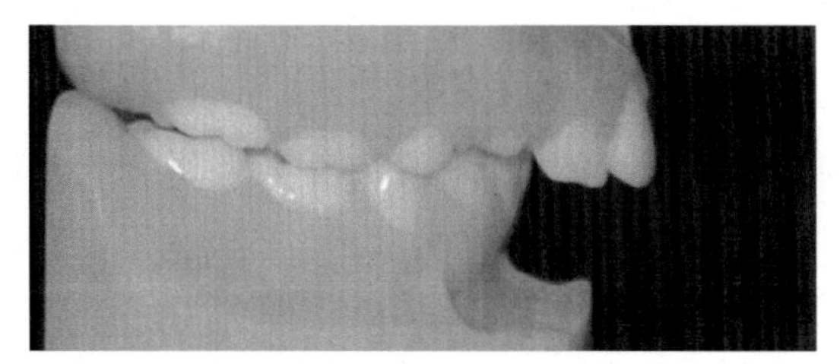

Fig. 10.3 Angle class II/1 dentition.

the protruded incisors through accident or periodontal damage. The double bite may also contribute to the development of arthropathy in these patients.

ANGLE CLASS II/2

The mesiobuccal cusp of the upper first molar is positioned mesially of the buccal groove of the lower first molar. The upper incisors are retroinclined.

Steeply inclined front and canine teeth are indicative of this type of malocclusion. The overjet is reduced, so that commonly there is contact of the front teeth at the end of closure. Another common symptom is deep overbite so that the lower incisors contact the palate and may cause significant tissue damage (Fig. 10.4).

Aetiology

Patients classified as Angle class II division 2 frequently show hypertrophic perioral facial and masticatory muscles. This strong musculature is responsible for the retroclination of the incisor teeth. These muscles also play a role in the development of a dental and skeletal deep overbite. An alternative explanation might be the lack of support of the front teeth that leads to an overeruption of the incisors. Like class II/1 patients, the influencing endogenous and exogenous factors are difficult to differentiate.

Clinical implications

In contrast to type II/1 patients who do not necessarily suffer from functional deficiencies, these patients develop arthropathy more frequently. Due to the steeply inclined incisor teeth the physiological protrusion-oriented function is reduced. This might lead to an unphysiological load of the joint structures with development of clicking noises and arthropathy. Furthermore, the lack of contact between the upper and lower incisors due to retrusion of the jaw can cause an increase of muscle tone in the craniocervical region. From an aesthetic point of view these patients show a concave profile with a prominent nose.

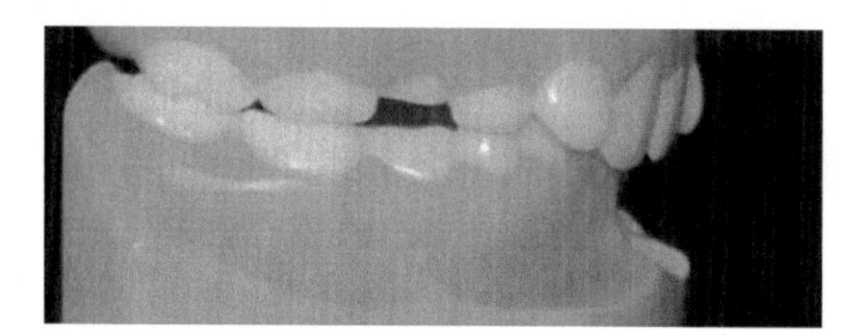

Fig. 10.4 Angle class II/2 dentition.

ANGLE CLASS III: UNDERBITE

The mesiobuccal cusp of the upper molar is positioned distal to the buccal groove of the lower molar (Fig. 10.5).

Various different manifestations of progenia can be distinguished:

- Anterior crossbite: Reverse overjet can be caused by incorrect positioning of the incisor alveolae, even with a neutral jaw base relationship.
- Progenic forced bite: Occlusal interference at the end of occlusion forces the patient to move the jaw ventrally to avoid the interference of occlusion. The base of the jaw can be neutral.

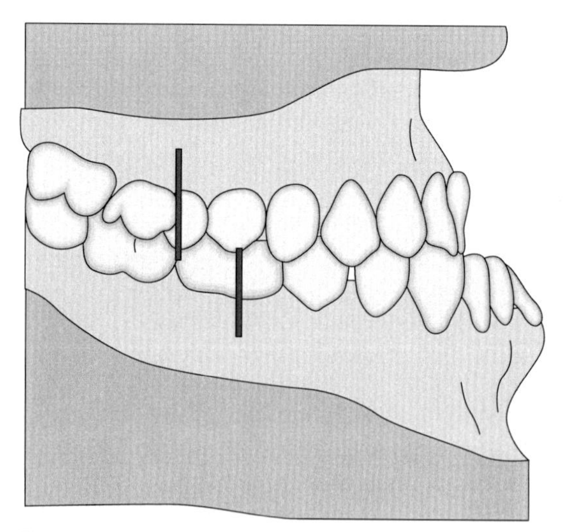

Fig. 10.5 Angle class III dentition.

- Pseudoprogenia: In this case the maxilla is underdeveloped whereas the mandible has developed normally. There is a maxillary sagittal and transverse developmental deficiency with incongruent dental arches, reflected by the occlusion.
- Progenia: The maxilla is normally developed, whereas the mandible is overdeveloped and adopts a mesial bite.

Any of these variants may also appear as mixed clinical pictures.

Aetiology

Genetic factors play an important role for the development of some of the types of progenia. As with class II/1, the skeletal causes of progenic dentition demonstrate an endogenous influence. The family history will help to detect such influences. A well-known example is the 'Habsburg jaw', the prognathic mandible of the Habsburg imperial family, consisting of macrogenia and micrognathia with malocclusion of the side incisors.

Congenitally missing teeth, early loss of teeth and cleft lip/palate can inhibit growth of the upper jaw.

Dentoalveolar symptoms (e.g. progenic forced bite) point towards exogenous factors. Differentiation of these factors can be difficult.

Clinical implications

If class III is compensated, meaning that the upper incisors are massively protruded, the lower front is retruded and there is strong contact between the upper and lower incisors; this may lead (as with class II/2) to a forced distal displacement of the mandible.

Large gaps between the dental arches may disrupt mandibular positioning and lead to problems with the associated articulations and muscles.

In well-compensated class III malocclusion problems are generally aesthetic rather than functional.

OTHER TYPES OF DYSGNATHIA

COVER-BITE/DEEP BITE

Cover-bite malocclusion is characterized by retroinclination of the front and an overbite exceeding 3 mm, which may be so severe as to traumatize the palate. Deep positioning of the maxillary front with neutral molar positioning is called cover-bite, whereas with distal occlusion it is called Angle class II/2. The aetiology and clinical implications of both variants of this malocclusion are similar. Functional free space is limited, with consequences as shown in Figures 10.6 and 10.7.

OPEN BITE

Absent tooth contact in occlusion is characteristic of an open bite. Two clinical variations are distinguished: absent contact of the lateral teeth and of the front teeth. If the incisor teeth and canine teeth do not touch it is called an anterior open bite; a lateral open bite refers to the premolar and molar teeth.

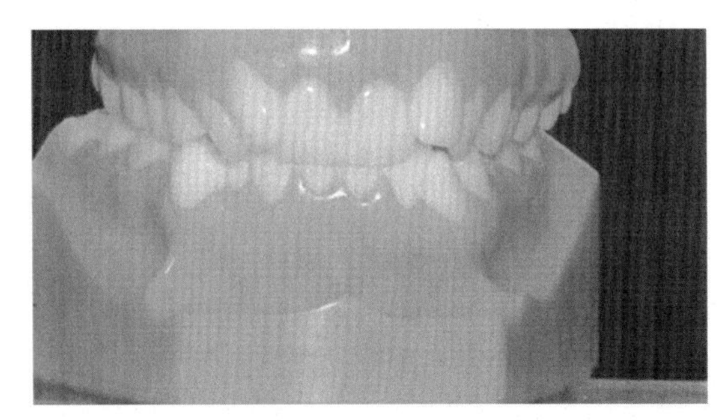

Fig. 10.6 Cover-bite.

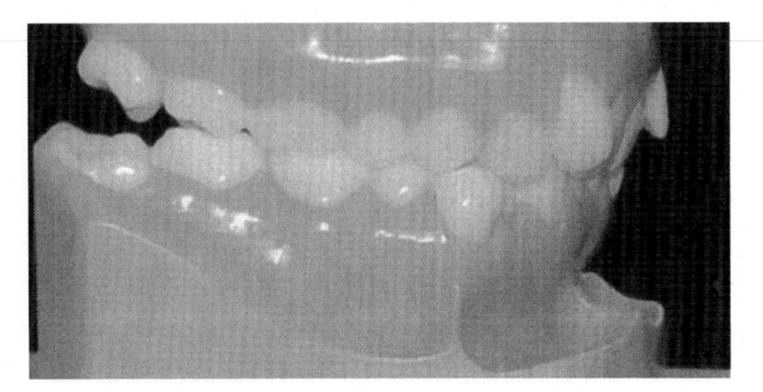

Fig. 10.7 Deep bite.

Aetiology

Again endogenous and exogenous factors are distinguished. Exogenous influences relevant for the development of an open bite are sucking habits, use of pacifiers, tongue thrust, biting of the cheeks and infantile swallowing. The structural open bite is characterized by a dolichofacial viscerocranium and is caused predominantly by genetic factors. Some diseases such as rickets have also been shown to cause deformities that might lead to an open bite.

Clinical implications

An open bite reduces the functions of biting and chewing. Frequently associated symptoms due to the lack of overbite are speech dysfunctions (e.g. sigmatism). Furthermore, the teeth are loaded in an unphysiological manner: some teeth might suffer from overuse or misuse due to habits and dysfunctions. Most patients perceive the open bite as disabling for aesthetic reasons.

CROSSBITE/LATEROGNATHIA

Crossbite, in which one or more lower molars overlap the vestibular surface of an upper molar, is one of the commonest molar occlusal abnormalities. Anything from a single tooth pair to all molar pairs may be affected. Crossbite often occurs in conjunction with laterognathia, displacement of the mandible towards the side of the crossbite. Signs of laterognathia include central deviation with otherwise symmetrical dental arches and lateral offset of the chin away from the centre of the face.

Aetiology

Crossbite with laterognathia is caused by functional influences in many cases. For example, mouth breathers frequently show an underdeveloped upper arch of teeth, especially in the transverse plane. With the tongue lying in a low position, discrepancies between the normally developed lower jaw and the narrow upper jaw become obvious. In occlusion the jaw is shifted to one side to improve the contact position of the teeth. As for all types of dysgnathia the aetiology of the crossbite can be influenced by various endogenous and exogenous factors, and differentiation of these is difficult.

Clinical implications

A crossbite resulting from a single dentoalveolarly malpositioned tooth or a symmetrical bilateral posterior crossbite without mandibular shift may remain without any symptoms. However, laterognathia may have an impact on the joint due to the asymmetric position of the mandible.

Besides the above mentioned malocclusions, malpositioning of single teeth may also limit physiological occlusion, thereby provoking craniomandibular disorders. Insufficient prosthetic or conservational treatment should also be considered where relevant.

ORTHODONTIC EXAMINATION AND TREATMENT

TREATMENT GOALS

The main goal of treating patients suffering from chronic pain syndromes and craniomandibular disorders is to detect and remove the malocclusion which is thought to have an influence on the symptoms and contribute to its resistance to therapy. The provision of an occlusal splint should guide the mandible into a physiological position and eliminate malocclusion After a sufficient stabilization phase it may be possible to adjust the position of the splint into the patient's normal occlusion.

HISTORY AND PHYSICAL EXAMINATION

Initially a detailed history is taken followed by a thorough physical examination. The clinical examination includes palpation of the relevant muscles, manual examination (e.g. following the method of Bumann), a neurological examination and functional observation of occlusion and the condition of the teeth. Magnetic resonance imaging can be helpful in confirming the clinical diagnosis.

Manual functional analysis assists in diagnosis of problems of the TMJ and masticatory musculature. The jaw needs to be investigated for adaptation, compensation and loading vectors if a specific diagnosis is to be determined. Manual orthopaedic techniques are useful here (Bumann & Lotzmann 2000).

Active and passive movements of the joints are assessed for pain and range of motion. The joint itself is examined by the application of compression and translatory movements under compression. Passive compression mainly stresses the bilaminar zone of the TMJ and therefore assesses the load of the joints. Traction and translation are used to assess the joint capsule. In addition to palpation of the masticatory musculature, isometric tests are used to detect asymmetry of strength or lesions of the opening/closing muscles of the jaw. Clicking on opening and/or closing of the mouth is documented regarding quality and timing and potential change after application of manipulation. Any abnormalities are documented on the assessment form.

OCCLUSAL SPLINTS

Occlusal splints are removable instruments, generally made of plastic and intended for temporary use. They are used to adapt the interocclusal contact pattern and thereby change mandibular position and function.

Occlusal splints should sit comfortably without causing stress. They should be small and not damage the gums. There should be equal contact with the molar teeth and front/cuspid guidance. This should be checked regularly and adjusted if necessary. After starting splint use, wearing it all day long may lead to a brief increase in symptoms, which should subside after a few days. There should not be any extreme increase in muscle tone or trigger points. Wearing the splint should not cause any craniomandibular or craniocervical dysfunction.

A great variety of splints have been proposed in the literature. Lotzmann (1998) categorizes the types by their indications:

- Relaxation splints: Are used to normalize muscle tone. The lateral splint surface is smooth so that the jaw can move freely and occlusion is symmetrical. The splint has to ensure posterior clearance upon protrusive anterior and lateral excursions.
- Repositioning splints: Are used to achieve repositioning of discs that are partially or totally displaced anteriorly at maximum intercuspidation. The therapeutic position of this splint is always anterior of maximal intercuspidation and in a craniodorsal position in which the disc–condyle relationship is correct. Repositioning splints should not be used for persistent disc dysfunctions, adaptation of the bilaminar zone or for patients who do not perceive the symptoms as disabling.
- Decompression splints: Are used for TMJs that suffer dorsal or cranial compression if muscles, ligaments or joint capsule prevent articular release. The compressed structures are treated with manual therapy techniques while the splint supports and stabilizes occlusion. The splint will need regular adjustments.
- Stabilizing splints: Are used to stabilize treatment effects achieved in terms of lower jaw positioning and to ensure symmetric occlusion. In contrast to relaxation splints, this appliance shows impressions for the molars to achieve optimal positioning of the mandible. Similar to the relaxation splint, the stabilizing splint is provided with a movement control of the canines. Stabilization splints will need regular adjustments throughout the course of treatments.

When making the occlusal splint the condyles should be in a central position in the fossae. In this position, with a correct disc–condyle relationship, the condyles should be in the furthest possible anterior–superior position in the glenoid fossa. Furthermore, the joint structures should not be loaded and the articular disc should bind the articular condyles together with the articular eminence of the fossae. Tooth contact in this position is defined as the retral contact position. In most cases this position is different from maximal intercuspidation. The retral contact position is the desired reference position for splint adjustment.

There are a number of methods available to find a patient's retral contact position, for example manual bite-taking, mainly using wax. The mandible is moved into the retral reference position by the therapist, but without using pressure. Skilled practitioners can obtain reproducible results this way. However, it can often be difficult to obtain satisfactory results using this method in patients with strong muscle bracing.

The advantage of an instrumental functional analysis is documentation of reproducibility. Adjustments of the splint can easily be performed by relying on the measured and documented data.

One type of instrument commonly used is the Gerber registration. Movements of the mandible guided by the masticatory muscles are documented on a plate. An electronic device has been developed (IPR by Prof. Vogel) using a standardized pressure on the registration plate.

A further instrument for the analysis of jaw function is paraocclusal axiography. The method used depends on the therapist's personal preference. The data obtained are transferred to an articulator in which the occlusal splint is manufactured by a laboratory. The splint should show even contact of the molar teeth on occlusion; during excursions posterior clearance is required.

The occlusal splint should be worn throughout the day and only taken out for hygienic procedures. This way the negative influences of malocclusion are reduced to a minimum.

PHYSIOTHERAPEUTIC TREATMENT

Following an interdisciplinary approach for the treatment of CMD patients the orthodontic procedures should be supported by physiotherapy techniques for the involved structures. During the course of treatment the influence of manual therapy techniques will normalize TMJ function so that the splints will need regular adjustment (Storm 2000). The orthodontist should therefore check the splints after each physiotherapy session and make adjustments for fit if necessary.

Since most physiotherapy practices are not at the same location as the orthodontist it has been found useful to supply the patient with a temporary splint made of silicone for travel to the orthodontist's practice. This will stabilize the treatment result until the orthodontist adapts the splint to the new situation. After a few treatments the function of the craniomandibular system will return to normal so that no more changes of jaw position are to be expected and no more adjustments of the splint become necessary.

At this point, if the patient is free of symptoms and physiotherapist and orthodontist agree on a physiological function, a decision needs to be taken as to whether the splint should be replaced by natural occlusion (Fig. 10.8).

FINAL THERAPY

Generally there is always the possibility of grinding the teeth to an optimal occlusion, to implement restorative or prosthetic changes or to intervene with a combined orthodontic–surgical procedure. A detailed analysis of the choices, depending on the state of individual teeth, occlusion and jaw, will guide the decision-making process.

Some cases of early contact, particularly those involving prosthetic dentition, can often be treated easily using grinding therapy. If more substantial alterations are required, replacement prostheses may be considered.

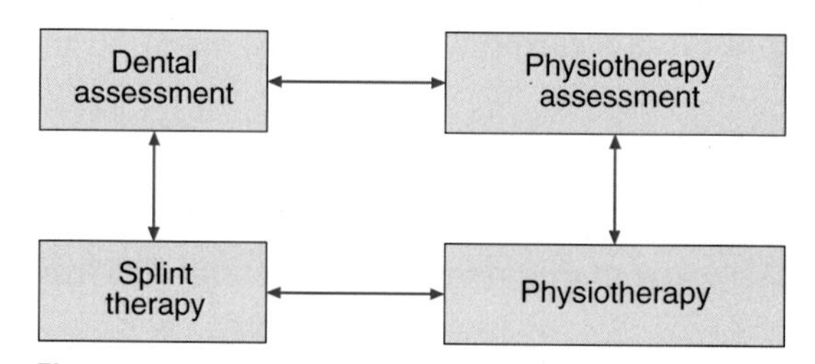

Fig. 10.8 Orthodontic model. A specialized dentist and specialized physiotherapist work together to reach a consensus.

Orthodontics represents the treatment of choice for caries-free dentition without prostheses. The difference between initial dentition and the desired standard of occlusion is rarely so severe that changes can only be effected surgically.

Outlook

Some authors voice objections to irreversible invasive therapies compared to conservative methods since they have not yet been established scientifically (Stohler & Zarb 1999). They argue that the aetiology of CMD cannot be identified clearly enough to support a curative approach. Therefore they recommend reversible procedures for craniomandibular dysfunctions (Greene 2001).

Some studies suggest that occlusal factors do not carry as much weight as was previously assumed (Seligmann & Pullinger 1991a, 1991b, 1996, Clark et al 1999, Kahn et al 1999, De Boever et al 2000, Pullinger & Seligmann 2000). It has also been pointed out that while occlusal abnormalities occur with the same frequency in men as in women, craniomandibular dysfunction occurs more commonly in women (LeResche 1997, Kahn et al 1999).

Occlusion and the craniomandibular system are only ever a part of the picture for therapy of patients with craniofacial and craniocervical dysfunction. Several symptoms, including headache, facial pain, neck ache, tinnitus and dizziness, may be caused by the dysfunction or may indeed be a cause of it. Patients with chronic pain must be assessed for craniomandibular dysfunction and if necessary interdisciplinary therapy must be initiated.

Studies show the interdisciplinary approach for patients with craniomandibular disorders to be the most successful. The results confirm that the simultaneous combination of occlusal splint and manual therapy is superior to other methods (splints followed by manual therapy, splints exclusively, manual therapy exclusively and a control group that did not receive any treatment) (Storm 2000).

Other explanatory approaches propose that successful application of occlusal splint therapy is due to discrete relief of painful musculature of the TMJs because of direct positional change of the mandible, rather than through 'centralisation' of the mandible (Turp 2003).

The interdisciplinary approach with an individual management adapted for every patient is recommended by a number of authors (Clark et al 1990, Garafis et al 1994, De Leeuw et al 1995). Occlusion is just one of several aspects to be considered in the complex pattern of craniomandibular dysfunction. Because of the current paucity of scientific data and frequent technical difficulties in implementation, long-term and irreversible occlusal therapy should be carried out with caution and only in specific cases.

Clarification of other, potentially more serious explanations should always be borne in mind.

References

Angle E H 1913 Die Okklusionsanomalien der Zähne. Meusser, Berlin

Balters W 1964 Die Wirbelsäule aus der Sicht des Zahnarztes. Zahnärztl Mitt 9:408

Bumann A, Lotzmann U 2000 Manuelle Funktionsanalyse und Funktionsdiagnostik und Therapieprinzipien. Thieme, Stuttgart

Capurso U, Perillo L, Ferro A 1992 Cervical trauma in the pathogenesis of cranio-cervico-mandibular dysfunction. Minerva Stomatologica 41:5

Clark G T, Seligman D A, Solberg W K, Pulling A G 1990 Guidelines for the treatment of temporomandibular disorders. Journal of Craniomandibular Disorders, Facial and Oral Pain 4:80

Clark G T, Tsukiyama Y, Baba K, Watanabe T 1999 Sixty-eight years of experimental occlusal interference studies; what have we learned? Journal of Prosthetic Dentistry 82:704–713

De Boever J A, Carlsson G E, Klineberg I J 2000 Need for occlusal therapy and prosthodontic treatment in the management of temporomandibular disorders. Part I. Occlusal interferences and occlusal adjustment. Journal of Oral Rehabilitation 27:367–379

De Leeuw R, Boering G, Stengenga B, de Bont L G 1995 Symptoms of temporomandibular joint osteoarthrosis and internal derangement 30 years after non-surgical treatment. Cranio 13:81

Esposito V, Leisman G, Frankenthal Y 1993 Neuromuscular effects of temporomandibular joint dysfunction. International Journal of Neuroscience 68:205

Fink M, Wahling K, Stiesch-Scholz M, Tschernitschek H 2003 The functional relationship between the craniomandibular system, cervical spine, and the sacroiliac joint: a preliminary investigation. Cranio 21(3):202–208

Garafis P, Grigoriadu E, Zarafi A, Koidis P T 1994 Effectiveness of conservative treatment for craniomandibular disorders: a 2-year longitudinal study. Journal of Orofacial Pain 8:309

Greene C S 2001 The etiology of temporomandibular disorders: implications for treatment. Journal of Orofacial Pain 15:93

Huggare J A, Raustia A M 1992 Head posture and cervicovertebral and craniofacial morphology in patients with craniomandibular dysfunction. Journal of Craniomandibular Practice 10:173

Kahn J, Tallents R H, Katzberg R W, Ross M E, Murphy W C 1999 Prevalence of sental occlusal variables and intraarticular temporomandibular disorders: molar relationship, lateral guidance, and nonworking side contracts. Journal of Prosthetic Dentistry 82:410–415

Kaufman R S 1980 Case reports of TMJ repositioning to improve scoliosis and the performance by athletes. New York State Dental Journal 46:206

Kopp S, Plato G 1995 Pilotstudie zur Beeinflussung der Unterkieferlage durch den funktionellen Zustand der HWS. Manuelle Medizin 33:38

Kopp S, Plato G 1996 The influence of manual therapy on the 3-D-position of the mandible. European Journal of Orthodontics 18:527

Kopp S, Plato G 2001 Kiefergelenk: Dysfunktionen und Schmerzphänomene aus der Sicht interdisziplinärer Diagnostik und Therapie. Kieferorthop 15:55

LeResche L 1997 Epidemiology of temporomandibular disorders: implications for the investigation of etiological factors. Critical Reviews in Oral Biology and Medicine 8:291–305

Lotzmann U 1998 Prinzipien der Okklusion, 5th edn. Neuer Merkur, Munich

Makofsky H W, August B F, Ellis J J 1989 A multidisciplinary approach to the evaluation and treatment of temporomandibular joint and cervical spine dysfunction. Journal of Craniomandibular Practice 7:205

Plato G, Kopp S 1996 Das Dysfunktionsmodell. Manuelle Medizin 34:1–8

Pullinger A G, Seligmann D A 2000 Quantification and validation of predictive values of occlusal variables in temporomandibular disorders using a multifactorial analysis. Journal of Prosthetic Dentistry 83:66–75

Rocabado M 1983 Biomechanical relationship of the cranial, cervical, and hyoid regions. Journal of Craniomandibular Practice 1:62

Schopf P 2000 Kieferorthopädie, Bd 1 und 2. Quintessenz, Berlin

Schöttl W 1991 Die kraniomandibuläre Regulation: interdisziplinäre Betrachtung des neuromuskulären Reflexgeschehens. Hütig, Heidelberg

Seligmann D A, Pullinger A G 1991a The role of functional occlusal relationships in temporomandibular disorders: a review. Journal of Craniomandibular Disorders, Facial and Oral pain 5:265–279

Seligmann D A, Pullinger A G 1991b The role of intercuspal occlusal relationships in temporomandibular disorders: a review. Journal of Craniomandibular Disorders, Facial and Oral Pain 5:95–106

Seligmann D A, Pullinger A G 1996 A multiple stepwise logistic regression analysis of trauma history and 16 other history and dental co-factors in females with temporomandibular disorders. Journal of Orofacial Pain 10:351–361

Slavicek R 2000 Das Kauorgan. Funktionen und Dysfunktionen. Gamma Med Wiss Fortbildungs Ges

Stohler C S, Zarb G A 1999 On the management of temporomandibular disorders: a plea for a low-tech, high-prudence therapeutic approach. Journal of Orofacial Pain 13:255

Storm J 2000 Einfluss zahnärztlicher und manualtherapeutischer Behandlungsmaßnahmen auf die Unterkieferposition und Kiefergelenkbefunde. Dissertation, Universität Kiel

Turp J C 2003 [Myoarthropathy of the temporomandibular joint and masticatory muscles. Pain therapy management and relaxation instead of aggressive surgery.] MMW Fortschritte der Medizin 145(19):33–35

Chapter 11

Craniomandibular contribution to craniocervical dysfunction: management with the aid of neuromuscular splints

Manfred Hülse, Brigitte Losert-Bruggner

CHAPTER CONTENTS

INTRODUCTION

The number of patients suffering from headaches, neck or back pain, together with other dysfunctions such as dizziness, cochlear disorders, tinnitus, vasomotor rhinitis, pharyngeal paraesthesia (globus), concentration difficulties and functional heart symptoms appears to have been increasing steadily over the past few years. On assessment, many of these patients show craniomandibular and craniocervical (occiput, axis to atlas, C3) dysfunctions (Türp 1998, Pilgramm et al 1999, Peroz et al 2000, Peroz 2001, Schorr-Tschudnowski 2001). Effective craniocervical or craniomandibular treatment frequently relieves these complaints. Initially the obvious relationship between craniocervical/mandibular disorders and headaches, dizziness and cochlear complaints including tinnitus (Chole & Parker 1992, Vernon et al 1992, Cooper & Cooper 1999, Peroz 2001), pharyngeal paraesthesia and vocal problems were considered only empirically (Keersmaekers et al 1996, Hülse et al 1998, Meyer 2000, Peroz 2001). Dentists focused their treatment on the craniomandibular region whereas manual therapists, orthopaedic surgeons and ear, nose and throat specialists took care of the craniocervical tissue without recognizing the close relationship of these two regions and hence the requirement for a coordinated approach.

More recent studies have shown interactions between these two systems and demonstrated how craniomandibular dysfunction might influence physiological function of the craniocervical system (Lossert-Bruggner 1998, 2003, Schöttl 2001a, Hülse & Lossert-Bruggner 2002, Hülse et al 2003). Targeted assessment of patients will detect craniomandibular or craniocervical dysfunctions in the majority of cases, even if patients are not aware of pain or functional limitations. Any additional stress such as an infection or 'lying awkwardly' or even a procedure at the dentist may lead to symptoms in the dysfunctional region and thereby reveal hidden structural deficiencies (Losert-Bruggner 2000). If treatment management only focuses on one of the two systems, recurrent symptoms are likely and long-term outcomes tend to be insufficient.

It is generally difficult to distinguish which system became dysfunctional first. This is important for surgeons and insurance assessors, as it can explain why a simple distortion of the neck might be followed by a craniomandibular dysfunction (CMD); or the inverse: being hit on the jaw may cause craniocervical dysfunctions (CCD) either by causing the neck to turn rapidly or by producing a CMD that is followed by a CCD due to reflex mechanisms. Only very rarely will one observe tooth or mandibular abnormalities that are not accompanied by dysfunctions of the craniocervical region (Fig. 11.1).

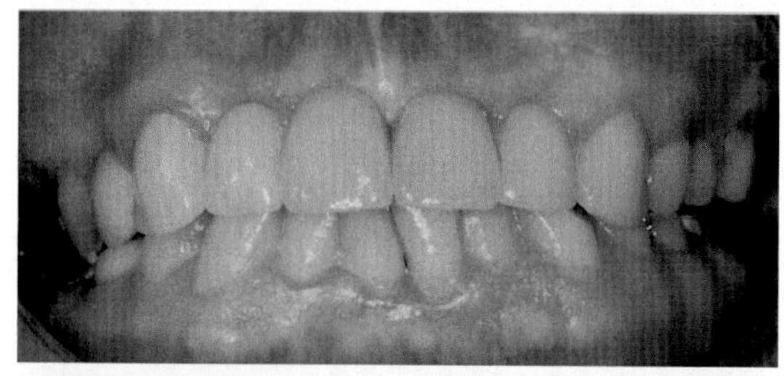

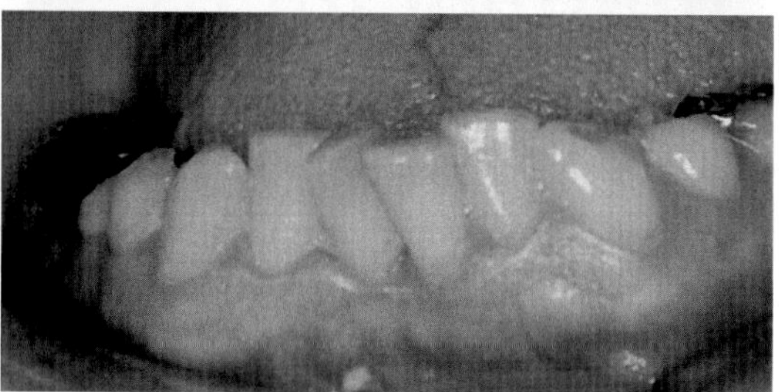

Fig. 11.1 Typical signs of oral dysfunction: overbite, narrow mandibular front, abrasions, chipped teeth. A narrow lower jaw and overbite are clear signs of a retral position of the mandible. Overbite and retral shift of the mandible are the most common oral dysfunctions which are known to cause stress on the craniomandibular and craniocervical systems.

Even patients whose teeth have been orthodontically regulated to an optimum position and who are not aware of any symptoms might show dysfunctions on assessment. This is to be expected whenever there is a neuromuscular imbalance of masticatory, neck and head muscles, even though teeth and jaw are proportional and well developed (Fig. 11.2).

A typical posture is shown in Figure 11.2b. The ventral muscles of the neck are phasic muscles with a tendency to weaken in an unphysiological situation. The dorsal neck muscles are tonic muscles with a tendency to shorten. If this type of muscle imbalance is not treated it will present itself as a head-forward posture. The overbite additionally contributes to the shortness of the dorsal and the weakness of the ventral muscles (Hülse et al 2001, 2003).

Since a CMD might cause a CCV, and a CCV might cause a CMD with positional dysfunction of the mandible, both systems will need to be assessed and treated.

This chapter will focus on the typical clinical features of craniomandibular dysfunctions. Methods to detect muscle imbalance of the masticatory, neck and head muscles will be described, as these are then useful during assessment of occlusion.

The central question for bite-taking should be: In which position should the mandible lie so that it will not cause irritation of the muscles, nerves, blood vessels, ligaments, jaw or craniocervical system? An agreement on the

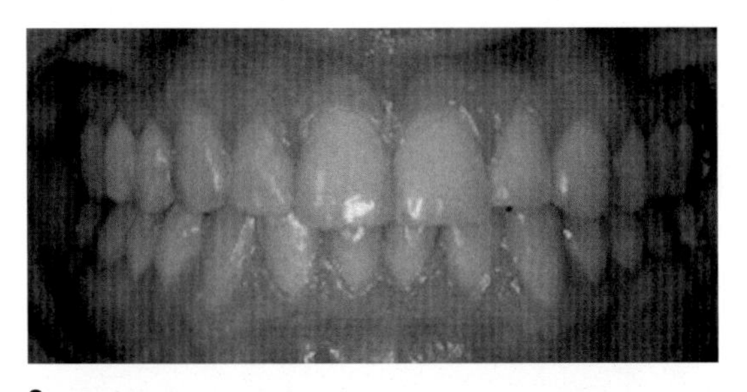

a

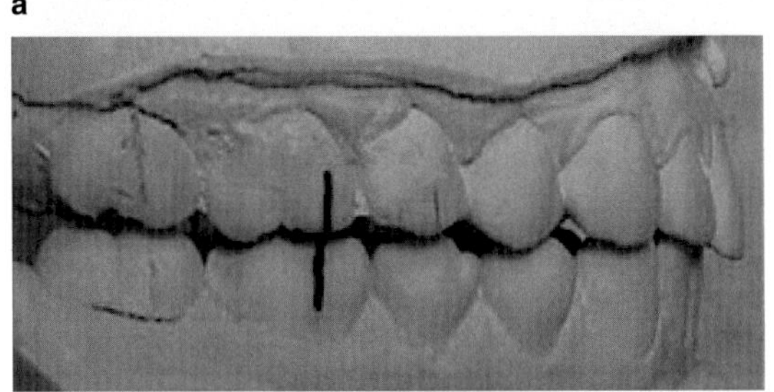

c

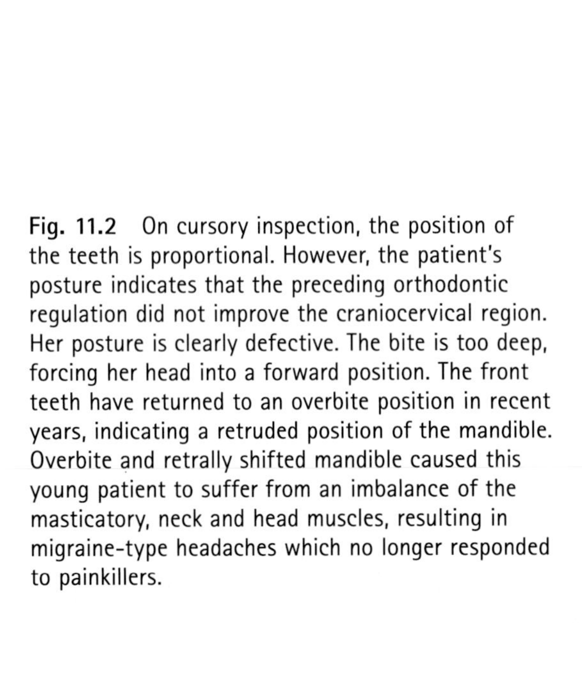

Fig. 11.2 On cursory inspection, the position of the teeth is proportional. However, the patient's posture indicates that the preceding orthodontic regulation did not improve the craniocervical region. Her posture is clearly defective. The bite is too deep, forcing her head into a forward position. The front teeth have returned to an overbite position in recent years, indicating a retruded position of the mandible. Overbite and retrally shifted mandible caused this young patient to suffer from an imbalance of the masticatory, neck and head muscles, resulting in migraine-type headaches which no longer responded to painkillers.

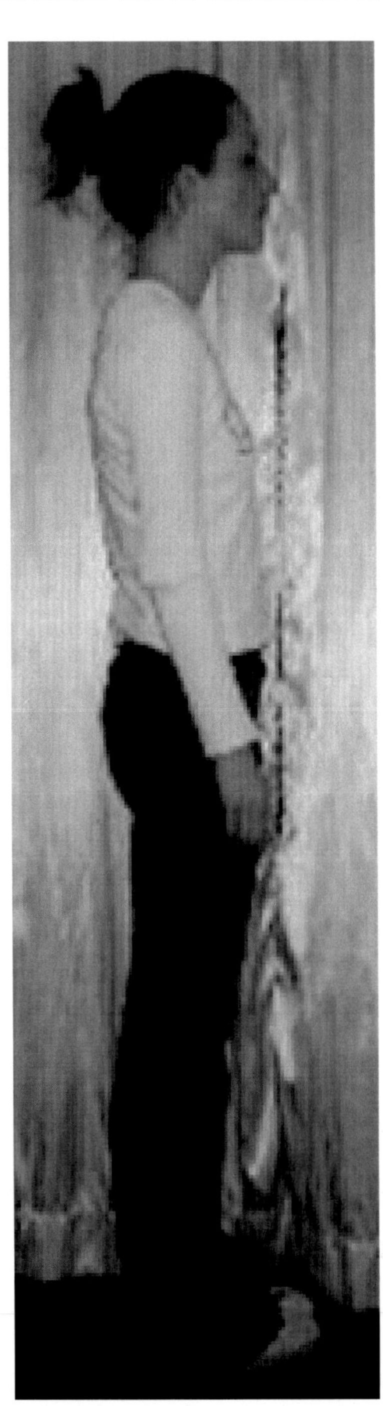

b

optimum position often requires interdisciplinary cooperation of dentist and manipulative physiotherapist.

For an explanation of the different interaction models of the craniocervical and craniomandibular regions, see Chapter 5. If you want to know more about the clinical patterns of CMD, read Chapter 8 first.

THE ROLE OF ELECTROMYOGRAPHY IN THE DIAGNOSIS AND THERAPY OF CMD AND CCD

The reciprocal relationship between the craniocervical and craniomandibular regions and the clinical pattern of CMD will not be expounded upon here as these are dealt with in detail in Chapters 5 and 8.

Albert Einstein defined complexity as 'that which we do not understand'. Dentists and manual therapists involved in the assessment and treatment of facial pain, headaches and craniomandibular dysfunctions will often see pain syndromes where structural causes are difficult to identify. The more we know about CMD and its various presentations the more the dentist will have to assess whether successful management of the problem requires the aid of a co-therapist from another medical discipline. The dentist will also have to decide whether the co-therapist needs to be involved even before starting medical interventions. This decision is sometimes difficult and electromyographic procedures for the neck, masticatory and cranial muscles have been shown to be valuable in the detection and differential diagnosis of craniomandibular dysfunction (Hülse et al 2003). Furthermore, the electromyography parameters might be used as objective reproducible indicators of change within the course of the pathology and the success of the treatment: 'If it has been measured, it is a fact; if it has not been measured, it is an opinion' (Jankelson 1990, Losert-Bruggner 2000).

RESTING EMG

Resting EMG measures the tension of masticatory, cranial and neck muscles while the mandible is at rest. The EMG indicates how well the patient is capable of active muscle relaxation or how effective manual therapy and other techniques are at influencing muscle tension. These are decisive criteria for aligned bite-taking and are also essential for mandibular adaptation using splints. Physiological mandibular position is optimal when the tone of the masticatory muscles is decreased.

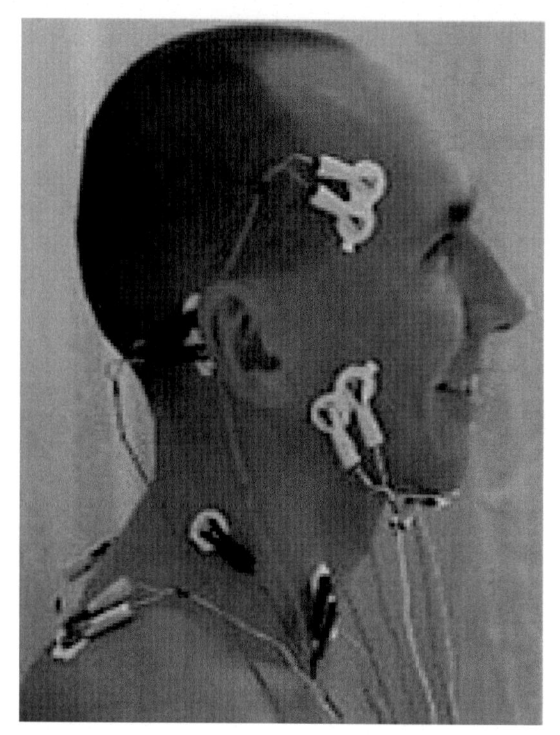

Fig. 11.3 Placement of electrodes for the EMG. Temporalis anterior (LTA, left; RTA, right) and posterior neck muscles (LTP, left; RTP, right), masseter (LMM, left; RMM, right), digastricus anterior (LDA, left; RDA, right) and posterior neck muscles (LDP, left; LDA, right), sternocleidomastoideus (LSM, left; RSM, right), trapezius (LTR, left; RTR, right).

Since clinical muscle tests are not a reliable measurement tool, electromyographic procedures may be used to determine the degree of muscle relaxation. The following muscles should be assessed (Fig. 11.3): temporalis anterior and posterior, masseter, digastricus anterior and posterior neck muscles, sternocleidomastoideus and trapezius. Electromyography also allows for the assessment of other muscles but the muscles mentioned are the ones mainly involved in CMD and CCD.

An example of a resting EMG is outlined in Case study 1.

Case study 1

Mr MH, aged 32 years, presented with a history of tinnitus, neck, back and shoulder pain, craniomandibular complaints and headaches.

The initial resting EMG shows increased activity of masticatory, cranial and neck muscles. After 45 minutes of low-frequency electrotherapy (TENS), distinct relaxation of all muscle groups is observed. Based on this positive result no other interventions were needed for diagnostic and therapeutic bite-taking. Figure 11.4 shows the initial resting EMG (Fig. 11.4a) and after 45 minutes of TENS therapy (Fig. 11.4b).

FUNCTIONAL EMG

Muscle force and quality of occlusion

Measuring the muscle force of the masseter and anterior temporal muscles helps to assess the quality of the occlusion. Strong and symmetrical activity of these muscles points towards a good mandibular position and occlusion of tooth surfaces. If the muscles are weak and muscle force is asymmetrical, occlusal dysfunctions are likely. If the bite force cannot be increased by placing thin pieces of cotton on the lateral teeth, this suggests a weakened masticatory system. The bite force is therefore an important diagnostic parameter for assessing the success of treatment with splint and/or grinding therapy. Any increase in muscle force and symmetry indicates an improvement and shows that the problem can be potentially influenced by the chosen treatment.

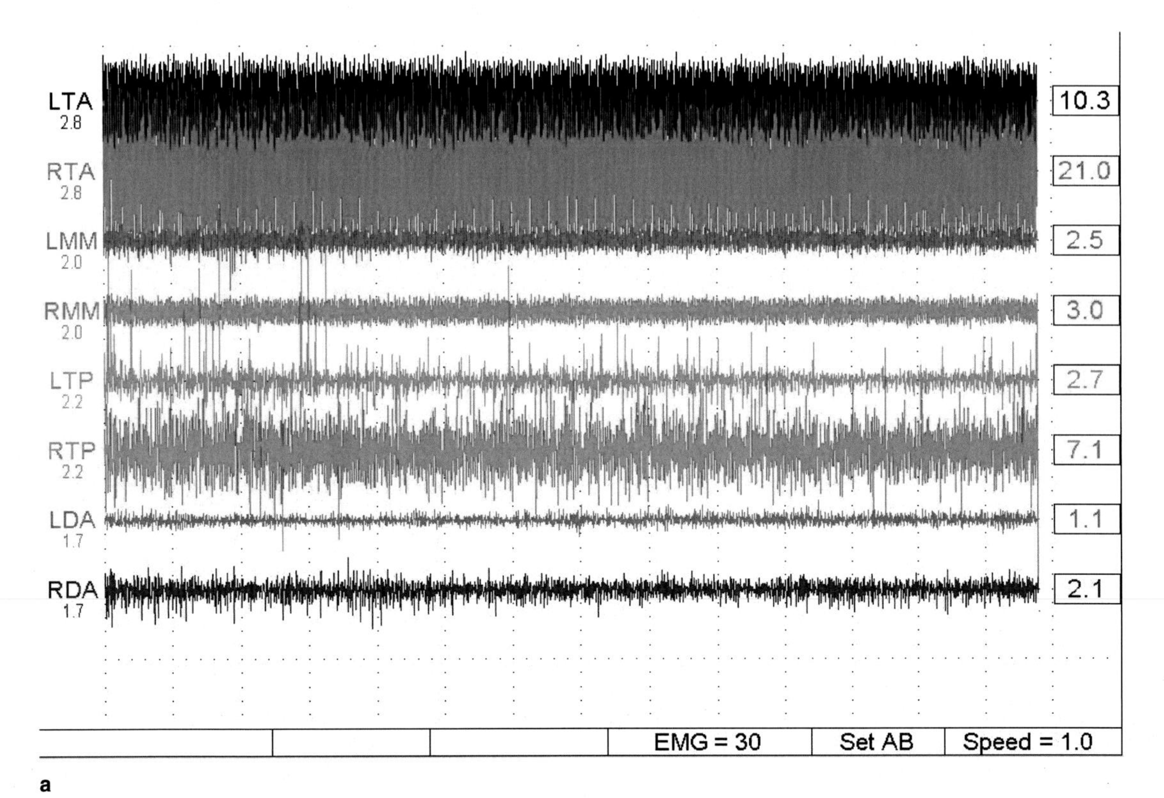

a

Fig. 11.4 EMG-assessment of Case study 1 (Patient MH). The distinct relaxation of all involved muscles enabled bite-taking for neuromuscular mandibular adaptation.
a EMG before treatment. High tension of masticatory, neck and head muscles.
b EMG after 45 minutes of low-frequency TENS therapy on the masticatory muscles.

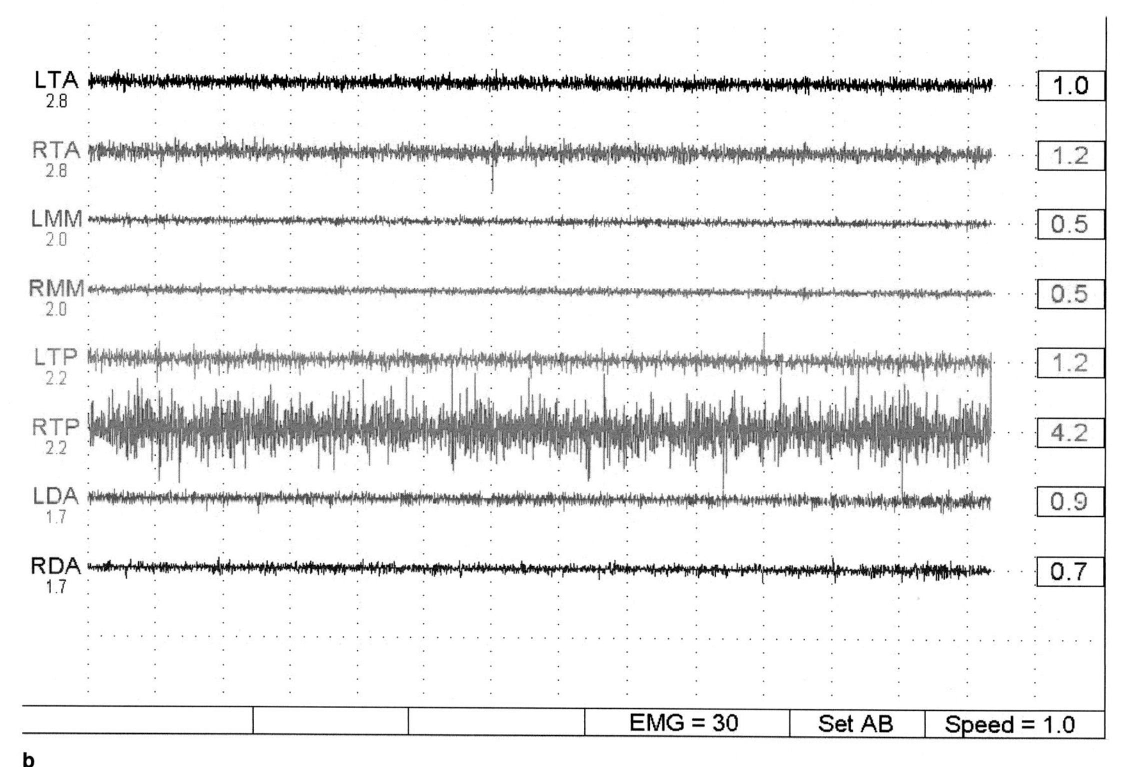

b

Fig. 11.4—cont'd

Symmetry of muscle contraction

The symmetry of muscle contraction of the masseter and anterior temporalis muscles is an important indicator for the quality of the occlusion and the mandible/cranial relationship. If all the muscles are activated at the same time this indicates a good occlusal relationship. If the muscles are activated in an irregular pattern this might indicate an occlusal dysfunction. The muscle activation pattern may also guide the process of identification of the location of the malocclusion and is therefore helpful prior to grinding therapy.

In conclusion, it can be said that electromyographic imaging is helpful in assisting the diagnosis and treatment of craniomandibular and craniocervical dysfunctions. During manual therapy treatment of craniocervical dysfunctions or during neuromuscular management of the masticatory muscles, efficiency of the interventions can be assessed and decisions about treatment options can be supported.

MANDIBULAR KINESIOGRAPHY AS A SUPPORTING METHOD FOR THE DIAGNOSIS AND THERAPY OF CMD AND CCD

A detailed description of the possibilities of mandibular kinesiography would exceed the remit of this chapter; however, the most important movement recording options for the mandible will be described below.

Mandibular kinesiography using, for example, the technology of the company Myotronics (www.myotronics.com) records the movement of the middle front teeth. A magnet fixed on these teeth conducts its magnetic field onto an outer frame that is connected to a computer which records any movement of the jaw (Fig. 11.5). Bradykinesia and dyskinesia become clearly visible. Dysfunctions can be analysed and integrated into overall management.

You may note that the young female patient shown in Figure 11.5 is holding her tongue between her teeth (Fig. 11.5a). Frequently patients use their tongue to prevent malcontact of the teeth and deep bite. The position captured coincidentally on this photograph represented exactly the neuromuscularly adapted jaw position that was achieved later on in the treatment. Recordings of the end of range movements of the mandible (Fig. 11.6) were based on the following questions:

- How far can the patient open the mouth? How far can the patient move the mandible anteriorly and laterally?
- Is the movement inhibited by joint limitations?
- Is the quality of movement influenced by potential muscle imbalances?
- Are any movements limited or impossible due to innervation problems of the masticatory system?

RECORDING THE RESTING POSITION BEFORE AND AFTER NEUROMUSCULAR RELAXATION OF THE MASTICATORY MUSCLES

The resting position of the mandible indicates the distance that needs to be regulated by, for example, splints. The difference between dental occlusion and resting position of the mandible, the so-called interocclusal distance, should be around 1.5–2 mm. If the distance is greater than 2 mm after relaxation of the muscles, an intervention is indicated. On swallowing, the teeth make contact. A human being swallows more than 2000 times a day. If the mandible has to move, say, 4 mm instead of 2 mm, unnecessary muscle force is required. To reduce this strength requirement, the jaw musculature needs to be pulled upwards, such

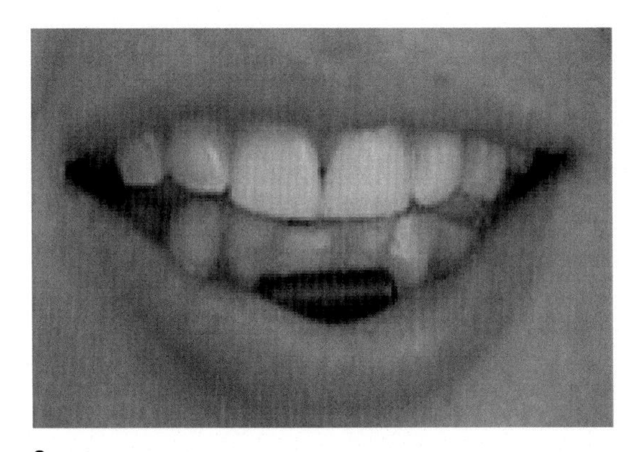

a

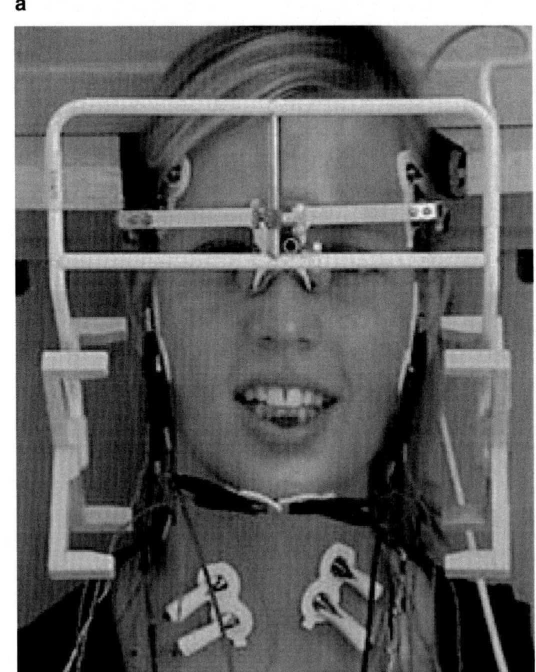

b

Fig. 11.5 Mandibular kinesiography (Myotronics system). The position of the magnet in the centre of the mandible is detected by detectors in the outer frame. This is connected to a computer which records and projects movement onto a screen. The frame is very light (170 g) to prevent it from interfering with muscle activity. Using kinesiography in combination with electromyography is extremely helpful in determining neuromuscular mandibular position adaptation.

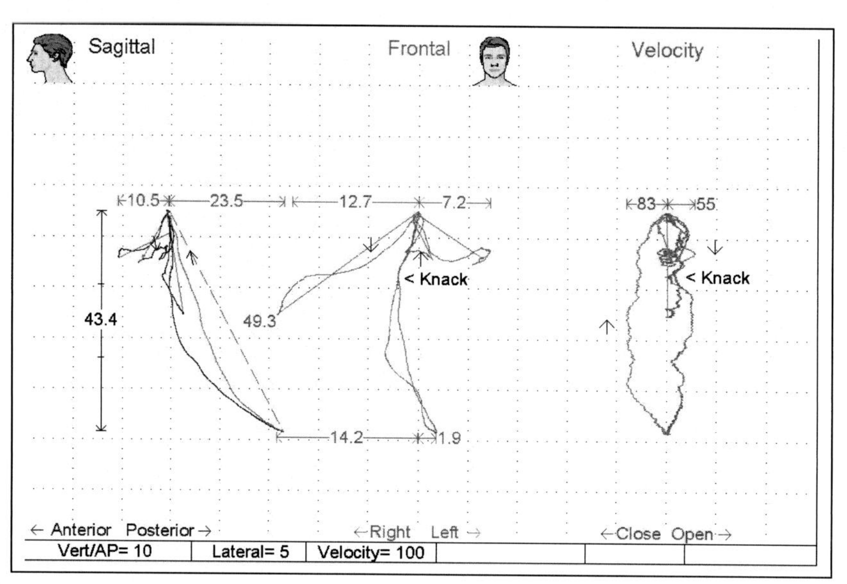

Fig. 11.6 Recorded end of range mandibular mobility (maximum opening, maximum lateral movement and protrusion). Left graphic gives a view from the side, the middle graphic from the front. The right graphic is the velocity curve of the mandible during maximal mouth opening. The movement to the left is significantly decreased. Abnormal deviations are recorded on opening. When the craniomandibular 'click' occurs, the motion curve shows a deceleration of speed. Opening and closing are not performed along the same path, a common indicator of a retral position of the mandible.

that the required tooth contact can be made with less effort and more ergonomically. Thus the jaw muscles always shorten so that a relaxed muscle length can no longer be achieved.

COMPARING THE HABITUAL MOVEMENT PATTERN OF THE MANDIBLE WITH THE MOVEMENT PATTERN AFTER NEUROMUSCULAR RELAXATION

Figure 11.7 shows a comparison of relaxed mandibular movements and the resting position after relaxation of the masticatory, head and neck muscles compared with the habitual closing movement.

Mandibular kinesiography might also help to detect craniomandibular and craniocervical dysfunctions. It provides important information about the type and direction of the treatment approach and about neuromuscular mandibular adaptation in relation to the upper jaw.

THE OCCLUSAL PLANE OF THE MAXILLA AND ITS RELATIONSHIP TO OTHER BODY PLANES

The occlusal plane determines the harmony between the craniomandibular and pelvic regions. If this plane stands at a certain angle towards the base of the skull no dysfunctions of the neuromuscular system are to be expected (Saxer & Czech 1997, Schöttl 2001a). As the sutures are not twisted, the cranium is freely mobile, so that cerebrospinal fluid can circulate freely. The cranium is a compliance system. It will adapt to exogenous forces (e.g. a splint) and may also influence the intracranial structures such as the brain and the cerebrospinal fluid (Oudhof 2001, von Piekartz 2001).

The ideal occlusal plane runs parallel to the 'hamulus-papilla-incisiva plane' (HPI plane). It is determined by three anatomical reference points on the upper jaw. These parts of the upper jaw are not subject to resorption. They remain unchanged throughout life and are

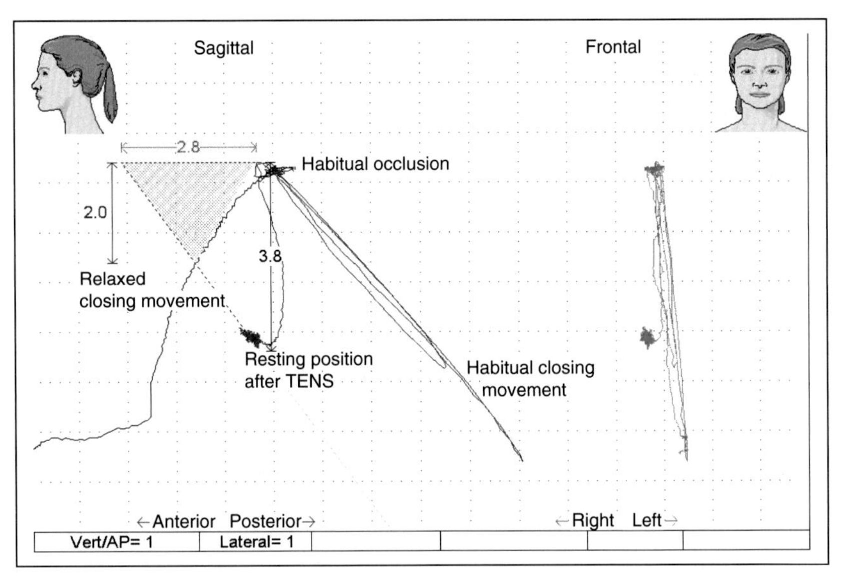

Fig. 11.7 Comparison of neuromuscular relaxed movement path of the mandible with that of habitual mandibular closure. It is clearly visible how the mandible is aiming for a contact position with the upper jaw that is 2.9 mm further anterior. The interocclusal distance after relaxation indicates a raising of the bite by approximately 2 mm. In the frontal plane habitual and relaxed movement patterns are fairly similar.

therefore ideal to indicate the physiological occlusal plane (Figs 11.8 and 11.9).

FUNCTIONAL INVESTIGATION TO CONFIRM UNINHIBITED INTERACTION BETWEEN THE CRANIOMANDIBULAR AND CRANIOCERVICAL REGIONS

Coincidence of a craniomandibular dysfunction and a functional craniocervical dysfunction is very high. Diagnostically, the important question is whether CMD is an attendant symptom to the craniocervical dysfunction and will therefore resolve following successful manual therapy, or whether it is the lead cause of symptoms and is itself causing the craniocervical dysfunction. In general, if a successfully treated craniocervical dysfunction relapses (say three times) within a few weeks, craniomandibular dysfunction should be treated by a specialist.

The same problem is faced by dentists: craniocervical dysfunction often leads to incorrect positioning of the mandible. If splint

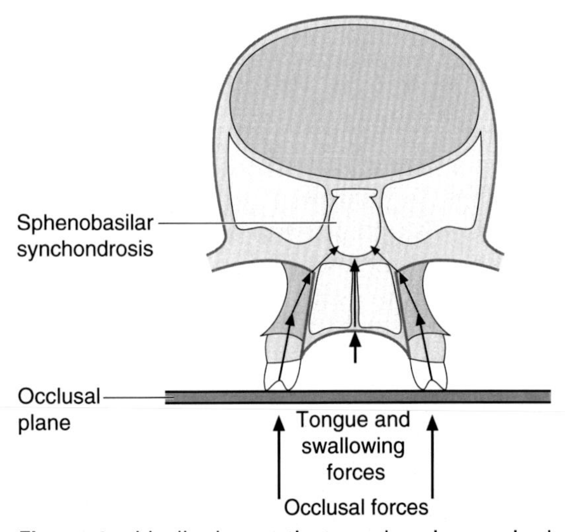

Fig. 11.8 Ideally the masticatory plane is organized symmetrically to the skull base, so that the forces which occur on biting and chewing meet at the sphenoidal synchondrosis. This enables free mobility of the skull sutures and circulation of cerebrospinal fluid. The system can breathe.

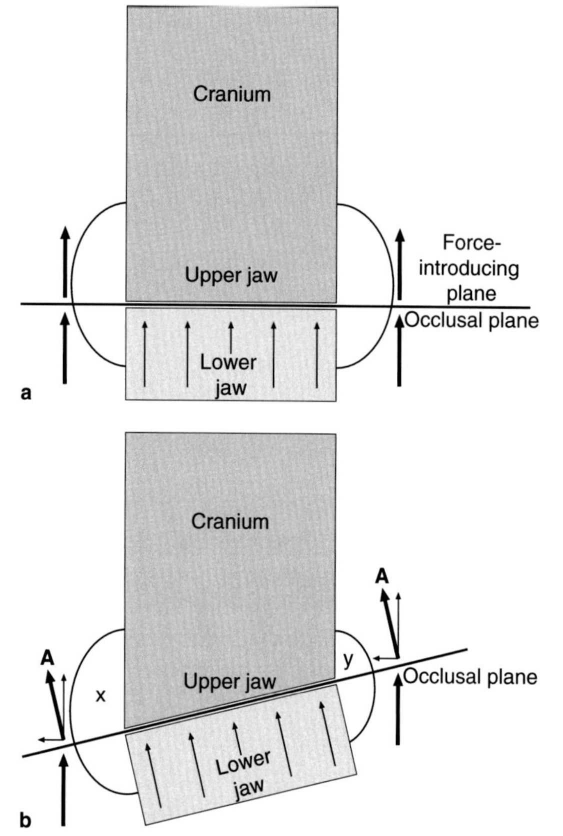

Fig. 11.9 Diagram of forces that occur on biting in symmetrical and asymmetrical occlusal planes. Asymmetrical occlusal planes cause unphysiological loading on the base of the skull. The sutures twist and mobility is impaired. This can inhibit the circulation of cerebrospinal fluid.

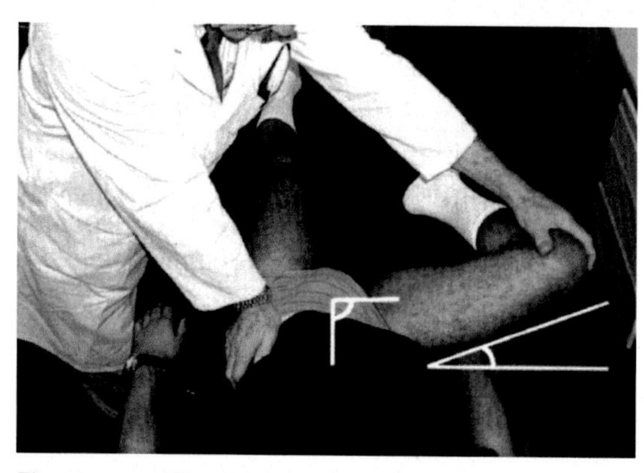

Fig. 11.10 Hip abduction test according to Patrick-Kubis and modified by Marx (Priener abduction test, PAT). The test is performed in 90° of hip flexion; the angle between upper thigh and bench is measured.

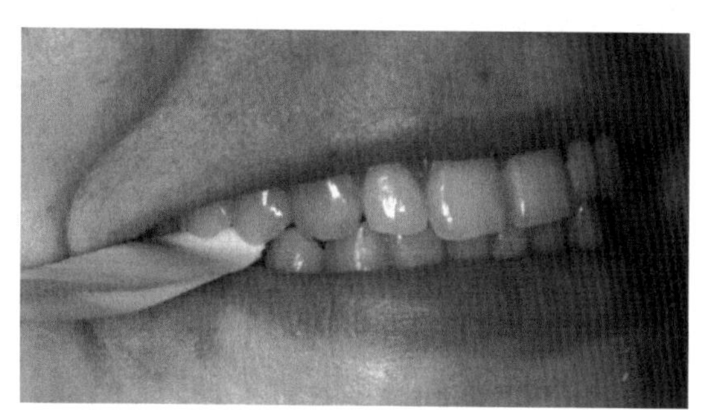

Fig. 11.11 Meersseman test.

treatment is initiated without prior treatment for the craniocervical dysfunction, the splint may establish a craniocervical dysfunction, and the overall clinical picture of CMD and craniocervical dysfunction will become more chronic.

HYPERABDUCTION TEST OF THE HIP

Introduction

Marx (2000) described a connection between arthropathy of the craniomandibular region and hip abduction. Hip abduction in his study was assessed by the Patrick-Kubis test, known to all manual therapists. This test is especially meaningful when applied as modified by Marx – the Priener abduction test (PAT, Fig. 11.10). In contrast to the original Patrick-Kubis test, in the PAT hip abduction is measured in 90° of flexion.

An impressive test to confirm CMD is the Meersseman test. The patient bites on between one and four pieces of paper with the second premolar and the first molar teeth to equalize mandibular malpositioning (Fig. 11.11). This small increase, by equalizing the position, decreases stress on the craniomandibular system and hip abduction improves by a minimum of 15°, indicating that the two areas must be somehow connected.

The same phenomenon can be observed in occiput–atlas dysfunctions. After manual therapy treatment of the CCD, hip abduction again increases by at least 15° (Hülse & Hölzl 2003). It can be hypothesized that a positive PAT may indicate dysfunctions in the craniomandibular or craniocervical region. Suggestions for appropriate diagnostic procedures are described below:

Test method

- After a thorough manual therapy assessment of the craniocervical intervertebral movements, the Priener hip abduction test is performed in 90° of flexion under dental occlusion to the passive physiological end of range. Range of motion and quality of the movement are assessed (Hülse et al 1998). The angle between thigh and bench is documented (the smaller the angle, the more range of motion) as well as the type of dysfunction (soft/hard).
- Meersseman test: Put two strips of paper (e.g. clean typing paper) on the second premolar and the first molar teeth and ask the patient to bite on the paper with one side of the jaw. It takes only two to four strips of paper to significantly reduce this irritation. If hip abduction increases by at least 15°, CMD is likely.
- Compare the results of the PAT without paper. The initial results should be repeated.
- Manual therapy treatment of the CCD: If the hip itself is not dysfunctional, hip abduction should improve significantly. Even in pronounced hip inflammation, the improvement should be clearly visible.
- Repeat the PAT with paper as described above. If CCD was treated successfully and the jaw position was influenced during the treatment, hip abduction will decrease by 15° or more.
- Final control of the PAT: Optimum range of motion should be observed similar to results after manual therapy intervention. This check is necessary to confirm that the final craniomandibular irritation (bite on paper) has not reactivated the craniomandibular and craniocervical dysfunction.
- If craniocervical mobility is reduced, the patient is asked to clench their teeth together 10 times. If the PAT is positive, this shows that even a slight craniomandibular irritation is enough to reactivate the dysfunction and dental treatment is essential. In contrast, if the PAT remains stable this indicates that craniocervical dysfunction is the dominant component of the craniomandibular disorder and that manual therapy alone promises to be successful (Fig. 11.12).

Why this test?

The clinical relevance of this test for the dentist is that it may help to decide whether the patient will need manual therapy treatment prior to the splint fitting procedure. Without this test there is a risk of fitting the splint with a functionally inappropriate mandibular position. The manual therapist, however, should repeat this test a few days after treatment to determine if a CMD has redeveloped after a short period of time, or whether it can be concluded that the CMD was simply a concomitant symptom of the craniocervical dysfunction. The manual therapist may also obtain indications for correct fitting of the splint.

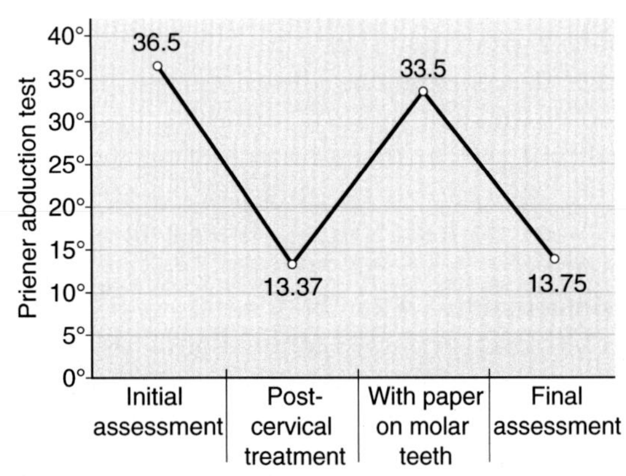

Fig. 11.12 The Priener abduction test after cervical spine manipulation and after the Meersseman test.

DIZZINESS AFTER GENERAL ANAESTHESIA – A CASE STUDY

General subjective examination

A 32-year-old lady, Mrs CU, had gallbladder surgery 3 years ago. Immediately after the operation she experienced disabling dizziness. She described the quality of the dizziness as 'asymmetrical'. It was not perceived as vertigo but rather as a feeling of insecurity and swaying. The symptoms were accompanied by blurred vision and a loss of sight. The dizziness was always there, increased after standing for a long period and decreased when lying down. The patient said that the symptoms became even worse when she opened her mouth wide. She complained of weekly intense headaches which were diagnosed as occipital neuralgia. She also complained of tension headaches. Physiotherapy interventions initially increased the symptoms. Additionally, she had pain at the 5th and 6th thoracic vertebrae and pain in the right knee. Since the onset of symptoms the patient has suffered from disturbed sleep. CT and MRI of the cranium and of the neck did not detect any obvious changes. Since puberty she has experienced repetitive headaches which increased just prior to the onset of menstruation.

A peripheral equilibrium dysfunction was excluded after a videonystagmographic investigation. While testing for vestibulospinal reactions she tested positive in the 'Unterberger' procedure: when walking on the spot in a darkened room, she repeatedly turned 100° to the right within 60 seconds (physiological limit: 60° to the right and 40° to the left). The acoustic reflex threshold audiogram showed normal hearing; brainstem audiometry was also normal and excluded dysfunctions of midbrain and brainstem.

On intervertebral examination a dysfunction of occiput/atlas in the transverse direction (left > right) and a general stiffness of axis/C3 on the left was found. The Priener abduction test showed a mobility deficit of 35° of the right and 40° of the left hip.

Manual therapy for CCD normalized the Priener abduction tests to 10° bilaterally and the rotation in the Unterberger test was no longer demonstrated. Subjectively she experienced the first symptom-free period for 5 months. Subsequently, the symptoms returned in a lower intensity. The second manual therapy achieved three symptom-free days. The craniomandibular area was then assessed and an appointment with a dentist agreed.

Special dental subjective examination

The patient showed narrow mandibular front teeth with abrasions, as well as an extensive history of dental procedures on her lateral teeth in the maxilla and mandible.

Excessive tension of the masticatory, neck and cranial muscles was observed and treated with a combination of low-frequency TENS of the masticatory muscles and manual therapy of the craniocervical dysfunction. An impaired relationship of condyles and disc as well as degenerative changes and capsulitis were found.

Additionally, a slight overbite (Shimbashi dimension 16 mm) and a clear retral position of the mandible were diagnosed. Neuromuscular relaxation of the masticatory, neck and cranial muscles was achieved by manual therapy of the craniocervical dysfunctions and TENS of the masticatory muscles. It was clear that the mandible was now aiming towards a more ventral contact with the upper jaw; however, the teeth there did not fit together. To be able to eat, the masticatory muscles, especially the anterior temporalis muscle, are forced to pull the mandible backwards, away from the physiological position (Jankelson 1990). This will also occur on swallowing, a procedure that depends on the teeth supporting each other. Since human beings swallow about 2000 times a day, it becomes very difficult to achieve relaxation of the masticatory muscles. The mandible will be maintained in the retral position to provide the required contact of the teeth. This may be followed by neuromusculoskeletal changes of more caudal parts of the body.

Course of treatment

A splint was fitted in a neuromuscularly adjusted position. Prior to the fitting procedure the patient was treated with craniocervical manual therapy and low-frequency TENS of the masticatory muscles. It is extremely important to achieve neuromuscular relaxation prior to fitting the splint, otherwise the patient will not be able to achieve a correct position for the splint and an unphysiological and unhelpful splint will result.

From the day the splint was fitted, the patient did not experience any further dizziness. A few weeks later the headaches occurred only occasionally, the pain in the neck was a lot better, the pain in the knee was gone and the tinnitus had reduced in frequency. She also slept well with her splint. Initially the splint was worn at all times apart from when eating. After 10 weeks the splint wearing times were reduced to a few hours during the day and at night, with a steady reduction of the number of hours the splint was worn. For the past 2 years she had only worn the splint at nights. Her situation is stable and the symptoms have not returned.

Conclusion

This patient is not an unusual example. The seeming cause of the symptoms – the gallbladder operation – cannot explain the dizziness and pain described. An explanation might be that the patient was positioned in head reclination for the intubation during the anaesthetic that resulted in the craniocervical dysfunction. It is quite possible that a clinically silent dysfunction existed long before the surgery. The jaw positioning suggests that the CMD had existed symptom-free for a long time. Only the additional stress due to the head position during anaesthesia increased the craniocervical and craniomandibular dysfunction to a point where it finally became symptomatic.

This case study underlines how CMD and functional CCD sometimes exist without causing any symptoms and how comparably small stimuli may produce the symptom pattern described above with dizziness, headaches, cochlear paraesthesia, blurred vision, vasomotor rhinitis, feeling of globus, and also changes in blood pressure and heart rhythm.

The wide range of symptoms shows that there is no clearly defined symptom pattern for CMD and CCD. Joint mobility and muscle function can usually be predicted after successful treatment (either CCD or CMD) but the reaction of concomitant vegetative symptoms remains unpredictable.

SUMMARY

- This chapter shows that interdisciplinary cooperation will frequently be the only truly successful approach to CMD presenting with a complex set of symptoms.

References

Chole R A, Parker W S 1992 Tinnitus and vertigo in patients with temporomandibular disorder. Archives of Otolaryngology, Head and Neck Surgery 118:817

Cooper B C, Cooper D L 1999 Das Erkennen von otolaryngologischen Symptomen bei Patienten mit temporomandibulären Erkrankungen. ICCMO (International College of Cranio-Mandibular Orthopedics) 6:40

Hülse M, Hölzl M 2003 Nachweis der Wirksamkeit einer modifizierten Atlasimpulstherapie nach Arlen. Manuelle Medizin 41:453

Hülse M, Losert-Bruggner B 2002 Der Einfluss der Kopfgelenke und/oder der Kiefergelenke auf die Hüftabduktion. Manuelle Medizin and Osteopathic Medizin 40:97

Hülse M, Neuhuber W L, Wolff H D 1998 Der kraniozervikale Übergang. Springer, Berlin

Hülse M, Losert-Bruggner B, Kuksen J 2001 Schwindel und Kiefergelenkprobleme nach HWS-Trauma. Manuelle Medizin and Osteopathic Medizin 39:20

Hülse M, Losert-Bruggner B, Schöttl R 2003 CMD, CCD und neuromuskulär ausgerichtete

Bisslagebestimmung. Dental Praxis 20:195
Jankelson R 1990 Neuromuscular dental diagnosis and treatment. Ishiyaku EuroAmerica, St Louis
Keersmaekers K, De Boever J A, Van Den Berghe L 1996 Otalgia in patients with temporomandibular joint disorders. Journal of Prosthetic Dentistry 5(1):72
Losert-Bruggner B 1998 Therapieresistente Beschwerden in der großen Zehe und im Daumen durch Blockaden im Kieferbereich. Paracelsus Report 6:28
Losert-Bruggner B 2000 Therapieresistente Kopfschmerzen, Probleme im Bereich der HWS, Schwindel, Augenbrennen und Tinnitus können ihre Ursache im Zahnsystem haben. Zeitschrift für Physiotherapie 52:1923
Losert-Bruggner B 2003 Nächtliche Stabilisierung des Halswirbelsaulenbereiches durch Schnarcherschienen bei kraniozervikalen Dysfunktionen. Somno Journal 3:15
Losert-Bruggner B, Schöttl R, Zawdadzki W 2003 Neuromuskulär ausgerichtete Bisslagebestimmung mit Hilfe niedrigfrequenter TENS-Therapie. GZM 8:12
Marx G 2000 Über die Zusammenarbeit mit der Kieferorthopädie und Zahnheilkunde in der Manuellen Medizin. Manuelle Medizin 38:342
Meyer F 2000 Kasuistik. HNO Highlights 4:8
Oudhof H A J 2001 Schädelwachstum und Einfluss von mechanischer Stimulation. In: von Piekartz H J M (ed.) Kraniofaziale Dysfunktionen und Schmerzen. Thieme, Stuttgart, p 1
Peroz I 2001 Otalgie und Tinnitus bei Patienten mit CMD. HNO 49:713–718
Peroz I, Kirchner K, Lange K P 2000 Kraniomandibuläre Dysfunktionen bei Tinnituspatienten. Deutsche zahnärztliche Zeitschrift 55:694
Pilgramm M, Rychlik R, Lebisch H et al 1999 Tinnitus in der Bundesrepublik Deutschland. HNO Aktuell 7:261
Saxer T, Czech C G 1997 Das Accu-Liner-System nach JE Carlson. ICCMO Brief 4; 1:34
Schindler H 1994 Die propriozeptive Wirkung von Aufbissschienen. Scriptum zu einem Vortrag beim ITMR-Symposium, Erlangen
Schorr-Tschudnowski M 2001 Dogmatisches vertiefen und Undogmatisches diskutieren. Manuelle Medizin and Osteopathic Medizin 39:137
Schöttl R 2001a Die Analyse und Korrektur der Kauebene im Artikulator. GZM-Praxis und Wissenschaft 2:18
Schöttl R 2001b Physiologie und Applikation der Niederfrequenz-TENS. Dental Praxis 5/6:165
Türp J C 1998 Zum Zusammenhang zwischen Myoarthropathien des Kausystems und Ohrenbeschwerden. HNO 46:303
Vernon J, Griest S, Press L 1992 Attributes of tinnitus, associated with the temporomandibular joint syndrome. European Archives of Otorhinolaryngology 249:93
von Piekartz H J M 2001 Merkmale des Schädelgewebes als Grundlage zur Erkennung, Untersuchung und Behandlung klinischer Muster. In: von Piekartz H J M (ed.) Kraniofaziale Dysfunktionen und Schmerzen. Thieme, Stuttgart, p 21

Chapter 12

Muscular dysfunction and pain in the craniofacial and craniomandibular region: recommendations for examination and treatment

Di Andriotti, Harry von Piekartz

CHAPTER CONTENTS

INTRODUCTION

The examination and treatment of muscular dysfunctions or muscular imbalances is not new. The importance of muscular dysfunction in various pain syndromes, and the types of pain they may cause, has been demonstrated scientifically. Pain may cause changes in muscle recruitment but it is also believed that incorrect use of the musculature may result in imbalances that can eventually cause pain (Comerford & Mottram 2001, Sahrmann 2001).

For many years abnormal movement patterns and postures have been recognized and described by clinicians treating musculoskeletal pain (Janda 1994, O'Sullivan et al 1997, Hodges 1999, Richardson et al 1999, Jull 2000, Comerford & Mottram 2001, Sahrmann 2001). Changes in activity and motor control have been observed as increases in activity in some muscle groups while other groups are inhibited, lengthened or weakened. These recruitment changes may result in changes of joint movements or, in other words, changes in the dynamic stability of a joint. Gibbons et al (2001) describe stability as central nervous system modulation of efficient low threshold recruitment and the integration of local and global muscle systems. Much research has been done on this loss of joint control in areas of the body such as the lumbar spine, cervical spine and knee (Stokes & Young 1984, Voight & Wieder 1991, Hides et al 1994, Hodges & Richardson 1996, O'Sullivan et al 1997, Wadsworth & Bullock-Saxton 1997, Dangaria & Naesh 1998, Richardson et al 1999, Jull 2000, Cowan et al 2001). However, minimal published information exists regarding the craniofacial and craniomandibular regions.

Loss of joint control may leave patients open to microtrauma that could eventually lead to pain and pathology (Panjabi 1992, Cholewicki & McGill 1996, Comerford & Mottram 2001, Sahrmann 2001). If we consider the chronicity of many pain problems, it should be noted that although pain and dysfunction are related, the pain may resolve but the dysfunction will often persist (Richardson et al 1999). This has been shown to predispose to recurrence of symptoms (Wiemann et al 1998) and so underlines the requirement for specific, well-targeted rehabilitation programmes to recruit the relevant fibre populations of the correct muscles and to re-establish the correct muscle timing and movement pattern, even though pain may no longer be a problem.

Since the craniofacial and craniomandibular areas have not been covered in any detail as yet, an overview of the scientific literature specific to this region is given here, with hypotheses as to the possible muscular dysfunctions that may occur and the specific rehabilitation programmes that may be applied. The chapter is divided into two parts: the first is a brief general overview of current biomedical and clinical knowledge about muscle dysfunction; the second part will attempt to apply this knowledge to the craniofacial and craniomandibular regions.

MUSCLE DYSFUNCTION

Muscle dysfunction can be diagnosed in both the local and global muscle systems (Bergmark 1989, Comerford & Mottram 2001). Their functions are listed in Table 12.1. The local muscles

Table 12.1 Muscle function and characteristics

Local stabilizers	Global stabilizers	Global mobilizers
↑ Muscle stiffness to control segmental motion Controls the neutral joint position Contraction = no/minimum length change therefore does not produce range of motion Activity is often anticipatory (or at the same instant) to functional load or movement to provide protective stiffness prior to motion stress Activity is independent of direction of movement Continuous activity throughout movement Proprioceptive input re: joint position, range and rate of movement	Generates force to control range of motion Contraction = eccentric length change therefore control throughout range especially inner range ('muscle active = joint passive') and hypermobile outer range Low load deceleration of momentum (especially axial plane: rotation) Activity is direction dependent	Generates torque to produce range of motion Contraction = concentric production of movement (rather than eccentric control) Concentric acceleration of movement (especially sagittal plane: flexion/extension) Shock absorption for load Activity is direction dependent Non-continuous activity (on/off phasic pattern)

are deep and are responsible for control of articular translation and intersegmental motion. Their activity is independent of direction and is often anticipatory to movement to provide protective joint stiffness during motion. The local muscles control local segmental stability. These muscles do not change length significantly during normal functional movements. The global muscles, on the other hand, are responsible for alignment and range of motion. They change length significantly during functional movements, with concentric shortening to produce range of motion, isometric co-contraction to maintain position or alignment and eccentric lengthening to decelerate movement and protect against excessive range of motion. The global muscles control single-joint stability and multi-joint dynamic stability during functional movements. All the global muscles are direction dependent and, as such, are influenced by antagonistic muscle activity. Neither the local nor global muscle systems in isolation can control functional stability but a fine coordination of the two is necessary.

LOCAL MUSCLE SYSTEM DYSFUNCTION

Local muscle system dysfunction presents in four ways (Comerford & Mottram 2001) and the apparent inhibition appears to be secondary to pain:

- Uncontrolled segmental translation: Excessive intersegmental accessory or gliding movement in one or more directions that is no longer efficiently controlled by the local muscle system.
- Segmental change in cross-sectional area: With MRI, CT and ultrasound imaging, local stability muscles have been observed to lose their cross-sectional area within 24 hours of the onset of pain which, because this change occurs so quickly, must be attributed to muscle inhibition and not muscle atrophy (Richardson et al 1999).
- Altered patterns of motor recruitment: The normal tonic recruitment pattern of the local stabilizing muscles may change to become more phasic or 'on/off' in the presence of pain.
- Altered 'timing' of motor recruitment: The normal anticipatory or preparative activity (or tone increase) of local muscle recruitment has been seen to be delayed in the presence of pain.

GLOBAL MUSCLE SYSTEM DYSFUNCTION

Global muscle system dysfunction has to do with alterations in length and force relationships (active or passive) between the different global muscles. It presents in three ways (Comerford & Mottram 2001).

Changes in muscle length

Alteration of length–tension characteristics reflect habitual use or misuse (Gossman et al 1982, Richardson & Sims 1991, Wiemann et al 1998), i.e. muscles adapt to the demands or restrictions placed on them. They may also adapt to protect the nervous system (Elvey 1986). They become longer or shorter by increasing or decreasing the number of sarcomeres in series or, when overloaded, they respond by increasing the number of sarcomeres in parallel and the amount of connective tissue proteins. Therefore, everyday activities can strongly influence relative strength and length of muscles. Repetitive loading activities or sustained postures, especially those maintained in faulty alignments or in end of range positions, can induce changes in the length of the muscles and of the supporting tissues. These changes alter the relative participation of synergists and antagonists and, eventually, the movement pattern. A lengthened muscle can generate more tension than a muscle of normal length, particularly when contracting in outer range or in stretch positions, but may have difficulty and test weak in the shortened or inner range position because the myofilaments (actin and myosin) may be excessively overlapped. Even though these muscles may appear stronger they are no longer able to control the joint eccentrically through its entire range, especially in the shortened ranges that may be necessary for normal functional movements (Sahrmann 2001) (Fig. 12.1).

Changes in recruitment patterns

In altered recruitment patterns (imbalance) between synergistic and antagonistic muscles (Janda 1983, 1994, O'Sullivan et al 1998, Jull et al 1999, Sahrmann 2001), muscles at the same joint can be synergists for one movement and antagonists for another. One synergist may lengthen or be inhibited while the other maintains its normal length or is shortened. Therefore, clinically, we observe a consistent dominance of recruitment of one of the muscles in a force couple or of one of the counterbalancing synergists. Thus, the movement may be 'pulled' in the direction of the dominant synergist and no longer be balanced. At a segmental level this means that the instantaneous axis of rotation of the joint no longer remains centred but may be pulled towards the dominant component of the force couple. Altered recruitment patterns contribute to changes in muscle dominance and therefore in muscle length and strength.

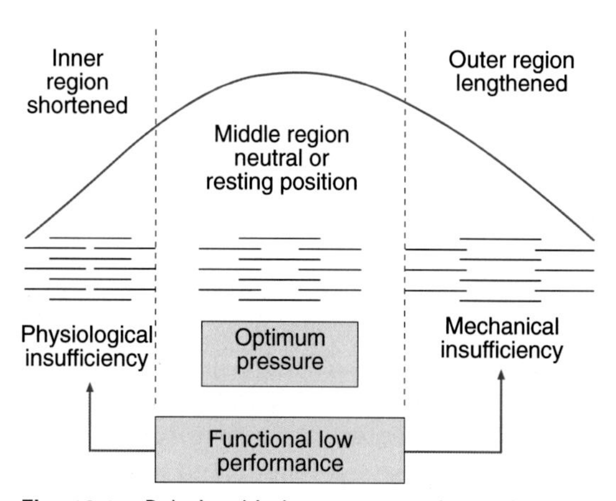

Fig. 12.1 Relationship between muscle tension and range of movement

Changes in muscle strength

Relative stiffness in one direction and relative excess flexibility in the other direction (Woolsey et al 1988, Hamilton & Richardson 1998, Jull et al 1999, Sahrmann 2001) is defined as the change in tension per unit of change in length. An increase in the stiffness of joints and muscles in one area can be a factor in the development of compensatory motion in adjacent joints or areas and can therefore contribute to musculoskeletal pain syndromes. Hypertrophy increases the amount of connective tissue protein and of contractile elements and therefore increases muscle stiffness or the muscle's resistance to passive elongation. The hypothesis is that motion will occur earlier at the joint or region with the lesser degree of stiffness or where there is more flexibility compared to the 'stiffer' joint or region. Under normal circumstances there should be an automatic stabilizing action to control the compensatory relative flexibility, but if that does not occur, the region or segment with too much uncontrolled movement is susceptible to microtrauma and eventually pain and pathological changes.

There is no answer as to which of these changes comes first. Sahrmann (2001) feels they are relatively concurrent. From the research it appears evident that pain changes recruitment patterns but it is also easy to imagine that muscle length and/or strength changes, originating from overuse and misuse, may, eventually, cause microtrauma, pathology and pain and therefore be considered a contributing factor.

PROPOSED MODELS TO EXPLAIN MOTOR RESPONSES TO PAIN

In the clinical situation, in patients with pain due to craniomandibular dysfunction (CMD), Mongini et al (1989) found smaller and slower movements during mastication whereas Möller et al (1984) have shown a significantly longer duration of the masticatory cycle. Lund et al

(1991) drew attention to the fact that comparable findings of slower movements with less EMG activity in the agonist phase and more EMG activity in the antagonist phase could also be observed during other dynamic motor tasks. Based on this they have formulated the 'pain-adaptation' model to explain the interaction between muscle pain and muscle coordination.

This model strongly contrasts the 'vicious cycle' model hypothesized by Travell et al (1942) and Johansson and Sojka (1991) that suggests that pain causes muscles to become hyperactive. This model would seem to apply more to the acute muscle pain phase.

Hodges and Richardson (1997, 1999) and Jull (2000) present a new model called the 'neuromuscular activation' model that describes altered patterns of neuromuscular control of muscles that perform key synergistic functions to stabilize the spine and major peripheral joints. This model appears to provide an important insight into the chronic state when selective control and activation of specific muscles has been lost. Unfortunately, these models only explain the motor consequences of pain and possible chronification of many musculoskeletal pain problems but do not provide any explanation for the origin of pain.

In studies of muscle recruitment in the lumbar spine (O'Sullivan et al 1997, Richardson et al 1999), in the cervical spine (Jull 2000) and in craniofacial muscles (Ro & Capra 2000, Wang et al 2000) it has been shown that pain changes the recruitment patterns. Thus, there is no doubt that these adaptive muscle imbalances, or flexibility in one direction such as a give (uncontrolled movement), can, in some cases, be the cause of pain and pathological changes, and consequently compensate for other restrictions.

If these muscle imbalances are not corrected following elimination of pain there will be a tendency to chronification, or there may be a recurrence. This view is also supported by Comerford and Mottram (2001) and Sahrmann (2001).

MOVEMENT DYSFUNCTION CAUSED BY MUSCLE DYSFUNCTION

Movement dysfunction or reduction in the quality of the movement may present at two different levels (Comerford & Mottram 2001) or simultaneously:

- Articular
- Myofascial.

At the articular level, the dysfunction presents as abnormal accessory movements, either restricted or too lax. At a myofascial level, in functional movements, it is observed as abnormal myofascial extensibility and recruitment. This loss of quality of movement results in abnormal functional or physiological movements. Articular and myofascial dysfunctions commonly occur together. The inability to dynamically control the articular and the myofascial dysfunction at a mobile segment may present as uncontrolled movement or 'give', which is usually associated with, or the result of, a loss of motion or a 'restriction' at the same level or at an adjacent articular or myofascial level (Table 12.2). Often the give may develop to compensate for a restriction in order to maintain normal function.

For example, in the temporomandibular joint (TMJ) complex, the right TMJ could develop an abnormal anterior or lateral translation to maintain function because there is restriction in the left TMJ. Alternatively, within the same joint, an increased anterior translation could develop to compensate for a restricted condylar head rotation in jaw depression.

The give occasionally develops because an excessive range of movement is habitually performed as may be the case in singers or when a position is habitually maintained either actively or passively in abnormal alignment or in an end of range position. An example could be hours of violin playing (Kovero & Könönen 1996) or of using a telephone with the jaw in laterotrusion. This could result in true shortening (loss of sarcomeres) of a particular muscle that holds the joint towards the end of range

Table 12.2 Articular myofascial instability and shortening

	Articular	Myofascial
Instability	Local stability muscle integration to control intersegmental motion (tonic recruitment)	Global stability muscle training to control range of motion (tonic recruitment)
Shortening	Mobilization of segmental articular restriction	Inhibit overactivity and regain extensibility of myofascial length

position and the lengthening of the antagonist muscle and/or the passive structures such as the ligaments and capsule.

A common posture seen in patients with craniofacial and craniomandibular pain syndromes is that of a forward head posture with an increased craniocervical angle and a forward inclination of the neck on the trunk. This is often accompanied by a scapula that is in an inferiorly rotated position. Certain working postures (computer work, driving) or recreational postures (cycling, rowing or overhead ball sports) predispose to this posture. A forward head posture may also be observed when there is impaired nasal breathing in order to maintain adequate airway space (Ono et al 1998, Zepa et al 2000) or to compensate for a hyperkyphotic (Zepa et al 2000) or stiff, flat thoracic spine.

Clinically, we often see a compensatory segmental give into extension in the midcervical spine when there is restricted jaw depression and the flexibility in the upper cervical spine in extension is less than the flexibility in the midcervical area. This may result in repetitive microtrauma and the eventual onset of cervical symptoms. When the mandibular musculature and the TMJ are given more proprioceptive input by asking the patient to lightly touch the teeth together, the extension will often occur more correctly throughout the entire cervical spine. This mandibular stability seems to increase cervical segmental control as is typically seen in patients with an Angle class II malocclusion (Fig. 12.2).

The give may even be unrelated to habitual movements and postures, but may be the result of direct trauma to the jaw damaging the temporomandibular ligaments and contributing to translational instability. Some authors suggest that a TMJ instability can also be the direct result of a whiplash injury; however, there is much controversy in this area (McKay & Christensen 1999). Clinically, extreme cases are seen in patients that have had a whiplash injury, especially when pain has been present

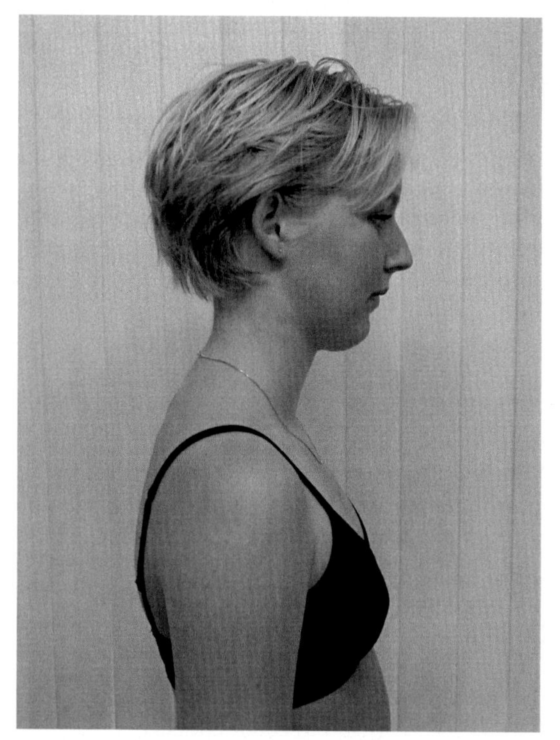

Fig. 12.2 Profile of a patient with Angle class II malocclusion: note protraction of the shoulders and increased anteroposition of the head.

for a long time. Since pain is known to cause inhibition in the local stabilizers it seems more probable that it develops as a secondary consequence after cervical trauma when, through the convergence of the trigeminal nerve and the upper three cervical nerves in the trigeminocervical nucleus (Kraus 1988), pain leads to altered proprioception and craniomandibular muscular inhibition.

What is evident is that the craniocervical and craniomandibular regions are mechanically and neurophysiologically interrelated and a change in one area causes a reaction in the other area, thus positions or movements in one area will change the other (see Chapter 5).

SITE OF THE STABILITY DYSFUNCTION

When considering movement dysfunction, the site of the dysfunction must be established. In the movement system, the site of greatest give or the site of the greatest compensation is the 'site of stability dysfunction'. This is the uncontrolled segment or region of give where the myofascial, articular, neural or connective tissue structures are abnormally loaded or stressed and therefore this becomes the most likely site of the source of symptoms and pathology of a mechanical origin.

For example, in the case of an anterior dislocation of the disc without reduction on the right, when opening the jaw the mandible will likely deviate to the right and there will be a give or an excessive movement in the left TMJ anteriorly and medially. The left TMJ will therefore be the site of the stability dysfunction, i.e. it will be the site of the give and of eventual pain and pathology even though the cause, in this case, would be a restriction in the right TMJ. In this same scenario, there could also be a posterior give of the right condylar head with the addition of pain in the right TMJ. Thus the right TMJ would also be the site of the stability dysfunction. For the same restriction, two common compensations may occur. The site (or compensation) that has the least efficient control is the one more likely to be painful and to be the clinical priority. The second uncontrolled give would be a risk for future problems but not a priority for this patient at the present moment. However, the restriction could be the same for both and be a clinical priority.

Another example could be in habitual eccentric closing positions or when there is loss of the posterior teeth which should provide a mechanical spacer; the mandible may drift posteriorly or laterally to accommodate the position and possibly irritate the highly nociceptive retrodiscal area causing symptoms. In this case the give will be into the posterior or lateral direction without being a compensation for any restriction and the TMJ will be the site of the stability dysfunction and the site of the symptoms.

The direction of give relates to the direction of uncontrolled motion which results in abnormal tissue stress or strain. This relates to the direction of pain-provoking movements or of static holding. It is important not only to find the site of give but also the direction of give in order to develop a specific rehabilitation programme.

FUNCTIONAL CLASSIFICATION OF MUSCLES

A clinically useful model of muscle classification has been developed (Mottram & Comerford 1998, Comerford & Mottram 2001). This functional classification divides muscles into three groups:

- Local stabilizers
- Global stabilizers
- Global mobilizers.

The functions of these muscles are considered in Table 12.3.

Many studies have been done to determine the function of the muscles of mastication in the normal situation but few during dysfunction. Before attempting to establish a functional classification that can almost exclusively be based on what is seen clinically, it would be

Table 12.3 Characteristics of muscle dysfunction

Local stabilizers	Global stabilizers	Global mobilizers
Motor control deficit associated with delayed timing or low threshold recruitment deficiency Reacts to pain and pathology with altered recruitment ↓ Muscle stiffness and poor segmental control Loss of low threshold control of joint neutral position	Muscle active shortening ≠ joint passive (loss of inner range control) If hypermobile, poor control of excessive range Poor low threshold tonic recruitment Poor eccentric control Poor rotation dissociation	Loss of myofascial extensibility – limits physiological and/or accessory motion (which must be compensated for elsewhere) Overactive low threshold, low load recruitment Reacts to pain and pathology with spasm/overactivity

useful to explore what is found in the literature to date.

TEMPOROMANDIBULAR JOINT DYSFUNCTION

The TMJ cannot be thought of in isolation since there are two joints that must move in close relation with each other and both must also move in close relationship to the cervical spine, the hyoid bone and to the occlusion. On the working (loaded) side, where the food is crushed between the upper and lower molars, stability of the TMJ is required. The condyle must be controlled in the temporomandibular fossa against the biting force produced by the closing muscles. On the contralateral, non-working (unloaded) side, the condyle has to move widely and smoothly in a medioanterior direction. In addition, there must be coordinated and controlled movements of the articular disc relative to the condyle to allow smooth movements of the mandible.

Some investigators (Isberg-Holm & Ivasson 1980, Farrar & McCarty 1983, Solberg 1986, Huang et al 2005) consider that muscle tension or spasm is responsible for the change in the disc–condyle relationship. Toller (1974) suggested that uncoordinated contraction of the upper and lower heads of the lateral pterygoid muscle causes a hesitation in meniscal glide. This momentary hesitation or 'sticking' of the disc results in clicking and is eventually responsible for the TMJ dysfunction.

Wilkinson and Chan (1989) also suggest a mechanism of disc displacement involving the superior pterygoid muscle that, with sustained contraction, may prevent the disc from gliding posteriorly and rotating backward on the condyle with the retrusive condylar movement after the protrusion. These investigators suggest that protrusion associated with parafunctional clenching or the protrusive component of chewing, possibly associated with forceful chewing while eating tough foods, may lead to sustained activity of the superior pterygoid muscle. Once this has developed, smooth jaw opening and closing is associated with a change in the linear relationship between disc translation and rotation.

Contrarily, Hiraba et al (2000) demonstrated that the disc is rigidly attached to the condyle by the lateral structures, and when the superior head of the lateral pterygoid was pulled forward in a cadaver dissection, the disc did not displace anteriorly but became fixed onto the condyle. When it was released, it rolled backwards, suggesting that the role of the superior head of the lateral pterygoid is to stabilize the condyle in the temporomandibular fossa against the posterior slope of the articular eminence. The force pulling the condyle posteriorly, as generated by the jaw-closing muscles, particularly the temporal muscle, can thus be resisted. These authors postulate that the superior head controls the relative positional relationship between the disc and the condyle.

Quinn (1995) suggests that the suprahyoid and anterior belly of the digastric muscle should produce a hinge movement in jaw opening of 50% and then the inferior head of the lateral pterygoid should complete the rest of the opening movement with the translation. In dysfunction it is often observed that the rotational part of the movement is limited and excessive translation may occur as compensation to maintain functional jaw opening, suggesting that the suprahyoids tend to be inhibited, changing the timing at the TMJ.

In the literature there is little consensus as to the mechanisms that cause craniomandibular dysfunction, which makes a focused rehabilitation difficult. However, when there is dysfunction, certain incorrect postures or movement patterns seem to prevail and therapy can be directed to correct these patterns.

DEGLUTITION

Deglutition or swallowing is pushing a bolus or saliva from the mouth to the pharynx. It is performed by the tongue. The tongue needs a stable base which is provided by the suprahyoid muscles that elevate the hyoid. In order to limit the elevation of the hyoid bone the infrahyoid muscles must also contract. The mandible must also be stable and this is provided by the contraction of the craniomandibular muscles or the jaw elevators which hold the mandible motionless in occlusion. With the contraction of the orbicularis oris muscles in response to food entering the mouth, contraction of the buccinators will flatten the cheeks and pull the pterygoid raphe forward, reducing the oropharyngeal space and danger of food accidentally passing into it. Relaxation of the orbicularis oris changes the role of the buccinator and the pterygoid raphe is pulled posteriorly, increasing the oropharyngeal space in order to facilitate swallowing, talking and singing. It is the stabilization of the mandible that permits the internal muscles of the pharynx to work.

Graf (1971) calculated the frequency of swallowing and concluded that we swallow once every 1–3 minutes. Bazzotti (1998) found that in swallowing there was almost no difference between mandibular movement time and electromyographic activity in pathological subjects compared to controls. In both groups digastric was more often the first muscle to fire and sternocleidomastoid was the last, suggesting that initially there is stabilization activity for the tongue, causing a certain ventral flexion action of the head and then the sternocleidomastoid fires to counterbalance and correct the head position. Since there was little difference found between the control group and the pathological group, Bazzotti concluded that this is because swallowing, like breathing, is physiologically vital and the body will always maintain this function at the cost of others. It will always reproduce a 'physiological pattern' even if, in pathology, this will require a muscular adaptation (for further information on swallowing dysfunction, see Chapter 14).

MUSCULAR FUNCTION

The following section will discuss the isolated functions of the masticatory muscles, particularly their role in normal functions such as eating, drinking, singing, speaking and kissing, with regard to the current literature. The muscles to be considered are shown in Figure 12.3.

Lateral pterygoid

In 1999 Murray et al (1999b) stated that, in their opinion, the lateral pterygoid is the only muscle capable of applying a range of force vectors directly to the jaw joints. In the literature, the superior head (SHLP) and the inferior head (IHLP) of the lateral pterygoid have inevitably been grouped together as a single muscle group; however in recent studies it seems evident that they do not have the same function (Widmalm et al 1987, Uchida et al 2001).

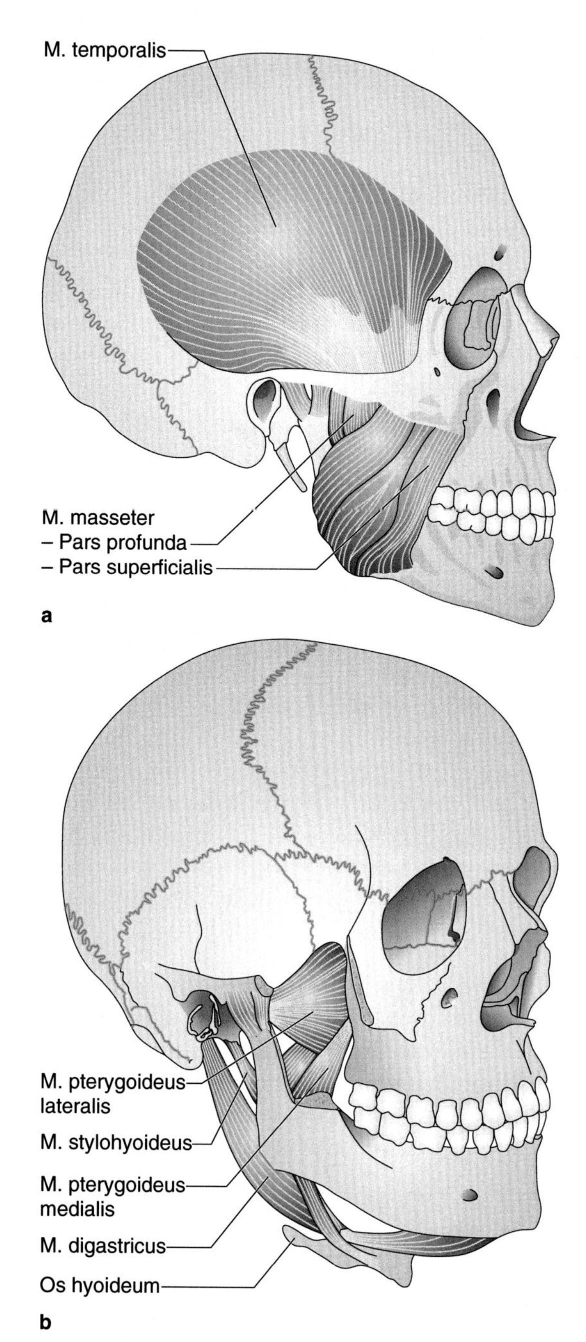

Fig. 12.3 The masticatory muscles.

The superior head is said to be a jaw elevator. However, Widmalm et al (1987) and Uchida et al (2001) consider it to be too close to the condyle to create a closing force vector of any significant magnitude and therefore its role appears to be more of a local stabilizer, keeping the condyle stable against the posterior surface of the articular eminence and thereby creating a fulcrum for the closing movement and maintaining the disc in contact with the condyle.

According to Hiraba et al (2000) it has a tonic background EMG activity of 5–32% maximal voluntary clenching (MVC) at rest which would reinforce the idea of a local stabilizer role.

Murray et al (1999a, 1999b, 1999c) and Phanachet et al (2001) agree that the IHLP, with its predominantly horizontal arrangement of fibres, is involved in the fine control of jaw movements in the horizontal plane at low force and is functionally heterogeneous.

Juniper (1984) noted that the inferior head is normally inactive. In patients with TMJ dysfunction and pain, however, it is active during mouth closing and clenching. He suggests that this can be explained as the IHLP taking over the stabilizing function that the SHLP can no longer perform.

Tay (1986) pointed out that the IHLP can establish a state of continuous spastic contraction, even in the mandibular rest position, in the case of an anteriorly subluxed disc that does not reduce. Widmalm et al (1987) found that the IHLP was particularly active when the jaw was pushed passively into retrusion as in the situation of an anteriorly subluxed disc. This could suggest that in dysfunction the SHLP is inhibited, as would be a local stabilizer, and that the IHLP becomes hyperactive to compensate, much as a global mobilizer would do.

In a hypermobile TMJ, Quinn (1995) feels the give is in the anterior translation and caudal movement of the condyle. The suprahyoid and anterior belly of the digastric muscle should produce a hinge movement in jaw opening of 50% and then the IHLP should complete the rest of the opening movement with the translation. If the give is as Quinn states, then we would have an overdominance of the inferior head and an inhibition or inefficiency of the suprahyoid and digastric muscles. This give would eventually, over time, contribute to a lengthening in the posterior lamellae, permitting the disc to travel too far forward. Any inhibition of the SHLP would jeopardize the stability of the condyle in the fossa and of the disc onto the condylar head. In addition, an inhibition of the suprahyoids could cause changes in the hyoid position with resultant changes in swallowing and breathing patterns. As previously stated, these vital body functions will always be maintained if possible and be compensated for by a muscular adaptation elsewhere.

The work by Hiraba et al (2000) tends to confirm this hypothesis. They were able to demonstrate that the muscle activity of the SHLP appears to be primarily correlated to the rotation of the condyle and that of the IHLP to the anterior displacement. To permit the jaw to open, the SHLP, which had fixed the disc onto the condyle during the intercuspal position, must relax and allow the disc to rotate backwards around the condyle. After the rotation of the disc the condyle can rotate around the mediolateral axis and the activity of the IHLP can translate the condyle anteriorly. At maximum opening, the SHLP is completely relaxed and the inferior head is in maximum tension. Thus both the condyle and the disc are in the anterior-most position in relation to the maxilla (maximum anterior translation) although the disc is in the posterior-most position in relation to the condyle. During jaw closing, the inferior head decreases its activity to allow the condyle to return into the temporomandibular fossa whereas the SHLP becomes active to change the relative position of the disc to the condyle.

Raustia et al (1998), using CT to investigate symptomatic TMJs of long duration, found there was a significant loss in the density and size of the ipsilateral lateral pterygoid and masseter muscles. Shellehas (1989) found fatty replacement in MRI examinations in masticatory muscles in patients with TMJ problems. These changes suggest inhibition or disuse atrophy as can be seen in local and global stabilizers elsewhere in the musculoskeletal system (Stokes & Young 1984, Voight & Wieder 1991, Hides et al 1994, 1996, Hodges & Richardson 1996, Wadsworth & Bullock-Saxton 1997, Dangaria & Naesh 1998, Jull 2000, Cowan et al 2001). Recent studies show that the IHLP appears to have most EMG activity during lateral movements with the teeth together (Huang et al 2005).

Medial pterygoid

Medial pterygoid, a heavily pennated, thick, rectangular muscle, produces low force and velocity over a small excursion range. Its line of action is anteromedial. Little is known of recruitment changes in this muscle in the presence of pathology; however, like the inferior head of the lateral pterygoid, it primarily appears to control movement in the horizontal and anterior planes (Raustia et al 1998, Goto et al 2005). Therefore, in the light of its orientation and anatomy and until more is known, it may be classified as a global stabilizer.

Digastrics and suprahyoids

These muscles are fundamental for two vital functions of our bodies: swallowing and breathing. They have been shown to be active bilaterally in most movements of the jaw except elevation and protrusion (Widmalm et al 1988, Bérzin 1995, Castro et al 1998) and regardless of body position (Ormeño et al 1999).

The anterior belly of the digastric muscle increases the anteroposterior dimension of the oral pharynx during swallowing while the posterior digastric acts with the stylohyoid to prevent regurgitation of food after swallowing. The suprahyoids depress the mandible if the hyoid bone is stable. Absence or abnormality of these structures may seriously impair mandibular dynamics. The craniovertebral joints will maintain their normal position, and the TMJs will remain equally balanced towards the cranium through tensile forces produced by normal function of the supra- and infrahyoid muscles. The position of the hyoid bone is a reflection of the muscles, ligaments and fascia attached to it.

Widmalm et al (1988) found that the obliquus capitis superior and the digastric are often coactivated in jaw movements. Since the innervation of the anterior belly of the digastric is from the mandibular branch of the trigeminal nerve and the posterior belly is from the facial nerve, disturbances in either of these could cause muscular imbalance. They noted short bursts of high amplitude EMG activity during tooth gnashing in both digastric bellies and in obliquus capitis superior and from that they have hypothesized that bruxism (night grinding) can be the cause of symptoms of muscular hyperactivity in the suprahyoid and posterior neck region.

As many tongue muscles attach to the hyoid bone, any displacement of the tongue acts on the hyoid bone and on the hyoid musculature and, as noted previously, will have an effect on the cervical spine. The sternohyoid muscle and the anterior belly of the digastric muscle are active in protraction and right and left lateral movements of the tongue, especially when the tongue is placed on the soft palate (Derrick & Lapointe 1991) causing a forward movement of the hyoid bone. In tongue protraction the hyoid bone is displaced cranially.

Ormeño et al (1999) examined the EMG activity of the anterior temporalis and the suprahyoids while changing the body position and suggested that both the anterior temporalis muscle and the suprahyoids are involved in stabilizing the mandible. The suprahyoids are also active in elevation of the hyoid bone and larynx during swallowing. The infrahyoids resist elevation of the hyoid bone.

Sternocleidomastoid and masseter muscles

It has been demonstrated that there is a close relationship between the vestibular system and the neck musculature (Suzuki & Cohen 1964, Sumino & Nozaki 1977, Kraus 1988, Palazzi et al 1999) whereas visual input seems to show less significant changes (Miralles et al 1998). It is well known that the tonic neck reflex plays a key role in the achievement of head/neck posture. Kraus (1988) suggests that the tonic neck reflex is the primary neck proprioceptor contributing to the final neck/head posture.

In recent studies comparing the EMG activity of the sternocleidomastoid and masseter muscles in healthy subjects and in patients with myogenic cranio-cervical-mandibular dysfunction it was noted that there was a higher level of asymmetrical bilateral EMG activity of the sternocleidomastoid muscle observed in patients with craniomandibular dysfunction, with or without visual input (Miralles et al 1998, Santander et al 2000).

Svensson and Graven-Nielsen (2001), when discussing the masticatory muscles, state that in patients with TMJ pain there is only weak evidence in favour of an EMG increase and nothing that indicates that this increase can induce long-lasting pain in the masticatory muscles. There is, in fact, good evidence of a decreased agonist EMG activity and increased antagonist EMG activity during painful mastication. There is evidence of an inhibitory effect of nociceptive muscle afferents on alpha motor neurone activity and this could cause a lowered functional endurance and reduced capacity to work against load in attempts to protect a painful muscle. In fact, Wang et al (2000) found that when pain was induced experimentally by injecting hypertonic saline into the masseter muscle, the maximum bite force was significantly lowered.

There seems to be no measurement indicating that these parameters return to normal levels when the muscle pain is successfully treated. It has been suggested that there is a tendency for weak muscles to become painful and even to have active trigger points, and this would appear to be supported by the lack of significant increases in maximum EMG activity following treatment of patients with craniofacial pain (Whitty & Willison 1958, Lewit 1978).

Ono et al (1998) also demonstrated immediate inhibition of the masseter EMG activity when nasal breathing was interfered with. In addition, swallowing appears to facilitate bilateral inhibition of the masseter muscles before the onset of excitation of the infra- and suprahyoid muscles (Hiraoka 2004).

The sternocleidomastoid presents with the characteristics of a global mobilizer, tending to become dominant and hyperactive, whereas the masseter seems to be more of a global stabilizer of the mandible.

Temporal muscle

Isberg et al (1985) found the anterior temporalis muscle to be hyperactive when there was an anteriorly subluxed disc. The hyperactivity in the elevators would make it difficult for the condyle to move anteriorly and caudally to pass over the posterior part of the disc to re-establish the correct meniscal–condylar position. The temporal muscle is particularly active when there is extension of the head on the neck (Funakoshi & Amano 1973, Funakoshi et al 1976, Boyd et al 1987) as in a forward head position.

The temporal muscle presents more as a global mobilizer.

Table 12.4 shows recommendations for the functional classification of the primary muscles involved in craniomandibular and craniofacial dysfunction. More research needs to be done in this area to verify this classification.

OTHER POSSIBLE CONTRIBUTING FACTORS

Among the possible contributing factors that can influence muscle function in the craniomandibular and craniofacial regions are:

- Occlusal disharmony
- Parafunctions
- Trigger points
- Posture
- Nasal airway obstruction
- Hormonal changes
- Proprioception and pain.

These will be discussed briefly in the following text.

Occlusal disharmony

Since the jaw elevators do not have Golgi tendon organs to create the normal inhibitory feedback system (Matthews 1975), the proprioceptive fibres from the periodontium in normal tooth contact play an essential role in the inhibition of elevator muscle activity and guide mandibular movements to close the jaw into the intercuspal position. It is thought that premature tooth contact or gross tooth loss results in inadequate recruitment to achieve the inhibition threshold (De Boever 1979). If the condyle is displaced posteriorly due to a loss of the posterior teeth, this loss of tooth contact could clinically explain hyperactivity or loss of inhibition of the masseter and temporalis muscles, leading to a TMJ dysfunction.

It has been shown that balanced bilateral electromyographic responses in the masticatory muscles could be changed to unbalanced after artificially creating a premature tooth contact, and that activity would return to normal after removing it (Funakoshi et al 1976).

In 1996 Obrez and Stohler showed that pain induced experimentally in the masseter muscle decreased the length of the protrusive

Table 12.4 Classification of muscles around the craniomandibular joint (TMJ)

Local stabilizers	Global stabilizers	Global mobilizers
Superior head of lateral pterygoid – TMJ	Inferior head of lateral pterygoid – TMJ	Inferior head of lateral pterygoid – TMJ
Suprahyoids – hyoid bone	Masseter – TMJ	Digastric – TMJ
Infrahyoids – hyoid bone	Orbicularis oris – lips	Temporalis – TMJ Medial pterygoid – TMJ Mentalis – lips

mandibular border movement (Gothic arch tracings), thereby changing the occlusion. They hypothesize that patients may exhibit significant limitations due to structural incongruities within the TMJ complex but that it must also be considered that pain itself could be the cause of the occlusal incongruence and not necessarily the result. They state that pain-induced changes in mandibular posture form the basis for the patient's perception of being disturbed by 'teeth not fitting together properly'.

Parafunctions

Parafunctions such as bruxism, nail biting, thumb-sucking, habitual eccentric closing positions of the jaw and possibly generalized joint hypermobility (reviewed by Westling & Helkimo 1992) are other possible causes of muscle imbalance and stress in the soft tissues around the craniomandibular region. The hyperactivity of a certain muscle group could cause it to become relatively less flexible (stiffer) while the antagonist group becomes relatively more flexible. In general, it is unbalanced muscular activity (right against left, agonist against antagonist or synergist against a different synergist) which leads to joint stress.

Parafunctions causing an overactivity in certain muscles and an overstretching of other muscles could possibly cause a nerve entrapment pain source (DuPont & Matthews 2000).

Trigger points

Friction (1985) noted that there are significantly more trigger points in patients with CMD than in patients without CMD. Efficacy studies of the treatment of trigger points confirmed the reduction of craniomandibular and craniofacial pain and positive effects on normal musculoskeletal function (Tschopp & Bachmann 1992, Hong 1994).

A reliable tool for obtaining information about the patient's masticatory system is an algometer (McMillan & Blasberg 1994, Farella et al 2000).

Clinical examples and histories show that symptoms such as pain during chewing, temporal and frontal pain, otalgia, eye pain, difficulty in swallowing and static or dynamic dysfunctions of coordination are the most common symptoms that can be evoked by trigger points (Friction 1985, Mongini 1999). Therefore it is important to consider craniomandibular trigger points and tender points when assessing posture. For further information, the reader is referred to the more comprehensive discussion of this subject in Chapter 9.

Posture

The craniomandibular region requires a stable musculoskeletal posture to perform its many regular functions. In a study carried out by Nobili and Adversi in 1996 they demonstrated that it is not only the craniocervical and mandibular postures that are important but also the total body posture. Afferent proprioceptive input comes from the plantar aspect of the feet and from all joints and muscles up to the cranium.

To date, much has been written about the effect of cervical posture on the craniomandibular region (Darling et al 1984, Goldstein et al 1984, Kylämarkula & Huggare 1985, Boyd et al 1987, Kraus 1988, Makofsky 1989, 2000, Gonzalez & Manns 1996) and this is covered in detail in Chapter 5.

Kraus (1988) describes three peripheral control mechanisms by which he feels the head posture is maintained:

- Vestibular system: Internal part of the hearing organ that functions as a balancing organ
- Ocular system: Spatial perception and proprioceptive ocular function that generates a synergistic activity between neck muscles and eye muscles
- Proprioceptive system of the neck: Neuromuscular spindles and the articular mechanoreceptors produce the tonic neck reflex and this latter mechanism is thought to provide the basic control of the craniocervical posture as it is the only one that can directly determine the angle formed between the head and the cervical spine.

Gonzalez and Manns (1996) have suggested a fourth peripheral mechanism:

- Interceptors monitoring adequate airflow: Breathing is a vital body function and the body will adapt in any way possible to preserve it. Other autonomous reflexes such as swallowing, coughing, sneezing or vomiting need adequate adjustment of breathing and craniocervical posture in order to function.

Swallowing, breathing, seeing and equilibrium are essential for our existence and will be preserved at the expense of all else.

In our activities of daily living, professionally or in sporting activities, there will often be sustained activities with the arms in front of the body that will predispose us to a forward head posture and downwardly rotated scapulae. This posture causes an overactivity of levator scapulae, rhomboids, pectoralis minor, sternocleidomastoid, scalenes and the superficial suboccipital extensors. The omohyoid muscle runs from the hyoid bone to the scapula so a downwardly rotated scapula will also directly affect the hyoid bone position and the hyoid musculature, possibly causing an inferior give of the hyoid.

Several authors have demonstrated that during craniocervical extension there is increased muscular activity, especially in the temporalis muscle and moderately in the masseter muscle, and increased viscoelastic tension in the suprahyoid muscles. These changes cause mandibular elevation and retrusion and have an effect on the trajectory of mandibular closure (Solow & Tallgren 1976, Goldstein et al 1984, Boyd et al 1987).

This posture could, in theory, 'lock down' or hold the upper cervical vertebrae either unilaterally in lateral flexion or bilaterally in extension which could contribute to a compensatory give of the mandible and the tongue. Derrick and Lapointe (1991) observed that when the occiput is extended on the neck the mouth opens and the mandible retracts and the tongue drops. This puts the SHLP and digastric in a lengthened position. When maintained in a lengthened position, the SHLP could adapt by increasing the number of sarcomeres in series and would no longer be able to work efficiently in its inner (shortened) range position to fulfil its role as a stabilizer of the condyle against the posterior slope of the articular eminence or stabilizer of the disc against the condylar head.

Tallgren and Solow (1984), while studying variations in the hyoid bone position, discovered that this position was controlled by two postural systems: changes of mandibular inclination and changes of the cervical and craniocervical posture. In order to achieve maximum mouth opening there must be at least 15° of posterior head movement; the hyoid bone must follow the head posteriorly and must also move inferiorly with jaw depression (Muto & Kanazawa 1994). If there is a limitation in one of these movements and function is to be maintained, then there will have to be a compensatory give in the cervical area or in the TMJ.

Recent publications have brought to light the close relationship between the position of the cranium on the neck, the mandibular position and the vertical occlusion dimension:

- Vertical occlusion dimension
- Craniocervical angle
- Retrognathia or prognathia.

VERTICAL OCCLUSION DIMENSION

Vertical occlusion dimension (VOD) is defined as the distance from the base of the nose to the base of the chin. Moya et al (1994) demonstrated that when using an occlusal splint of 4.0–5.5 mm thickness the increased VOD caused a significant craniocervical extension and a decrease of the lordosis in the cervical spine. Therefore the position of the jaw directly influences the cervical spine. The more the jaw is advanced anteriorly, the more the VOD is increased (Kraus 1988).

Urbanowicz (1991) concluded that a change in mandibular posture, specifically an increase in VOD, contributes to craniovertical extension, leading to suboccipital compression and upsetting the postural balance between the head and neck.

Darling et al (1984) found that the resting VOD was decreased in individuals with a forward head posture and was newly increased after correcting the head posture with physiotherapy. Therefore correction of the head and neck on the trunk will directly change the jaw position.

RETROGNATHIA AND PROGNATHIA

When analysing the relationship between internal derangements of the TMJ and facial growth disturbances, Shellehas (1989) found that, out of 60 patients that presented with retrognathia, 56 (93.31%) showed internal derangements of both TMJs. As mentioned previously, retrognathia is significantly associated with an extension of the head over the cervical spine which is always present in the forward head position. Retrognathia may be the give or the site of compensatory stability dysfunction in a forward head posture.

Solow (1992) showed that certain patients had a backwardly inclined upper cervical column, a small craniocervical angle, reduced posterior mobility of the TMJ and an increased prognathism. On the contrary, others presented with a large craniocervical angle, an upright position of the upper cervical column, increased posterior mobility of the TMJ and retrognathia. Thus the position of the mandible has a direct influence on the cervical spine.

In agreement with these findings, Nobili and Adversi (1996) found that in patients with an Angle class I occlusion the posture was baricentric, in Angle class II malocclusion patients it was anteriorly displaced and in patients with an Angle class III malocclusion it was posteriorly displaced. The correlation between body posture and the occlusion was statistically significant.

In conclusion, the correlation between the mandible, cranium, cervical spine and the hyoid bone together as part of the whole body has been demonstrated (see Chapter 5). When there is dysfunction, which of these is the cause and which is the result is unknown and is probably different in each case. However, it is evident that the muscles and fascia controlled by the neural system play a significant role in maintaining equilibrium or balance.

Nasal airway obstruction

It is well documented that nasal obstruction is directly related to a forward head posture (Ormeño et al 1999). Since breathing is essential to life the body will adapt in whatever way is necessary to control the position of the cranium, mandible, lips and tongue with respect to the cervical spine in order to maintain an adequate airway. In order to be able to breathe through the mouth the mandible must be lowered, decreasing the tension in the suprahyoid muscles and allowing the hyoid to fall downwards and backwards and, in so doing, the pharyngeal air passage is reduced. Consequently, to maintain adequate air flow the head must assume a more forward and more extended position to passively pull the hyoid bone forward and upwards by tensioning the suprahyoid musculature.

Respiratory problems necessitate the use of the auxiliary respiratory muscles (sternocleidomastoid, scalenes) which, when overdominant, will tend to hold the lower cervical vertebrae in flexion and the upper cervical vertebrae in extension, signifying also that longus colli and semispinalis are no longer sufficiently controlling the cervical intersegmental movement.

Clinically, people with open-mouthed posture habits without any type of nasal airway obstruction demonstrate two essential characteristics (Schievano et al 1999):

- Lower lip everted, confirmed through visualization of the labial mucous membrane
- Tension in the chin region when the lips are closed, confirmed through visualization of wrinkle formation.

Schievano et al (1999) showed that in a nasal breather the EMG activity of orbicularis oris superior and inferior and mentalis at rest and in a closed lip situation should be the same. This suggests that the recruited motor units are similar in both situations. However, in the mouth breather, we see a greater number of units recruited to close the lips, possibly because of a hypofunction of the orbicularis oris muscles. To close the lips the mentalis muscles become hyperactive to compensate for the lack of activity of the orbicularis oris muscles, especially that of the orbicularis oris inferior. This muscle imbalance can also have implications for craniofacial and craniomandibular dysfunction. As in many recruitment dysfunction problems, Mathew et al (1982) noted that after an adenoidectomy the breathing pattern does not always return to normal and oral breathers may continue to breathe through the mouth even when the cause has been corrected. For more information about breathing patterns, craniofacial growth and posture, see Chapters 21 and 22.

Hormonal changes

Since pain itself is now recognized as one of the possible aetiologies of musculoskeletal dysfunction, more interest is being directed to the cause of pain. When looking at the prevalence rates for craniomandibular dysfunction, these have been shown to be lower among older subjects, and the initial onset in both males and females appears more likely to occur before the age of 50 than later in life (Hiltunen et al 1995). The frequency is higher for women of reproductive age than those in postmenopausal years (Von Korff et al 1988, 1991). LeResche et al (1997) further noted that the chances of seeking treatment is increased by 77% with the use of supplemental oestrogen in the postmenopausal years and by 19% in patients using oral contraceptives. Taking all this into consideration, there are sufficient grounds to conclude that oestrogen and nerve growth factor (a secretory protein) together may lead to an increased incidence of clinical muscle pain (Stohler 1997), including craniofacial and craniomandibular pain.

Proprioception and pain

Proprioceptive feedback can come from joints and ligaments as well as from muscles and skin. It is the key to informing the central nervous system of changes in position and movement and essential to the rehabilitation programme. The reprogramming of a correct movement pattern is dependent on proprioceptive feedback (Revel et al 1994, McPartland et al 1997, Jull 2000).

Boering (1966) reported on a number of anatomical studies that described end-organs of Ruffini, Vater–Pacini and Golgi found, in particular, in the lateral and laterodorsal part of the TMJ capsule and ligaments. These mechanoreceptors are thought to be involved in the proprioceptive mechanisms of the joint and therefore contribute to the control of function in the masticatory muscles. Clark and Carter (1985) blocked intramuscular proprioceptive input by giving anaesthetic blocks to muscle nerves. Loss of static position sense was observed whereas dynamic position sense was preserved.

Pain also seems to be responsible for changing this control of function. Experimentally induced pain alters kinaesthetic sensibility caused by irregularities of muscle spindle discharge (Ro & Capra 2000). This result is in agreement with Lund et al (1991) who conclude that pain changes the coordination of the movement during dynamic exercises. Harper and Schneiderman (1996), while comparing the reproducibility of the centric relation position and the condylar pathway in patients with TMJ internal derangement, found that there is a loss of ability to trace a constant path in opening and a loss of dynamic range of horizontal adaptation.

In summary, muscle dysfunction in the craniomandibular and craniofacial regions is a dominant functional occurrence of the musculoskeletal system and is influenced by a wide range of contributory factors. The therapist should be aware of the range of potential influences in order to distinguish between them if required.

REHABILITATION PROPOSALS FOR THE CRANIOFACIAL AND CRANIOMANDIBULAR REGIONS

Goals

Specific goals necessary to create a rehabilitation programme for a muscular dysfunction include increasing proprioceptive awareness, facilitating correct coordination, controlling a newly acquired range of movement and increasing inner range low load control and eccentric outer range control.

To establish a rehabilitation programme for each patient a thorough assessment must be made to determine where there is a specific articular give or restriction and/or a myofascial give and restriction. Since the global muscle system is direction specific, it is important to establish the direction in which the symptoms are provoked. What are the movements or positions that are provoking the symptoms and where is the site of the dysfunction? As not all of the gives and restrictions encountered will be clinically relevant for each patient, a clinical reasoning process is necessary to determine clinical priority.

Once this has been established there are four main treatment principles important for correcting a muscle imbalance:

- Control of the neutral position
- Dynamic control of the direction of the stability dysfunction – mobilizing the give and restriction
- Global stabilizer control through range
- Extensibility of the global mobilizers.

CONTROL OF THE NEUTRAL POSITION

It is especially important for the patient suffering from craniomandibular or craniofacial pain to be aware of the daily habits, positions and movements that are causing the give and stressing articular, neural or muscular tissue. The simple act of paying attention to these and minimizing the load on the affected structures will decrease peripheral pain and thereby central nervous system afferent input and will immediately give positive results. Therefore, an essential part of the rehabilitation programme must be aimed at identifying and eliminating the contributing factors and it sometimes becomes necessary to work with a dentist or speech therapist.

Joint restrictions must be mobilized using techniques such as passive joint mobilization; however, the new joint mobility must be controlled and coordinated with a well-designed exercise programme or it will again be lost. The patient's awareness or proprioceptive sense of where or how they are moving is essential to re-establish central nervous system control. If an articular restriction is present, correct muscle recruitment is difficult. From the evidence in the literature it appears quite possible that a muscle dysfunction in the craniomandibular and craniofacial area can be a predisposing factor for pain; however, pain can also be the direct cause of an altered muscle recruitment, altered joint mechanics and further pain.

'Red dot' system

The 'red-dot' system (Comerford & Mottram 2001) is a useful learning tool to stimulate the memory and help patients become aware of their mandibular position, muscular tension and habits. The red dots are placed in common locations within the patient's occupational and recreational environment. Whenever a red dot is sighted, the patient must note the position of the mandible at that moment and then relax the jaw into a mandibular rest position and properly position the tongue. This must be maintained for at least 10 seconds while continuing the daily activity and breathing calmly through the nose. This can be repeated three to five times whenever a red dot is sighted.

Mandibular rest position and tongue position

The mandibular rest position is one of good alignment with the teeth slightly apart and the lips lightly closed; there should be no tension in the lips or chin. The tongue should be in a relaxed, neutral position just behind the upper teeth, not on the floor of the mouth or pushed upward onto the palate. Kraus (1988) prefers the term *upright postural position of the mandible* (UPPM) as it implies the essential interrelationship of the jaw, head and neck in the upright position; therefore, when referring to this complete scenario – including the jaw, head, neck, scapula and tongue position – the term UPPM will be used.

Rocabado (1983) has always advocated that the tip of the tongue should be maintained against the palate with a slight pressure and states that, in this way, the masticatory muscle activity is at a minimum. Carlson et al (1997) have challenged that theory with EMG studies which show that the temporalis and the suprahyoid muscle activity is actually increased with the tongue on the roof of the mouth. Muscle activity in the masseter muscle remained unaltered in the different tongue positions. The tongue drops to the floor of the mouth when the head is in a forward head position, the scapulae are downwardly rotated and the mandible is held forward. These authors believe that if we gradually instruct the patient to bring the cervical spine, scapulae and the mandible into a more corrected or neutral position, then the tongue will take its natural relaxed position with the proper minimal muscular activity of the local stabilizers. The key is probably having a complete postural correction and therefore, as soon as this can be integrated by the patient, the visualization of the red dot should stimulate a complete postural correction.

Correction of the neutral position or control of the neutral position with minimal effort as often as possible and in as many varied positions as possible is one of the key elements of the rehabilitation programme. It is imperative that this be carried over into functional positions or stressful moments of the day that are known to the patient. As the description says, 'the neutral position is a mid-position and therefore not an end of range or forced position'. The neutral position is not always the ideal or perfect position but it is the mid-position for the individual patient.

Scapular neutral position (Mottram 1993)

Starting position and method

Sitting or standing with the centre of gravity well placed over the feet or the ischial tuberosities and with the weight of the arm in an unloaded position against gravity. Place the index finger of the right hand across the pectorals onto the left coracoid process.

Exercise

Ask the patient to lift the coracoid up and posteriorly away from the finger and hold the position 10 times for 10 seconds without pain or fatigue. Ideally, both shoulders are corrected together; however, beware of thoracic or lumbar extension compensating for correct scapular movement. The desired movement is scapular upward rotation and not depression or protraction of the scapula.

Aim

The aim is to recruit a low tonic contraction in the trapezius and serratus anterior muscles and to unload the levator scapula and rhomboid muscles and, thus, the upper cervical spine.

Cervical neutral position (Jull 2000)

Starting position and method

Sitting in cervical extension with the posterior aspect of the head and the scapulae against the wall but not the sacrum (beware not to be in end of range cervical extension) or standing with the centre of gravity well placed over the feet and the scapulae in a neutral position.

Exercise

Lengthen the cervical spine by sliding the head up the wall (upper cervical flexion) to achieve a neutral position (take care not to be in end of range flexion). The patient should be taught to palpate to ensure that the superficial neck flexors are not compensating for the deep neck flexors (take care not to move into low cervical flexion). Hold the contraction 10 times for 10 seconds while breathing calmly without pain or fatigue.

Aim

The aim is to recruit a low load tonic contraction of the deep neck flexors and not the superficial muscles such as the sternocleidomastoid, scalenes or hyoid muscles and unload the pathology caused by a head forward position.

Hyoid bone neutral position

Starting position and method

Sitting or standing in UPPM with the mouth slightly open, the therapist places the index finger and thumb on either side of the hyoid bone and asks the patient to maintain the hyoid bone in that position: 'Don't let me move it.'

Control of the neutral position
The patient maintains the position for 10 seconds as the therapist gives slight resistance to the left or right. The patient is then instructed to do this independently.

Aim
The aim is to recruit a low load tonic contraction of the supra- and infrahyoid muscles (Fig. 12.4).

Mandible neutral position

Starting position and method
Sitting or standing in UPPM with the mouth slightly open, the therapist places the index finger and thumb on either side of the mandible and asks the patient to maintain the mandible in that position: 'Don't let me move it' (Fig. 12.5).

Control of the neutral position
The patient maintains the position for 10 seconds as the therapist gives slight resistance to the left, right, cranially or caudally. The patient is instructed to do this independently.

Aim
The aim is to recruit a low load tonic contraction of the medial pterygoid, temporalis and masseter muscles.

> **!** All of the low load tonic work is to be performed with the tongue and mandible in a correct position and the lips relaxed. This should be carried over to a variety of functional positions throughout the day and becomes the basis of the 'red dot' system.

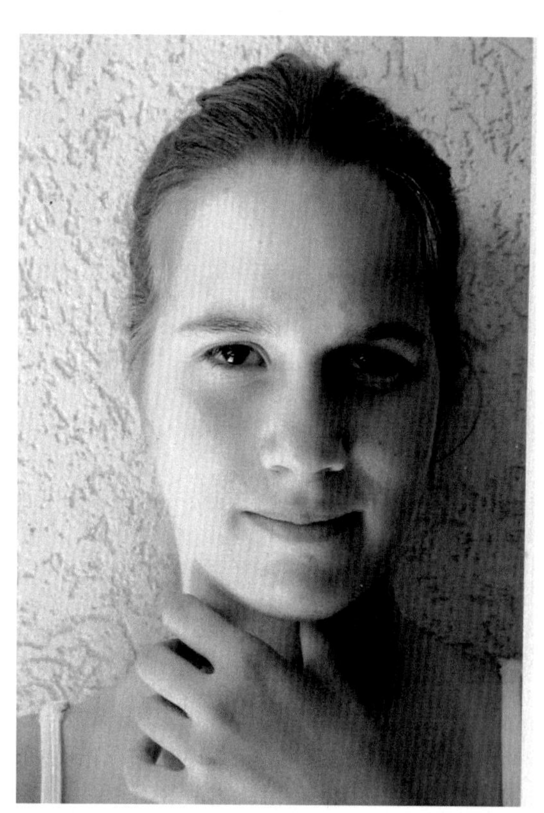

Fig. 12.4 Hyoid bone, neutral position. The patient is asked to gently resist the pressure on the hyoid bone.

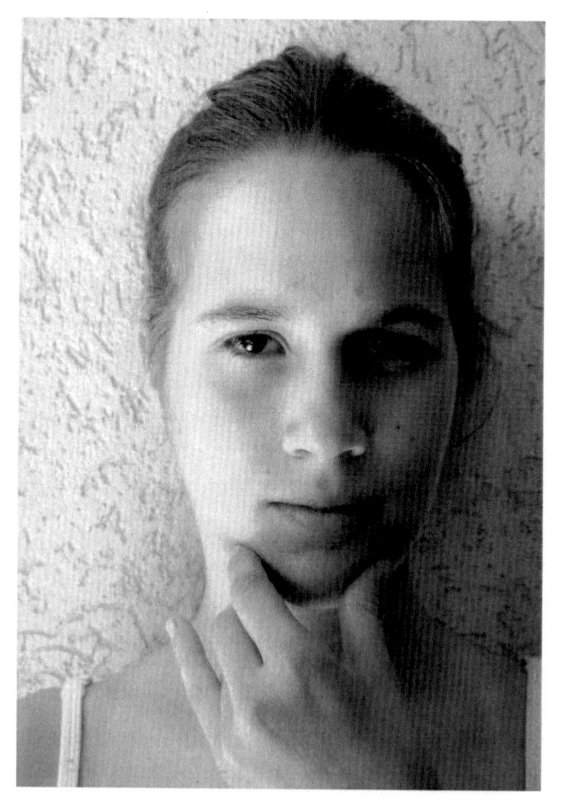

Fig. 12.5 Mandibular neutral position. The patient is asked to gently resist the displacement of the mandible.

DYNAMIC CONTROL OF DIRECTION AND THROUGH RANGE CONTROL

The aim is to correct the imbalance in the global muscle system. Dynamic control of direction aims to change the recruitment pattern. By controlling the give when the patient is used to moving, and mobilizing the restricted movement direction when the patient is not used to moving, and, therefore, dissociating the movements, we will challenge the patient's control of the neutral position and their proprioceptive sense. Proprioception is essential for higher central nervous system control and correct movement patterns. Controlling the movement in the pain-provoking direction helps to unload the affected structures, controls symptoms and gives the patient the power of knowing they can control their own symptoms.

In the presence of dysfunction global stabilizers become long and inhibited. The main role of a global stabilizer is to eccentrically control movement throughout its entire range, especially in rotation, but the challenge comes mostly in inner range positions. Through range control it uses inner range holding to improve eccentric control.

Thoracic

Starting position and method

Sitting or standing in UPPM, ask the patient to place a finger on the sternum and lift the sternum towards the ceiling without retracting the shoulders or extending in the lumbar spine.

Control of direction

Lift the sternum slowly 20 times while breathing calmly, three to four times per day. Take care not to move the pelvis forward.

Through range control

With the sternum elevated, hold for 10 seconds while breathing calmly and without fatigue or pain. Repeat 10 times.

Aim

The aim is to recruit a low load tonic contraction of the thoracic multifidi to segmentally move the thoracic spine without permitting lumbar, cervical or mandibular movement and to improve eccentric control from thoracic extension to flexion.

Cervical

Starting position and method

In sitting or standing in UPPM, ask the patient to lightly place both hands on the mandible near the TMJs to ensure that there is no movement or clenching and slowly move the cervical spine into flexion, extension, lateral flexion or rotation or any combination of these movements specific to the patient's functional problem. The patient must go only to the point where they are able to control the movement with *minimal effort* (and not with a co-contraction rigidity) and the movement must be without symptoms.

In extension, ensure that the patient is using a correct movement pattern and not simply giving into midcervical extension. They must have a smooth arc of extension and not a folding at the C4–C5 or C5–C6 level. Giving in one region to rehabilitate another region is not useful. Any give should be protected and controlled. In rotation, again the pattern should be correct, with a slight lateral flexion component coming only at the end of the rotation range and there should be no chin poking (upper cervical extension). If the proper pattern is difficult for the patient, try initiating by asking them to lightly touch the teeth together to increase proprioceptive feedback which seems to enhance a more correct pattern. As the pattern is learned, the teeth touching can be eliminated.

Control of direction

Repeat the movement 20 times, three to four times per day without compensation or co-contraction rigidity.

Through range control

At the end of the range of movement, hold the contraction for 10 seconds against a slight manual resistance (not more than 30% MVC to ensure a tonic, low load recruitment) while breathing calmly, without fatigue, compensation or symptoms. Repeat 10 times, three to four times daily (Fig. 12.6).

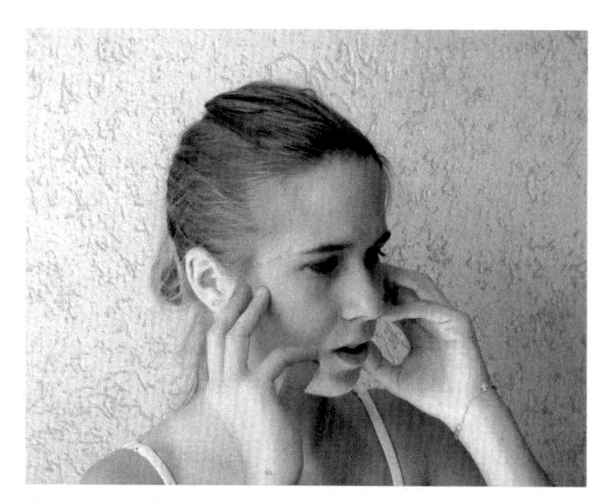

Fig. 12.6 Cervical spine movement. The patient is asked to move the thoracic spine without compensating this movement elsewhere.

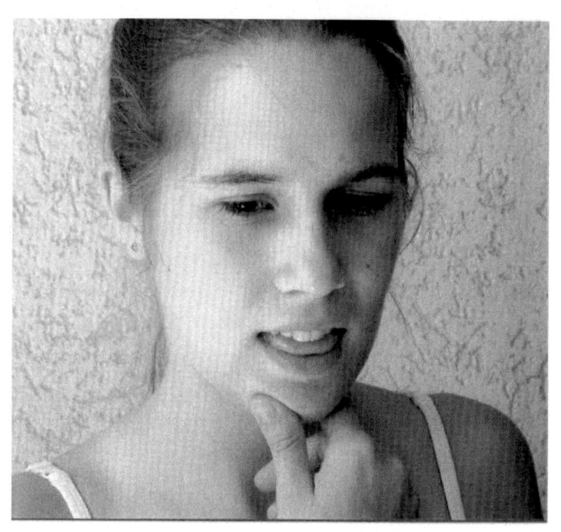

Fig. 12.7 Mandibular movement. The patient is asked to move the mandible without compensating this movement elsewhere.

Aim

The aim is to facilitate a new recruitment pattern, to challenge the control of neutral of the mandible and to increase inner range strength and control.

Mandible

Starting position and method

Sitting with the head against the wall in the cervical neutral position or standing in UPPM. Initially, a 'pressure biofeedback unit' as described by Jull (2000) can be used under the cervical spine to assist correct participation of the deep neck flexors in a supine or sitting position. Using the wall and/or a mirror as feedback to control any cervical movement or any deviation of the mandible, ask the patient to move the mandible slowly into depression, retraction, protraction or laterotrusion or any combination of these movements as indicated by the patient's movement problem. Beware of compensation of the superficial neck flexors, a give into cervical extension or co-contraction rigidity (Fig. 12.7).

Control of movement direction

Repeat the movement 20 times, three to four times daily with control, minimal effort and without symptoms or clicking.

Through range control

In the end of range position, hold against a slight manual resistance (not more than 30% MVC to ensure a tonic, low load recruitment) for 10 seconds while breathing calmly, without fatigue, compensation or symptoms. Repeat 10 times, three to four times daily.

Aim

The aim is to facilitate a new recruitment pattern of the mandible, trying to re-establish the kinaesthetic sensibility and challenge the control of neutral of the cervical spine. This is especially important if the joint is free passively but the patient cannot coordinate the correct movement pattern or if the patient needs to acquire proprioceptive awareness of a newly attained mobility.

Tongue

Starting position and method

In sitting or standing in UPPM with the mouth slightly open, ask the patient to place one index and thumb on the hyoid bone to facilitate proprioception and the other on the chin to control mandibular movement. Move the tongue slowly into the direction of the stability dysfunction: protrusion, retrusion, laterally, onto the hard palate, onto the soft palate, touching the molars to the right or left, or touching the upper incisors to the right or left (Fig. 12.8).

Control of movement

Repeat the movement 20 times, three to four times daily without symptoms, fatigue or compensation.

Through range control

In the end of range position, hold for 10 seconds while breathing gently and without fatigue or symptoms. Repeat 10 times, three to four times daily.

Aim

The aim is to facilitate a new recruitment pattern of the tongue and increase inner range strength and control, and to challenge the control of neutral of the cervical spine, mandible and hyoid bone.

Controlling the temporomandibular joint

Instability and hypermobility, in the literature, are often used as synonyms meaning that a joint moves more than a standard range. For certain professions or sports hypermobility is required and will not necessarily be an instability. As long as the entire range can be eccentrically controlled by the global and local stabilizers the joint is functionally stable and pain-free. For example, in the TMJ, singers often need more than the usually accepted standard of mobility and this can be functionally stable, without pain or clicking.

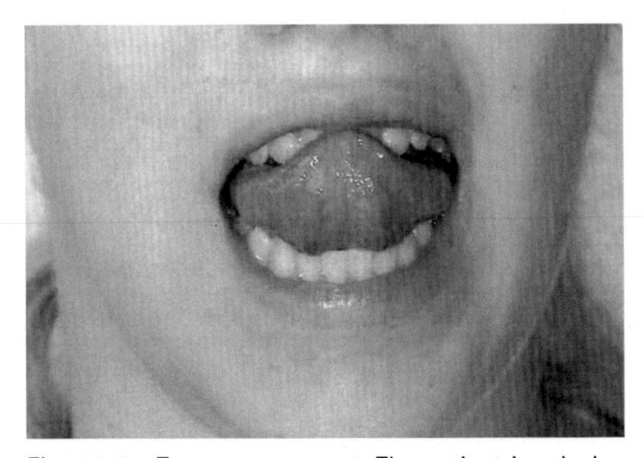

Fig. 12.8 Tongue movement. The patient is asked to move the tongue without compensating this movement elsewhere.

Clinical instability is orthopaedically well defined as being glide tests or ligament stress tests which are positive in at least one direction. The passive supporting system is no longer completely intact. A *functional instability* is when the person is unable to control the dynamic stability of the joint with the active muscle system. Someone can be clinically unstable but be functionally stable because the muscular system is able to compensate for the ligamental laxity. For more information about instability in general, see Chapter 6.

Clinically, in a hypermobile joint where the jaw depression exceeds 50 mm, we may see an articular give mostly into an anterior and medial direction. Difficulties in coordinating retrusion are also common. On palpation, the condylar head is felt to go anteriorly and caudally to the eminence. This is often accompanied by a terminal clicking and pain. Schulte (1988) states that if the hypermobility persists for a long time, hyperactivity develops in one or both lateral pterygoids and ultimately hypertrophy is seen on CT scans. The musculature probably attempts to control the hypermobility by a co-contraction rigidity.

EXTENSIBILITY OF THE GLOBAL MOBILIZERS

After determining that the accessory movements in all directions of both TMJs are free, it is then necessary to regain correct control of the dynamic stability of the craniomandibular region.

Facilitation of craniomandibular rotation (global control)

Starting position and method

Sitting in UPPM, the patient is asked to place the tip of the tongue on the soft palate, to pull the mandible backwards and, while maintaining it there, to open the mouth in a straight line without deviation (Fig. 12.9).

Control of movement direction

Repeat the movement 20 times, three to four times daily without symptoms, fatigue or compensation.

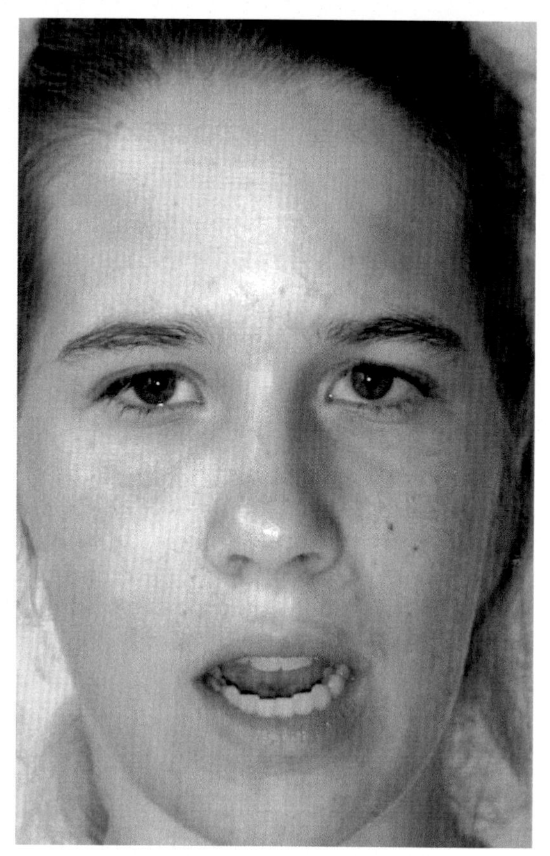

Fig. 12.9 Facilitation of craniomandibular rotation. The patient is asked to touch the soft palate with the tongue, move the mandible backwards and open the mouth without deviation.

Through range control
Hold in the end of range position for 10 seconds without compensation or signs of fatigue and repeat 10 times, three to four times per day.

Aim
The aim is to regain the inner range control of the digastric and suprahyoid muscles and reciprocally inhibit the IHLP.

The other clinical pattern that we see is a hypomobile joint with or without difficulty in controlling protraction. On palpation the condylar head does not move sufficiently into anterior translation and often the patient will compensate by giving into cervical extension to maintain sufficient mouth opening.

After assessing and treating the accessory movements of both TMJs and of the cervical spine to ensure that they are free, it is necessary to regain control of the newly acquired range.

Facilitation of mandibular anterior translation (local control)

Starting position and method
Sitting in UPPM, the patient is asked to position the tongue in front of the central incisors under the upper lip and to maintain it there while opening the mouth as far as possible. Be careful not to allow an upper or midcervical extension. If there is a deviation of the mandible to one side, the starting position of the tongue is moved slightly to the contralateral side in front of the canine teeth before opening the jaw.

Control of movement direction
Repeat the movement 20 times, three to four times daily without symptoms, fatigue or compensation.

Through range control
Maintain this position for at least 10 seconds without compensation or signs of fatigue and repeat 10 times, three to four times per day.

Aim
The aim is to regain the inner range control of the IHLP and the reciprocal inhibition of temporalis and masseter.

To facilitate the exercise programme, self-massage of the hyperactive muscles and trigger point release should be integrated from the beginning. Passive joint mobilizations that are considered necessary should be carried out by the therapist to permit correct muscle recruitment. All of the exercises should be done without symptoms and always reinforcing the correct postural position for the cervical spine, scapulae and the general alignment of the body over the weight-bearing points.

Conclusions

Muscle dysfunction in the head and neck region can be a contributing factor to head, neck and face pain. Therefore a muscle imbalance orientated rehabilitation programme of the craniomandibular and craniofacial regions should be considered. It should be an integral part of the patient's treatment and management concept, rather than standing on its own.

Early intervention is suggested to reduce nociceptive input by reducing the load on the affected structures and controlling the dynamic stability, thereby reducing potential motor control dysfunctions and further pain. Collaborative clinical reasoning and early introduction of exercises aimed at maintaining correct motor control patterns integrated into the activities of daily living may be of considerable importance in the prevention of chronic pain in the cranial, facial and mandibular regions.

References

Bazzotti L 1998 Mandible position and head posture: electromyography of the sternocleidomastoids. Journal of Craniomandibular Practice 16(2):100

Bergmark A 1989 Stability of the lumbar spine. A study in mechanical engineering. Acta Orthopaedica Scandinavica 230(60):20

Bérzin F 1995 Electromyographic analysis of the sternohyoid muscle and anterior belly of the digastric muscle in jaw movements. Journal of Oral Rehabilitation 22:463

Boering G 1966 Temporomandibular joint arthrosis: an analysis of 400 cases. Stafleu and Tholen, Leiden

Boyd C H, Slagle W F, MacBoyd C, Bryant R W, Wiygul J P 1987 The effect of head position on electromyographic evaluations of representative mandibular positioning muscle groups. Journal of Craniomandibular Practice 5(1):51

Carlson C R, Sherman J J, Studts J L, Bertrand P M 1997 The effects of tongue position on mandibular muscle activity. Journal of Orofacial Pain 11(4):291

Castro H A L, Resende L A L, Bérzin F, König B 1998 Electromyographic analysis of superior belly of the omohyoid muscle and anterior belly of the digastric muscle in mandibular movements. Electromyography and Clinical Neurophysiology 38:443

Cholewicki J, McGill S 1996 Mechanical stability in the in vivo lumbar spine: implications for injury and chronic low back pain. Clinical Biomechanics 11(1):1

Clark G T, Carter M C 1985 Electromyographic study of human jaw-closing muscle endurance, fatigue and recovery at various isometric force levels. Archives of Oral Biology 30:563

Comerford M J, Mottram S L 2001 Movement and stability dysfunction – contemporary developments. Manual Therapy 6(1):31

Cowan S M, Bennell K L, Hodges P W, Crossley K M, McConnell J 2001 Delayed onset of electromyographic activity of vastus medialis obliquus relative to vastus lateralis in subjects with patellofemoral pain syndrome. Archives of Physical and Medical Rehabilitation 82:183

Dangaria T R, Naesh O 1998 Changes in cross-sectional area of psoas major muscle in unilateral sciatica caused by disc herniation. Spine 23(8):928

Darling D W, Kraus S, Glasheen-Wray M B 1984 Relationship of head posture and the rest position of the mandible. Journal of Prosthetic Dentistry 52(1):111

De Boever J 1979 Functional disturbances of the temporomandibular joint. In: Zarb G, Carlsson G (eds) Temporomandibular joint function and dysfunction. Mosby, St Louis, p 193

Derrick L J, Lapointe H 1991 Demystifying the temporomandibular joint. Orthopaedic Division Newsletter Sept/Oct:23

DuPont J S, Matthews E P 2000 Orofacial sensory changes and temporomandibular dysfunction. Journal of Craniomandibular Practice 18(3):174

Elvey R 1986 Treatment of arm pain associated with abnormal brachial plexus tension. Australian Journal of Physiotherapy 32:225

Farella M, Michelotti A, Steenks M H et al 2000 The diagnostic value of pressure algometry in myofascial pain of the jaw muscles. Journal of Oral Rehabilitation 27:9

Farrar W B, McCarty W L 1983 A clinical outline of temporomandibular joint diagnosis and treatment. Walker Printing, Alabama, p 119

Friction J R 1985 Myofascial pain syndrome of the head and neck: a review of clinical characteristics of 164 patients. Oral Surgery, Oral Medicine, Oral Pathology 60:615

Funakoshi M, Amano N 1973 Effects of the tonic neck reflex on the jaw muscles of the rat. Journal of Dental Research 52:668

Funakoshi M, Fujita N, Takehana S 1976 Relations between occlusal interference and jaw muscle activities in response to changes in head position. Journal of Dental Research 55:634

Gibbons S G T, Mottram S L, Comerford M J 2001 Orthopaedic Division Review Sept/Oct:1

Goldstein D F, Kraus S L, Williams W B, Glasheen-Wray M B 1984 Influence of cervical posture on mandibular movement. Journal of Prosthetic Dentistry 52(3):421

Gonzalez H E, Manns A 1996 Forward head posture: its structural and functional influence on the stomatognathic system, a conceptual study. Journal of Craniomandibular Practice 14(1):71

Gossman M R, Sarhmann S A, Rose S J 1982 Review of length-associated changes in muscle. Physical Therapy 62(12):1799

Goto T K, Yahagi M, Nakamura Y et al 2005 In vivo cross-sectional area of human jaw muscles varies with section location and jaw position. Journal of Dental Research 84(6):570–575

Graf H 1971 Il bruxismo. CONA 5(1):143

Hamilton C, Richardson C 1998 Active control of the neutral lumbopelvic posture: a comparison between back pain and non back pain subjects. Vienna, Austria: 3rd Interdisciplinary World Congress on Low Back Pain and Pelvic Pain

Harper R P, Schneiderman E 1996 Condylar movement and centric relation in patients with internal derangement of the temporomandibular joint. Journal of Prosthetic Dentistry 75(1):67

Hides J A, Stokes M J, Saide M, Jull G A, Cooper D H 1994 Evidence of lumbar multifidus wasting ipsilateral to symptoms in patients with acute/subacute low back pain. Spine 19(2):165

Hides J A, Richardson C A, Jull G A 1996 Multifidus muscle recovery is not automatic after resolution of acute, first episode low back pain. Spine 21(23):2763

Hiltunen K, Schmidt-Kaunisaho K, Nevalainen J, Narhi T, Ainamo A 1995 A prevalence of signs of temporomandibular disorders among elderly inhabitants of Helsinki, Finland. Acta Odontologica Scandinavica 53:20

Hiraoka K 2004 Changes in masseter muscle activity associated with swallowing. Journal of Oral Rehabilitation 31(10):963–967

Hiraba K, Hibibo K, Hiranuma K, Negoro T 2000 EMG activities of the two heads of the human lateral pterygoid muscle in relation to mandibular condyle movement and biting force. Journal of Neurophysiology 83(4):2120

Hodges P W 1999 Is there a role for transversus abdominis in lumbo-pelvic stability? Manual Therapy 4(2):74

Hodges P W, Richardson C A 1996 Inefficient muscular stabilisation of the lumbar spine associated with low back pain: a motor control evaluation of transversus abdominis. Spine 21(22):2640

Hodges P, Richardson C 1997 Contraction of the abdominal muscles associated with movement of the lower limb. Physical Therapy 77:132

Hodges P, Richardson C 1999 Altered trunk muscle recruitment in people with low back pain with upper limb movement at different speeds. Archives of Medical Rehabilitation 80:1005

Hong C Z 1994 Lidocaine injection versus dry needling to myofascial trigger points. American Journal of Physical Medicine and Rehabilitation 73:256

Huang B Y, Whittle T, Murray G M 2005 Activity of inferior head of human lateral pterygoid muscle during standardized lateral jaw movements. Archives of Oral Biology 50(1):49–64

Isberg A, Widmalm S, Ivarsson R 1985 Clinical, radiographic and electromyographic study of patients with internal derangement of the temporomandibular joint. American Journal of Orthodontics 8(6):453

Isberg-Holm A, Ivasson R 1980 The movement pattern of mandibular condyles in individuals with and without clicking. A clinical and cineradiographic study. Dento-maxillo-facial Radiology 9:59

Janda V 1983 Motor learning impairment and back pain. FIMM Proceedings, Zurich

Janda V L 1994 Muscles and motor control in cervicogenic disorders: assessment and management. In: Grant R (ed.) Physical therapy of the cervical and thoracic spine, 2nd edn. Churchill Livingstone, Edinburgh, p 195

Johansson H, Sojka P 1991 Pathophysiological mechanisms involved in genesis and spread of muscular tension in occupational muscle pain and in chronic musculoskeletal pain syndromes: a hypothesis. Medical Hypothesis 35:196

Jull G 2000 Deep cervical flexor muscle dysfunction in whiplash. Journal of Musculoskeletal Pain 8(1/2):143

Jull G, Barrett C, Magee R, Ho P 1999 Further clinical clarification of the muscle dysfunction in cervical headache. Cephalalgia 19(3):179

Juniper R P 1984 Temporomandibular joint dysfunction: a theory based upon electromyographic studies of the lateral pterygoid muscle. British Journal of Oral and Maxillofacial Surgery 22:1

Kovero O, Könönen M 1996 Signs and symptoms of temporomandibular disorders in adolescent violin players. Acta Odontologica Scandinavica 54(4):271

Kraus S L (ed.) 1988 Cervical spine influences on the management of TMD. In: Temporomandibular joint disorders: management of the craniomandibular complex. Churchill Livingstone, New York

Kylämarkula S, Huggare J 1985 Head posture and the morphology of the first cervical vertebra. European Journal of Orthodontics 7:151

LeResche L, Saunders K, Von Korff M R, Barlow W, Dworkin S F 1997 Use of exogenous hormones and

risk of temporomandibular disorder pain. Pain 69:153
Lewit K 1978 The contribution of clinical observation to neurobiological mechanisms in manipulative therapy. In: Korr I (ed.) The neurobiologic mechanisms in manipulative therapy. Plenum Press, New York
Lund J P, Donga R, Widmer G, Stohler C 1991 The pain adaptation model: a discussion of the relationship between chronic musculoskeletal pain and motor activity. Canadian Journal of Physiology and Pharmacology 69:683
Makofsky H W 1989 The effect of head posture on muscle contact position: the sliding cranium theory. Journal of Craniomandibular Practice 7(4):286
Makofsky H W 2000 The influence of forward head posture on dental occlusion. Journal of Craniomandibular Practice 18(1):30
Mathew O P, Abu-Osba Y K, Thach B T 1982 Influence of upper airway pressure changes on genioglossus muscle respiratory activity. Journal of Applied Physiology 52:438
Matthews B 1975 Mastication. In: Lavelle C (ed.) Applied physiology of the mouth. John Wright, Bristol, p 209
McMillan A S, Blasberg B 1994 Pain–pressure threshold in painful jaw muscles following triggerpoint injection. Journal of Orofacial Pain 8(4):384
McKay D C, Christensen L V 1999 Electrognathographic and electromyographic observations on jaw depression during neck extension. Journal of Oral Rehabilitation 26:865
McPartland J M, Brodeur R R, Hallgren R C 1997 Chronic neck pain, standing balance and suboccipital muscle atrophy: a pilot study. Journal of Manipulative and Physiological Therapeutics 20:24
Miralles R, Valenzuela S, Ramirez P et al 1998 Visual input effect on EMG activity of sternocleidomastoid and masseter muscles in healthy subjects and in patients with myogenic cranio-cervical-mandibular dysfunction. Journal of Craniomandibular Practice 16(3):168
Möller E, Sheikholeslam A, Lous I 1984 Response of elevator activity during mastication to treatment of functional disorders. Scandinavian Journal of Dental Research 92:64
Mongini F, Tempia-Valenta G, Conserva E 1989 Habitual mastication in dysfunction: a computer based analysis. Journal of Prosthetic Dentistry 61:484
Mongini F 1999 Muscle disorders in headache and face pain. Thieme, Stuttgart, p 29
Mottram S L 1993 Dynamic stability of the scapula. Manual Therapy 2(3):123
Mottram S L, Comerford M 1998 Stability dysfunction and low back pain. Journal of Orthopaedic Medicine 20(2):13
Moya H, Miralles R, Zuniga C et al 1994 Influence of stabilization occlusal splint on cranio-cervical relationships. Part I: Cephalometrical analysis. Journal of Craniomandibular Practice 12:47
Murray G M, Orfanos T, Chan J C Y, Wanigaratne K, Klineberg I J 1999a Electromyographic activity of the human lateral pterygoid muscle during contralateral and protrusive jaw movements. Archives of Oral Biology 44:269
Murray G M, Phanachet I, Hupalo M, Wanigaratne K 1999b Simultaneous recording of mandibular condylar movement and single motor-unit activity at verified sites in the human lateral pterygoid muscle. Archives of Oral Biology 4:671
Murray G M, Phanachet I, Klineberg I J 1999c Electromyographic evidence for functional heterogeneity in the inferior head of the human lateral pterygoid muscle: a preliminary multi-unit study. Clinical Neurophysiology 110:944
Muto T, Kanazawa M 1994 Positional change of the hyoid bone at maximal mouth opening. Oral Surgery, Oral Medicine, Oral Pathology 77(5):451
Nobili A, Adversi R 1996 Relationship between posture and occlusion: a clinical and experimental investigation. Journal of Craniomandibular Practice 14(4):274
O'Sullivan P B, Twomey L, Allison G 1997 Evaluation of specific stabilising exercises in the treatment of chronic low back pain with radiological diagnosis of spondylosis or spondylolisthesis. Spine 22(24):2959
O'Sullivan P, Twomey L, Allison G 1998 Altered abdominal muscle recruitment in back pain patients following specific exercise intervention. Journal of Orthopaedic and Sports Physical Therapy 27(2):114
Obrez A, Stohler C S 1996 Jaw muscle pain and its effect on gothic arch tracings. Journal of Prosthetic Dentistry 75:393
Ono T, Ishiwata Y, Kuroda T 1998 Inhibition of masseteric electromyographic activity during oral respiration. American Journal of Orthodontics and Dentofacial Orthopedics 113(5):518
Ormeño G, Miralles R, Loyola R et al 1999 Body position effects on EMG activity of the temporal and suprahyoid muscles in healthy subjects and in patients with myogenic cranio-cervical-mandibular dysfunction. Journal of Craniomandibular Practice 17(2):132
Palazzi C, Miralles R, Miranda C 1999 Effects of two types of pillows on sternocleidomastoid EMG activity in healthy subjects and in patients with myogenic cranio-cervical-mandibular dysfunction. Journal of Craniomandibular Practice 17(2):202

Panjabi M 1992 The stabilising system of the spine. Part II. Neutral zone and instability hypothesis. Journal of Spinal Disorders 5(4):390

Phanachet I, Wanigaratne K, Whittle T, Uchida S, Peeceeyen S, Murray G H 2001 A method for standardizing jaw displacements in the horizontal plane while recording single motor unit activity in the human lateral pterygoid muscle. Journal of Neuroscience Methods 105:201

Quinn J H 1995 Mandibular exercises to control bruxism and deviation problems. Journal of Craniomandibular Practice 13(1):30

Raustia A M, Oikarinen K S, Pyhtinen J 1998 Densities and sizes of main masticatory muscles in patients with internal derangements of temporomandibular joint obtained by computer tomography. Journal of Oral Rehabilitation 25:59

Revel M, Minquet M, Gergoy P, Vaillant J, Manuel J L 1994 Changes in cervicocephalic kinaesthesia after a proprioceptive rehabilitation programme in patients with neck pain: a randomised controlled study. Archives of Physical and Medical Rehabilitation 75:895

Richardson C A, Sims K 1991 An inner range holding contraction. An objective measure of stabilising function of an antigravity muscle. 11th International Congress of World Confederation for Physical Therapy, London, p 831

Richardson C, Jull G, Hides J, Hodges P 1999 Therapeutic exercise for spinal stabilisation: scientific basis and practical techniques. Churchill Livingstone, London

Ro J Y, Capra N F 2000 Modulation of jaw muscle spindle afferent activity following intramuscular injections with hypertonic saline. Pain 92:117

Rocabado M 1983 Arthrokinematics of the temporomandibular joint. Dental Clinics of North America 27:573

Sahrmann S A 2001 Diagnosis and treatment of movement impairment syndromes. Mosby, St Louis

Santander H, Miralles R, Pérez J et al 2000 Effects of head and neck inclination on bilateral sternocleidomastoid EMG activity in healthy subjects and in patients with myogenic cranio-cervical-mandibular dysfunction. Journal of Craniomandibular Practice 18(3):181

Schievano D, Rontani R M P, Bérzin F 1999 Influence of myofunctional therapy on the perioral muscles. Clinical and electromyographic evaluations. Journal of Oral Rehabilitation 26:564

Schulte W 1988 Conservative treatment of occlusal dysfunctions. International Dental Journal 38:28

Shellehas K P 1989 MR imaging of muscles of mastication. American Journal of Roentgenology 154:658

Solberg W K 1986 Temporomandibular disorders: management of internal derangement. British Dental Journal 60:379

Solow B 1992 Cervical and craniocervical posture as predictors of craniofacial growth. American Journal of Orthodontics 16:86

Solow B, Tallgren A 1976 Head posture and craniofacial morphology. American Journal of Physical Anthropology 44:417

Stohler C S 1997 Masticatory myalgias. Emphasis on the nerve growth factor-estrogen link. Pain Forum 6:176

Stokes M, Young A 1984 Investigation of quadriceps inhibition: implications for clinical practice. Physiotherapy 70(11):425

Sumino R, Nozaki S 1977 Trigemino-neck reflex: its peripheral and central organization. In: Anderson D J, Matthews B (eds) Pain in the trigeminal region. Elsevier/North-Holland Biomedical Press, Amsterdam, p 365

Suzuki J, Cohen B 1964 Head, eye, body and limb movements from semicircular canal nerve. Experimental Neurology 10:393

Svensson P, Graven-Nielsen T 2001 Craniofacial muscle pain: review of mechanisms and clinical manifestations. Journal of Orofacial Pain 15(2):117

Tallgren A, Solow B 1984 Long term changes in hyoid bone position and cranio-cervical posture in complete denture wearers. Acta Odontologica Scandinavica 42:257

Tay D 1986 The role of closed packed positions in the pathogenesis of temporomandibular joint internal derangements. Annals of the Academy of Medicine 15(3):418

Toller P A 1974 Opaque arthrography of the temporomandibular joint. International Journal of Oral Surgery 3:17

Travell J G, Rinzler S, Herman M 1942 Pain and disability of the shoulder and arm. Treatment by intramuscular infiltration with procaine hydrochloride. Journal of the American Medical Association 120:417

Tschopp K, Bachmann R 1992 Das temporomandibuläre Myoarthropathiesyndrom – eine häufige Ursache für Gesichtsschmerzen. Schweizerische Rundschau für Medizin Praxis 81:468

Uchida S, Whittle T, Wanigaratne K, Murray G M 2001 The role of the inferior head of the lateral pterygoid muscle in the generation and control of horizontal mandibular force. Archives of Oral Biology 46:1127

Urbanowicz M 1991 Alteration of vertical dimension and its effect on head and neck posture. Cranio 9(2):174

Von Korff M, Dworkin S F, LeResche L, Kruger A 1988 An epidemiologic comparison of pain complaints. Pain 32:173

Von Korff M, Wagner E H, Dworkin S F, Saunders K W 1991 Chronic pain and use of ambulatory health care. Psychosomatic Medicine 53:61

Voight M, Wieder D 1991 Comparative reflex response times of vastus obliquus and vastus lateralis in normal subjects and subjects with extensor mechanism dysfunction American Journal of Sports Medicine 19:131
Wadsworth D J S, Bullock-Saxton J E 1997 Recruitment patterns of the scapular rotator muscles in freestyle swimmers with subacromial impingement. International Journal of Sports Medicine 18:618
Wang K, Arima T, Arendt-Nielsen L, Svensson P 2000 EMG-force relationships are influenced by experimental jaw-muscle pain. Journal of Oral Rehabilitation 27:394
Westling L, Helkimo E 1992 Maximum jaw opening capacity in adolescents in relation to general joint mobility. Journal of Oral Rehabilitation 19:485
Whitty C, Willison R 1958 Some aspects of referred pain. Lancet 2:226–231
Widmalm S E, Lillie J H, Ash M M 1987 Anatomical and electromyographic studies of the lateral pterygoid muscle. Journal of Oral Rehabilitation 14:429
Widmalm S E, Lillie J H, Ash M M 1988 Anatomical and electromyographic studies of the digastric muscle. Journal of Oral Rehabilitation 15:3
Wiemann K, Klee A, Startmann M 1998 Fibrillar sources of the muscle resting tension and therapy of muscular imbalances. Deutsche Zeitschrift für Sportmedizin 49(4):111
Wilkinson T, Chan E K K 1989 The anatomic relationship of the insertion of the superior lateral pterygoid muscle to the articular disc in the temporomandibular joint of human cadavers. Australian Dental Journal 34:315
Woolsey N B, Sahrmann S A, Dixon L 1988 Triaxial movement of the pelvis during prone knee flexion. Physical Therapy 68:827
Zepa I, Hurmerinta K, Kovero O et al 2000 Association between thoracic kyphosis, head posture, and craniofacial morphology in young adults. Acta Odontologica Scandinavica 58(6):237

Chapter 13

Neuromusculoskeletal plasticity of the craniomandibular region: basic principles and recommendations for optimal rehabilitation

Renata Horst

CHAPTER CONTENTS

INTRODUCTION

This chapter proposes an integrative neuro-orthopaedic concept encompassing biomechanics and neurophysiology to approach the way the central nervous system (CNS) organizes individual movements.

The chapter consist of three parts: the first part discusses the neurobiological background, the second part explains the basic fundamentals of the approach and the last part describes treatment procedures in detail using two case studies.

The paradigm of the 1980s and early 1990s of physiotherapy was that passive mobilization of joint structures was sufficient to restore normal function. However, restoring function is more than just mobilizing joint structures; there is evidence that a goal is needed during activation of muscles to accomplish function.

Function may be defined as the complex activity of the entire organism with the aim of accomplishing a specific task. Optimal function entails behavioural strategies that are needed to reach a task-oriented goal within a relevant environmental context (Shumway-Cook & Woollacott 2001).

Muscle activation and joint mobilization should take place during a meaningful exercise in an environmental situation that is relevant to the patient. Performing structural treatment during a functional and goal-oriented activity promotes movement learning. The effect on articular, muscular and neural structures while the patient is carrying out functional activities can open up completely new treatment modalities for the therapist.

NEUROBIOLOGICAL MECHANISMS: A BASIS FOR MODERN REHABILITATION

Basic principles and mechanisms which are fundamental for neuromusculoskeletal plasticity as a treatment concept in rehabilitation are summarized as follows:

- Plasticity:
  - Neural
  - Muscular
- Skeletal
- Protective mechanisms
- Inhibition and habituation
- Reciprocal innervation
- Subcortical and cortical organization of movement.

PLASTICITY

Plasticity is the ability to adapt to functional demands.

When tasks vary or environmental conditions change, then variability in patterns of interconnections within the sensory and motor system, as well as changes in the effectiveness of neural connection, are required for learning (Kandel et al 2000). Plasticity can be divided in neural, muscular and arthrogenic.

Neural plasticity

There are many collateral connections within the brain allowing variability according to behavioural needs (Edelman 1987).

Muscle synergies needed to perform a functional task are referred to as volitional or functional synergies (Umphred 2001).

Bernstein (1967) referred to the 'degrees of freedom' of joints, questioning how these are organized by the CNS. Today synergies are considered to be variable and are thought to be organized subconsciously according to task and environmental demands. Shumway-Cook and Woollacott (2001) define synergy as a functional coupling of groups of muscles which act together as a unit (synonym: coordinative structure).

A muscle that is needed within a synergy to enable the performance of a specific activity may also take part in a different synergy to carry out a different function.

Grasping a glass which stands upright on a table will require the activation of a different synergy than if the glass is upside down. If the glass were standing upright and a person were to use the same synergy as when it is upside down, one would say that the movement is abnormal. However, it may be very normal for that person if weakness or pain creates the necessity to reach the goal in this manner. Here again, the need for change will cause adaptation.

An example of a synergy can be seen on opening the mouth to eat, when the depressors and protractors of the mandible are usually activated and the neck extensors stabilize the head, eccentrically (Clark et al 1993). The neck extensors work concentrically to move the maxilla away from the mandible, thereby opening the mouth (Zuniga et al 1995).

This is in fact the movement strategy employed throughout evolution prior to hominids becoming upright. If you fix the mandible with both hands at the chin and then attempt to open the mouth you will notice that this is only possible through extending the head (see Chapter 5).

Specific areas of the brain control different parts of the body. It has been shown that Broca's area and the surrounding areas on both sides of the sulcus lateralis control not only speech, but also the mouth and face region, as well as mimicry of facial expressions (Calvin & Ojemann 1994). This makes sense, since many functional activities of daily living involve the interconnection of hand–mouth coordination, such as eating, speaking and writing. One just needs to look at the homunculus to see how close together the representations of mouth, face and hand regions lie (Dudel et al 1996) (Fig. 13.1).

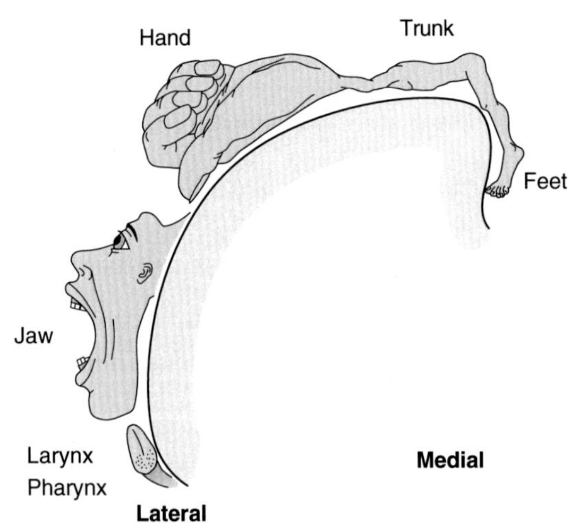

Fig. 13.1 Somatotopic representation of the motor cortex (reproduced with permission from Dudel et al 1996).

Leroi-Gourhan (1995) explains that the development of speech and hand function occurred at the same time during evolution. He hypothesizes that since the hands were no longer needed for quadruped locomotion, they were able to be used for other manipulative functions. As quadrupeds we were dependent on the mouth for grasping, as are many animals. With the development of the hand for manipulative functions the mouth gained the opportunity to develop a new function – speech.

According to use, receptors demonstrate plasticity, causing synaptic transmission to become stronger or weaker. If certain body parts are not used – due to weakness, pain or even fear of movement – then the cortical map representations will also change.

Merzenich et al (1984) showed in experiments with monkeys that, in this case, neighbouring areas take over these sites (Fig. 13.2). Ramachandran and Blakesee (2001) showed that hand amputees feel their individual fingers on the face.

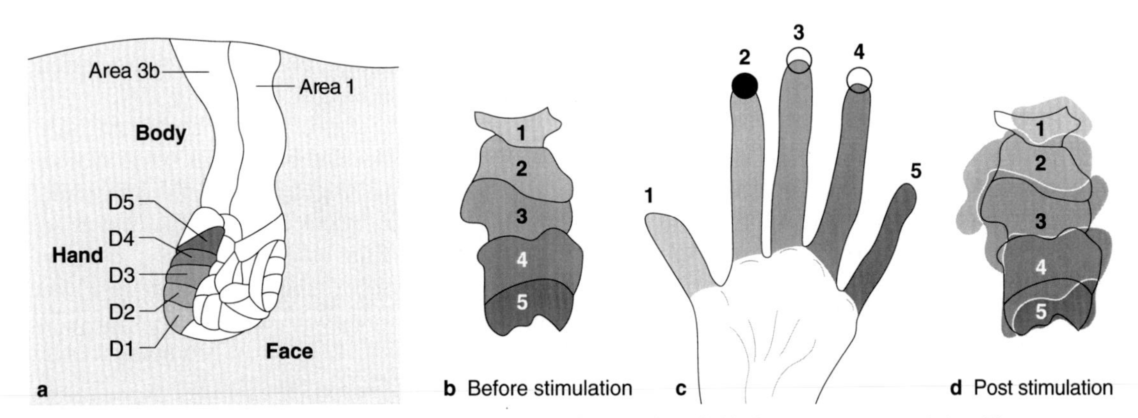

Fig. 13.2 Reorganization of the somatosensory receptive cortical fields in response to training. The representation of the fingers which were used more increased in contrast to those which were used less (reproduced with permission from Merzenich et al 1984).

a Somatosensory zones 1 and 3b for the left brain in oblique view (receptive fields for the fingers of the right hand, D1–D5).
b Receptive fields before training.
c Right hand and skin surface as represented in the relevant cortical zones. The fingers marked with a circle were used for training.
d Receptive fields after training.

Phantom pain can be explained by this, since the afferent information is misinterpreted. Ramachandran developed a box into which amputees put their intact hand. The box contained a mirror so that when the amputee placed the amputated limb alongside it looked as if they had two hands. In this way the amputee was able to minimize phantom pain (Ramachandran & Blakeslee 2001).

Visualizing body parts obviously enhances cortical representation. Even imagining muscle contractions can result in an increase in maximal voluntary contraction (see also Chapter 1).

Yue and Cole (1992) performed a study in which subjects imagined muscle contractions over a 4-week period. They showed more maximal voluntary contraction than those who did no training, although less than those who had actually trained physically. The same central structures that are activated during the performance of motor actions are activated during mental training (Pascual-Leone et al 1995). Even the use of visual imagery to plan a movement invokes the same patterns of activity in the premotor and posterior cortical areas as those that occur during performance of the movement (Krakauer et al 2000).

Passive mobilization of the temporomandibular joint may be more effective if the client envisions opening the mouth to bite into an apple while being mobilized. Since the necessary postural adjustments for this task can only be organized with the trunk in an upright position it may be best to choose this as a starting position for treatment.

Muscular plasticity

In addition to neural changes, muscles and other soft tissues adapt according to functional demands and use. If muscles are not used, in most cases, they will become atrophic. Training will, of course, cause them to grow in size again.

The fibre type may also change. With increasing age, the ratio of fibre types becomes more phasic at the expense of tonic fibres. Some diseases also cause change in the types of muscle fibre.

It was long believed that it was not possible to change slow twitch fibres into fast twitch fibres with training. Unexpectedly, however, some evidence was found in sprinters to suggest that this is possible (Andersen et al 2000). During their resistance training period the amount of slow twitch fibres diminished. Two months after resistance training, they attained the same amount of phasic fibres as they had had prior to starting training. The astonishing thing was that they acquired double the amount of fast twitch fibres 3 months later (Andersen et al 2000).

Muscles must be able to change their length according to the demands of the activity and the environment. For eccentric control, which is required for postural adjustments, it is necessary that they have the structural elasticity needed for this.

Immobility leads to stiffness, which appears to be caused by changes in tendon and connective tissues such as water loss and collagen deposition (Van den Berg 2000). Animal studies have shown that immobilization in shortened positions causes loss of sarcomeres, which results in shortening and increased stiffness (Tabary et al 1972, Williams & Goldspink 1978, Witzmann et al 1982).

Muscle stiffness is defined by the force required to change the length of a resting muscle (Dietz & Berger 1983).

Coordinated, skilful movements not only require that task-related muscles be activated, but also require appropriate agonist recruitment. However, if the cortical representation has changed, this cohesive process may be impaired. Excessive contraction may result as an adaptive strategy in the attempt to gain more control, which, in turn, promotes loss of motor control and causes stiffness.

Bone adaptation

Changes in bone mass occur according to changes in the pressure put upon it. Astronauts who have been in space for a long period lose bone mass (Netter 1987). If too much pressure is put on joints osteophytes develop. The same principle applies to the growth of the skull (Oudhof 2001). More pressure on the skull causes more growth and asymmetry (Proffit 1993).

Even the shape of our skull has changed during the course of evolution. The jaw has become smaller and Broca's area – where manipulation of the tongue, face and hand muscles is coordinated – has become much larger (Leroi-Gourhan 1995) (Fig. 13.3). Here again functional demands have led to adaptation over time.

Structures can only take over the function for which they have been trained. Bones can only take on loads that they are used to. They grow and remodel in response to external forces exerted by the soft tissue (Rocabado & Iglash 1991). This is why it is important for the therapist to know what activities the client needs to perform in daily life.

The patient's occupational demands must also be considered. It makes a difference if the strategies needed are mainly in sitting or during heavy weight-bearing activities. Thus the choice of rehabilitation should be in a functional position that provides optimal input for the somatosensory cortex which in turn influences the motor system as needed for function.

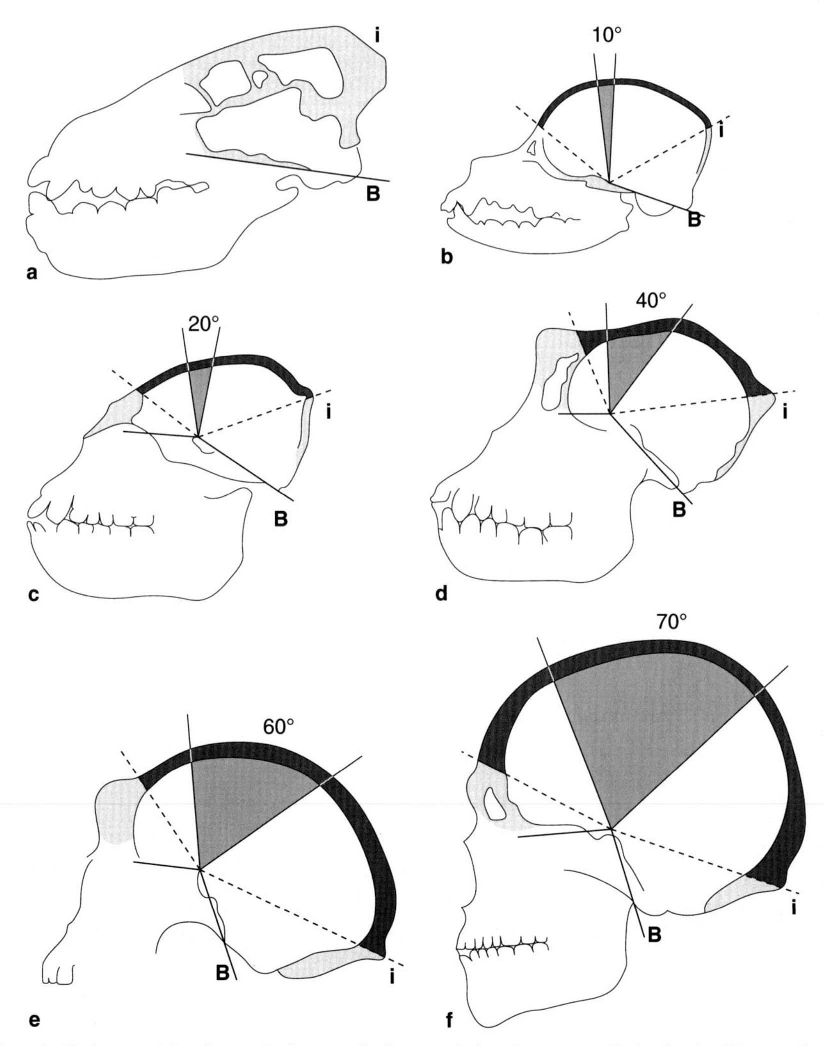

Fig. 13.3 The skull changed its form during evolution and development of the brain. The surface of the cortex in the frontoparietal region became larger as time went on (reproduced with permission from Leroi-Gourhan 1995).

PROTECTIVE MECHANISMS

When danger threatens an organism, the limbic system is alerted. A number of reactions occur automatically when the autonomous nervous system is triggered by a subcortical nucleus (amygdala) with the aim of protecting the organism (Le Doux 1996).

As already discussed, muscles will alter their activity according to changing demands. If protection of a body part is necessary for healing to occur, then the muscles will try to 'freeze' the painful and damaged body parts. The tongue, lips and teeth constantly feedback information which enables central pattern generators to choose the best chewing stroke. As soon as an efficient chewing pattern that minimizes damage to any structure is found, it is repeated and learned (Okeson 1996).

Why are protective mechanisms learned?

Biochemical changes also occur with the aim of protecting painful body parts against excessive movement. The concentration of hyaluronic acid decreases, leading to less joint play. Matrix production also decreases, leading to less capsular mobility. In addition, connective tissue becomes less mobile due to activation of myofibroblasts (Van den Berg 2000).

Even within the blood, changes occur. It has a lower concentration of oxygen and more carbon dioxide. It also becomes more acidic (Van den Berg 2000). This leads to less nutrition for the nerves and causes pain mechanisms to continue. Pain mediators such as bradykinin, prostaglandin and serotonin are produced and transported within the nervous system (Le Doux 1996, Squire & Kandel 1999).

Repeated harmful stimuli or even fear of these will keep these changes going and temporal summation may facilitate hypersensitivity within the entire nervous system (Butler 2000). Serotonin is a necessary neurotransmitter for long-term memory (Le Doux 1996, Squire & Kandel 1999). This explains why it is so difficult to abandon the changes brought about by the protective mechanism which were sensible at the time of injury but which are no longer needed after healing.

INHIBITION AND HABITUATION

Habituation is defined as a decrease in responsiveness that occurs as a result of repeated exposure to a non-painful stimulus (Shumway-Cook & Woollacott 2001).

Repeated application of stimuli that are not harmful or do not cause fear of pain lead to biochemical changes in synapses in different parts of the nervous system which can promote reorganization (Butler 2000). The organism adapts to these inputs over time and habituation occurs (Kandel et al 2000). The CNS becomes desensitized.

Desensitization based on the same system is used to treat allergy patients, using homeopathic doses of the allergen that causes the immune system to overreact. These small doses give the organism a chance to get used to these stimuli and adapt. Experience has shown that if movements which were painful are performed in a manner that the patient can cope with without fear, then these movements can be repeated.

RECIPROCAL INNERVATION

Reciprocal innervation is task specific (Pearson & Gordon 2000).

During fast goal-oriented voluntary movements the CNS activates a triphasic muscle activation pattern (Beradelli et al 1996, Ghez & Krakauer 2000) (Fig. 13.4). First the agonists of the target movement are activated (acceleration phase). Shortly before reaching the target, the antagonists contract to decelerate, after which the antagonists fire a second time to stabilize the end position.

Executing a voluntary movement in a given direction using concentric agonist activity requires that the antagonists 'know' what to do at each moment. Depending on the task, the antagonists may have to relax or may have to maintain co-contraction. Gravity determines whether the antagonists have to control the movement eccentrically.

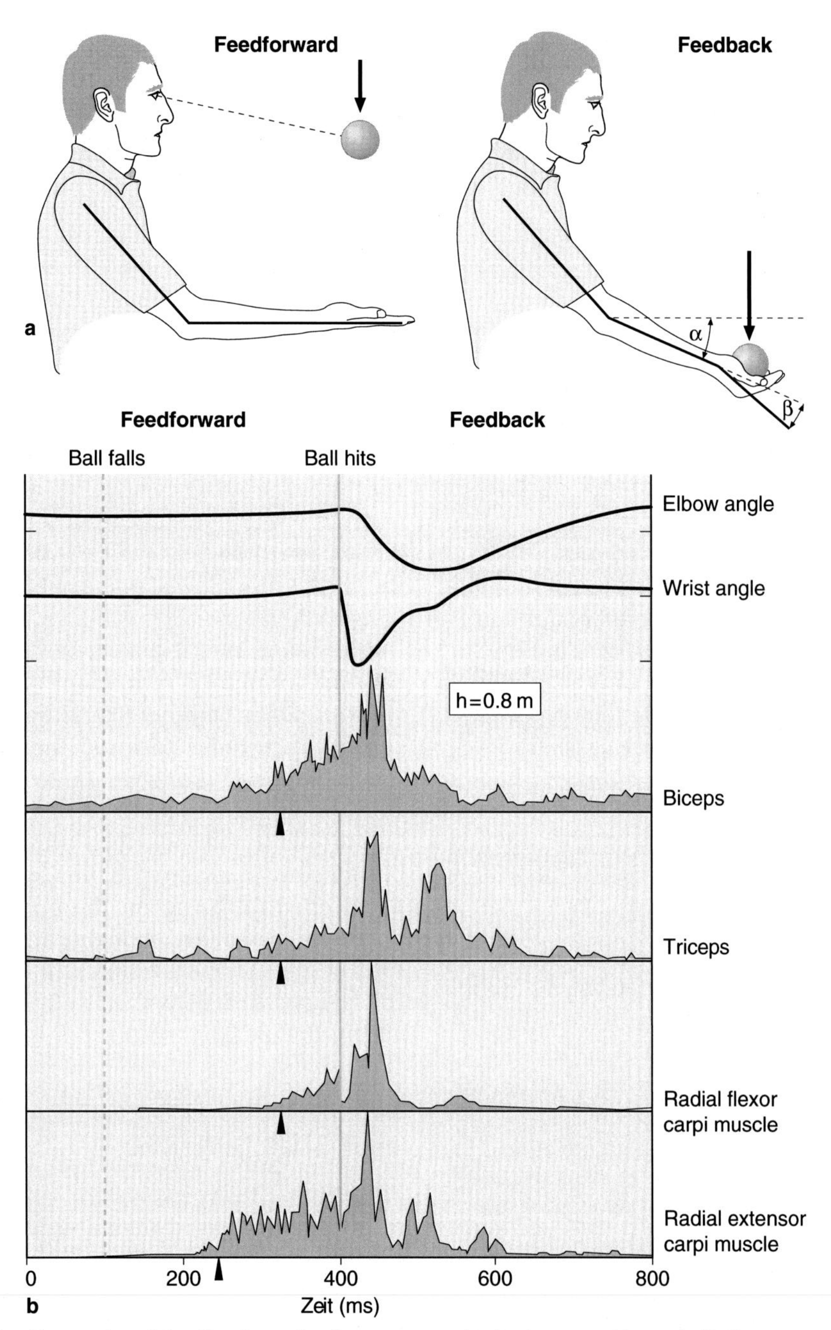

Fig. 13.4 Feedforward and feedback mechanisms are required when catching a ball. Co-contraction is needed before the ball reaches the hand and afterwards (reproduced with permission from Ghez & Krakauer 2000).

a Starting position for the ball experiment. The therapist drops the ball from a height of 80 cm.

b Average responses of a person catching the ball. The upper part of this graphic shows the angle at the elbow and wrist. The lower part shows EMG activity of relevant muscles.

Example 1

Different types of movement require different information. Feedforward plays a major role in quick movements, which can be understood as a neural process based entirely on the brain's knowledge and calculations regarding the planned movement (Berry et al 1995). The movement is too quick for feedback to play an important part.

Sensory feedback is necessary, however, to create the brain's model of the movement in the first place and this process contributes to the acquisition of new motor skills (Rosenbaum 1991).

Feedback is also needed for making corrections, especially if unpredictable changes occur during the execution of a movement. When moving the hand to the mouth to eat something, the biceps brachii must contract concentrically and the triceps brachii must allow the motion to occur (reciprocal innervation).

Example 2

When catching a ball, both the biceps and triceps must co-contract, and do so before the ball is caught as well as afterwards, even though it is the biceps that gets stretched due to the weight of the ball (Ghez & Krakauer 2000). This coactivation of biceps and triceps, before the ball is actually caught, is dependent on visual information (feedforward). The impact of the ball provides proprioceptive information so that the biceps can react (feedback). Anticipation of the destabilization also causes the triceps to contract.

Information required by the antagonists of a particular movement is supplied through the interneurone connections within the spinal cord and these receive their input from corticospinal and other descending pathways (Pearson & Gordon 2000).

The movement target will determine the form of reciprocal innervation, i.e. whether the antagonist which inhibits the target movement-performing musculature is inhibited or coactivated.

The same can be observed in the craniomandibular region: when opening the mouth, mouth-closing muscles such as the masseter, temporal, suprahyoid and lateral pterygoid are also activated through reciprocal innervation.

Changing environmental conditions may also influence reciprocal innervation. If the goal is to stabilize the arm on a table when perturbation occurs on the other arm, then the triceps brachii will contract. If the goal is to stabilize the arm in the air when holding a cup during perturbations on the other arm, then the triceps brachii will not contract (Pearson & Gordon 2000).

One could hypothesize that, during a goal-oriented voluntary movement when antagonists should normally relax, they may instead coactivate in order to avoid movements that have been painful or still are. In this way, the need for protection could be fulfilled.

If opening the mouth to eat or speak has been a painful experience, this experience has a powerful influence on the elevators of the mandible, which are suddenly inhibited. This kind of memory behaviour can have enormous consequences for activities needed for function within the orofacial region.

SUBCORTICAL AND CORTICAL ASPECTS OF MOTOR CONTROL

The central nervous system controls movements both voluntarily and involuntarily (Ghez & Krakauer 2000) (Fig. 13.5). Distal muscles are controlled cortically, i.e. distal body parts move in a goal-oriented fashion and require cognitive, visual and acoustic information. The paths for these run laterally within the anterior horn of the spinal cord and often have very few synaptic connections. To some finger muscles there may only be one synaptic connection. This is why we can move our fingers so quickly and skilfully. On the contrary, proximal muscles are controlled subcortically. These

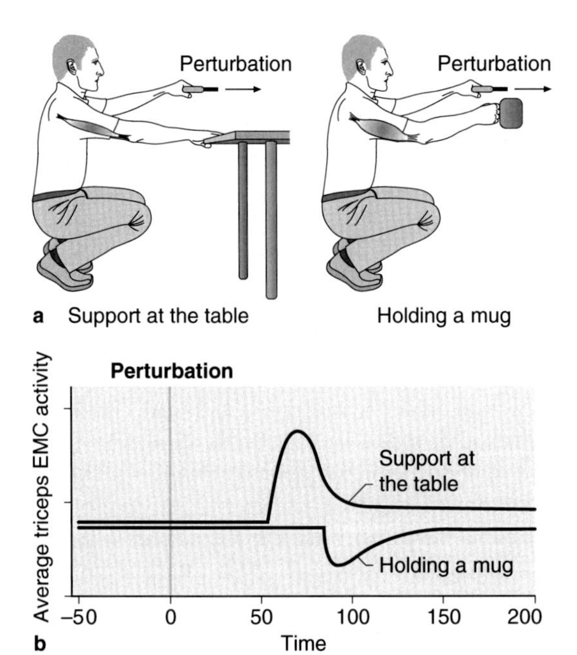

Fig. 13.5 Reciprocal innervation is task specific. The triceps is active when the hand is placed on a table; however, it remains silent when holding a cup, although all other conditions remain the same (reproduced with permission from Ghez & Krakauer 2000).

paths run more medially in the anterior horn of the spinal cord and have many synaptic connections. This is why muscles of the head and neck region can interact with muscles of the pelvic and sacral region for quick postural adjustments.

Since proximal muscles as well as eccentric control needed for postural adjustments are controlled subcortically, they require proprioceptive information. Proximal muscles are activated proactively during goal-directed movements. For example, the trunk must be stable before the arm moves towards an object, just as the head must be stable before tongue and mouth motions for speech and swallowing can occur. If the mandible is hypomobile then these functions cannot be executed. The temporomandibular joint then becomes the fixed point of the movement which leads to stiffness and pain within this region.

Neuromuscular control of joint stability is also dependent on proprioceptive information. If tension in joint capsules and ligaments increases, then receptors within these structures will transfer information to the spinal cord, activating an automatic spinal reflex to activate joint stabilizing muscles (Pollack 2000).

The ligaments and muscles function synergistically in stabilizing, for example, the shoulder. Experiments have shown that the axillary nerve takes up afferent information from the joint capsule of the shoulder and causes activation of the rotator cuff. If this nerve is cut then the rotator cuff remains inactive upon stimulation (Guanche et al 1995).

In order to activate stabilizing muscles of the neck and head as needed for functional activities it is important that the upper and lower cervical spine are aligned and the trunk and head are in an upright position. Head and trunk stability is required for mobility of the temporomandibular joint as needed for eating and speaking.

What does this mean for the craniomandibular region?

In summary, the following basic principles of rehabilitation can be formulated:

- Postural control is organized subcortically and needs to be automated for optimal function.
- Active manual techniques for the temporomandibular and craniofacial region, or intraoral techniques (e.g. for the tongue), may have a beneficial effect on other body regions, especially the cervical spine and trunk.
- If this stability cannot be organized automatically, then more proprioceptive information may be needed during the execution of these functions.
- Using proprioceptive feedback, such as having the patient try to activate muscles against a tactile resistance applied by the therapist, will not enable the organization of postural control as needed for functional activities.

- For this, proprioceptive information must be applied during the simultaneous execution of voluntary functional mouth and tongue activities.

BASIC PRINCIPLES FOR TREATMENT AND FURTHER MANAGEMENT

The use of appropriate treatment techniques during the execution of functional activities can support correct acquisition of such activities. Concurrent active pain management is instigated if the patient is pain-free during these activities. The therapist's main goal, therefore, is to influence structures so that functional activities can be performed without the patient feeling pain.

INFLUENCES OF PERIPHERAL AND CENTRAL MECHANISMS

Since immobilization causes so many undesired changes, it is essential that it be no longer than necessary for healing to occur. Preventing stiffness and contracture (peripheral events) and encouraging cortical representation (central mechanisms) are the main therapeutic goals at this time. When structural healing occurs the patient has to be encouraged to learn that the protective mechanisms are no longer needed.

Facilitation of meaningful activities

As protective mechanisms can be considered as physiological adaptive strategies needed for protection of the injured structures, the therapeutic goal is to facilitate meaningful activities during which necessary proprioceptive and/or cognitive information may be applied, rather than merely inhibiting these compensatory activities at a structural level.

Example 3

If a thyroid tumour has been growing for some time, the neck muscles (e.g. sternocleidomastoid) may be stiff on the opposite side to allow more room for the tumour. Rather than just passively stretching the muscle while lying in supine, it may be more effective to activate the contralateral sternocleidomastoid by asking the patient to look upward towards the stiff side. This leads to reciprocal innervation. At the same time, manual lengthening of the stiff structure applies tactile information so that the sternocleidomastoid 'knows' what to do during this activity. Having the patient look in a specific direction gives them the necessary visual information and doing so while seated will provide them with the necessary proprioceptive information so that the required muscle synergies needed for postural control may be activated. The sternocleidomastoid muscle is believed to be the prime muscular source of proprioceptive input relative to orientation of the head in space (Zuniga et al 1995).

Facilitation of face muscles by simple verbal instructions, such as asking the patient to consciously lift the eyebrows or to lift the corners of the mouth to smile, may be less effective than causing a situation in which the patient may feel surprised or happy, or combining these muscle expressions with sounds, such as: 'oh', 'ah' or 'wow'. Facilitating the facial muscles while the patient is lying supine does not result in the same gravitational forces acting on the face as usually experienced when performing functional activities for real.

Avoidance of predominantly cognitive/affective influences

Fear of pain may have an even more detrimental influence on the course of therapy than pain itself (Butler 2000). The patient needs to learn to cope with pain and consider it as a normal reaction to the healing process during the (sub)acute phase of injury. Systematic, repeated, pain-free movements reduce fear of movement, in particular with centralized pain patterns. Knowledge of functional anatomy and biomechanics, wound healing processes, pain mechanisms and good communication skills are essential for optimal patient management.

As representations in the sensory and motor cortices appear to change in response to pain it is a very important treatment goal to facilitate the representation of these body parts. The brain must be familiar with the movements, i.e. they must make sense. Performing movements without a context will probably lead to fear and further activation of protective mechanisms.

Active versus passive movement

Since different areas of the brain are activated if movements are executed passively or actively, it may be preferable when learning to perform actions actively to at least imagine them being performed actively during passive execution.

Passive movements activate the contralateral primary and secondary somatosensory cortex whereas active movements activate other areas needed for planning and coordination of functional synergies such the basal ganglia, cerebellum and the premotor cortex (Taub et al 1993).

Reciprocal innervation, as mentioned above, is task specific. It would therefore make sense to have a goal in mind when moving rather than just being moved passively. The starting position is also a controversial issue; for example, grasping a glass while lying on the side is not very realistic, since swallowing isn't easy in this position either.

One might argue that gravity exerts a different effect in side-lying, so that elevating the arm should be easier since elevation in this position does not require force against gravity. Notwithstanding the fact that no movement against gravity is required, the overall picture still seems more difficult as postural control is different in side-lying from that in standing.

As already discussed, the entire head and trunk control is activated in a feedforward manner, even by the mere thought of grasping for an object. However, as this control is not required in side-lying, a different motor strategy is employed than the one needed in 'real life'.

Hands-on versus hands-off

A further debate concerns hands-on versus hands-off approaches. In fact, the question may be easily answered by reviewing the neuroanatomical aspects and considering how the CNS organizes voluntary motions.

During the execution of voluntary movements or the attempt to move towards a goal, distal body parts should be facilitated with visual and/or acoustic information, whereas proximal body parts should obtain adequate proprioceptive information. For example, good qualitative mouth opening without give (e.g. mid-cervical extension) can be promoted by functional movements, such as bringing the hand to the mouth as if eating, for which the eyes follow the movement of the hand.

Proprioceptive information may be supplied by using tactile stimuli such as facilitation, mobilization or the use of appliances, for example the use of a spatula against the teeth during testing or treatment (see Chapter 8). Orofacial activities such as yawning, chewing, talking, singing and kissing may need to be facilitated in patients with new splints to enable the brain to form an optimal response to this new information.

The isolated application of tactile stimuli without conscious and goal-orientated movement on the part of the patient does not support this learning process.

Tactile stimuli may also have a psychological effect. Touching an adapted area can demonstrably reduce the production of stress hormones which promote degenerative changes of the hippocampus (Meaney et al 1995). The hippocampus is an important structure of the limbic system which is concerned with storage of memories among other functions (Le Doux 1996). Combining daily movements with touch (facilitation) so that these are felt to be positive can also promote learning processes. The positive psychological effect of touch should therefore not be undervalued.

SUMMARY

- Joint movements can be neuromuscularly controlled through mobilization or stabilization of joint complexes during a normal movement.
- Either mobility or stability, or in some cases both, may be required for a particular movement.
- Movement components that are unconsciously organized should be facilitated proprioceptively, whereas movement components that are consciously organized should be facilitated through visual stimulation or mental visualization of the movement.
- Facilitation through sensory input depends on the individual's sensory deficiencies and biomechanical and neuromuscular conditions that are relevant for the functional movement.

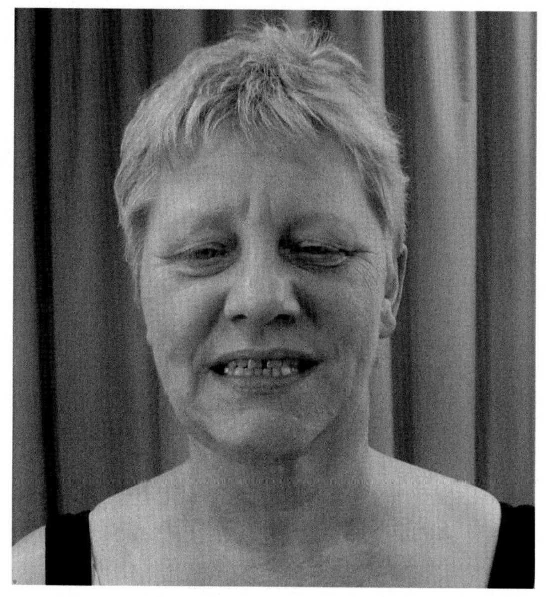

Fig. 13.6 A 52-year-old patient with facial and shoulder pain. The patient has problems chewing and a class III mesial bite.

CASE STUDIES

Details of the investigation and treatment of the two following case studies are only given in brief, and are therefore incomplete. The main aim is to demonstrate the application of the principles described above.

Case study 1

A 52-year-old female presented with facial and shoulder pain. Past history shows that she was provided with a dental prosthesis for her lower teeth 5 years ago. After 1 year it had to be renewed. The patient has problems chewing and still has a mesial bite (Angle class III) (Fig. 13.6). She is a waitress and must carry plates in external rotation. Six months ago she started experiencing shoulder pain and a gradual decrease in range of movement. Six weeks ago, she had a synovectomy and mobilization under general anaesthesia.

Physical dysfunctions

Overhead activities with the right arm are not possible. She can carry plates, but not without pain. During palpation, the muscles of the craniomandibular region are painful, especially the masseter and lateral pterygoid on the right side. The same was found in the digastric and omohyoid muscles on the same side.

Treatment

Reciprocal innervation for the sternocleidomastoid (Fig. 13.7)

Starting position and method

The patient is seated and is asked to look upwards towards her right eyebrow. This causes lateral flexion of the cervical spine to the left and rotation to the right. The therapist stands on the left side of the patient and stabilizes the right clavicle and sternum caudally with the left hand, while the right hand applies proprioceptive information for lengthening of the muscle

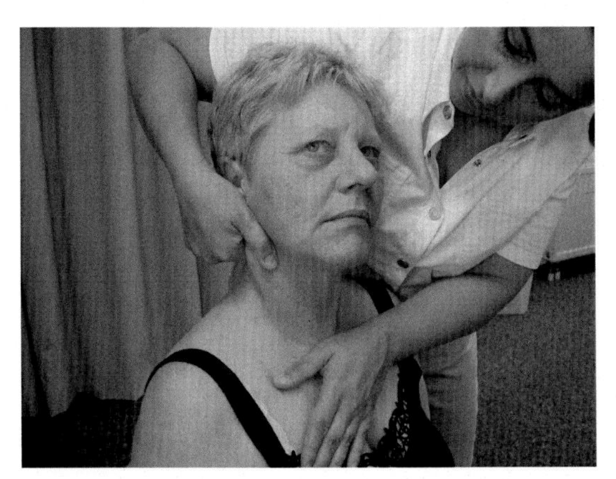

Fig. 13.7 Reciprocal innervation of the sternocleidomastoid muscle.

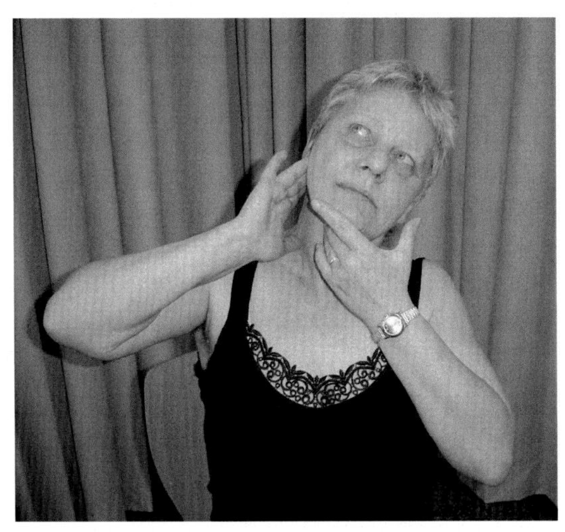

Fig. 13.8 Reciprocal innervation of the digastricus venter posterior muscle.

belly. The therapist should monitor the patient's chin, so that not too much extension between C0 and C1 occurs.

While still seated, the patient is again asked to look upwards toward her right eyebrow while fixating her hyoid bone with her left hand and mastoid process with her right hand (Fig. 13.8). This causes lateral flexion of the cervical spine to the left and rotation to the right, during which lengthening of the right digastric muscle occurs. The patient's fingers give proprioceptive information during lengthening of the muscle belly.

Eccentric activation of the masseter muscle (Fig. 13.9)

Starting position and method

With the patient seated, the therapist stands on the patient's left side and fixes the zygomatic bone with the right hand. The patient is asked to open her mouth, during which traction is applied by the therapist's left hand which is placed on the chin. This activity can be accompanied by having the patient depress her tongue, pushing it against the lower teeth. Care must be taken that the patient's head is not pulled towards the therapist, as this would cause lateral flexion.

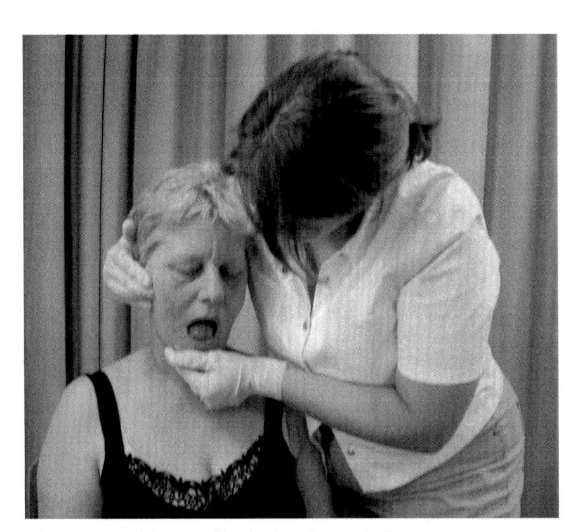

Fig. 13.9 Eccentric activation of the masseter muscle.

Eccentric activation of the lateral pterygoid muscle (Fig. 13.10)

Starting position and method

While sitting, the patient stabilizes her head with her left hand while actively mobilizing her tongue to the right. This mobilizes the mandible to the right. This activity may also be executed while the therapist applies pressure towards the muscle belly with the

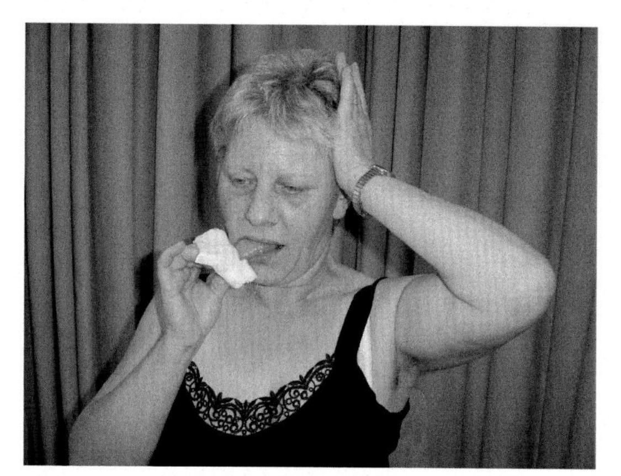

Fig. 13.10 Eccentric activation of the lateral pterygoid muscle.

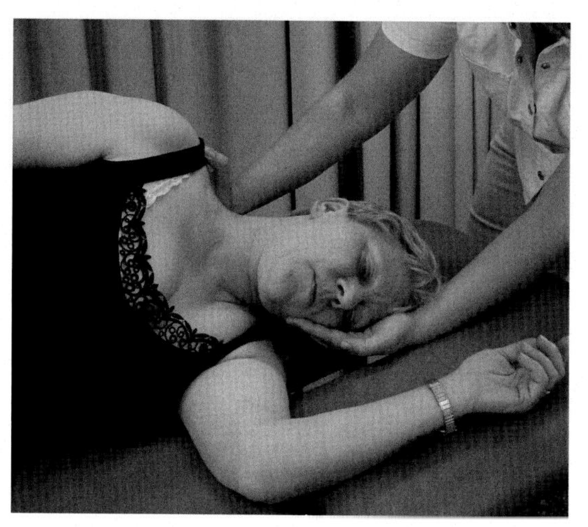

Fig. 13.11 Eccentric activation of the omohyoid muscle.

right index finger. The therapist's left hand stabilizes the patient's upper jaw.

Eccentric activation of the omohyoid muscle (Fig. 13.11)

Starting position and method

The patient lies on her left side with the head and neck in partial lateroflexion to the left. The patient is asked to push the tip of her tongue into her left cheek for which the therapist gives tactile information with the left index finger. This stabilizes the hyoid bone. During active depression of the shoulder the therapist facilitates caudal movement of the superior angle of the scapula with the right hand, giving proprioceptive information for lengthening of the muscle belly.

Assessment before and after treatment (after six sessions)

The occlusion judged by the patient and the dentist remained unchanged. External rotation of the shoulder for grasping over and behind the head, as well as for carrying plates was improved. Palpation of the craniomandibular muscles was less painful.

Hypothesis and a retrospective analysis

Malocclusion causes changes in neuromuscular activity. For example, the digastric muscle is under constant tension, placing the hyoid bone into a more cranial position. With this, more tension is placed on the omohyoid muscle. This, in turn, causes protraction of the shoulder, so that subacromion compression occurs, especially on elevation of the arm and external rotation, which the patient needs for her job. The majority of proprioceptive information originates from the craniocervical and craniomandibular regions and enters the CNS (Schupp 2000). Because of the changes in length and elasticity of these muscles, other proprioceptive information relating to the position of the scapula is also transmitted.

Conclusion and further procedures

It may be worth considering whether these results can be maintained if the situation with the dental prosthesis is not dealt with. As long as malocclusion remains, inadequate proprioceptive information will be a predisposing factor for impaired function of the craniofacial region.

Further thought should be given to shoulder mobilization under anaesthesia. Since experiencing painless movements is so essential for motor learning to take place, it may be worth considering having the patient awake and aware of what is happening during mobilization. If she sees the results, this visual experience could help her to plan her movements better and to organize functional synergies as needed for various tasks. Another possibility could be to record the operation on video. Knowledge of results is one of the main criteria for motor learning, as is knowledge of performance (Schmidt & Lee 1999). Using the visual system aids planning and organization of goal-oriented movements and helps the patient gain knowledge of performance and of results. Giving appropriate proprioceptive information while doing these goal-oriented movements also facilitates this learning process.

Case study 2

A 59-year-old female patient has a 20-year history of migraine headaches accompanied by facial pain on the left side. Eight years ago she had root canal treatment. Eight teeth were extracted, after which her migraine headaches became rarer. She now has a diagnosis of soft tissue rheumatism and has a swollen temporomandibular joint about two or three times a year. She wears a dental prosthesis which does not fit when the joint is swollen.

Physical dysfunction

The patient's main problem is that she still has frequent facial pain. Rotation of her head and neck towards the left is limited as is her mouth opening.

Treatment

Neurodynamic mobilization of the hypoglossal nerve

Starting position and method

The patient is seated. The therapist stands on her right side and stabilizes the head so that the craniocervical region is in lateroflexion of the cervical spine to the right. Active and passive flexion was severely restricted in this patient. The tongue is mobilized towards the right with a gauze pad (Fig. 13.12). In this position of the head, the left hypoglossal nerve is under less tension (for more information on the hypoglossal nerve, see Chapter 18).

Inhibition of facial pain

Starting position and method

The patient is seated with her hand placed comfortably on a table. The therapist mobilizes the scar tissue of the patient's thumb without pain (Fig. 13.13).

Distraction of the temporomandibular joint (Fig. 13.14)

Starting position and method

With the patient seated, two mouth spatulas are placed between her left molars. She presses her chin upwards with her right hand while stabilizing her head with her left arm with the intention to press her front teeth together. This causes distraction at the temporomandibular joint.

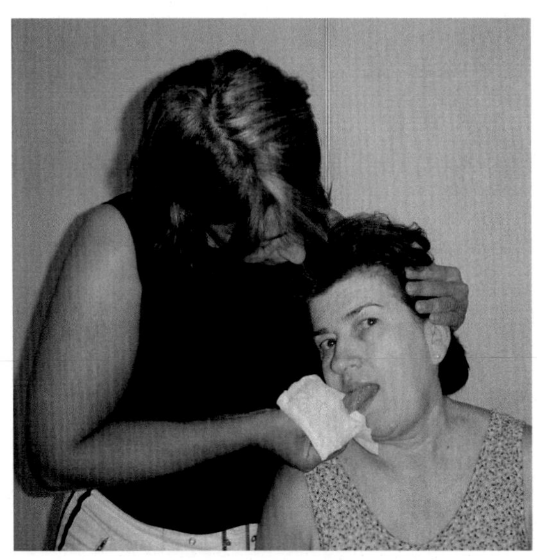

Fig. 13.12 Neurodynamic mobilization of the left hypoglossal nerve in a 59-year-old patient with chronic migraine and left-sided facial pain.

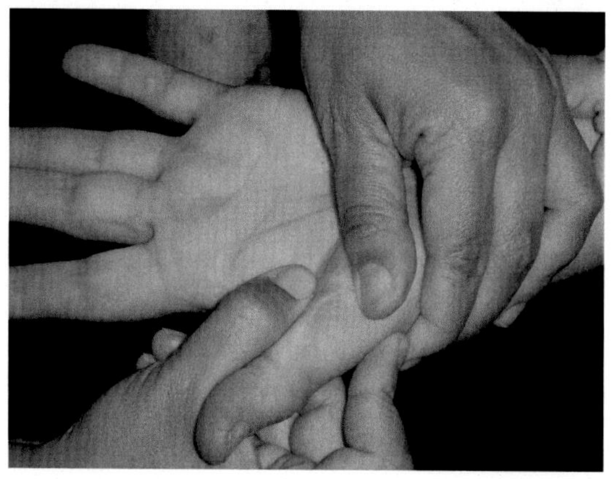

Fig. 13.13 Repression of facial pain. The therapist performs a painless mobilization of the nerve tissue at the thumb.

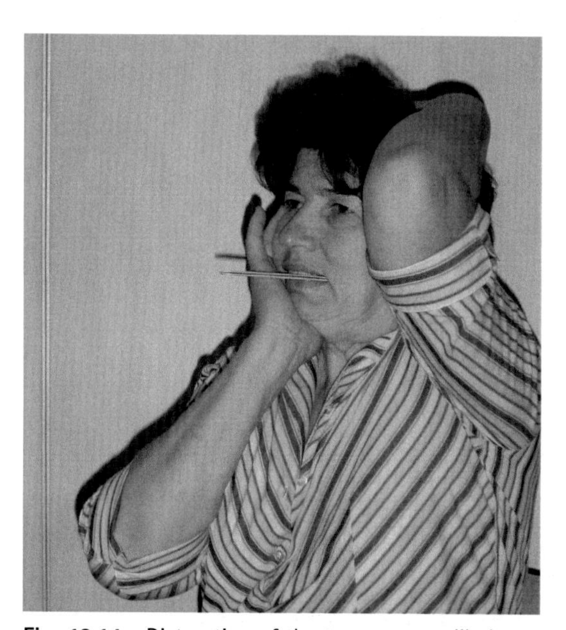

Fig. 13.14 Distraction of the temporomandibular joint.

Reciprocal innervation of the scaleni and infrahyoid muscles and mobilization of the hypoglossal nerve (Fig. 13.15)

Starting position and method

The patient is in supine and asked to activate lateral flexion to the right to provide a fixed point for the head and neck. In addition, she presses the tip of her tongue into her right cheek to provide a fixed point for her hyoid bone. The therapist gives her tactile information for the direction of the tongue with the right index finger. During exhalation, the therapist mobilizes the first and second rib as well as the sternum with the left hand caudally. During inspiration, the therapist continues to apply pressure in a caudal direction. The auxiliary breathing muscles are activated in their maximal lengthened position.

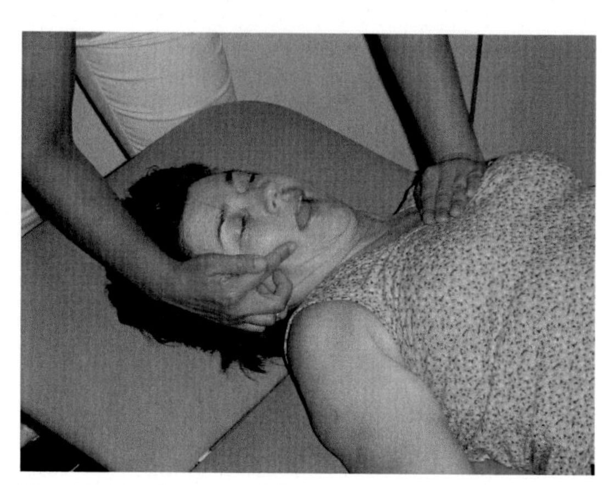

Fig. 13.15 Reciprocal innervation of the scaleni and infrahyoid musculature and mobilization of the hypoglossal nerve.

Assessment before and after treatment

Prior to treatment, the neurodynamic test for the hypoglossal nerve reproduced typical facial pain over the left eyebrow. After treating the scar on the thumb this pain disappeared immediately, and left rotation of the cervical spine improved from 45° prior to treatment to 80° afterwards.

Retrospective analysis and hypothesis

Since cortical representation of painful body parts diminishes and neighbouring areas overlap, it may be that the representation area of the face has been replaced by the hand. Treatment of the thumb led to a reduction in facial pain.

Reciprocal innervation of the scaleni and sternocleidomastoid as well as the infrahyoid muscles leads to increased cervical rotation. Due to their activation in lengthened position, actin and myosin connections have changed, thus reducing stiffness and leading to more optimal neurodynamics of the hypoglossal nerve.

SUMMARY

- It is sensible to consider several treatment options for craniomandibular dysfunction. Neural and muscular interrelationships as well as functional issues enable the therapist to consider several options for dealing with the patient's problem.
- The neural and muscular connections as well as the functional relationships allow the therapist to choose different ways to attend to the patient's deficits. Rather than it being a choice of techniques it should be a choice of input systems, which, in turn, depends on the patient's individual potentials and needs, as well as the therapist's neurophysiological knowledge as to how movements are planned and organized.
- Biomechanical and biomedical knowledge as to how compensation strategies evolve and are learned helps the therapist choose alternative ways to facilitate functional activities.
- Management of quality of life at a functional level should be the dominant therapy goal, rather than merely influencing the quality of movement at a structural level.
- Interdisciplinary work with professionals from different fields is necessary to provide optimal management of patients with craniomandibular and related functional problems.

References

Andersen J L, Schjerling P, Saltin B 2000 Muscle, genes and athletic performance. Scientific American 283(3):48

Beradelli A M, Hallett J C, Rothwell R et al 1996 Single-joint rapid arm movements in normal subjects and in patients with motor disorders. Brain 119:661

Bernstein N 1967 The coordination and regulation of movement. Pergamon, London

Berry M M, Standring S M, Bannister L H 1995 Nervous system. In: Bannister L H, Berry M M, Collins P, Dyson M, Dussek J E, Ferguson M W J (eds) Gray's anatomy, 38th edn. Churchill Livingstone, Edinburgh

Butler D 2000 The sensitive nervous system. Noigroup Publications, Adelaide

Calvin W H, Ojemann G A 1994 Conversations with Neil's brain: the neural nature of thought and language. Addison-Wesley, Reading, MA

Clark G T, Browne P A, Nakano M, Yang Q 1993 Co-activation of sternocleidomastoid muscles during maximum clenching. Journal of Dental Research 72:1499

Dietz V, Berger W 1983 Normal and impaired regulation of muscle stiffness in gait: a new hypothesis about muscle hypertonia. Experimental Neurology 79:680

Dudel J, Menzel R, Schmidt R 1996 Neurowissenschaft. Vom Molekül zur Kognition. Springer, Heidelberg

Edelman G M 1987 Neuronal Darwinism: the theory of neuronal group selection. Basic Books, New York

Ghez C, Krakauer J 2000 The organisation of movement. In: Kandel E R, Schwartz J H, Jessell T M (eds) Principles of neural science, 4th edn. McGraw Hill, New York

Guanche C, Knatt Th, Solomonow M, Lu Y, Baratta R 1995 The synergistic action of the capsule and the shoulder muscles. American Journal of Sports Medicine 23:301

Kandel E R, Schwartz J H, Jessell T M 2000 Principles of neural science, 4th edn. McGraw Hill, New York

Krakauer J W, Pine Z M, Ghilardi M F, Ghez C 2000 Learning of visuomotor transformations for vectorial planning of reaching trajectories. Neuroscience 20(23):8916

Le Doux J 2000 The emotional brain. Touchstone, New York

Leroi-Gourhan A 1995 Hand und Wort. Suhrkamp, Frankfurt

Meaney M J, O'Donnell D, Rowe W et al 1995 Individual differences in hypothalamic-pituitary-adrenal activity in later life and hippocampal aging. Experimental Gerontology 30(3–4):229

Merzenich M M, Nelson R J, Stryker M P, Shoppmann A, Zook J M 1984 Somatosensory cortical map changes following digital amputation in adult monkey. Journal of Comparative Neurology 224:591

Netter F H 1987 The Ciba collection of medical illustrations, Vol. 8, Musculoskeletal system. Part 1: Anatomy, physiology and metabolic disorders. CIBA-Geigy Collection, Summit NJ

Okeson J P 1996 Orofacial pain: guidelines for assessment, classification, and management. Quintessence, Chicago

Oudhof H A J 2001 Schädelwachstum und Einfluss von mechanischer Stimulation. In: von Piekartz H J M (ed.) Kraniofaziale Dysfunktionen und Schmerzen. Thieme, Stuttgart, p 1

Pascual-Leone A, Dang N, Chen L G et al 1995 Modulation of muscle responses evoked by transcranial magnetic stimulation during the acquisition of new fine motor skills. Journal of Neurophysiology 74:1037

Pearson K, Gordon J 2000 Spinal reflexes. In: Kandel E R, Schwartz J H, Jessell T M (eds) Principles of neural science, 4th edn. McGraw Hill, New York

Pollack R G 2000 Role of shoulder stabilization relative to restoration of neuromuscular control and joint kinematics. In: Lephart S M, Fu F H (eds) Proprioception and neuromuscular control in joint stability. Human Kinetics, Champaign, IL

Proffit W R 1993 Contemporary orthodontics. The development of orthodontic problems. Mosby Year Book, St Louis, p 139

Ramachandran V S, Blakeslee S 2001 Die blinde Frau, die sehen kann. Rowohlt, Reinbek

Rocabado M, Iglash A 1991 Maxillofacial pain, musculoskeletal approach. J B Lippincott, Philadelphia

Rosenbaum D A 1991 Human motor control. Academic Press, San Diego, CA

Schmidt R A, Lee T D 1999 Motor control and learning: a behavioral emphasis. Human Kinetics, Champaign, IL

Schupp W 2000 Schmerz und Kieferorthopädie Eine interdisziplinäre Betrachtung kybernetischer Zusammenhänge. Manuelle Medizin Kieferorthopädie 38:322

Shumway-Cook A, Woollacott M 2001 Motor controls. Williams and Wilkins, London

Squire L R, Kandel E R 1999 Gedächtnis Die Natur des Erinnerns. Spektrum Akademischer Verlag, Heidelberg

Tabary J C, Tabary C, Tardieu G et al 1972 Physiological and structural changes in the cat soleus muscle due to immobilisation at different lengths by plaster casts. Journal of Physiology 224:231

Taub E, Miller N E, Novack T A et al 1993 Technique to improve chronic motor deficit after stroke. Archives of Physical Medicine and Rehabilitation 74:347

Umphred D A 1995 Neurological rehabilitation. Mosby, St Louis

Van den Berg F 2000 Angewandte Physiologie für Physiotherapeuten, Bd. 1. Thieme, Stuttgart

Williams P E, Goldspink G 1978 Changes in sarcomere length and physiological properties in immobilized muscle. Journal of Anatomy 127:459

Witzmann F A, Kim D H, Fitts R H 1982 Hindlimb immobilization: length-tension and contractile properties of skeletal muscle. Journal of Applied Physiology 53:335

Yue G, Cole K J J 1992 Strength increases from the motor program: comparison of training with maximum voluntary and imagined muscle contractions. Journal of Neurophysiology 67:1114–1123

Zuniga C, Miralles R, Mena B et al 1995 Influence of variation in jaw posture on sternocleidomastoid and trapezius electromyographic activity. Cranio 13(3):157–162

Chapter 14

The neurocranium: assessment and treatment techniques

Harry von Piekartz

CHAPTER CONTENTS

INTRODUCTION

This chapter will discuss how the therapist can examine the patient with craniofacial dysfunction through the use of passive movements. It is described in an open thinking model and is divided into three parts, which will be discussed in the following order:

- Introduction to the nature of passive movements which can be applied in the craniofacial region
- A general introduction to techniques and the reasoning behind them
- More detailed techniques from each neurocranial bone region.

DEFINITIONS AND GUIDELINES FOR PASSIVE MOVEMENTS

Passive movements (movements which are performed actively by the therapist) as manual skills play a large part in the assessment and treatment of the craniomandibular and craniofacial regions.

Aspects of these passive movements, which are the basis of these guidelines, are:

- Types of passive movement
- Dose
- Normal response.

For documentation, specific abbreviations will be presented and advice for the interpretation of pain responses during investigation will be given.

TYPES OF PASSIVE MOVEMENT

Passive movements can be divided into two basic types:

- Physiological movement: Movement that could otherwise be performed actively by the patient.
- Accessory movement: Movement that cannot be performed actively by the patient, but which can be performed by another person. Accessory movements are necessary for normal physiological joint movements. For example, lateral transverse movement of the mandible cannot be actively performed but is a movement which is necessary in order to be able to open the mouth.

> **!** Both physiological and accessory movements are possible in the craniomandibular region, but only accessory movements in the cranium.

Definition of cranial accessory movements

It is important to define the terminology used to describe movement. In the literature many descriptions are given. For example, biomechanical systems define movement in relation to three imaginary axes through the body which are labelled X, Y and Z (Boyling et al 1994). The anatomical system defines movements in three planes, namely sagittal, coronal and horizontal. All movements can be defined as translation and/or rotation in any of these three planes. Clinically it is not known precisely what happens biologically or mechanically when accessory movements are applied to the cranial bones. Grieve stated: 'We do not know what the application of passive movements does on the living human body. The only thing we can say is that it influences tissues and biological mechanism, nothing more' (Grieve 1995). Grieve's statement can be interpreted as showing that passive movements are not only restricted to physical changes of body tissue but that they also influence the whole person. This would mean that the value of placebo may not only be unilateral. This could be used by therapists in a positive way in patient management. Accessory movements of craniofacial bone tissue could be expected to have a similar effect. Therefore we have to define the accessory movements as follows:

- In which *direction* is the accessory movement applied by the therapist?
- Which *grade* of movement is to be used?
- What *changes* are possible in response to the technique (in terms of signs and symptoms)? This should be achieved through a constant process of (re)assessment of clinical evidence (Yen & Suga 1982, Reynolds 1987).

Definition of the direction of the accessory movements

The direction of movement in which the therapist applies pressure is simple to understand and to describe, without having to use difficult analyses of movement direction around the artificial axes of biomechanical models (van der Bijl 1986). You are free to use this model to assist in the interpretation of clinical patterns, but it is not obligatory. For example, osteopaths use a biomechanical model to describe the classic sphenobasilar dysfunction, which occurs when the sphenobasilar (spheno-occipital) joint is fixed in a flexion position (Cottam 1984, Margulies et al 1990). In the author's opinion such biomechanical hypotheses provide one basis from which to make a clinical diagnosis (Yen & Suga 1982). There are other hypotheses to explain the changes that therapists see in the clinic.

Reassessment using active, flexible and non-dogmatic thought processes allows the therapist to assess which examination techniques are most relevant for each individual patient (Yen & Suga 1982, Reynolds 1987). It is clinically useful to use the biomechanical axes to determine the direction of the accessory movements. Some advantages of this are (Fig. 14.1):

- Biomechanical and anatomical knowledge is of secondary importance compared to an analysis of the response to the techniques.
- Artificial axes on the cranium are simple to visualize.
- Angulations and modification of the accessory movement can be described more easily.

The possible axis co-ordinates are:

- The Y-axis is a longitudinal axis with longitudinal movements to cranial and caudal and rotation to left and right.
- The Z-axis is a sagittal axis with anterior–posterior movement and posterior–anterior movement; rotations are to the left and the right.
- The X-axis is a transverse axis. Transverse movement to medial and lateral and rotations to anterior and posterior are possible (Fig. 14.2).

Accessory movements of the craniomandibular region

These are discussed in detail in Chapter 8.

1. Transverse laterally	lat.
2. Transverse medially	med
3. Longitudinal caudal	caud
4. Longitudinal cranial	cran
5. Anterior–posterior	
6. Posterior–anterior	
7. Rotation about X-axis (transverse axis)	transv, (x), transv or (x)
8. Rotation about y-axis (longitudinal axis)	long., (y), long. or (y)
9. Rotation about z-axis (sagittal axis)	sag., (z), sag. or (z)

Variation by angulation of these movements is possible

Fig. 14.1 General accessory movements and their abbreviations.

GRADES OF PASSIVE MOVEMENTS

The grades of passive movements described by Magarey (1988), Maitland (1986), Jones et al (1994) and Maitland et al (2001) can be applied to the cranium (Christensen 1967, Reynolds 1987). Passive movements of a joint may be considered to begin at a defined point (A) and end at a defined point (B) with normal resistance to movement occurring between the two, i.e. through range. The grades of movement can be defined as:

Grade I: A small amplitude movement in the resistance-free range

Grade II: A large amplitude movement within the resistance-free range (R_1 = first resistance)

Grade III: A large amplitude movement into resistance

Grade IV: A small amplitude movement into resistance.

Grade III and IV movements are of the same strength but of different amplitude (Fig. 14.3).

For more detailed information the reader is referred to the work of the above-mentioned authors. All movement analyses of passive

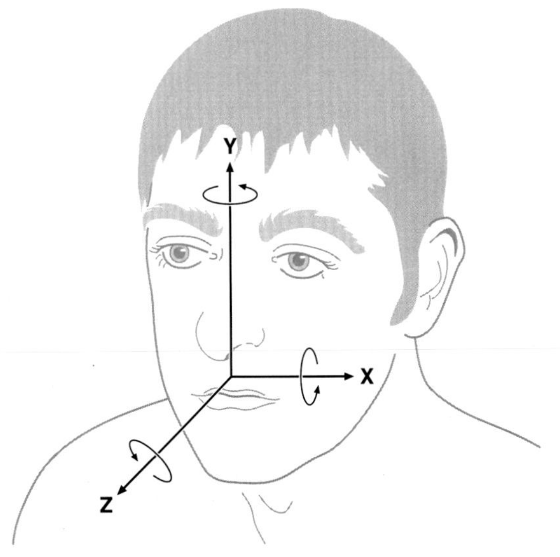

Fig. 14.2 The three virtual rotation axes of the head: longitudinal (Y), sagittal (Z), and transverse (X).

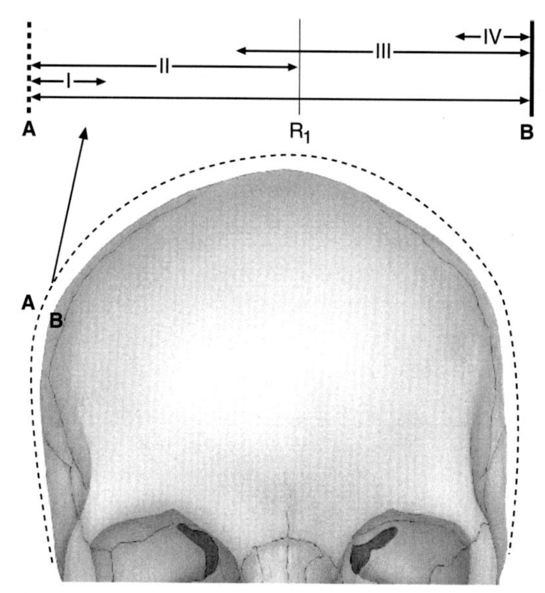

Fig. 14.3 Grades of movement that can be applied to the cranium. The natural compliance of craniofacial tissue allows early resistance (R_1) and a small range of motion (AB line) during general passive movements. In this model the AB range is 3 mm. A: dotted line: start of passive movement. B: dashed line: end of passive movement.

movements on different joints have their own qualities. For example, posterior–anterior movement of the shoulder differs in range, onset and progression of resistance (R) and end-feel to that of the posterior–anterior movement of the thoracic spine. Likewise the cranium has its own particular qualities.

POTENTIAL CHANGES IN SIGNS AND SYMPTOMS FOLLOWING ACCESSORY MOVEMENTS

Because you never know for each individual patient exactly what the effects of cranial tissue mobilization will be, it is useful to describe the movement directions, starting positions and grades. Whether the technique chosen for an individual patient is valuable depends on reassessment of the signs and symptoms. This is then the clinical evidence for this technique on this patient (Yen & Suga 1982, Reynolds 1987). Once the patient's reaction to the technique is clear, a decision can be made about dosage (grade and movement) of the accessory movement that will be used to progress treatment.

NORMAL RESPONSES DURING ASSESSMENT OF THE CRANIUM BY ACCESSORY MOVEMENTS

The range of motion of cranial facial bone tissue examined by accessory movements is very small and different qualities can be recognized. In the following paragraphs the possible qualities are briefly described, seen in a person without symptoms:

- Range of movement
- Onset of resistance
- Local pain:
  - No local pain at end of range
  - Strong accumulating or increasing pain
  - Local pain at the onset of resistance.

Range of movement

From the literature it is known that cranial bones have only a small range of movement (a few millimetres) and that this will vary in relation to the location of the movement and age of the subject (Retzlaff et al 1975, Enlow 1982, Oudhof 1982). Clinical observation is that the range of motion varies from 0–1 mm (e.g. occipital–parietal region) to 0–5 mm (e.g. occipital–sphenoidal region).

Onset of resistance

The resistance to passive movement in every direction on the cranium usually starts early. Therefore a grade II accessory movement is difficult to perform and examination and treatment of these joints is mostly with grade III or IV (see Fig. 14.3).

Local pain

The experience of many therapists on individuals without symptoms in the head region follows four general patterns that are principally input-based mechanisms (nociceptive and peripheral neurogenic):

- No pain at end range: Often seen in the most mobile articulations such as occiput–sphenoid, nasofrontal and frontal–zygomatic regions.
- Strong accumulating pain during the manoeuvre and a decrease directly after the manoeuvre: Seen in regions with a small range and a strong accumulative resistance during the manoeuvre. Some examples are the occiput–parietal, petrosal–temporal and zygomatic–maxillary regions.
- Pain at the onset of first resistance (R_1), which increases together with increasing resistance: This can be more of an iatrogenic cause. Perhaps the contact of your hands is uncomfortable or the technique is performed too quickly and results in pain and spasm with a strong accumulating character during increased range. You have to assess firstly the rhythm and secondly the starting position of the applied accessory movement. A slower rhythm of examination (one manoeuvre longer than 2 seconds) can change the pain behaviour. If it is still the same you should change points of contact, for example thumb techniques during movement of the parietal–parietal and temporal–parietal regions.

CRANIOFACIAL INVESTIGATION AND PAIN CLASSIFICATION

Therapists need to consider that the pain they are evoking does not necessarily arise from the tissue under the hands. Input-based mechanisms (e.g. nociceptive and peripheral neurogenic mechanisms) have the tendency to have a local, on/off pain pattern accompanied by clear dysfunctions (Gifford 1998). The other side of the spectrum are those patients without clear dysfunctions and a diagnosis such as stomatodynia (pain in the mouth), atypical odontalgia, or atypical facial or idiopathic orofacial pain. These can be categorized as mainly processing and/or output mechanisms (Okeson 1996, Gifford 1998, Butler 2000, Woda 2000). Therefore passive craniofacial techniques are a valuable instrument for:

- Confirmation of the dominant classification of pain from which the patient is suffering
- Explaining sensitivity and secondary hyperalgesia to the patient in order to reduce the patient's fear or hypochondriac thoughts (this strategy can be very helpful for further management strategies, i.e. processing)
- Helping the patient to understand that not every stimulus on the head has to increase the symptoms.

For a more philosophical background, see Chapter 1.

ABBREVIATIONS FOR RECORDING

Because most of the 14 craniofacial bones (see Chapter 2) are easily palpable with many possible passive movement directions, is it important to make frequent short recordings of findings.

In addition, adequate recording gives you the opportunity of 'learning by doing' and thus recognizing clinical patterns retrospectively (Christensen 1967, Schon 1983, Reynolds 1987). Therefore, simple additional abbreviations for the cranial bones are required. Clinically the skull bones can be defined into two groups: the coupled bones and the uncoupled bones. Recommended abbreviations are shown in Table 14.1.

The uncoupled bones form the skull base and the coupled bones are situated to the left and right of the base. For the uncoupled bones the side which is examined can be described as left (L) or right (R). You can draw a line under the bone which is examined or treated for convenience. The next step is recording the signs and the symptoms and, lastly, the grades. Some general examples of recording are given:

- Physical examination (P/E)

  —•—►$_{lat}$ $\underline{O}$/S 1/2 restrict. P↑↑ IV

  Transverse movement to lateral of the occipital bone while holding the sphenoid bone is approximately half as stiff in comparison with the other side, and reproduces symptoms at grade IV of passive accessory movement.

Table 14.1 Functional classification and notation: recommended abbreviations for the central (I) and paired (II) bones

	Abbreviation
I	
Parietal bone	P
Temporal bone	T
Petrosal bone	Pe
Zygomatic bone	Z
Maxillary bone	M
Nasal bone	N
Palatine bone	Pa
Lacrimal bone	La
II	
Occipital bone	O
Sphenoid bone	S
Ethmoid bone	E
Frontal bone	F
Vomer	V

↻ P_R/F_V P↑ IV

On rotation of the right parietal bone to the right about the transverse axis relative to the frontal bone, resistance to grade IV movement is no different from that on the opposite side. However, the beginning of symptom onset is observed with a grade IV movement.

- Therapy (Rx)

Rx ◄—•—►$_{caud}$ P/P II 2″

A longitudinal caudal movement for 2 minutes at grade II is applied to the right parietal bone while stabilizing the left parietal bone.

For more information on abbreviation and recording, see Butler (2000) and Maitland et al (2001).

GENERAL TECHNIQUES FOR THE NEUROCRANIUM

In this part of the chapter the main general cranial bone techniques are discussed. For general topographical details and clinical comments on the different bones the reader is referred to the specific techniques in Chapter 15. For the purposes of this text, the starting position of all general techniques is that the patient lies supine on the plinth and the therapist stands or sits on the right side of the plinth. Any glasses, non-fixed dental prostheses and pocket contents are removed before starting the techniques.

WHAT IS MEANT BY GENERAL TECHNIQUES AND WHAT ARE THE INDICATIONS FOR THEM?

General techniques mean:

- First 'screening tests' by manual application which gives an idea about which region of the cranium may be relevant for the patient's problem. The parameters that can be measured are stiffness and response of the patient.
- The techniques are based on subtle changes in the compliance and stress of cranial tissue as further described in this chapter under specific techniques. Therefore these tests are applied to different regions in different directions. They are the techniques with which you start and have the following functions:
  - To obtain a general impression about conditions such as severity, irritability and pain
  - To supply information about which region has (relevant) dysfunction related to the patient's symptoms and to provide a platform with which to examine that region with more specific techniques
  - To allow the patient to get used to cranial techniques in general.

In most cases five general techniques are necessary to get an impression of the condition of the neurocranium (Fig. 14.4):

- Compression techniques for the occipito-frontal region
- Compression technique for the occipital region
- Compression and distraction of the frontal region

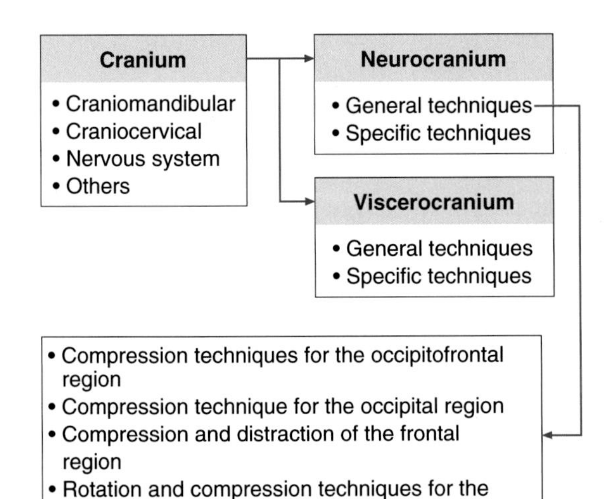

Fig. 14.4 General techniques of the neurocranium.

- Rotation and compression techniques for the temporal region
- Compression and distraction of the parietal region.

Compression techniques for the occipitofrontal region

Starting position and method

The patient lies supine and the therapist is seated to the right of the patient with the right hand resting on the plinth. The therapist holds the patient's occipital bone with the tips of the fingers on the left side. The therapist's left hand is placed on the frontal bone, keeping both elbows flexed, thus maintaining contact with the trunk. The therapist applies increasing pressure with the left hand posteriorly while at the same time moving the right hand anteriorly in the opposite direction, thus increasing pressure on the cranium. The therapist grasps with the whole volar side of both hands so that the pressure is evenly distributed (Fig. 14.5).

The same starting position can be used for the traction technique. The therapist starts with the hands in the same position, makes an anterior movement with the left hand (avoiding squeezing the thumb and fingers together), then makes a posterior movement with the right hand.

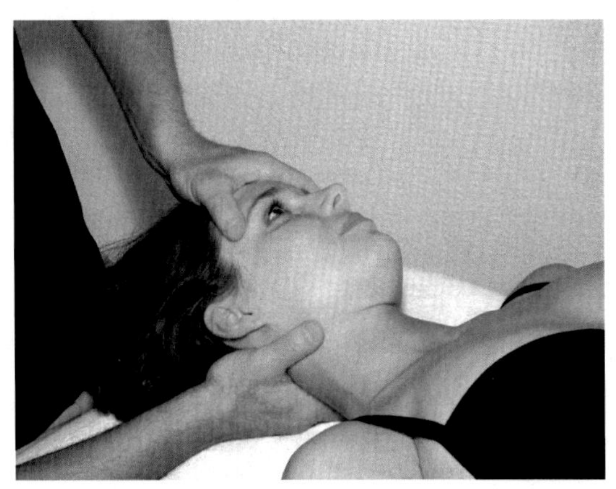

Fig. 14.5 General compression technique in the occipital–frontal region.

If the therapist has gained insufficient information, but still has the feeling that this general technique might be relevant, variations in the direction of movement might be chosen:

- Diagonal movements of the frontal and occipital bones
- Transverse movements of the occipital or frontal bone
- Rotations around the sagittal, longitudinal and transverse axes.

ANGULATION (DIAGONALS)

Changes of the axis and the position on the two bones during these occipital–frontal techniques may also change stress levels throughout the cranium and cause other responses. In the clinic, the following two diagonals are used most frequently:

- With one hand on the *left* lateral side of the occipital bone, the other hand grasps the *right* part of the frontal bone.
- With one hand on the *right* lateral side of the occipital bone, the other hand grasps the *left* part of the frontal bones (Enlow 1982).

This diagonal technique is frequently an appropriate and harmless technique in the examination and treatment of babies and young children with (secondary) plagiocephaly. Differences noticed with the hands, resistance and sometimes (non-verbal) responses are easy to observe. It is often used as one of the first treatment techniques.

TRANSVERSE MOVEMENT FROM RIGHT TO LEFT, WITH EMPHASIS ON THE OCCIPITAL REGION

Starting position and method

Once the patient is lying comfortably in a supine position with the head resting on the plinth, the therapist takes the occipital bone in the right hand as for the compression technique. This time the forearm needs to be perpendicular to the lateral side of the occipital bone. The therapist first increases the pressure from the right hand by holding the right hand steady and moving the body, followed by the right arm and right hand in the transverse direction.

TRANSVERSE MOVEMENT TO RIGHT WITH EMPHASIS ON THE FRONTAL REGION

Starting position and method

In the same starting position, the therapist places the left hand touching the patient's frontal bone with the left forearm perpendicular. Without increasing the tension in the forearm, the therapist rotates the trunk from left to right so that the grip tightens in both hands.

ROTATION ABOUT A SAGITTAL AXIS

Starting position and method

With the patient in supine position and the hands still holding the occipital and frontal bones, the therapist applies a rotary force around the sagittal axis with the thenar and hypothenar eminencies of the left hand on the lateral sides of the frontal bone. The therapist moves the fingers of the right hand downwards, rotating to the right. For rotation to the left, the movement is reversed.

These rotation techniques can be combined. For example, the occiput can be rotated to the right while the frontal bone is rotated to the left, or both can be rotated simultaneously to the same side.

ROTATION ABOUT A LONGITUDINAL AXIS

Starting position and method

With the patient lying supine, comfortable and relaxed, with the head resting on the plinth, the therapist holds the frontal bone with the volar side of the left hand, cradling the occipital bone in the right hand. By shifting the body weight to the left, rotation to the left is performed. There should be no increase in pressure through the thumbs or index fingers.

> **!** The same technique can be used for rotating the occiput to the right. Alternatively, it is possible to combine movements to move the occipital bone to the right while simultaneously moving the frontal bone to the left. To rotate in the opposite direction it is easier to start with reversed hand positions.

ROTATION ABOUT A TRANSVERSE AXIS

Starting position and method

For this approach it is necessary to rotate the frontal bones around an imaginary axis which runs through both temporal bones. The therapist's trunk is slightly flexed and the right shoulder is slightly elevated and protracted. Control is maintained by anchoring the elbow to the trunk and keeping a firm hold with the right forearm on the patient's occipital bone. These principles should be maintained for posterior rotation. The therapist should hold the trunk in slight extension with the shoulder slightly depressed. From this position it is possible to perform occipital bone movements with or without frontal bone movements, rotating to the left or right.

COMBINATION OF TECHNIQUES USING ROTATION ABOUT AN AXIS

Starting position and method

A combination of techniques with rotation around axes is also possible. For example, rotation to the right around the transverse axis of the frontal and occipital bone or rotation around the longitudinal axis may both reproduce the patient's symptoms. A combination of these two movements may be applied to provoke symptoms where it is considered appropriate.

ROTATION OF THE TEMPORAL REGION

Starting position and method

With the patient lying supine and comfortable on the plinth, the therapist rests the forearms on the plinth and holds the dorsolateral side of the patient's temporal bone directly behind the ear canal with the right hand. The therapist places the little or ring finger of the right hand in the external auditory canal and the thumb of the same hand on the temporal part of the pars squamosa. The middle and index fingers of this hand should rest on the upper and lower sides, respectively, of the zygomatic process of the temporal bone. The same procedure takes place with the left hand and the left temporal bone.

It is now possible to initiate rotation around the transverse axis towards posterior and anterior, comparing stiffness and responses. The therapist must be careful that the movements come from the trunk and that the lower arms stay perpendicular on the lateral side of the head. When the pressure is spread over all fingers the patient does not feel a local pressure of the fingers. In this starting position other movement directions are possible, such as longitudinal caudal or cranial, anterior–posterior or posterior–anterior (Fig. 14.6).

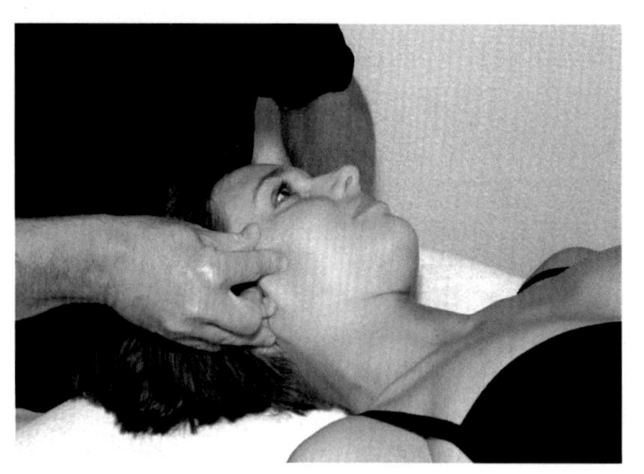

Fig. 14.6 General technique: rotation about a transverse axis in the temporal region.

General compression technique for the occipital region

Starting position and method

With the patient lying supine, comfortable and relaxed, the therapist sits at the patient's head, elbows resting on the plinth. The therapist positions their cupped hands so that the patient's head is resting in them and then contacts the occipital bone, taking care not to contact the petrosal bone. Slight pressure is applied simultaneously via both thenar eminences, avoiding extraneous movement and increased pressure on the neck muscles. The therapist slightly adducts both upper arms, keeping the trunk in slight flexion to avoid creating increased tension.

If the responses are minimal, rotating around the transverse and sagittal axes may provide more information (Fig. 14.7).

> **!** Anatomically speaking, these types of technique can be used to influence the hypoglossal canal and the foramen magnum. In the clinic, patients have often reported that this technique is beneficial for dorsal and frontal headaches, saying that it gives them a 'relaxed feeling'. Osteopaths have advocated direct manoeuvres for the occipital bone as a key relaxation technique. The techniques may also influence changes in the behaviour of mandibular depression movements, particularly during craniomandibular dysfunction or pain. After sustained pressure the patient will often show latent autonomic reactions such as sweating, a warm feeling, dizziness or changes in breathing patterns. This is seen particularly after craniocervical and craniofacial traumas such as post-whiplash, or pain following fractures in the neurocranium.

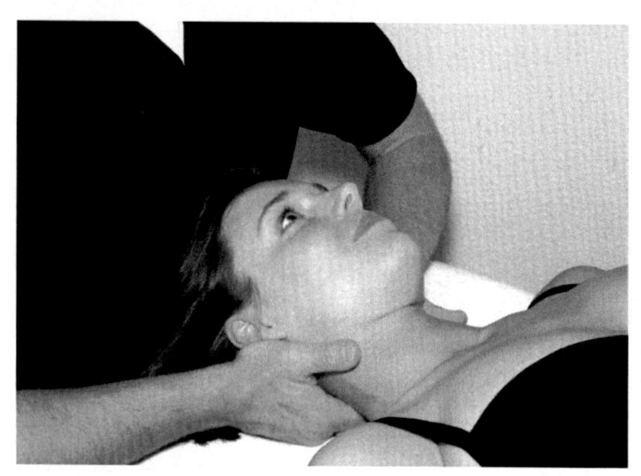

Fig. 14.7 General compression technique in the occipital region.

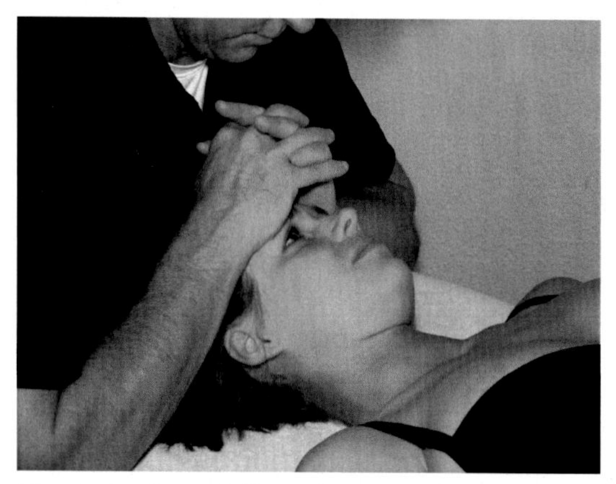

Fig. 14.8 General distraction technique in the frontal region.

Distraction of the frontal region

Starting position and method

The patient lies supine, comfortable and relaxed with the head resting on the couch. The therapist is seated behind the patient, with the trunk making slight contact against the patient's head. Both elbows are flexed and are resting on the plinth. The thenar and hypothenar eminences of both hands contact the frontal bone. To ensure a good grip, a slight pronation of both hands is made to take up the 'slack' of the skin. In this position the therapist tries to initiate a movement in the posterior–anterior direction whereby the elbows move a little over the table towards the patient's head. Variations of these movements are compression (anterior–posterior) and rotations around the sagittal and transverse axes.

> **!** The experience of patients is that this technique relieves dull headaches, and causes a general relaxed feeling in frontal sinus pain, often independent of the diagnosis. Therefore the frontal traction technique and its variations can often be used as a first treatment to reduce pain and to allow the patient to get used to this type of treatment (Fig. 14.8).

Compression and distraction of the parietal region

Starting position and method

The therapist sits behind the patient, who is lying comfortably in supine on the plinth. The therapist slightly flexes the trunk so that the sternum faces the highest point of the sagittal suture. With both forearms in pronation, perpendicular to the lateral sides of the cranium, the therapist takes the parietal bones in both hands. The therapist then moves the hands slowly towards the middle of the patient's body, ensuring that the pressure is evenly distributed between both hands.

For traction, the therapist slowly moves the trunk toward anterior while at the same time trying to move both hands laterally. Both hands keep contact with the parietal bones during the manoeuvre. During compression, the trunk is moved approximately 10° dorsally so that a bilateral movement medially can be initiated with both hands. Rotation around a transverse axis is a good alternative if nothing relevant is found.

> **!** It is known that general movements in the parietal regions can produce latent autonomic reactions. Responses such as dizziness, sweating, quick temperature changes or feelings of relaxation for several seconds or even minutes are not uncommon (Fig. 14.9).

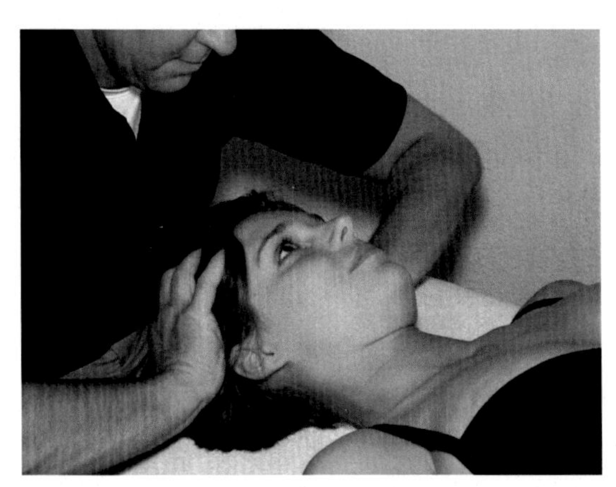

Fig. 14.9 General techniques: distraction and compression in the parietal region.

FURTHER STEPS TO FOLLOW AFTER THE GENERAL TECHNIQUES

How much dysfunction is present and the degree of symptoms, as well as the mental and physical capacity of the patient, are important factors which help the therapist to decide which pilot treatment or specific techniques to choose.

Pilot treatment

A pilot treatment can be viewed as a test treatment to see if the craniofacial dysfunction and symptoms can be influenced by one or more general techniques. Reassessment after more than 24 hours usually provides the answer as to the relevance of the chosen techniques (Maitland et al 2001).

Age, irritability of the problem and time pressure are factors influencing the choice for a pilot treatment. For example, during the first examination of a restless young child a specific examination has no use. A 58-year-old female patient with a fear of dizziness gets a mild increase of her symptoms during the first examination. In this case it is wise to leave the specific techniques alone and choose a standard craniofacial technique to try to reduce the dizziness.

Specific techniques

'Specific' here means 'more detailed' and 'local' means passive movements of a specific cranial bone structure where clear (relevant) dysfunction and symptoms are suspected to originate. In general:

- One cranial bone will be held, usually in the starting position, as described during the general techniques.
- Different movement directions of different adjacent cranial bones will then be examined.

For example, during assessment using general techniques, a patient with headache following a skull floor fracture has asymmetrical stiffness and pain responses from the occipital region. As there is enough time, the history is stable and an irritable situation is not present, the therapist decides to examine the patient further using specific accessory movements of the parietal, temporal and sphenoid region stabilizing the occipital bone. The therapist plans to make a pilot treatment of one or more movement directions to provoke the most dysfunctions and/or symptoms.

It is important to emphasize here that the therapist had already undertaken the general techniques before performing these 'specific' techniques and has a good understanding of the pain state of the patient's problem. Some of the more common specific techniques are discussed in the following section.

SPECIFIC TECHNIQUES OF THE NEUROCRANIUM

Some further points need to be emphasized regarding the special neurocranial treatment techniques already discussed in Chapter 13.

The starting position for the majority of techniques is with the patient lying supine and the therapist sitting or standing on the right-hand side of the plinth. Glasses, non-permanent dental prostheses and pocket contents should be removed. Six cranial bones and their anatomical relation to neighbouring bones will be pointed out. The connections are not described as 'sutures', 'junctions' or 'joints' but as 'regions' because the manual techniques influence different cranial tissue, not just the sutures (for more information on this subject, see Chapter 1).

Before the starting position and the method, the clinical relationship is exposed in a topographical map (Fig. 14.10). This means that the lines which are connected with the cranial bone being discussed are correlated with the topographical position of the connected bone. Thick lines refer to clear or relevant connections which are often used in practice for examination or treatment. Thin lines do not indicate that this technique is not important, but rather that these techniques are ones that may be important to the individual patient. Therefore, clinical reasoning and clinical evidence will indicate whether or not the technique is appropriate. The main techniques are also summarized in Figure 14.11.

Not all techniques are described but only those which are most used in daily practice. When you understand the basic principals, you can invent new techniques yourself, thus opening a door for the recognition of new clinical patterns. These patterns can be a basis for further management of the patient.

The occipital, sphenoid, temporal, petrosal, frontal and parietal regions of the neurocranium can be considered for the specific techniques and will be described. The main accessory movements for these bones will be covered below and, where necessary, cross-referenced.

THE OCCIPITAL REGION

In many ways this is one of the most important bones in the skull. From embryological studies it is known that the shape and growth of the cranial bones are directly and indirectly dependent on that of the occipital bone (Oudhof 2001). This bone is connected to other bones such as the sphenoid, temporal and parietal bones in the neurocranium. The occipital bone forms the base of the skull and, together with the other bones, in particular the sphenoid, it becomes the source of the main foramina, namely the lacerated and the jugular foramina.

The foramen magnum and the hypoglossal canal are formed exclusively by the occipital bone. In addition, the internal layers of the dura mater insert into the inner surface of the occipital bone, leaving only the cranial bone with a direct connection via the synovial joint to the cervical spine via the occipital condyles

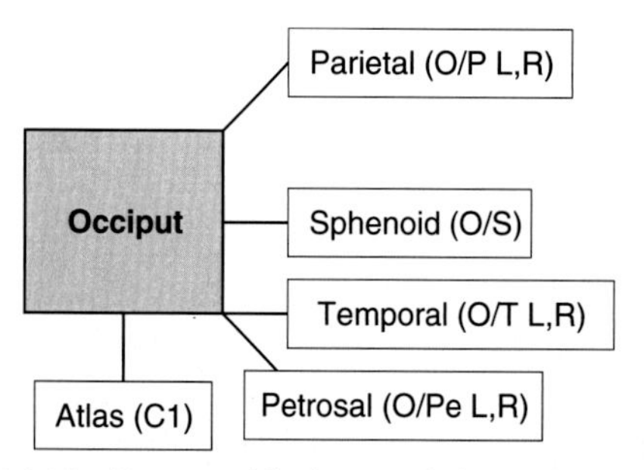

Fig. 14.10 Topographical map of the occipital bone (O). During specific techniques the occipital bone is in the centre. Ventral-cranial is connected with the parietal bone (P), in the middle with the sphenoid (S), and ventral with the temporal bone (T) and the petrosal bone (Pe).

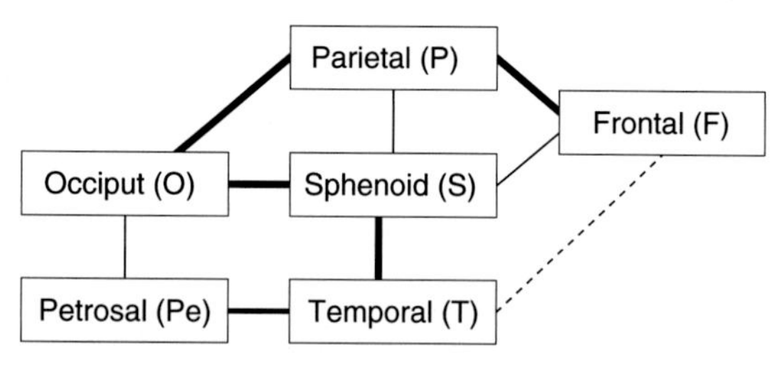

Fig. 14.11 Functional connections and their relevance during neurocranial assessment.

(see Chapter 2). It is because of these direct connections to the atlas that many ventral and dorsal neck muscles insert into the occipital bone (Williams et al 1989). For further information, see Chapters 5 and 12.

Examination of occipital bone junctions can occur at the following regions:

- Occipital–cervical region (O–C_1)
- Occipital–sphenoid region (O/S)
- Occipital–temporal region (O/T)
- Occipital–petrosal region (O/Pe)
- Occipital–parietal region (O/P).

Occipital–atlas region (O–C_1): occipital movements against C1

STRUCTURAL DIFFERENTIATION

Some of these smooth, passive accessory movements can provide very useful tools for structural differentiation between cranium and cervical spine, particularly when there is a dominant input mechanism (nociceptive or peripheral neurogenic).

Starting position and method

For this technique it is essential for the patient to lie in a comfortable supine or prone position. If the prone position is adopted, the patient will need to rest the forehead on overlapping palms of their hands to avoid rotation in the neck. The spine should be in a neutral mid-flexion/extension position. Discussion of the prone position is included here because the cervical spine is so often examined in this position in the clinic.

The therapist sits or stands cranially to the patient's head. With the index finger and thumb of the right hand, the therapist holds the transverse processes of the patient's atlas. With the left hand, the therapist grasps the whole occipital bone without touching the cervical spine. The forearms should be in supination and both forearms held parallel.

In this position the therapist can perform any accessory movements for the occipital bone. During the manoeuvre the fingers of the left hand on the atlas must remain motionless to avoid movement of the occipital–atlas joint. The manoeuvre is initiated from the thrust of the body which is transferred through the left hand without moving the fingers.

CRANIOFACIAL MORPHOLOGY, HEAD POSTURE AND THE FIRST CERVICAL VERTEBRA

The craniocervical area in humans and other animals is a marvellous example of function following form and form following function (Proffit 1993). For example, the relationship between craniofacial morphology and head posture has been demonstrated by Solow and Tallgren (1976) and Huggare (1987). One such example is that of greater upper cervical head extension. Experimental studies on animals have reported a significant correlation between head posture and anomalies of the first vertebra which were craniocaudally wider (Huggare 1987, Kylämarkula 1988). The same pattern is seen in children with tonsils who have a greater head extension due to different respiratory behaviour and therefore atypical craniofacial growth (Linder-Aronson & Woodside 2000, Fig. 14.12).

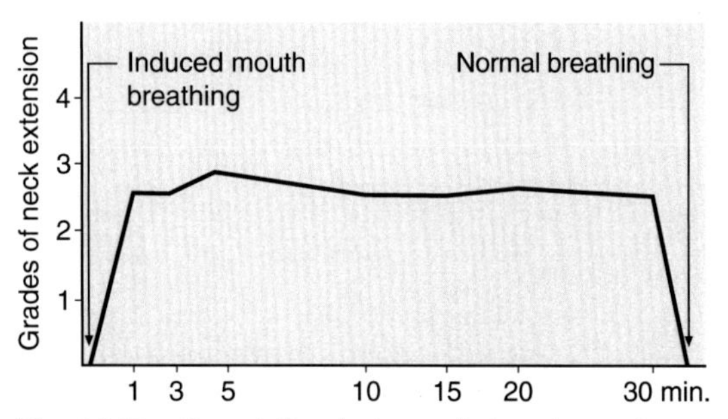

Fig. 14.12 Correlation between induced mouth breathing and changed head posture in 12 healthy probands. The graph shows that EMG activity of the suprahyoid muscles and head extension is increased by an average of two to three grades with induced mouth breathing. The process is reversible if normal breathing (without nasal obstruction) is restored after 30 minutes. This supports the hypothesis that prolonged extension of the head influences the face, the mandible and craniocervical growth (reproduced with permission from Linder-Aronson & Woodside 2000).

Muscle imbalance in the head region also seems to encourage compensation in the morphology of the upper cervical vertebrae and cranium (Avis 1959, Kylämarkula 1988). Indeed, it has been found that craniofacial dysfunction influences the growth patterns in prepubertal children. Such imbalance is a possible predictor for some growth characteristics and can lead to a predisposition for other dysfunctions.

Some key points from this are:

- Morphological compensation may occur in this area in relation to normal and/or abnormal functioning.
- Morphological changes in the vertebrae may produce abnormal signs and symptoms during manual examination, not only of the upper cervical spine region but also of the neurocranium (Maitland 1986, Gonzalez de Dios et al 1998).

Morphological abnormalities can also be an expression of early abnormal stress-transducer forces (Wagemans et al 1988, Oudhof 2001). This may be due to external forces or stressors such as splints and/or sustained pressure, such as the wearing of a helmet. Passive movements can influence these abnormal stress transducer forces. In fact, passive accessory and intervertebral movements of the upper cervical spine as well as accessory movement of the cranium can be useful in detecting relevant dysfunction and pain. This in turn might also highlight the need for further management.

ABNORMAL CRANIOCERVICAL AREAS IN THE NEWBORN AND FURTHER CONSEQUENCES FOR DEVELOPMENT

A complex of symptoms in newborn babies is often described in the literature under different diagnoses, such as newborn scoliosis (Mau & Gabe 1981, Slate et al 1993), 'moulded' baby syndrome (Good & Walker 1984), habitual unilateral supine position (Palmèn 1984), squint baby syndrome (Ruige et al 1993) and TAC syndrome (turned head, adducted hip, truncal curvature; Hamanishi & Tanaka 1994).

Symptoms of this syndrome could be plagiocephaly (without synostosis), torticollis, 'bat ear', scoliosis and limited hip abduction with or without defective foot position.

Plagiocephaly caused by deformity with the same symptoms described above is often increased because babies are placed in their cots lying on their backs, in preference to side lying or prone postures, as a safeguard against cot death (de Jonge & Engelberts 1987, Ratliff-Schaub et al 2001, Ozawa & Takashima 2002).

Buchmann et al (1992) indicated in an epidemiologic study that one-third of newborns in a random population have an asymmetrical range of movement in the atlantocranial and atlantoaxial joints. Often their shape is also abnormal. The asymmetry may remain or increase, but in most cases it is self-correcting.

If the asymmetry remains, this can influence the function of the cervical spine or the hips, and also motor development. Buchmann et al (1992) and Biedermann (2001) established the KISS syndrome, a craniocervical functional impairment, as a kinematic imbalance caused by suboccipital loading. Biedermann identified some characteristic clinical patterns from the evaluation of typical radiological findings and questionnaires in a group of 100 babies. Craniovertebral functional impairments were often accompanied by symptoms such as torticollis, cranial scoliosis, flat dorsal head with unilateral swelling of the facial soft tissue, acute sensitivity of the neck, opisthotonos and C-shaped scoliosis of the spine (Neufeld & Birkett 2000).

Risk factors appear to be:

- Trauma to the upper cervical spine during birth, which may be caused by assisted delivery
- Prolonged expulsion phase
- Injuries occurring in early childhood (Biedermann 1995, Krous et al 2001).

In the eighteenth century Nicolas Andry, a very important figure in general orthopaedics, was already using gross craniofacial manoeuvres for young children with torticollis (Andry 1741). General manual therapy and osteopathic literature from the last three decades has described the relevance of manual treatment for this region to reduce dysfunction and symptoms as described above. For example, a clear link has been found in newborn and young children between atlantocranial and atlantoaxial joints and asymmetry in the cranium due to a type of scoliosis (Meissner 1992). Manual therapy of the upper cervical spine was said to influence the pathogenesis of torticollis and scoliosis. Biedermann's interviews with patients (Biedermann 1996) and long-term radiological studies (Meissner 1992) were used as a gold standard.

Frymann (1983) undertook a classic study showing different types of morphological change in the neurocranium during the first 24 hours after birth in asymptomatic newborn babies. Frymann found that during manual examination, different types of stress were observed on the occipital, temporal and parietal bones when craniocervical dysfunction was present. Frymann suggested that this abnormal stress-transducer in the cranium can lead to 80% of the body being predisposed to further symptoms which children will often go on to develop. As therapists, however, we need to be aware that not all asymmetry in the neurocranium and atlantocranium leads to symptoms. Buchmann et al (1992) advocate reassessment after short- and long-term treatment of each patient to provide clues as to the relevance of the dysfunction.

OCCIPITAL CONDYLE FRACTURE AND CRANIOFACIAL PAIN

Standard x-rays of the skull and cervical spine after head injury with an occipital fracture usually show soft tissue injuries (Alker et al 1978, Hanson et al 2002). After removing the cervical collar, palpation of the occipitocervical region, active flexion, extension and touching the lateral area of the head can be painful. Rotations are generally pain-free (Stroobants et al 1994, Kaushik et al 2002). Such an individual, who on first impression is a reasonably straightforward post-traumatic patient, will often visit a therapist specializing in the neuromusculoskeletal system for treatment.

Where this clinical pattern is recognized, and the atlantocranial differentiation and movement of the occiput are extremely painful, further examination and diagnosis is indicated (Capobianco et al 2002). A final diagnosis of a possible avulsion fracture of the occipital condyle can only be made with high resolution CT (Miltner et al 1990, Stroobants et al 1994). Passive movements are not indicated in such a case.

NON-INVASIVE AND POSTOPERATIVE TREATMENT OF AN ATLAS FRACTURE

A fracture of the atlas is a serious injury with important diagnostic traps. The type of fracture indicates whether an operative or non-invasive treatment is needed (Grob & Magerl 1987). Cranial nerve paralyses are exceptionally rare with atlas fractures, but have been described in the literature (Henche et al 1994). The glossopharyngeal (IX), vagus (X) and accessory (XI) nerves, and especially the hypoglossal (XII) nerve, appear to be susceptible to damage from atlas fractures at the base of the skull (Zielinski et al 1982, Aebi & Nazarian 1987, Capobianco et al 2002, Kaushik et al 2002, Muthukamar 2002).

Some clinical studies show a significant correlation between atypical craniofacial pain and other diagnosed symptoms following atlas fractures. Trauma to the neck and cranial region varies in impact and direction. Post-traumatic symptoms can also differ. Common symptoms in post-whiplash patients such as minor neck pain and headaches, burning eye pain, pressure on the throat, dysphasia, etc. without clear CT or MRI findings lead one to suspect that a minor neuropathy in one of the cranial nerves described could be producing the symptoms. In this situation it will be necessary to examine the craniocervical and craniofacial areas, together with the neurodynamics of the cranial nerves, to clarify the diagnosis.

INFANTILE CEREBRAL PALSY AND THE CRANIOCERVICAL REGION

Many practitioners from a variety of fields agree that the current definition for cerebral palsy (CP) – 'an irreversible sensory–motor dysfunction caused by early brain damage' (Cano et al 2001) – needs to be made more specific (Flehming 1979, Biedermann 1995). Of all children seen in the clinic with output mechanism changes such as behaviour changes, asymmetrical muscle tone or motor retardation, 20% are diagnosed as having CP. Modern ultrasound and MRI techniques now used as the gold standard show that only 1% of these cases have any real cerebral damage (Largo 1986, Biedermann 1996). Dysfunctional atlantocranial and atlantoaxial joints (Buchmann et al 1992, Lohse-Busch & Kraemer 1994), as well as abnormal stress and strain on the neurocranium, is found to be significantly higher in these children (Frymann 1983).

Two main features are:

- Cerebral afferent input is the most important requirement for cerebral development in newborn babies (Flehming 1979, Buchmann & Bülow 1989).
- The most measurable afferent proprioceptive signal originates from the craniocervical region: head stabilization is a complex process involving the interaction of vertebral, visual and proprioceptive reflexes (Schor et al 1988).

One possible hypothesis is that abnormal afferent stimulation from the craniocervical region (which stimulates abnormal effects in the brain) exaggerates abnormal output mechanisms, creating aberrant movements and forces. This leads to irregular learning behaviour which in turn has consequences for later neuromotor development (Lohse-Busch & Kraemer 1994, Biedermann 1995). Passive movements such as mobilization and manipulation of the upper cervical junction can normalize the control mechanisms from motor and vegetative systems (Buchmann et al 1992, Lohse-Busch & Kraemer 1994). Cranial techniques may reduce stress in the caudal tissue, encouraging normal cranial nervous tissue movement and influencing fluctuations in the cervical fluid and altering hyperactivity in the nervous system (Frymann 1983).

The key message here is that adequate hands-on management of infantile cerebral palsy in this region is a new area to consider. These cranial techniques as described above can be good non- invasive, painless techniques for this purpose, in conjunction with other treatment strategies. For more detailed information about children, cranial techniques and motor problems, see Chapters 19 and 20.

Occipital–sphenoid region (O/S)

Starting position and method

With the patient lying in a comfortable supine position, the therapist sits or stands at the patient's head. The therapist cups the occipital bone in the right hand, the elbow resting on the plinth. The therapist holds the greater wings of the sphenoid bone between the tips of the thumb and index finger of the left hand, steadying the left forearm against the trunk during movement of the occipital bone to prevent extraneous movement.

In this position it is possible to perform any of the accessory movements. Transverse movements and rotations around the sagittal and longitudinal axes are simple to perform and very valuable clinically. In order to move in the anterior–posterior direction, the therapist will need to rotate the patient's head at a 30–40° angle with the right hand and hold the occipital bone perpendicular. When applying longitudinal cranial movements, this position sometimes provides a comfortable alternative (Fig. 14.13).

SPECIFIC TECHNIQUES

The occipital–sphenoid region is often one of the first regions that should be examined using specific techniques. Some reasons for this might be:

- The relatively long duration of suture mobility which can be a source of dysfunction and pain. Researchers have varying opinions about the age at which union of the sutures occurs.
- The sphenoid bone and its foramina are responsible for the majority of skull growth, which can predispose to changes in cranioneurodynamics (Chapters 2, 17 and 18).

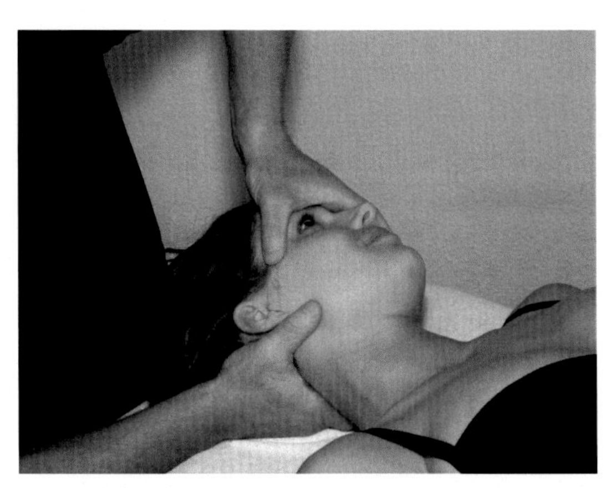

Fig. 14.13 Accessory moments of the occiput while holding the sphenoid bone with the head in 30° of rotation.

- General signs and symptoms can be traced to deformation or dysfunction in this region, with consequences for neighbouring bones and foramina. The jugular foramen which is formed by the temporal and occipital bone at the skull base is a case in point. The jugular vein drains blood from the cranial vault, while cranial nerves IX, X and XI pass through the same foramina. Symptoms such as problems with the gag reflex, abnormal taste at the back of the tongue, problems speaking and swallowing, vagus symptoms such as cranial arrhythmia, digestive problems and abnormal sternocleidomastoid and trapezius tone may be closely related to obstructed flow of intracranial fluids (Patten 1995, Zuniga et al 1995). The manual technique for the occipitosphenoid region is therefore considered as the sixth screening test for the cranium.

Occipital–temporal region (O/T)

Starting position and method

With the patient lying comfortably on their back, the therapist sits or stands at the patient's head with the left hand in supination. The therapist cups the patient's occipital bone in the palm of the left hand and rotates the patient's head approximately 30° laterally. The right index, middle and little fingers grasp the cranial and ventral part of the temporal bone; the hand should remain perpendicular to the temporal bone and supinated.

From this position any accessory movements described below are possible, always being careful to prevent shift or glide movements of the neck and head.

Occipital–parietal region (O/P)

Starting position and method

The patient should be lying in a comfortable supine position with the therapist sitting at the end of the plinth, cupping the patient's occipital bone with the supinated right hand. The therapist holds the left parietal bone by positioning the left lower arm in pronation, with the point of the elbow supported on the plinth, steadying the proximal third of the right forearm against the trunk. This is important to avoid unnecessary tension in the hands.

From this position it is possible to produce any accessory movements by moving the body. There should be no increase in pressure from the fingers in the left hand on the parietal bones during the manoeuvre.

AN ALTERNATIVE IN PRONE

Starting position and method

For this technique, it is best if the patient lies prone with their hands under the forehead. If this is uncomfortable, have the patient lie prone, arms at the side, with a rolled-up towel under the forehead to reduce pressure from the plinth. The therapist stands at the patient's head with the hands pronated and forearms perpendicular to each other. The therapist takes the parietal bones in the left hand with the medial side of the left elbow resting on the plinth, then, with the right hand resting on the plinth, the therapist cups the occipital bone without touching the other hand or the lambdoid suture. This alternative position is easier for anterior–posterior or posterior–anterior movements and rotations.

Any accessory (but particularly longitudinal and transverse) movements are easy to perform in this position. If the technique is uncomfortable for either therapist or patient, it can be done standing at the side. The hand contact points are the same, except the forearms do not rest on the plinth as before.

POSTERIOR–ANTERIOR MOVEMENTS USING A LOCALIZED THUMB TECHNIQUE

Sometimes it is useful to examine or treat with localized techniques, for example in the presence of extracranial scar tissue or craniosynostosis in a specific area. The author has also seen patients following cerebral concussion where significant changes in signs and symptoms were observed after sharp local pain was treated with localized techniques. Here posterior–anterior manoeuvres with angulations and longitudinal movements can usefully be applied.

Starting position and method

The patient lies in a prone position with the arms by the sides and a rolled-up towel under the forehead. The therapist stands at the patient's head, the exact position depending on the area to be examined. Both thumbs should be touching the desired location on the occipital bone, adjacent to the lambdoid suture. The therapist spreads the fingers over the lateral sides of the parietal and occipital bones, building up pressure slowly using an oscillatory movement by moving the trunk rather than adding flexion via the thumbs or fingers. Trunk movements help to prevent localized pain.

Accessory movements are now possible by angling the body and holding the patient's head steadily in position against the trunk. The therapist can vary the emphasis by focusing on the occiput in order to change the symptom response.

LONGITUDINAL MOVEMENTS

Starting position and method

For this technique the patient lies in a comfortable supine position with the therapist sitting or standing at the head end. The therapist places the thumbs slightly flexed, longitudinally and crossed on the lambdoidal suture, with the other fingers resting on the occipital and parietal bones.

For a longitudinal movement in upwards direction with compression on the bone connections, the therapist flexes the interphalangeal joints of the left hand. Simultaneous movement of the opposite thumb will produce greater compression.

An extension of this movement of the interphalangeal joint of the right thumb will produce longitudinal movement downwards while the left thumb movement will add a decompression.

These local techniques can be useful in producing symptoms which help to compare the left and right sides of the skull in terms of local symptoms. For example, 'spot' pain can be compared in this way with traumatic neck and skull problems such as contusion syndromes, contusion in the cervical spine, whiplash and consolidated skull fractures.

A NOTE ON PLAGIOCEPHALY AND POSTURE

Symptoms such as deformity, torticollis, adduction restrictions of the hip and scoliosis are suggestive of plagiocephaly and are significantly more common in children with preferential posture, particularly babies up to the age of 6 months (de Jonge & Engelberts 1987, de Jonge 1992, Gonzalez de Dios et al 1998). Boere-Boonekamp and van der Linden-Kuiper (2001) conclude that the resting position of the child after the first week of life, as well as the feeding method adopted, contributes significantly to risk factors in plagiocephaly. They concluded retrospectively that, of one-third (32%) of babies who were treated, more than 50% still had residual movement restrictions and associated symptoms after 1 year, though consequences in later years are unknown. Neufeld and Birkett (2000) suggest starting with posture reposition techniques (posture changes) and physiotherapy at an early stage to reduce the dysfunction as soon as possible. Should this management prove ineffective, a helmet or band may be implemented (Neufeld & Birkett 2000, Losee & Mason 2005). Symptoms in schoolchildren such as frequent severe migraine, torticollis, neck stiffness with periodic adolescent scoliosis, concentration disturbances, motor retardation, craniomandibular malformations and face asymmetry may all be expressions of unrecognized dysfunction of the cranium or craniocervical junctions early in the child's life (von Piekartz 2001, Spermon Marijnen & Spermon 2001). Such symptoms provide a valid reason for further examination and treatment of the cranium and craniocervical region.

THE SPHENOID BONE

General qualities

The sphenoid bone is at the base of the skull, wedged between the frontotemporal and occipital bones. It has a central body as well as greater and lesser wings. The lateral side of the greater wing is easy to palpate, which makes it ideal for examination and/or treatment.

In the literature, opinions differ as to the age at which sphenoid–occipital bones fuse. One author states that they are completely fused by the age of 25, whereas others describe cranial movement still occurring into old age (Enlow 1982, Proffit 1993).

The joint complexes and functional connections of the sphenoid bone are as follows (Fig. 14.14):

- Spheno-occipital region (S/O)
- Sphenofrontal region (S/F)
- Sphenotemporal region (S/T)
- Sphenoparietal region (S/P).

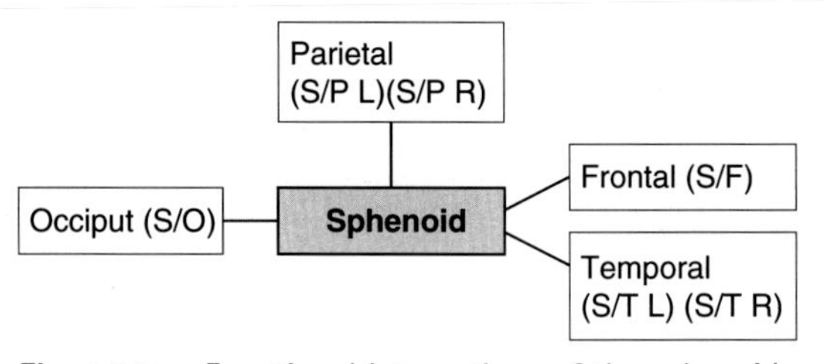

Fig. 14.14 Functional interactions of the sphenoid region.

Spheno-occipital region (S/O)

Starting position and method

Start as for the technique that moves the occipitosphenoid region, except that this time the occiput is held and the sphenoid is moved.

The patient lies comfortably in supine and the therapist sits or stands at the end of the plinth. The therapist cups the occipital bone in the right hand, the elbow resting on the plinth. Holding the greater wings of the occipital bone between the tips of thumb and index finger of the left hand, the therapist steadies the left forearm against the trunk during movement of the sphenoid bone to prevent extraneous movement.

> **!** Once again, it is important that it is the body and not the hands that create the movement. Apart from anchoring the forearm against the trunk, concentrating on the thumb, index and middle fingers will help with this. Watch that the distance between the two fingers is always the same, avoiding any increase in tone in the hand muscles. The patient should be asked to indicate if there is any increase in localized pressure from the fingers.

ALTERNATIVE PROPOSAL FOR ASSESSMENT OF A PATIENT WITH A BIG HEAD AND/OR A THERAPIST WITH SMALL HANDS

The therapist's hands might be too small to grasp both lateral sides of the greater wings of the sphenoid bone. In this case it is proposed that the patient's head be rotated approximately 40° away (in this case to the left) from the therapist with a supporting pillow on the left side of the patient's face.

The therapist sits on the right side of the patient as during the standard technique and places the thumbs softly on the right lateral side of the sphenoid bone. The right hand supports the left side of the occipital bone. In this position the therapist initiates the transverse movement of the sphenoid region towards the left.

BILATERAL THUMB TECHNIQUE

The second alternative technique that can be used in appropriate situations, for example if the patient cannot tolerate the head being touched, is the bilateral thumb technique.

Starting position and method

The patient lies supine and the therapist sits on the short end of the plinth. Both of the lower arms rest on the couch in supination. The therapist grasps the occipital bones as with the general occiput compression. The pads of both thumbs contact both greater wings of the sphenoid. Rotation around all three axes is possible but also anterior–posterior and posterior–anterior movement without too much pressure from either thumb. The therapist should be aware of increasing unilateral pressure during performance of the movement. The patient should be asked to indicate any increasing local pressure under the thumbs.

Sphenofrontal region (S/F)

Starting position and method

The patient should be lying comfortably in supine with the therapist sitting or standing at the head end. The therapist holds the whole of the frontal bone in the pronated left hand, with the thumb adjacent to the sphenofrontal suture and the index, middle and ring fingers on the other side (Fig. 14.15). The therapist anchors the left elbow against the body to prevent further movement of the head, while holding the greater wings of the sphenoid bone with the thumb and index finger of the right hand with the forearm in pronation.

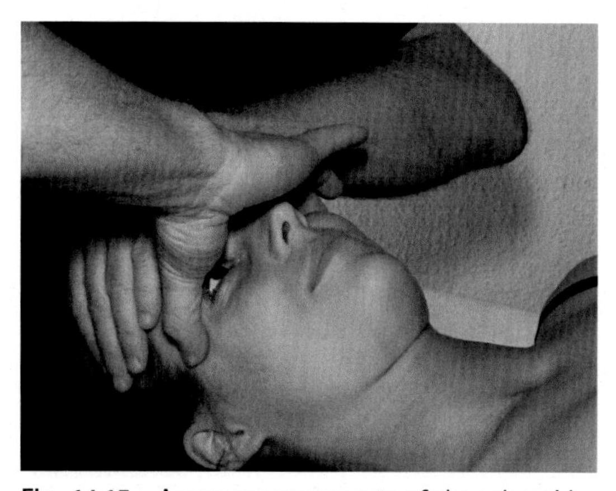

Fig. 14.15 Accessory movements of the sphenoid bone while holding the frontal region.

All accessory movements for the sphenoid bone can be performed from this position. The therapist should increase pressure slowly, avoiding provocation of localized pain at the contact points of the thumb and index finger.

AN ALTERNATIVE METHOD FOR UNILATERAL LONGITUDINAL CRANIAL MOVEMENT OF THE SPHENOID BONE

This is a clinically useful technique that can be used for undefined (atypical) facial pain which has a relative local projection. The method is intraoral.

Starting position and method

The patient should lie in a comfortable supine position, close to the edge of the plinth with their head turned to the left. The therapist sits at the side so that the trunk is touching the parietal and temporal bones on the right-hand side. The therapist takes the skull in the left hand, with the fingers holding the temporal bone above the zygomatic bone. The proximal two-thirds of the left index finger should be holding onto the greater wing of the sphenoid so that the finger can be flexed at the interphalangeal joints. With the right hand supinated, the therapist puts the little finger inside the patient's mouth on the external surface of the pterygoid process, slightly extending the interphalangeal joint of the little finger while guiding the little finger upwards. The therapist should avoid applying extra pressure through the other fingers.

This technique can be used as an alternative if the bilateral thumb technique produces too much local 'pressure' pain. It also gives an idea of the range of movement and is most useful in the presence of unilateral symptoms. It is also easier to hold the index, ring and little fingers on the frontal bone and to move the sphenoid with the middle finger when not totally satisfied about the outcome.

DEFORMATION OF THE FRONTAL REGION BY IMPACT AND SUSTAINED POSITIONS

Studies of frontal and occipital impacts conclude that there is a relatively large stress/pressure factor and shear distribution on the cranium and hence, the brain (Sano et al 1969, Chu et al 1994). This could explain why, during passive movements, symptoms are often reproduced in the occipital and neck region. It might also explain why, after cerebral contusion, patients will sometimes react with severe symptoms when treated with a minor passive application on the frontal and/or occipital bone. With this in mind it is important to assess the treatment dose carefully. Extreme deformities such as frontal plagiocephaly where there is flattening on one or more sides of the cranium are often seen at birth. Minor forms are usually neglected and can be seen in old age (Hansen & Mulliken 1994, Besson et al 2002).

Plagiocephaly and ocular torticollis occur together in 1 in 300 births (Dunn 1974). Slate et al (1993) reported in their research that more than 50% of these children have C1–C2 subluxations with no other neurological deficit. All patients in the group had positional skull moulding, with consistent flattening of the contralateral occipital parietal region as well as the ipsilateral fronto-orbital region, relative to the side of the torticollis. The atlas was rotated forward on the side opposite to the torticollis. Conservative non-surgical treatment produced favourable results, and if the child was under 1 year old positioning in helmet moulding was also successful (Ripley et al 1993, Neufeld & Birkett 2002).

There is as yet a scarcity of studies that have considered the relationship between minor plagiocephaly and the manifestation of head–neck symptoms.

Craniofacial and craniocervical treatment using passive movements might be helpful in changing the signs and symptoms in this patient group. The author proposes either or both of the following examination and treatment techniques, coupled with assessment of the craniocervical region:

- Compression techniques on the ipsilateral occipital bone and contralateral frontal bone of the flattened side
- Distraction techniques for the contralateral occipital bone and the ipsilateral frontal bone of the flattened side.

VERTICALIZATION OF THE MANDIBLE

Longitudinal radiocephalometry in children with mandibulofacial dysostosis (MFD) shows that progressive cranial basilar kyphosis places abnormal stress on the sphenofrontal suture. This allows less opportunity for verticalization of the mandible and hence is followed by abnormal growth of the mandible and associated dysfunction of the airway (Schlenkler et al 2000; see also Chapter 22). Such an extreme craniofacial growth pattern can exist in minor forms and apply the same extreme pressure to the sphenofrontal region (Cordasco et al 1999). Abnormalities such as unilateral growth of the mandible, airway dysfunction and long-term sinusitis complaints might indicate the need for cranial mobilization. As always, it is prudent to heed contraindications and respect the necessary precautions.

Frontal bone movement can also be beneficial in assessment and treatment of the following clinical patterns:

- General dull headache symptoms with an autonomic output component
- Facial dysfunction or pain after cranial trauma or operations in the area, e.g. cystectomy for chronic sinusitis, hypophysectomy or intracranial nasal operations
- Frontal sinusitis symptoms. Several factors influence the frontal sinus morphology: These include craniofacial configuration and the width of the frontal bone in relation to the intracranial pressure (Brown et al 1984, Bracard et al 1987).

Sphenotemporal region (S/T)

This technique has enormous clinical value. It can be an effective technique for treating subjective tinnitus, bruxism and non-infectious earache. It can also be applied in trying to change the diameter of the unilateral skull foramina which might result from neural container dysfunction in the cranial nervous tissue (as described in Chapter 17).

Starting position and method

The patient lies supine and comfortable on the plinth with the head rotated 20–30° to the left. The therapist holds both greater wings of the sphenoid bone between the left index finger and thumb, keeping the left forearm parallel to the torso. The therapist pronates the right hand and places it on the temporal bone, with the right thumb resting on the dorsolateral side of the temporal bone, directly behind the external auditory canal. The little finger of the right hand should be in the external auditory meatus and the middle and ring fingers of this hand lie adjacent to the sphenoid–temporal region so that this region can be accentuated when necessary.

From this position it is possible to perform any of the accessory movements for the sphenoid bone. The longitudinal movement is transmitted through the forearm via the little finger holding the pterygoid process. The index finger of the left hand needs to be flexed during the manoeuvre to support this action.

Sphenoparietal region (S/P)

This connection is relatively small and is connected to the sphenotemporal and frontosphenoid joints (see Chapter 2).

Starting position and method

The patient lies supine and comfortable on the plinth. With the tip of the thumb and index finger of the left hand, the therapist holds both parietal bones adjacent to the sphenoid–parietal region. The right index finger should be resting on the left part of the greater wing of the sphenoid, adjacent to the sphenoid–parietal region; the right thumb should be resting on the greater wing of the sphenoid on the right hand side.

From this position any accessory sphenoid movements are possible. The therapist should ensure that the distance between the thumb and index finger on the sphenoid remains constant and should try not to increase the tone of the hand muscles. The patient should be asked to indicate if the grip becomes uncomfortable at any stage of the process.

THE TEMPORAL BONE

The temporal bone forms the lateral side of the neurocranium and is connected to the petrosal, parietal, sphenoid and occipital bones of the cranium. The temporal fossa connects to the head of the mandible to form the temporomandibular joint (TMJ).

The way in which the TMJ interacts with the temporal bone has great influence on the growth and shape of the skull (Oudhof 2001; see Chapter 2). It is possible to see from the kind of sutures found in the temporal bone how many different forces have an input towards its function (see Chapter 2). The temporoparietal and temporosphenoid connections are described in the literature as being still mobile in old age and can be palpated as follows (Fig. 14.16):

- Temporoparietal region (T/P)
- Temporozygomatic region (T/Z)
- Temporopetrosal region (T/Pe)
- Temporosphenoid region (T/S)
- Temporo-occipital region (T/O)

Movement of the temporal bone against neighbouring bones

Starting position and method

With the patient lying supine and comfortable on the plinth, the therapist rests the forearms on the plinth and holds the dorsolateral side of

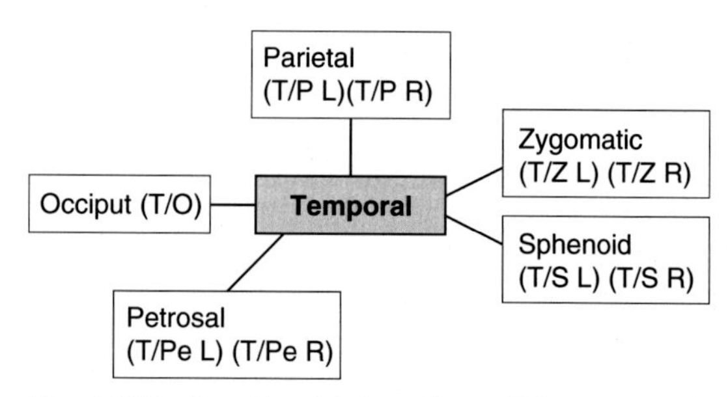

Fig. 14.16 Functional interactions of the temporal region.

the temporal bone directly behind the auricle with the right hand. The therapist places the right little or ring finger in the external auditory canal and the thumb of the same hand on the temporal planum of the pars squamosa. The middle and index fingers of this hand should rest on the upper and lower sides, respectively, of the zygomatic process of the temporal bone. The therapist holds the neighbouring bone whose connection is to be examined in the left hand.

The following positions can be adopted by the therapist for the relevant region:

- Temporoparietal region: With the left hand in pronation, hold the parietal bone with the whole palm of that hand, the thumb lying along the temporoparietal suture (Fig. 14.17a).
- Temporosphenoid region: With the webspace of the left hand parallel to the coronal suture, hold the greater wing of the sphenoid bone between the left thumb and left middle or ring finger, as described for the occipitosphenoid region.
- Temporozygomatic region: Rotate the patient's head 30° away from the side to be examined. Hold the zygomatic bone between the index finger and thumb of the left hand (Fig. 14.17b).
- Temporo-occipital region: With your left hand in supination, hold the occipital bone in the palm of this hand. Move the patient's head into slight extension in order to relax the soft tissue of the upper cervical spine. Rest the right index and middle fingers on the temporal bone ventromedially to the mastoid process on the side to be examined.
- Temporopetrosal region: With the patient's head rotated 50° away from the side to be examined, sit to the patient's left with the torso slightly flexed. The left arm should be parallel with the patient's body while holding the patient's mastoid process between the flexed left index finger and thumb.

It is possible to make any of the accessory movements for the temporal bone from these positions. The rotations around a transverse axis are produced by pronating or supinating the forearm; otherwise the movements are initiated from the trunk. For a more efficient movement during the lateral transverse movement, it is necessary to hook the slightly flexed right ring finger in the external auditory canal while the middle and index fingers squeeze the zygomatic process. Even pressure on the temporal bone is maintained by keeping the fingers equidistant.

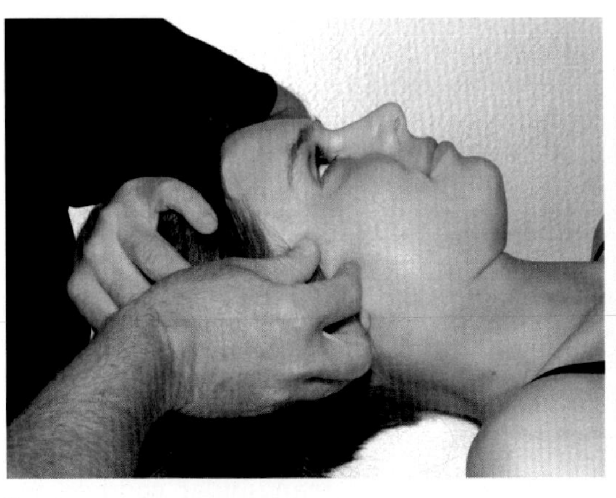

a

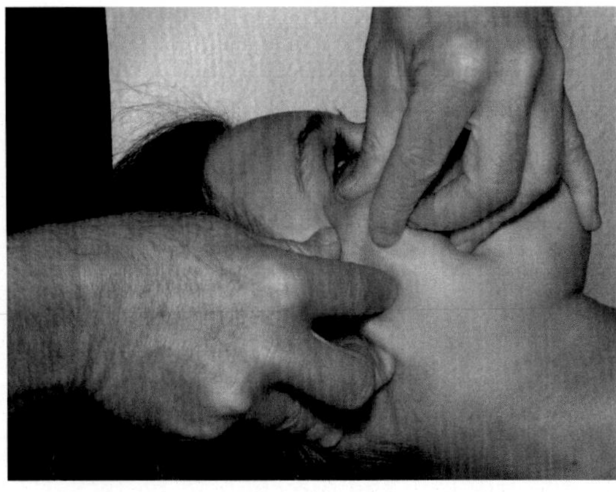

b

Fig. 14.17 Movement of the temporal bone.
a Movement of the temporal bone in the standard position as described during the general techniques and holding in this case the parietal bone.
b Movement of the temporal bone with fixed zygomatic bone.

Movement of neighbouring bones against the temporal bone

Starting position and method

The starting positions for the techniques are as described above, only this time the therapist's right hand holds the temporal bone and the left changes according to the junction being examined.

From that position the right hand stays on the temporal bone while the left initiates the movement towards the direction to be examined. Clinically this technique is more used than others, perhaps because it presents greater clinical advantages, such as its large area and its relative flexibility into old age (Oudhof 2001). An exception to this is the temporoparietal region discussed in more detail below.

Temporoparietal region (T/P)

There are a few main techniques that are often used in the clinic for this region. These are longitudinal movements up and down using compression and distraction, rotations about the longitudinal, transverse and sagittal axes and anterior–posterior or posterior–/anterior movements.

Starting position and method

The patient lies in a comfortable supine position with the head rotated 30° to the left, the therapist sitting to the right of the patient's head. The therapist rests the palm of the left hand on top of the skull with the middle and index fingers on the parietal bone distal to the parietotemporal region. The hypothenar eminence of the right hand should be over the pars squamosa with the fingers facing towards the face. The therapist's right middle finger is touching the zygomatic process while the little finger of that hand is touching the mandibular angle (see Fig. 14.17a).

The temporal movement must be initiated from the trunk in the direction to be tested. Slight counter-pressure should be applied in the opposite direction to emphasize the squeeze action of the pars squamosa (the temporoparietal region).

VARIATIONS FOR LONGITUDINAL MOVEMENTS IN COMPRESSION AND DISTRACTION

This technique uses six fingers, three from each hand, to perform the movements.

Starting position and method

The patient lies comfortably in supine, with the therapist standing or sitting to the left of the patient's head, which is rotated approximately 30° to the left. With the three middle fingers of the right hand, the therapist holds the squamosa of the temporal bone just below the parietotemporal region. The therapist grasps the spaces between the fingers of the right hand with the middle fingers of the left hand to link hands and hold the suture on the parietal bone. The forearms should be parallel to each other.

The movement is produced by slightly extending the distal and interphalangeal finger joints and slightly abducting the forearms, ensuring that the patient's head remains stable and that the fingers do not dig in and feel uncomfortable.

A localized thumb technique can also be used to carry out the procedure. The principle is the same except that the thumbs are kept parallel to each other and extend and flex the interphalangeal thumb joints to produce distraction and compression of the parietotemporal joint.

THE TEMPORAL BONE IN RELATION TO THE HEAD OF THE MANDIBLE AND SKULL GROWTH

The temporal bone and the mandibular condyle are seen together as an important growth centre for the development of the facial skeleton and the mandible. During normal oral function such as eating, talking, chewing, licking, lapping and sucking there is a constant articular contact of mandibular condyle and temporal bone which influences the shape and strength of the skull by remodelling and reabsorption of bone tissue (Akahane et al 2001). In Enlow's (1982) words: 'The growth of the mandible and its functional agents is a special product of all different regional functional agents of growth control acting on it to produce the topographical complex shape of the mandible and the face as a whole'. In other words, the mandible takes its form from the stress transducers in the cranium but the forces from the mandibular head on the temporal bone also influence the shape and form of the cranium. Schellhas et al undertook an interesting study in 1992 using radiography and tomography to investigate temporomandibular joint degeneration in 100 patients without previous mandibular fractures. Results revealed three factors:

- The chin deviated more often to the side where more degeneration was apparent.
- An unstable occlusion caused facial skeletal changes.
- The mandibular condyle and the temporal bone tended to be smaller on the degenerated side.

This is also confirmed by other research (Nerder et al 1999). Other abnormal forces on the temporal region are seen due to minor injuries to the facial–oral region. Many injuries might result in possible development of malfunctioning in remote areas of the cranium. These include injury that occurs during birth such as from forceps delivery or long drawn-out births, or in childhood sporting and car accidents, or even after oral and dental surgery (Frymann 1983, Biedermann 1995). This is why it is so important to be aware of any historical injuries that might relate to the onset of symptoms. This can be confirmed by checking to see if the patient has facial asymmetry with abnormal positioning and movement patterns of the head of the mandible in the glenoid fossa. In such cases there is usually subluxation with local pain. In addition, abnormal craniomandibular signs with aberrant signs on accessory movement of the temporal bone will often be found. In this case it is possible to change signs in the craniomandibular region after accessory movements to the temporal bone (Case study 1).

Case study 1

A 16-year-old female with deep earache and burning eye pain on the right side presented complaining about clicking in her left temporomandibular joint. She said she sometimes experienced local pain around her right auriculotemporal region. She had been treated by an orthodontist who prescribed splints which she said did not help her symptoms.

Manual examination consisted of slight transverse compression medially on the temporal bone as she opened her mouth. The deep earache changed, she had more range of movement on the right, and the temporomandibular joint clicking had gone. Treatment of the right temporal bone was an important factor in further treatment of her cranium, relieving her symptoms considerably (Fig. 14.18).

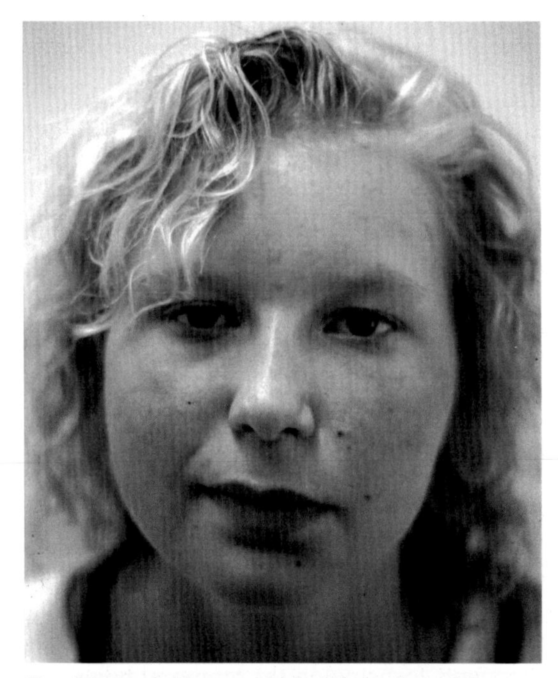

Fig. 14.18 A 16-year-old female patient with a craniomandibular dysfunction and asymmetric craniofacial growth.

Related structures and specific clinical patterns

We know from functional anatomy that the dural membrane and all the cranial nerves except for the olfactory (I), optic (II) and accessory (XI) nerves touch the temporal bone (Counter 1989, Lang 1995, Wilson-Pauwels et al 2002). The dural membrane also contains all the organs of balance including the three semicircular canals in each temporal bone (Patten 1995, Wilson-Pauwels et al 2002). Thus, malfunctioning of the temporal bone can result in changes in these tissues and might be expressed as symptoms in the absence of clear organic abnormalities. An example of this is seen in the literature where facial paralysis, hearing loss, vertigo, craniofacial pain and trismus after cranial trauma is often described (Avrahami 1994, Hickham & Cote 1995). Bower and Cotton (1995) reported that children with unexplained vertigo as well as middle ear pain and migraine symptoms often show abnormal pressure on the brain which appears related to the temporal bone in CT scans. Also relevant anatomically is the fact that the facial canal is a relatively long canal through which the facial nerve runs for several centimetres, giving it a predisposition to development of facial neuropathies (Lang 1995, Patten 1995).

In cases of diabetes, after radiotherapy in the region (Guida et al 1990) and where there are temporal haemangiomas (Eby et al 1992) the facial nerve is often involved and hemifacial spasm and facial paresis can follow. Minor changes in pathodynamics can be attributed to modest temporal dysfunction which can in turn provoke physical dysfunction of the facial nerve. Fundamental literature in this area appears to be sparse. We can conclude that symptoms such as oral and facial pain, craniomandibular dysfunction, non-infective earache, dizziness, vertigo, tinnitus and minor cranial nerve symptoms can be related to the functioning of the temporal bones. Significant changes in symptoms may be noticed after two to four treatments focusing on the temporal bones. If the symptoms remain the same or increase, wise action dictates that the patient be referred to a neurosurgeon or neurologist for further diagnosis.

Eagle's syndrome

Eagle's syndrome is a common name for a series of clinical symptoms arising from an elongated styloid process (Babler & Persing 1985, Jung et al 2001, Murtagh et al 2001). Frequent presentations occur after tonsillectomy, with nerve irritation (particularly the hypoglossal nerve) and where there is impingement on either external or internal arteries. Other symptoms will often appear, for example some throat, glossodynia and craniofacial pain (Chien et al 1991, Prasad et al 2002, Renzi et al 2005), temporal headache with pain in the craniomandibular region, ear soreness, voice changes, pain in the masseter muscle, restricted mandibular openings or lock jaw, sinusitis, tinnitus, excessive lacrimation and bloodshot eyes (Ozawa et al 1995, Wong et al 1995). There is a dearth of literature available about the percentage of relapse and patients who either fail to improve or experience persistent postoperative symptoms.

For minor presentations of Eagle's syndrome as might be seen in patients who experience some postsurgical pain, a 'hands-on' approach using passive movement of the temporal bone and hyoid could be combined with an assessment of neurodynamics of the hypoglossal nerve to relieve pain.

Zaki et al (1996) support conservative management of patients' symptoms where the styloid process is found to be elongated. A patient who experiences painful and limited jaw opening can become symptom-free. While this suggests that the styloid process is a painful dynamic structure it also indicates its ability to adapt to passive movements, potentially useful knowledge for us as therapists (Zaki et al 1996). For more information about the neurodynamics of the hypoglossal nerve, see Chapter 17 (Fig. 14.19).

Contraindications

The most common symptoms that present from dural defects in the temporal bone are

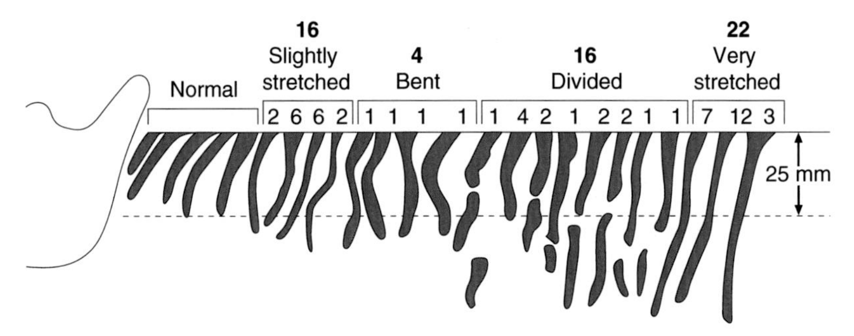

Fig. 14.19 Variation of the shape of the styloid process. A summary of 1771 panoramic radiographs revealing various degrees of elongation of the styloid process (after Corell & Wescott 1982). Depending on the shape and form, an abnormal interface of the glossopharyngeal nerve may develop, which can cause a (minimal) neuropathy.

unilateral ear 'fullness', pain in the temporal region and mild hearing loss which can be reproduced during manual examination. Some examples include:

- Ruptures of the arachnoid membrane or penetration of the brain due to a defect in the protective dura which manifests as cerebrospinal fluid leakage as in otorrhoea or otorhinorrhoea (Montgomery 1993).
- Tumours that mimic temporomandibular joint disorders and temporal pain or infratemporal space pathology.

Keith and Glyman (1991) assert that patients with these types of tumour are often treated for temporomandibular dysfunction and are subsequently diagnosed as suffering some kind of pathology of the infratemporal space. A patient who presents with these symptoms and fails to improve after treatment using passive movements should be referred for further diagnosis.

THE PETROSAL BONE

Another area which can be examined is the petrosal bone region. This chapter describes the petrosal region separately from the temporal bone region because of different patterns that are seen clinically. In the anatomical literature there is still debate as to whether or not the petrosal bone belongs to the temporal bone (Zielinski & Sloniewski 2001) (Fig. 14.20).

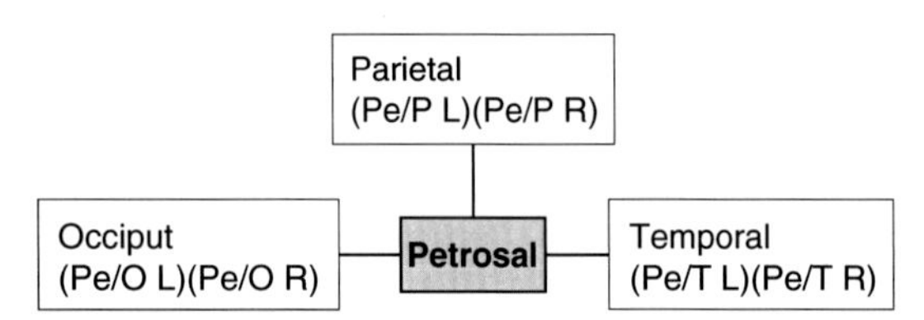

Fig. 14.20 Functional interactions of the petrosal region.

General qualities

The petrosal bone is connected to the temporal bone at the temporopetrosal sutures, to the parietal bone at the parietopetrosal sutures, the occipital bone at the occipitopetrosal sutures and with the sphenoid bone at the sphenopetrosal sutures. It differs from the temporal bone in the following ways (Fig. 14.21):

- It is part of the chondrocranium. Together with the occipital, sphenoid and ethmoid bones, the nasal bones and the pterygoid process the petrosal bone is developed from cartilage (Enlow 1982; see also Chapter 2).
- It may be responsible for signs and symptoms other than those arising from the temporal bone. As a therapist it helps to bear in mind that during movements other bones are also moving but to a lesser degree.

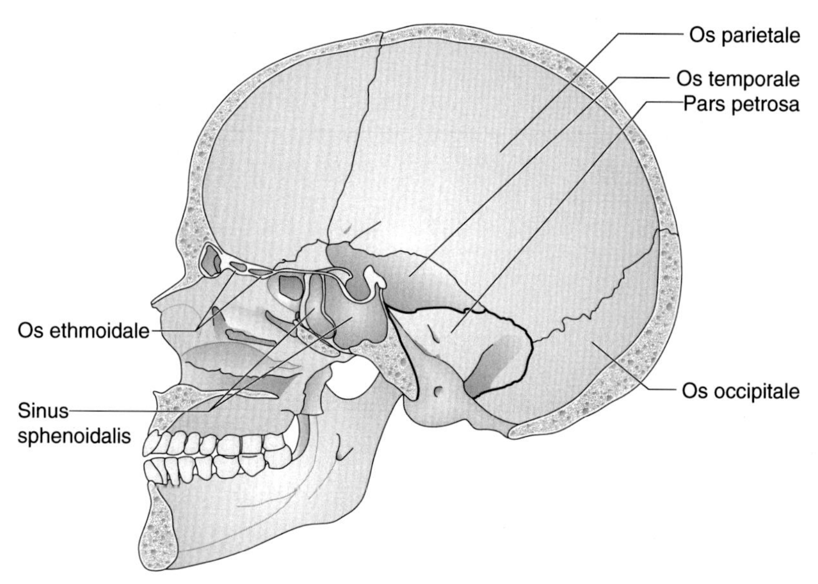

Fig. 14.21 The petrosal region in relation to other structures.

A general technique for movement of the petrosal region

The aim of the general technique is to gain information about the mobility, type and behaviour of symptoms provoked. This technique makes it possible to gain a quick impression of the relevance of the petrosal bone to the problem. If this is considered relevant, further examination will be needed.

Starting position and method

With the patient lying in a comfortable supine position, the therapist sits at the patient's head, resting both forearms on the plinth perpendicular to the lateral side of the mastoid process. The therapist takes the dorsal part of the mastoid process between the flexed index fingers with the thumb resting ventrally to the mastoid process.

In this position general movements (e.g. rotation, posterior–anterior and transverse movements) are possible and provide the required general information about the petrosal bone. Avoid pressing with tips of fingers and especially tips of thumbs, as this can cause a small irritation of branches of the vagus and facial nerves (Fig. 14.22).

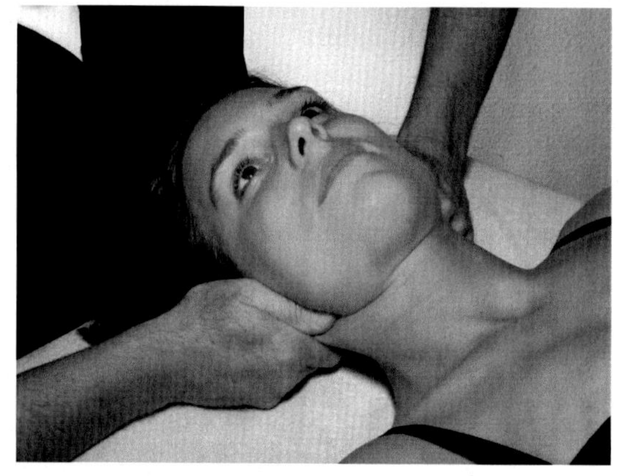

Fig. 14.22 General technique for influencing the left and right petrosal region.

Movement of the petrosal bone against neighbouring bones

Starting position and method

The patient lies comfortably in supine with the head rotated approximately 30° to the left. The therapist stands on the other side of the plinth with the left forearm parallel to the patient's body and perpendicular to the caudal side of the mastoid process of the petrosal bone. The right hand grasps that bone which is a part of the region to be examined. For example:

- The temporal bone (Pe/T): Hold the thumb of the right hand in front of the external acoustic meatus; the other fingers contact the rest of the temporal bone.
- The parietal bone (Pe/P): Hold the parietal bone slightly distal to the parietopetrosal joint with the right middle and ring fingers.
- The occipital bone (Pe/O): Cup the occipital bone with the right hand in pronation.
- The sphenoid bone (Pe/S): Take the lateral border of the greater wing of the sphenoid between the right index finger and thumb, as described as above.

The therapist holds the ventral side of the mastoid process with the flexed left index finger, on the dorsal side to maintain a comfortable grasp, keeping the left forearm perpendicular to the petrosal bone. The movement is produced by the thrust of the body. During examination and treatment the therapist should not increase the pressure between the index finger and thumb in order to keep the patient's head steady.

Any accessory movement is possible in this position. The lateral transverse movement is relatively difficult, and for the medial transverse movement the forearm must be positioned at a perpendicular angle to the lateral side of the right mastoid process. The thumb technique as described above for the parietal–parietal region can be used in the same way.

Movement of the neighbouring bones against the petrosal bone

To complete the examination it is sometimes necessary to move the region further once some dysfunctional aspect has been recognized. For the petrosal bone region the following combinations are possible:

- Temporopetrosal region (T/Pe) – this region is also discussed in the section on the temporal bone
- Parietopetrosal region (P/Pe)
- Occipitopetrosal region (O/Pe).

Starting position and method

With the patient lying supine with the head rotated about 30° to the left, the therapist stands on the left-hand side with the pelvis leaning against the plinth. The therapist holds the petrosal bone with the thumb and index finger of the left hand, keeping the left forearm perpendicular, and resting the right elbow on the right side of the plinth.

- For the right parietal bone, the whole surface of the parietal bone is taken in the right hand. From here it is possible to do longitudinal posterior movements and cranial rotations around the sagittal, frontal and longitudinal axes, as well as medial transverse movements.
- For movement of the temporal bone against the petrosal region, the right hand should be positioned as for moving the temporal bone. Thus, the right ring finger would move dorsal to the external auditory canal, the right middle finger would be in the external auditory canal and the right index finger would be on the zygomatic process of the temporal bone, as would the right thumb.
- For the occipital bone movement the right forearm is on the plinth perpendicular to the occipital bone and cups around the occipital bone. Transverse movements and rotations around all axes of the occipital bone are possible.

THE PETROSAL BONE AND PLAGIOCEPHALY

Symptoms may not be so clearly recognizable where patients with minor plagiocephaly have associated abnormal forces happening in the asterion region, causing a deeper and more complex bone matrix. The area of involvement includes, distally, mainly the lambdoid suture but also the parietopetrosal, occipitopetrosal and proximal squamosal sutures (Jimenez et al 1994). In a study of this phenomenon most patients showed that there was progressive involvement of the skull base, anterior shifts of the ear on the ipsilateral side and compensatory molar protrusion (Matson & Crigler 1969).

Petrosal bone movement is one of the most important areas to examine and treat in the skull for the above reasons (Enlow 1982, Oudhof 2001). Minor neurodynamic changes in the cranial nerves can be caused by petrosal bone movements, along with changes in neighbouring structures such as temporal bone blood vessel changes (Enlow 1982, Patten 1995). Cranial nerves that might be affected could include the facial nerve (VII), the vagus nerve (X), the accessory nerve (XI) and the hypoglossal nerve (XII) (Leonetti et al 1993). Special facial nerve neuropathies and palsies can be complications of petrosal traumas, especially fractures (Kawamoto & Ikeda 2002, Lee & Halcrow 2002). Symptoms such as local pain, dysphagia, voice changes, hearing loss, tinnitus, otorrhoea, trismus, and unilateral headaches might indicate the need for further examination of this region. As a therapist you need to be convinced that there is no serious pathology in the region before you treat it with these techniques. It is possible, for instance, that you may be looking at a case of parotid neoplasm, a tumour that produces similar signs and symptoms as individual cranial neuropathies (Hoyt 1989).

Finally, many structures have connections to the petrosal bone, such as petrosal nerves and the superior and anterior margins of the internal fissure of the auditory canal for the endolymph area (Khosla et al 1994, Zielinski & Sloniewski 2001, Schulknecht & Graetz 2005).

THE FRONTAL BONE

The frontal bone is one of the largest skull bones, the others being the parietal bones. It is connected to the maxilla, as well as the nasal, zygomatic, sphenoid and parietal bones. The general compression and distraction technique for the fronto-occipital region of the cranium is described earlier in this chapter.

Signs and symptoms in the frontal region can be examined at the following regions:

- Frontosphenoid region (F/S)
- Frontonasal region (F/N)
- Frontoparietal region (F/P)
- Frontomaxillary region (F/M)
- Frontozygomatic region (F/Z).

Techniques for the frontal bone against three neighbouring bones are discussed. The F/S, the F/N and the F/P will be covered in this section, while the other two, F/M and F/Z, are covered in Chapter 16.

Frontosphenoid region (F/S)

Starting position and method

The patient lies in a relaxed supine position with glasses etc. removed. The therapist sits behind the patient's head with the left hand cupped to envelop the surface of the frontal bone. To enable optimum emphasis on the frontosphenoid region, the therapist places the tip of the right thumb or middle finger on the greater wing of the sphenoid. It is important to avoid squeezing when holding the frontal bone in the left hand, and to flex the left elbow and fix it against the trunk.

The therapist moves the whole body slightly towards the side to be examined without changing the position of the elbow. This position is particularly advantageous for sustained techniques and allows any accessory movements required (Fig. 14.23).

Frontonasal region (F/N)

The frontonasal region is a functional connection of the calvarium to the facial skeleton. Although it does not directly belong to the orbit, the frontonasal region plays an important embryological part in the history of the facial bones of the orbital region (Hoyt 1989). Treatment of this region often has the effect of reducing orbital pain and hence plays a pivotal

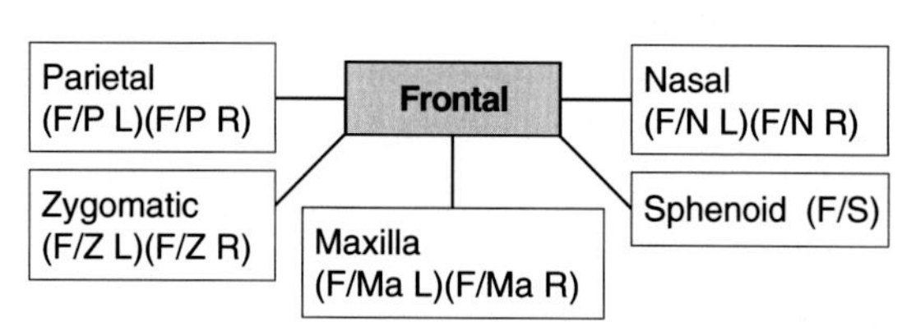

Fig. 14.23 Functional interactions of the sphenoid region.

role in the treatment of the orbital and sinus regions.

The patient can use this technique advantageously at home as a reassessment tool together with automobilization techniques.

Starting position and method

The patient lies comfortably in supine. The therapist sits to the patient's right with the underarm parallel to the patient's sternum. The therapist controls the frontal bone with the left hand so that the index finger and thumb hold the frontonasal region. The right index finger and thumb are able to move the nasal bone in different accessory positions from this point (Fig. 14.24).

Movements such as longitudinal caudal and cranial rotation around the sagittal, longitudinal and transverse axes to perform distraction and compression techniques and transverse lateral movements are all possible from this position. The pressure needs to build up slowly without causing any local pain of the contact points. The patient's head should be held steady with the left hand.

ANATOMICAL PROBLEMS OF THE FRONTONASAL REGION

Movement of the frontonasal region may produce general local pain. This will often be the case where there is minor erosion of the skull base caused by nasopharyngeal carcinoma and chronic sinusitis (Cheung et al 1994, Enepekides & Donald 2005). This type of pathological change may also indicate involvement of cranial nerves III and VI (Sham et al 1991). If the clinical features do not fit and as a therapist you are not convinced about the cause of the problem, the patient should be referred to a specialist for further diagnosis. CT scanning and x-ray are better suited for providing a more complete diagnosis.

Patients with a minor frontonasal dysplasia or a palate disorder are not usually seen by a neuro-ophthalmologist because of the relative moderate severity of their symptoms which might include sinusitis, ocular defects or other dysfunctional symptoms such as strabismus and diplopia. However, these patients should first be assessed by a neuro-ophthalmologist (Roarty et al 1994, Marcharc et al 2002). Hypertelorism (an abnormal distance between two paired organs) with a minor midline facial defect such as is seen in broad nasal root and nasal bifidity can lead to nasal airflow changes and oral dysfunction because of the abnormal craniofacial morphology. Affected individuals often complain of typical craniofacial pain, sinusitis and tiredness (Okeson 1996, 2005). Experience shows that passive movements can contribute to change in airflow and possibly to related symptoms in the head and neck region with this patient group.

Signs of rapid growth of the temporonasal and nasal regions can provide helpful clues during assessment and reassessment. These may take the form of enlargement of the frontal sinus or the patient may just have a subjective feeling of stenosis. Normal airflow should make a full low sound while sharp, high breathing suggests a stenosis (Björk 1955).

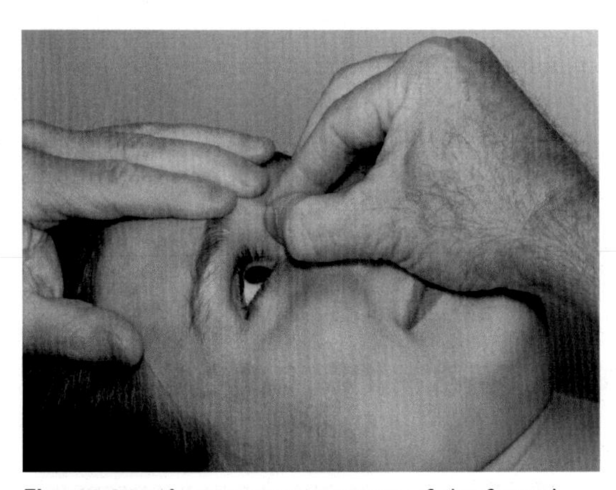

Fig. 14.24 Accessory movements of the frontal bone. The nasal region is fixed by the index finger and thumb.

Frontoparietal (coronal) region (F/P)

The coronal suture is a large suture in the frontoparietal region created by the parietal bones and the frontal bone. This suture is the main focus for techniques in this area. The general techniques will be covered first, followed by some local thumb techniques.

Starting position and method

The patient lies in a comfortable supine position with the head rotated about 30° to the left. For the convenience of the patient and the therapist, the patient can support the head by putting the left hand under the head. The therapist sits on the side to be examined with the plinth adjusted to the optimum height.

With the left hand in pronation, the therapist cups the whole parietal bone from the lateral side. The left little finger and hypothenar eminence should be parallel to the coronal suture. The therapist grasps the frontal bone with the right hand from the lateral side. As can be seen from Figure 14.25, the right thumb is parallel to the coronal suture without touching the fingers of the other hand.

Any accessory movement for the parietal bone can be made from this point with a movement from the body. The thrust of the trunk is transmitted through the arms and hands so that the left hand does not move at all.

LONGITUDINAL THUMB TECHNIQUE MOVING IN A DOWNWARD DIRECTION

Thumb techniques such as this, and the one described for the temporoparietal region, are particularly useful for longitudinal movements downwards, anterior–posterior and posterior–anterior movements and transverse movements medial to the frontal bone. These techniques can be used to treat persistent local symptoms, for example contusion patients who continue to suffer from headaches in this area and whose symptoms may be due to craniosynostosis of the coronal suture or scar tissue following trauma or surgery.

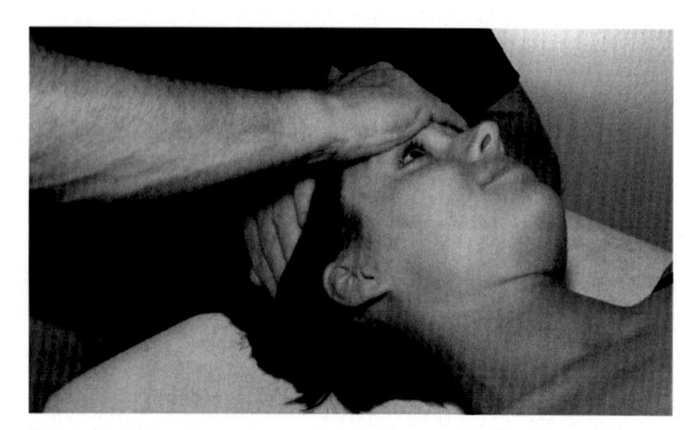

Fig. 14.25 Accessory movement of the frontal bone with the parietal region fixed.

Starting position and method

With the patient lying in a comfortable supine position, the therapist sits at the patient's head and holds the frontal bone with two-thirds of the volar side of the left hand, resting the left thumb pad on the frontal bone adjacent to the coronal suture. The fingers of the right hand and the right thumb contact the right parietal bone near the coronal suture.

During the manoeuvre the cranium is held with the last four fingers of the right hand and a slight counter-pressure is added in the cephalic region as both thumbs perform the longitudinal movement. Finger movement should be avoided and the patient advised to indicate if the pressure feels uncomfortable or increases too quickly.

ANTERIOR–POSTERIOR AND POSTERIOR–ANTERIOR THUMB TECHNIQUES

These are relative compression and distraction techniques for the coronal suture. The advantage of these techniques is that the therapist can emphasize pressure on the parietal or the frontal bone, or on both, using the same starting position.

Starting position and method

The patient lies in a comfortable supine position with the head rotated about 40° to the left and a rolled-up towel supporting the head. Sitting at the end of the plinth, the therapist places the left thumb on the parietal bone and the right thumb on the frontal bone in a cross-grip, perpendicular to the coronal suture. The interphalangeal joints are slightly flexed and the other fingers are spread over the top of the calvarium to keep the thumbs stable.

Only the thumbs are active during the movement, the fingers simply hold the patient's head steady. By flexing and extending the interphalangeal joints of both thumbs, anterior–posterior and posterior–anterior movements can be performed, as long as the thumbs do not lose contact with the parietal bone. Movement can also proceed with both thumbs on the frontal or parietal bones to provide further information.

ASSESSMENT OF THE FRONTAL REGION

It is often noticed that assessment of the frontal region is the most relevant for patients who present with the following:

- A relatively wide cranium which is anteriorly proportionately shorter than posteriorly.
- A growth dysfunction, particularly seen in children who have a relatively flat occiput and prominent frontal bone in the sagittal plane (Marchac et al 2002).
- In cases of diffuse frontal head symptoms, local pain in the nasal region, pseudo-sinusitis and autonomic reactions in the face such as sweating, blushing or a feeling of eye pressure (Fig. 14.26).

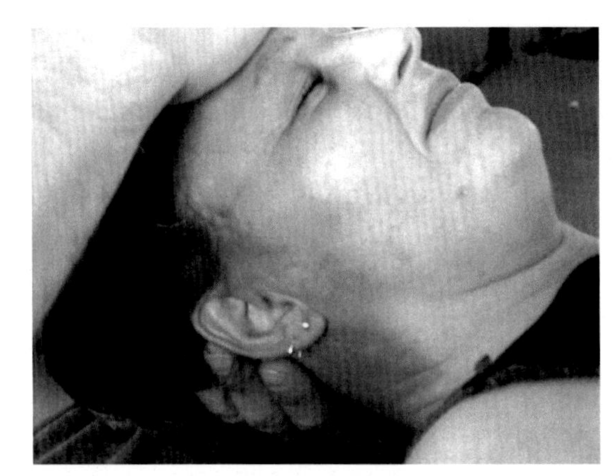

Fig. 14.26 A 36-year-old patient after a mandibular fracture with localized reddening and sweating in the right craniocervical and craniomandibular regions. The symptoms appeared several minutes after the use of general frontoparietal techniques.

THE PARIETAL REGION

Together the parietal bones form the largest expanse of the neurocranium and are connected to the temporal, frontal, occipital and sphenoid bones. As the only structure in the calvarium they are coupled bones which form a joint, the parietal–parietal or P/P region. In anatomy textbooks this connection is known as the 'sagittal suture' and has the ability to adapt to pressure changes into old age (Fehlow et al 1992, Oudhof 2001).

The regions and their neighbouring bones are:

- Parietoparietal region (P/P)
- Parietotemporal region (P/T)
- Parietofrontal region (P/F)
- Parieto-occipital region (P/O)
- Parietosphenoid region (P/S).

We will now discuss the parietoparietal region, focusing on its unique construction and clinical value, and cross-referencing the connections to neighbouring bones (Fig. 14.27).

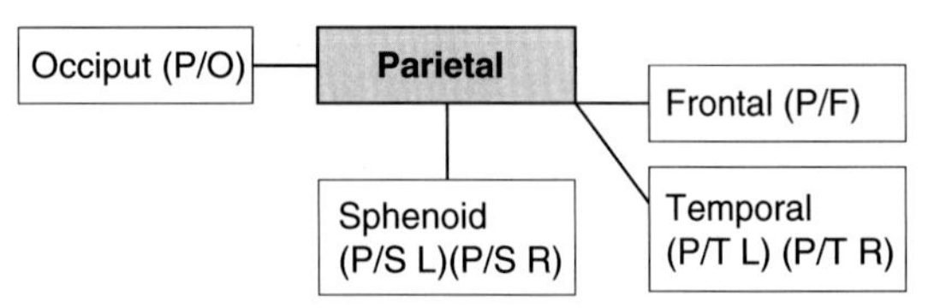

Fig. 14.27 Functional interactions of the temporal region.

Parietoparietal region (P/P)

Because this joint has a particularly long suture, averaging 12–15 cm in adults, many techniques are possible. There are general techniques which influence the whole joint as well as localized thumb techniques, emphasizing one part of the joint as appropriate.

A GENERAL LONGITUDINAL TECHNIQUE TOWARDS CAUDAL

Starting position and method

With the patient lying in a comfortable supine position, the therapist sits at the end of the plinth with the elbows flexed at a 90° angle and the forearms level with the patient's head. The therapist rests the medial side of the right elbow against the trunk and orientates by palpating the sagittal suture. The therapist then grasps the left parietal bone with the whole hand and supinates the left forearm so that the thumb points to the front. The same procedure applies to the right-hand side. The radial sides of both thumbs and thenar eminences should be touching each other and, at that precise point, lying over the sagittal suture.

The torso should be rotated slightly to the left so that the therapist can move backwards and forwards with the right parietal bone. Without moving the hands at all it is possible to move the trunk to transmit the movement through the right hand and arm. Only a slight movement is needed, since the range of movement is small and a larger thrust will produce cervical torsion (Fig. 14.28).

A VARIATION USING LOCALIZED LONGITUDINAL CAUDAL THUMB MOVEMENT

Starting position and method

The patient lies supine on the plinth. Using both hands, the therapist grasps both parietal bones as described in the last technique and spreads the fingers of both hands around the lateral sides of the parietal bones. The left and right thumbs should be touching each other close to the sagittal suture, the left thumb on the left parietal bone and the right thumb on the right parietal bone.

The procedure is the same as for the more general technique (see above) only now the therapist moves by slowly flexing the torso. Excessive local pressure can be avoided by slightly flexing the interphalangeal joints in the thumbs. The advantage of this thumb technique is that it makes it possible to feel along the sagittal suture to localize the abnormal sites in this region and reproduce symptoms.

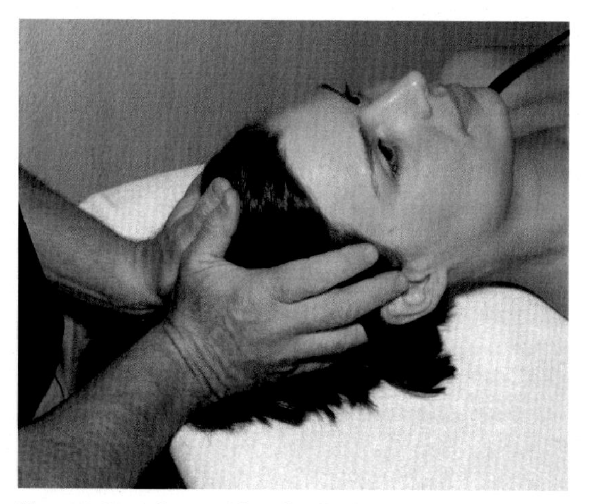

Fig. 14.28 General longitudinal movement of the right parietal region with a small body movement to the left.

ROTATION OF THE RIGHT PARIETAL REGION AROUND THE TRANSVERSE AXIS

This technique may be applied for a number of reasons:

- It is easily performed
- There is a large surface area to work with
- Patients often say that it relaxes them.

Starting position and method

With the patient lying comfortably supine on the plinth, the therapist takes the parietal bones in both hands so that the fingers are spread over the lateral sides of both bones as in the longitudinal thumb movement described above. The thumbs should be next to the sagittal suture.

The rotation is initiated by slightly moving the trunk towards the patient's head, ensuring that the pressure at the points of contact remains constant. Anchoring the elbow against the trunk will help to avoid extraneous forearm movement. If an anterior rotation is to be performed it is easiest to pronate the right hand, hold it against the lower end of the parietal bone, just above the temporoparietal suture. The fingers of the right hand should be pointed in the direction of the trunk and covering the whole right parietal bone.

Follow these principles for movement and rotation around the sagittal and longitudinal axes.

A LOCALIZED COMPRESSION AND DISTRACTION TECHNIQUE FOR THE PARIETOPARIETAL REGION

This technique can be used where the patient has localized symptoms such as regional headaches or local stiffness after a skull operation.

Starting position and method

With the patient lying comfortably supine on the plinth, and sitting behind the patient, the therapist takes the parietal bones in both hands with the fingers spread, crossing the thumbs and placing them perpendicular to the part of the sagittal suture region that is to be examined.

The therapist squeezes the sagittal suture region with the thumbs, activating the interphalangeal joints of both thumbs and ensuring that the pressure is evenly distributed and remains constant.

This technique is also used for distraction in the parietoparietal region when the opposite of compression is desired.

A GENERAL POSTERIOR–ANTERIOR TECHNIQUE FOR THE PARIETOPARIETAL REGION

When symptoms are localized more in the dorsal region of the head or when pressure on the cranium in daily life such as lying supine provokes symptoms, the movement/stress on the cranium needs to be in a posterior–anterior direction.

Starting position and method

The patient lies comfortable and supine towards the right-hand side of the plinth with the head rotated approximately 60° to the left. The therapist supports the left side of the patient's head with the left hand, elbows pointing behind. Pronating the right forearm, the therapist holds the patient's right parietal bone in the right hand.

The trunk is rotated to the left to initiate the technique; however, if the patient complains of neck pain due to excessive rotation in the cervical spine, the rotation is slackened to take it out of pain. The right forearm should be kept perpendicular to the dorsal side of the patient's head. This is possible because the patient is placed on the right side of the plinth, providing sufficient room to move.

If the patient complains of local dorsal head symptoms, or there are indications of dorsal trauma or (sub)occipital surgery, a local posterior–anterior technique can be useful either as an examination or a treatment technique.

A LOCALIZED POSTERIOR–ANTERIOR TECHNIQUE

Starting position and method

The patient should be lying in a comfortable supine position for this technique. Sitting at the patient's head, the therapist holds both sides of the parietal bone in the spread fingers of both hands, crossing the thumbs and holding them perpendicular to the part of the sagittal suture to be examined (lambda region). The thumbs are moved without increasing the pressure of the fingers or moving the patient's head.

GROWTH PATTERNS OF THE PARIETAL REGION

The lambdoid suture is a paired structure that connects the sagittal suture superiorly to the parietomastoid and occipitomastoid sutures along the cranial base. This suture facilitates posterior skull growth via the growth of the occipital bone. In particular the posterior part of the parietal bone, and hence the other skull bones, receive a growth impulse (Enlow 1982, Oudhof 2001, Aalami et al 2005).

Abnormality or synostosis of the lambdoid suture results in localized flattening of the dorsal side of the skull due to abnormal cranial forces (van der Kolk & Carson 1994). Lambdoid synostosis was rare until recently when minor occipital and parietal deformities have become more common, perhaps influenced by dysfunction in early development. In most cases surgery is indicated (Albright et al 1999, Christophis et al 2001, Anderson & David 2005).

A patient presenting with flattening to one side of the head and abnormal signs on examination, particularly any suggestion of physical dysfunction of the parietal bone region, would be a candidate for treatment in this area (Case study 2). Premature closure of the suture

Case study 2

An 8-year-old boy has been complaining of headaches and difficulty concentrating at school for 2 years. The school doctor and the child physiotherapist reported that his height and motor development were significantly retarded. The neurologist could not find a real pathology and diagnosed the boy as having 'migraine'. When he was 6 years old he received medication (sumatriptan) which reduced his headache some of the time, but not always. In the last year the headache was progressive (more easily exacerbated with more background headache often present) and motor development was static. During manual physical examination of the craniocervical and craniofacial region a minor scaphocephaly with facial asymmetry (right facial region smaller than left, see Fig. 14.29a–c) was noted, and the sagittal suture was hard, stiff and painful during palpation. A right C0–C2 craniocervical dysfunction, which was painful during examination, was noted. Furthermore, possibly relevant functional impairments were also noted.

Mainly craniofacial hands-on therapy, especially of the parietal bones and their connections, and mobilization of the cervical dysfunction once a week for the first month and once every 2 weeks for the next 2 months, together with continuing sensomotor training by the child physiotherapist, eliminated the headache and increased concentration. The child's mother says that he plays more outside with his friends and laughs more than before. He no longer needs medication.

During inspection after 3 months it was clear to see that the craniofacial asymmetry and the cervical dysfunction were reduced and the general tone of his muscles was also reduced (Fig. 14.29d–f). Retrospectively it is fair to conclude that the craniofacial and craniocervical dysfunction was relevant for his problem and that treatment by passive movements in this area clearly changed his signs and symptoms.

between the parietal bones or the sagittal suture restricts mediolateral growth of the cranial vault which then presents longer and more ovoid in shape than normal (Kohn et al 1994). Known as scaphocephaly, this is the most common form of craniosynostosis, seen more often in men than in women (Cohen 1986). Although abnormal stress on the bones influences facial morphology (Kreiborg & Pruzansky 1981), the literature is less clear about how it affects development at the skull base (Babler & Persing 1985, Babler 1989). A patient may show signs and symptoms originating in the parietal region as well as in the facial and cranial bones. In this case it is wise to examine these regions also. It should be noted that intelligence deficiencies are not always present (Hwang et al 2002).

Neurological complications and craniosynostosis

With craniosynostosis, neurological differences may present loud and clear, or they may be much less obvious in their presentation.

Clear complications of premature craniosynostosis might be:

- Neuraesthenic disorders, especially headaches and vertigo
- Slight mental retardation
- Schizophrenic and depressive psychoses
- Early changes in cerebrovascular diseases
- Disorders of the cranial nerves
- Epileptic seizures (Magge et al 2002).

The sagittal and coronal sutures have been particularly well investigated (Schmid 1969, Fehlow et al 1992). Both reported that impairment of the frontal lobe, possibly caused by some of the symptoms listed above, resulted in shortening of the anterior cranial fossa and thus led to craniosynostosis.

Pertschuk and Whitaker (1985) studied 43 children between the ages of 6 and 13 years with various craniofacial anomalies caused by craniosynostosis compared with a control group. As might be expected, the symptomatic

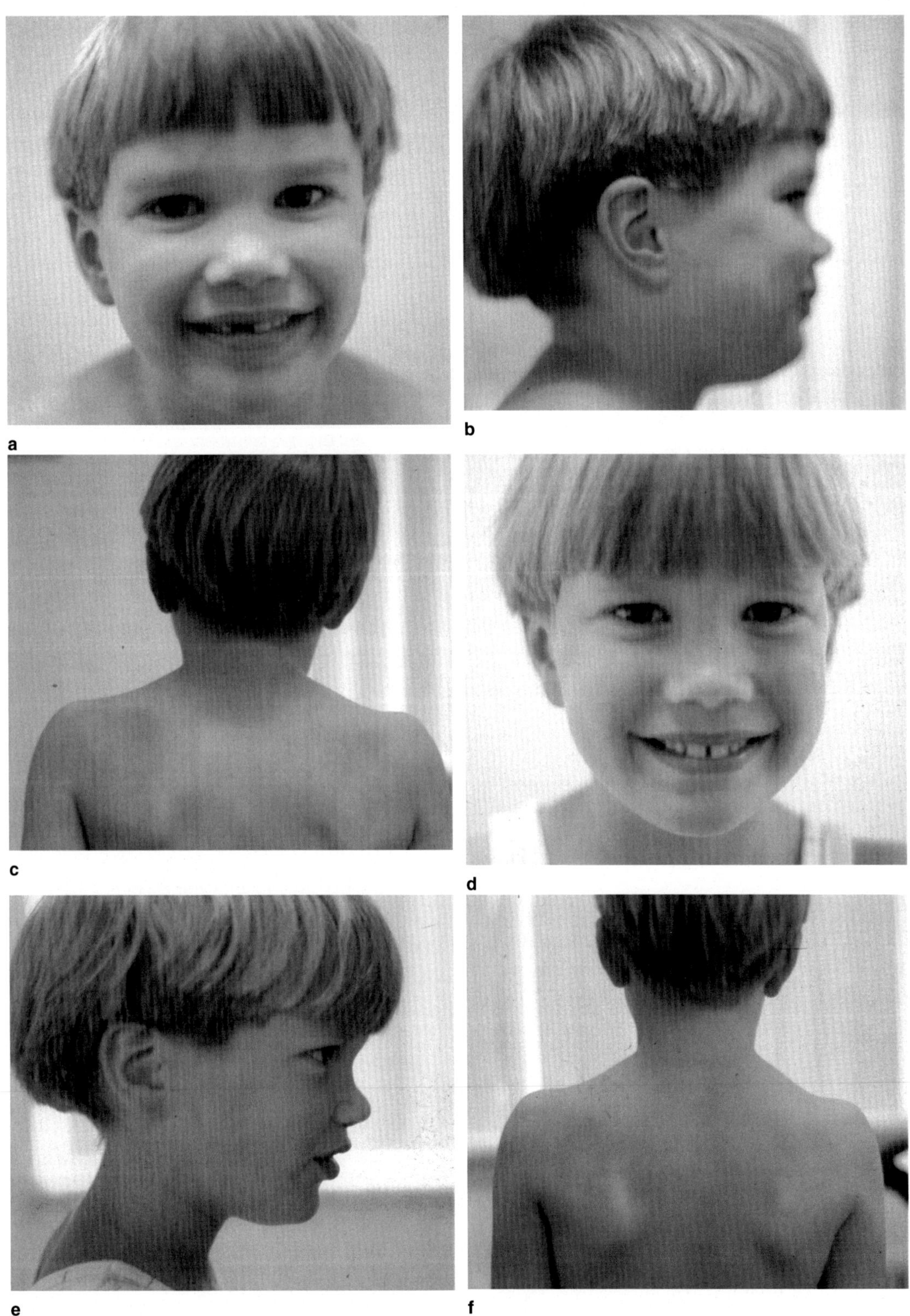

Fig. 14.29
a 8-year-old boy with headache and concentration disturbances.
b Slight sagittal synostosis with facial asymmetry.
d–f Craniofacial asymmetry, cervical dysfunction and general tone of the neck musculature reduced on treatment.

children tended to have poorer self-image, greater anxiety during examination and were more generally introverted. Their parents reported that the children had more frequent negative social encounters and displayed more hyperactive behaviour at home. Teachers also reported more disruptive classroom behaviour. In Italy, Giuffre et al (1978) also found behaviour disorders among children with craniosynostosis. Barrit et al (1981) found that teasing at school often led to a refusal to attend school in South Australian children with scaphocephaly. Hence it is important for therapists to be aware of the physical, mental and social implications both during and after treatment for these problems. The assessment of mental dysfunction can be very helpful. Such tests might include learning, behaviour and concentration indices alongside craniofacial tests (Virtanen et al 1999, Speltz et al 2004).

When it is possible to ameliorate symptoms in the craniocervical region with parieto-occipital techniques, passive movements with a large amplitude (grades II and III) often prove to be more successful than sustained pressure. Sustained pressure can sometimes provoke a latent reaction such as neck stiffness or dorsal headache, even if the patient has not complained of pain at the time of treatment.

The lambda region and fusion

The lambda region is enormously flexible even into middle age, and appears to ossify in different ways (Matsumara et al 1993). At around 40–45 years of age it starts to fuse with neighbouring bones, leaving irregular sutures between them. This might explain why large passive movements may work better than pressure techniques in patients under 50. In the author's experience general techniques on the parietal region are most useful in treatment for sympathetic dominant symptoms such as dull, deep, undefined dizziness, cap headache, vertigo and/or bilateral arm symptoms. This is particularly prevalent with bilateral techniques performed over a longer duration (minutes) and using minimal pressure.

SUMMARY

- In this chapter the main accessory movements in the region of the neurocranium are discussed. The word 'regions' and not 'sutures' or 'joints' is used deliberately because it is believed that during application of passive movements in the craniofacial region, more than just sutures or joints are influenced. Literature and research data support this premise.
- With this starting point of multistructural influences related to the different shifts in pain mechanisms it is realistic to assert what exactly happens during the application of different techniques on the neurocranium. Therefore at the end of each technique section main contraindications and different clinical patterns based on clinical experience and literature are discussed.
- This chapter should give the reader the impression that these (in the author's opinion oft neglected) categories of patients also have a good chance of being influenced by the use of these techniques.
- Clinical patterns and positive changes during and after the treatment have to be observed. If not, the therapist has to stop and refer the patient to another specialist for further diagnosis.
- Good evidence-based knowledge in manual therapy in the craniofacial region is still lacking. Standardization of tests and techniques, which we try to start with in this chapter, as well as the gathering of clinical data, open doors for further basic research.

References

Aalami O O, Nacamuli R P, Salim A et al 2005 Differential transcriptional expression profiles of juvenile and adult calvarial bone. Plastic and Reconstructive Surgery 115(7):1986–1994

Aebi A, Nazarian S 1987 Klassifikation der Halswirbelsäulenverletzungen. Orthopäde 16:27

Akahane Y, Deguchi T, Hunt N 2001 Morphology of the temporomandibular joint in skeletal class III symmetrical and asymmetrical cases: a study by cephalometric laminography. Journal of Orthodontics 28:119

Albright A, Pollack I, Adelson P, Solot J 1999 Outcome data and analysis in pediatric neurosurgery. Neurosurgery 45:101

Alker G, Oh Y, Leslie E 1978 High cervical spine and craniocervical junction injuries in fatal traffic accidents. Orthopedic Clinics of North America 9(4):1003

Anderson P J, David D J 2005 Late results after unicoronal craniosynostosis correction. Journal of Craniofacial Surgery 16(1):37–44

Andry N 1741 In: Wessinghage D (ed.) L'Orthopédie ou l'art de prévenir et de corriger dans les enfants les difformités du corps. Schattauer, Stuttgart

Avis V 1959 The relation of the temporal muscle to the form of the coronoid process. American Journal of Physical Anthropology 17:99

Avrahami E 1994 CT of intact but nonfunctioning temporomandibular joints following temporal bone fracture. Neuroradiology 36:142

Babler W 1989 Relationship of altered cranial suture growth to the cranial bone and midface. In: Persing J, Edgerton M, Jane J (eds) Scientific foundations and surgical treatment of craniosynostosis. Williams & Wilkins, New York, p 87

Babler W, Persing J 1985 Alterations in cranial suture growth associated with premature closure of the sagittal suture in rabbits. Anatomical Record 211:14A

Barrit J, Brooksbank M, Sipson D 1981 Scaphocephaly: aesthetic and psychosocial consideration. Developmental Medicine and Child Neurology 23:183

Besson A, Pellerin P, Doual A 2000 Study of asymmetries of the cranial vault in plagiocephaly. Journal of Craniofacial Surgery 13:664

Biedermann H 1995 Manual therapy in newborn and infants. Journal of Orthopedic Medicine 17:2

Biedermann H 1996 KISS-Kinder. Ursachen, (Spät-)Folgen und manualtherapeutische Behandlung frühkindlicher Asymmetrie. Ferdinand Enke, Stuttgart

Biedermann H 2001 Primäre und sekundäre Schädelasymmetrie bei KISS-Kindern. In: von Piekartz H J M (ed.) Kraniofaziale Dysfunktionen und Schmerzen. Untersuchung, Beurteilung und Management. Thieme, Stuttgart, p 45

Biedermann H 2004 Manual therapy in children. Churchill Livingstone, Edinburgh

Björk A 1955 Cranial base development. American Journal of Orthodontics 41:198

Boere-Boonekamp M M, van der Linden-Kuiper L T 2001 Positional preference: prevalence in infants and follow-up after two years. Pediatrics 107:339

Bower C M, Cotton R T 1995 The spectrum of vertigo in children. Archives of Otolaryngology, Head and Neck Surgery 121:911–915

Boyling J, Palastanga N, Jull G, Lee D, Grieve G 1994 Grieve's modern manual therapy. Churchill Livingstone, Edinburgh

Bracard A, Sakka R, Roland J 1987 Effects des contrainets intracraniennes sur le developpement des sinus frontaux. Bulletin de l'Association des Anatomistes 71:31

Brown W, Molleson T, Chin T 1984 Enlargement of the frontal sinus. Annals of Human Biology 11:221

Buchmann J, Bülow B, Pohlmann B 1992 Asymmetrien in der Kopfgelenkbeweglichkeit von Kindern. Manuelle Medizin 30:93

Buchmann J, Bülow B 1989 Asymmetrische frühkindliche Kopfgelenkbeweglichkeit. Bedingungen und Folgen. Manuelle Medizin 30:126-129

Butler D 2000 The sensitive nervous system. Noigroup Publications, Adelaide

Cano A, Fons F, Brines J 2001 The effects on offspring of premature parturition. Human Reproduction Update 7:487

Capobianco D, Brazis P, Rubino F, Dalton J 2002 Occipital condyle syndrome. Headache 42:142

Cheung Y K, Sham J, Cheung Y L, Chan F L 1994 Evaluation of skull base erosion in nasopharyngeal carcinoma: comparison of plain radiography and computed tomography. Oncology 51(1):42–46

Chien C, Kuo W, Juan K 1991 Elongated styloid process syndrome. Kao Hsiung I Hsueh Ko Hsueh Tsa Chih 7:663

Christensen L 1967 Facial pain from the masticatory system induced by experimental bruxism. A preliminary report. Tandae gebladet 74:175

Christophis P, Junger T, Howaldt H 2001 Surgical correction of scaphocephaly: experiences with a new procedure and follow-up investigations. Journal of Craniomaxillofacial Surgery 29:33

Chu C, Lin M, Huang H, Lee M 1994 Finite element analysis of cerebral contusion. Journal of Biomechanics 27:187

Cohen M 1986 Perspectives on craniosynostosis. In: Craniosynostosis: diagnosis, evaluation

and management. Raven Press, Stratford-on-Avon, p 21
Cordasco G, Cicciu D, Lo Giudice G, Matarese G, Nucera R, Mazza M 1999 Kinesiographic investigations in children with increased nasal airways resistance. Bulletin du Groupement International pour La Recherche Scientifique en Stomatologie et Odontologie 41:67
Correll R, Wescott W 1982 Eagle's syndrome diagnosed after history of headache, dysphasia, otalgia and limited neck movement. Journal of the American Dental Association 104:491
Cottam C 1984 Cranial manipulations roots references. Coraco, Los Angeles
Counter R 1989 A colour atlas of temporal bone surgical anatomy. Wolfe Medical Publications, New York
de Jonge G 1992 Zijligging als slaaphouding voor zuigelingen ontraden. Tijdschrift voor Jeugdgezondheidszorg 24:72
de Jonge G, Engelberts A 1987 Naar preventie van Wiegedood. Tijdschrift voor Jeugdgezondheidszorg 19:91
Dunn P 1974 Congenital sternomastoid torticollis: an intrauterine deformity. Archives of Disease in Childhood 49:825
Eby T, Fisch U, Makek M 1992 Facial nerve management in temporal bone hemangiomas. American Journal of Otology 13:223
Enepekides D, Donald P 2005 Frontal sinus trauma. In: Stewart M (ed.) Head, face and neck trauma: comprehensive management. Thieme, New York, p 26–39
Enlow D 1982 Handbook of facial growth. W B Saunders, Los Angeles
Fehlow P, Fröhlich W, Misge W et al 1992 Neuropsychiatrische Begleitsymptome bei Saethe-Chatzen-Syndrom. Fortschrift fur Neurology und Psychiatry 60:66
Flehming I 1979 Normale Entwicklung des Säuglings und ihre Abweichungen. Thieme, Stuttgart
Frymann V 1983 Cranial osteopathy and its role in disorders of the temporomandibular joint. Dental Clinics of North America 27:595
Gifford L 1998 Whiplash: science and management. Fear-avoidance beliefs and behaviour. Topical Issues of Pain, NOI Press, Adelaide
Giuffre R, Vagnozzi R, Savino S 1978 Infantile craniosynostosis. Acta Neurochirurgica 44:40
Gonzalez de Dios J, Moya M, Jimenez L, Alcala-Santaella R, Carratala F 1998 Increase in the incidence of occipital plagiocephaly. Revista de Neurologia 27:782
Good C, Walker G 1984 The hip in the moulded baby syndrome. Journal of Bone and Joint Surgery 66B:491
Grieve G 1995 'Quote'. Lausanne: On a lecture at the IFOMT Manual Therapy Congress
Grob D, Magerl F 1987 Stabilisierung bei Frakturen von C1 und C2. Orthopäde 16:46
Guida R, Finn D, Buchalter I et al 1990 Radiation injury to the temporal bone. American Journal of Otology 11:6
Hamanishi C, Tanaka S 1994 Turned head – adducted hip – truncal curvature syndrome. Archives of Disease in Childhood 70(6):515
Hansen M, Mulliken J 1994 Frontal plagiocephaly. Clinics in Plastic Surgery 21(4):543–553
Hanson J, Deliganis A, Baxter A et al 2002 Radiologic and clinical spectrum of occipital condyle fractures: retrospective review of 107 consecutive fractures in 95 patients. AJR American Journal of Roentgenology 178:1261
Henche H, Lücking C, Schumacher M 1994 Atlasfrakturen mit Parese kaudaler Hirnnerven. Eine Fallbeschreibung. Zeitschrift für Orthopädie und ihre Grenzgebiete 132:394
Hickham M, Cote D 1995 Temporal bone fractures. Journal of the Louisiana State Medical Society 147:527
Hoyt D 1989 The role of the cranial base in normal and abnormal skull development. In: Persing J, Edgerton M, Jane J (eds) Scientific foundations and surgical treatment of craniosynostosis. Lippincott, Williams and Wilkins, Philadelphia, p 58
Huggare J 1987 A roentgenocephalometric study of head posture and craniofacial morphogenesis in the cold environment of northern Finland. Thesis. Oulu. Proceedings of the Finnish Dental Society, p 83
Hwang K, Lee D, Lee S, Lee H 2002 Roberts syndrome, normal cell division, and normal intelligence. Craniofacial Surgery 13:390
Jimenez D, Barone C, Argamaso R et al 1994 Asterion region synostosis. Cleft Palate-Craniofacial Journal 31:136–141
Jones H, Jones M, Maitland G 1994 Examination and treatment by passive movements. In: Grant R (ed.) Physical therapy of the cervical and thoracic spine. Churchill Livingstone, New York
Jung T, Tschernitschek H, Bremer B, Borchers L 2001 Styloid process: radiograph and craniomandibular dysfunction (CMD). Schweizer Monatsschrift für Zahnmedizin 111:701
Kaushik V, Kelly G, Richards S, Saeed S 2002 Isolated unilateral hypoglossal nerve palsy after minor head trauma. Clinics in Neurology and Neurosurgery 105:42
Kawamoto H, Ikeda M 2002 Evaluation of greater petrosal nerve function in patients with acute peripheral facial paralysis: comparison of soft palate electrogustometry and Schirmer's tear test. Acta Otolaryngology Suppl 546:110
Keith D, Glyman M 1991 Infratemporal space pathosis mimicking TMJ disorders. Journal of

the American Dental Association 122: 59–61
Khosla V, Hakuba A, Takagi H 1994 Measurements of the skull base for transpetrosal surgery. Surgical Neurology 41:502
Kohn L, Vannier M, Marsh J, Cheverud J 1994 Effect of premature sagittal suture closure on craniofacial morphology in a prehistoric male Hopi. Cleft Palate-Craniofacial Journal 31:385
Kreiborg S, Pruzansky S 1981 Craniofacial growth in premature craniofacial synostosis. Scandinavian Journal of Plastic and Reconstructive Surgery 15(3):171–186
Krous H, Nadeau J, Silva P, Blackbourne B 2001 Neck extension and rotation in sudden infant death syndrome and other natural infant deaths. Pediatric and Developmental Pathology 4:154
Kylämarkula S 1988 Growth changes in the skull and upper cervical skeleton after partial detachment of neck muscles. An experimental study in the rat. Journal of Anatomy 159:197
Lang J 1995 Skull base and related structures, brain and cranial nerves. Schattauer, Stuttgart, p 72
Largo R 1986 Frühkindliche Zerebralparese: epidemiologische und klinische Aspekte. Deutsches Ärzteblatt 88:1133
Lee G, Halcrow S 2002 Petrous to petrous fracture associated with bilateral abducens and facial nerve palsies: a case report. Trauma 53:583
Leonetti J, Smith P, Anand V et al 1993 Subtotal petrosectomy in the management of advanced parotid neoplasms. Otolaryngology Head and Neck Surgery 108(3):270–276
Linder-Aronson S, Woodside D 2000 Excess face height malocclusion etiology, diagnosis and treatment. Quintessence, Carol Stream, IL
Lohse-Busch H, Kraemer M 1994 Atlastherapie nach Arlen – heutiger Stand. Manuelle Medizin 32:153
Losee J E, Mason A C 2005 Deformational plagiocephaly: diagnosis, prevention, and treatment Clinics in Plastic Surgery 32(1):53–64, viii
Magarey M 1988 The first treatment session. In: Grieve G (ed.) Grieve's modern manual therapy. Churchill Livingstone, Oxford, p 661
Magge S, Westerveld M, Pruzinsky T, Persing J 2002 Long-term neuropsychological effects of sagittal craniosynostosis on child development. Journal of Craniofacial Surgery 13:99
Maitland G 1986 Vertebral manipulation, 5th edn. Butterworth-Heinemann, Oxford
Maitland G, Hengeveld E, Banks K, English K 2001 Vertebral manipulation, 6th edn. Butterworth-Heinemann, Oxford
Marchac D, Arnaud E, Renier D 2002 Frontocranial remodeling without opening of frontal sinuses in a scaphocephalic adolescent: a case report. Journal of Craniofacial Surgery 13:698
Margulies S, Thibault L, Gennarelli T 1990 Physical model simulations of brain injury in the primate. Journal of Biomechanics 23:823
Matson D D, Crigler J F Jr 1969 Management of craniopharyngioma in childhood. Journal of Neurosurgery 30(4):377
Matsumura G, Uchiumi T, Kida K et al 1993 Development studies on the interparietal part of the human occipital squama. Journal of Anatomy 182:197
Mau H, Gabe I 1981 Die sogenannte Säuglingsskoliose und ihre krankengymnastische Behandlung. Thieme, Stuttgart
Meissner J 1992 Skoliosetherapie und Atlastherapie. Orthopädie Praxis 6:397
Miltner E, Kallieris D, Schmidt G et al 1990 Verletzungen der Schädelbasiskondylen bei tödlichen Straßenverkehrsunfällen. Zeitschrift für Rechtsmedizin 103:523
Montgomery W 1993 Dural defects of the temporal bone. American Journal of Otology 14:548
Murtagh R, Caracciolo J, Fernandez G 2001 CT findings associated with Eagle syndrome. AJNR American Journal of Neuroradiology 22:1401
Muthukumar N 2002 Delayed hypoglossal palsy following occipital condyle fracture – case report. Journal of Clinical Neuroscience 9:580
Nerder P, Bakke M, Solow B 1999 The functional shift of the mandible in unilateral posterior crossbite and the adaptation of the temporomandibular joints: a pilot study. European Journal of Orthodontics 21:155
Neufeld S, Birkett S 2000 What to do about flat heads: preventing and treating positional occipital flattening. Axone 22:29
Okeson J 1996 Orofacial pain: guidelines for assessment, classification and management. Quintessence, Chicago
Okeson J 2005 Bell's orofacial pains, 6th edn. Quintessence. Chicago
Oudhof H 1982 Sutural growth. Acta Anatomica 112:58
Oudhof H 2001 Skull growth in relation to mechanical stimulation. In: von Piekartz H, Bryden L (eds) Craniofacial dysfunction and pain, assessment, manual therapy and management. Butterworth-Heinemann, Oxford
Ozawa Y, Takashima S 2002 Developmental neurotransmitter pathology in the brainstem of sudden infant death syndrome: a review and sleep position. Forensic Science International 130(Suppl):S53–59.
Ozawa T, Hasegawa M, Okaue M et al 1995 Two cases of symptomatic elongated styloid process. Journal of Nihon University School of Dentistry 37:178
Palmèn K 1984 Prevention of congenital dislocation of the hip. The Swedish experience of neonatal

treatment of hip joint instability. Acta Orthopaedica Scandinavica Suppl 208:1

Patten J 1995 The cerebellopontine angle and the jugular foramen. In: Neurological differential diagnosis, 2nd edn. Springer, London, p 61

Pertschuk M J, Whitaker L A 1985 Psychosocial adjustment and craniofacial malformations in childhood. Plastic and Reconstructive Surgery 75(2):177

Prasad K, Kamath M, Reddy K, Raju K, Agarwal S 2002 Elongated styloid process (Eagle's syndrome): a clinical study. Journal of Oral and Maxillofacial Surgery 60:171

Proffit W R 1993 Contemporary orthodontics, 2nd edn. Mosby Year Book, St Louis

Ratliff-Schaub K, Hunt C, Crowell D et al 2001 Relationship between infant sleep position and motor development in preterm infants. Journal of Developmental and Behavioral Pediatrics 22:293

Renzi G, Mastellone P, Leonardi A, Becelli R, Bonamini M, Fini G 2005 Basicranium malformation with anterior dislocation of right styloid process causing stylalgia. Journal of Craniofacial Surgery 16(3):418–420

Retzlaff E, Michael D, Roppel R 1975 Cranial bone mobility. Journal of the American Osteopathic Association 74:138

Reynolds J 1987 The skull and spine. Seminars in Roentgenology 23:168

Ripley C, Pomatto J, Beats S et al 1993 Treatment of positional plagiocephaly utilising the cranial remodelling othosis (doc). Oaxaca, Mexico: 5th International Congress of the International Society of Craniofacial Surgery

Roarty J, Pron G, Siegel-Bartelt J et al 1994 Ocular manifestations of frontonasal dysplasia. Plastic and Reconstructive Surgery 93:25

Ruige M, Palmans E, Vles J 1993 Hoofdzaken en kopzorgen bij plagiocefalie. Tijdschrift voor Kindergeneeskunde 61:24

Sano K, Nakamura M, Hirakawa K, Masuzawa H 1969 Mechanism and dynamics of closed head injuries. Neurologia Medico-Chirurgica 9:21

Schellhas K P, Piper M A, Omlie M R 1992 Facial skeleton remodeling due to temporomandibular joint degeneration: an imaging study of 100 patients. Cranio 10(3):248

Schlenker W, Jennings B, Jeiroudi M, Caruso J 2000 The effects of chronic absence of active nasal respiration on the growth of the skull: a pilot study. Am Journal of Orthodontics and Dentofacial Orthopedics 117:706

Schmid R 1969 Kraniostenose beim Kind. Schweizer Archiv für Neurologie, Neurochirurgie und Psychiatrie 105:55

Schon D 1983 The reflective practitioner: how professionals think in action. Basic Books, New York

Schor R, Kearney R, Dieringer N 1988 Reflex stabilization of the head. In: Peterson B, Richmond F (eds) Control of head movement. Oxford University Press, Oxford, p 141

Schuknecht B, Graetz K 2005 Radiologic assessment of maxillofacial, mandibular, and skull base trauma. European Radiology 15(3):560–568

Sham J, Cheung Y, Ckay D et al 1991 Cranial nerve involvement and base of the skull erosion in nasopharyngeal carcinoma. Cancer 68:422

Slate R, Posnick J, Armstrong D, Buncic J 1993 Cervical spine subluxation associated with congenital muscular torticollis and craniofacial asymmetry. Plastic and Reconstructive Surgery 91(7):1187–1195; discussion 1196–1197

Solow B, Tallgren A 1976 Head posture and cranio-facial morphology. American Journal of Physical Anthropology 44:417

Sommering S 1839 Von Bau des menschlichen Körpers. Voss, Berlin

Speltz M L, Kapp-Simon K A, Cunningham M, Marsh J, Dawson G 2004 Single-suture craniosynostosis: a review of neurobehavioral research and theory. Journal of Pediatric Psychology 29(8):651–668

Spermon-Marijnen, Spermon J 2001 Manual therapy movements of the craniofacial region as a therapeutic approach to children with long-term ear disease. In: Von Piekartz H, Bryden L (eds) Craniofacial dysfunction and pain, assessment, manual therapy and management. Butterworth-Heinemann, Oxford

Stroobants J, Fidlers L, Sorms J et al 1994 High cervical pain and impairment of skull mobility as the only symptoms of an occipital condyle fracture. Journal of Neurosurgery 81:137

van der Bijl G 1986 Het individuele functiemodel in de manuele therapie. Uitgeversmaatschappij de Tijdstroom BV

van der Kolk C, Carson B 1994 Lambdoid synostosis. Clinics in Plastic Surgery 21:575

Virtanen R, Korhonen T, Fagerholm J, Viljanto J 1999 Neurocognitive sequelae of scaphocephaly. Pediatrics 103:791

von Piekartz H 2001 Features of cranial tissue as a basis for clinical pattern recognition, examination and treatment. In: von Piekartz H, Bryden L (eds) Craniofacial dysfunction and pain, assessment, manual therapy and management. Butterworth-Heinemann, Oxford

Wagemans P A, van de Velde J P, Kuijpers-Jagtman A M 1988 Sutures and forces: a review. American Journal of Orthodontics and Dentofacial Orthopedics 94(2):129

Williams P, Warwick R, Dyson M, Bannister L 1989 Gray's anatomy, 37th edn. Churchill Livingstone, Edinburgh

Wilson-Pauwels L, Akesson E, Stewart P, Spacey S 2002 Cranial nerves in health and disease, 2nd edn. Decker, London
Woda A 2000 A unified concept of idiopathic orofacial pain: pathophysiological features. Journal of Orofacial Pain 14:196
Wong E, Lee G, Mason D 1995 Temporal headaches and associated symptoms relating to the styloid process and its attachments. Annals of the Academy of Medicine, Singapore 24:124
Yen E, Suga D 1982 Immunohistochemical localization of type I and type III collagen in calvarial suture. Journal of Dental Research 61(SI):183
Zaki H, Greco C, Rudy T, Kubinski J 1996 Elongated styloid process in a temporomandibular disorder sample: prevalence and treatment outcome. Journal of Prosthetic Dentistry 75:399
Zielinski P, Sloniewski P 2001 Virtual modelling of the surgical anatomy of the petrous bone. Folia Morphologica 60:343
Zielinski C, Gunt S, Deeb Z 1982 Cranial nerve palsies complicating Jefferson fracture. Journal of Bone and Joint Surgery 64A:1382
Zuniga C, Miralles R, Mena B et al 1995 Influence of variation in jaw posture on sternocleidomastoid and trapezius electromyographic activity. Cranio 13(3):157–162

Chapter 15

The viscerocranium: examination and treatment guidelines

Harry von Piekartz

CHAPTER CONTENTS

INTRODUCTION

The terminology and classification of the skull was discussed in Chapters 1 and 2. In general, the face can be divided into three functional regions for the purposes of clinical investigation:

- The orbital region
- The zygomatic region
- The maxillary region.

Why consider these divisions of the facial skeleton?

Two arguments support making these distinctions:

- From the phylogenetic and ontogenetic point of view the viscerocranium develops later than the calvaria (Oudhof 2001).
- Clinical experience shows that sensory responses to passive movements differ between these different regions: the neurocranium responds mainly with diffuse, deep responses; the viscerocranium responds with local, sharp and largely superficial responses. The neurocranium is also frequently responsible for reactions and symptoms elsewhere in the body which are more associated with increased output tendencies such as vegetative reactions and/or regulation (or dysregulation) of tone. The

viscerocranium generally reacts with clear symptoms that are well localized in the face.

It is therefore practical to divide the face into three regions when starting a therapeutic investigation using passive techniques. An impression of which region is most responsible for the symptoms can thus be formed rapidly.

When comparing the responses of the neurocranium and viscerocranium to passive movements, it will be observed that, in the case of the neurocranium:

- Deep, diffuse pain with an extrasegmental character is observed.
- Large amplitude passive movements (grade II or III) provoke the responses in most cases.
- The responses during passive movements are cumulative or only appear after a latency period of seconds to minutes.
- Autonomic and motor responses are frequently provoked.

By comparison, in the case of the viscerocranium:

- Local, sharp and superficial pain is often observed.
- Passive movements of small amplitude in resistance (grade IV) usually provoke responses.
- The responses can be provoked more frequently during passive movements.
- The responses are most usually manifested in the craniofacial region.

The next part of the chapter is divided into two parts. The first part will describe the general techniques of the three regions. The second part discusses in detail the most important specific techniques of every region (Fig. 15.1).

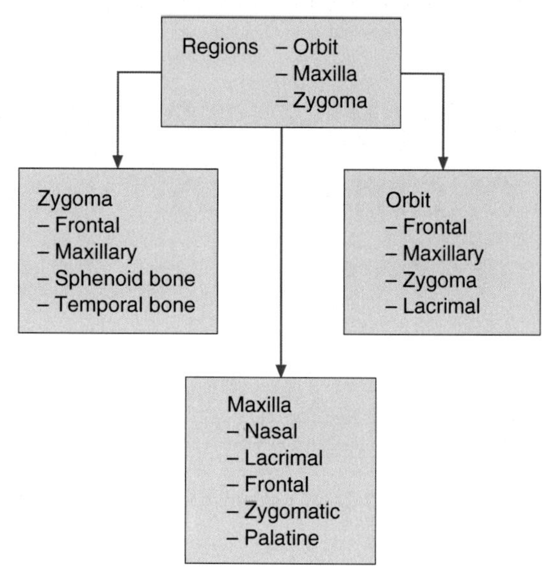

Fig. 15.1 Functional interrelationships of the viscerocranium (facial skeleton).

THE ORBITAL REGION

Relevant anatomy

A SHORT REVIEW OF THE ANATOMY

The orbital region is like a pyramid with four sides. The orbit is formed superficially by the following bones:

1. Roof: orbital part of the frontal bone; lesser wing of sphenoid bone
2. Lateral border: zygomatic and frontal bones
3. Medial border: ethmoid bone; lacrimal bone; sphenoid bone
4. Base: greater wing of sphenoid, palatine and ethmoid bones.

Foramina – including the optic canal (optic nerve II) and anterior and posterior ethmoid foramen (ethmoid nerves) – are formed by the orbital region.

The regions we can influence directly with passive movements are:

- Zygomatic maxillary region (Z/M)
- Frontomaxillary region (F/M)
- Lacrimal maxillary and lacrimal frontal region (La/M, La/F)
- Sphenopalatine region (S/Pa)
- Frontozygomatic region (F/Z) (Fig. 15.2).

General techniques for the orbit

General techniques principally change the stress-transducer system around the orbit and

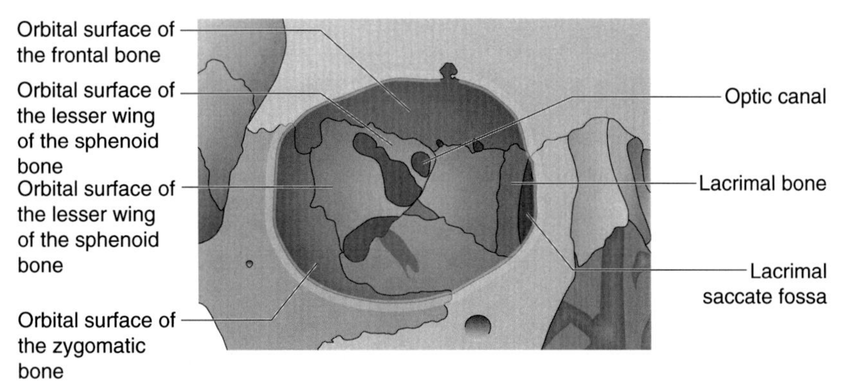

Fig. 15.2 The right orbit: overview of the facial bones forming the right orbit and their connections.

therefore compression and distraction techniques are the ones to use initially.

General compression

STARTING POSITION AND METHOD

The patient lies supine and is comfortable and relaxed. The therapist sits at the patient's head facing the cranial side. The thumbs and index fingers of both hands are placed around the orbital margin, with the right thumb on the right orbit and the left thumb on the left orbit, as shown in Figure 15.3. The other fingers are spread out on the cranium and control the facial bones. The index finger is on the maxilla medial to the maxillary foramen and the middle finger is on the inferior border of the zygoma. Both thumbs and index fingers are moved towards the centre of the orbit. The therapist's forearms are parallel and do not really move.

The technique is based on a fine action which requires precise coordination of all the fingers as much as possible. The patient should not experience any uncomfortable local pressure of the fingers.

General distraction

For the general distraction technique the same hand position as above is used, but the thumbs and index fingers are very carefully hooked just inside the inner rim of the orbit. During the movement the fingers are moved from the centre of the orbit laterally to allow a general widening of the orbit without an uncomfortable increase in pressure.

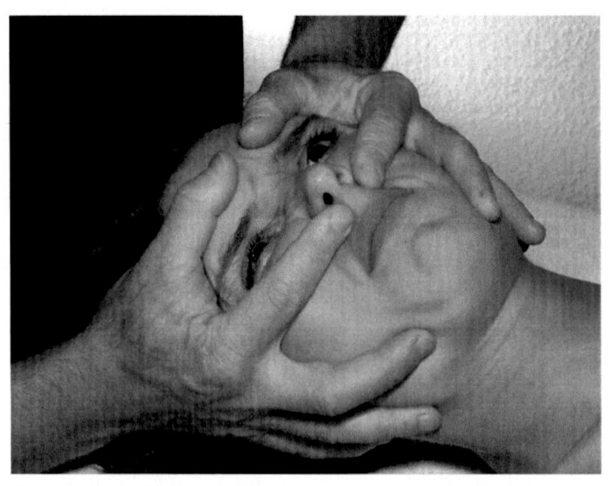

Fig. 15.3 General bilateral compression of the orbit.

THE ZYGOMATIC BONE

Introduction

The zygomatic bone has a functional relationship with the maxilla, temporal and frontal bones (see Fig. 15.2). They influence each other directly through stress and movement (Schwenzer & Ehrenfeld 2002). An impression of the zygoma and its connections can be gathered using the following two general techniques

General extraoral bilateral technique

STARTING POSITION AND METHOD

The patient lies supine and is comfortable and relaxed. The therapist sits at the patient's head and rests both forearms on the plinth which has been adjusted to a convenient height. The thumb, index and middle fingers of both hands touch and lightly pinch respectively the lateral border of the orbit, and the superior and inferior part of the zygoma bilaterally (Fig. 15.4). In this position all accessory movements of the zygoma are possible, and left/right comparisons are easy to assess. The movement is a small smooth movement from the wrist without movement of the forearm. The distance between the three fingers always stays the same and care is taken that no extra pressure is added when performing this movement.

The general extraoral technique gains information about signs and symptoms arising from the zygomatic region. It also gives an indication about the difference in mobility of the left and right sides. Together with observation of the viscerocranium it gives a good impression of the position, prominence and shape of the zygomatic bone. It also helps to ascertain information about the general mobility of the cranium, perhaps because of the prominent role of the zygomatic bone during facial growth (Bentley et al 2002a). When this technique suggests symptoms arising from the zygomatic region then unilateral techniques are the next step in the examination.

Unilateral technique (anterior–posterior) movement

STARTING POSITION AND METHOD

The patient lies supine and is comfortable and relaxed. The therapist sits at the patient's head and rests the left hand on the occipital region of the head. The right hand is in pronation and the part of the hand between the thenar and hypothenar eminences contacts the highest point of the zygomatic bone. If convenient, the volar side of the right fingers can make contact with the dorsal side of the left hand to provide better control while performing the manoeuvre (Fig. 15.5).

The therapist's right elbow is slightly flexed and the sternum is perpendicular to the right zygomatic bone. In this position a slow oscillatory movement can be initiated from the body. During the movement you should be aware that there is a small natural neck movement as a result of the anterior–posterior movement on the zygomatic bone. Therefore, do not fix the cervical spine or the patient may feel too much local pressure.

This clinically valuable technique is often used during examination and treatment of patients with severe irritable symptoms or long-term persistent stable midface complaints after facial trauma and long-term sinusitis.

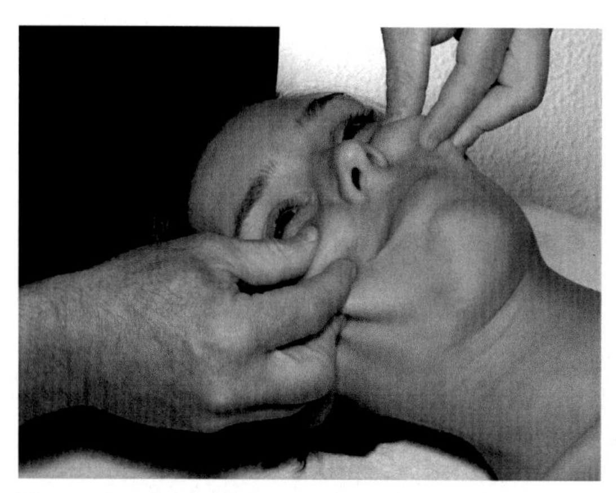

Fig. 15.4 General bilateral zygoma technique (rotation around the sagittal axis).

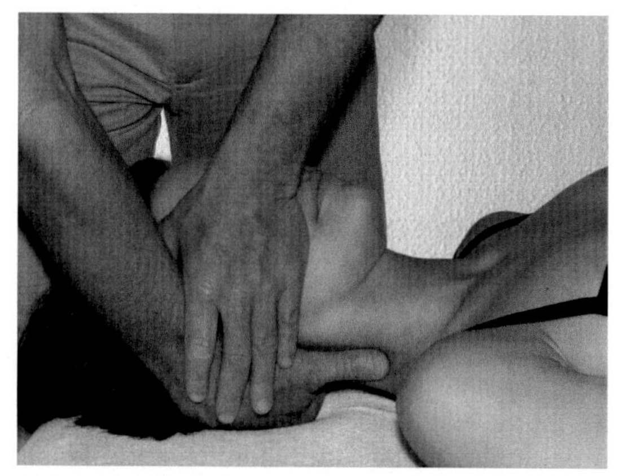

Fig. 15.5 General unilateral technique for the zygomatic bone (anterior–posterior movement).

Many patients in this category experience this pain as a 'pleasant' pain. In addition, it has shown clinical efficacy in patients with respiratory problems with nasal obstruction and associated difficulties.

THE MAXILLA

Introduction

The maxilla is connected to the frontal, zygomatic, lacrimal and sphenoid bones. The maxilla is a coupled bone and forms a suture between left and right (the intermaxillary suture) which is partly intra- and partly extraoral. Intraorally, the maxilla also forms part of the hard palate – the palatine bone.

All standard accessory movements are possible. The general techniques can be divided into general bilateral and unilateral intraoral techniques.

General bilateral intraoral technique

General intraoral techniques of the maxilla can best be accomplished by movements such as rotation (longitudinal and sagittal axes), longitudinal movements and transverse movements.

The aim is to establish whether the signs and symptoms are more dominantly provoked from the maxillary region or from the orbit or zygomatic region.

STARTING POSITION AND METHOD

The patient lies supine, comfortable and relaxed. The plinth is at the height of the therapist's iliac crest. A small towel against the contralateral side of the patient's head can be useful, especially during rotation and transverse movements. The web space of the left thumb and index finger spans the frontal bone and fixes the right lateral border of the frontal bone or fixes both sides of the greater wing of the sphenoid. This depends on which region is to be examined: the maxillofrontal or maxillosphenoid. The left thumb and index finger are placed left and right intrabuccally on the maxilla above the teeth (Fig. 15.6). The therapist leans gently against the plinth with the trunk and fixes the medial side of the right elbow against the trunk, enabling a leaning position over the patient. During the movement the therapist makes a slow trunk movement in the direction of the mobilization, preventing a forearm–hand movement.

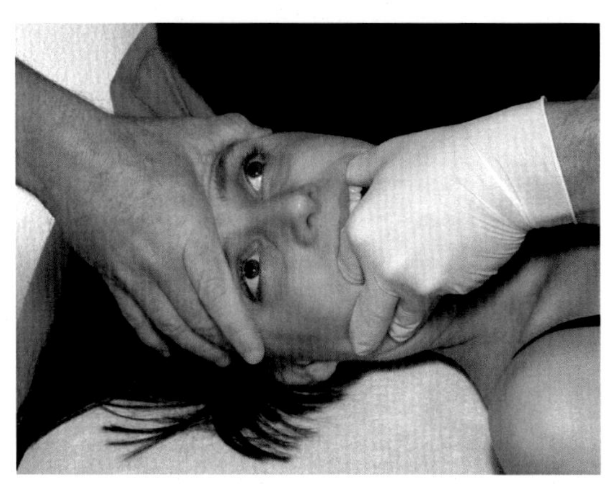

Fig. 15.6 General bilateral intraoral technique of the maxilla.

The distance between the right thumb and index finger stays the same without increasing local pressure on the bones. When the maxilla is too small on the lateral side, the longitudinal movement to caudal can be better accomplished using a unilateral technique.

Stiffness, pain and reproduction of symptoms are often noted during and after performing the general maxillary technique. These responses are often interpreted as malocclusions, craniomandibular dysfunctions, neuropathic pain from the maxillary nerve and maxillary sinusitis.

SPECIFIC TECHNIQUES FOR THE ORBIT, ZYGOMATIC AND MAXILLARY REGIONS

THE ORBIT

The orbit is formed by the following main regions:

- Zygomaticomaxillary region (Z/M)
- Frontomaxillary region (F/M)
- Lacrimal region:

  - Lacrimal frontal region (La/F)
  - Lacrimal maxillary region (La/M)
- Sphenopalatine region (S/Pa)
- Frontozygomatic region (F/Z).

Both bone partners can be moved separately or together and will be discussed in the following text.

Zygomaticomaxillary region (Z/M) (extraoral)

STARTING POSITION AND METHOD

The patient lies supine, and is comfortable and relaxed. The therapist palpates the right zygomaticomaxillary suture with the right index finger, and then fixes the zygomatic bone with the right thumb, index and middle fingers. The left hand palpates the maxilla with the thumb and index finger, either extra- or intraorally. The most commonly used and clinically relevant movements are:

- Longitudinal caudal, cranium
- Rotation around the sagittal and transverse axes
- Transverse movement in medial and lateral direction.

Frontomaxillary region (F/M)

STARTING POSITION AND METHOD

The patient lies supine and relaxed with a small towel under the occipital protuberance (inion) to prevent shifting of the head. The head is rotated 30° towards the therapist. The therapist is seated at the patient's head on the opposite side, with the plinth adjusted to a convenient height. The left thumb and index finger contact the frontal bone; the right thumb and middle finger contact the frontal process of the maxillary bone lateral to the nose. The right index finger palpates the region during the movement.

The most common movements for performing this position are compression, distraction in a longitudinal direction, transverse movements to one side and rotations around the sagittal, frontal and transverse axes.

Patients with signs and symptoms including ventral nose pain, symptoms of chronic sinusitis (e.g. abnormal airflow), nose bleeding, post-traumatic conditions following surgery (e.g. septum reconstruction) and with no other underlying pathology may be indicated for passive movements of this region (Younis et al 2002).

Lacrimal frontal and lacrimal maxillary region (La/F, La/M)

STARTING POSITION AND METHOD

Both these regions are dealt with here because they have nearly the same hand position – only the localization of palpation differs. The patient lies in a comfortable and relaxed position. The therapist sits beside the plinth on the left-hand side facing the patient's head. For the lacrimal frontal region the medial side of the pad of the right index finger contacts the lacrimal bone; the left thumb and index finger hold the frontal bone (Fig. 15.7). For the lacrimal maxillary region the right index finger contacts the lacrimal bone and the left index finger contacts the maxillary bone. The fingertips are pointed in the opposite direction and lie adjacent to each other. For the lacrimal bone, slight longitudinal, anterior–posterior and rotational movements around the longitudinal axis are performed. The longitudinal movement of the lacrimal bone is a flexion/extension movement of the therapist's interphalangeal joints. Rotation around the longitudinal axis is a rotation of the index finger around its own axis. The same standard movements can be performed for the maxillary and frontal bone with the lacrimal bone fixed and stabilized, ensuring that there is no increase in pressure on the regions that are fixed.

It is possible that during examination of this region the nasolacrimal canal (Fig. 15.8), which transports waste products from the eye to the nose and mouth, is influenced, and that patients with longstanding pressure in the medial orbital region or eye divergence problems without clear pathology can be improved by this technique. Mechanical and neurological reflex stimuli can influence the production of tears by the lacrimal system. Objective and subjective orbital pressure can be reduced (Wagner & Lang 2000).

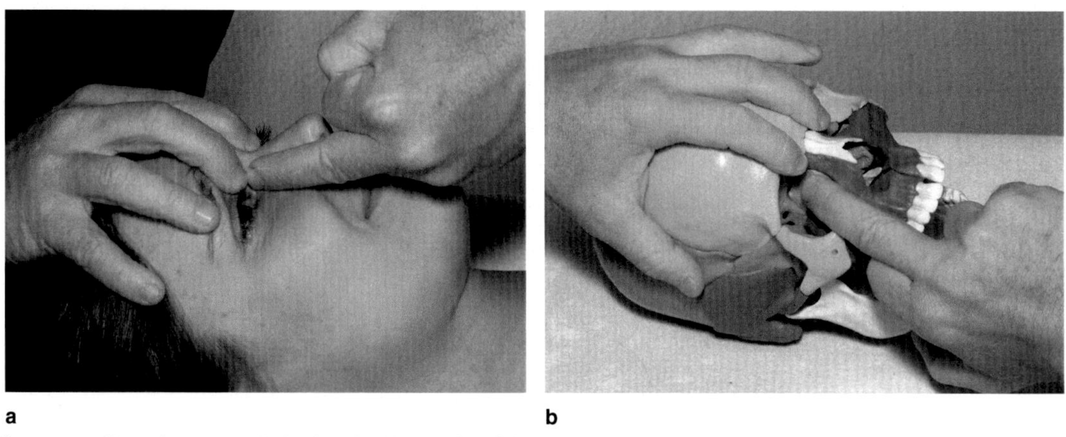

a b

Fig. 15.7 Rotation around the longitudinal axis of the lacrimal bone while holding the maxilla with index finger and thumb.

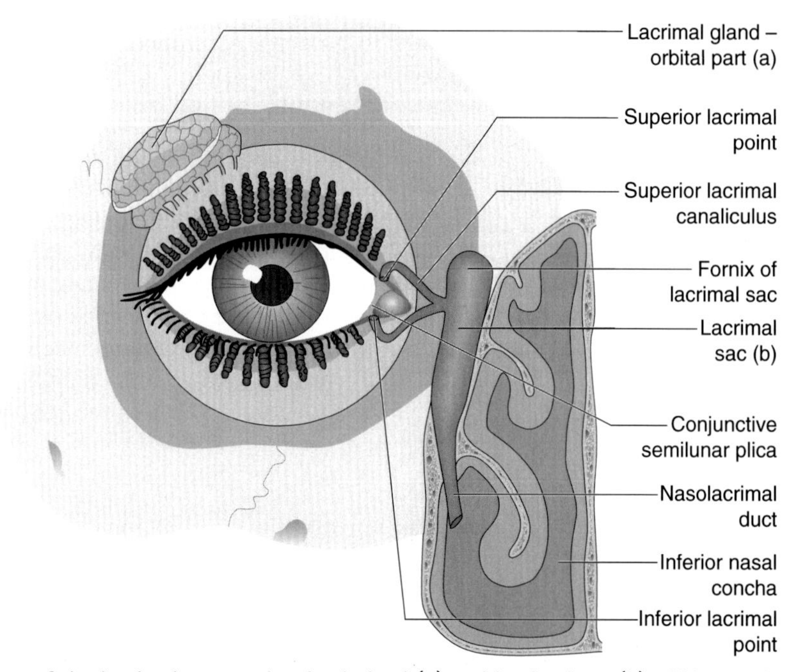

Fig. 15.8 Course of the lacrimal system. Lacrimal gland (a) and lacrimal sac (b) will be mechanically and neuroreflexively stimulated by, among others, medial orbit techniques.

This technique is suitable for patients with facial paresis and dry eyes. The motor activities responsible for secretion of tears from the lacrimal glands are less controlled. Lacrimal facilitation can be a positive contribution to the recovery of the normal water balance of the orbital region (Wagner & Lang 2000).

Sphenopalatine region (S/Pa)

The palate is directly connected with the sphenoid bone. The most dorsal part (soft palate) has a direct connection with part of the sphenoid which is also the insertion point of the superior head of the lateral pterygoid muscle and the inferior head of the medial pterygoid muscle (William et al 1989). The palatine process and the sphenoid bone together form the caudal dorsolateral part of the orbital fossa.

STARTING POSITION AND METHOD

The patient lies supine and is comfortable and relaxed. The therapist sits or stands beside the plinth on the right side, facing the patient. The therapist holds the patient's sphenoid with the index finger and thumb of the left hand. The right index finger or right little finger is intraoral on the dorsolateral side of the hard palate.

The therapist presses slowly with the right index or little finger on the palate, trying not to increase local pain. The hard palate and the soft palate can be influenced. The soft palate is normally locally sore. The therapist must take care that, during the manoeuvre on the maxilla, the pressure on the sphenoid does not increase. Accessory movements towards longitudinal cranial, transverse lateral, rotation around the longitudinal axis and combinations of these are possible.

As the spheno-occipital region has a direct connection to the sphenopalatine region, assessment of the spheno-occipital region during and after passive movements of the palate is sensible and useful (see Chapter 14). This technique may influence the spheno-palatine ganglion which influences cerebral circulation (Hardebo & Elner 1987).

The sphenopalatine ganglion is an important structure for the function of the autonomic nervous system of the face; it is also believed to be important in atypical facial pain (Klein et al 2001). Ganglion blockade is therefore often used with moderate success (Brown 1997), as well as for other body regions (Quevedo et al 2005).

Anatomically, direct influences of the foramen rotundum (mandibular nerve), foramen ovale (maxillary nerve), foramen palatum (palatum major), canal caroticus, caroticus, plexus sympaticus, carotid artery, and the medial and lateral pterygoid muscles are possible. Bilateral signs and symptoms such as a 'pressure' in the head, bilateral burning pain in the eyes, tinnitus, dizziness and changes of skin colour ('red spots') without clear pathology are the commonest clinical signs that may require prompt treatment with these techniques.

The above are extremely effective techniques for patients with bruxism or general sympathetic type symptoms in the head region and frontal symptoms in the nasofrontal region.

Muscular function may change (increase of tone), for example because of parafunctions such as bruxism or bracing, together with pulsing pain in the temporal and orbital regions of the same side. This reacts well to passive movements of this region. The result is a reduction in muscle tone which clearly indicates a parafunctional clinical pattern.

Precautions

The clinician has to be aware that changes of symptoms (e.g. tinnitus, retro-orbital headache) by passive movements can be a sign of arteriovenous malformation (AVM) of the anterior cranial fossa (Friedmann et al 2001, Shin et al 2002). Such signs often lead to spontaneous infracerebral haemorrhage (Stewart & Soparkar 2005). This pathology has been reported sporadically since the first report by Lepoire et al (1963); however, since the advent of new radiology techniques the pathology and clinical presentation have been more frequently described (Gerschman et al 1979). Further precautions are required in the event of an extreme increase of symptoms and to latency reactions with a long duration. Referral to a specialist for further diagnosis is, in the author's opinion, the best clinical decision.

Frontal plagiocephaly

Neurosurgical research has shown the importance of the transducer system, the forces of the sphenofrontal suture (in the orbital region) and of the frontal plagiocephaly syndrome (an asymmetrical skull deformity due to premature synostosis of a coronal hemisuture). Much of the stress in the region of the lateral orbital pillar and the pterion gives rise to a set of facial and cranial deformities which vary according to the predisposition and topography of the synostosis (Bentley et al 2002b). The most extreme frontal plagiocephalies may need a bilateral orbitofrontal nasal osteotomy to give a better chance of normalization (Reinhart et al 1998). How the abnormal pressure during face asymmetry in the orbital region relates to symptoms in minor clinical presentation is at present unknown.

It is not uncommon for smooth passive movements in the frontonasal and frontosphenoidal region to invoke strong symptomatic reactions in some patients. In the clinical setting it is often noticed that smooth passive movements in the frontonasal and frontosphenoidal regions provoke extreme symptoms with a short duration. In most cases the patient has a history of craniofacial symptoms but these are decreased or gone completely. Some examples are facial pain after an old fracture together with headache, long-term chronic conjunctivitis with facial pain, sinusitis with general headache (poorly localized) and unilateral burning eye pain after concussion. The reaction to the first examination or treatment is often more severe than the following treatments.

The major influence on facial growth comes from the orbital region

In growth studies it is seen that particular bones (frontal, zygomatic and maxillary bones) undergo a direct displacement in relation to each other, especially during adolescence. This is regulated by the sutures of the orbit (Enlow & Hunter 1996, Bentley et al 2002a). Ophthalmological studies show the correlation between the growing eye and its exertion of a mechanical influence on the morphogenesis of the orbit. It is hypothesized that the extent to which the development of the eye influences the skull depends on the relationship between the intensive growth rates of the orbit, the optic nerve and the eye (Coulombre & Grelm 1958, Wohlrab et al 2002). These relationships have already been shown in studies on chickens and monkeys. However, it is known that the same tendency of asymmetrical growth of the orbit is observed in other cranial regions as seen in young children with an underdeveloped eye (Limborgh & Tonneyck-Müller 1976, Bentley et al 2002a). In the author's opinion, a young patient with a small orbit and associated symptoms and signs of eye problems has the potential to change the symptomatic response following passive movements in the orbital region. Orbital changes caused by passive movement might also prevent changes in neurodynamics of the optic nerve. In this group of patients, children as well as adults, eye movements are in a different direction and are not balanced. Treatment by passive movements together with active eye movement as a reassessment tool and/or target tissue activity is often needed and useful.

Anatomical variation of the orbit

Not only morphological but also anatomical variations can influence eye function; this has been seen with craniofacial malformation due to trigonocephaly – premature closure of the orbit followed by oculomotor imbalance (Denis et al 1994, Schneider et al 2000). Each oculomotor muscle is covered by a sheath at the origin of the ligaments. The ligaments insert at the edge of the orbit. The shortest ligament belongs to the lateral rectus muscle. It is inserted on the external orbital edge and wall in the region of the frontozygomatic bones (Proffit 1993). For example, minor strabismus symptoms with an abnormal shape of the orbit can be an indication for orbital assessment, especially the frontozygomatic region (Fig. 15.9), and neurodynamic testing of cranial nerves III, IV and VI.

Three-dimensional computed tomography studies of apes and humans show large skull deformations (particularly in the zygomatic bone) during different phases of the chewing process. This is particularly noticeable at the zygomatic/maxillary suture (displacement of maxilla and zygoma) which reacts strongly to orthodontic splints. These skull deformations arise from normal forces during chewing and

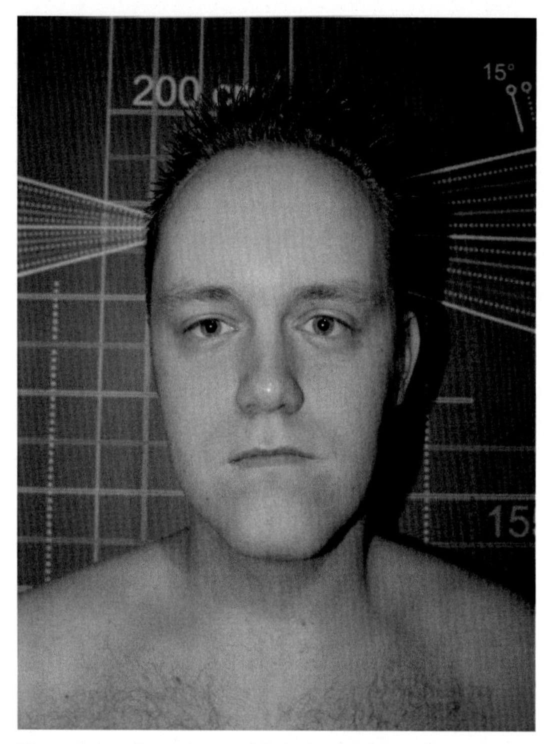

Fig. 15.9 A 25-year-old patient with unilateral headache, strabismus caused by a congenital dominant right eye dysfunction. Note the small right orbita, the flat right zygoma region and the assymmetry of the lower face (left mandibula part is 1.6 cm smaller than the right one).

occlusion. Abnormal unilateral biting or abnormal mouth habits can change the stress transducer component in the face, particularly in the orbital region, and can predispose to signs and symptoms in later life (Fuchs & Scott 1973, Schneider et al 2000, Azimi et al 2003). The therapist may often notice that patients with orofacial pain with dominant craniomandibular symptoms have a wide orbit and a more prominent zygomatic bone. This is a possible sign to be considered alongside the patient's symptoms.

Fractures in the region of the orbit

That the orbital region is important for the function of the sinuses is seen retrospectively after surgery for maxillofacial trauma. Miniplates in the frontozygomatic region, for example, result in a large frontal sinus (Reher & Duarte 1994, Gasparini et al 2002). Clinically this region is relevant if frontal sinus changes are indicated.

Orbital floor fractures together with orbital floor fissures in the zygomatic–maxillary and naso-ethmoidal suture lines are most commonly seen after a midfacial trauma (Peter et al 1994, Lauer et al 1996, Sargent & Rogers 1999, Haug et al 2002). Entrapment of the infraorbital nerve is often seen as a complication and is often decompressed by plastic surgery in extreme 'blow-in' fractures (Gruss & Mackinnon 1986, Antomyshyn & Gruss 1989, Read & Sires 1998, Sakavicius et al 2002). Trauma in the midface with or without fractures and fissures seems to have an enormous impact on the orbital bones (Fig. 15.10). This could be a broad explanation for the large number of patients with post-traumatic head injuries that complain about long-term facial pain. Subjective thickness of the eye region, numbness or burning eye pain, dry or wet eyes (often together with craniomandibular or upper cervical symptoms) are often found. From a clinical point of view it is felt that many of these post-traumatic symptoms are nociceptive, peripheral neurogenic and can be changed by smooth movement and pressure changes of the orbital region, together with neurodynamic assessment and treatment.

It is known that the infraorbital nerve is often involved in orbital trauma (Read & Sires 1998, Benoliel et al 2001). In these cases care is required with techniques with longstanding effects as reactions may only appear after a latent period. This latency could be due to peripheral neuropathic reactions of the infraorbital nerve. Palate techniques in such cases often give a release of the symptoms and are prognostically better when release of symptoms takes place during the palate treatment.

The superior orbital fissure and cranial nervous connective tissue

The superior orbital fissure is a canal that lies between the greater and lesser wings of the

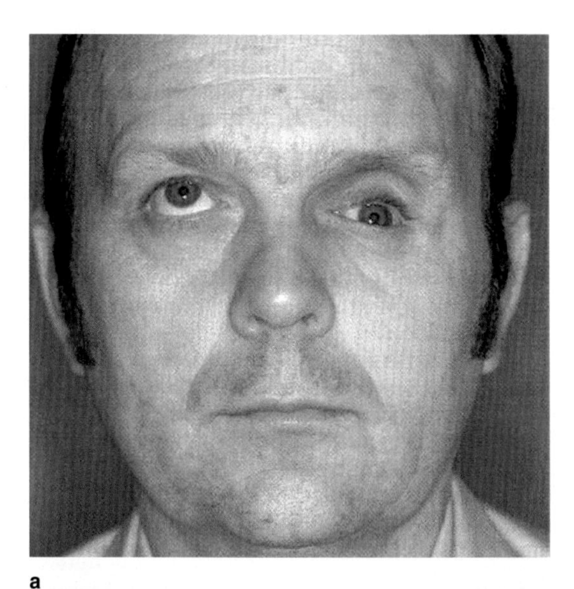

a

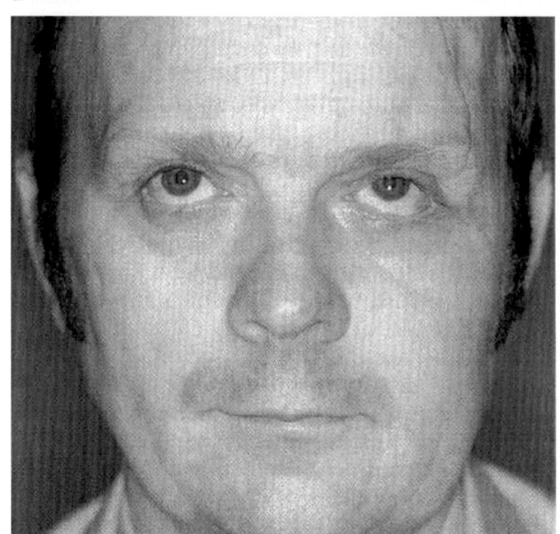

b

Fig. 15.10
a A patient 7 days after fracture of the left zygomatic bone and left orbit. Clinical pattern of endophthalmitis, lowered position of the left eyeball, diplopia and functional deficit of the rectus inferior muscle.
b The same patient several months after surgical repositioning of the zygomatic bone, orbitoplasty and correction of the position of the left eye. Facial symmetry and eye function have been restored. This patient may still have postoperative orbital pain and visual problems (reproduced with permission from Schwenzer & Ehrenfeld 2002).

sphenoid bone lateral to the optic canal. It contains the third, fourth and sixth cranial nerves and the branches of the ophthalmic division of the fifth cranial nerve. Most of the venous drainage from the orbit passes through this fissure within the superior ophthalmic vein (Morard et al 1994, Haug et al 1999, Fukai et al 2001). The nerves and supraorbital veins have tight adhesions with structures such as the dura mater and the orbital connective tissue (Housepain et al 1982, Austermann 2002). These anatomical facts may explain the clinical pattern seen in, for example, a patient with deep eye pressure or pain change on upper cervical flexion or extension which can change the cranial neurodynamics. The same effect is often seen during frontal, zygomatic and or sphenoid bone movements. In addition, divergence of the eye and diplopia can, in the author's experience, be changed quickly by orbital treatment techniques, especially on patients with a history of head and neck trauma.

SPECIFIC TECHNIQUES OF THE ZYGOMA REGION

The main regions discussed are the:

- Zygomatic–maxillary region (Z/M)
- Zygomatic–temporal region (Z/T)
- Zygomatic–frontal region (Z/F).

Intraoral unilateral techniques of the zygomatic maxillary, temporal and frontal regions

The advantage of intraoral techniques is that they have a local effect and, like the maxillary sinus, teeth, mouth and the orbit, can cause local pain during passive movements.

The main accessory movements (e.g. longitudinal, transverse lateral and rotational) can be very effective.

STARTING POSITION AND METHOD

The patient lies supine, and is comfortable and relaxed. The therapist sits or stands at the patient's head, on the left side. The right hand grasps the right zygomatic bone by placing the right thumb and index finger on the cheek outside the mouth and the left index finger intrabuccally to allow examination of the zygomatic–temporal region. For the frontozygomatic region, the right thumb and index finger are on the frontal bone. For the zygomatic–maxillary region the left index finger and right thumb are on the maxilla intraorally (Fig. 15.11).

For all movements it is important that the distance between the right index finger and the right thumb remains the same. The therapist's right elbow is directed laterally for all accessory movements. During the manoeuvre, the therapist should ensure that there is no movement of the head. If the right index finger is uncomfortably large for the patient, then use the right middle or little finger.

Extraoral unilateral techniques for the zygomatic bone

The starting position and method are the same as described above, the sole exception being that the therapist grasps the zygomatic bone extraorally with the right index finger and thumb. These techniques are useful when intraoral procedures are unacceptable because of pain, during intraoral infection or spasm like trismus. A disadvantage can be that facial soft tissue changes can hinder these extraoral techniques and further intraoral examination is necessary.

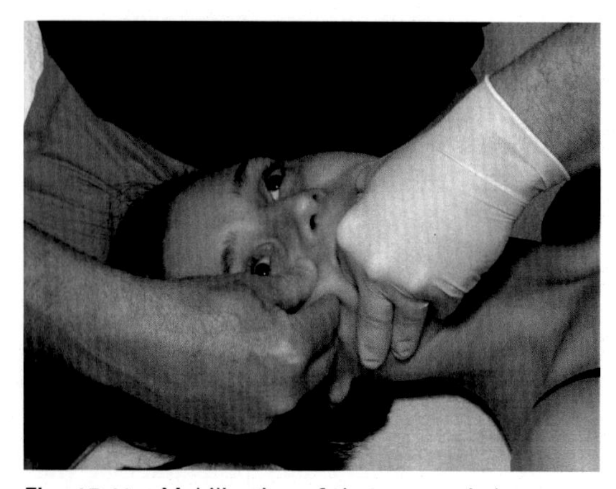

Fig. 15.11 Mobilization of the zygomatic bone with an intraorally fixed maxillary bone.

Movement of neighbouring bones against the zygomatic bone

Another possibility for treatment of the zygomatic region is moving the neighbouring bones against the zygomatic bone. The starting position is the same as described above. The therapist needs to decide on an intra- or extraoral technique and fixes the zygomatic bone while mobilizing the frontal, temporal or maxillary bones.

Growth pattern of the zygomatic bone, maxilla and the maxillary sinus

The different growth rates of the facial ecto- and endocranial regions which form the sinuses at different ages depend on genetics and stress-transducing forces on the facial bones (Bear & Harris 1969). The zygomatic and maxillary bones play an important role in this development during adolescence (Ngan 2002). Although expansion of the maxillary sinus in normal subjects results in a significant change in cranial vault length, the maxillary and zygomatic bones predominantly change the shape of the face (Babler & Persing 1982, Persing et al 1994, Tsai 2002). Orthodontic experiments show that orthopaedic interventions (splints) change the histology of the maxilla and shape of the sutures and contours of the face (Enlow & Hunter 1966). Observations from animal experiments and human studies indicate that there is a close correlation between the growth of the maxilla and the mandible (Lux et al 2002). Artificial synostoses of the orbital (frontonasal and frontopremaxillary) sutures in animal experiments imply that the growth in length of the mandible follows that of the maxilla (Xenakis et al 1995, Arens et al 2002, Dargaud et al 2002).

In the clinical setting, head–neck facial pain patients are often seen with the following patterns:

- Differences in length of the mandibular ramus
- Shortened maxilla on one side
- Nasal airflow changes

- Subjective sinusitis symptoms
- Craniomandibular symptoms, e.g. shift during mouth opening, popping, clicking with or without pain
- Past orthodontic treatment (Fig. 15.12).

Maxillary assessment can often change signs and symptoms in that region, and shows a good prognosis, especially when during a maxillary technique symptoms such as unilateral air stenosis or pain change after a few (in average less than five) sessions.

Undiagnosed facial pain in children

Children (adolescents) who have already been seen by different specialists (neurologists, ophthalmologists, ENT surgeons, dentists, orthodontists, etc.) but without being given a clear diagnosis are particularly indicated for this treatment method (Macfarlane et al 2002). Most of these individuals are diagnosed with headache of unknown origin, chronic tension headache, craniomandibular dysfunction, (pseudo)sinusitis, facial pain or symptoms of concussion syndromes (Harley 2001).

Youngsters who have had to wear orthodontic stabilizing splints for several years belong to another category (Needleman et al 2000, Bergius et al 2002). It is not unusual for this category of patients to have a highly sensitive maxilla during passive movements.

That the maxilla is an important region for facial growth which responds strongly to the stress transducer system and can cause facial dysfunction is described in the literature. For example, Nakamo (1993) proved, using dogs, that a vertical sustained traction of the teeth induces a vertical deformation of the maxilla,

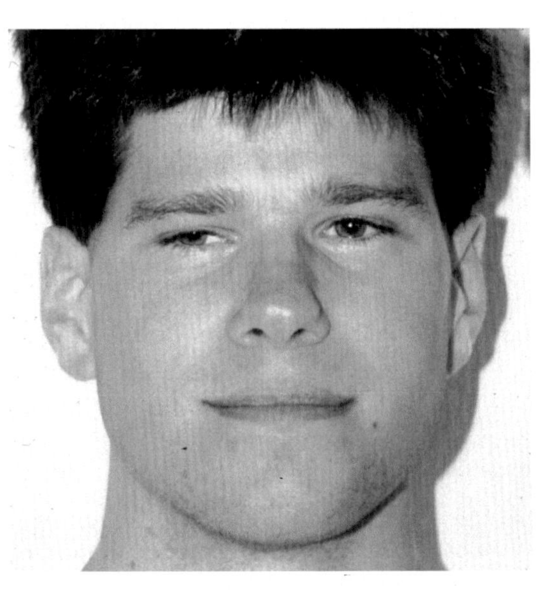

a

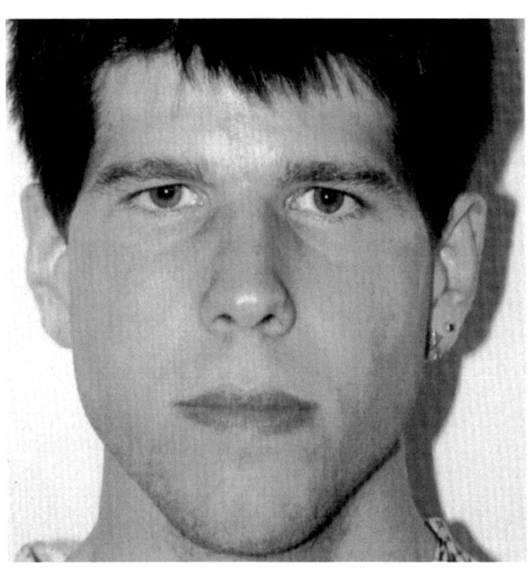

b

Fig. 15.12 Craniofacial growth model of 25-year-old monozygotic twins. The difference in form and size of their faces is particularly interesting.

a Hans has persistent and inconsistent headache in the frontotemporal area of the ear, which started at age 7, the onset coinciding with a middle ear inflammation and occasional maxillary sinusitis, dominantly on the left-hand side. From that time until he was 15 there were recurrent episodes of inflammation, particularly on the left. Head and ear pain persist to this day.

b Ron, his elder by 20 minutes, had no inflammation or related problems in infancy. Examination of the brothers showed that Hans had a clear craniofacial dysfunction but Ron did not. Hans' right orbit is smaller, the zygomatic bone is less prominent and the right mandibular ramus is approximately 1.2 cm shorter than the left. The right ear is higher. Manual therapy of the zygomatic and maxillary bones reproduces his symptoms. Both regions play an important role in this case.

the neighbouring bones and the mid-palate suture. Baumrind et al (1983) showed in humans that maxillofacial deformity is the result of abnormal force on the maxilla. Currently, there is little relevant literature about the behaviour of pain or other symptoms related to orthodontic treatment. For this reason the therapist must be aware of atypical facial symptoms in this group of patients and can use the maxilla and neighbouring bones for examination and treatment. Further maxillary techniques should be used after zygomatic–maxillary fractures, during neuropathic pain of the maxillary nerve, phantom pain after tooth extraction, and pain after orthodontic treatment, face surgery or trauma.

THE MAXILLA

Intra- or extraoral investigation of the following areas is possible:

- Maxillofrontal region (M/F)
- Maxillozygomatic region (M/Z)
- Maxillosphenoid region (M/S)
- Palatine region (Pa)
- Intermaxillary region (M/M)
- Palatomaxillary region (P/M).

Techniques for the maxillofrontal and zygomatic regions are discussed in the section on orbital techniques; techniques for the maxillosphenoid and palatine regions are detailed here.

Maxillosphenoid region (M/S)

STARTING POSITION AND METHOD

The patient lies supine and is comfortable and relaxed. The therapist sits or stands at the right side of the patient. The therapist's left index finger and thumb grasp both greater wings of the sphenoid bone, as well as grasping the maxillary bone intraorally with the right index finger and thumb, just as in the general technique for the maxilla. The right elbow is perpendicular to the patient's face to prevent extraneous movement such as rotation of the maxilla around all three axes, longitudinal and transverse movements (see Fig. 15.6).

> **!** Once again, it is important that it is the body and not the hands that create the movement. Apart from anchoring the forearm against the trunk, concentrating on the thumb, index and middle fingers will help with this. The therapist should ensure that the distance between the two fingers on each hand remains the same, avoiding any increase in tone in the hand.

Unilateral maxilla technique

When unilateral dysfunctions and symptoms are suspected, the therapist can focus techniques on that side of the maxilla.

STARTING POSITION AND METHOD

The patient lies supine, comfortable and relaxed. The plinth is at the height of the therapist's iliac crest. A small towel against the contralateral side of the patient's head can be useful, especially during rotation and transverse movements. Flexing the trunk to facilitate bending over the patient, the therapist grasps the medial border of the lateral wall of the maxilla with the right thumb intraorally. The right index finger contacts the lateral part of the maxilla and the upper teeth. The right lower arm is in slight pronation, parallel with the patient's sternum. The position of the left hand depends on which region is to be examined:

- The maxillofrontal region: The left index and middle fingers contact the frontal bone on the medial border of the orbit.
- The maxillosphenoid region: The left index finger and thumb contact the greater wings of the sphenoid as described in the standard technique.
- The maxillozygomatic region: The left thumb, index and middle fingers are placed perpendicular on the zygomatic bone.

Movements such as longitudinal to cranial and caudal, transverse to lateral and medial, and rotations on all three axes can easily be performed. During the movement a slow trunk movement in the direction of the mobilization prevents a right forearm–hand movement. The distance between the right thumb and right index finger stays the same without increasing tension.

THE PALATINE REGION

Introduction

The palatine is formed by two bones – the maxilla and the palatine – and is connected by three sutures: the intermaxillary, interpalatine and palatomaxillary sutures. Together they are called the 'crucifix suture' (William et al 1989) because of the crucifix form of these sutures (Fig. 15.13). In addition, it is richly innervated by branches of the maxillary nerve which runs through six foramina (incisive fossa, two greater and two smaller palatine foramina). In this chapter we shall discuss the intermaxillary, interpalatine and palatomaxillary regions (Fig. 15.13).

Intermaxillary region

STARTING POSITION AND METHOD

The patient lies supine, and is comfortable and relaxed with a small rolled towel in the neck (occipitoparietal region) to stabilize cervical extension when the mouth is open. Facing the patient, the therapist's left thumb and index finger cups the frontal bone. For performing the technique with the right hand, the therapist can choose between a one finger, two finger or two thumb technique, depending upon the size of the patient's oral cavity, the size of the therapist's fingers and the spread of symptoms (unilateral/bilateral).

One finger technique

The pad of the right index finger touches the palate on one side. The forearm and hand are in supination and the middle finger leans or supports the right index finger. Movements such as longitudinal with or without angulation and transverse to lateral with little resistance are indicated.

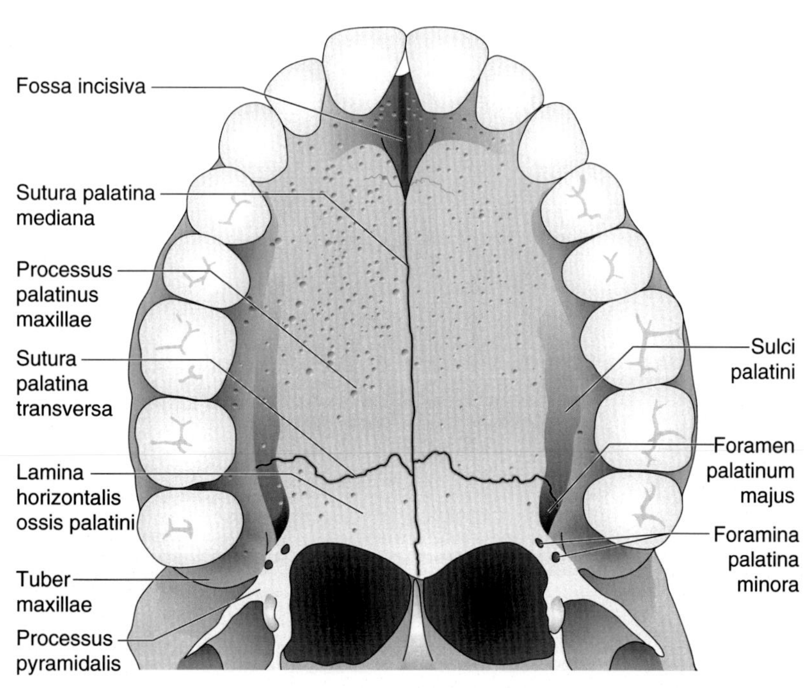

Fig. 15.13 Overview of the palate region. Note the 'cross' which is formed between the intermaxillary, interpalatine and palatomaxillary sutures.

Two finger technique

This technique can be performed in two ways: intraorally (Fig. 15.14) and intrabucally (lateral from teeth and medial from cheeks). For the intraoral technique the forearm and hand are in supination and the right middle and index fingers make contact with the right and left sides of the palate, respectively. For the intrabuccal technique two-thirds of the surface of the right index finger and thumb are placed on both lateral sides of the maxilla. General compression (bilateral transverse to medial) and rotation around the different axes are ideal techniques for this grip.

Two thumb technique

A stronger distraction technique (bilateral transverse movement laterally) can be accomplished by placing the two thumbs intraorally (Fig. 15.15). The pads of the thumbs contact the ipsilateral sides of the hard palate and the forearms are in the midline so that the interphalangeal joints of the thumbs are flexed. The middle and index fingers of both hands are able to palpate other regions during the movement (e.g. the nasofrontal region).

The best available intraoral movements are transverse laterally and medially, longitudinal to cranial, anterior–posterior and posterior–anterior. When the therapist wants to move one part of the palate, for example with the middle finger, the index finger tries to fix the other side of the palate. The forearm stays in supination without extra movement. A more intensive movement is produced when both fingers move in opposite directions, such as with the transverse movement. During this technique the left hand tries to hold the frontal region to prevent movement of the head. The pressure of the right middle and index fingers increases slowly, trying not to change the contact points (the pads), otherwise the stress within the palate complex changes. The intrabuccal position provides the option to perform a bilateral transverse movement to medial (recompression of the intermaxillary region). During this technique the patient can emphasize the movement by strongly increased pressure of their upper lip muscles.

The interpalatine region

STARTING POSITION AND METHOD

The starting position and method is the same as for the intermaxillary region except that the fingers or thumbs contact the palatine region. Be aware that pressure on the soft palate can provoke a swallowing reflex (Wilson-Pauwels et al 2002). An alternative is to use both little fingers instead of the middle and index fingers.

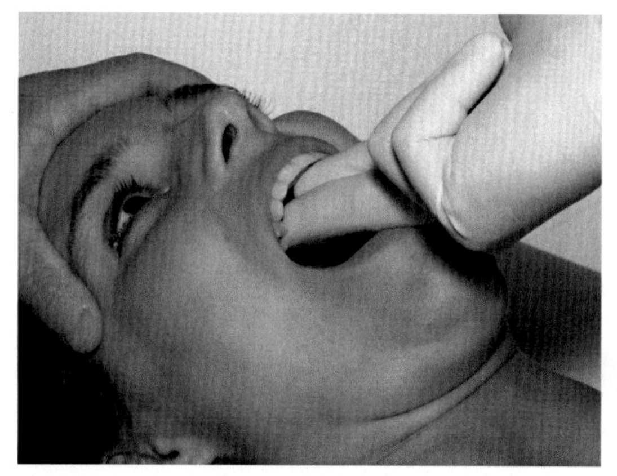

Fig. 15.14 Two finger technique in the intermaxillary region.

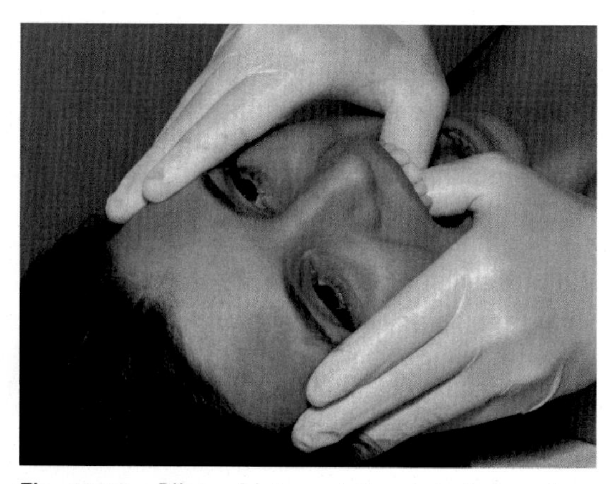

Fig. 15.15 Bilateral intraoral thumb technique for the palate region.

The palatomaxillary region

STARTING POSITION AND METHOD

The starting position and method is the same as for the intermaxillary region. The two finger technique is an easy technique to perform and generally comfortable for the patient, with the therapist touching the palate with the right index finger and the maxilla with the right middle finger. The palpation between the hard (maxilla) and soft palate (palate) is not difficult to differentiate. The soft palate has less resistance and is locally more sensitive than the hard palate. Distraction (abduction of both fingers), compression (adduction of both fingers) and rotation techniques around a longitudinal axis of one of the two fingers are the most commonly performed movements in this area.

Alternatively, for distraction and compression, the left hand can be held around the maxilla, intra- or extraorally, and the distraction and compression performed using the index, middle, ring or little finger. The choice depends on the shape and size of the patient's oral cavity. The therapist should ensure that the right hand is in supination without extra contact with other intraoral tissue. This can be prevented by only moving the chosen finger by interphalangeal extension for distraction and interphalangeal flexion for compression.

Palate and physical structure

The facial skeleton, including the palate, can take a number of different physical forms, reflecting (possibly abnormal) craniofacial morphology (Subtelny 2000, Arens et al 2002). For example:

- The palate is round and symmetrical in normal, symmetrical craniofacial growth (Fig. 15.16b).
- A child who breathes mainly through the mouth develops a rather narrow midface and has a narrow, flat and symmetrical palate (Linder-Aronson & Woodside 2000) (Fig. 15.16c).
- Patients with retrognathia corresponding to Angle class I type 1 have a steep, small and

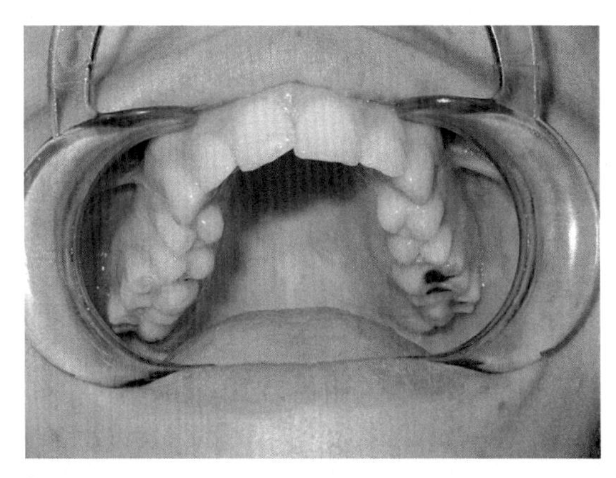

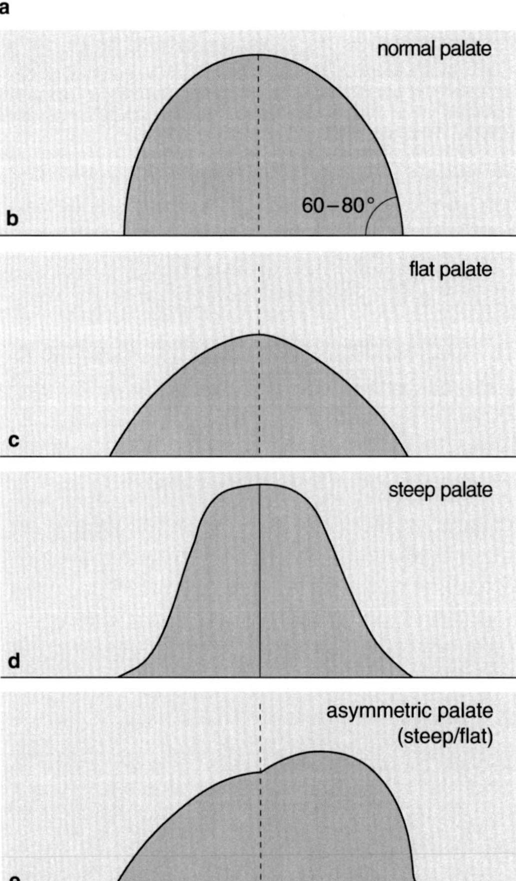

Fig. 15.16 Palate shapes and their clinical patterns.
a The therapist can judge the shape of the palate by standing in front of the patient and looking into the patient's open mouth from below.

symmetrical palate which appears as if the tongue is projected forward (Fig. 15.16d).

- An asymmetric palate (flat or steep) is often associated with an external factor causing growth disturbances, such as prolonged catarrh or middle ear inflammation during growth (Fig. 15.16d) (Harley 2001).

These clinical patterns can assist the therapist in deciding whether it is important to examine and/or treat the palate.

Palate forms and their clinical patterns

These forms are generally recognizable if the therapist stands in front of the patient and inspects the palate from below (Fig. 15.16a).

NORMAL PALATE

The palatal arches are symmetrical, and the middle of the tongue has enough space to stretch against the uppermost edge of the rim of the palatal arch. There is no need to exert an anterior pressure of the tongue to make more space (Fig. 15.16b).

FLAT PALATE

The lateral tongue angle diverges from the parallel line. The angle of the lateral part of the palate is clearly smaller than 60/70° with the horizontal plane, and the side of the tongue no longer contacts the palate. This is often seen in patients with a poorly developed midface or in mouth breathers. This condition is also commonly seen in patients with marginal prognathia because the midface has not developed proportionately with age (Fig. 15.16c).

STEEP PALATE

The distance between one side and the other is smaller and the upper surface of the palate is too steep, so that the middle part of the tongue cannot move aside. In the majority of cases, the tongue is protruded and there is retrognathia (Fig. 15.16d).

ASYMMETRICAL PALATE

Many combinations of palatal forms are possible: steep/normal, flat/normal, steep/flat. Figure 15.16e shows a steep right palate with a flat left palate, which is often seen in patients with chronic sinus conditions or in patients following middle ear inflammation during a growth phase.

Influences on the midface structures

Anatomically, palate techniques can directly influence the vomer and indirectly the perpendicular plate of the ethmoid bone (Breitsprecher et al 1999). The interpalatine techniques particularly influence the vomer–sphenoid connection because of the large movement of vomer and the small distance between the soft palate and the sphenoid bones (Ortiz Monasterio et al 1996, Subaric & Mladina 2002).

Therefore symptoms due to airflow changes (sinusitis), frontal headache, craniomandibular dysfunction, malocclusion, neuropathies of palate nerves and neurological patients with speech and swallowing problems can, in the author's opinion, be positively influenced by these techniques.

Palate and forces

Orthodontically, large orofacial splints which influence the face, particularly the maxilla and palate, can be used to direct the growth pattern. Maintenance of extraoral lateral pressure on the maxilla or crossbite corrections of the maxilla with splints is followed by palate plane alteration and exerts different forces on other facial regions (Ricketts 1960, Merrifield & Cross 1970, Van Harberson & Myers 1978, Bernhart et al 2000).

A therapist who works with palate treatment can change forces or stress which is transformed throughout the whole face. In the study of Merrifield and Cross (1970) it was shown that the zygomatico- and frontomaxillary sutures were the most common areas where forces are adapted during long palate stress (Booy et al 2000).

In clinical experience some atypical facial pain, especially in the nose region, often changes during or after palate movements. Sometimes during subjective examination, patients mention that extreme long pressure against the palate reduces their symptoms (Fig. 15.17).

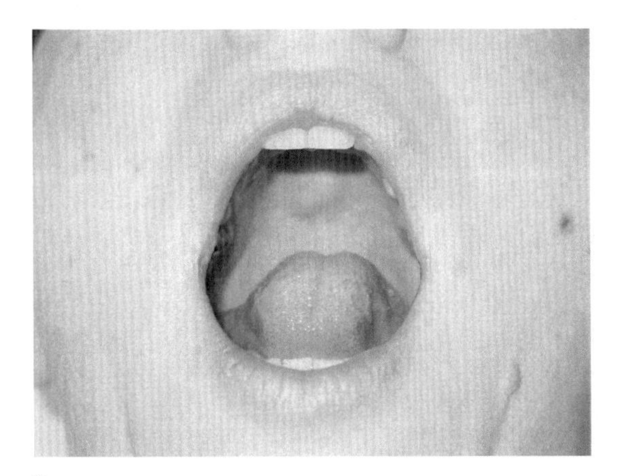

a

b

Fig. 15.17

a Woman with exostosis of the intermaxillary region which is responsible for her headache and tinnitus. Compression of the maxilla provokes her headache, distraction reduces it. Longitudinal movements to cranial around the exostosis produce a local sharp pain.

b Profile of the same patient. Note reduced maxillofacial growth.

Together with assessment and treatment with cranioneurodynamic techniques, optimal results can be achieved (see Chapters 18 and 19).

Palate and growth

Results from experiments on rhesus monkeys (*Macaca mulatta*) suggest that sutures of the midface, in particular the transverse palatine suture, may be important in the bony development of the palate during growth (Kremenak et al 1967, Ross 1987, Lehman et al 1990). Midfacial prognathism, deformities such as maxillary hypoplasia, and malocclusion (class III occlusal relationship) can be the result of palate anomalies (cleft palate) (King 1993, Rothstein & Yoon-Tarlie 2001). Minor examples of these craniofacial abnormalities and craniofacial symptoms may be changed by palate mobilization, especially using lateral and medial movement of the palate. The explanation for the change in symptoms and the craniofacial anomalies may be stress transducing forces (Oudhof 2001).

Hearing loss in infants with craniofacial anomalies is often seen (Downs & Silver 1972, Feinmesser & Tell 1976, Jones 1988, Proffit 1993). Auditory brainstem responses (ABRs) show significantly different results in young children with cleft lip and/or palate abnormalities or external ear anomalies (Jones 1988, Friede 1998). Previous investigations have reported that otitis media with effusion is commonly or virtually universally present in children with unrepaired cleft palate (Paradize & Bluestone 1974, Helias et al 1988, Friede 1998). This was investigated in young children (within the first year after birth). Most authors in this specialist field are convinced that young children with craniofacial anomalies represent an otologic and audiologic emergency (Coplan 1987, Fria et al 1987). In the clinic and from the literature it is known that minor craniofacial anomalies (e.g. minor palate abnormality) may be related to ear dysfunction and pain in older children. Generally two to four sessions are needed to change chronic eye and ear pain and/or sinusitis symptoms without clear pathology. Palate assessment and treatment can be very useful in patients with dysphagia and headache with no clear pathology (Jones 1988).

Palate and the nervous system

Minor neuropathies of the branches of the maxillary division of the trigeminal nerve in the region of the greater palatine foramen are not uncommon (Shane 1975, Shankland 2001). Deep burning oral or cheek pain can be one of the major symptoms (Meechan et al 2000). The published descriptions of the position of palatine foramen in the adult human skull have not been consistent (Ajmani 1994). Therefore, palpation with the tip of the little finger is useful to orientate where the nerve is running to prevent compression of these nerves by passive movements in the posterolateral border of the palate. Together with neurodynamics of the trigeminal nerve, signs and symptoms in the cheek region caused by a cranial neuropathy can be changed.

The sphenopalatine ganglion

The sphenopalatine ganglion (SPG) is a mechanosensitive parasympathetic ganglion that lies in the roof of the pterygopalatine fossa (Fig. 15.18) (Shankland 2000). It is intimately connected with the fifth and seventh cranial nerves and the sympathetic nervous system (Hardebo & Elner 1987, Klein et al 2001). In the early part of the 20th century, Sluder reported the potential importance of the SPG in the mediation of headaches, facial neuralgia, earache and 'lower-half' headache (Sluder 1908). Ruskin (1946) and Scudds et al (1989, 1995) described the use of SPG blocks using lidocaine in patients with chronic muscular pain syndromes in the face. Nowadays microsurgery techniques are improved and SPG blocks have moderate to good results in atypical facial pain patients (Klein et al 2001). The literature and clinical studies describe sympathetic regions in the palate which often arise during SPG blocks.

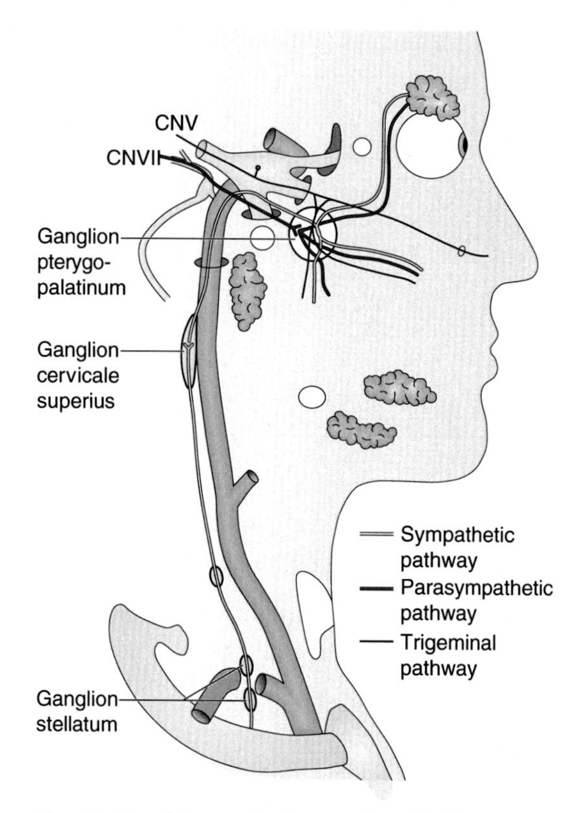

Fig. 15.18 Sphenopalatine ganglion (SPG): topography and its neural connections (modified after Klein et al 2001).
Afferent to the SPG:

- Sensory fibres of the maxillary nerve of the trigeminal nerve (CN V)
- Parasympathetic fibres via the petrosal nerve of the facial nerve (CN VII)
- Sympathetic fibres via the internal carotid plexus and the deep fibres of the petrosal nerve.

Efferent fibres of the SPG:

- Nerve fibres running to the nasal cavity, palate, upper larynx and lacrimal gland. Other branches of the maxillary nerve lie in close proximity.

Abnormal sweating in the head region, changes of muscle tone of the masticatory muscle, abnormal saliva production and tinnitus are changes that are not uncommon. In addition, neuropathic trigeminal pain without secondary hyperalgesia or allodynia reacts well to palate treatments. To influence the region of the SPG it is necessary to bring the finger in a posterolateral direction towards the posterior wall of the hard palate. When the local pressure is too painful one has to position the fingers a little more medially. If this technique is performed too quickly, immediate (para)sympathetic reactions may be produced, such as watering of the eyes, a sudden feeling of warmth throughout the head or dizziness and brief tinnitus.

AFFERENTS TO THE SPG

- Sensory fibres of the maxillary nerve from the trigeminal nerve (V).
- Parasympathetic fibres of the facial nerve (VII) via the petrosal nerve.
- Sympathetic fibres via the plexus of the internal carotid artery and the deep petrosal nerve.

EFFERENTS FROM THE SPG

These include fibres which run to the nasal cavity, palate, upper larynx and the tear gland. Other branches of the maxillary nerve are found in the vicinity (modified after Klein et al 2001).

Palate and posture

Unfavourable forces on the palate result from undesirable habits such as thumb sucking, protracted dummy use, abnormal tongue pressure, etc. These can disturb not only the developmental dynamics of teeth, joints and adjacent soft tissues but also influence the position of the head and the vertebral column (Duyzings 1959). Several authors have reported the necessity of the normal reposition of tongue against the palate (Rocabado 1992, Coste et al 1999, Ono et al 2000, Battagel et al 2002). Together with the position of the orbicularis oris muscles and the external masticatory muscles, this equilibrium of forces is essential for optimal maxillofacial growth and development (Kraus 1994, Ozbek et al 1998). Assessment and treatment (using passive movements) of the palate in children with bad postures, abnormal maxillofacial or craniofacial growth and bad habits could be a wise action. Together with treatment of the facial muscles and stimulation of the palate by passive movements, the somatosensory cortex receives new information which may contribute to normal maxillofacial development and posture (Morales 1991, Ramachandran & Blakesee 2000).

It can also been used for educational purposes. The patient can break bad orofacial habits and stimulate new functions of the orofacial region. Together with attention paid to the rest of the body, posture can be positively influenced.

SUMMARY

- This chapter describes the main viscerocranial accessory movements. Relevant comments are based mostly on clinical features and literature.
- The quality of sensory responses to passive movements in the facial region are different (more local and severe) in comparison with the neurocranium. Accessory movements of the cranium are easy to integrate into daily practice and can be used for assessment, treatment, to prove relevant dysfunction and for further management.

References

Ajmani M 1994 Anatomical variation in position of the greater palatine foramen in the adult human skull. Journal of Anatomy 184:635

Antomyshyn O, Gruss J 1989 Blow-in fractures. Plastic and Reconstructive Surgery 84:20

Arens R, McDonough J, Corbin A et al 2002 Linear dimensions of the upper airway structure during development: assessment by magnetic resonance imaging. American Journal of Respiratory and Critical Care Medicine 165:117

Austermann K 2002 Frakturen des Gesichtsschädels (Mittelgesichtsfrakturen) In: Schwenzer N, Ehrenfeld M (eds) Spezielle Chirurgie, Zahn-, Mund-, Kiefer-, Heilkunde, Bd. 2. Thieme, Stuttgart, p 339

Azimi C, Kennedy S, Chitayat D et al 2003 Clinical and genetic aspects of trigonocephaly: a study of

25 cases. American Journal of Medical Genetics 1(2):127
Babler W, Persing J 1982 Experimental alteration of cranial suture growth: effect on the neurocranium, basic cranium and midface. In: Dixon A, Garnat B (eds) Factors and mechanisms influencing bone growth. Liss, New York, p 333
Battagel J, Johal A, Smith A, Kotecha B 2002 Postural variation in oropharyngeal dimensions in subjects with sleep disordered breathing: a cephalometric study. European Journal of Orthodontics 24:263
Baumrind S, Korn E, Isaacson R et al 1983 Quantitative analysis of the orthodontic and orthopedic effects of maxillary traction. American Journal of Orthopedics 84:384
Bear H, Harris J 1969 A commentary on the growth of the human brain and skull. American Journal of Physical Anthropology 30:39
Benoliel R, Eliav E, Tal M 2001 No sympathetic nerve sprouting in rat trigeminal ganglion following painful and non-painful infraorbital nerve neuropathy. Neuroscience Letters 297:151–154
Bentley R, Sgouros S, Natarajan K, Dover M, Hockley A 2002a Normal changes in orbital volume during childhood. Journal of Neurosurgery 96:742
Bentley R, Sgouros S, Natarajan K, Dover M, Hockley A 2002b Changes in orbital volume during childhood in cases of craniosynostosis. Journal of Neurosurgery 96:747
Bergius M, Berggren U, Kiliaridis S 2002 Experience of pain during an orthodontic procedure. European Journal of Oral Science 110:92
Bernhart T, Vollgruber A, Gahleitner A, Dortbudak O, Haas R 2000 Alternative to the median region of the palate for placement of an orthodontic implant. Clinical Oral Implants Research 11:595
Booy A, Dorenbos J, Tuinzing D 2000 Surgically assisted maxillary expansion. Nederlands Tijdschrift voor Tandheelkunde 107:213
Breitsprecher L, Fanghanel J, Metelmann H et al 1999 The influence of the muscles of facial expression on the development of the midface and the nose in cleft lip and palate patients. A reflection of functional anatomy, facial esthetics and physiology of the nose. Anatomischer Anzeiger 181:19
Brown C 1997 Sphenopalatine ganglion neuralgia. Practical Periodontics and Aesthetic Dentistry 9(1):99
Chaconas S, Caputo A, Davis J 1976 The effects of orthopedic forces on the craniofacial complex utilizing cervical and headgear appliances. American Journal of Orthodontics 69(5):527–539
Coplan J 1987 Deafness: ever heard of it? Delayed recognition of permanent hearing loss. Pediatrics 79:206
Coste A, Lofaso F, d'Ortho M et al 1999 Protruding the tongue improves posterior rhinomanometry in obstructive sleep apnoea syndrome. European Respiratory Journal 14:1278
Coulombre A, Grelm E 1958 The role of the developing eye in the morphogenesis of the avian skull. American Journal of Physical Anthropology 16:25
Dargaud J, Lamotte C, Dainotti J, Morin A 2001 Venous drainage and innervation of the maxillary sinus. Morphologie 85:11
Denis D, Genitori L, Bardat J et al 1994 Ocular findings in trigonocephaly. Graefe's Archive for Clinical and Experimental Ophthalmology 232:728
Downs M, Silver H 1972 The ABCD's to hear: early identification in nursery, office, and clinic of the infant who is deaf. Clinical Pediatrics 11:563
Duyzings J 1959 Dento-maxillare, faciale, craniale en cervicale orthopedie. Nederlands Tijdschrift voor Tandheelkunde 66:695
Enlow D, Hans M 1996 Essentials of facial growth. Saunders, Philadelphia
Enlow D, Hunter S 1966 A differential analysis of sutural and remodeling growth in the human face. American Journal of Orthodontics 8:216
Feinmesser M, Tell L 1976 Neonatal screening for detection of deafness. Archives of Otolaryngology 102:297
Fria T, Paradise J, Sabo D, Elster B 1987 Conductive hearing loss in infants and young children with cleft palate. Journal of Pediatrics 111:84
Friede H 1998 Growth sites and growth mechanisms at risk in cleft lip and palate. Acta Odontologica Scandinavica 56:346
Friedman J A, Pollock B E, Nichols D A et al 2001 Results of combined stereotactic radiosurgery and transarterial embolization for dural arteriovenous fistulas of the transverse and sigmoid sinuses. Journal of Neurosurgery 94:886
Fuchs P, Scott D 1973 Holographische Interferometrie zur Darstellung von Verformungen des menschlichen Gesichtsschädels. SMFZ/RMSO 83
Fukai J, Terada T, Kuwata T et al 2001 Transarterial intravenous coil embolization of dural arteriovenous fistula involving the superior sagittal sinus. Surgical Neurology 55:353
Gasparini G, Brunelli A, Rivaroli A, Lattanzi A, De Ponte F 2002 Maxillofacial traumas. Journal of Craniofacial Surgery 13:645
Gerschman J, Burrows G, Reade P 1979 Chronic orofacial pain. In: Bonica J, Liebeskind J, Albe-Fessard D (eds) Advances in pain research and therapy. Raven Press, Philadelphia, p 317
Gruss J, Mackinnon S 1986 Complex maxillary fractures: role of buttress reconstruction and immediate bone graft. Plastic and Reconstructive Surgery 78:9
Hardebo J, Elner A 1987 Nerves and vessels in the pterygo-palatine fossa and symptoms of cluster headache. Headache 27:528

Harley E 2001 Ear pain in children. Journal of the National Medical Association 93:195
Haug R, Nuveen E, Bredbenner T 1999 An evaluation of the support provided by common internal orbital reconstruction materials. Journal of Oral and Maxillofacial Surgery 57:564
Haug R, Van Sickels J, Jenkins W 2002 Demographics and treatment options for orbital roof fractures. Oral Surgery, Oral Medicine, Oral Pathology, Oral Radiology, and Endodontics 93:238
Helias J, Chobaut J, Mourot M, Lafon J 1988 Early detection of hearing loss in children with cleft palates by brainstem auditory response. Archives of Otolaryngology and Head and Neck Surgery 114:154
Housepain E, Trokel S, Yakobrec F, Hilal S 1982 Tumors of the orbit. In: Youmans J (ed.) Neurological surgery. Saunders, Chicago, p 3024
Jones R 1988 Smith's recognizable pattern of human malformation. Saunders, New York, p 216
King A 1993 Differential growth among components of the palate in rhesus monkeys (Macaca mulatta). Cleft Palate Craniofacial Journal 30:302–308
Klein R, Burk D, Chase P 2001 Anatomically and physiologically based guidelines for use of the sphenopalatine ganglion block versus the stellate ganglion block to reduce atypical facial pain. Cranio 19(1):48
Kraus S 1994 Temporomandibular disorders, 2nd edn. Churchill Livingstone, New York
Kremenak C, Huffman W, Olin H 1967 Growth of maxilla in dogs after palate surgery II. Cleft Palate Journal 50:1488
Lauer S, Snyder B, Rodriguez E, Adamo A 1996 Classification of orbital floor fractures. Craniomaxillofacial Trauma 2:6
Lehman R, Douglas B, Husami T 1990 One stage closure of the entire primary palate. Plastic and Reconstructive Surgery 86:675
Lepoire J, Montaut J, Renard M 1963 Recurrent meningitis caused by a congenital osteomeningeal fistula of the anterior fossa revealed by an injury. Annales Médicales de Nancy 22:1497
Limborgh J, Tonneyck-Müller I 1976 Experimental studies on the relationships between eye growth and skull growth. Ophthalmologica 173(3–4):317–325
Linder-Aronson S, Woodside D 2000 Excess face height malocclusion, etiology, diagnosis and treatment. Quintessence, Chicago
Lux C, Starke J, Rubel J, Stellzig A, Komposch G 2002 Visualization of individual growth-related craniofacial changes based on cephalometric landmark data: a pilot study. Cleft Palate Craniofacial Journal 39:341
Macfarlane T, Kincey J, Worthington H 2002 The association between psychological factors and oro-facial pain: a community-based study. European Journal of Pain 6:427
Meechan J, Day P, McMillan A 2000 Local anesthesia in the palate: a comparison of techniques and solutions. Anesthesia Progress 47:139
Merrifield L, Cross J 1970 Directional forces. American Journal of Orthodontics 57:435
Morales R 1991 Die Orofaziale Regulationstherapie. Pflaum, München
Morard M, Tcherekayev V, de Tribolet N 1994 The superior orbital fissure: a microanatomical study. Neurosurgery 35(6):1087–1093
Nakamo H 1993 Cephalometric study on the influence of vertical traction of teeth on maxillofacial bones in young dogs. Tohoku Journal of Experimental Medicine 169:289
Needleman H, Hoang C, Allred E, Hertzberg J, Berde C 2000 Reports of pain by children undergoing rapid palatal expansion. Pediatric Dentistry 22:221
Ngan P 2002 Maxillary protraction. American Journal of Orthodontics and Dentofacial Orthopedics 122:13A
Ono T, Otsuka R, Kuroda T, Honda E, Sasaki T 2000 Effects of head and body position on two- and three-dimensional configurations of the upper airway. Journal of Dental Research 79:1879
Ortiz Monasterio F, Molina F, Sigler A, Dahan P, Alvarez L 1996 Maxillary growth in children after early facial bipartition. Journal of Craniofacial Surgery 7:440–448
Oudhof H 2001 Skull growth in relation to mechanical stimulation. In: von Piekartz H, Bryden L (eds) Craniofacial dysfunction and pain, assessment, manual therapy and management. Butterworth-Heinemann, Oxford
Ozbek M M, Memikoglu T U, Gogen H, Lowe A A, Baspinar E 1998 Oropharyngeal airway dimensions and functional-orthopedic treatment in skeletal Class II cases. Angle Orthodontist 68(4):327
Paradize J, Bluestone C 1974 Early treatment of the universal otitis media of infants with cleft palate. Pediatrics 53:48
Persing J, Gampper T, Margan E, Wolcott P 1994 Experimental expansion of the maxillary sinus. Journal of Craniofacial Surgery 5
Peter K, Prauter W, Seidl R 1994 Ästhetische Schnittführungen in der Traumatologie des Mittelgesichts. HNO 42:488
Proffit W R 1993 Contemporary orthodontics, 2nd edn. Mosby Year Book, St Louis
Quevedo J P, Purgavie K, Platt H, Strax T E 2005 Complex regional pain syndrome involving the lower extremity: a report of 2 cases of sphenopalatine block as a treatment option. Archives of Physical and Medical Rehabilitation 86(2):335–337

Ramachandran V, Blakesee S 2000 Phantoms in the brain. Probing the mysteries of the mind. William Morrow, New York
Read R, Sires B 1998 Association between orbital fracture location and ocular injury: a retrospective study. Journal of Craniomaxillofacial Trauma 4:10
Reher P, Duarte G 1994 Miniplates in the frontozygomatic region. An anatomic study. International Journal of Oral and Maxillofacial Surgery 23:273
Reinhart E, Reuther J, Collmann H et al 1998 Long-term outcome after corrective surgery of the neuro- and viscerocranium of patients with simple and syndrome-related premature craniosynostosis. Suppl 1. Mund-, Kiefer- und Gesichtschirurgie 2:44
Ricketts R 1960 The influence of orthodontic treatment and facial growth and development. Angle Orthodontist 30:103
Rocabado M 1992 Maxillofacial growth and development. In: Proceedings of the Manual Therapy Congress, Edinburgh
Ross R 1987 Treatment variables affecting facial growth in unilateral cleft lip and palate repair of the cleft lip. Cleft Palate Journal 24:45
Rothstein T, Yoon-Tarlie C 2001 Dental and facial skeletal characteristics and growth of males and females with class II, division 1 malocclusion between the ages of 10 and 14 (revisited) – part I: characteristics of size, form, and position. American Journal of Orthodontics and Dentofacial Orthopedics 120(5):541
Ruskin S 1946 The control of muscle spasm and arthritic pain through sympathetic block at the nasal ganglion and the use of the adenylic nucleotide. American Journal of Digestive Diseases 13:311
Sakavicius D, Kubilius R, Sabalys G 2002 Post-traumatic infraorbital nerve neuropathy. Medicina (Kaunas) 38:47
Sargent L, Rogers G 1999 Nasoethmoid orbital fractures: diagnosis and management. Journal of Craniomaxillofacial Trauma 5:19
Schneider E, Bogdanow A, Goodrich J, Marion R, Cohen M Jr 2000 Fronto-ocular syndrome: newly recognized trigonocephaly syndrome. American Journal of Medical Genetics 93:89–93
Schwenzer N, Ehrenfeld M 2002 Spezielle Chirurgie: Erkrankungen der Nerven im Mund-Kiefer-Gesichts-Bereich. Thieme, Stuttgart
Scudds R, Trachsel L, Luckhurst B, Percy J 1989 A comparative study of pain, sleep quality and pain responsiveness in fibrositis and myofascial pain syndrome. Journal of Rheumatology 19:120–126
Scudds R, Janzen V, Delaney G, Heck G 1995 The use of topical 4% lidocaine in spheno-palatine ganglion blocks for the treatment of chronic muscle pain syndromes: a randomized controlled trial. Pain 62:69
Shane S 1975 Principles of sedation, local and general anesthesia in dentistry. Quintessence, Chicago, p 173
Shankland W 2000 The trigeminal nerve. Part I: An over-view. Cranio 18:238
Shankland W 2001 The trigeminal nerve. Part III: The maxillary division. Cranio 19:78
Shin M, Kawamoto S, Kurita H et al 2002 Retrospective analysis of a 10-year experience of stereotactic radio surgery for arteriovenous malformations in children and adolescents. Neurosurgery 97:779
Sluder G 1908 The role of the sphenopalatine ganglion in nasal headaches. Journal of Medicine 27:8
Stewart M, Soparkar C 2005 Orbital fractures. In: Stewart M (ed.) Head, face and neck trauma: comprehensive management. Thieme, New York, p 59–68
Subaric M, Mladina R 2002 Nasal septum deformities in children and adolescents: a cross sectional study of children from Zagreb, Croatia. International Journal of Pediatric Otorhinolaryngology 63:41
Subtelny J 2000 Early orthodontic treatment, maxillary jaw malocclusions. Quintessence, Chicago, p 3
Tsai H 2002 Cephalometric characteristics of bimaxillary dentoalveolar protrusion in early mixed dentition. Clinical Pediatric Dentistry 26:363
Van Harberson A, Myers D 1978 Midpalatal suture opening during functional posterior crossbite correction. American Journal of Orthodontics 74(3):310–313
Wagner P, Lang G 2000 Lacrimal system. In: Lang G (ed.) Ophthalmology. Thieme, Stuttgart, 2:49
William P, Warwick R, Dyson M, Bannister L 1989 Gray's anatomy. Churchill Livingstone, Edinburgh, p 355
Wilson-Pauwels L, Akesson E, Stewart P, Spacey S 2002 Cranial nerves in health and disease, 2nd edn. B C Decker, Hamilton, Ontario
Wohlrab T, Maas S, de Carpentier J 2002 Surgical decompression in traumatic optic neuropathy. Acta Ophthalmologica Scandinavica 80:287
Xenakis D, Rönning O, Kanomad T, Helenius H 1995 Reactions of the mandible to experimentally induced asymmetrical growth of the maxilla in rat. European Journal of Orthodontics 16:15
Younis R, Lazar R, Anand V 2002 Intracranial complications of sinusitis: a 15-year review of 39 cases. Ear Nose and Throat Journal 81:636

Chapter 16

The cranial nervous system: assessment and treatment basics

Harry von Piekartz

CHAPTER CONTENTS

INTRODUCTION

In recent decades the interest of physiotherapists and manual therapists in the movement behaviour of the nervous system, including its response to movement, has increased greatly and it has become difficult to imagine daily physiotherapy practice without it.

This chapter will give an overview of the anatomical (patho)biology of the peripheral nervous system only. In combination with the results from current research this will form the basis for the development of cranioneurodynamic tests.

THE CRANIAL NERVOUS SYSTEM AS A PART OF THE PERIPHERAL NERVOUS SYSTEM

Clinicians often need to be reminded that the cranial nerves belong to the peripheral and not to the central nervous system. The following definition may clarify this:

> All afferent fibres and of the nervous system, that arrive from outside the dorsal horn or the brain stem nucleus, belong to the peripheral nervous system (Butler 2000, Hu 2001).

This includes the peripheral nerves of the extremities and the trunk as well as the cranial nerves and the dural tissue within the spine and the cranium. This becomes obvious when the skull is opened and the spine is dissected (von Hagen 1997). It will be noticed that the nerve roots, the spinal and cranial ganglions as well as the spinal and cranial dura are almost identical regarding their anatomical constitution and a differentiation into cranial and spinal nervous tissue is practically impossible (Murzin & Goriunov 1979).

Anatomical and physical features

The features and anatomical similarities of the spinal and the cranial nervous tissues may be summarized as follows.

CONSTITUTION OF THE CONNECTIVE TISSUE

The cranial nerve consists of three layers, the same any other peripheral nerve: the epineurium, the endoneurium and the perineurium. These are formed like a tube (Fig. 16.1) that provides mechanical protection and nourishes the nerve (Cornelius 2002). Sunderland (1978) estimates that the connective tissue forms 21–81% of the peripheral nervous system. This also allows for a movement of the peripheral nerve by sliding the layers intraneurally against each other (Millesi 1986). This potential expansion provides the opportunity to adapt neurodynamically at places where there is limited space such as within the facial canal, the cerebellopontine angle and the foramina at the base of the skull (Breig 1960, Lang 1995).

INNERVATION

Nervous tissue is richly innervated and is therefore sensitive to pain. The craniofacial meninges are dominantly innervated by the trigeminal nerve. The posterocranial fossa (the dorsal part of the neurocranium) is innervated

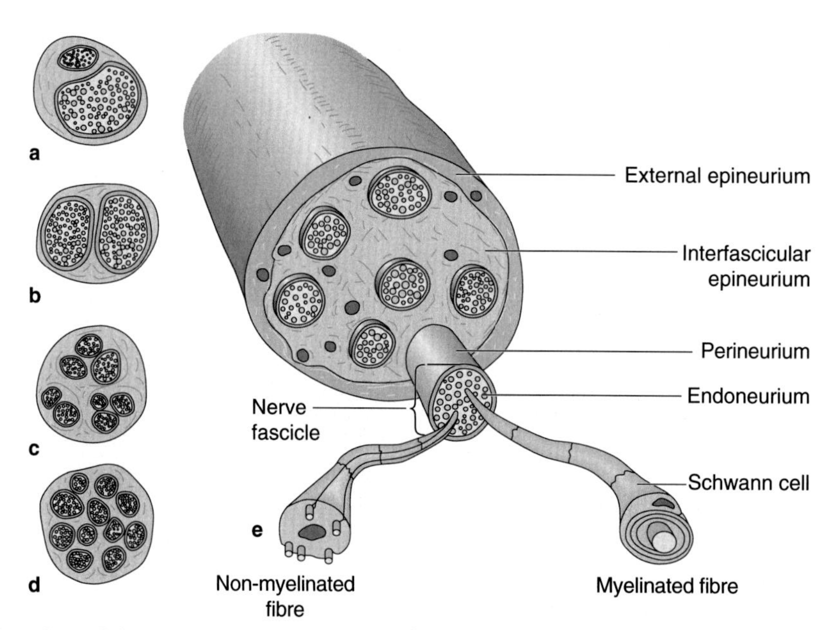

Fig. 16.1 Overview of the nervous connective tissue (after Schwenzer & Ehrenfeld 2002). The microstructure (modified from Brandt & Mackinnon 1997) shows that the axons are surrounded by connective tissue. The cross-section shows various structure types:
a Cross-section of a nerve with monofascicular structure.
b Cross-section of a nerve with oligofascicular structure.
c Cross-section of a nerve with grouped polyfascicular structure.
d Cross-section of a nerve with non-grouped polyfascicular structure.
e Components of a peripheral nerve.

by the sinovertebral nerves that run through the foramen magnum of the upper three cervical segments (Bogduk 1988). The cranial dura shows a significantly greater innervation than the spinal dura. This fact explains, for example, the mechanisms of dural headaches and the intensive pulling and pushing extrasegmental (craniocervical) pain which occurs during active craniocervical flexion (von Piekartz 2001, Davies 2003). The connective tissue that surrounds the cranial nerves is innervated in the same manner as the connective tissue of other peripheral nerves:

- Intrinsic innervation: This is provided by local axonal branches that perforate and innervate the connective tissue (Hromada 1963, Thomas & Olsson 1984). These branches are also called *nervi nervorum* and it is assumed that they play an important role in neurogenic inflammation (Sauer et al 1999). Neurogenic inflammation of the mandibular nerve following tooth implantation in older age is an increasingly common phenomenon (Janssen 2000). A physiologically reduced jaw increases the chance of nerve branch irritation due to the implanted metal that leads to a neurotoxic reaction of the inferior alveolar nerve and causes orofacial symptoms like orofacial dysfunctions and movement restrictions (Janssen 2000).
- Extrinsic (vasomotor) innervation: This is provided by the autonomic nervous system of the adjoining perivascular plexi (Thomas & Olsson 1984). Okeson (1996) indicates that patients with migraine-type headaches also show a higher prevalence of minimal cranial neuropathies that may become symptomatic.

FLUIDS

The nervous system contains large amounts of fluids such as cerebrospinal fluid (CSF) and the cytoplasm of peripheral nerves called axoplasm. The CSF protects the nervous system and the cranium against acceleration. This 'pillow of water' surrounding the nervous system in the cranium and the spinal cord also provides the nervous system with oxygen and nutrients, resorbs carbon dioxide and other waste products and is then transported away by the veins (Westmoreland et al 1994). After cranial trauma and inflammatory processes in the meninges (e.g. encephalitis), an impaired flow of CSF is frequently observed. The consequences for the local trophic situation may include dural headaches (Davies 2003, Inoue et al 2003), cervical movement restrictions and growth dysfunctions of the neurocranium and the viscerocranium (Murzin & Goriunov 1979, Wagemans et al 1988). Lumbar dural puncture causes craniodural traction with a decreased cerebellopontine angle and stress/pressure on the blood vessels and cranial nerves (Patten 1995).

PLASMA

Plasma is a fluid that is five times more thixotropic (viscous) than water. The most important function is communication with its target tissue and supporting anabolic and catabolic metabolism of the target tissue (Delcomyn 1998, Medeiros & Moura 2003). A more extensive overview is found in Butler (2000).

AXOPLASMATIC TRANSPORT

It is known that dysfunctional axoplasmatic transport and a change in depolarization of the cranial nerves influences the constitution of the connective tissue and the function of the target tissue (Lundborg 1988, Cornelius 2002).

Adhesions due to previous surgery or to trauma may therefore predispose to impaired axoplasmatic transport. For example, scarring due to facial trauma or surgery may impair vascular and axoplasmatic microcirculation and thereby result in poor function of the target tissue (Schumann & Hyckel 2002) (Fig. 16.2).

The therapist should be aware that body movements assist the dynamic function of the CSF (Nicholas & Weller 1998). Axoplasmatic movements are also positively influenced by range-of-motion movements (ROM) which optimize the transport of proteins and nerve growth factor (NGF) (Ochs & Jersild 1984, Dahlin & McLean 1986, Nicholas & Weller 1988, Elvey 2001). On this basis it is sensible, in certain cases, to include passive and active cranial neurodynamic tests in rehabilitation programmes.

BLOOD SUPPLY

Neurones are well supplied with blood vessels, which run both within and outside the nerve (Lundborg 1988, Butler 2000). They are adapted for elongation and retraction and can cope with unusual forces such as compression and distortion (Gifford 1998). They supply the nervous tissue with oxygen and metabolic substances to support normal function. The studies of Dommisse (1994) showed that the nervous system requires a large amount of oxygen: although the brain and spinal cord account for only 2% of body weight, they absorb approximately 20% of oxygen from the circulation.

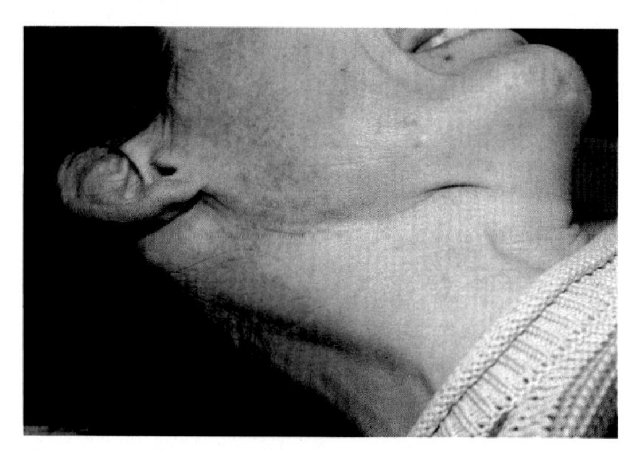

Fig. 16.2 Patient with a suprahyoid scar and adhesions of branches of the hypoglossal nerve. After 15 minutes of speaking she suffers from dysphagia and dysarthria (Photograph by Paul Kubben).

Intrinsic blood vessel structure consists of a longitudinal and a transverse system. The transverse system permeates the perineurium because it does not contain a barrier to diffusion and osmosis, and therefore provides optimal vascularization of the perineurium. The advantage of this arrangement is that normal macrolevel functional movements act as a vascular pumping mechanism as proposed for the spinal canal by Brieg (1978) (Fig. 16.3).

The same arrangement is also found within the cranium. Furthermore, the cranial nerves within the cranium have a relatively long distance to travel to the transitional regions, are often bundled and frequently encounter

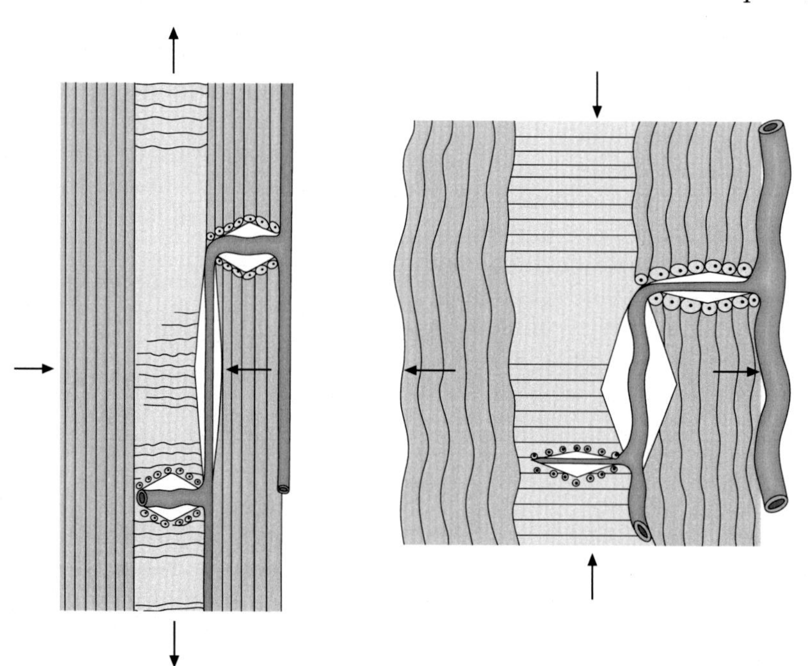

Fig. 16.3 Macroscopic model showing the effect of normal deformation of the intra- and extraneural blood vessels on nerve movement. The transverse and longitudinal blood vessels close and open rhythmically during movement increasing the blood flow within the nerves (modified from Breig 1978).

bottlenecks (von Piekartz 2001). This also applies in a narrow sense to blood vessels. Poor vascularization due to (minimal) compression and neurogenic inflammation in a critical intracranial area may have minor or major consequences for cranial cerebral function. The best-known critical area is the vascular compression at the cerebellopontine angle and the sinus cavernosus (Fig. 16.4).

GANGLIA

The cell bodies of the primary neurones are generally positioned outside the central nervous system in the sensory ganglia. The dorsal root ganglia of the spinal nervous system show the same structure as the cranial ganglia but are generally smaller and are easily missed (von Piekartz 2001, Wilson-Pauwels et al 2002). They are very mechanosensitive and may produce neurotransmitter substances after orthodrome and antidrome stimulation, which may cause or maintain neurogenic inflammation (Sugawara et al 1996). This usually occurs after long-term compression or abnormal pressure with movement. Examples of ganglia which may cause a neuropathic disorder are the trigeminal ganglion, the vestibular ganglion, the ganglion oticum and the ganglion pterygopalatinatum (for anatomical background, see Chapter 2).

In summary, the cranial nervous tissue is very similar anatomically and physiologically to the rest of the peripheral nervous system.

Reaction to movement

The anatomic construction of the peripheral nervous system seems to be particularly adapted to movement (Breig 1978). The cranial nervous system shows three adaptation mechanisms:

POSITION OF THE MOVEMENT AND LOCALIZATION OF THE NERVOUS TISSUE

The upper cervical flexion–extension axis is ventral to the brainstem (Rossitti 1993, von Piekartz 2001). Since most of the cranial nerves originate at the dorsolateral side of the brainstem – the V to XII – cranial nerves need to adapt the most (Breig 1960, Rossitti 1993).

ADAPTATION BY SLIDING, ELONGATION AND COMPRESSION

Normally, sliding, elongation and compression occur in combination. One example is the spinomedullary angle which increases by between 1 and 32° (average 14°) on craniocervical flexion. Upper cervical flexion increases the spinomedullary angle by an average of 14° (6–32°). Doursounian et al (1989) showed in dynamic MRI that the medulla oblongata

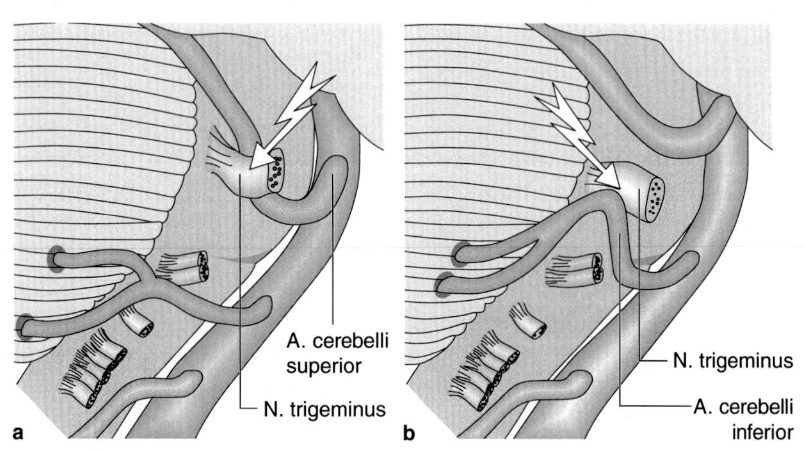

Fig. 16.4 Pathophysiology of idiopathic trigeminal neuralgia according to Janetta. The trigeminal nerve is compressed within the cerebellopontine angle by (a) the arteria cerebelli superior and (b) the arteria cerebelli inferior (modified from Cornelius 2002).

moves upwards and that the dorsal part becomes longer (elongation). Pericranially the lingual nerve (branch of the mandibular nerve) elongates on mouth opening by an average of 8 mm (Schlessel et al 1993).

CONNECTION TO THE SURROUNDING TISSUES

The human body does not show a uniform tissue adaptation to movement as, for example, does a rubber band. As the neuraxis and the peripheral nerves contain various amounts of connective tissue and are of different widths as well as having various connections to their surrounding tissues (Sunderland 1978, Lundborg 1988), different mechanical forces occur. Where the nervous system cannot adapt to movement it will compensate by pressure or pulling (Breig 1978, Shacklock 1995). Areas where the nervous system is tightly connected to the surrounding tissue are predisposed as contributing areas to neuropathic changes (Butler 2000).

The neuraxis of the craniocervical region will serve as an example. The dura is connected dominantly at the insides of the vertebral bodies of the second and third vertebrae, but not as much to the atlas. Tight connections are found at the intercranial part of the occiput and the foramen magnum (Lang 1995, Patten 1995). One can imagine the pulling forces that occur on flexion of the rather heavy (5–8 kg) head, especially given the 2–3 cm elongation of the craniocervical neuraxis from the occiput to C7 and the 1.5-fold decrease in craniocervical diameter from occiput to C6 (Breig 1960).

Other regions with tight connections that may predispose to neuropathies are those around the major occipital nerve within the occipital fascia, around the auriculotemporal nerve within the temporal fascia (Lang 1995) and the superior laryngeal nerve (branches of the vagus nerve) within the neck fascias (Gavilán et al 2002).

Cranioneurodynamics

Shacklock (1995) introduced the term 'neurodynamics' to describe mechanical and biological mechanisms and their interactions.

Cranioneurodynamics refers to neurodynamics occurring topographically in the face, the neck and the head (von Piekartz 2001). It includes all neural tissues of the craniofacial and the craniocervical region down to the third cervical vertebra. Although it is difficult to discriminate clinically, based on anatomical, biomechanical and empirical assessments that form the basis for current neurodynamic tests, it seems logical to use C3 as a cut-off point. As described above, anatomical and clinical studies confirm the tremendous neurodynamic adaptation capacities during upper cervical flexion and extension (Janetta 1976, Breig 1978, Barba & Alksne 1984, Doursounian et al 1989). It is observed clinically that upper cervical flexion (occiput–C3) is an important cranioneurodynamic testing manoeuvre. Therefore it makes sense to define the topography of the cranial nervous system from C3 upwards.

Neural pathodynamics and pain mechanisms

Chapter 1 describes how an injury to the peripheral nervous system causes an increased nociceptive input. The type of nociceptive afference depends on the localization and structure of the peripheral nerve. Two main categories apply:

- Sensory ends of the connective tissue of an unhealthy, injured peripheral nerve such as an inflamed cranial dura or an irritation of the perineurium of the lingual nerve after an implantation (Cornelius 2002).
- Abnormal depolarization and spontaneous impulses of peripheral nerves. This phenomenon is known as *abnormal impulse generating sites* (AIGS) or *ectopic pacemakers* and will be described later in this chapter (Devor 1994).

Both categories may be involved in the development of neuropathic pain and result in the typical clinical picture of peripheral neuropathy (Devor 1996). Pathophysiological changes of peripheral nerve tissue are the prerequisite for increased nociceptive inputs from the peripheral nervous system. Some facts about the cranial nervous tissue are described in the following.

Pathophysiology of the cranial nervous system

Healthy movement behaviour of the cranio-neural tissue shows mechanical features including elongation, sliding and compression in combination with optimal physiology (vascularization, axoplasmatic transport) (Shacklock 1995). This is not always the case. Abnormal forces or physiological changes, for example diabetes mellitus or serious blood pressure abnormalities, may impair the balance. This will lead to pathophysiological and pathomechanical changes in the nerve (Powell & Meyrs 1986, Dyck et al 1990). Shacklock introduced the term 'neural pathodynamics' that includes both mechanical *and* physiological changes (Shacklock 1995).

Abnormal longstanding forces, by changing the pressure on the nerve, may lead to a lack of circulation and cause degenerative changes of the nerve. This is not necessarily associated with neurogenic inflammation or pain (Olmarker et al 1995). This process is enforced and symptoms are enhanced when more than one pressure change has taken, or is taking place. If the circulation is impaired in multiple sites and axoplasmatic transport is dysfunctional the nerve becomes unhealthy and will eventually degenerate or fibrose (Lundborg 1988, Patten 1995, Wilbourn & Gilliat 1997). Other criteria are:

- The status of the nervous system before the abnormal mechanical load occurred
- The frequency, quality and intensity of forces acting on the craniofacial region, which may be subdivided as follows:
  - Direct acting forces, e.g. abnormal traction and compression
  - Long-term pressure, e.g. of the lower part of the spectacles' frame on the point of exit of the maxillary nerve from the infraorbital foramen
  - Repetitive mechanical forces, e.g. subluxation of the head of the mandible on mouth movements such as speaking and chewing which causes rhythmic stress to the trigeminal ganglion which is less than 1 cm from the temporomandibular joint (von Piekartz 2001), or entrapment of the glossopharyngeal nerve between the stylomandibular ligament and the mandible on swallowing (Shankland 1995)
  - Long-term compression. Neurogenic dysfunction and pain due to compression caused by scar tissue after maxillofacial surgery is an unpleasant side effect that is often difficult to treat adequately (Schumann & Hyckel 2002, Schwenzer & Ehrenfeld 2002). Small scars due to periauricular acne may also lead to minimal neuropathy of branches of the facial nerve and the vagus nerve later in life (Gavilán et al 2002).

Abnormal impulse generating sites (AIGS)

The above-mentioned mechanical processes may lead to degenerative changes of the nerve such as sprouting, demyelinization, ephatic transmission (abnormal cross-talk of two axons) and/or neuromas that may result in spontaneous and long-term abnormal nerve impulses. This type of impulse is called an ectopic pacemaker or abnormal impulse generating site (Devor & Seltzer 1999, Mongini 1999).

The structures that are principally responsible for AIGS are ion channels, which are produced and transported by spinal and cranial ganglia. Ion channels are small protein molecules that arise in proximity to neurogenic trauma sites and provoke a depolarization of the degenerative area (directed by the ganglion), potentially leading to further ectopic impulses (Devor & Seltzer 1999, Waxman 2000). The extent of depolarization is influenced by temperature changes, cytokines, catecholamines (e.g. adrenalin), inactivity and mechanical stress (Devor 1994, Bennet 1999, Butler 2000). This explains how a spontaneous increase in symptoms may be caused by a dominantly neurogenic source.

AIGS that may cause peripheral neurogenic pain have been identified in the cranial nervous tissue. Examples include the following:

As already mentioned, the cranial dural tissue is innervated more thoroughly by the N. recurrens than the spinal dural tissue (Kumar et al 1996). The severe, often spontaneous pain that occurs due to scarring of the cranial dural tissue and the high concentration of nerve irritating substances lead to the assumption that AIGS are very active in these structures (Schlessel et al 1993).

Ephatic transmission has been shown to be indicative for trigeminal neuralgias (Fromm & Sessle 1991). Abnormal cross-talks cause a lowering of the stimulus threshold in the neighbouring axons (Fields & Rowbotham 1993). This will eventually lead to a sensitization of the dorsal horn where the secondary neurones, the wide dynamic range (WDR) cells, play an important role in the processing of sensory stimuli to the craniofacial region. A gentle touch to the face will result in increased firing of the WDR neurones. The nervous system will perceive the information as a normally generated noxious stimulation (Dubner et al 1987, Schlessel et al 1993). Classically this will occur during an idiopathic trigeminal neuralgia but may also be caused by minor trauma such as a tooth extraction or a minimal (sports) injury to the face (Zakrzewska 1995, Butler 2000).

Other increased or spontaneous electrogenic activities are found in various ganglia (e.g. the trigeminal ganglion). These activities are also called *ignitions* (Rappaport & Devor 1994) (Fig. 16.5). A minor injury along the trigeminal nerve facilitates the AIGS in a local group of the trigeminal ganglion. If the activities are supported by neighbouring neurones due to stimulation of peripheral sensitized zones in the skin or muscle, spontaneous long-term impulses may occur leading to long-term and/or spontaneous neuralgic pain (Mongini 1999). Similar phenomena have been described for the glossopharyngeal nerve, the major occipital nerve and the maxillary nerve. This may explain diagnoses such as idiopathic glossopharyngeal neuralgia, occipital neuralgia and burning pain in the mouth (Mongini 1999).

Pathobiological changes resulting in dysfunction and pain

Figure 16.6 gives an overview of the topics in this section. Long-term (minimal) mechanical changes such as compression or distraction lead to vascular changes and ischaemia. Neurogenic inflammation may also be part of the morphological changes of the nerve. This will eventually influence the function of the nervous tissue, leading to the status of an 'unhealthy neurone'. As such, pathodynamic changes in combination with the sensitization of the nervous system will have consequences for the functioning of the target tissue (Hasue 1993, Gifford 1998).

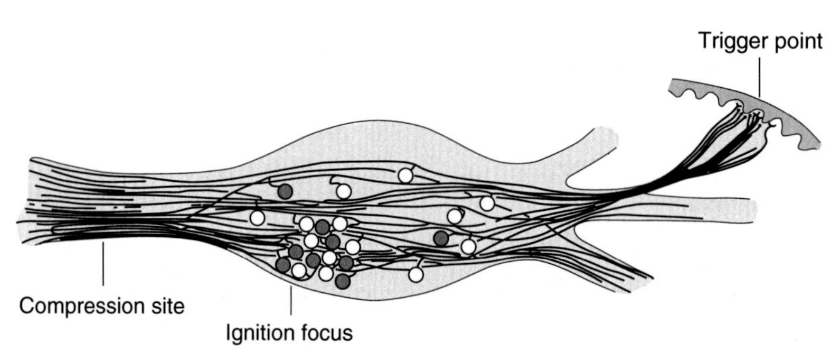

Fig. 16.5 The trigeminal ganglion: ignition hypothesis according to Rappaport and Devor (1994). Dark circles: ectopic excitation of a focal group of axons from the trigeminal ganglion following a minor trauma of a trigeminal branch. Light circles: neighbouring neurones that are excited by peripheral stimulation.

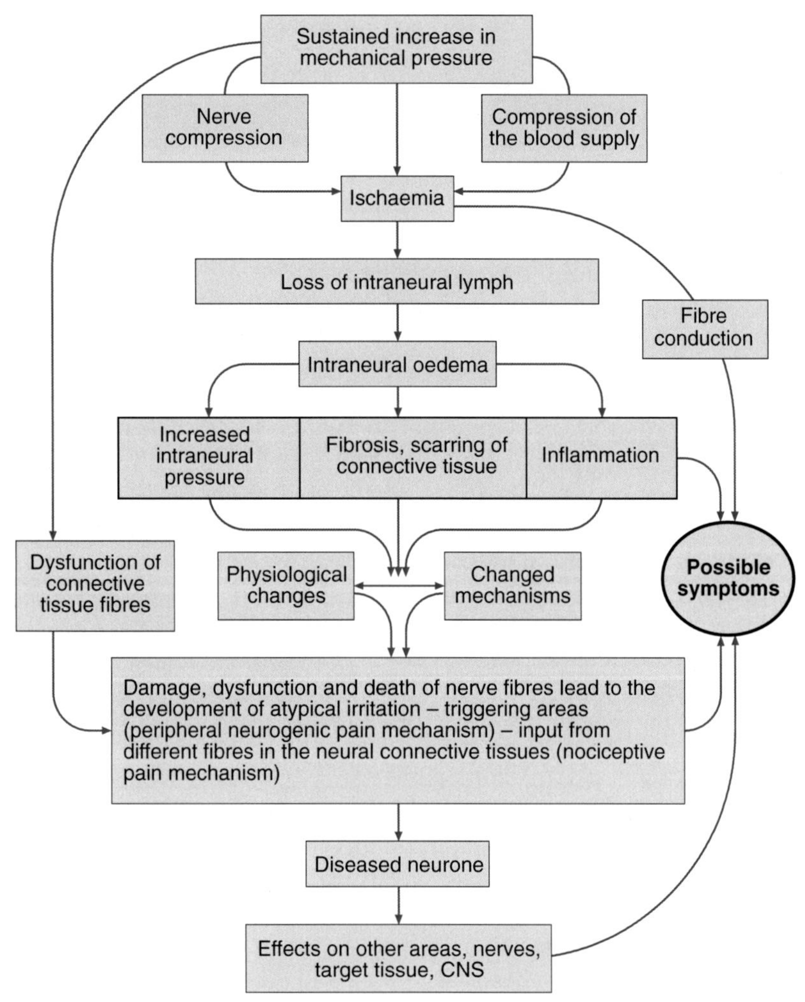

Fig. 16.6 Pathobiological effects of a (minimal, long-term) compression to a peripheral nerve (modified from Gifford 1998).

Modern neurodynamics and evidence-based practice (EBP)

The increasing importance of evidence-based practice has led to a number of research projects about neurodynamic tests. These can be summarized as follows.

Most studies are based on an anatomical and/or clinical model (Selvaratnam et al 1994). Kleinrensink et al (2000), for example, examined cadavers to assess the movement behaviour of nervous tissue in the upper extremities. Coppietersen (2001) used submaximal pain (P1 = onset of sensory response) and the onset of resistance (R1) as parameters, while Hall et al (1998) studied the behaviour of the nervous tissue more effectively in an end of range situation using the parameter of muscular reflex activity (first spasm, S1).

The reliability of normative neurodynamic test studies such as straight leg raising (SLR), slump and upper limb neurodynamic test (ULNT) is controversial. These studies commonly rely on intratester reliability which is generally between medium and good (Matheson 2000). Currently authors are using various techniques to standardize the test methods and to assess intratester reliability (Huck 2000, Matheson 2000). Practically this implies that the therapist will need to standardize the test each time and eliminate external variables such as temperature, equipment, verbal information, etc.

A neurodynamic test is generally not a useful diagnostic test (a test that minimalizes the probability of clinical signs in healthy individuals as well as in the pathological group). To put it simply, after one testing procedure the therapist will not be able to determine whether or not the patient suffers from a neuropathy, and will certainly be unable to describe the localization and extent of the dysfunction. The original testing paradigm of neural tissue testing relied on the mobilization of (mainly peripheral) nerves and dural tissue. Pathobiologically it was performed to detect a neuropathy. Current knowledge of the central nervous system and its afferent inputs has shown that the wide variety of responses to afferent inputs has a considerable influence on the organism's reaction. This is expressed as different types of pain (primary and secondary hyperalgesia) and different output reactions such as motor excitations and inhibitions (Butler 2000, Sterling et al 2001). The challenge now is to put the knowledge of pain mechanisms and biopsychosocial theories together with the neurodynamic test results. This way of thinking requires a new approach to test validation and is still at a very early stage of development (Butler 2000).

There are still insufficient effect studies that compare neurodynamic mobilization with, or integrate it with, other therapy methods. The assessed population is often very small (usually between 10 and 20 participants) and the measurements vary from R1 (onset of resistance), to P1 (onset of pain). Discussions about appropriate assessment concepts and inclusion/exclusion criteria are lively and exciting (Butler 2000).

In summary, it is impossible at the present time to make a definite statement on the effects of neural mobilization.

Implications for clinical practice

It is quite understandable that inveterate theorists may regard neurodynamic tests as irrelevant and utterly useless due to their low reliability, the lack of accuracy and their undemonstrated efficacy.

Does that mean that neurodynamic tests are useless and without practical value? It has been shown in clinical practice that neurodynamic tests support the decision-making process when forming hypotheses about dysfunctions, sources and pain mechanisms. Furthermore, it is not uncommon for a therapeutic method that follows the neurodynamic concept to be appropriate for the clinical situation. The following explanations are found in the literature:

- The therapist recognizes a clinical pattern from the results of the subjective and physical examination (see Chapter 3).
- The results of other neural tests such as conduction tests and palpation increase the probability of a potential neuropathic problem (Gifford 1998, Butler 2000).
- If the symptoms and/or other responses (e.g. the conduction test results, palpation and neurodynamic tests) to treatment of the neural connective tissue (the structures surrounding the peripheral nerve) change, the likelihood increases that the health of a nerve plays a role in this particular patient (von Piekartz 2001).

In his book, Butler (2000) presents the essential features of a positive test and its relevance for the discussion. It is fundamental that the therapist recognizes the following two values whenever it comes to clinical decisions:

- A positive tests that indicates a neurogenic source shows various features including the reproducibility of symptoms, differences between left and right, support of subjective and physical data and the potential for structural differentiation (Butler 2000). This does not imply that the test is also relevant for the particular syndrome.
- The relevance of a test is connected to function and the improvement of function. The

central question in the event of improvement of a neurodynamic test is whether the patient's functionality has improved as well. For example, a patient suffers from toothache and the dentist is not convinced there is any inflammation. The neurodynamic test for the mandibular nerve is positive. If, in neck flexion, laterotrusion towards the pain-free side is restricted by comparison to the affected side, the toothache will be reproduced, and then reduced in extension. Two treatment sessions including active and passive laterotrusion to the symptom-free side with and without upper cervical flexion decreases the intensity and frequency of the toothache significantly. The laterotrusion shows an increased range of motion and does not reproduce the symptoms any longer. Retrospectively it may be said that the mandibular laterotrusion showed a positive (selective) influence on the mandibular nerve and reduced the neuropathic pain (toothache).

The development of cranioneurodynamic tests

The neurodynamic tests described in Chapter 17 are based on anatomical knowledge, the literature, clinical evidence and – where possible – on research results. Current research focuses only on the cranial neural tissue in general and not so much on its individual movement behaviour. Only anatomical studies confirm the probability of intra- and pericranial nerve entrapments. Case studies frequently claim that non-diagnosed pain has a neuropathic aetiology. To the author's knowledge, only one pilot study exists that focuses on the cranial nervous tissue. It concerns benchmark values and the reliability of the tests for the mandibular nerve (von Piekartz 2001). The standardization of neurodynamic tests as presented in Chapter 17 presents material for discussion and needs to be evaluated for its (clinical) relevance and ultimately for its reliability and validity.

SUMMARY

This chapter gives an overview of current biomedical understanding of peripheral nervous tissue, especially the cranial nervous tissue.

The main statements are:

- There are many anatomical similarities between cranial brain tissues and the rest of the peripheral nervous system.
- They both show the same reactions to movement.
- Neurodynamic tests for the cranial nervous tissue are traditionally based on the anatomical, biomechanical, clinical and – if possible – current research results.
- Knowledge about normal and pathological movement behaviour of cranial nervous tissue and the influences conservative treatment techniques may have is still insufficient.

References

Barba D, Alksne J F 1984 Success of microvascular decompression with and without prior surgical therapy for trigeminal neuralgia. Journal of Neurosurgery 60(1):104

Bennet G J 1999 Does a neuroimmune interaction contribute to the genesis of painful peripheral neuropathies? Proceedings of the National Academy of Sciences USA 96:7737

Bogduk N 1988 Innervation and pain patterns of the cervical spine. In: Grant R (ed.) Physical therapy of the cervical and thoracic spine. Churchill Livingstone, New York, p 1

Brandt K, Mackinnon S 1997 Microsurgical repair of peripheral nerves and nerve grafts. In: Aston S J, Beasley R W, Thornme C H M (eds) Grabb and Smith's plastic surgery, 5th edn. Lippincott-Raven, Philadelphia, p 79

Breig A 1960 Biomechanics of the central nervous system. Almqvist and Wiksell, Stockholm

Breig A 1978 Adverse mechanical tension in the central nervous system. Almqvist and Wiksell, Stockholm

Butler D 2000 The sensitive nervous system. Noigroup Publications, Adelaide

Coppietersen M 2001 Physical examination and treatment of neurogenic disorders of the upper quadrant – a manual therapeutic perspective. Thesis, Catholic University, Department of Biomedical Sciences, Leuven, Belgium

Cornelius C 2002 Erkrankungen der Nerven im Mund-Kiefer-Gesichts-Bereich. In: Schwenzer N, Ehrenfeld M (eds) Spezielle Chirurgie. Thieme, Stuttgart, p 55

Dahlin L B, McLean W G 1986 Effects of graded experimental compression on slow and fast axonal transport in rabbit vagus nerve. Journal of the Neurological Sciences 72:19

Davies J R 2003 Post dural puncture headache. Anaesthesia 58:398

Delcomyn F 1998 Foundations of neurobiology. W H Freeman, New York

Devor M 1994 The pathophysiology of damaged nerves. In: Wall P D, Melzack R (eds) Textbook of pain, 3rd edn. Churchill Livingstone, Edinburgh, p 79

Devor M 1996 Pain mechanisms and pain syndromes. In: Campbell J N (ed.) Pain 1996 – an update review. Course syllabus. IASP Press, Seattle, p 103

Devor M, Seltzer Z 1999 Pathophysiology of damaged nerves in relation to chronic pain. In: Wall P D, Melzack R (eds) Textbook of pain, 4th edn. Churchill Livingstone, Edinburgh

Dommisse G F 1994 The blood supply of the spinal cord and the consequences of failure. In: Boyling J, Palastanga N, Jull G, Lee D, Grieve G (eds) Grieve's modern manual therapy, 2nd edn. Churchill Livingstone, Edinburgh

Doursounian L, Alfonso J M, Iba-Zizen M T et al 1989 Dynamics of the junction between the medulla and the cervical spinal cord: an in vivo study in the sagittal plane by magnetic resonance imaging. Surgical and Radiologic Anatomy 11:313

Dubner R, Sharav Y, Gracely R H, Price D D 1987 Idiopathic trigeminal neuralgia: sensory features and pain mechanisms. Pain 31:23

Dyck P J, Lais A C, Gianni C et al 1990 Structural alterations of nerve during cuff compression. Proceedings of the National Academy of Sciences USA 87:9828

Elvey B 2001 Peripheres Nervensystem. In: Van den Berg F (ed.) Angewandte Physiologie; Therapie, Training, Tests. Thieme, Stuttgart, p 463

Fields H L, Rowbotham M W 1993 Neuropathic pain: mechanisms and medical management. 7th World Congress on Pain. IASP Press, Seattle, p 369

Fromm G H, Sessle B J 1991 Trigeminal neuralgia: current concepts regarding pathogenesis and treatment. Butterworth-Heinemann, Boston, p 1

Gavilán J, Herranz J, DeSanto L W, Gavilán C 2002 Rationale and anatomical basis for functional and selective neck dissection. In: Functional and selective neck dissection. Thieme, Stuttgart

Gifford L 1998 Neurodynamics. In: Pitt-Brooke J, Reid H, Lockwood J, Kerr K (eds) Rehabilitation of movement: theoretical basis of clinical practice. Saunders, London, p 159

Hall T, Zusman M, Elvey R 1998 Adverse mechanical tension in the nervous system? Analysis of straight leg raise. Manual Therapy 3:140

Hasue M 1993 Pain and the nerve root. An interdisciplinary approach. Sine 18:2053

Hromada J 1963 On the nerve supply of the connective tissue of some peripheral nervous system components. Acta Anatomica 55:343

Hu J W 2001 Neurophysiological mechanisms of head, face and neck pain. In: Vernon H (ed.) The craniocervical syndrome. Butterworth-Heinemann, Oxford, p 31

Huck S 2000 Reading statistics and research. Addison Wesley Longman, New York

Inoue T, Cohen-Gadol A A, Kraus W E 2003 Low-pressure headaches and spinal cord herniation. Case report. Journal of Neurosurgery 98 (1 Suppl):93

Janetta P J 1976 Microsurgical approach to the trigeminal nerve for tic douloureux. In: Krayenbühl H P, Maspes E, Sweet W (eds) Progress in neurological surgery, Vol. 7. Karger, Basel, p 180

Janssen H 2000 Sensibilitätsstörungen nach Implantation im Unterkiefer (Eine retrospektive Studie). Aus der Klinik und Poliklinik für Mund-, Kiefer- und Gesichtschirurgie. Direktor: Professor Dr. Dr. H. Niederdellmann, Klinik und Poliklinik für Zahn-, Mund- und Kieferkrankheiten der Universität Regensburg

Kleinrensink G J, Stoeckart R, Mulder P G H et al 2000 Upper limb tension tests as tools in the diagnosis of nerve and plexus lesions. Clinical Biomechanics 15:9

Kumar R, Berger R J, Dunsker S B, Keller J T 1996 Innervation of the spinal dura: myth or reality? Spine 21:18

Lang J 1995 Skull base and related structures. Atlas of clinical anatomy. Schattauer, Stuttgart

Lundborg G 1988 Nerve injury and repair. Churchill Livingstone, Edinburgh

Matheson J W 2000 Research and neurodynamics: is neurodynamics worthy of scientific merit: In: Butler D (ed.) The sensitive nervous system. Noigroup Publications, Adelaide, p 342

Medeiros F A, Moura F C 2003 Axonal loss after traumatic optic neuropathy documented by optical coherence tomography. American Journal of Ophthalmology 135:406

Millesi H 1986 The nerve gap: theory and clinical practice. Hand Clinics 2:651

Mongini F 1999 Headache and facial pain. Thieme, Stuttgart, 2:12

Murzin V E, Goriunov V N 1979 Study of strength of fixation of dura mater to the cranial bones. Zhurnal Voprosy Neirokhirurgii Imeni 4:43
Nicholas D S, Weller R O 1988 The fine anatomy of the human spinal meninges. Journal of Neurosurgery 69:276
Ochs S, Jersild R A Jr 1984 Calcium localization in nerve fibers in relation to axoplasmic transport. Neurochemical Research 9(6):823
Okeson J P 1996 Neuropathic pains: behavior of neuropathic pains. In: Bell's orofacial pains, 5th edn. Quintessence, Chicago, p 403
Olmarker K, Blomquist J, Stromber J et al 1995 Inflammatogenic properties of nucleus pulposus. Spine 25:665
Patten J (ed.) 1995 The spinal cord in relation to the vertebral column. In: Neurological differential diagnosis, 2nd edn. Springer, London, p 247
Powell H C, Meyrs R R 1986 Pathology of experimental nerve compression. Laboratory Investigation 55:91
Rappaport Z, Devor M 1994 Trigeminal neuralgia: the role of self-sustaining discharge in the trigeminal ganglion. Pain 56:127
Rossitti S 1993 Biomechanics of the pons-cord tract and its enveloping structures: an overview. Acta Neurochirurgica 124(2–4):144–152
Sauer S K, Bove G M, Averbeck B et al 1999 Rat peripheral nerve components release calcitonin gene-related peptide and prostaglandin E2 in response to noxious stimuli: evidence that the nervi nervorum are nociceptors. Neuroscience 92:319
Schlessel D A, Rowed D W, Nedzelski J M, Feghali J G 1993 Postoperative pain following excision of acoustic neuroma by the suboccipital approach. Observations on possible cause and potential amelioration. American Journal of Otology 14:491
Schumann D, Hyckel P 2002 Weichteilverletzungen, Verbrennungen und Narben. In: Schwenzer N, Ehrenfeld M (eds) Spezielle Chirurgie. Thieme, Stuttgart, p 367
Schwenzer N, Ehrenfeld M (eds) 2002 Plastische und wiederherstellende Mund-Kiefer-Gesichts-Chirurgie. In: Spezielle Chirurgie. Thieme, Stuttgart, p 403
Selvaratnam P, Matyas T, Glasgow E 1994 Noninvasive discrimination of brachial plexus involvement in upper limb pain. Spine 19:26
Shacklock M 1995 Neurodynamics. Physiotherapy 81:9
Shacklock M 2005 Clinical neurodynamics. A new system of musculoskeletal treatment. Elsevier, Edinburgh
Shankland W E 1995 Craniofacial pain syndromes that mimic temporomandibular joint disorders. Annals of the Academy of Medicine, Singapore 24:83
Sterling M, Jull G, Wright A 2001 The effect of musculoskeletal pain on motor activity and control. Journal of Pain 2:135
Sugawara O, Atsuta Y, Iwahara T et al 1996 The effects of mechanical compression and hypoxia on nerve roots and dorsal root ganglia. Spine 21:2089
Sunderland S 1978 Nerves and nerve injuries, 3rd edn. Churchill Livingstone, Edinburgh
Thomas P K, Olsson Y 1984 Microscopic anatomy and function of the connective tissue components of peripheral nerve. In: Dyck P J, Thomas P K, Lambert E H et al (eds) Peripheral neuropathy, 2nd edn. Saunders, Philadelphia
von Hagen G 1997 Körperwelten: Einblicke in den menschlichen Körper. Die Deutsche Bibliothek – CIP Einheitsaufnahme
von Piekartz H J M (ed.) 2001 Neurodynamik des kranialen Nervengewebes (Kranioneurodynamik). In: Kraniofaziale Dysfunktionen und Schmerzen. Untersuchung – Beurteilung – Management. Thieme, Stuttgart, p 115
Wagemans P A H M, Velde van de J P, Kuijpers-Jagtman A 1988 Sutures and forces: a review. American Journal of Orthodontics and Dentofacial Orthopedics 94:129
Waxman S G 2000 The neuron as a dynamic electrogenic machine: modulation of sodium-channel expression as a basis for functional plasticity in neurons. Philosophical Transactions of the Royal Society of London 355:199
Westmoreland B F, Benaroch E E, Daube J R et al 1994 Medical neurosciences, 3rd edn. Little Brown, Boston
Wilbourn A J, Gilliat R W 1997 Double-crush syndrome: a critical analysis. Neurology 49:21
Wilson-Pauwels L, Akesson E J, Stewart P A, Spacey S D 2002 Cranial nerves in health and disease, 2nd edn. Decker, London
Zakrzewska J M 1995 Trigeminal neuralgia: do we know the cause? Saunders, London, p 40

Chapter 17

Assessment and treatment of cranial nervous tissue

Harry von Piekartz

CHAPTER CONTENTS

INTRODUCTION

This chapter gives an overview of the physical examination of cranial nervous tissue. It starts with a short revision of relevant neuroanatomy. Conduction and target tissue tests, palpation and neurodynamic tests are then described in detail. The goal is to standardize neurodynamic tests for cranial nervous tissue. The tests are relatively simple to use during examination and treatment. Related literature, clinical features and some clinical examples are provided to outline some ways to integrate the new material and put theory into practice. For treatment management rationales and pain mechanisms related to cranial nervous tissue, see Chapters 18 and 19.

CLASSIFICATION

In the literature, cranial nerves are mostly classified in relation to anatomy, embryology and neurophysiological functions (Wilson-Pauwels et al 2002). In this chapter a classification is suggested which is clinically easy to use during neurodynamic testing. The tests are built on global movements of cranial nervous tissue in order to gain an impression of the tissue dysfunction without too much loading on specific tissues. Neurodynamics of cranial nervous tissue can be divided into three main categories:

- The first category is the most fundamental, giving the therapist the first clues to cranio-neurodynamic dysfunction. These tests are *passive neck flexion* and *neck extension*.
- Tests of the cranial nerves which are mostly used in the clinic belong to the second category. These tests are relatively simple and can be used to screen a broad spectrum of patients with cranial dysfunction. These are the tests of the trigeminal (V), facial (VII), accessory (IX) and hypoglossal (XII) nerves. These will be also called the 'key' cranial nerves.
- The other cranial nerves (the third category or 'particular' cranial nerves) are less important but are encountered in certain specific pathologies. The tests are for the olfactory (I), optic (II), oculomotor (III), trochlear (IV), abducens (VI), vestibulocochlear (VIII), glossopharyngeal (IX) and vagus (X) nerves.

The relationship and the amount of time in the clinic between the different categories are considered in Figure 17.1. In this chapter, cranio-neurodynamic and conduction tests and the palpation of all categories will be discussed.

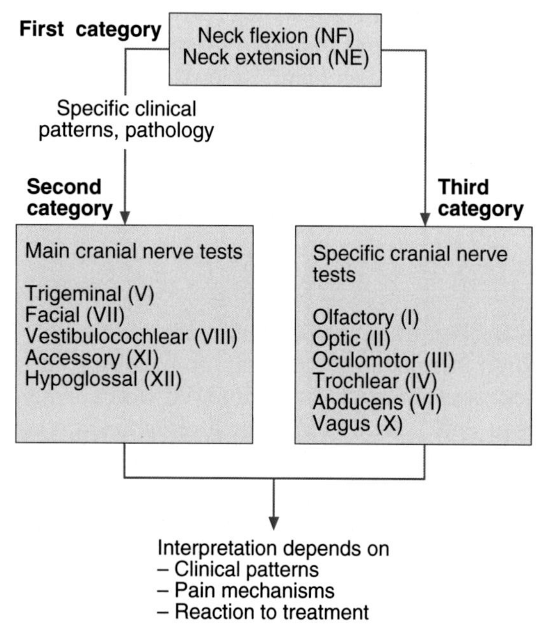

Fig. 17.1 Proposed categories to assess cranial tissue.

Note: The starting point during all tests is with the therapist positioned at the head of the plinth and the right cranial nervous tissue is tested.

EXAMINATION OF THE CRANIAL NERVOUS TISSUE: FIRST CATEGORY

PASSIVE NECK FLEXION (PNF)

Introduction

Historically, this test was used to help diagnose meningitis (O'Connel 1946). More recently it has also been used for other purposes. Neurosurgeons, for example, use passive sustained neck flexion to alleviate stress on specific intracranial tissue during suboccipital surgery (Doursonian et al 1989). Cadaver studies show what therapists have hypothesized in practice: that passive neck flexion moves the meninges in the lumbar spine, as well as moving and tensing the sciatic tract (Breig 1976, Jannetta 1990).

The last decade has seen development of studies on neurodynamics of cranial tissue during lateroflexion in addition to other tests (see Chapter 16). In all cadaver studies and also in clinical computed tomography/magnetic resonance imaging (CT/MRI) studies (Penning 1968, Doursonian et al 1989), it is clear that upper cervical flexion is specifically responsible for creating marked amounts of elongation, sliding and compression of the cranial nervous tissue in the dorsal region of the cranium. In addition, the prepontine and premedullary spaces appear to become narrower in flexion whereas during extension the diameter of the spinal cord in the craniocervical region is 3–5 mm larger (Breig 1960).

Using magnetic resonance imaging, Doursonian et al (1989) found in 18 asymptomatic subjects that the spinomedullary angle from neutral to flexion changes on average 14° (range 1–32°) (Fig. 17.2a).

Passive neck flexion is an oft-forgotten standard neurodynamic test for examining the musculoskeletal system. For the therapist who sees patients with craniofacial dysfunction and

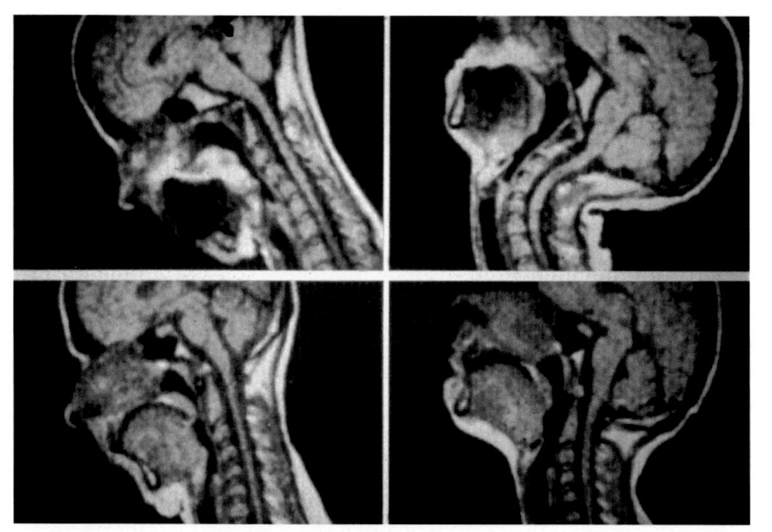

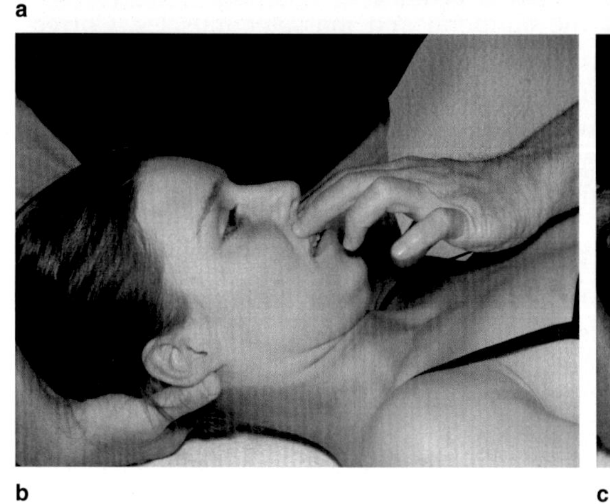

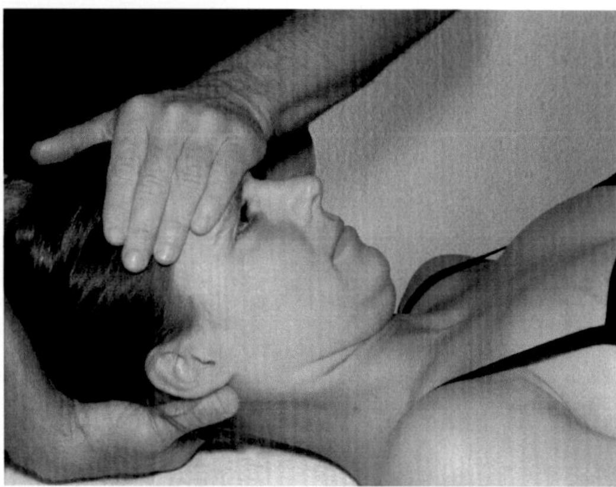

Fig. 17.2 a Magnetic resonance imaging (MRI) of the cervical spine in neutral and upper cervical flexion. Note the changes at the dorsal side of the brainstem (upper right). b and c Variations of passive neck reflection.

pain, this test is extremely important as a basic test before going on to examine cranial nervous tissue further.

The neck flexion described here is a standard test for detailed examination of the cranial nervous tissue. For the general neurodynamic test related to the musculoskeletal system, see the work of Butler (2000).

Starting position and method

The patient lies supine, preferably without a pillow but without extension of the head. The patient's arms are by the sides and the legs are together. The patient's mouth should be slightly open so that the masticatory muscles are relaxed and the tip of the tongue is visible. The right hand of the therapist cups around the occipital bone. The middle and/or ring finger of the right hand makes contact with the dorsal part of the parietal bone and the lower arm rests on the table. The left hand makes contact with the maxillary region with the middle and index fingers under the nose without grasping the mandible to make the test more comfortable for the patient and to exclude possible unpleasant reactions during the test (Fig. 17.2b). In this starting position the mandible is prevented from unnecessary mechanical stress. An alternative way of testing passive neck flexion, especially in hypersensitive tissue in this area, is to position the left hand on the forehead (Fig. 17.2c).

Both hands make a smooth simultaneously coupled movement around an artificial axis in the dorsocaudal region of the cranium so that a head-on-neck movement is performed. During the passive neck flexion care should be taken that the patient does not actively assist the manoeuvre. The fingers placed on the maxilla can guide the patient's movements in the required direction, for example lateroflexion, rotation or upper cervical flexion, so that an optimal movement is achieved. Furthermore, this grip enables the therapist to obtain verbal and non-verbal information. Some of the non-verbal clues to cranial tissue involvement might concern the eyes, tongue, mandible and mimic musculature.

EYES

- Widened pupils during the test can indicate physical dysfunction of cranial tissue in the dorsal intracranial region or result from a sympathetic reaction (Butler 2000).
- Abnormal reactions such as diplopia or extreme deviation of one eye can be relevant.
- A common pattern of lateralization of one eye – called exotropia (Lang 2000) – is often seen in chronic whiplash patients who can exhibit neuropathic changes of the intracranial tissue during flexion of the cervical spine. In addition, the dura and cervical spine should be considered as possible sources of abnormal eye position and movements (Brown 1995, Gorman 1995a, 1995b).
- Sometimes nystagmus is seen during flexion. It may be necessary to rethink a diagnosis if, on examination, there is strong resistance or spasm in the neck extensors at the same time as nystagmus. Benign tumours in the middle ear can cause these kinds of symptoms (Lang 1995). Furthermore it gives a reason to examine the neurodynamics of the vestibulocochlear nerve for clues that suggest an extreme pathology.

THE TONGUE

Lateral deviation or fasciculation of the tongue during or at the end of the passive neck flexion can be a relevant sign for possible physical dysfunction, especially of the hypoglossal nerve. If there are no obvious indications of abnormal changes it is possible to further monitor lateral deviation by asking the patient to put their tongue out, or to apply a spatula to the lateral side of the tongue (see 'Hypoglossal nerve', p. 489).

MANDIBLE

The mandible may laterally deviate or even protrude during passive neck flexion. This can be an abnormal habit but also an antalgic movement adaptation of the mechanical interface tissue of the longest branch of the mandibular nerve, the lingual nerve (Arzouman et al 1993, Jacobson et al 1998). The therapist needs to be aware of any changes in the tone of the masticatory muscles, especially parts of the temporal and masseter muscles. Correction of the mandibular deviation will often increase the tone of these masticatory muscles which means that this deviation is a relevant protective deformity (Maitland et al 2001, von Piekartz et al 2001).

FACIAL MUSCLES

It is not uncommon for patients' facial expression to change during neck flexion without this being painful. Some superficial nerve branches in the face can be involved or facial expression can be a sign of serious intracranial pathodynamics where the facial nerve is a contributing factor (see below for the facial nerve test).

Comment

Neck flexion has to be seen as the basic standard test not only in a more acute state of tissue injury but also in chronic ongoing pain states where relevant physical dysfunction of the nervous system is suspected. Once neck flexion has been tested it is possible to proceed to a specific cranial neurodynamic test, where it is necessary to add further neurodynamic manoeuvres (Fig. 17.3). Some variations may be:

- Addition of lower cervical flexion, lateroflexion or rotation during or at the end of the manoeuvre.
- A change in the order of movement, e.g. first loading in lateroflexion and then in flexion.

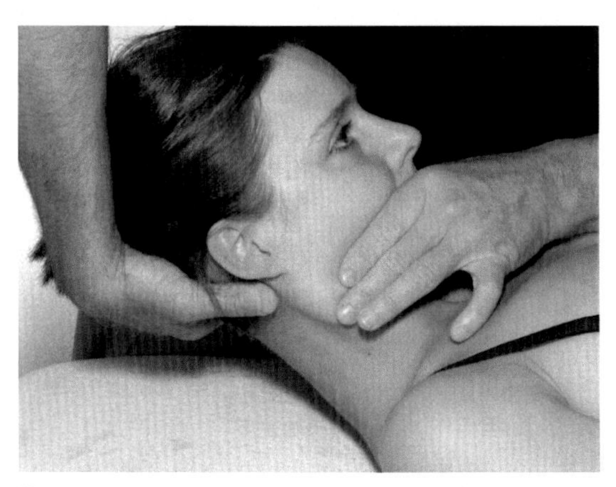

Fig. 17.3 Neck flexion with lower cervical flexion.

Lower cervical flexion (flexion of the cervicothoracic region) can sometimes be very useful to include initially to obtain more loading on the cranial nervous tissue. This can be especially useful in patients with an antalgic forward head posture where the flexion position provokes the head symptoms.

- Addition of standard neurodynamic tests for the rest of the body such as straight leg raising (SLR), the upper limb neurodynamic test (ULNT), or the slump test (Elvey 1986) (Case study 1).

Case study 1

A 26-year-old man presents with tinnitus and a dull right unilateral facial ache which increases during computer work. His screen was on the right side of his desk.

During testing of the sensitivity of the craniofacial structures, neck flexion together with lateroflexion to the left was a little bit tight but did not provoke the 'dull' ache. During slump in neck flexion plus lateroflexion to the left the frequency of the tinnitus changed and the dull facial pain slowly decreased. The patient avoided upper cervical extension.

It is evident from this test that a more detailed examination of the cranial nervous tissue is required using the slump test.

PASSIVE NECK EXTENSION (PNE)

Neck extension is a test that is less of a routine test than neck flexion but can give useful information (Grant 1988, Butler 1991). The neural and neural-innervated tissue of the dorsal intracranial and upper cervical regions shows a tendency to glide caudally on passive extension (Schlessel et al 1993). Passive extension can be useful as a basic cranial neurodynamic test if extension is observed as a relevant sign during the subjective examination. For example, post-whiplash patients or hemiplegics (both groups having upper cervical extension) often present.

STARTING POSITION AND METHOD

The starting position is similar to the neck flexion starting position with a change to the positioning of the hand cupping the occiput and the left hand touching the frontal region. The right forearm is in supination, with the hand cupping the occipitoparietal region. It is usually more convenient if the treatment plinth is raised slightly for this manoeuvre and the therapist kneels beside the patient. The neck is then extended from a previously flexed position.

Comment

Some variations are possible and the same kind of non-verbal signs may be present. An awareness of changes in other structures such as the cervical spine, vertebral artery and the sympathetic ganglions chains is useful here. Structural differentiation related to neck extension alone is difficult (Bogduk 1982, Fukui et al 1996). Further tests are required to assess the possible sources.

CRANIOCERVICAL DYSTONIA AND THE ASSESSMENT OF PNF AND PNE

Neck flexion and extension are often severely restricted or painful in patients with neurological pathology, and particularly in patients with craniocervical dystonia. Dystonia is not described as a pathology but as a neurological syndrome that is recognized by sustained muscle contraction, repetitive movements and abnormal posture (Fahn 1988). In the last 10 years dystonia in the head and neck region has been attributed to different diagnoses, for example cranial dystonia, cervical dystonia, cervical–facial dystonia and otomandibular dystonia (Csala & Deuschl 1994). This is due to the variety of areas of localization and the combination of symptoms. Nowadays the term is more generalized as a clinical pattern called craniocervical dystonia (CCD) which is more widely recognized by therapists from different disciplines (Jankovic et al 1991, Tarsy 1998).

From a neuroscientific approach it is known that the primary cause of CCD is neurobiological changes in the basal ganglion which might be genetic or acquired. Table 17.1 gives a general overview of the classification incidence and gender-specific incidence of CCD.

CCD is often accompanied by pain which is dominantly nociceptive and/or peripheral neurogenic. This can lead to primary and secondary hyperalgesia which can have an effect on conditioned reflexes of increase of muscle tone and spasm (Wall & Melzack 1994, Okeson 1995, Ertekin et al 2002). During this increase in muscle tone, there is a risk of neuropathies of nerves directly contacting these muscles because of changes of the neural container. The occipital, accessory (IX) and the trigeminal (V) nerves are most frequently involved (Thompson & Carroll 1983, Nook 1985). Some general features seen in CCD are accompanied by pain during treatment and examination of passive neck flexion, extension and lateroflexion (Case study 2).

Table 17.1 General overview of the classification incidence and gender incidence of craniocervical dystonia

Focal dystonias	Incidence per million	Sex ratio (male:female)
Cranial		
Ocular dystonia	n.i.	n.i.
Essential blepharospasm	5	4:3
Mandibular dystonia	n.i.	n.i.
Lingual dystonia	n.i.	n.i.
Pharyngeal dystonia (spasmodic dysphagia)	n.i.	n.i.
Spasmodic dystonia (inner laryngeal dystonia)	3	2:2
Outer laryngeal dystonia	n.i.	n.i.
Cervical		
Spasmodic torticollis (cervical dystonia)	11	2:9
Torticollis/retrocollis	8	3:5
Laterocollis/anterocollis	2	n.i.
Segmental dystonias		
Blepharospasm/oromandibular dystonia (Meige's syndrome)	3	1:3
Other combinations of facial and neck dystonias	n.i.	n.i.
Generalized dystonias		
Generalized dystonia with craniocervical symptoms	n.i.	n.i.

After Casala & Deutschl (1994)
n.i., not investigated.

Case study 2

A 52-year-old female patient had a car accident 5 years ago. She suffered a head injury and was in a coma for 3 weeks. During the rehabilitation period she slowly developed neck stiffness, headaches and started with bruxism and grinding. The neurologist gave her the diagnosis 'chronic whiplash'. Her clinical pattern of physical examination reflects, in the author's opinion, the general signs that are seen in patients with CCD:

- During testing her pain was mostly provoked by passive correction.
- During testing spasm of the antagonist was increased (in this case, the deep neck extensors during flexion).
- Hypertrophy of the sternocleidomastoid muscle (Fig. 17.4).
- Upper cervical flexion was restricted and through range passive neck extension and flexion were without pain but with resistance.
- Neck stiffness and headaches were changed during movement.
- Range of active movement was increased and spasm in the masticatory muscles (masseter) was lessened.

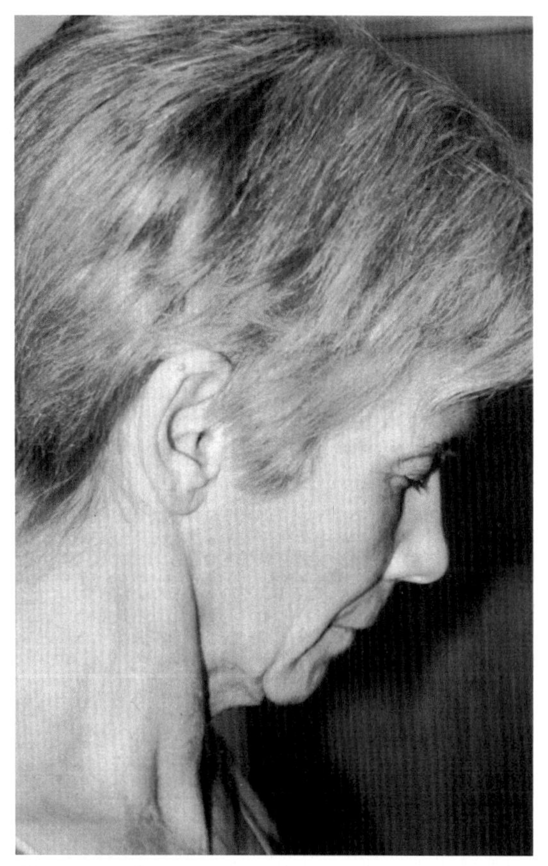

Fig. 17.4 Flexion restriction in a cervical dystonia patient.

Why, in some cases, using simple through range movement, can the symptoms change for a period? It is possible to hypothesize about why a peripheral nociceptive barrage can contribute to dystonia.

- A long-term nociceptive barrage leads to spinal motor reflex phenomena in order to protect the involved tissue. The muscle tone increases although there is a minimal load on the nervous tissue.
- A small amount of afferent information to the nervous system leads to simple motor patterns (Wall 1999).

Motor output scenarios are influenced by a multitude of factors, such as conditioned reflexes resulting from primary or secondary hyperalgesia, or by controlled reactions, influenced by higher levels such as basal ganglia and other brain regions.

Therefore passive pain-free movements give the patient an opportunity to perceive their environment, past experience, thoughts and feelings and may (in some cases dramatically) change the clinical patterns of these symptoms. These phenomena can open new doors for further rehabilitation and management.

Once an impression has been gained about upper cervical extension and flexion, a clinical choice must be made about the next nerve test. The second category tests include:

- Trigeminal nerve (V)
- Facial nerve (VII)

- Glossopharyngeal nerve (IX)
- Accessory nerve (IX)
- Hypoglossal nerve (XII).

EXAMINATION OF THE CRANIAL NERVOUS TISSUE: SECOND CATEGORY

THE TRIGEMINAL NERVE (V)

Because the trigeminal nerve is the major sensory nerve and one of the largest nerves of the head region, the functional neuroanatomy is divided into three parts; first the general anatomy is described, followed by detailed neuroanatomy of the individual branches and finally the neurodynamic tests.

General anatomy

The trigeminal nerve emerges on the mid-lateral surface of the pons and has sensory and motor roots. It runs over a prominence of the petrous temporal bone and forms the sensory ganglion (trigeminal ganglion) in the trigeminal 'cave' in the floor of the middle cranial fossa. The trigeminal 'cave' is surrounded by the sphenoid, the ventral part of the dorsum sellae of the sella turcica, and parts of the dura. The major divisions of the nerve are the ophthalmic division (V_1), maxillary (V_2) and mandibular (V_3) (Patten 1995, Wilson-Pauwels et al 2002).

OPHTHALMIC NERVE (V_1)

Relevant functional anatomy

The ophthalmic nerve is sensory, runs medial to the trochlear nerve (IV) and divides into three branches before entering the orbital fissure: the frontal, the lacrimal and the nasociliary nerves.

The frontal nerve travels next to the lateral section of the orbital fissure of the frontal bone, medial to the lacrimal nerve and lateral to the trochlear nerve. The lacrimal nerve reaches the orbit more laterally and runs to the lacrimal gland together with the lacrimal artery. The nasociliary nerve runs medially through the medial wall of the orbit via the anterior ethmoid foramen. As it passes through the foramen, it is renamed the anterior ethmoidal nerve (Shankland 2001a) (Fig. 17.5).

Neurodynamic test

The cervical spine is moved into upper cervical flexion and left lateroflexion to load the entry branches of the trigeminal nerve more in the brainstem area. The eyes are moved caudally for the frontal nerve, medially for the lacrimal nerve and laterally for the nasociliary nerve. Cranial movements can be added (e.g. to the frontal bone) which influence the neural container of the frontal branches. In the orbital region the sphenoid, lacrimal, ethmoid and nasofacial bones surround the nasociliary nerve; the zygoma, lacrimal and maxillary bones form the bony guides for the lacrimal nerve.

STARTING POSITION AND METHOD

The patient lies comfortably relaxed in a supine position, with the therapist at the head of the patient. The left hand cups around the dorsal side of the head with the forearm resting on the table. The right hand grasps around the laterofrontal side of the head in such a position that the middle, index and ring fingers can make contact with the upper, medial and lateral part of the orbit respectively (Fig. 17.6a).

The therapist moves the patient's head into upper cervical flexion and left lateroflexion using a slight movement of the trunk without extra compression of the dorsal side of the head by the left hand. The right hand guides the head movement without putting extra pressure on the orbit. The eyeball movement can then be performed using the right index finger which contacts the cranial tip of the eyeball.

- By shaft rotation of the index finger the eyeball moves caudally (Fig. 17.6b).
- For the orbit, the right index finger grasps around the orbital wall and gives small distractions and/or compressions.

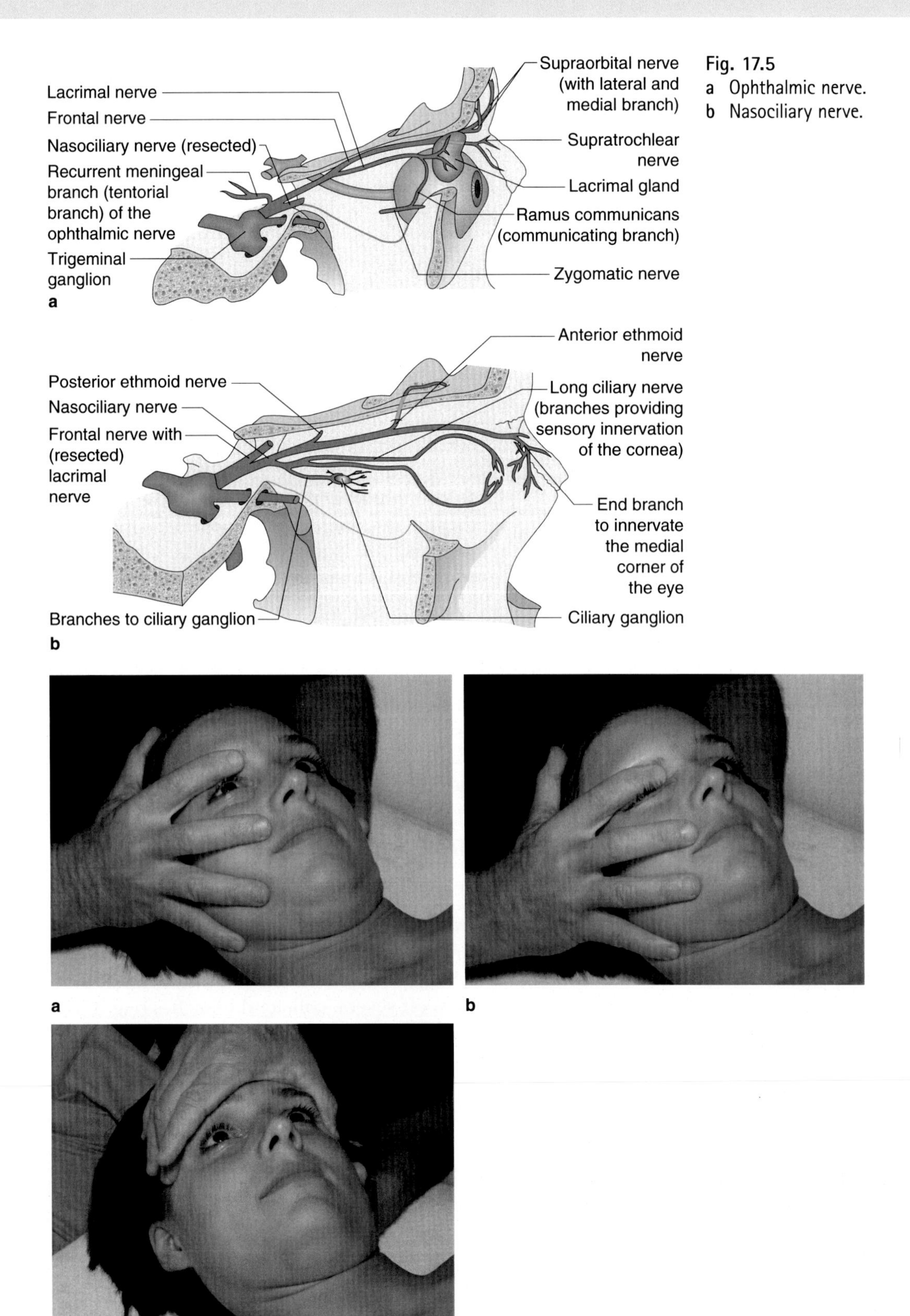

Fig. 17.5
a Ophthalmic nerve.
b Nasociliary nerve.

Fig. 17.6a–c Neurodynamic test for the ophthalmic nerve.

- For various accessory movements of the sphenoid bone, the right thumb contacts the right great wing and the right index finger the left great wing. These can then be moved in different accessory directions (Fig. 17.6c).
- Accessory movement of the frontal bone such as rotation around different axes as described in Chapter 15.

Palpation

The frontal branches of the ophthalmic nerve can be palpated in the ophthalmic foramen of the frontal bone (Fig. 17.7). A slight upper flexion and contralateral flexion of the head produces more loading for structure differentiation. During palpation in this position, symptoms are often more severe and occasionally patients will press on this spot to reduce symptoms.

Comment

SENSORY DISTRIBUTION

Because of the rich sensory distribution of the ophthalmic division the author must stress the need for awareness of the possible high level of nociceptive afferent barrage in the nervous system. This can have a quick normalizing effect in reducing symptoms, but can also result in a strong disturbance of pain mechanisms (Shankland 2001a). The intensity and duration of testing and treatment must be based on careful retrospective assessment and reassessment of the patient.

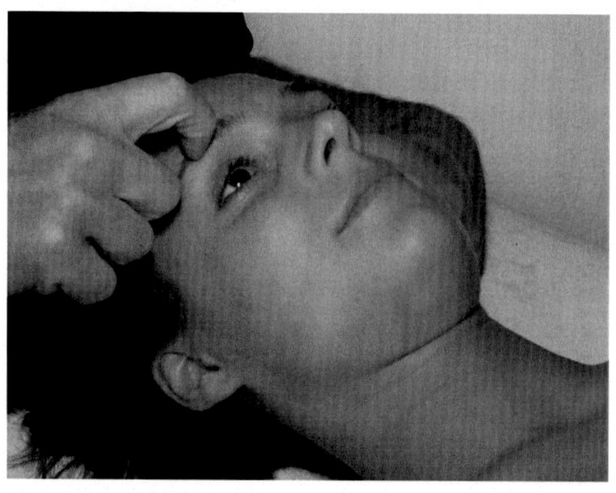

Fig. 17.7 Palpation of the ophthalmic nerve in the ophthalmic foramen.

EYE PAIN AND DYSFUNCTION

Manifestations of eye pain and eye dysfunction, such as accommodation dysfunction, diplopia and minor strabismus, will often present together clinically. Tiredness, post-traumatic neck syndromes or pain elsewhere in the body may be noted together with these problems. In microsurgical anatomical studies of the trigeminal nerve it was reported that the ophthalmic nerve leaves the superior orbital fissure. A considerable amount of ophthalmic nerve tissue is situated lateral to the cavernous sinus and maintains direct contact with the oculomotor and trochlear nerves, and together they pass through the superior orbital foramina (Umansky & Nathan 1976, Lang 1983, Soeira et al 1994, Pareja et al 2002, Tucker & Tarlov 2005). When considering minor cranial neuropathies it appears that the narrow mechanical interface (orbit and the other nerves) can influence the pathophysiology. For many patients who fit into this clinical pattern, neurodynamic testing and treatment of this nerve, together with the oculomotor and trochlear nerves and the orbit, are useful.

MAXILLARY DIVISION (V_2)

Relevant functional anatomy

The maxillary nerve runs directly to the foramen rotundum of the greater wing of the sphenoid. As it exits the foramen rotundum it gives off several collateral branches (Fig. 17.8):

- The zygomatic nerve: This nerve pierces the frontal process of the zygomatic bone. A second branch, the zygomatic temporal nerve, traverses the lateral part of the orbit.
- The infraorbital nerve: This nerve passes through the infraorbital foramen of the maxilla.
- The palatine nerves: These originate in the hard and soft palate (foramen palatinum) (Shankland 2001b, Wilson-Pauwels et al 2002).

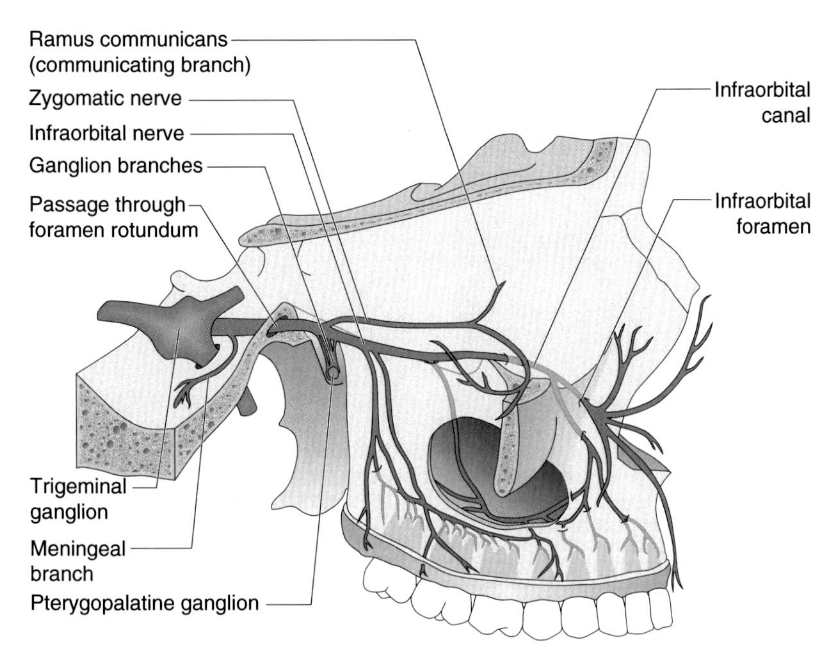

Fig. 17.8 Maxillary nerve.

Neurodynamic test

An upper cervical flexion and contralateral lateroflexion load the nerve branches around the brainstem. Eye movement must be added medially and caudally for the zygomatic temporal branch of the maxillary nerve. Cranial movement can change the environment from the zygomatic facial branches by moving the zygoma. The infraorbital branches are influenced by maxillary movements and the palate does the same for the palatine branches.

STARTING POSITION AND METHOD

The patient lies supine and is comfortable and relaxed. The therapist sits beside the patient's head, holding the head with the left hand. The right index and middle fingers are positioned on the lateral side of the eyeball while the palm of the right hand makes contact with the temporal bone region. Contact with the zygoma, maxilla and palate is possible using the same technique, so that passive movement of these areas can be performed easily.

The therapist moves the patient's head using a slight trunk movement in upper cervical flexion and contralateral flexion. A medial caudal eye movement is produced by flexing the right index and middle fingers with the palm of the hand over the temple (Fig. 17.9a). For accessory movements of the zygomatic bone, the right thumb and index finger contact the zygoma. Intraoral maxilla and palate techniques can also be added as described in Chapter 15. The therapist moves the elbow towards the patient's front to enable an accessory movement of the zygoma, maxilla and palate. To test the palate the most general approach is via longitudinal cranial movements (Fig. 17.9b) and for the zygoma and maxilla rotation around the transverse axis.

Palpation

The infraorbital area is easy to palpate at the infraorbital foramen (Fig. 17.10). Find the nerve with the most resistance and twang back and forth as if it were a guitar string. Use the same principles for the zygomatic branches on the frontal process. 'Loading' the nerve more by upper cervical flexion and contralateral eye movement can change symptoms during palpation and might be a valuable source of information.

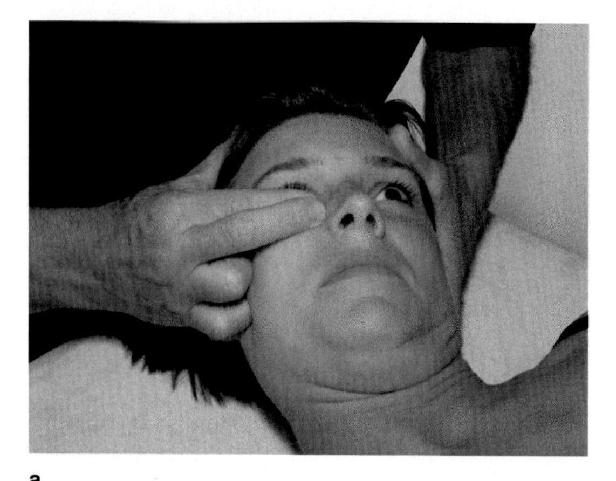

a

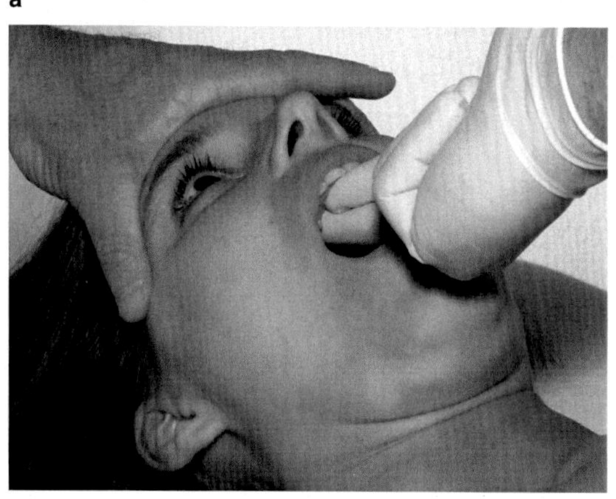

b

Fig. 17.9 Neurodynamic test of the maxillary division.

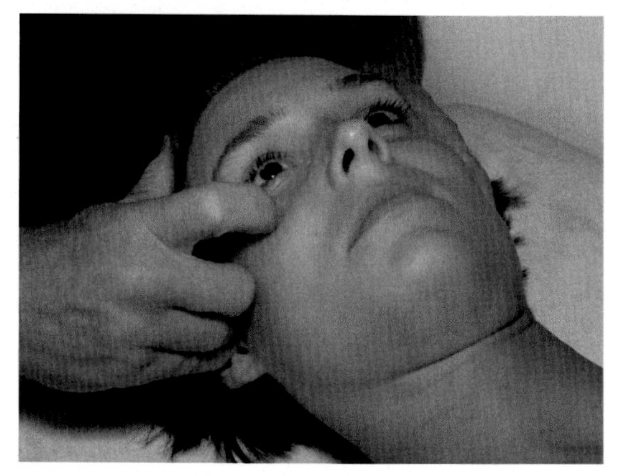

Fig. 17.10 Palpation of the maxillary branches around the intraorbital foramen.

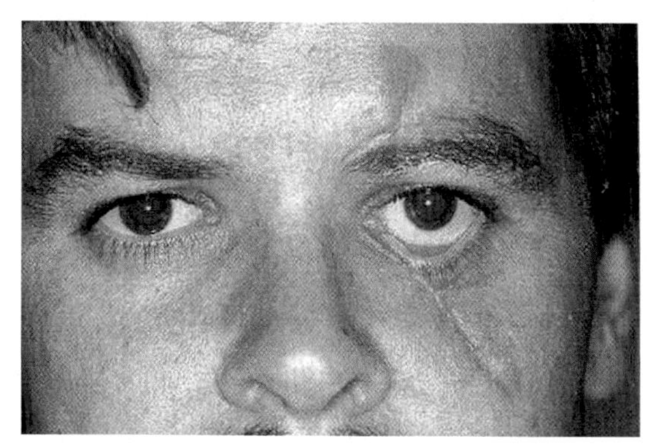

Fig. 17.11 Infraorbital scar tissue and bony changes following a maxillary fracture (reproduced with permission from Lang 2000).

Comment

TRAUMA IN THE ORBITAL REGION

Signs and symptoms which can be changed by neurodynamic testing in this region are often seen in post-traumatic disorders such as fractures of the infraorbital wall or superior wall of the maxillary sinus (Fig. 17.11). Developmental and growth abnormalities of the palate such as tooth-related problems (toothache without tooth decay), maxillary sinusitis and abnormal signs may be reproduced by other neurodynamic tests from the extremities such as ULNT, SLR or slump.

MINOR ENTRAPMENTS OF OPHTHALMIC AND MAXILLARY BRANCHES

The 'pair of glasses' syndrome describes the effect of wearing glasses that are too heavy or tight around the infraorbital, nasal rami and ethmoidal branches. Subjective signs such as hyperalgesia and sharp pain in the nasal eye region and maxilla are often described (Stefan 1994, Shankland 2001a, Schwartz-Arad et al 2004). Wearing tightly fitting diving goggles can lead to pathomechanical changes in the supraorbital and supratrochlear nerves and may bring on neuralgia. Using a stethoscope can often lead to neuropathy in the region of the auricularis magnus nerve when the stethoscope is worn around the neck for a long time. Reddy et al (1987) and others describe that after approximately 10 minutes of compression of the nerve by the stethoscope, symptoms such as a burning feeling or pins and needles can develop (Costen 1934, Shankland 1995).

MANDIBULAR DIVISION (V_3)

Relevant functional anatomy

The mandibular nerve (V_3) travels laterally from the trigeminal ganglion through the foramen ovale, which is a hole approximately 1 cm in diameter and 2–3 mm in length located in the greater wing of the sphenoid (Fig. 17.12). Because of the variety of branches it gives off as it exits, different neurodynamic loading is possible.

- Buccal nerve: A motor branch of the mandibular nerve, the buccal nerve runs a deep course through the cheek to the masseter and pierces the lateral pterygoid muscle.
- Lingual nerve: This nerve runs downwards along the mandible from the trigeminal ganglion, through the lateral pterygoid muscle, then somewhat deeper on the medial pterygoid muscle, ending in several skin branches.
- Auriculotemporal nerve: A branch of the mental nerve which runs below the head of the mandible to the ventral part of the acoustic meatus.
- Mental nerve: This nerve enters the mandibular foramen into the mandibular canal which has a length of approximately 4–6 cm. Within the canal some branches run to the lower teeth. The end of the nerve pierces the mental foramen.

Neurodynamic test

Upper cervical flexion and contralateral lateroflexion of the cervical spine is the first manoeuvre for changing neurodynamics around the brainstem. Depression (approximately 1.5 cm) and contralateral deviation of the mandible are needed for the lingual and mental nerves. For the buccal and auriculotemporal branches transverse movements medially and/or laterally are added. Sphenoid movements can influence the foramen ovale through which the mandibular nerve runs.

STARTING POSITION AND METHOD

The patient lies comfortably relaxed in a supine position with the head over the plinth, with the hands on the abdomen. The therapist grasps with both hands around the occiput region. Both thumbs are on the angle of the mandible and the therapist's stomach supports the patient's head without compression (Fig. 17.13a). The patient has to relax the mandible. The patient is asked to bring the tip of the tongue against the palate with a small mouth opening, followed by relaxing the tongue back again into the floor of the mouth, whereby the mandible stays in this position (a mouth opening from an average of 1.5 cm measured from the upper to the lower incisors).

For the upper cervical spine a head-on-neck movement of the patient (Fig. 17.13b) is made about an imaginary transverse axis which runs through the first two vertebrae. The second movement is a lateroflexion of the upper cervical spine (head-on-neck movement), whereby the imaginary sagittal axis also runs between the first and second vertebrae (Fig. 17.13c). The therapist guides both movements with the hands and performs the movements by a trunk movement in the direction that is being examined. Both movements are performed in maximal permitted resistance and/or pain to ensure optimal loading of the intracranial tissue which is necessary for the testing of the extracranial branches of the mandibular nerve. In this position, lateropulsion or lateral shift away (here to the left) has to be executed. The patient's head is held in this combined upper flexion position using the left hand. The right hand moves slowly to the right side of the mandible and the right index finger is positioned on the superior part of the mandible whereby the metacarpal joint lies under the right corner of the mouth. The right middle finger contacts the mandible inferiorly so that the right side of the mandible is covered by these two fingers.

Before the manoeuvre, the therapist should check if the patient's mouth is still relaxed and the tongue is still on the floor of the mouth. If not, the patient is asked to relax the mandible

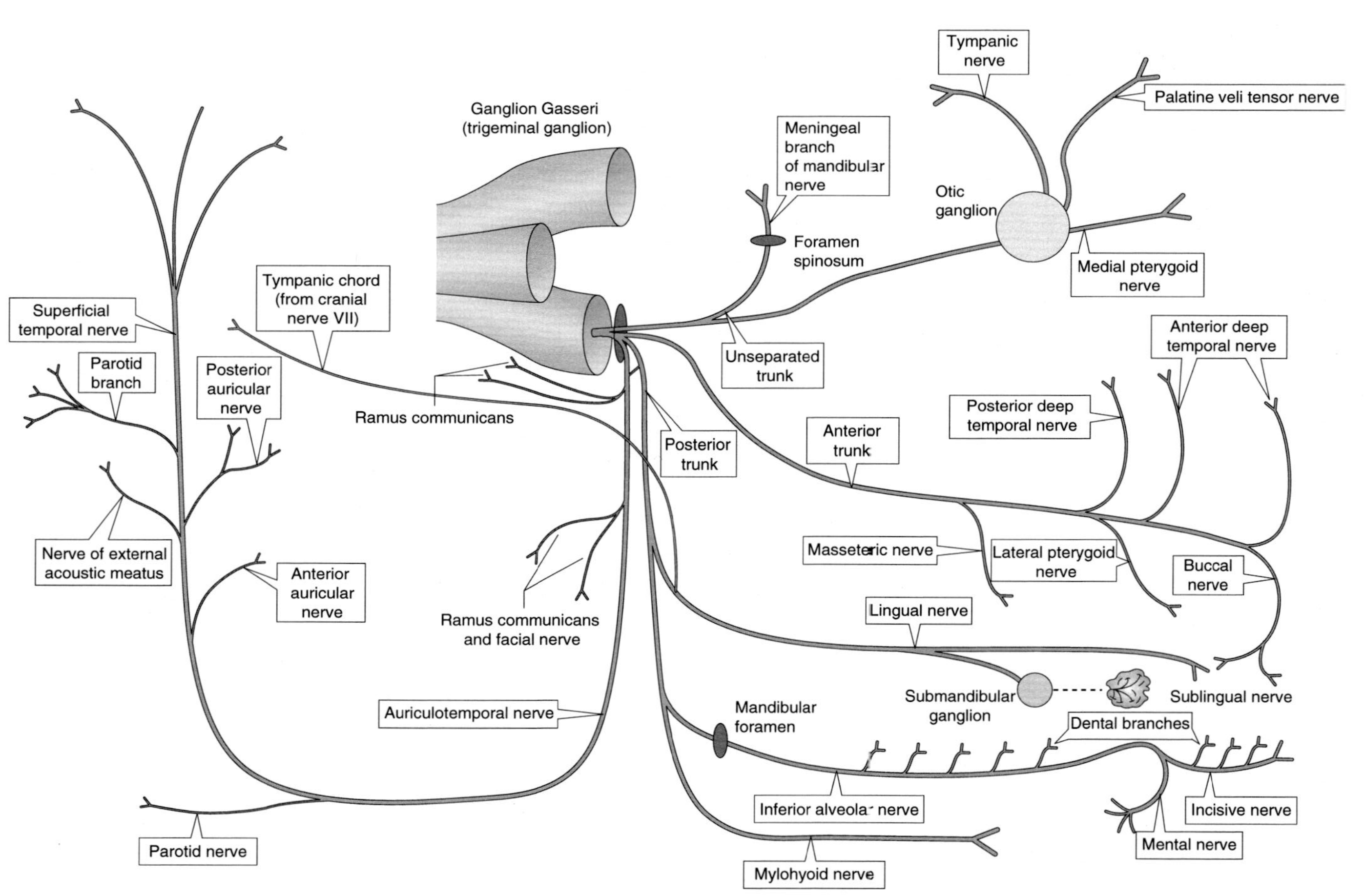

Fig. 17.12 Mandibular nerve (reproduced with permission from Shankland 2001c).

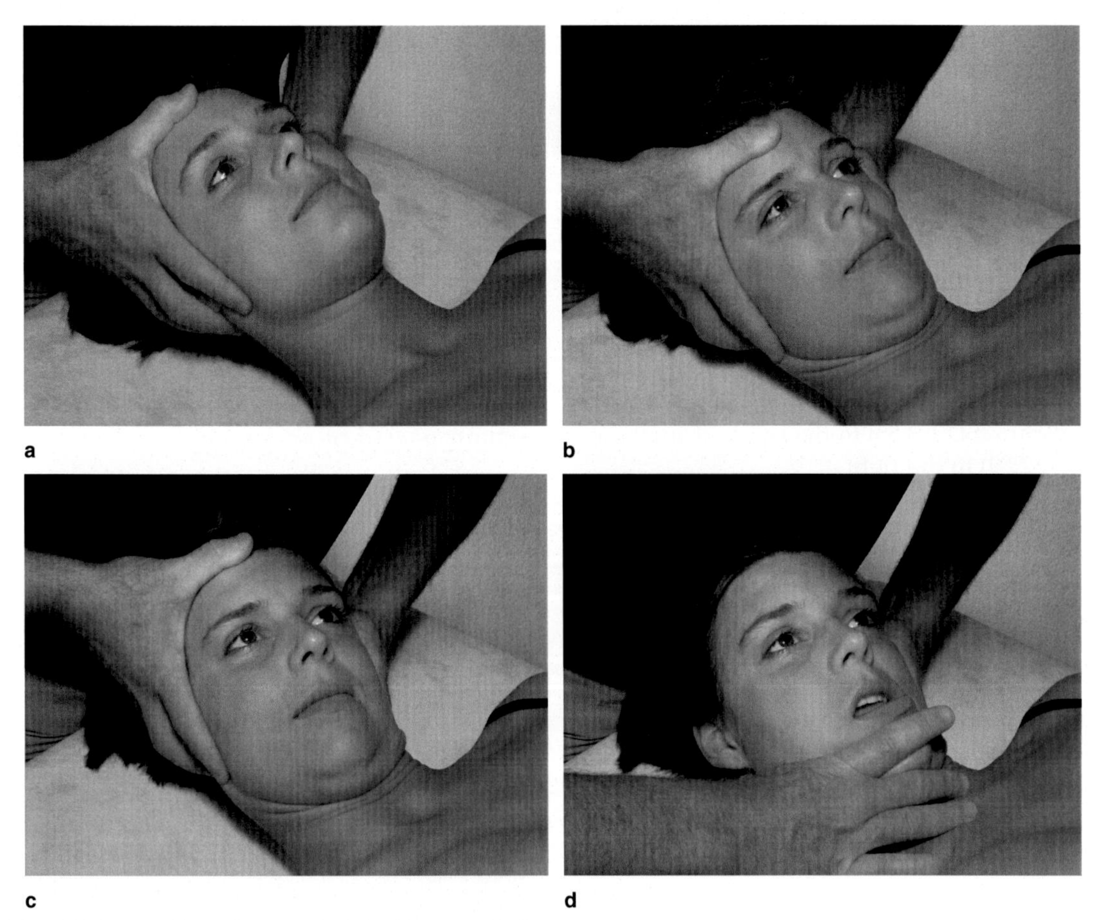

Fig. 17.13a–d Neurodynamic test for the mandibular nerve.

by taking the tip of the tongue back against the palate followed by relaxing the tongue on the floor of the mouth. If this has been checked, lateropulsion to the left can be carried out. Be mindful that lateropulsion is a curving, not a linear movement.

Lateropulsion is performed by a small body movement without increasing pressure in the right hand or underarm (Fig. 17.13d). The qualities that can be noted are types of resistance, end-feel, noises, range of movement and symptoms that can be reproduced.

An alternative method of influencing the neurodynamics is to move the head on the mandible, for example a transverse movement medially or accessory movements of the sphenoid bone such as transverse or rotation around a sagittal axis.

REFERENCE VALUE AND RELIABILITY OF THE NEURODYNAMIC TEST OF THE MANDIBULAR NERVE

The test was undertaken using laterotrusion of the mandible in a combined position of craniocervical flexion and lateroflexion to the other side. It was performed on 50 volunteers (26 asymptomatic and 24 patients with a whiplash-associated disorder) and the range of the laterotrusion, localization, intensity and quality of the sensory responses were measured. Some major results were discussed (von Piekartz et al 2001).

The intraclass correlation coefficient for the intertester reliability of the mandible's laterotrusion in neutral (without flexion and lateroflexion of the craniocervical region) was 0.72 to the left and 0.79 to the right. In neurodynamic position this was 0.77 and 0.90, respectively, which means that the intertester reliability was good to excellent (Haas 1991).

Range of movement of lateropulsion

The range of movement of lateropulsion was measured using an electronic calliper between the midline of the upper and lower incisors. The extent of lateropulsion with 2 cm mouth opening was, on average, 22.31 mm (SD ± 2.48) to the left, and 22.44 mm to the right (SD ± 2.37) in asymptomatic probands. This was significantly smaller in the patient group, at 19.88 mm (SD ± 3.55) to the left, and 20.02 mm (SD ± 2.89) to the right.

Symptoms and intensity

As with other neurodynamic tests (Kenneally 1985), the proposed neurodynamic test reproduced classic sensory reactions:

- 61.5% (16 of 26 volunteers) experienced a 'pulling' feeling no further than the mandibular angle, with an average score on the visual analogue scale (VAS) of 1.89 (SD ± 0.45).
- 38.5% (10 of 26 volunteers) informed the examiners of a 'deep pressure' in the auriculotemporal region, approximately 1 cm from the middle of the head of the mandible (von Piekartz et al 2001). The score on the VAS was 2.01 (SD ± 0.28).

COMMENT

The therapist has to interpret these results with caution because of the small group which was tested and because more than just the nervous system was tested (von Piekartz et al 2001). Because the intertester reliability is good, this manoeuvre can be used together with other data collected from the subjective and physical examination for interpretation and decision-making within the therapist's clinical reasoning processes (Jones et al 2002).

Palpation

LINGUAL NERVE

The lingual nerve is situated on the medial dorsal side of the mandible, up to 1 cm caudal to the head of the mandible on the superior part of the medial pterygoid muscle. The best approach is to relax the soft tissue around the mandible using a slight ipsilateral lateroflexion in upper cervical extension and a slight depression of the jaw (approximately 1 cm). In this position the ipsilateral little or ring finger with supination of the forearm can try to palpate the nerve and its branches. Many anomalies have been described (Isberg et al 1987). For confirmation of the 'right spot', the author usually uses a sensitizing movement of the head and neck using upper cervical flexion (Fig. 17.14a).

INFERIOR ALVEOLAR NERVE

Several small branches run through the mental foramen approximately 1.5 cm laterally from

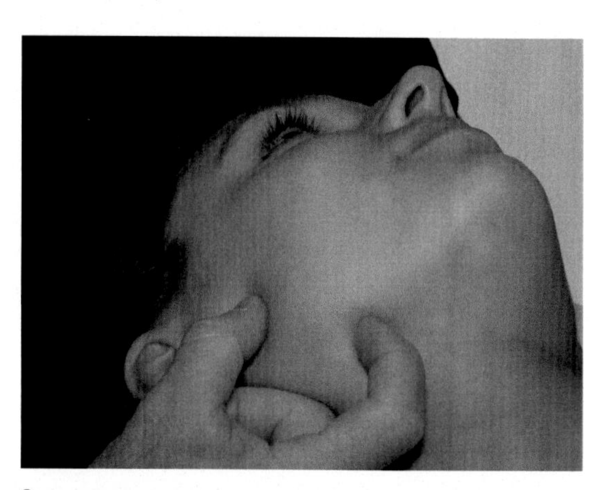

a

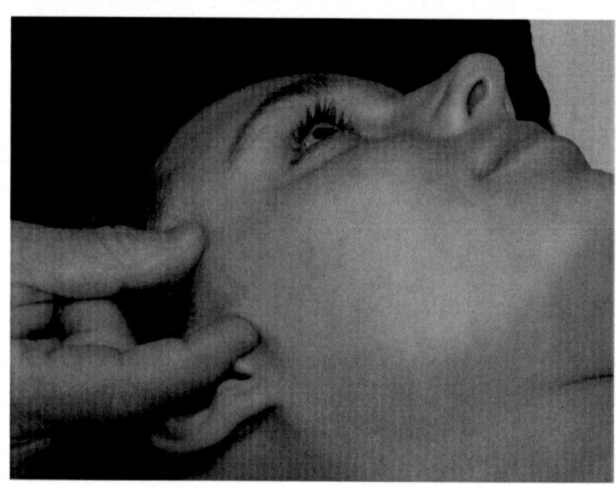

b

Fig. 17.14 Palpation of the mandibular branches.
a The lingual nerve.
b The auriculotemporal nerve.

the midline. Palpation with the index finger is possible, especially when the patient opens their mouth and the therapist holds the mandible in lateropulsion to the other side. The therapist can often feel superficial branches on the palate below the lower incisors.

AURICULOTEMPORAL NERVE

The tip of the index finger is placed 0.5 cm in front of the acoustic meatus and behind the head of the mandible. With the patient's mouth slightly open, it is often easy to 'twang' this nerve (Fig. 17.14b).

Conduction tests of the trigeminal nerve

PURPOSE

The purpose of the conduction tests of the trigeminal nerve is to:

- Differentiate between a peripheral lesion and a dysfunction in the brainstem
- Determine whether the motor weakness is uni- or bilateral, and whether of lower or upper motor origin (Spillane 1996)
- Get an idea at which level the target tissue needs to be examined or treated.

ASSESSMENT OF THE AFFERENTS

Corneal reflex

The fibres most sensitive to compression or distortion appear to be those fibres responsible for the corneal reflex. The earliest sign during a dysfunction but also in pain (e.g. vasomotor headaches) is often an impaired or absent corneal reflex (Patten 1995, Wagner & Lang 2000, Matharu & Goadsby 2003). To assess the corneal reflex, hold the patient's lower eyelid down as far as possible. It must be the cornea, and not the lids, fluid or even the conjunctiva that is stimulated. Have the patient look up as far as possible and, with a piece of cotton wool twisted to a point, touch either side of the pupil (Spillane 1996) to differentiate a problematic area. Problems might be suspected where the patient immediately flinches. This can be double checked by testing another area of the eye where the response is normal, i.e. the patient neither flinches nor hesitates, after which it will be possible to again test the problem area (Patten 1995, Wilson-Pauwels et al 2002).

ASSESSMENT OF THE EFFERENTS

The motor function of the temporal muscles, masseters and pterygoid and the joint reflex are discussed in the following text.

Muscle palpation

The masseter muscles can be palpated 0.5 cm towards the angle of the mandible while the patient clenches the jaw. The muscles can be compared bilaterally as they stand out as hard lumps. At maximal closure the therapist can hold the tip of the index and middle fingers medially to the lateral jaw line to palpate the distal part of the muscle belly of the medial pterygoid muscle.

Sensory function

The dermatomes should be examined with the patient's eyes closed.

- Soft touch: This tests large diameter myelinated nerves. With a camel-hair brush, a small piece of cotton or the tip of a handkerchief, brush the examined area lightly. The patient should be able to identify softer quality of touch associated with a more localized area, as well as the direction and onset of the movement (Fig. 17.15a).
- Pin prick: This tests small diameter myelinated and non-myelinated nerves. A sterile needle or a sharp dental explorer is needed for the examination of the head. The ability to localize the stimulus is recorded as well as the patient's assessment of the intensity in relation to the other side and the rest of the body.
- Temperature: This tests small diameter nerves. Take two small pieces of cotton and place one in a bowl of hot water and the other in a bowl of iced water. Bring one of the pieces approximately 0.5 cm in front of the face. The patient has to register the decrease or increase in temperature. If unable to do so, a lower or upper motor neurone pathology is hypothesized (Spillane 1996). The therapist needs to be

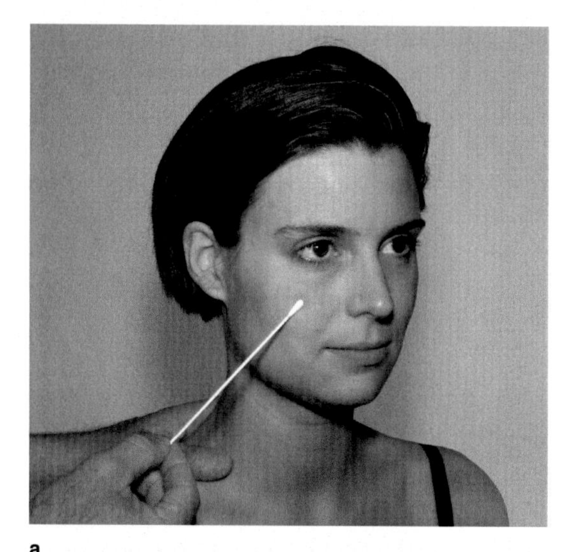
a

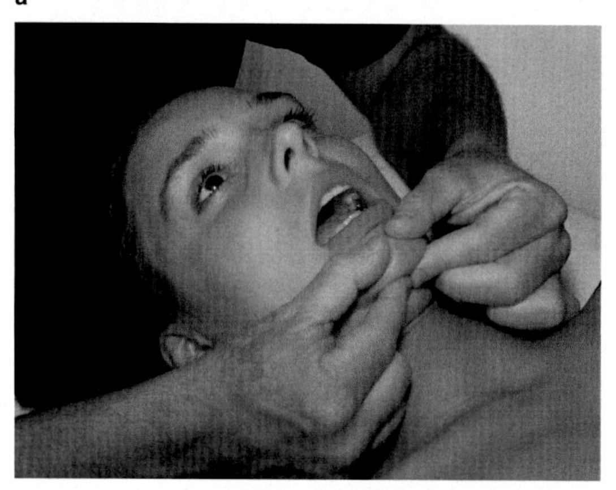
b

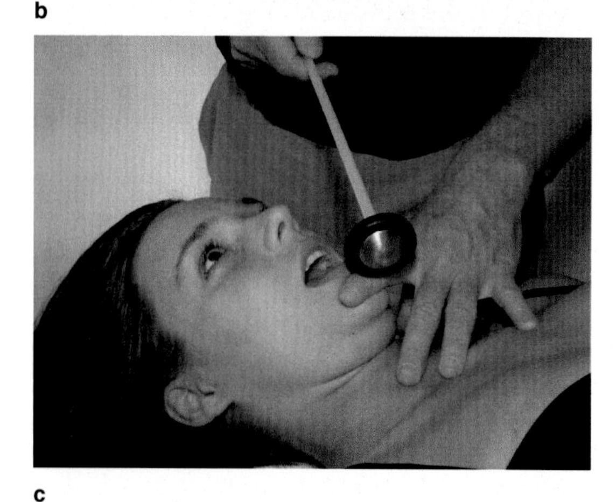
c

Fig. 17.15 Conduction test of the trigeminal nerve.
a Testing sensitivity with cotton bud.
b Isometric testing of the masticatory muscles.
c The jaw jerk test using a reflex hammer.

aware that this clinical pattern can be mimicked by craniomandibular dysfunction in which an inhibition is noted on examination of the masticatory muscles (Patten 1995). One way to differentiate is by changing the neurodynamics of the trigeminal nerve or the upper limbs to determine possible changes in muscle tone.

Isometric tests

For isometric depression and elevation of the mouth, have the patient place the tip of the tongue against the tip of the palate, opening the mouth just far enough to maintain contact with the palate. In adults this is usually about 2 cm. When this degree of openness is reached, the patient should relax the tongue onto the floor of the mouth. This position allows maximum isometric contraction.

For elevation, the therapist takes the patient's chin between the index and middle fingers of both hands (Fig. 17.15b). For depression, maintain this position and hold both thumbs under the patient's chin, asking them to open and close the mouth slowly. After 2–3 seconds of isometric contraction it is possible to test recruitment function by 'breaking' the contraction (Maitland et al 2001, Watanabe & Watanabe 2001, Aizawa et al 2002). Some therapists repeat this test three times. If the masticatory group tests weak on the right-hand side, the jaw will be easily pushed across to that side when tested (Patten 1995). Spasm and fasciculations might also be present. Any or all of these clinical events during break contraction might strengthen the suspicion of conduction dysfunction of the trigeminal nerve.

The jaw jerk

According to Spillane (1995), the jaw jerk is often sadly ignored by therapists even though it offers a plethora of information about conduction in the trigeminal nerve. To administer this test, place the left index finger on the patient's chin while the middle, ring and little fingers rest on the patient's chest in the vicinity of the sternoclavicular joint. With a percussion hammer, tap downward on the index finger (Fig. 17.15c).

Responses

- A sudden slight closing of the jaw which can be detected by the palpating finger(s) is the normal response (Wilson-Pauwels et al 2002). Sometimes, as with other reflexes, no response is observed.
- Jaw reflex appears exaggerated and even jaw clonus can be found in the event of an upper motor neurone lesion above the level of the pons (Fukuyama et al 2000, Aramideh & Ongerboer de Visser 2002).
- Clonus or a trismus reaction has been seen during facial oral dysfunction after radiotherapy for cancer or for severe pain.

An exaggerated jaw reflex, in combination with exaggeration of reflexes in the arms and legs is not necessarily directly related to pathology (Spillane 1996). For the therapist it can be used as a reassessment.

Sometimes it can be useful to perform the tests in neurodynamic loading of the cranial nervous tissue. A more exaggerated jaw reflex is seen in cases of undefined cranial facial pain in upper cervical flexion and lateroflexion away from the examined side.

Table 17.2 gives a general overview of the physical examination options for the trigeminal nerve.

Comment

MANDIBULAR NERVE PATHOLOGY

Rich variation of sensory branches in the craniofacial region and motor innervation of the masticatory muscles suggest that neuropathies can be influenced by neurodynamic changes in the trigeminal nerve. These include orofacial pain, CMD, tinnitus, vertigo, eye and ear aches, atypical facial pain and other neuropathies such as trigeminal neuralgia or tic douloureux (Okeson 1995, Zakrzewska 1995, Chong & Bajwa 2003). Some examples where dynamic changes in the nerve might change symptoms from a minor trigeminal neuropathy might include the following.

Widespread projection of primary afferents of the first neurone in the trigeminal brainstem complex (Fields 1990, Sessle 1993)

Direct loading of the nerve branches can create neurophysiological and neurobiological changes in the caudal nucleus of the trigeminal brainstem complex and the possibility of convergence with other neurones, for example from the cervical spine (Hu et al 1981, Okeson 1995).

Ectopic discharges that occur at the sites of nerve injury

These were shown to increase mechanosensitivity and chemosensitivity of the nerve as observed by Devor and colleagues (Devor et al 1993, Devor 1996). Rappaport and Devor (1994) note that remyelination of the trigeminal ganglion is the first sign of damage to the rest of the trigeminal nerve. This reminds us that we must be alert to the nature of morphological changes. Pathophysiological processes such as the setting up of a circuit between excitatory and inhibitory synapses that continues indefinitely, or so-called autorhythmic firing, starts in the trigeminal ganglion and sets off the whole activity, especially in the mandibular division (Connor 1985). Pain or other symptoms may affect all of the three divisions of the trigeminal nerve. In their study of 8124 patients with craniofacial pain, White and Sweet (1969) noted that 32% had trigeminal nerve involvement with the mandibular nerve dominant and that 17% had mixed disturbances. Zakrzewska and Nally (1988) found that pain was reduced in patients with craniofacial pain by cryotherapy to the peripheral nerve branches, particularly the branches of the mandibular nerve.

The difference between the functional anatomy and the neurodynamics of the mandibular nerve branches

This alone might provide a clue to symptoms that present in this area. The auriculotemporal, inferior alveolar and lingual nerves have three main differences as compared to the other nerve divisions.

Table 17.2 Overview of the physical examination options for the trigeminal nerve (V)

Trigeminal nerve (V)	Neurodynamic tests	Palpation	Conduction tests
Ophthalmic division (V_1)	Craniocervical: Upper cervical flexion Contralatera lateroflexion Craniofacial: Sphenoid Lacrimal Eye movements: Caudal Medial Lateral	Foramen ophthalmicum (supraorbital)	
Maxillary division (V_2)	Craniocervical: Upper cervical flexion Contralateral lateral flexion Craniofacial: Maxillary Zygoma Sphenoid Palatinum Eye movements: Medial Lateral	Infraorbital foramen	
Mandibular division (V_3)	Craniocervical: Upper cervical flexion Contralateral lateroflexion Craniofacial: Sphenoid Mandible: Depression Contralateral laterotrusion Transverse head of mandible	Mandible: Angle (lingual nerve) Mental foramen (inferior alveolar nerve) Ventral ear (auriculotemporal nerve)	Afferents: Muscle palpation Sensory function: - light touch - pin prick - temperature Efferents: Isometric tests Mandibular reflex

1. All three have longer extracranial branches than the other cranial nerves (Wilson-Pauwels et al 2002).
2. They have many more extracranial tunnels, anastomoses and fixation points, and thus must adapt to the resulting dynamic interface (Leblanc 1995). A spasm of the pterygoid medial and pterygoid lateral from a craniomandibular dysfunction is an example of how the lingual nerve can influence neuropathy (Isberg et al 1987). Another is the case of mandibular growth spurts in youth, where the inferior alveolar nerve and the lingual nerve must adapt vertically and horizontally, respectively (Enlow 1986). The intraosseous anterior loop of the inferior alveolar nerve is another oft-forgotten branch where functional neuroanatomy and dynamics might be implicated. It extends beyond the mental foramen, and

anatomical and radiological studies show that variations in this branch are relatively common, with the average length being 6.95 mm and consistent findings of a 2 mm loop (Misoh & Crawford 1990, Sadiq et al 2003).

3. The final factor, along with the above anatomical attributes which might realistically provide some insights into mandibular nerve neuropathies, is the enormous range of movement of the craniomandibular joint to which, at 50–60 mm maximum opening, the mandibular nerve has to adapt (Palla 1998).

TRIGEMINAL NEURALGIA

Numerous theories based on clinical and experimental data have been put forward to explain this rare condition of severe paradoxical pain with a unilateral localization limited to a zone innervated by the trigeminal nerve.

Attacks of pain are triggered by local stimuli to one or more parts of the face or oral or nasal cavity. Sometimes allodynia or hyperalgesia can occur during routine testing with cotton wool or a pin (Gerschman et al 1979, Sweet 1988, Zakrzewska 1995, Göbel 1997, Wilson-Pauwels et al 2002). For detailed classification of cranial neuropathies, see the Headache Classification Committee of the International Headache Society (Olesen 1988), the International Association for the Study of Pain (Merskey & Bogduk 1994) or others such as the Maxwell classification (Maxwell 1990). The International Headache Society (IHS) has classified neuralgias into two categories according to their aetiology:

- Neuralgias associated with compression of the nerve root or systemic causes are considered 'symptomatic neuralgias'.
- Neuralgias of unknown cause are called 'idiopathic neuralgias' (Olesen 1988).

The most common causes of symptomatic neuralgias described in the literature are middle and posterior cranial fossa tumours (Nguyen et al 1986, Bullit et al 1987, Puca et al 1995, Barret et al 2002), multiple sclerosis plaques (Jannetta 1976, Okeson 1995, Quinones-Hinojosa et al 2003) and aneurysms (Kerber et al 1972, Wilson et al 1980).

It is not uncommon that in radiographic and neurosurgical literature vascular compression as a possible cause of idiopathic trigeminal neuralgia is observed and described (Jannetta 1976, Roberts et al 1979, Sens & Higer 1991, Ciftci et al 2004).

Retrospectively, good results are seen when decompression of the superior cerebellar artery, the inferior cerebellar artery or the basilar artery in the prepontine space or the pontine angle are performed (Jannetta 1976, Roberts et al 1979, Badwin et al 1991, Sens & Higer 1991). Decompression of the sensory root of the dural sleeve and the motor root also produce good results (Gardner & Miklos 1959, Saunders et al 1971, Leblanc 1995).

On the other hand, several authors have suggested that neurovascular compression is a normal anatomical variation and is not responsible for trigeminal neuralgia (Morley 1985, Hamlyn & King 1992). Conditions such as chronic vascularization disturbances and early denervation may also be contributors (Sunderland 1948, Hamlyn & King 1992). From the literature we can conclude that the pathophysiological and pathomechanical mechanisms of the trigeminal nerve in the middle and posterior cranial fossa are still poorly understood (Kerr & Lysak 1964, Gelson et al 1994, Robinson et al 2004). Experience, empirical data and clinical evidence from microneurosurgery can give the therapist some ideas about how it may be possible to treat and try to change pathodynamics caused by trigeminal neuralgia (see also Case study 3).

- The intracranial blood vessel in the pontine angle and mechanical interfaces: Head movement changes the load and contact of cranial nerves and blood vessels in the pontine angle. Different positions of the head and neck can change the symptoms when the pain has a peripheral neurogenic character.
- Type of head movement and position: Jannetta (1976) used upper cervical neck flexion and Barba and Alksne (1984) used

Case study 3

In Figure 17.16a, the 32-year-old patient is in an unloaded position of the trigeminal nerve tissue (upper cervical extension and ipsilateral lateroflexion). By loading the right side (upper cervical flexion and contralateral lateroflexion) of the head (Fig. 17.16b), tone in the muscles of facial expression as well as the masticatory muscle increased and the patient experienced a shooting, stabbing pain in his right cheek and mandible. Pathodynamics of the trigeminal nerve was assumed.

Treatment of neurodynamics changed the symptoms of this patient, although the cause remained unclear. The pain started several months after a tooth extraction and there were to date no neurological signs. Management of the trigeminal nerve, passive mobilization of the occipital and sphenoid bones and a home programme reduced his pain by more than 50% on a visual analogue scale. In addition, scores of physical and social functions of the Facial Disability Index showed significant changes after 6 weeks. Before treatment of the trigeminal nerve, this patient had only temporary relief with acupuncture but no other (para)medical treatment.

Therapists must ask themselves how many patients with trigeminal neuralgia could be helped with neurodynamic and cranial techniques, including patients with atypical facial pain or with mild symptoms of trigeminal neuralgia (Feinmann 1990, Zakrzewska 1995), who have not been diagnosed as such, but for whom the cause is nevertheless a pathophysiological change such as deafferentation (Loeser 1984), reversed double crush (Upton & McComas 1972) or changed mechanical interfaces (Breig 1976, Leblanc 1995, Butler 2000).

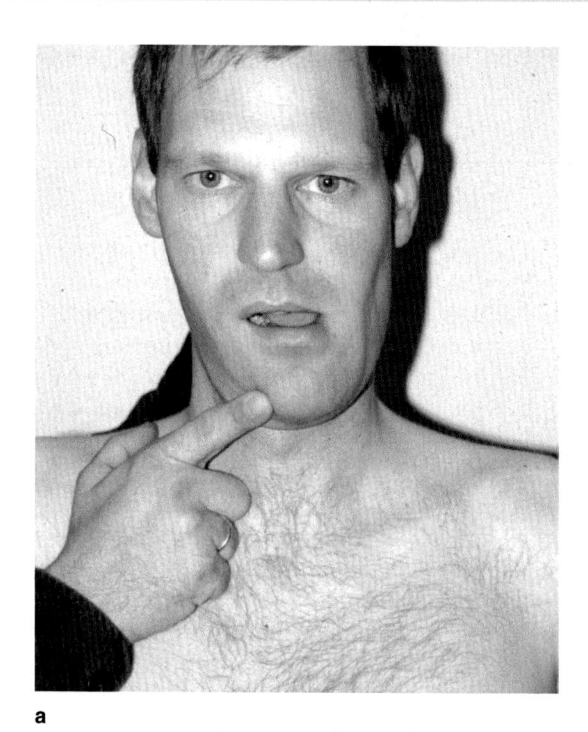

a

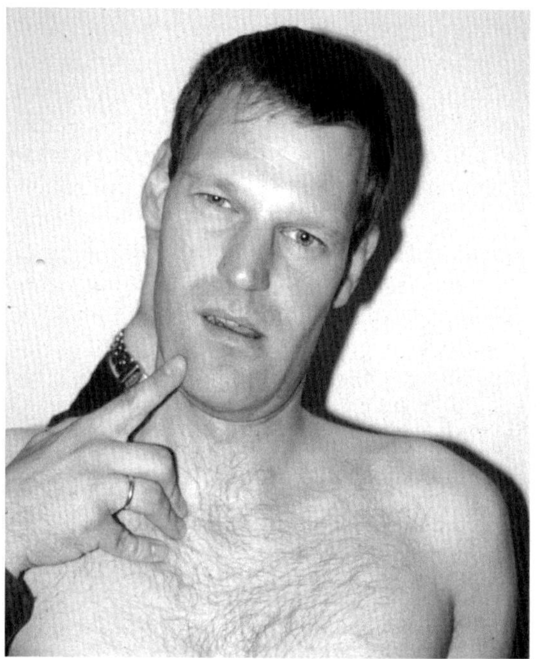

b

Fig. 17.16 Patient with pain from trigeminal tissue.
a Position without pain.
b Correction of the head to the other side, an on/off pain reaction with burning pain from the right head of mandible to the chin.

upper cervical lateroflexion to decompress the blood vessels in the region of the pontine angle during surgery.

- The cranium as an abnormal mechanical interface which causes the neuropathy: Breig (1976) discovered that 75% of nine groups of 24 patients with trigeminal neuralgia demonstrated an impingement phenomenon in the foramen rotundum on lateroflexion to the contralateral side. Jannetta (1976, 1990), Barba and Alksne (1984) and Jannetta and Bissonette (1985) confirmed this during neurosurgical procedures.

INFERIOR ALVEOLAR NERVE NEUROPATHIES FOLLOWING MANDIBULAR IMPLANTS

The last decade has seen a trend towards mandibular implants posterior to the mental foramen. This has increased the incidence of a neuropathy of the inferior alveolar nerve in the mandibular canal (Zarf & Schmidtt 1990, Kieser et al 2005). The incidence of postoperative reversible hypoaesthesia is in the range of 10–39% and that of irreversible hypoaesthesia is between 4 and 19% (Ellies 1992, Janssen 2000). A retrospective study by Janssen (2000) found out that in both groups 66% of patients in the reversible and irreversible groups were moderately to strongly inhibited in general daily life activities: eating (47%), drinking (32%), speaking (55%) and kissing (24%). Although these studies could not show whether the implants were the cause of the neuropathy, they do appear to be a concomitant factor for craniofacial dysfunction and pain.

Neurodynamic tests (in this case of the mandibular nerve), palpation of the nerve branches and conduction tests give the therapist an impression of the health and sensitivity of the cranial nervous tissue in this region. Depending on what is found, the following clinical decisions may be made:

- Careful neural container techniques such as active and passive mobilization of the mandible, treatment of the pterygoid lateral and medial muscles or skin techniques in the region of the mental foramen where the mental nerve exits, etc.
- Active mobilization of the mandibular nerve. Movements of the mandible (laterotrusion to the other side) will be assessed in different positions of the craniocervical region such as upper cervical flexion and lateroflexion.
- Target tissue exercises such as mechanical and thermal stimuli on the chin and lower lip with a warm and cold cotton wool ball, together with functional exercises of the orofacial muscles, will produce an optimal stimulation of the somatosensory cortex of the orofacial region.

FACIAL NERVE (VII)

Relevant functional anatomy

Cranial nerve VII emerges from the brainstem dorsolateral to the pons and has four components (see Chapter 2) which run laterally and enter the internal auditory meatus of the temporal bone together with the vestibulocochlear nerve (VIII). This meatus leads to the facial canal of the temporal bone which runs laterally for approximately 2 cm, then turns 90° (geniculum), runs posteriorly/inferiorly for 5 cm and terminates at the stylomastoid foramen, located behind the base of the styloid process. A further six branches are formed which run in the facial muscles and are relatively superficial. These branches are the temporal nerve, the zygomatic nerve, the mandibular nerve, the buccal nerve, the cervical nerve and the posterior auricular nerve (Fig. 17.17).

Neurodynamic test

The cervical spine is positioned in upper cervical flexion, contralateral lateroflexion and ipsilateral rotation to get more load on the branches directly extracranial which run parallel with the sternocleidomastoid muscle.

It is possible to influence the auditory meatus and facial canal through temporal bone accessory movements. Petrosal bone movement changes the stylomastoid foramen region.

Branches that innervate the mimic muscles

Temporal branches
Pterygopalatine ganglion
Zygomatic branches
Greater petrosal nerve
Outer facial nerve with geniculate ganglion
Tympanic chord
Stylomastoid foramen
Posterior auricular nerve
Lingual nerve
Parotid gland
Buccal branches
Mandibular marginal branch
Cervical branch

Fig. 17.17 Facial nerve.

Moving the mandible into depression and in contralateral laterotrusion reaches the buccal ramus of the mandibular nerve. Contraction of the ipsilateral mimic musculature creates compression tension on the side being investigated. To reach the cervical branch a longitudinal caudal movement of the hyoid bone is used.

STARTING POSITION AND METHOD

The patient is comfortable in a relaxed position lying supine. The therapist sits on the short side of the plinth facing the patient's head, with both forearms resting on the plinth which has been adjusted to a convenient height. Both hands cup around the occipital region without extreme compression of the cranium. An alternative position is to place the left hand on the occipital region and the right hand on the frontal bone when nasal or orbital regions are to be examined or treated.

The therapist moves their body minimally with both forearms on the plinth for upper cervical flexion, lateroflexion away and ipsilateral rotation of the head (Fig. 17.18a).

Movement of the temporal or petrosal bone can be added by moving the right hand in the same position to the lateral side of the head to make contact with the bones as described in Chapter 14 (Fig. 17.18b).

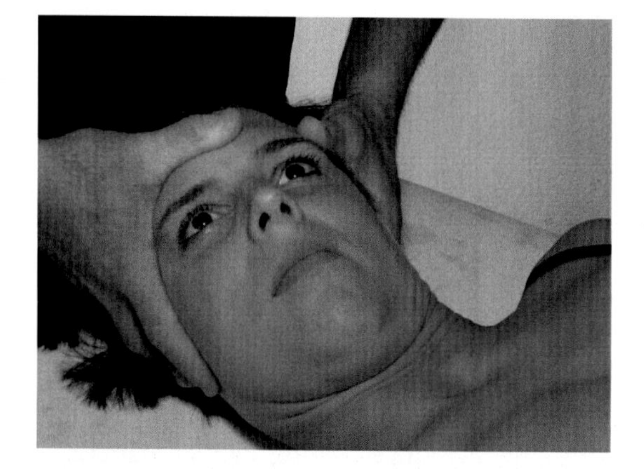

a

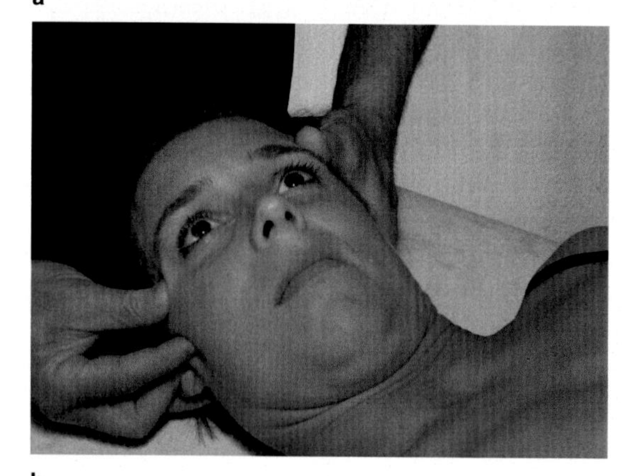

b

Fig. 17.18a–e Neurodynamic tests for the facial nerve.

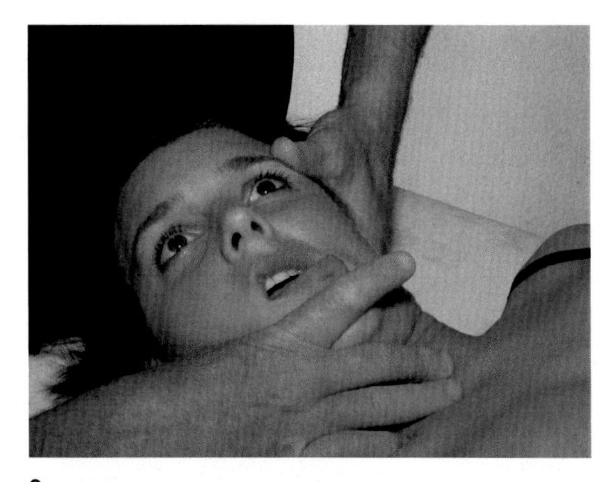
c

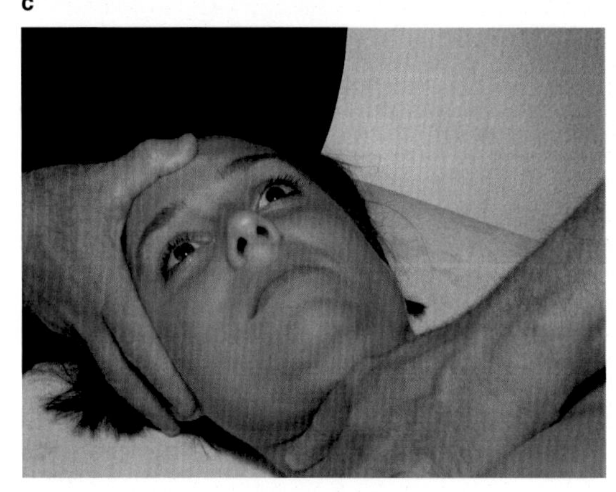
d

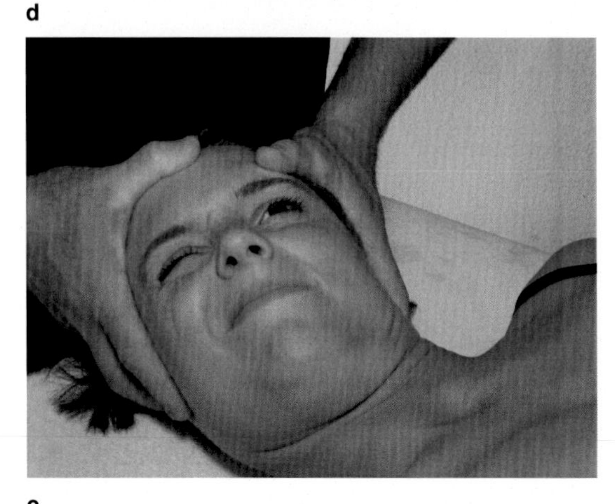
e

Fig. 17.18a–e—cont'd

For the craniomandibular movement, the right hand grasps around the lateral side of the mandibular angle, whereby the right index finger lies on the superior part and the middle finger contacts the inferior part of the chin. In this position it is possible to perform a slight depression and lateral deviation of the mandible to the left to emphasize the mandibular buccal branch (Fig. 17.18c).

When hyoid movement is needed, the right index finger and thumb grasp around the hyoid and perform the longitudinal movement towards caudal (Fig. 17.18d). Active movement of the facial muscles by the patient can be initiated in any position to change neurodynamics (Fig. 17.18e).

Palpation

Palpation of the facial nerve is on the one hand easy because it runs relatively superficially and has many branches. On the other hand it is difficult because it has different types of anastomoses (Miehlke et al 1979). Therefore it is essential to be sure that a nerve is being palpated. Twanging of the nerve in different neurodynamic positions often gives a good indication as to whether or not the therapist is on the facial branch. The relatively large extrapetrosal branches of the facial nerve (e.g. the posterior auricular, zygomatic, buccal and mandibular branch) are easily palpable and easy to treat. To 'preload', the patient's head is positioned in slight upper cervical flexion and contralateral lateroflexion and ipsilateral rotation. The contralateral hand holds this position by grasping around the top the head.

- Palpating the posterior auricular branch: The tip of the right thumb tries to palpate the ventral side of the petrosal bone from caudal to cranial (Fig. 17.19a). The branch usually lies 5–18 mm on this trajectory in the direction of the external acoustic meatus. The nerve can be followed dorsally on the occipital bone whereby the thumb can remain in the same position.

The following nerves can be palpated more easily with the right index or middle finger

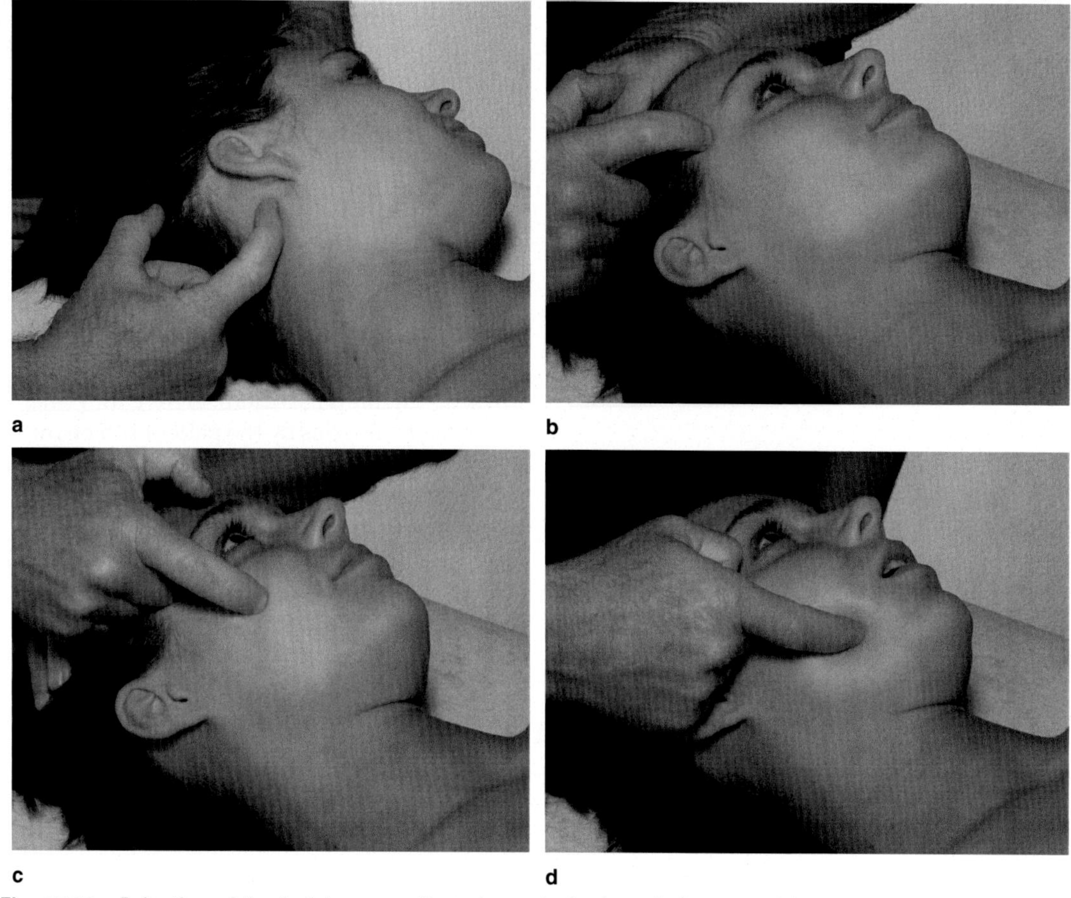

Fig. 17.19 Palpation of the facial nerve: **a** Posterior auricular branch; **b** temporal branch; **c** buccal branch; **d** mandibular branch.

because they are relatively small and run on a hard surface.

- The temporal branch can be palpated craniolaterally to the orbicularis oculis muscle (lateral from the eyebrow) (Fig. 17.19b).
- Palpation of the zygomatic branch is possible on the superior border of the zygomatic bone and lateral to the orbicularis oculis muscle. Anastomoses of the nerve often run through and over the mimic muscles.
- The buccal branch runs under the zygomatic bone and over the buccal muscle. Palpation can be performed by placing a slight pressure on the nerve against the inferior side of the zygomatic bone and its course followed by light twanging with the index and middle fingers (Fig. 17.19c). When considering treatment, the one or two finger technique may be chosen, depending on the individual anatomy of the patient and/or the desired effects of the techniques.
- The mandibular branch can be palpated ventrally to the parotid gland on the masseter muscle. The masseter muscle can be contracted by unilaterally clenching the teeth, followed by palpation with the index and middle fingers in the direction of the jaw line. The easiest place to palpate this nerve is on the ventral side of the muscle belly (Fig. 17.19d). Once convinced about the localization of the nerve, the masseter can be relaxed and the examination continued or treatment started.

As various anomalies of the extrapetrosal branches have been described, the therapist should be aware that they can never be certain which nerve is being palpated. The therapist needs to make a clinical decision regarding the general physical and subjective characteristics of the nerve as these become apparent during the different manoeuvres.

Conduction tests

The purpose of the tests is to detect the uni- or bilateral strength of the muscles of facial expression, the corneal reflex and to detect changes of taste and secretion.

TESTING THE MUSCLES OF FACIAL EXPRESSION

During the subjective examination the therapist inspects the patient's face for asymmetry and abnormal movements. To evaluate the muscles of facial expression the following instructions can be given:

1. 'Show the teeth' (Fig. 17.20a): The therapist notes the symmetry of the nasolabial folds.
2. 'Open the mouth' (Fig. 17.20b): The nasolabial folds are compared. Deviation of the jaw due to craniomandibular dysfunction can overshadow a pseudoweakness of muscles of facial expression.
3. 'Close the eyes, screw them up tightly, then open them again' (Fig. 17.20c): Assessment of eye muscles.
4. 'Frown, wrinkle the forehead and raise the eyebrows' (Fig. 17.20d): Tests the frontal muscle.
5. 'Show the teeth and open the mouth at the same time' (Fig. 17.20e): Assessment of platysma.

When facial/oral dysfunction is present, tests 1, 3 and 4 are the most appropriate. If the symptoms are due to a neurogenic dysfunction (due to changes of the neural containers, such as compression in the facial canal or swelling of neighbouring muscles) then neurodynamic components of the facial neurodynamic test (especially lateroflexion and rotation), the subjective symptoms and the tests of the muscles of facial expression will change. For example, a burning eye pain together with a minor closing dysfunction of the eye is respectively worse in slight upper cervical extension, ipsilateral lateroflexion and contralateral rotation.

The efferent motor branches of the facial nerve are responsible for the corneal reflex, and are discussed together with the trigeminal nerve.

ASSESSMENT OF TASTE

Best discrimination is possible using the four primary tastes, i.e. sweet, salt, sour and bitter. The tests are carried out with sugar, salt, vinegar and quinine. The patient sticks out the tongue and closes the eyes and the therapist applies the fluid substances on the anterior part of the tongue for 2–3 seconds. After each test the patient has to swill out the mouth with water and tells the therapist which of the primary tastes was perceived. In addition, the activity of the facial muscles has to be inspected during the test.

ASSESSMENT OF SECRETION

The submandibular and sublingual glands can be tested by sensory stimulation with lemon

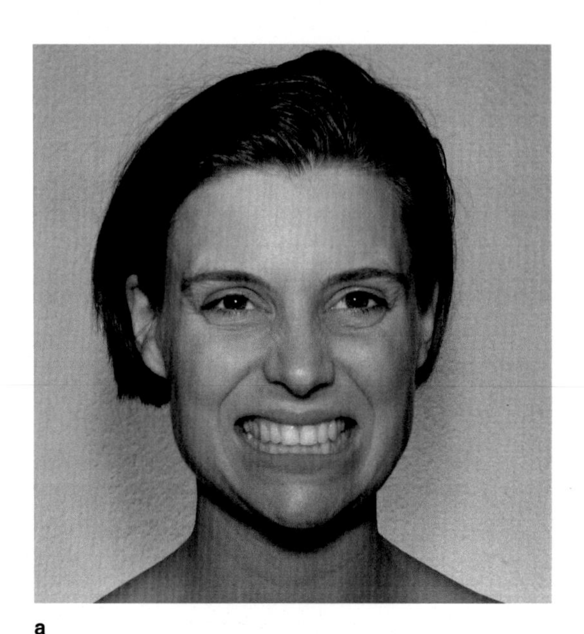

a

Fig. 17.20a–e Functions of the facial nerve.

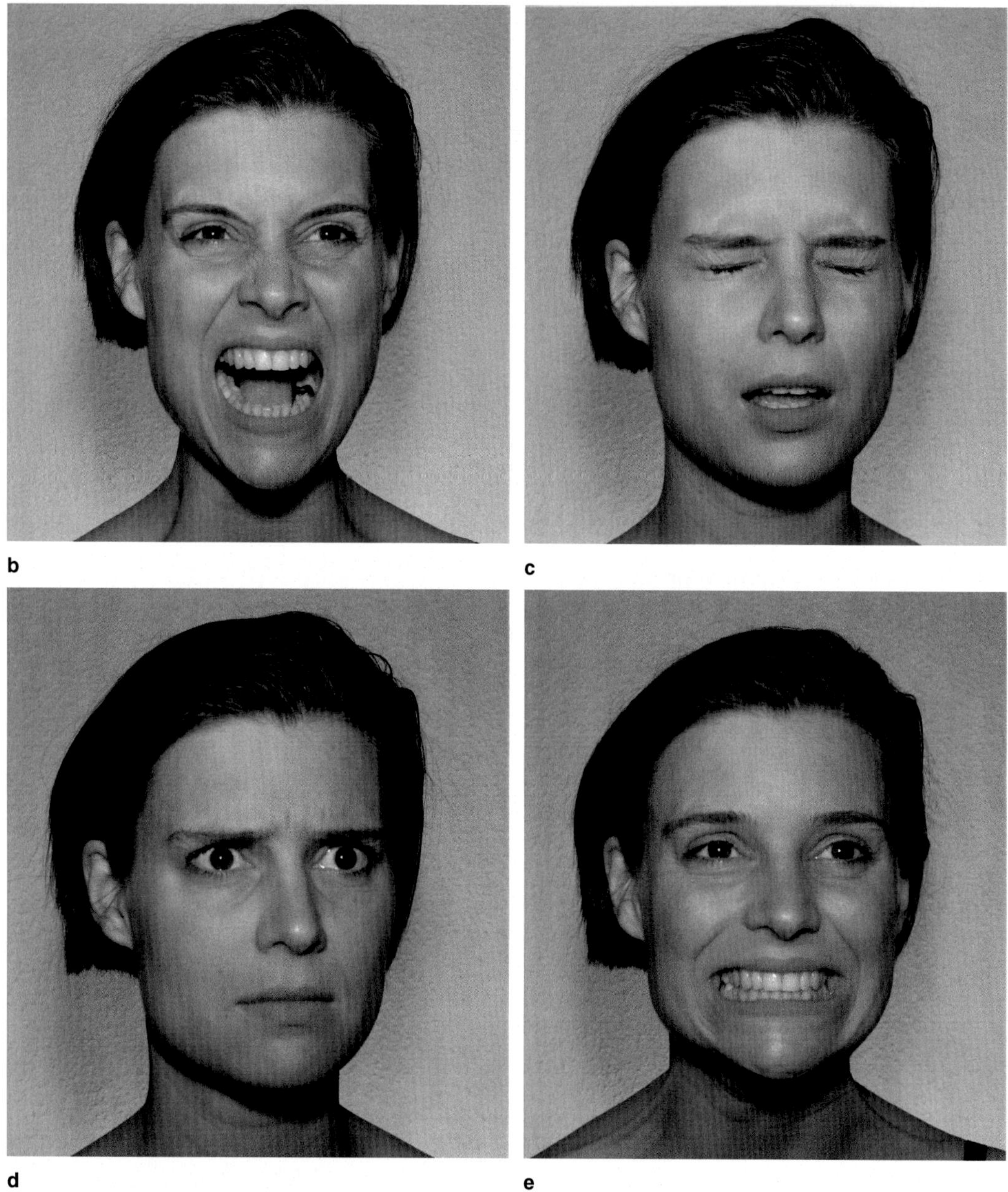

Fig. 17.20a–e—cont'd

sweets or by milking these glands by soft pressure using the index and middle fingers. Saliva secretion is observed at the opening of the duct and the patient detects an increase of fluid in the mouth.

Lacrimal gland dysfunction commonly presents itself in the form of eye dryness or a sandy, gritty feeling in the eye. A good impression can be obtained by placing a small electric fan 5–10 cm in front of the patient's eyes and blowing perpendicularly in the open eyes for 10–20 seconds. After the test check how the patient is feeling and compare the resultant secretions left and right by milking the gland

0.5 cm under the eyes. These results should then be compared with those in neurodynamic positions when the therapist considers there to be neurodynamic changes of the peripheral branches of the facial nerve.

Table 17.3 gives a general overview of the physical examination options for the facial nerve.

Comment

IS NEURODYNAMICS OF THE FACIAL NERVE USEFUL IN REHABILITATION?

Testing in functional positions such as sitting and standing is more comparative, especially for patients with neurological facial paresis. An example of a patient with hemiparesis and facial paresis is given in Figure 17.21. The patient has an upper motor neurone lesion (UMNL). In addition, lower motor neurone lesion (LMNL) components may play a role in his facial motor dysfunction with regard to articulation and eating. In an unloaded position of the facial nerve (upper cervical extension, lateroflexion towards and rotation away from the examined side), facial muscle contraction can be of better quality and the dysfunction therefore reduced (Fig. 17.21a). Palpation of the buccal nerve stimulates the activity even more (Fig. 17.21b). More loading (cervical flexion, lateroflexion away and rotation towards the examined side) gives the same patient less expression.

These neurodynamic principles are useful for treatment by mobilization as well as integration into neurological exercise therapy. Cranial nerves are richly innervated by their own nerves, termed nervi nervorum, and by the autonomic nervous system that regulates the vascularization of these nerves (Hromada 1963). Changes of the neural container because of spasm of the mimic muscle due to chronic pain (Kruschinski et al 2003) and neurological diseases (facial paresis) can change the physiological mechanisms of the nerve (pathodynamics) and can be a source of symptoms (Butler 2000). Alleviating pain and normalizing tone of the muscles of facial expression using neurodynamic movements can, in the author's opinion, be a reason why the symptoms of patients with orofacial pain and facial paresis can be changed.

HEMIFACIAL SPASM

The IASP describes hemifacial spasm as a progressive condition which, if not treated, characteristically results in unilateral tonic contraction of the facial muscles. Ipsilateral

Table 17.3 Overview of the physical examination options for the facial nerve (VII)

Neurodynamic tests	Palpation	Conduction tests
Craniocervical:	Temporal ramus	Testing of facial muscles
Upper cervical flexion	Mandibular ramus	Assessment of taste
Contralateral lateroflexion	Posterior auricular ramus	Assessment of secretion
Craniofacial:	Buccal ramus	
Temporal	Zygomatic ramus	
Petrosal		
Mandible:		
Depression		
Laterotrusion		
Hyoid:		
Transverse movements		
Facial muscles:		
Tensing		
Relaxing		

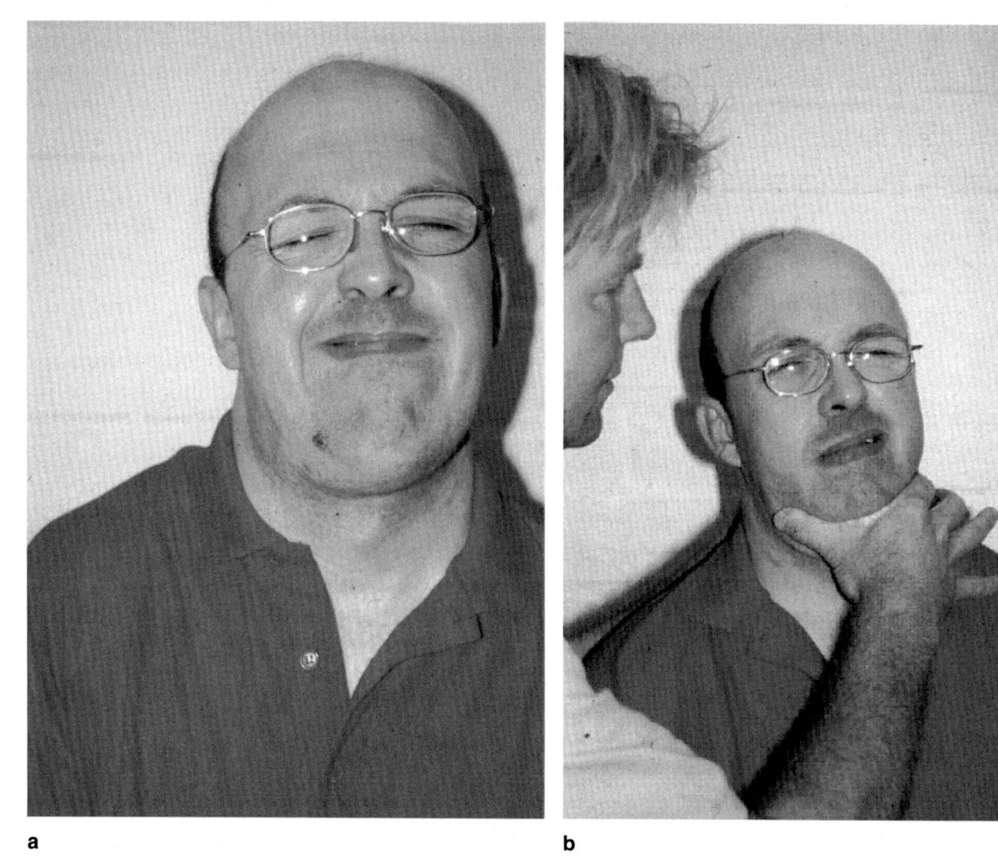

a b

Fig. 17.21 Rehabilitation of a patient with facial paresis: a In an unloaded position of the cranial nervous tissue (upper cervical extension, lateroflexion towards the same side and elevation of the shoulder); less inhibition of the facial muscle is seen than in a correct middle position (b).

facial weakness is possible (Merskey & Bogduk 1994). The pain is present ipsilaterally and has the features of trigeminal neuralgia. Most of the patients have compression or distortion of the relevant cranial nerve or abnormal blood vessels (Lang & Kessler 1991, Shenouda et al 2005). Microvascular decompression (MVD), mainly in the cerebellopontine angle (Jannetta 1970, 1980a, Iwakuma et al 1982, Born 2002), is the obvious therapy. However, this can often be a complication of vestibular nerve injury (Sekiya et al 1991). Spasm and lateral spread of antidromic activity can be recorded by electromyographic stimulation (EMS) techniques during MVD (Møller & Jannetta 1985, 1987).

Slight mechanical stimulation of the vessels around the nerve and the nerve itself evokes EMG activity (Howe et al 1977, Oge et al 2005), such as opening of the dura or the arachnoid decreases EMG activity, probably by the change in intracisternal volume and/or pressure on the nerves (Møller 1988). From this knowledge we learn that the facial nerve and its direct connections such as dura and arachnoid are extremely mechanosensitive when compromised by abnormal intracranial mechanical interfaces. Pathophysiological changes such as axon plasma flow changes, cross-talk, fibrosis, etc. of the cranial nerves are possible signs that the spasm and/or pain are still present (Zochodne et al 1997).

> **!** When there is a slow progressive weakness or spasm on one side of the face it is wise to refer the patient to a specialist for further diagnosis. Cranioneurodynamics should be an advance warning here. On the other hand, neurodynamics, and in particular neck movement, may make an effective contribution to changing the pathodynamics of the facial nerve and its immediate surroundings after surgical decompression for hemifacial spasm. To the best of the author's knowledge, there is no basic literature about investigation and treatment through cranioneurodynamics after facial surgery.

PERIPHERAL FACIAL PARESIS

In Europe, 1 in 5000 people suffers from acute facial paralysis. For children younger than 10 years, the frequency is 1 in 20 000 (Verjaal 1955, Miller 1967, Devriese 1986). Patients can suffer from different residual symptoms after a peripheral facial paralysis. These may include reduced activity of the facial muscles, which leads to problems while eating, drinking, speaking and with facial expression, and results in further contractures and synkinesis (signs of denervation) (Beurskens 1990, Beurskens et al 1994a, 1994b, Beurskens & Burger-Bots 1995). A rehabilitation programme is indicated when the patient complains about residual symptoms which do not recover naturally after 1–2 years. They can still have considerable synkinesis, even when the facial nerve has not suffered very severe nerve damage (Peitersen & Andersen 1966, Mündnich et al 1973, Huffmann 1979, Barat 1983, Beurskens et al 1987, von Eck 1989, Beurskens & Burger-Bots 1995). As literature studies show no consensus about treatment of facial paralysis patients, no conclusions about the outcome can be drawn (Peitersen & Andersen 1966, Huffmann 1979, Beurskens et al 1994a, 1994b, Beurskens & Burger-Bots 1995). Eighty-five per cent of all studies recommend rehabilitation in the form of exercise therapy, massage and biofeedback (Daniel & Guitar 1978, Boussons & Voisin 1984, Devriese 1986, Liebenstund 1989, Beurskens et al 1994a, 1994b, Kvale et al 2003). A particularly functional form of rehabilitation, known as 'mime therapy', was developed by Jan Bronk, a mime actor in Amsterdam (Devriese & Bronk 1977). The therapy is based on the central theme of mime and its reciprocity as a concept for positive feelings and functional movements (Beurskens et al 1994a, 1994b):

- Typical clinical findings related to cranial neurodynamics are that, during specific mime exercises of the face, the patient unloads the facial nerve using slight extension, ipsilateral lateroflexion and contralateral rotation. Furthermore, slight elevation of the shoulder and flexion of the ipsilateral arm leads to unloading of the neural structures. This is seen more obviously during active exercise of the most strongly affected area as well as during exercises for decreasing synkinesis.
- A nice addition to mime therapy and other exercise methods is to use this unloaded position of the nervous system and especially that of the facial nerve together with neurodynamic techniques. This can have the advantage of changing afferent–reafferent information and the pathophysiology of the facial nerve (Hromada 1963, Miehlke et al 1979, Barat 1983, Leduc & Decloedt 1989). One method is to start with painless cranioneurodynamics then reassess the tone and synkinesis and continue with active exercise in the unloaded position to stimulate only the desired facial activity. If the patient has only mild paralysis in a neutral head position, the therapist can add neurodynamic components to make the exercise more difficult.
- Local facilitation techniques of the peripheral facial branches provide the patient with a better circulation, more relaxation of the facial muscles and greater awareness of the face (Liebenstund 1989, Beurskens 1990, Beurskens & Burger-Bots 1995). Another direct technique to influence the tone,

improve local trophic conditions and facilitate the paralysed muscles is local neuropalpation or neural mobilizations (Butler & Gifford 1998). Good techniques in the length direction of the different superficial branches of the facial nerve are possible and can have a positive physiological contribution to the local peripheral branches. This can influence peripheral neurogenic symptoms such as burning pain, inhibition of the muscle and reduced tone (Woolf & Salter 2000).

Clinically these clear motor output mechanisms are often confirmed in the facial nerve. In cases of long-term facial paresis or an extracranial pathology, surgery can also lead to minor dysfunction of the cranial nerves without clear electrodiagnostic change (Huffmann 1997, Okeson 1995). Examples such as capsulitis of the temporomandibular joint, inflammation of the salivary glands, cystectomy in the ear region or symptoms following a blow to the face often cause local trophic changes which are easily treatable with neurodynamics and local palpation mobilization techniques. Perpendicular twang techniques are a good option to treat local signs and symptoms (Butler 1991, Butler & Gifford 1998). In addition, facilitation of the paralysed muscle group is possible using palpation techniques that are simple, cost little time and can easily be integrated into neuro-orthopaedic concepts. For the different types of facial paralysis, refer to the specialist literature (Patten 1995).

FACIAL NERVE ANASTOMOSES

Neurosurgeons have long been interested in the facial nerve because of its anatomical variety, particularly in the plexus formation of the lateral region of the face (Borucki et al 2002, Guntinas-Lichius et al 2006). It has been proven that facial paralysis can be successfully overcome with neural repair to part of the hypoglossal nerve tissue in facial nerve anastomosis. This results in improved facial muscle function (Miehlke et al 1979). Miehlke and colleagues developed a systematic classification for the types of anastomoses that are possible clinically (Fig. 17.22). The most frequently used surgical procedures prescribed for various injuries – otosurgical and parotid operations – may actually cause damage to the facial nerve. This occurs because nerve anastomoses can create particularly vulnerable points given the mechanical forces produced at the cross-section of the junction (Nisch 1973, Breig 1976, Miehlke et al 1979, Hammerschlag et al 1987, Mackinnon & Dellon 1988, Kwan et al 1992, Iriarte Ortabe et al 1993, Butler & Gifford 1998, Verberne et al 2003).

Studies of intraoperative electrophysiological monitoring of cranial nerves show that the facial nerve has a special feature: a small amount of traction or compression of the nerve may generate ectopic impulses producing relevant detectable EMG discharges from the facial muscles (Møller & Jannetta 1985, 1986, 1987, Harner et al 1986, Armon & Daube 1989, Nelson & Phillips 1990, Brown & Veitch 1994). This could explain the damage that occurs to the facial nerve during surgery.

It is very likely that some minor pathophysiological changes or neuropathies influence signs and symptoms after minor trauma or surgery to the face. It is possible to elicit clues from the patient's history during subjective examination. For example, information about a 'spontaneous' onset of facial pain or dysfunction might lead to clues that will help the therapist develop an appropriate treatment strategy. In such cases it is useful to examine the cranial nerves, especially the facial nerve, together with palpation of the facial nerve branches and the anastomosis. Small superficial pain spots are often found around the anastomosis when compared to the other areas. Treatment by neural palpation to the anastomosis, together with neurodynamic facial nerve techniques, can change signs and symptoms dramatically in such cases.

ATYPICAL FACIAL PAIN

Atypical facial pain, which carries the synonyms of atypical facial neuralgia, idiopathic facial pain and chronic facial pain, is a persistent facial pain that does not have the characteristics of the cranial neuralgias, is not

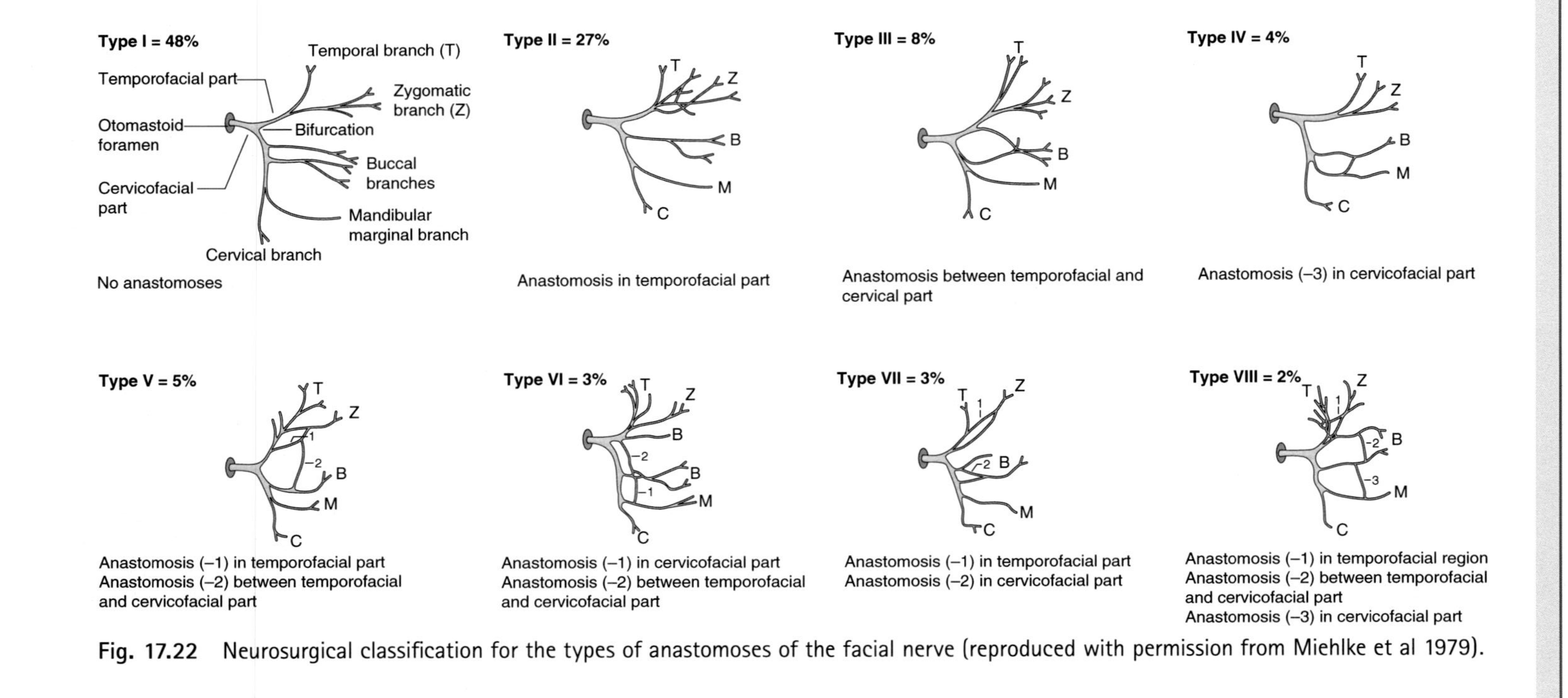

Fig. 17.22 Neurosurgical classification for the types of anastomoses of the facial nerve (reproduced with permission from Miehlke et al 1979).

associated with the physical signs and does not demonstrate organic causes in the definition put forward by the IHS (Olesen 1988, Zakrzewska 2002). The diagnosis is often used when the cause is unknown and all terminology has been exhausted (Mock et al 1985).

The characteristic symptoms are pains of different intensity, varying from unilateral pain to pain affecting the whole face. This worsens continually or episodically, is enhanced by stress and often connected with pain elsewhere in the body (Box 17.1). The most commonly used word from McGill's pain questionnaire is 'nagging'; 'shooting' and 'sharp' are used less frequently. This was shown in an investigation of 195 patients with facial pain (Zakrzewska & Feinmann 1990). This type of pain commonly presents with facial arthromyalgia (temporomandibular dysfunction), atypical dental pain and/or oral dysaesthesia (Harris 1996). On the assumption that the cause is dental, 75% of patients undergo unnecessary dental treatment (Mock et al 1985). These patients often have a long history of pain without clear onset and complain of increasing pain after craniofacial surgery (Zakrzewska & Feinmann 1990). The physical examination is often unremarkable and without neurological signs (Zakrzewska 1995, Peschen-Rosin 2002).

This clinical pattern suggests that deafferentation and centralization play an important role in the pathophysiology (Loeser 1984), although physical signs such as 'cramp' in muscles and blood vessels are reported. Management proposals start with reassurance and careful explanation about surgical intervention (Feinman 1990). Up to half of the patients may experience relief of symptoms with reassurance together with simple analgesics (Zakrzewska 1995).

Treatment with neurodynamics and craniodynamics within an overall management is as yet not suggested for atypical facial pain as it is for other atypical pain syndromes such as those of the shoulder or low back (Butler & Gifford 1998). Butler and Gifford (1998) and Butler (2000) recommend general mobilization techniques of the peripheral nervous system combined with neurodynamic techniques for the facial nerve, as well as pain-free local palpation techniques to change peripheral nociception and the biochemistry of the central nervous system. In the author's opinion, this is a good approach. Together with explanation and cooperation with other disciplines, therapists may make a contribution to the amelioration of these symptoms which affect between 25 and 45% of all patients with chronic facial pain (Agerberg & Carlsson 1972, Zakrzewska 2002).

Box 17.1 Characteristic symptoms of atypical facial pain

- Varying severity and character of pain
- Varies from unilateral to localized to the whole face
- Continuous with sharp exacerbations
- Provoked by stress
- Relieved by appropriate treatment
- Often associated with pain elsewhere in the body

After Zakrzewska (1995).

Tinnitus

DEFINITION AND PREVALENCE

Tinnitus is a relatively common auditory symptom, defined as the aberrant perception of sound in the region of the ear and/or head in the absence of an external source of stimulation (Chan & Reade 1994). In the industrialized world, the prevalence of constant or temporary tinnitus in adults older than 17 years is 35–45%. For those affected, this has a considerable effect at the activity and participation level. In 0.5% of this group the tinnitus is decompensated, i.e. life quality is extremely restricted by symptoms such as concentration and sleeping disturbances, reactive depression and fear (Tyeler 2000).

TYPES OF TINNITUS AND EXPLANATION MODELS

Tinnitus is not a disease, just the ability to hear sounds generated by the auditory (hearing)

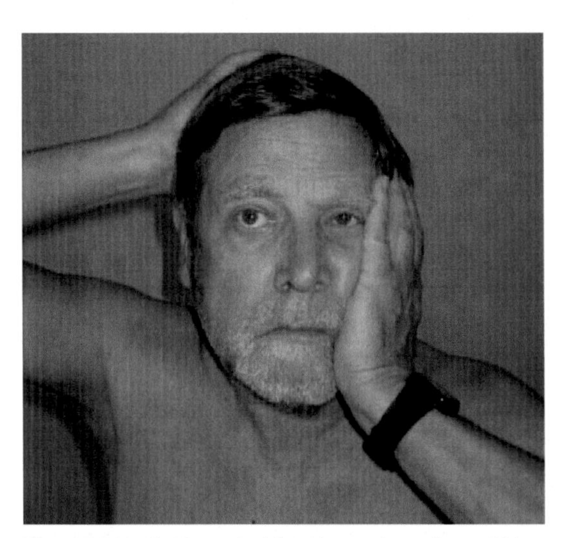

Fig. 17.23 A 58-year-old patient who reduces his tinnitus by own manual pressure on his cranium. What is the mechanism behind it?

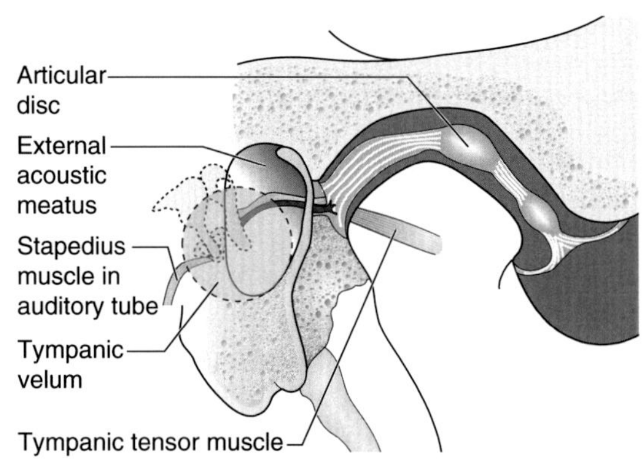

Fig. 17.24 Anatomical connection of the temporomandibular joint and the middle ear. Medioposterior superior fibroelastic tissue part of the joint capsule and the meniscus, attaching onto the neck of the malleus of the middle ear (after Pinto 1962 and designed by Bekkering (2006)).

system. This is evidence of compensatory mechanisms that are part of its normal function (Jastreboff & Hazell 2004). Mostly it is classified as subjective (non-auditory) or objective (clear pathology) tinnitus (Bush 1987, Ganz 1989, Ash & Pinto 1991, Chole & Parker 1992).

Subjective tinnitus is the most common and disturbing form of the condition (Ganz 1989, Chan & Reade 1994). It can be a seriously debilitating disorder for which a clinical solution may not be available. Different explanations in fundamental research and literature suggest that subjective tinnitus is more of a functional disorder of the inner ear caused by several structures (LePage 1993).

Three valid models to explain subjective tinnitus are introduced:

- Anatomical/structural
- Neurophysiological
- Cognitive and affective mechanisms.

Anatomical/structural tinnitus

Examples of structures responsible are the temporomandibular joint, wear to the roof of the temporomandibular joint socket (Costen 1937) and the eardrum (Shapiro & Truex 1943, Sicher 1948, 1955, Zimmerman 1959). Recruitment of the masticatory musculature and muscles in the inner ear also contribute (Dolowitz et al 1964, Malkin 1987, Hazell et al 1993). Nerve branches such as the auriculotemporal nerve and the chorda tympani (Costen 1956, Capps 1962, Vernon et al 1992) and occlusal abnormalities (Shapiro & Truex 1943, Goodfriend 1947, Kopp 1979, Boero 1989) are also indicated.

Embryological correlations (Frumker & Kyle 1987, Cohen & Perez 2003) between ear and mandible, also known as otomandibular structures, are proposed as an important trigger of tinnitus (Hardell et al 2003). Pinto's ligament, which is a fibroelastic tissue arising from the medioposterior superior part of the temporomandibular joint capsule and the meniscus and attaching onto the neck of the malleus, is an example of an otomandibular structure (Pinto 1962, Ash & Pinto 1991; Fig. 17.24). During movement of the jaw this ligament pulls on the malleus which triggers the vestibulocochlear nerve and therefore can change the qualities of the frequency of the tinnitus. Stress on this ligament during a craniomandibular dysfunction causes load on the middle ear structures and affects the depolarization of the vestibulocochlear nerve. This may be why, in some tinnitus patients, protrusion or extreme laterotrusion changes the frequency heard.

Neurovascular compression such as the cerebelli inferior in the posterior fossa (Jannetta 1980, Meaney 1993, Meansey 1994, Tikkakoski 2003) is mentioned (Jannetta 1980b, Meaney et al 1993, Meansey et al 1994, Tikkakoski et al 2003). The middle ear receives its nutrition by osmosis and diffusion from the neighbouring blood vessels. This means that a small compression of the main arteries to the middle ear, or changes of the blood vessel tone by autonomic dysregulation, can cause an ischaemic situation which influences the function of the stapedial velopalatine muscle which is also connected to the middle ear (Xu & Xiong 1999).

Neurophysiological model

The literature can be divided into two parts. The first has a strong input character, which means that nociception of unhealthy tissue from capsule, muscle and peripheral nervous tissue is directly related to the tinnitus. Here, a comparison with facial nerve neuropathy is interesting. For example, abnormal contraction of the stapedial muscle (which is innervated by the facial nerve) and facial nerve pathology have often been described (Badia et al 1994). Watanabe et al (1974) reported eight patients with tinnitus who could influence it by facial expression. Yamamoto et al (1985) reported 20 patients with temporary tinnitus secondary to either facial nerve paralysis or spasm. Facial paralysis and facial neuropathy change the stapedius muscle activity (intermittent or sustained spasms: Bischoff et al 1989, De Souza et al 1994). Marchiando et al (1983) described cases of tinnitus due to stapedial muscle contractions in patients with no concomitant facial nerve disorders. Cases of tinnitus during hemifacial spasm are often reported and are possibly due to anomalies of blood vessels in the posterior fossa or the facial nerve root close to the brain (Janetta 1980b, Badia et al 1994).

The second part of the literature is predominantly about processing mechanisms, particularly the brainstem. An excellent literature review about this has been carried out by Levine et al (2003). Tinnitus in the absence of other hearing complaints shares several clinical features, such as:

- An associated somatic disorder of the craniofacial and/or craniocervical region
- Localization of tinnitus to the ear ipsilateral to the somatic disorder
- No disturbance of balance
- No abnormalities on neurological examination.

In these cases, which are quite common, Levine hypothesized the role of the disinhibition of a brainstem nucleus, the *ipsilateral dorsal cochlear nucleus* (DCN). Disinhibition of this nucleus has consequences for the perception of acoustic information in the brain which can be interpreted as tinnitus (Jastreboff et al 1994, Abel & Levine 2004, Kaltenbach et al 2004).

Model of cognitive and affective mechanisms

In the last decade, central mechanisms have been recognized as causes of tinnitus alongside the traditional medical models. It has been shown that emotional and cognitive concepts can cause functional impairments that are related to tinnitus (Goebel 1997):

- In the brain, tinnitus can be considered as a new signal without a memory. For the brain it has, therefore, no cognitive meaning or complementary value (Robson 2002). This is understood as part of a cognitive/affective clinical picture. Coping strategies such as fear of irreversible damage to the ear, belief in a brain tumour or mental illness are not uncommon (Jastreboff 1990). In short, tinnitus can be perceived as life threatening and cause both hyperacusis and phonophobia. Hyperacusis means that daily sounds (traffic, kitchen, children, etc.) are excessively amplified. This is often accompanied by phonophobia, in which the patient has an excessive fear of daily environmental noise, and worries that these might damage hearing and cause further problems such as headache, fatigue and vertigo (Hazell 2001).

- The worst effect of tinnitus is usually the distress which increases with time, rather than the tinnitus itself (Goebel 1997). The intensity of unpleasant sensation is dependent on the strength of emotional influences (limbic system) and the body's autonomic reaction (Jastreboff 1990). These effects could be headache, fatigue or dizziness. The intensity and quality of the sound is irrelevant (Hazell 2002). Figure 17.26 shows this model, based predominantly on central mechanisms (Jastreboff 1990, Jastreboff & Hazel 2004).

From this model we learn that a cognitive behaviour strategy such as retraining or explanation of benign causes of tinnitus can have a positive influence on the attitude to tinnitus in every patient. A specialized programme that has proved these effects is the tinnitus retraining therapy (TRT) based on the Jastreboff model (Robson 2002).

This means that the therapist can integrate craniofacial and cranioneural manual techniques with cognitive behaviour principles such as:

- A simple explanation about (central) mechanisms and the natural course of tinnitus.
- Positive reinforcement of small personal limitations that are directly related to tinnitus.
- Integration of pain management techniques such as 'distraction' or 'pacing'.
- Discussion and formulation of subsequent goals, together with a programme of controlling activity, all of which are related to the tinnitus.

Two types of tinnitus are recognized due to the modulation of nerves in the brainstem, namely craniocervical and otogenic tinnitus (Levine 1999).

CRANIOCERVICAL TINNITUS

Sensory input comes from:

- The craniofacial region via the trigeminal nerve (V) and the spinal trigeminal tract (STT).
- The outer and middle ear via the facial (VII), glossopharyngeal (IX) and vagus (X) nerves.

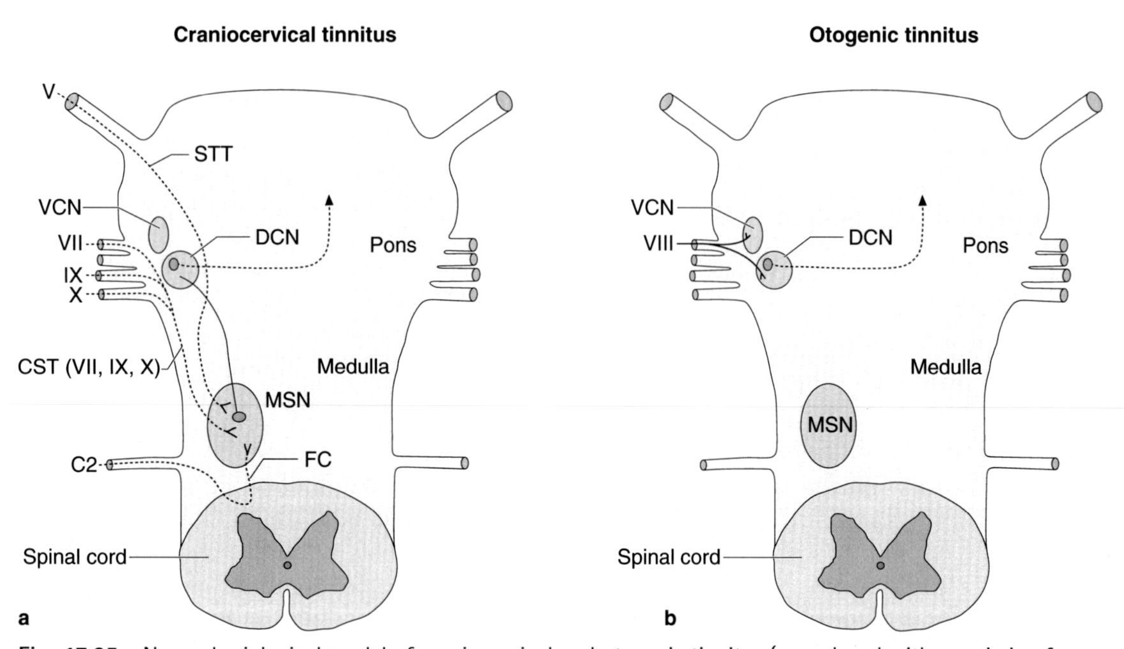

Fig. 17.25 Neurophysiological model of craniocervical and otogenic tinnitus (reproduced with permission from Levine 1999).

Table 17.4 Management suggestions for disinhibition of the dorsal cochlear nucleus (DCN)

Restoration of DCN inhibition	Reduction of DCN input
Electrical stimulation of the vestibulocochlear nerve (VIII)	Transect the output tract of DCN
Electrical or mechanical stimulation of somatic pathways	Lesion of the DCN

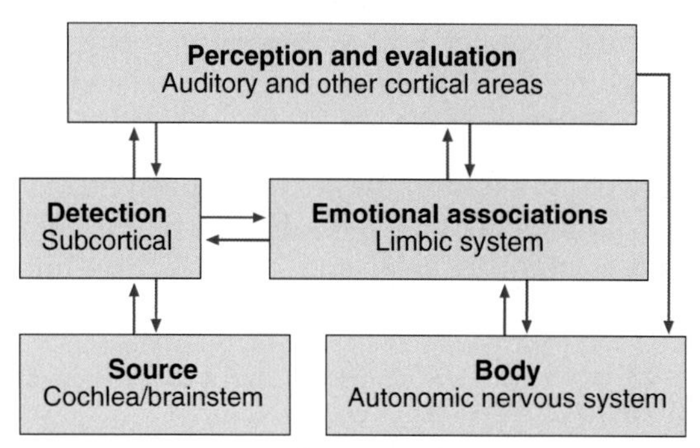

Fig. 17.26 Cognitive/affective model showing the possible consequences of tinnitus (reproduced with permission from Jastreboff 1990).

- The craniocervical region via the dorsal root.
- Fascicular nuclei of the somatosensory medulla (MSN). These converge to a common region in the lower medulla, the medullary somatosensory nuclei (MSN; Fig. 17.25). From here fibres project to the DCN and inhibition in the cortex arises.

OTOGENIC TINNITUS

The pathway of otic tinnitus is less complicated. A loss of input (spontaneous activity) from the auditory nerve (VIII) leads to impaired inhibition of the DCN.

Treatment suggestions from the dorsal cochlear nucleus disinhibition hypothesis are mentioned in Table 17.4.

For the therapist this means that:

- Manual therapy of the craniofacial and craniocervical regions can change the disinhibition of the DCN, thus reducing tinnitus.
- Treatment by cranioneurodynamics of the trigeminal (V), facial (VII), glossopharyngeal (IX) and the vagus (X) nerves can contribute to the restoration of the inhibition of the DCN.
- The effect of input for the vestibulocochlear nerve (VIII) through equilibrium and balance exercises should be assessed in each individual patient.

TINNITUS AND VERTIGO

In case studies and surveys, vertigo, dizziness and tinnitus are often associated with benign pathology such as acute vestibular dysfunctions (Vibert & Häusler 2003), Ménière's disease (Franz et al 1999), craniocervical dysfunction and trauma (Hulse 1994, Nagy & Pontracz 1997, Franz et al 1999, Kessinger & Boneva 2000, Alcantara et al 2002) or craniomandibular dysfunction (Williamson 1990, Chole & Parker 1992, Rubenstein 1993, Parker & Chole 1995, Lam et al 2001, Alcantara et al 2002).

Acoustic neuroma (vestibular schwannoma) which dominantly affects the vestibulocochlear nerve can also cause tinnitus together with vertigo. In this case there is a complex of symptoms including deep diffuse headache, facial nerve paresis, progressive hearing loss and/or sensitivity changes in the face (Baguley et al 1997, Matsuka et al 2000, Neff et al 2003). Due to this complication, it is advisable that the therapist refer the patient to a neurologist or ENT specialist as soon as it is clear that the patient's tinnitus and vertigo are not responding to treatment.

THE ROLE OF BALANCE EXERCISES FOR TINNITUS AND VERTIGO

Clinical experience has shown that balance exercises for perception and control of tinnitus can lead to clear improvements. However, there is a lack of effective studies in the literature, hence the following hypotheses:

- Auditory and vestibular afferents have the same projection on the somatosensory cortex (Ramachandran & Blakesee 1998). Overstimulation of vestibular branches filters and muffles the auditory cortex which changes the perception of tinnitus (Hazell 2002).
- As an overwhelmed somatic input inhibits the dorsal cochlear nucleus (DCN), the auditory cortex receives less stimulation and the tinnitus experienced will be reduced (Levine 1999, Abel & Levine 2004).
- Input from the head, face and neck region, such as balance exercises that do not provoke symptoms, changes the stimuli of the somatosensory cortex (distraction) and influences the activity of the auditory cortex (Ramachandran & Blakesee 1998).
- Systematic information regarding pathogenesis and natural course controls tinnitus and vertigo: most patients experience less tinnitus and vertigo during balance exercises. This phenomenon can be explained by an alertness that may have a positive influence on the patient's coping strategies, which in turn can lead to reduced fear and distress (Chatelier et al 1982, Jastreboff 1990, Goebel 1997).

The outcome of standardized balance tests before and after craniofacial techniques shows whether tinnitus and vertigo are related in the individual. More information about balance training can be found in the section about the oculomotor nerves and oculomotor rehabilitation below.

MANAGEMENT GUIDELINES FOR SUBJECTIVE TINNITUS

Besides management by operation, medication, orthodontic dental treatment, psychological intervention, injection, biofeedback, change of lifestyle, relaxation therapy, etc., examination and treatment of neurodynamics of the facial nerve, together with passive movements of neighbouring structures such as palate, sphenoid, petrosal, temporal and occipital bones and/or the craniomandibular region, are suggested (Chan & Reade 1994). Clinical experience with manual craniofacial and neurodynamic treatment shows that if one technique changes and/or reduces the frequency of the tinnitus, the prognosis is better.

- Equilibrium has to be examined and, if necessary, integrated into treatment and management. Some research shows that re-education and training of the patient's equilibrium makes the tinnitus more acceptable and enables the patient to control the problem better. Furthermore, balance exercises can be used as a kind of 'distraction' for the unpleasant sensations in the ear.
- In some cases it is useful to integrate cognitive strategies alongside manual craniofacial and cranioneurodynamic techniques. This is particularly the case when the manual therapy approach changes the tinnitus. The therapist can then provide the patient with positive feedback and an explanation as described under the cognitive/affective model.

The therapist must take account of a strong irritable and latency character of tinnitus in some patients. Examination and treatment has to be symptom-free initially. Depending on the reaction of the individual patient, the intensity may be increased. In most cases increasing the duration is more effective than increasing nerve loading. Experiments with facial nerve techniques combined with occipital and petrosal bone pressure medially provide the therapist with an opportunity to give input into the craniofacial region for a considerable period without provoking symptoms. If these techniques change the frequency of tinnitus together with other symptoms, adaptations of them can be used as home programmes and controlled regularly.

VESTIBULOCOCHLEAR NERVE (VIII)

Relevant functional anatomy

The vestibulocochlear nerve (Fig. 17.27) carries two kinds of specialized sensations: vestibular sensation (sense of equilibrium including posture and muscle tone) and auditory sensa-

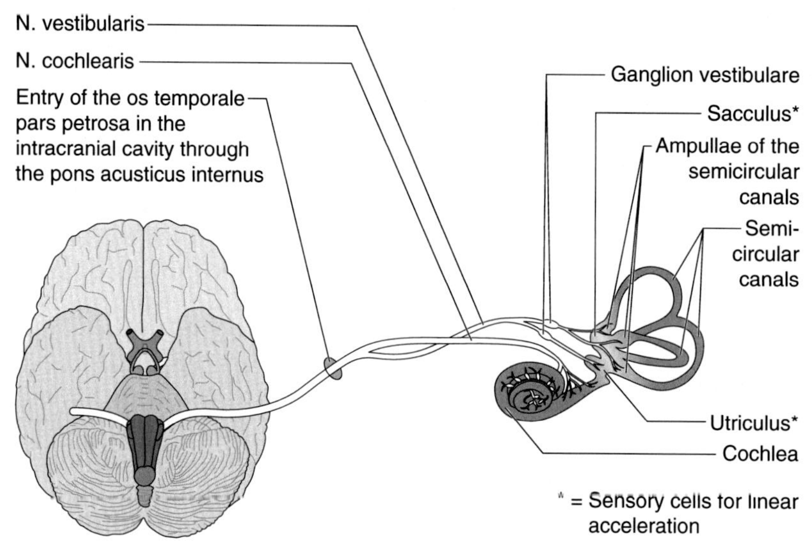

Fig. 17.27
Vestibulocochlear nerve.

tion from specialized sensory receptors in the inner ear. The vestibular nerve originates from the vestibular apparatus and runs for most of its length together with the auditory nerve which starts in the cochlea. Together they run laterally and are united in the petrosal foramen. From here they run together with the facial nerve from the inner side of the border of the temporal bone through the internal auditory meatus and the subarachnoid space. Together with the glossopharyngeal nerve they enter the lateral dorsal side of the brainstem (Silverstein & Jackson 2002).

Neurodynamic test

The neurodynamic test of the vestibulocochlear nerve is not really spectacular because the nerve runs 100% intracranially. If the history and the symptoms fit in with a possible dysfunction of the vestibulocochlear nerve, the proposed neurodynamic test together with neural container assessment can be performed. To load the nerve, upper cervical flexion and lateroflexion are necessary. Accessory movements of the petrosal, occiput, sphenoid and temporal bones can all influence the vestibulocochlear nerve which is intracranially connected with the lateral side of the cranium (temporal region).

STARTING POSITION AND METHOD

The patient lies supine, comfortably and relaxed. The therapist sits or stands on the right side of the patient's head. The left hand cups around the occipital bone which fixes upper flexion and lateroflexion. The right hand is free for influencing the petrosal and sphenoid regions. To change the temporal bone region, the starting position as described in the method needs to be changed.

For examination of the petrosal bone, bend over the patient and, with the thumb and the flexed index finger, grasp around the contralateral bone. Every accessory movement required can now be performed. Make sure that the head position does not change.

For movement of the occipitosphenoid region in this position, the therapist faces the patient. The left hand is in supination and cups the occipital bone. The right thumb and index finger grasp around the lateral side of the sphenoid bone (Fig. 17.28). In this position the main accessory movements of the occipitosphenoid region can be performed. The best position for access to the temporal bone is sitting above the patient's head. The left hand holds the required head position to load the cranial nervous tissue on the left side. With the right hand, grasp the temporal bone with the right middle finger in the ear

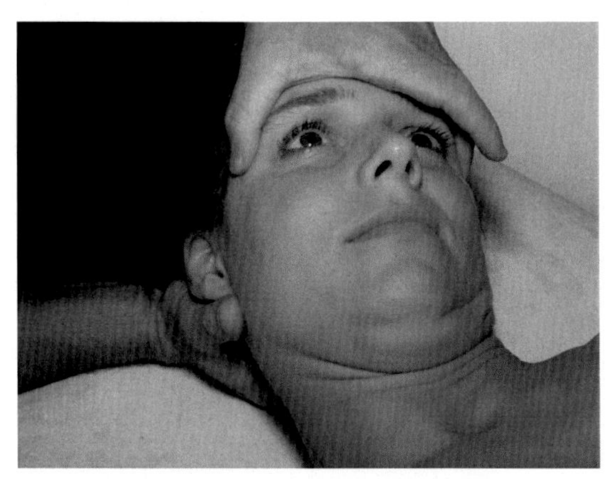

Fig. 17.28 (Part of the) neurodynamic test of the vestibulocochlear nerve. Sphenoid examination in craniocervical neurodynamic position.

canal, the right little finger on the petrosal bone and the auricular extension, and the right thumb on the region above the ear. All movements described in Chapter 15 may influence the symptoms which may come from pathophysiological changes of the vestibulocochlear nerve.

Palpation

The vestibulocochlear nerve runs 100% intracranially and is not palpable.

Conduction

The purpose of the conduction test is to reveal either a middle-ear hearing problem or reduced nerve activity. Balance impairments, if these originate from the labyrinth, vestibular nerve or the brainstem, are more dispersed and often have a predictable pattern. In this case the patient should be referred to an ENT specialist.

THE FUNCTION OF THE AUDITORY NERVE

Examination of hearing

The therapist gently rubs the tips of the index finger and thumb together 2–8 cm from the patient's ears and asks the patient if the sound produced is heard equally in each ear. If there is a loss or diminished response on one side, differentiation of the localization of the deafness can be achieved by a tuning fork using Rinne's and Weber's tests.

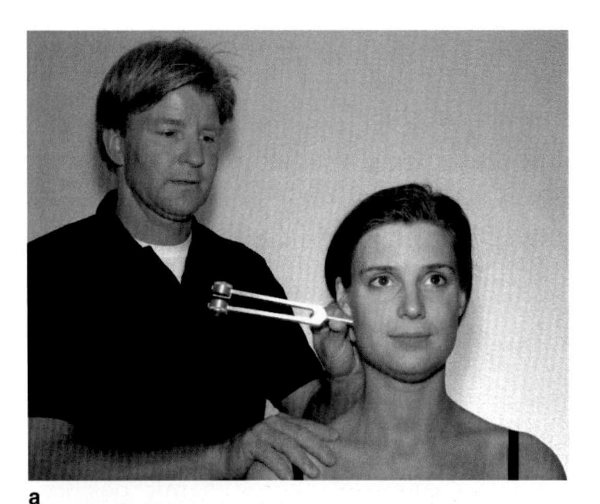

a

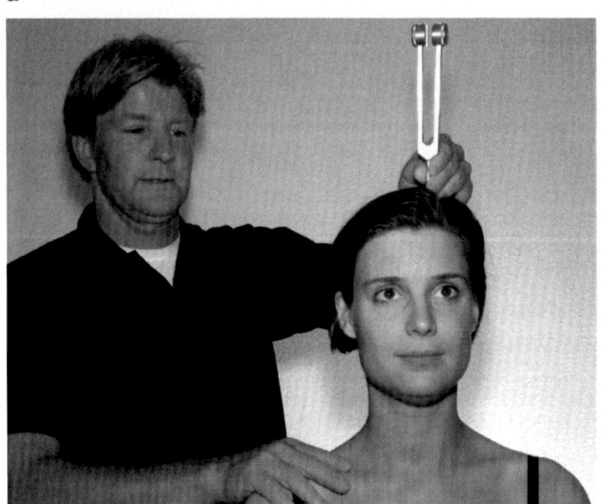

b

Fig. 17.29 Examination of auditory function using a tuning fork.
a Rinne test.
b Weber test.

The Rinne test

The therapist strikes a tuning fork, holds it near one external meatus, covering (± 2–3 cm) the other, and asks the patient if they can hear it.

The therapist then alternates the position of the tuning fork from the mastoid process to in front of the ear, until the note is no longer audible in any position (Fig. 17.29a). With normal conductivity, the tone can be heard longer in front of the ear than on the mastoid process (negative Rinne test). When the tuning fork can be heard for longer on the mastoid process than in front of the ear this is abnormal (positive Rinne test). This reaction indicates a hearing defect in the middle ear or neural hearing loss (related to the acoustic nerve). In this case the Weber test must be carried out.

The Weber test

The tuning fork is placed on the centre of the frontal bone (Fig. 17.29b). The patient is asked if they can hear the sound all over the head, in both ears or mainly in one ear. In nerve 'deafness' the sound appears to be heard in the normal ear but in chronic middle ear disease the sound is conducted to the normal ear.

- When changes of neurodynamic position alter the hearing during the Weber test, neurogenic dysfunction rather than middle ear disease is indicated.
- Hearing disturbance caused by the auditory nerve (VIII) together with conduction symptoms of the trigeminal (V) and facial (VII) nerves are probably due to lesions or pathodynamics of the cerebellopontine angle (Spillane 1996).
- Bilateral deafness during the Weber test may be due to bilateral middle ear disease or a central lesion (Spillane 1996).

On discovery of any of these clinical patterns, further assessment by a neurologist or otolaryngologist is imperative (Berghaus et al 1996, Halmagyi 2005). If no clear pathology is found, manual assessment of the craniofacial region can be an option (Berghaus et al 1996).

FUNCTION OF THE VESTIBULAR NERVE: EQUILIBRIUM TESTS WITH OR WITHOUT NEURODYNAMIC POSITION

Two legs standing test

Let the patient stand on two legs with a relatively small support base, i.e. feet together or one foot in front of the other (Fig. 17.30). In this position neurodynamic loading of the head is added. In the author's opinion upper cervical flexion is the best position. Passive neck flexion must always be assessed separately.

If symptoms such as vertigo, balance problems, falling, nystagmus and 'seeing stars' occur, the hypothesis is a conductive impair-

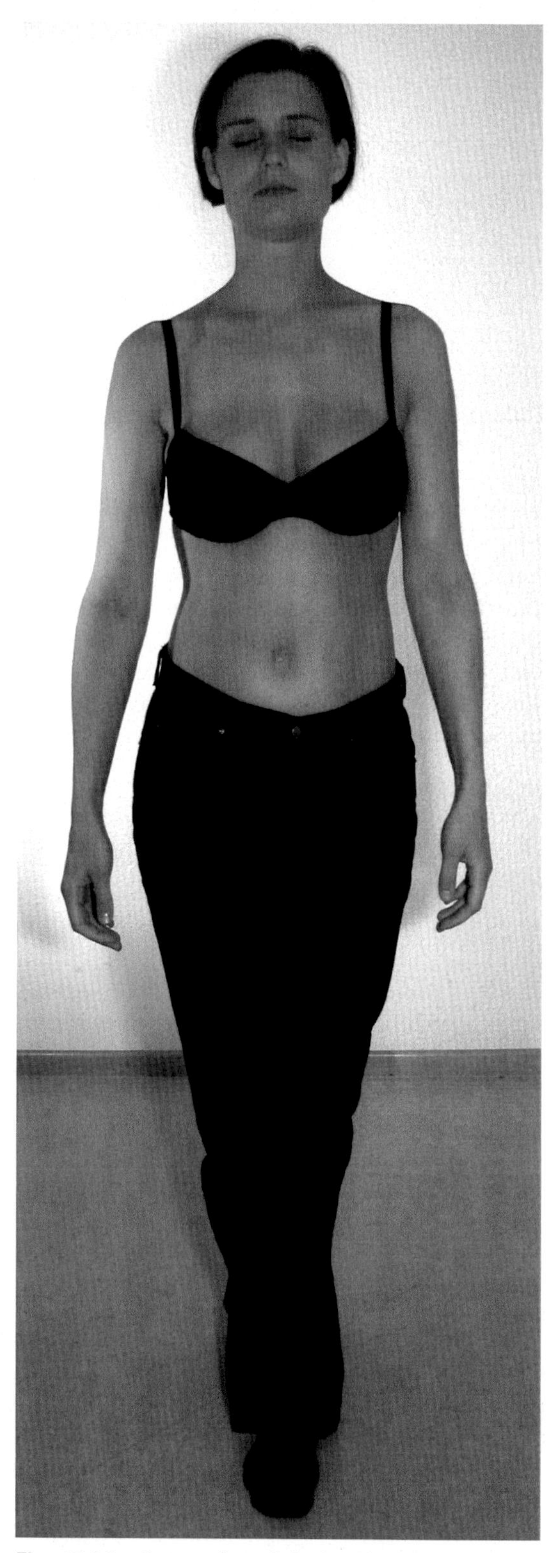

Fig. 17.30 Progression of the two leg standing test; here with one foot in front and one behind with the eyes closed.

ment of the vestibular (VIII) nerve. Lateroflexion to the other side can be helpful; however, this also influences the semicircular canals of the balance organ (Spillane 1996).

Other standardized balance tests such as the Romberg, Unterberger, rope dancer and Stern tests can be used. The head position can be varied, for example in upper cervical flexion or lateroflexion to the opposite side.

> **!** The therapist should be aware that the neurodynamics of the vestibular (VIII) nerve is not the only aspect affected. The capsule and endolymph in the semicircular canals of the labyrinth are also affected.

These stimulate input of the cochlear components and the vestibulocochlear nerve (Wilson-Pauwels et al 2002). If abnormal reactions such as stiffness or pain occur during the neurodynamic investigation, treatment without increase of vertigo or light-headedness is an option.

Re-examination of symptom behaviour and standardized balance tests can confirm or disprove the relevance of abnormal neurodynamic reactions. More information on balance tests and oculomotor rehabilitation is given in the section on the oculomotor system.

The rotation test

This is a test for the vestibular apparatus on both sides. The patient is seated in a swivel chair which is rotated ten times in 20 seconds. The patient's head is well supported and held in 30% flexion. Nystagmus, 'seeing stars' and falling to the ipsilateral side or an increase of tinnitus can be an indication of overstimulation of the labyrinth (Baloh et al 1984, Saadat et al 1995, Spillane 1996). As most nystagmus usually cannot be observed with the naked eye (Berghaus et al 1996), the therapist needs a pair of Frenzel glasses. This is an instrument with magnifying glasses and a small light on the inside. This magnifies the eyes so that eye movements can be seen more easily (Fig. 17.31).

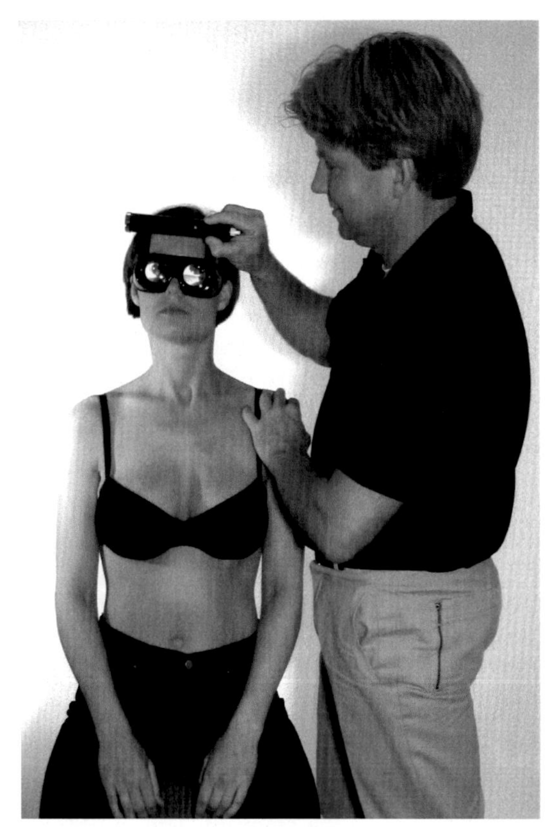

Fig. 17.31 Observation of nystagmus with Frenzel glasses after the rotation test.

The temperature test

This test is a general test for the vestibulo-ocular reflexes. Warm saline is placed in the ear. If it results in nystagmus, referral to a neurologist is indicated.

Comment

The vestibular nerve has a relatively long intracranial course and multifarious internal interactions with the vestibular muscles within the nervous system. Therefore there are numerous potential causes for light-headedness, vertigo, ear pain after middle ear inflammation and balance impairment. These could be impaired vascularization, metabolism, degenerative compression and neoplastic lesions of the vestibulocochlear brainstem complex (Torok & Kumar 1978, Mafee et al 1984, Schwaber & Whetsell 1992).

VASCULARIZATION

Recent magnetic resonance (MR) imaging reports show that inflammation in the areas of the anterior inferior cerebellar artery (AICA) and the posterior inferior cerebellar artery (PICA) reproduce signs and symptoms similar to vestibulocochlear nerve neuropathy (Nakayama et al 1989, Kido et al 1994, Laine & Underhill 2002). This is because these arteries supply the cerebellum, the lower part of the pons, the upper part of the medulla oblongata and the inner ear (Atkinson 1949, Naidich et al 1976). These arteries lie parallel to the flexion–extension axes and are influenced by upper cervical flexion and side flexion (Breig 1976, Jannetta 1990). This knowledge can be linked to the question of why, during and after upper cervical flexion and side flexion, symptoms such as dizziness, tinnitus and ear pain change, especially when a cranium technique of the sphenoid and/or occipital bone is added. Vascular occlusion disturbances due to compression because of anomalies and degeneration are possibly eliminated or lessened for a while during these gentle unloading techniques of the dorsal side of the cranium. This could be an alternative hypothesis as to why this happened (Breig 1960, 1976, Gorge 2001).

METABOLIC CHANGES

Viral infections can cause sudden dysfunction of cranial nerves. Ocular (Fuller et al 1989) and facial (Wechsler & Ho 1989) nerve involvement are clearly reported with increasing evidence. Temporal bone studies of patients during and after vestibular neuritis have highlighted maximal damage in the dural branches of the vestibular nerve where the changes are felt to be consistent with a viral aetiology. Several viruses (e.g. rubella, herpes simplex, reovirus, neurotrophic influenza and mumps) can infect the vestibular nerve and its environment (Davis 1993). In the past two decades, the human immunodeficiency virus (HIV) has been very evident, but the pathogenesis is currently unknown (Simpson & Bender 1988, Chaunu et al 1989, Grimaldi et al 1993). Grimaldi et al (1993) showed that, in a biopsy of the dural nerve of an HIV-1 seropositive man, the presence of perivascular inflammation (vasculitis) could be responsible for this HIV-1 associated cranial nerve neuropathy. Uneven disturbances of local ischaemia may explain the scattered occurrence of axon degeneration and segmental demyelination which contribute to destruction of the nerves (Nukada & Dick 1984). If a patient complains of sudden bilateral hearing loss, dizziness and/or a deep cranial pain of sudden onset, it may be wise to ask a neurologist or ENT specialist for a differential diagnosis. Whether the neurodynamics of cranial nervous tissue can change due to pathophysiology and mechanical scar tissue or adhesions which occur following a severe inflammation around blood vessels is still not clear.

TUMOURS

Acoustic neuromas, which account for 80–90% of cerebellopontine angle (CPA) tumours (Rowland 1989), are the most common of the posterior fossa tumours (Langman et al 1990). The tumour usually begins on the vestibulocochlear nerve in the CPA and the trigeminal and facial nerves are affected more often than other cranial nerves (Langman et al 1990, Normand & Daube 1994, Sanna et al 2003). A patient who presents with symptoms such as facial numbness, facial palsy, decreased corneal reflex and facial pain (Eisen & Danon 1974, Ylikoski et al 1981, Nager 1985, Fischer et al 1992), which increase with head correction into upper cervical flexion and contralateral lateroflexion, is not indicated for treatment by neurodynamics.

Needle electromyography of cranial nerves is used to diagnose the acoustic neuroma (Nager 1985, Harner et al 1987, Armon & Daube 1989, Normand & Daube 1994) and surgical removal (Fischer et al 1980, Cohen et al 1986, Glasscock et al 1986, Burchiel et al 1988, Shelton et al 1989) or stereotactic radiosurgery (Bederson et al 1991, Flickinger et al 1992, Linskey & Sekhar 1993, Ogunrinde et al 1994) will be the treatment of choice (Fischer et al 1980, Cohen et al 1986, Glasscock et al 1986, Burchiel et al 1988, Shelton et al 1989). On the other hand, an iatrogenic factor of surgery in the CPA may be vestibular and facial neuropathies (Flickinger et al 1992, Linksey & Sekhar 1993). In dogs it is proven that the caudal to posterior shift of the nerve trunk may avulse the vestibular nerve. Cranial neurodynamics performed passively or actively may be a good complementary therapy after cerebellopontine angle surgery.

DIZZINESS AND VERTIGO

Dizziness and vertigo are some of the most common symptoms for which a patient will consult a primary care therapist (Douglas 1993). *Dizziness* can be described in general terms, implying only the sense of a disturbed relationship to the space outside oneself (Smith 1990); *vertigo* can be described as the illusion of motion or position, either of the patient or the patient's environment (Adams & Victor 1985, Fowler & May 1985). They are often accompanied by other associated symptoms such as tinnitus, nausea, vomiting, nystagmus, perspiration, a sense of fear, diplopia, drop attacks, dysarthria, dysphagia, tiredness, etc. (Coman 1986, Oostendorp 1988, Hanson 1989, Douglas 1993, Roy 1994). Further detailed information about anatomy, pathophysiology, common differential diagnostic considerations and aetiology is reviewed in good fundamental literature in this domain and will not be discussed further here (Troost 1980, Gutmann 1983a, Oostendorp 1988, Patten 1995, Grant 1996).

For the therapist it can be interesting to note which head positions influence the dizziness in order to gain information about which structures are involved. For example, there are good clinical protocols for vertebral artery testing whereby the therapist gets an indication of the condition of the vertebrobasilar complex before manual therapy on the cervical spine is carried out (Maigne 1972, Gutmann 1983a, Maitland 1986, Aspinall 1989, Douglas 1993, Grant 1996).

Gutmann (1983b) argued that flexion and extension of the cervical spine have no influence on the narrowing of the vertebral artery. On the other hand, extension combined with cervical rotation produced occlusion of the vertebral artery whereas extension alone did not (Toole & Tucker 1960, Brown & Tatlow 1963). Krueger and Okazaki (1980) conclude that the occlusion of the vertebral artery was unpredictable during flexion and rotation of the cervical spine. Lateroflexion produces a small occlusion change and flexion, together with lateroflexion, has minimal influence on narrowing (Gutmann 1983b, Bolton et al 1990).

There are still patients who are dizzy in flexion and other positions combined with lateroflexion and any small amount of rotation, without a clear history of overstimulation of the proprioceptive system of the upper cervical spine (Terrett 1983). For example, symptoms during computer work, reading in bed with the hand on the lateral side of the face, putting on shoes, etc. whereby the patients feels that the head position and the movement influencing the dizziness may be cervicogenic in origin; however, another possibility could be pathophysiological changes of the vestibular nerve.

Vestibular neuritis is the second most common cause of vertigo. The superior division is mainly affected, including the afferent from the horizontal and anterior semicircular canals (SCC) (Fetter & Dichgans 1996). Upper cervical flexion and lateroflexion of the cervical spine change the pressure in the CPA and the vestibular nerve (Breig 1960, 1976, Jannetta et al 1984, Leblanc 1995). In some cases, where the patient provokes vertigo or dizziness in a flexed head position (or keeps the head in slight neck extension to prevent these symptoms), it could be useful to examine the neurodynamics of the cranial nerve tissue, especially that of the vestibulocochlear nerve. As treatment using neurodynamics often provokes reactions of severe dizziness or vertigo, the therapist must bear these facts in mind and is recommended to start without resistance in the direction of the neurodynamic position or to treat the cranial bones out of a loaded position (upper extension, ipsilateral lateroflexion of the head) without symptoms.

Generally, if the symptoms change, either during or after this test, this is a good indication for further examination and treatment. In the case of severe and irritable symptoms such as nausea and vomiting, tinnitus, vertigo, etc. it is best first to treat the petrosal or temporal bone in an unloaded position for the vestibulocochlear nerve. Studies show that mechanical impulses on the cranial bones activate the vertebral apparatus (Ito et al 1990, Halmagyi et al 1995, Manni et al 1996). On the other hand, in the author's opinion, otovestibular symptoms such as otalgia, sensitivity to loud noise or muffled hearing without underlying pathology such as infection, tumours, etc., react better to indirect techniques with little resistance (e.g. hard palate mobilization in or out of load position of the eighth cranial nerve).

Table 17.5 gives a general overview of the physical examination options for the vestibulocochlear nerve.

ACCESSORY NERVE (XI)

Relevant functional anatomy

The accessory nerve is a motor nerve consisting of a spinal and a cranial component (Fig. 17.32). The spinal component is derived from a number of upper cervical spinal nerve roots which arise from the five uppermost cervical segments and pass through the foramen magnum to access the skull. The cranial component is integrated into the peripheral distribution of the vagus nerve. Inside the skull, both these components join forces and exit through the jugular foramen. Once outside the skull they pass the styloid process medially. Some branches terminate in the sternocleidomastoid muscle. The nerve then crosses superficially to the posterior triangle of the neck, to the levator scapulae. This is the optimal point for palpation. Many anomalies are seen; for example, some branches meet above and run deep to the anterior edge of the trapezius to supply this muscle (Fig. 17.33). Many anoma-

Table 17.5 Overview of the physical examination options for the vestibulocochlear nerve (VIII)

Neurodynamic tests	Conduction tests
Craniocervical:	Auditory nerve:
Upper cervical flexion	Examination of hearing
Contralateral lateral flexion	Rinne's, Weber's test
Craniofacial:	Vestibular nerve:
Petrosal	Two leg standing test
Temporal	Other balance tests
Sphenoid	Rotation test
Occiput	Temperature test

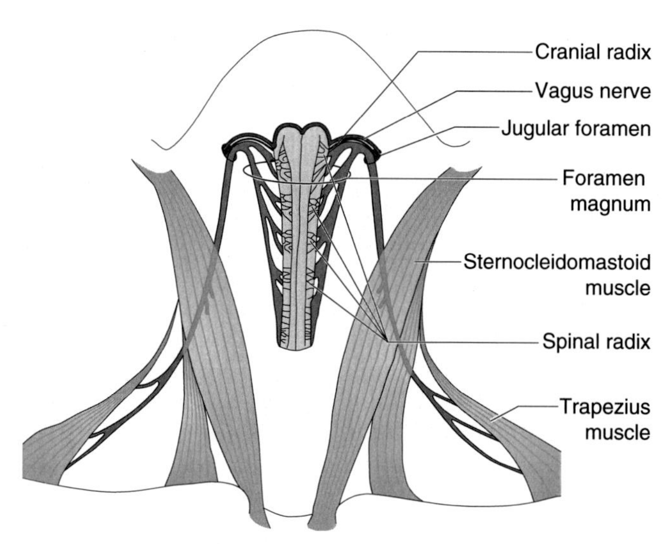

Fig. 17.32 Accessory nerve.

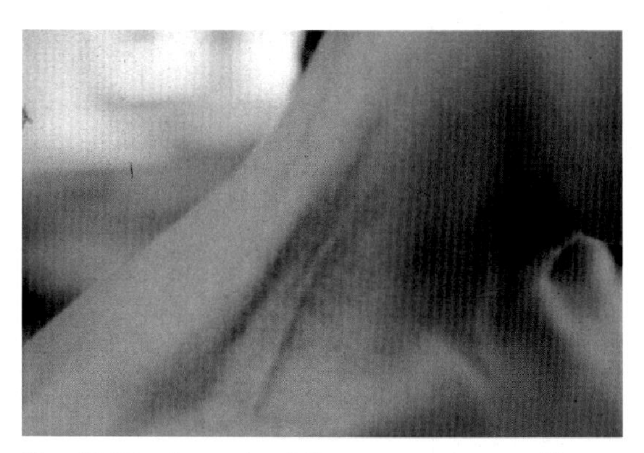

Fig. 17.33 Anomaly of the accessory nerve. The cervical branch does not run under the trapezius pars descendens muscle but instead into the supraclavicular region.

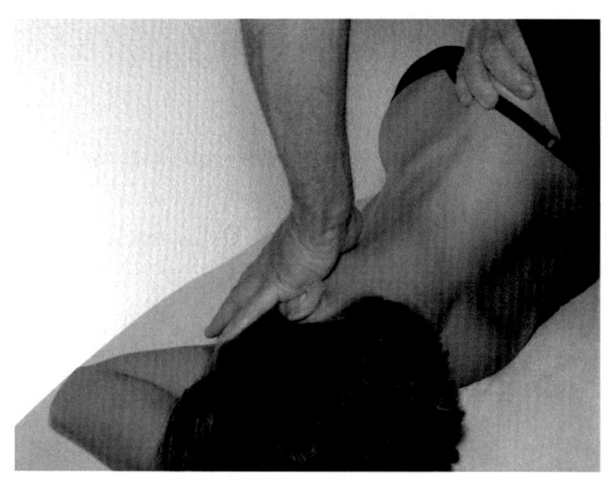

Fig. 17.34 Neurodynamic test for the accessory nerve.

lies and extra branches are seen superficially in the supraclavicular region and are predisposed to (minor) neuropathies (Mumenthaler & Schliack 1991, Wilson-Pauwels et al 2002).

Neurodynamic test

Upper and midcervical flexion and lateroflexion away change the neurodynamics of the intracranial tissue and upper extracranial tissue of the accessory nerve (Breig 1976). Deep cervical extension could be a challenge for accessory nerve tissue above and around the acromioclavicular joint. Cranial movements from occiput and/or sphenoid can be added, changing the jugular foramen. Depression and retraction of the shoulder are needed to change the neurodynamics of the extracranial part of the nerve.

STARTING POSITION AND METHOD

A side-lying position is best for this technique, with the patient's side to be examined uppermost. The patient's head should be positioned comfortably on the headrest, which should be set low (for lateroflexion to the opposite side). The lower elbow should be bent, and the hand may be under the head. The upper arm is behind the back, but without too much depression or retraction of the shoulder.

The therapist stands behind the patient, with the hip leaning on the plinth at the level of the patient's lumbar spine. The therapist cups the occipital region with the right hand and stabilizes the patient's ventral shoulder with the forearm. The therapist's left forearm can lean on the plinth, the left metacarpus is placed on the right zygomatic bone and the left thumb and index finger clasp the mandible. Upper cervical flexion and lateroflexion can be performed easily using this grip. The therapist then grasps the roof of the patient's shoulder with the right hand and performs a slight depression or retraction of the shoulder girdle. Rotation and extension of the thoracic spine should be prevented (Fig. 17.34).

To influence the lower part of this region (around the clavicle and acromioclavicular joint), the patient's head should be positioned in minimal flexion of the upper and midcervical spine and extension of the upper thoracic spine. Branches of the accessory nerve become visible and/or palpable ventromedial to the edge of the descending part of the trapezius muscle.

If necessary the patient can hold their head actively during the whole 'set up'.

Sometimes a classic reaction can be seen during the shoulder manoeuvres of the 'set up' procedure in the form of hyperextension of the neck and increased activity of the elevators of the masticatory system (the masseter and temporal muscles).

The neural container of the accessory nerve

In this position occipital movements against the sphenoid bone (especially the transverse movements) can be performed to influence the mechanical interface of the accessory nerve.

The therapist's right hand cups the occipital bone and the left index finger and thumb grasp around the greater wings of the sphenoid to perform the movement. The patient's head is in upper cervical flexion and contralateral lateroflexion, and the shoulder girdle fixed in retraction and depression as best possible by the therapist's forearm (Fig. 17.35).

Accessory movements, especially the unilateral posterior–anterior movements of the upper cervical segments C0–C3 in side-lying, are useful both to examine and to treat with or without neurodynamic positions (Fig. 17.36).

Palpation

The most superficial area of the accessory nerve is in the posterior triangle of the neck, where it also runs parallel to the fibres of the levator scapulae muscle. About 5 cm above the clavicle, the nerve crosses the anterior edge of the trapezius. In most cases, it is easily palpable parallel to, and sometimes under, the trapezius muscle (Fig. 17.37).

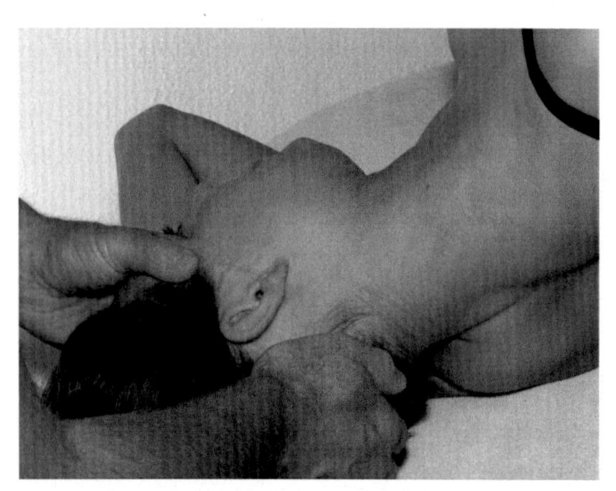

Fig. 17.35 Examination and treatment: starting position of the occiput in neurodynamic positioning of the accessory nerve.

Conduction

OBSERVATION AND PALPATION

During observation of the head and neck region, minimal asymmetry of the trapezius

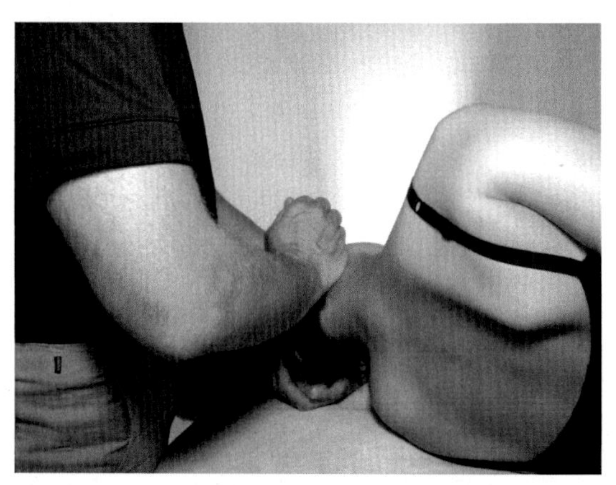

Fig. 17.36 Example of neural container treatment by unilateral movement of the upper cervical segments in side lying using the hypothenar eminence of the therapist's right hand (thumb techniques are also possible).

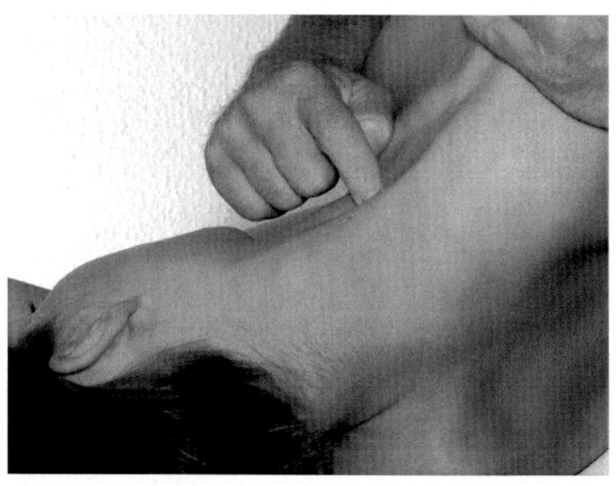

Fig. 17.37 Palpation of the accessory nerve under the trapezius muscle.

and sternocleidomastoid muscles may be related to conduction changes.

Palpation of the altered tone and sensory responses such as pain can support the hypothesis of an accessory nerve dysfunction.

MUSCLE TEST

Bilateral dysfunction indicates central problems of the nerve trunk. Unilateral weakness usually suggests problems in the branches of the accessory nerve. Resistive isometric tests for a couple of seconds should be carried out for each muscle.

Sternocleidomastoid muscle

For the sternocleidomastoid muscle the patient needs to lie supine with the head over the edge of the couch. Bring the head into slight extension of 20° with contralateral lateroflexion of 20–30° and ipsilateral rotation of 20–30°, so that the sternocleidomastoid is optimally engaged. During the isometric test, hold the hypothenar part of the left hand against the patient's chin and facilitate this combined movement to guard against other extraneous movements (Fig. 17.38).

M. trapezius pars descendens

The trapezius can also be tested in a supine position. Elevate the shoulder of the side to be tested and cup the thenar eminence of the right hand in supination around the scapula so that the acromion is in the palm of the hand. It may be easier to rest the elbow against the pelvis while performing this manoeuvre. Compare the left with the right side. Signs such as atrophy, spasm, fasciculation and pain should be noted. If it is possible to reproduce the symptoms, some neurodynamic components for the accessory nerve or for the extremities (e.g. ULNT or SLR) can be added. A change in symptoms signifies that the neurodynamic test is positive and suggests that further neurodynamic treatment is necessary.

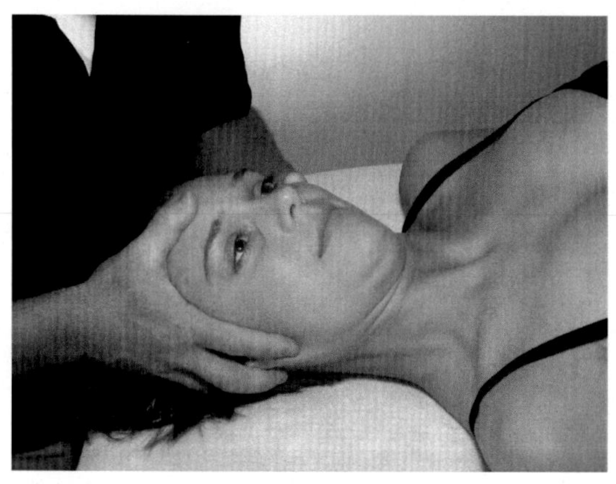

Fig. 17.38 Isometric test of the right sternocleidomastoid muscle.

Comment

ANASTOMOSES OF THE ACCESSORY NERVE

This nerve can have different anomalies (Lang 1995) and it is not uncommon for large branches to have anastomoses in the supraclavicular region which have signs of clear pathophysiological changes and can cause extreme local and remote pain during palpation. An example, proven by EMG-examination, is shown in Figure 17.33. The author's personal experience is that the amount and sequence of depression and retraction of the shoulder often plays an important role in recognizing changes in this nerve and its branches in the supraclavicular region. Only light palpation pressure is often needed to gain a response as described above (local or remote). You have to be aware that perpendicular local techniques under too much 'load' can frequently produce a latent reaction. Palpation along the nerve using the thumb, together with neurodynamics often changes dramatically the signs and symptoms in this region.

ISOLATED INJURIES AND DISEASES

Isolated accessory nerve injuries and diseases are rarely outlined in the literature; however, McCleary (1993) described possible isolated injuries to the vagus and accessory nerves after a fracture of the dens axis. Radiological research on the dens axis demonstrates that there is no subluxation or impingement directly on the nerves (Amyes & Anderson 1956, Dunn & Seljeskog 1986, Hammer 1991). It appears likely that the nerves are subjected to shearing or stretching forces. That there is recovery within a few months further supports this hypothesis (Evarts 1970, Hadley et al 1985). Unfortunately the quality of recovery has not been reported in any of these studies, nor the status at an annual follow-up.

Some case reports of whiplash-associated disorders (WADs) have shown that dysfunction of the accessory nerve can be a contributing factor to the patient's complaints (Bodner et al 2002). Possible causes can be the extreme stress on the neck which is generated during the traumatic event as well as oedema around the jugular foramen which is an important neural container of the accessory nerve (Gardiner et al 2002, Lachman et al 2002). An example of an unrecognized paresis and pain in a WAD patient is shown in Figure 17.39.

An isolated neuropathy of the accessory nerve is also presented as an iatrogenic factor in surgery when using a laryngeal mask airway (LMA). The LMA is a commonly used airway device for anaesthesia, laryngoscopy and cervical spine surgery to administer medication (Brain 1992, Thompsett & Cundy 1992). It appears that the neurovascular area near the hyoid contains branches of the accessory nerve which would be in close proximity to the LMA cuff. This may apply pressure to the accessory nerve when inflated (King & Street 1994). It is therefore essential that therapists are aware of minor accessory neuropathies in patients following head and neck surgery where an LMA may have been used.

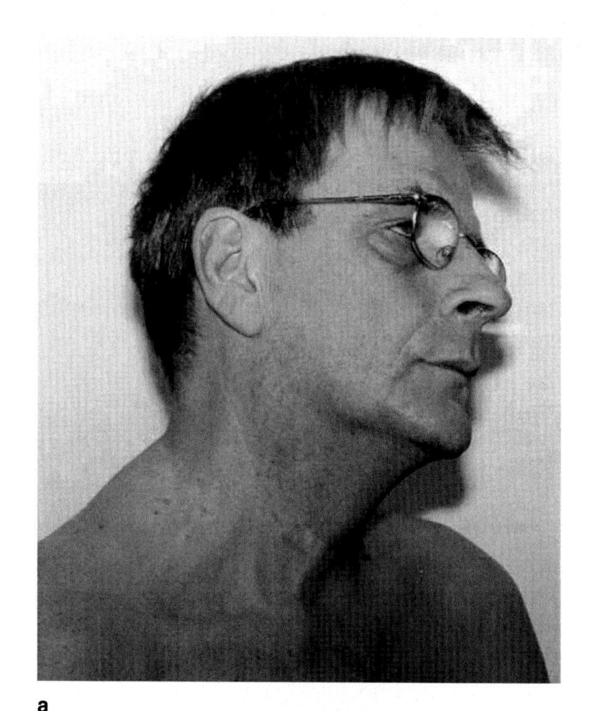

a

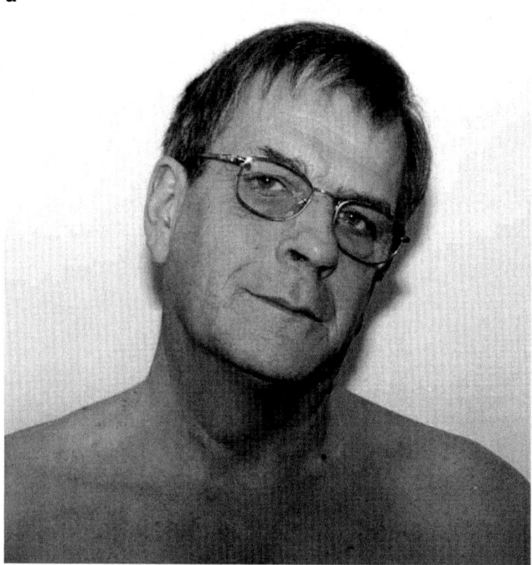

b

Fig. 17.39a–b A 55-year-old patient with torticollis due to paresis of the accessory nerve following a whiplash injury.

ACCESSORY NERVE AFTER NECK DISSECTION

Neck surgery for the treatment of head and neck cancers often causes a strong distraction or load on the accessory nerve (Villanueva 1977, Leipzig et al 1983, Remmler et al 1986, Van Wilgen et al 2003). During a radical neck dissection (RND), the main surgery for resection of tumours in the neck region, the accessory nerve is removed (Crile 1906, Skolnik et al 1967, Herring et al 1987). Decrease of trapezial function may lead to specific shoulder syndromes such as shoulder drop and scapula alata. The literature also mentions a diffuse, chronic, stabbing pain in the shoulder region (Ewing & Martin 1952, Nahum et al 1961, Hoaglund

& Duthie 1966, Short et al 1984, Mumenthaler & Schliack 1991, Salerno et al 2002). Using a modified neck dissection which is less invasive, the accessory nerve will, in the main, be preserved (Herring et al 1987, Wiarda & Wimmers 1988). It would appear that shoulder function will not be affected, provided there is no damage during the operation (Skolnik et al 1967, Short et al 1984, Remmler et al 1986).

A summary of literature suggests that pain and dysfunction in the accessory nerve following RND may be either temporary or long term (Bocca & Pignataro 1967, Skolnik et al 1976, Brandenburg & Lee 1981). Many rehabilitation programmes have been developed to alleviate the pain and preserve mobility and optimal muscle function, but pain is always the most difficult factor to treat in these cases (Nahum et al 1961, Anderson 1975, Saunders & Johnson 1975, Downie 1978, Johnson et al 1978, Dietz 1981, Gluckman et al 1983, Herring et al 1987, Wiarda & Wimmers 1988). All programmes suggest active and passive neck–shoulder mobilization, but without the integration of neurodynamic methodology. It may be a good idea to ensure that the neurodynamics of the accessory nerve are incorporated into such a programme to allow an optimal return of function to the nerve and its environment, prevent adhesions and reduce the risk of ectopic neural discharge (Brandenburg & Lee 1981, Short et al 1984, Devor 1994, Kitteringham 1996, Butler & Gifford 1998).

Table 17.6 gives a general overview of the physical examination options for the accessory nerve.

HYPOGLOSSAL NERVE (XII)

Relevant functional anatomy

The hypoglossal nerve is a somatic afferent nerve which supplies all intrinsic and extrinsic muscles of the tongue except the palatoglossus, which is supplied by the vagus (X). The nerve runs from the hypoglossal nucleus in the brainstem through the hypoglossal foramen in the occipital bone. After exiting the cranium, the hypoglossal nerve lies medial to cranial nerves IX, X and XI. It then runs laterally, abutting the posterior belly of the digastric muscle, where it can be palpated. From here it runs across the lateral surface of the hypoglossal and myohyoid muscles and supplies the tongue muscles (Mumenthaler & Schliack 1991, Wilson-Pauwels et al 2002; Fig. 17.40).

Neurodynamic test

For loading the intracranial tissue, upper cervical flexion and contralateral lateroflexion is executed. Occipital bone movements can be relevant because of the change of the hypoglossal foramen. Accessory movements of the hyoid, such as longitudinal towards caudal and lateral movement especially to the other

Table 17.6 Overview of the physical examination options for the accessory nerve (XI)

Neurodynamic tests	Palpation	Conduction tests
Craniocervical: Upper cervical flexion Contralateral lateroflexion with C1–C3 movement Craniofacial: Occiput Sphenoid Shoulder: Depression Retraction Accessory movements of the clavicle	Posterior triangle of the neck	Lengthening and static tests of sternocleidomastoid and trapezius pars descendens

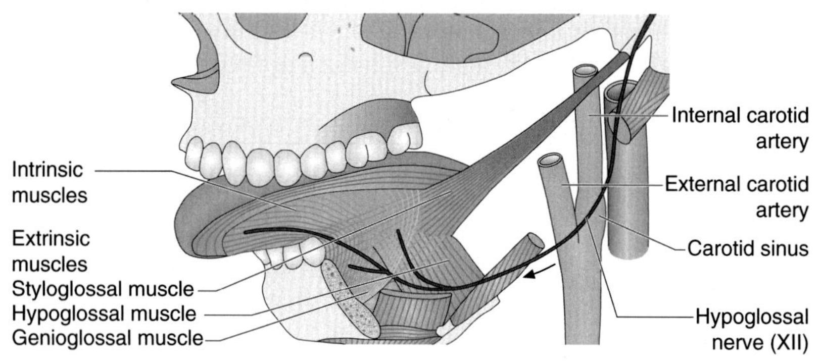

Fig. 17.40 Hypoglossal nerve.

side, change the loading of these branches. Tongue protrusion and lateral deviation affect the branches which innervate the tongue.

STARTING POSITION AND METHOD

The therapist sits or stands beside the patient who is lying comfortably in a supine position. The therapist cups the left hand around the dorsal side of the patient's head, leaving the other hand free to add the occipital bone, hyoid bone and tongue movements.

With the patient's head resting against it, the therapist's trunk provides enough force to create the desired movement to perform upper cervical flexion and contralateral lateroflexion. This movement is possible without increasing the tension in the left hand that is holding the head. The flexion should be smooth. The trunk can be used by contacting the right cranial region of the patient's head, fixing the right cranial region (Fig. 17.41a).

For occipital bone movement, the therapist grasps around the occipital bone with the right hand in supination and perpendicular to the patient's head. The main occipital movements such as transverse and longitudinal manoeuvres and rotations can be performed in this position. The thumb and index finger of the right hand contact the lateral side of the hyoid bone and can perform longitudinal caudal or lateral movements of the patient's hyoid bone (Fig. 17.41b). The therapist should ensure that it is a large arm movement from the shoulder rather than from the wrist or fingers. Simultaneously, active tongue movements can be added, especially during the occipital and hyoid bone examinations. Active tongue protrusion or lateral movements can be performed and can be guided using a spatula if required (Fig. 17.41c). The movement can also be performed passively by holding the tongue with the right index finger and thumb, maintaining a firm head hold and ensuring that there is no increase in pressure with the fingers on the patient's tongue.

Palpation

The optimal position for palpation of the hypoglossal nerve is in front of the common carotid artery, anteriorly above the corner of the hyoid bone and in front of the submandibular glands. Palpation can be achieved by holding the hyoid bone in a slightly neurodynamic position (mostly contralateral lateroflexion) with the thumb and index finger of the left hand and palpating the nerve with the right index or middle finger (Fig. 17.42).

Conduction tests

INSPECTION

Inspect the surface of the patient's tongue for wasting, weakness, deviations and involuntary movement. Light atrophy, wasting and fasciculation are best seen with the tongue lying on the floor of the mouth, as can inspection of surface, shape, position and movement of the tongue. Tongue movements should be quick and strong, and it should be possible to

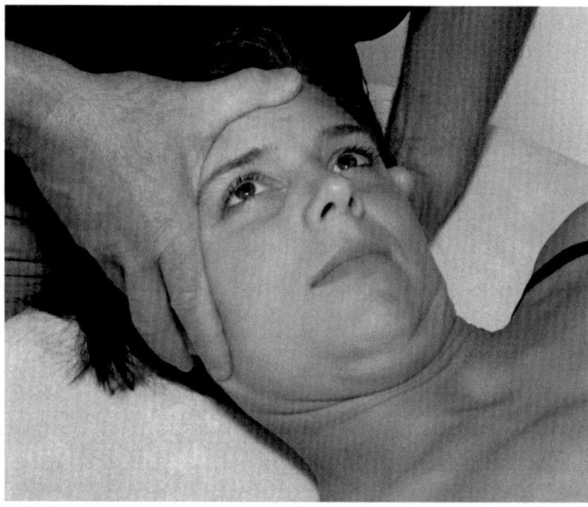
a

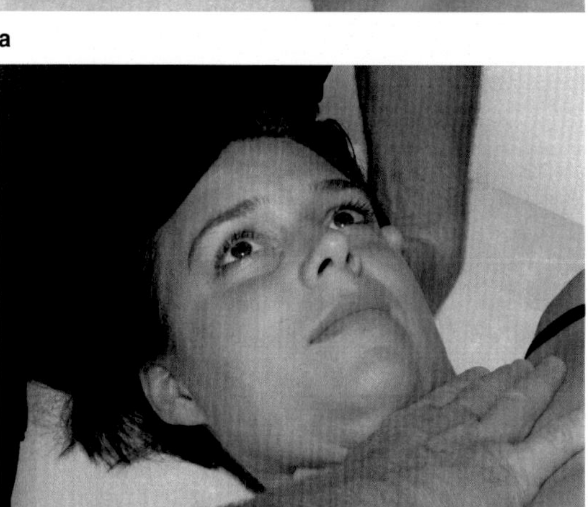
b

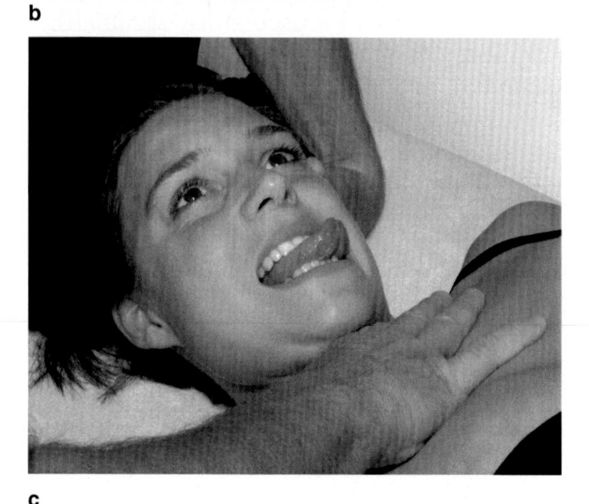
c

Fig. 17.41a–c Neurodynamic test of the hypoglossal nerve.

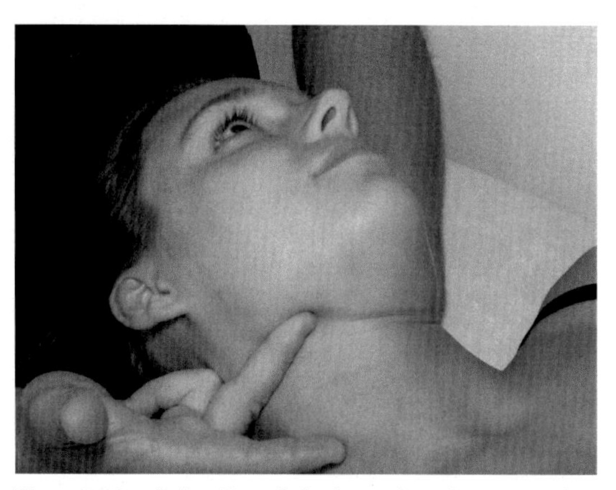

Fig. 17.42 Palpation of the hypoglossal nerve under the mandible, above the hyoid.

protrude the tongue a long way out of the patient's mouth.

MOTOR SYSTEM

The patient may have some speech difficulties with sounds such as N, T, D and L (Butler 2000). This may have already been recognized during questioning of the patient. If not, ask the patient to pronounce these letters clearly.

A normal tongue will show slight flickering activity when held out for longer than a few seconds (Pertes & Gross 1996). On attempted tongue protrusion, the tongue muscles on the weak side are unable to balance the forward push, resulting in deviation of the tongue towards the weak side. Patten makes the comment in his work that patients often do not notice this lopsided pattern (Patten 1995). To challenge the force of the genioglossus muscle (tongue), place a spatula on the lateral side of the tip of the tongue. The patient has to hold the tongue in this position during increasing lateral pressure (Fig. 17.43).

Neurodynamic components added during the tongue inspection as well as motor tests will give an idea of pathodynamic contribution. Minor pathology is challenged by isometric testing It is the author's experience that a combination of lateroflexion towards or away from the therapist with upper cervical flexion of the head will be most likely to change the motor behaviour.

Table 17.7 Overview of the physical examination options for the hypoglossal nerve (XII)

Neurodynamic tests	Palpation	Conduction tests
Craniocervical: Upper cervical flexion Contralateral lateroflexion Craniofacial: Occiput Hyoid Longitudinal and transverse movements Tongue Protrusion Laterotrusion	Above hyoid bone and below mandible	Inspection: Atrophy of the tongue Motor system: Speech Tongue movements Static tests tongue (spatula)

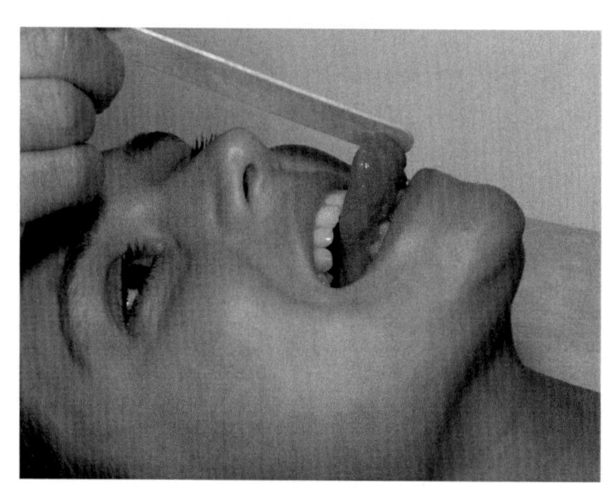

Fig. 17.43 Static test of the function of the tongue in a protruded position.

Table 17.7 gives a general overview of the physical examination options for the hypoglossal nerve.

Comment

Indications for using this neurodynamic test might be clinical patterns such as:

- Neck–tongue syndrome (Bogduk 1981)
- Lingual dysfunction when talking or singing
- Reflex activities such as problems swallowing, sucking and chewing
- Tongue pain where there is no clear indication of inflammation.

Since there is a strong relationship with the cervical spine with many loops between C0 and C2 and the hypoglossal nerve, it is highly recommended that the upper cervical spine be examined also (Bogduk 1981, Lang 1995).

HYPOGLOSSAL FACIAL NERVE ANASTOMOSIS (HFA)

Hypoglossal facial nerve anastomosis is one of the modern surgery techniques frequently performed to restore function after facial palsy, and secondary to surgical removal of CPA tumours (Kim et al 2003). Both animal and human studies demonstrate the enormous plasticity of the central nervous system after HFA. Axotomized hypoglossal motor neurones sprout into the facial plexus and re-innervate the facial musculature, stimulating reorganization of the hypoglossal nucleus (Salame et al 2002). In addition, heterotropic sprouting of the trigeminal neurones towards the hypoglossal motor neurones occurs (Willer et al 1993).

The advantages of HFA are:

- Improved facial tone with improved cosmetic results
- Intentional facial movements controlled by the tongue
- Protection of the eye
- Movements associated with physiological functioning of the tongue.

The disadvantages are:

- Hemiatrophy of the tongue
- Gross movements of the face and in some instances hypertonia of the face (Cusimano & Sekhar 1994, Linnet & Madsen 1995).

The published results of HFA are variable and continue to raise questions about indication, timing, surgical techniques and rehabilitation. Better results were recorded for younger patients (Willer et al 1993, Cusimano & Sekhar 1994, Kim et al 2003, Donzelli et al 2005). Neurodynamic rehabilitation for the hypoglossal nerve may be suggested where there is local nerve damage in the suprahyoid region. A combination of mobilization of the glossopharyngeal and facial nerves along with exercise for the facial muscles in and out of neurodynamic positions would be suggested. This may create possibilities for optimal plastic adaptation of the central nervous system resulting in restoration of the normal slide, glide and load functions of these nerves.

UPPER AIRWAY AIRFLOW MECHANISMS

Electric stimulation and stretching of the hypoglossal nerve and cervical nerve branches stimulates activity in the supra- and infrahyoid muscles, which in turn increases inspiratory airflow by decreasing airway collapsibility (Eisele et al 1995). In animal studies this expansion of the upper airway demonstrates an increase in respiratory volume (Wasicko et al 1990, Hida et al 1995). Possible indication for hypoglossal nerve treatment might be, for example, decreased airflow after throat surgery and radiotherapy. Hyperactivity of the supra- and infrahyoid muscles often occurs during syndromes such as hyperventilation, asthmatic bronchitis and subjective 'pressure' on the throat. It is possible to treat these problems and produce positive results by using neurodynamic techniques along with expiration manoeuvres to stimulate the phrenic nerve (Wasicko et al 1993). Hyoid techniques are particularly recommended.

HYPOGLOSSAL NERVE PALSY

Although these palsies are rarely seen, they usually show up in the clinic as signs rather than symptoms (Keane 1996, Hadjikoutis et al 2002). Abnormal mechanical interfaces including neuromas, compression in the hypoglossal canal and following occipital condyle fractures, neurological diseases such as strokes, multiple sclerosis, Guillain–Barré neuropathy, psychogenic trauma and surgery may be responsible for the slow onset of symptoms (Forssell et al 1995, Paley & Wood 1995, Voyvodic et al 1995, Keane 1996, Kobayashi et al 1996, Shiozawa et al 1996, Muthukumar 2002). These might comprise dysarthria, tongue atrophy and facial tone, hoarseness, swallowing dysfunction and pain.

If some of these localized symptoms are observed in the clinic in the absence of a differential diagnosis, it is reasonable to refer the patient to a neurologist or ENT specialist for further diagnosis. Where the diagnosis is clear-cut, applying neurodynamic techniques can be beneficial. In any event, 15% of all cases have a chance of complete or near complete recovery (Keane 1996).

SUMMARY

- This part of the chapter describes the examination and clinical patterns of the main cranial nervous tissue which is seen by the therapist based on the general anatomy and evidence-based and empirical knowledge.
- Cranioneurodynamics, conduction tests and palpation can make the hypothesis stronger that unhealthy cranial nervous tissue is related with the patient's problem, especially when the diagnosis is not clear.
- Cranioneurodynamics can be integrated very successfully in manual therapy approaches and neuro-orthopaedic rehabilitation programmes.
- It is essential to be aware that if a clinical pattern is not clear, examination and treatment must be stopped and further diagnosis obtained from a specialist such as a neurologist, otolaryngologist, orthodontist, etc.

EXAMINATION OF THE CRANIAL NERVOUS TISSUE: THIRD CATEGORY

INTRODUCTION

Physical examination of cranial tissue related to specific pathology and/or specific dysfunction and pain are described. The clinical decision to execute this test depends upon:

- Specific subjective, mostly isolated complaints that are classic for the related cranial nerve: A patient with hyposomy (reduced sensation of smell) after a skull floor fracture would be an indication to examine the olfactory nerve.
- The results of the cranioneurodynamic tests of the first and/or second category: For example, the patient complains of diplopia, and exotropia of the left eye is observed during upper cervical neck flexion. In such a case the clinician would be interested in the specific tests for the oculomotor system.
- Negative testing of the cranioneurodynamics of the first and second category: Nothing is found during testing but the hypothesis remains that cranial tissue is involved.

> **!** Before deciding to examine cranial nervous tissue of the second or third category, the first category should be tested. These influence the general cranial nervous tissue most strongly and can be considered as 'screening tests'.

The third category of cranial nerves opens doors for further examination and management when related clinical patterns are recognized. Relevant neuroanatomy, conduction–palpation tests and special neurodynamics tests are described in detail.

OLFACTORY NERVE (I)

Relevant functional anatomy

The olfactory epithelium is located in the roof of the nasal cavity and extends onto the superior nasal conchae and the nasal septum. It transverses the cribriform plate (ethmoid bone) and travels parallel to the optic nerve caudally from the limbic system to the dorsolateral side (cranial section) of the brainstem (Patten 1995, Wilson-Pauwels et al 2002; Fig. 17.44).

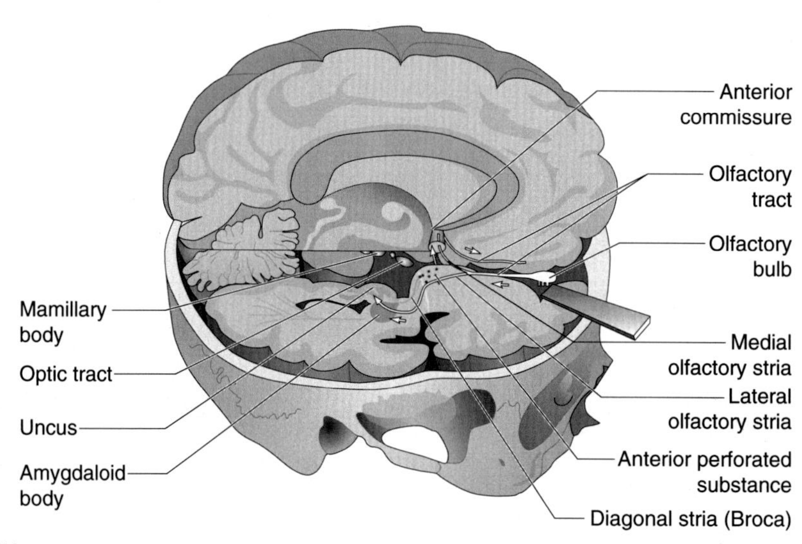

Fig. 17.44 Olfactory nerve.

Neurodynamic test

Upper cervical flexion and lateroflexion away from the side being examined produces neurodynamic changes of the olfactory nerves around the medulla oblongata. Movements of the orbital ethmoid bone, nasofrontal region and palate (nasal septum, conchae) can influence neural containers ventral to the medulla oblongata.

STARTING POSITION AND METHOD

The patient lies supine and comfortable in a relaxed position with glasses removed, if worn. The therapist sits at the end of the plinth, cupping the left hand around the occipital region of the patient's head.

With the right hand resting on the head/cranium, upper extension and/or contralateral/lateral flexion can be performed (Fig. 17.45). During and after testing of cervical movements, assessment and reassessment of changes to smell can be made by the hand in the caudal region by closing the nostril of the side that is not being examined. Facial techniques from the orbit (which is influenced by the ethmoid bone), the nasofrontal joint, the palate or combinations of both can then be added as described in Chapter 16.

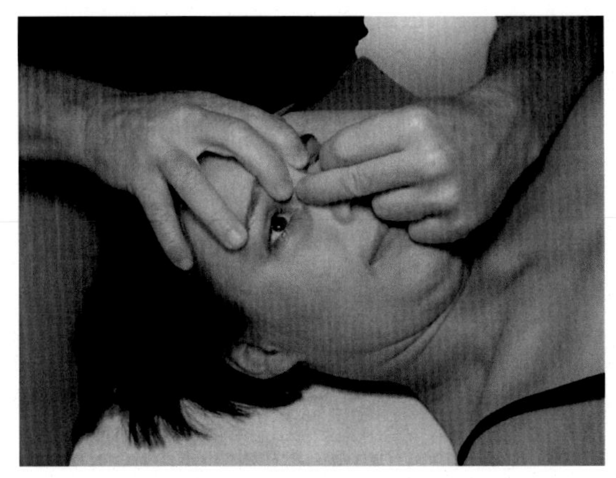

Fig. 17.45 Neurodynamic test of the olfactory nerve.

Table 17.8 gives a general overview of the physical examination options for the olfactory nerve.

Comment

OLFACTORY NERVE TRAUMA

The aetiology of anterior (rhinobasal) and posterior (otobasal) skull base fractures shows many physical and mental dysfunctions. Sensory disturbance of the temporal region, headache, concentration disorders, neurological changes, fear of heights and cranial nerve lesions are the most common post-traumatic symptoms (Kruse & Awasthi 1998). After 2 years the most common remaining symptoms of trauma are lesions and dysfunction of the olfactory nerve (70%), acoustic nerve (55%) and trigeminal nerve (45%) (Begall et al 1994). In 90% of patients with rhinobasal fractures, surgical treatment was necessary, with the main goal being to clear out the sinuses and repair the dural lesions (Stoll 1993). From clinical studies it is known that trauma to the dorsal part of the head can be related to smell disturbances more than visual disturbances (Brazis et al 1990, Kern et al 2000). Davis (1994) emphasizes the need for early mobilization of the nervous system and reanimation of face and mouth after traumatic and non-traumatic brain lesions as a prophylactic treatment to keep the nervous system as dynamic as possible.

Table 17.8 Overview of the physical examination options for the olfactory nerve (I)

Neurodynamic tests	Conduction tests
Craniocervical: Upper cervical flexion Contralateral lateroflexion	Smelling: Smelling of different odours
Craniofacial: Nasofrontal Palatinum	

It is possible that early treatment of cranial neurodynamics can contribute to optimal recovery and a reduction of symptoms after skull base fractures. The lack of published work in this area presents a challenge to therapists and researchers to get a better grip on these sometimes enormous problems at the activity and the participation level.

NEUROPATHY OF THE OLFACTORY NERVE WHERE THERE IS NO CLEAR DIAGNOSIS

Frontal region changes – such as abscesses, tumours, meningiomas in the floor of the anterior cranial fossa – can also cause olfactory neuropathies (Patten 1995). Postsurgery or post-skull fractures, especially anterior–posterior skull fractures parallel to the sagittal suture, can irritate olfactory fibres that cross the cribriform plate. Diffuse frontal–nasal headache and chronic sinusitis, combined with or without skull changes, can be caused by pathodynamics of the olfactory nerve.

Mostly the tests in flexion and lateroflexion of the cervical spine with relevant mobilization of palatinum and nasofrontal joints (sometimes combined) with the olfactory nerve in neurodynamic position (upper flexion and contralateral flexion) are the key techniques for changing the signs and symptoms related to the olfactory nerve.

Palpation

The olfactory nerve runs intracranially and is not palpable.

Conduction test

The purpose of the test is to determine unilateral or bilateral impairment of the sense of smell. Before the test, ensure that the airway is clear by compressing each nostril in turn and checking for the passage of air through the open one. Familiar odours such as coffee, almonds, chocolate, oil, lemon and peppermint can be presented to the patient to sniff in order to assess the sense of smell (Spillane 1996). There are scratch and sniff card sets available commercially for olfactory assessment. Each nostril is tested separately by occluding the opposite one and taking two good, but not overexuberant, sniffs. The patient can be asked:

- Do you smell anything?
- Can you identify the odour?
- Is the odour the same in each nostril?

A visual analogue scale is a reliable measure to get an impression of the subjective interpretation of these questions (Spillane 1996). The therapist should assess responses to the different odours separately.

OPTIC NERVE (II)

Relevant functional anatomy

Nerve fibres arise from cells of the retina and emerge posteriorly from the eyeball to leave the orbit through the optic canal, located in the lesser wing of the sphenoid bone. The branches of the optic nerve from each eye extend to the middle cranial fossa and meet to form the optic chiasma. These consist of a considerable amount of connective tissue (60–80%) and are richly vascularized (Lang 1995). These tracts continue posteriorly around the cerebral peduncle and terminate in the lateral geniculate body of the thalamus (Wilson-Pauwels et al 2002; Fig. 17.46).

Neurodynamic test

In an anatomical sense, upper cervical flexion and contralateral lateroflexion change the neurodynamics the most. Slight pressure on the eyeball can indirectly change the loading of the optic nerve. Accessory movements of the sphenoid, especially transverse and rotation movements, can influence the optic canal which acts as a neural container.

STARTING POSITION AND METHOD

The patient lies supine and comfortable in a relaxed position. The therapist sits at the end of the plinth and grasps the patient's head with

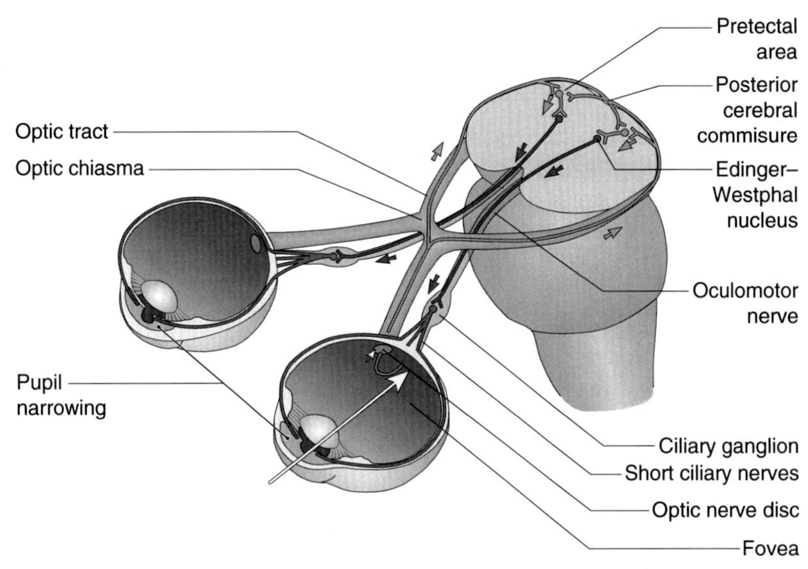

Fig. 17.46 Optic nerve.

both palms around the dorsolateral side of the cranium. Both hands simultaneously produce an upper cervical flexion without increasing the compression on the cranium. By executing a trunk movement around an imaginary transverse axis which runs through the optic chiasma, further lateroflexion away from the examined side is possible.

Clinically, some degree of lateroflexion of the craniocervical region is possible. In this position the tips of the index and middle fingers of the right hand can examine the eyeball pressure (Fig. 17.47). This requires care in order to avoid unnecessary discomfort. Eyeball pressure using two or three fingers can be applied while in this position to test for changes in signs and symptoms. Sometimes patients perform this to reduce their symptoms. The pressure applied is minimal, similar to that used during general manual lymph drainage techniques (30–50 mmHg). The pressure is a slowly increasing pressure because of the hypersensitivity of the eyeball. It has to be clear that there is no underlying pathology in the orbital region as this would be a contraindication.

An alternative way of influencing the neurodynamics of the optic nerve is by contacting the sphenoid bone using the left index finger and thumb on the major wings and examining the sphenoid bone in all directions in different cranioneurodynamic load positions, whereby the right hand initiates the movement of the neck.

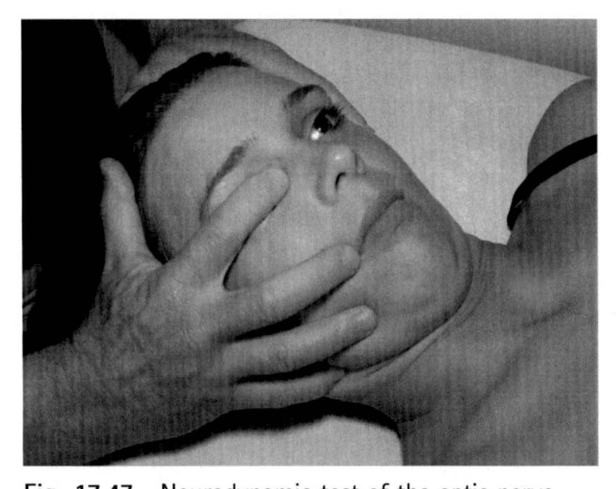

Fig. 17.47 Neurodynamic test of the optic nerve.

Palpation

Palpation of the intracranial optic nerve is not possible.

Conduction test

The purpose of the test is to measure the visual acuity and to chart visual fields and colour vision (Patten 1995).

VISION

A crude screening of visual acuity may be performed by asking the patient to read newsprint held at arm's length. Special cards for testing distance vision (Snellen-type charts) and near vision (Jaegar-type cards) are available commercially.

VISUAL FIELDS

This test for charting the visual fields is the most important test for assessing a possible dysfunction or lesion (Fig. 17.48).

- Face the patient at a distance of approximately 50 cm.
- Cover the patient's eye and also your own eye. Make sure you both have the opposite eyes closed.
- Bring a target object such as a pencil in the periphery at different angles and have the patient indicate when it comes into view.
- Now compare the patient's performance with your own assuming that yours is normal.

This crude diagnostic test can, if necessary, be improved upon using statistical perimetry by an ophthalmologist (Fig. 17.49).

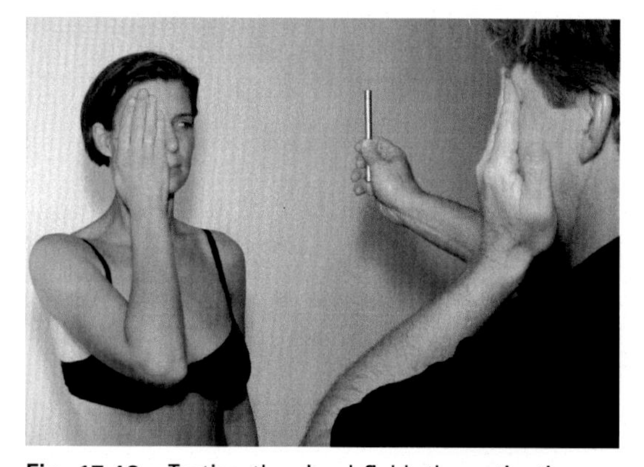

Fig. 17.48 Testing the visual field: the patient's right eye and the therapist's left eye are covered.

COLOUR VISION

Colour vision can be tested using a full colour spectrum chart. Any changes noted in the (primary) colours should raise an alarm suggesting pathology such as lesions of the pituitary (dorsal wall) or of the eyeball. Assessment of the conduction and neurodynamic tests should be carried out on each eye individually and must be compared with the other one. Abnormal findings require referral to neuro-ophthalmology specialist.

For detailed information about different representations of common visual field defects, refer to the specialist literature (Patten 1995, Wilson-Pauwels et al 2002).

PUPILLARY LIGHT REFLEX

A beam of light is shone directly on one pupil for several seconds and taken quickly away. This tests not only the optic nerve (the afferent pathway) but also the parasympathetic nerves which run with the oculomotor nerve (III).

When both nerves are intact, the examined pupil constricts (direct response) and the other eye will also constrict (consensual response) (Wilson-Pauwels et al 2002).

Table 17.9 gives a general overview of the physical examination options for the optic nerve.

Comment

OPTIC NERVE AND VASCULARIZATION

The optic nerve dura and the eye region are richly innervated by sympathetic fibres. The sympathetic component is derived from the superior cervical sympathetic ganglion or by communication with perivascular intracranial extensions. Trunk movements can often influence the sympathetic nervous system and can probably change cranial neurodynamics. This can cause disturbance of eye function (e.g. accommodation).

Horner's syndrome is a typical disorder that disturbs the vascularization of the eye. It is caused by paresis of the autonomic system of the lungs, thoracic or cervical spine or the cranium (Spillane 1996, Miura et al 2003). The clinical signs are:

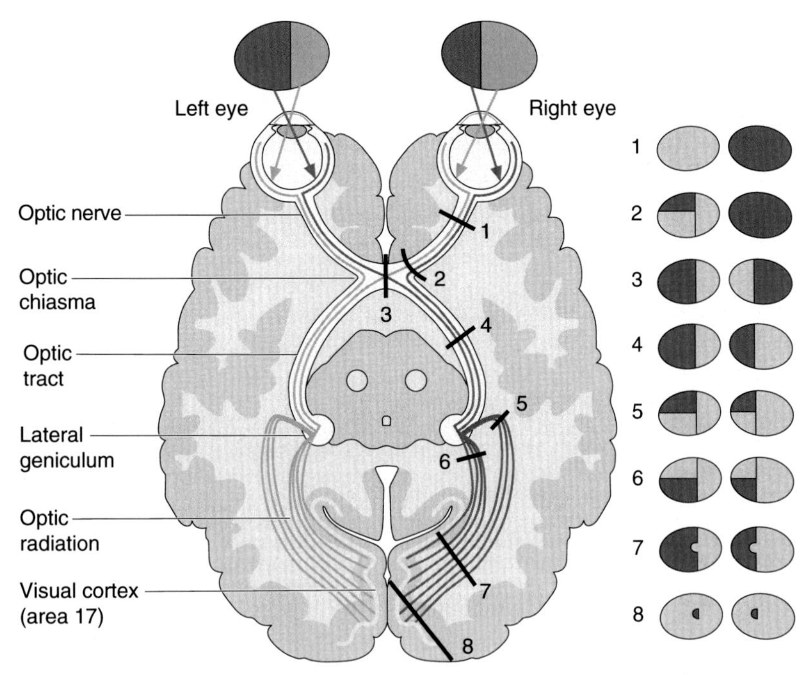

Fig. 17.49 Defects of the visual field associated with severe injury to the visual pathway.

Table 17.9 Overview of the physical examination options for the optic nerve (II)

Neurodynamic tests	Conduction tests
Craniocervical:	Visual activity:
Upper cervical flexion	Special cards (Shellens,
Contralateral flexion	Jargan type)
Eye:	Visual fields:
Compression	Pencil-distance test
Medial/lateral	Colour vision:
Craniofacial:	Colour spectrum chart
Sphenoid	Pupillary light reflex

- Ptosis (hingeing of the eyelid)
- Unilateral meiosis (constriction of the pupil)
- Enophthalmos (eye is retracted in the orbit) (Loewenfeld 1993, Butler 2000).

Reversed Horner's syndrome causes increased irritation of the autonomic nervous system with a intermittent or constant pupil dilatation (mydriasis) (Cross 1993, Butler 2000).

Monocular visual defects or scotomata, sometimes associated with headaches and neck pain, have been found to improve after spinal manipulation (Gorman 1996). Computerized static perimetry shows a significant improvement of optic nerve function measured before and after spinal treatment (Cross 1993). Neurodynamic changes in the craniocervical region and the optic nerve might be suspected where microvascular spasm presents in cerebral vascularization, for example in the eye and optic nerve (Langford-Wilson 1982, Spillane 1996).

THE OPTIC NERVE AND EYE PAIN

The clinical presentation of burning eye pain, periocular pain (especially with sympathetic symptoms such as facial sweating), incomplete Horner's syndrome, vasomotor headache and various cranial nerve deficiencies (nerves II–VI, in particular the trigeminal nerve) is described as the 'paratrigeminal' or Raeder's syndrome (Lang 2000). When this pattern or parts of this pattern presents, treatment will be in the form of flexion of the upper cranio-cervical region together with a technique for the eyeball. This may ease the symptoms immediately or after a period of time. Many abnormal signs, often consisting of sympathetic responses such as facial sweating or pulsating headache, may occur during cranial neurodynamics. The mandibular (V_3) and abducens (VI) nerves demand special attention. Purvin et al (2001) confirmed the importance of examination of cranial nerves during this pathology (Mokri 1982).

Eye pain can also be one of the main symptoms of an optic neuritis which is an inflammation of the optic nerve. It occurs more frequently in woman and in younger patients, 20–50 years old (Optic Neuritis Study Group 1991, Wilson-Pauwels et al 2002). Other symptoms include central visual loss, decreased visual acuity, altered colour vision perception and an afferent pupillary reflex defect. In most cases the symptoms are reversible (Lang 2000).

Cranioneurodynamic testing together with the information from the subjective examination can help clarify the clinical pattern and define the dysfunctions which can be the starting point for cranioneurodynamic treatment and further rehabilitation.

OPTIC NERVE AND THE DURA MATER

The meningeal layer is connected with the dural sheaths of the optic nerves and extracranial spinal cord nerves (Wolderberg et al 1994, Jiang et al 2001). Hence changes to the neurodynamics of the dura may lead directly to changes in the neurodynamics of the optic nerve. For example, dural puncture often causes post-dural puncture headaches and visual disturbances. This is possibly caused by a reactive vasospasm of the cranial and optic nerve arteries due to the anatomical brain displacement (Gobel et al 1990, Shearer et al 1995).

Primary meningioma (a slow-growing benign tumour) slowly invades the dura first. The optic nerve does not metastasize directly (Servodidio et al 1991). Many of the presenting signs, symptoms and clinical patterns are non-specific. The reduction in eyesight, visual field loss, limitation of eye movements, dull headaches and cervical spine problems (Jiang et al 2001) fit in with the direct link of pathodynamics of dura with optic nervous tissue. Awareness of these non-specific signs is essential, especially when a diagnosis is lacking or is not clear.

OPTIC NERVE AND THE CAVERNOUS SINUS

The optic nerve and the internal carotid artery lie in the cavernous sinus, make contact with the body wall of the sphenoid sinus and can easily be damaged during trauma (Aurbach et al 1991). Normally, intracranial cavernous haemangiomas are located in the frontal bone and temporal lobe. In many adults these haemangiomas are clinically silent (Manz et al 1979, Maitland et al 1982). Small cavernous haemangiomas within the intracranial anterior visual pathway are rarely found but present with dramatic visual changes and radiological findings (Corboy & Galetta 1989, Hassler et al 1989). These clinical features suggest that the mechanical interface of the optic nerve in the cavernous sinus (i.e. sphenoid bone, carotid artery) can influence the neurodynamics of the optic nerve (Kushen et al 2005). Optic nerve dysfunction due to neural container changes (cavernous sinus) suggests that sphenoid movement and changes of head position can change the load in the cavernous sinus region.

THE OCULOMOTOR SYSTEM: OCULOMOTOR NERVE (III), TROCHLEAR NERVE (IV) AND ABDUCENS NERVE (VI)

The motor function of the eyes (oculomotor system) together with the responsible cranial nerves – oculomotor (III), trochlear (IV) and abducens (VI) – will be discussed in the following paragraphs.

Relevant functional anatomy

OCULOMOTOR NERVE (III)

The oculomotor nerve has efferent somatic motor and visceral motor components that have their origins, respectively, in the oculomotor nucleus complex and the visceral motor nucleus (Edinger–Westphal nucleus) in the dorsocranial part of the brainstem. Outwith the brainstem the branches run through the oculomotor sulcus which is a part of the dorsum sellae (sphenoid bone). The nerve pierces the dura and enters the cavernous sinus. Together with the trochlear nerve (Lang 1995, Wilson-Pauwels et al 2002) it enters the orbit and splits into superior and inferior divisions. There they supply the levator palpebrae superior muscle and most of the oculomotor muscles, with the exception of the lateral rectus (VI) and superior oblique (IV). The main function is eyeball movements, i.e. adduction, cranial, cranial–medial, cranial–lateral and caudal–medial (Fig. 17.50).

TROCHLEAR NERVE (IV)

The trochlear nerve is a slender motor nerve supplying the superior oblique muscle, with its

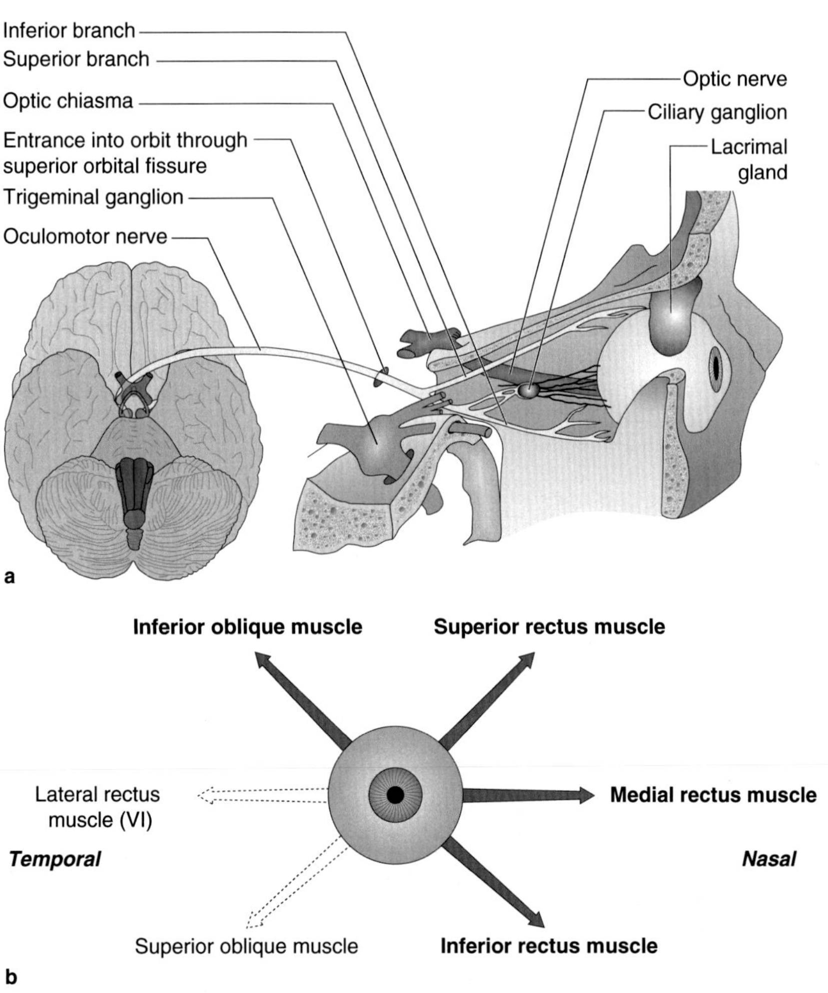

Fig. 17.50 The anatomy (a) and function (b) of the oculomotor nerve.

nucleus located in the tegmentum of the midbrain. Outwith the brainstem it crosses to the opposite side. It pierces the dura at the angle between the free and attached border of tentorium cerebelli and passes through the cavernous sinus along with cranial nerves III, V (sometimes V_2) and VI. At the end it enters the orbit and runs to the medial region of the orbit to reach the superior oblique muscle. Of the cranial nerves, the trochlear nerve is unique in four ways (Fig. 17.51):

- It is the smallest (2400 axons compared with approximately 1 000 000 in the optic nerve).
- It is the only nerve to exit from the dorsal aspect of the brainstem.
- It is the only nerve in which all of the lower motor neurone axons cross.
- It has the longest intracranial course (7.5 cm) (Wilson-Pauwels et al 2002).

ABDUCENS NERVE (VI)

The abducens nerve (VI) emerges from the anterior aspect of the brainstem caudal to the pons (medullopontine sulcus). It runs anteriorly and laterally to the subarachnoid space of the posterior fossa to pierce the dura that is lateral to the dorsum sellae. The nerve continues forward between the dura and the apex of the petrous bone where it takes a sharp right-angled turn over the apex of the bone to enter the cavernous sinus. Afterwards the nerve enters the orbit where it runs laterally to supply the lateral rectus muscle which abducts the eye (Fig. 17.52).

Neurodynamic tests

Upper cervical flexion and side flexion away from the testing side for the cervical spine are the first two movements that stress the nervous tissue in the dorsal side of the cranium.

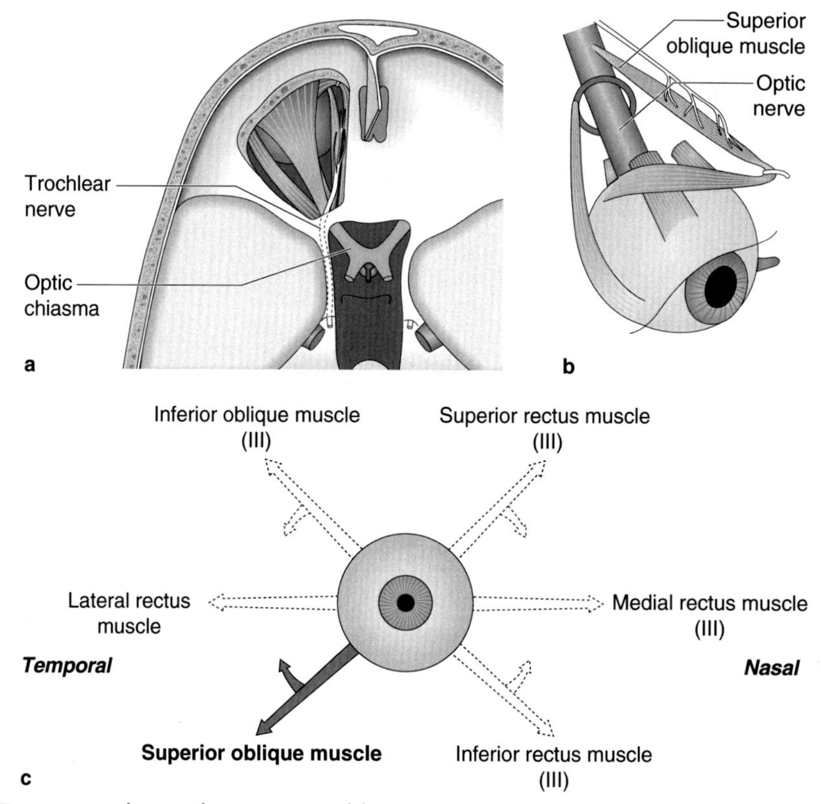

Fig. 17.51 The anatomy (a and b) and function (c) of the trochlear nerve.

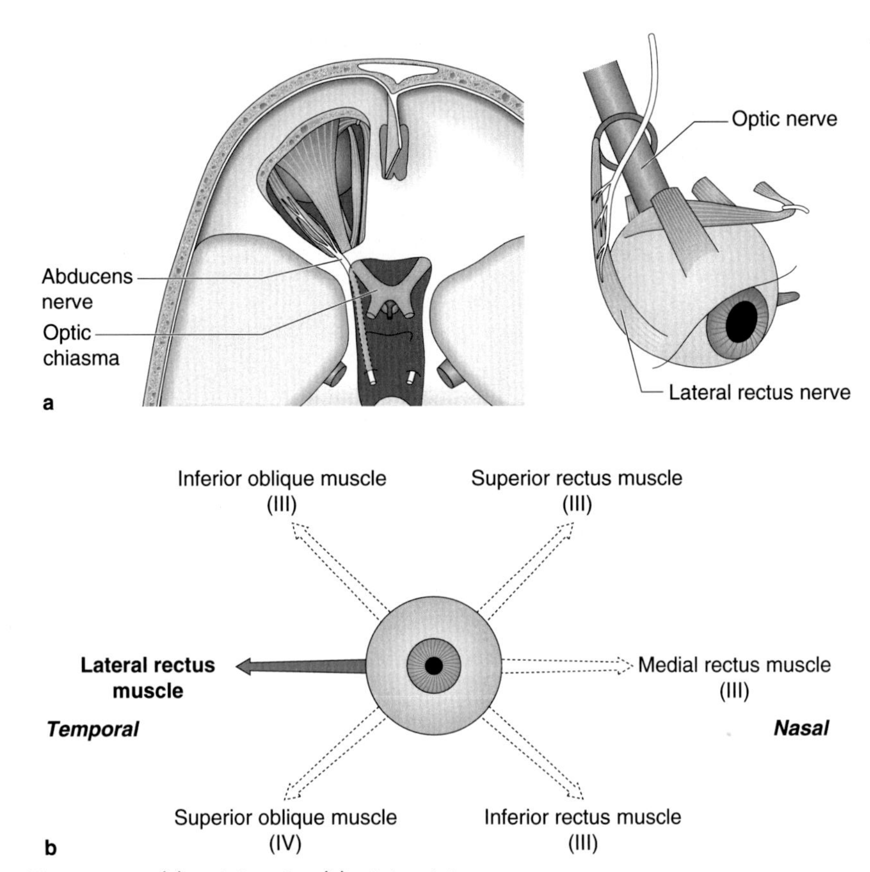

Fig. 17.52 The anatomy (a) and function (b) of the abducens nerve.

STARTING POSITION AND METHOD

The patient lies supine and comfortable in a relaxed position. The therapist sits beside the patient facing the head, forearm resting on the treatment table which has been adjusted to a convenient height. The left hand cups the dorsal side of the patient's head; the right hand contacts with one of the cranial bones (sphenoid, right temporal or petrosal bone) or eye region as described below.

After these two standard movements, slight differentiation between the three nerves is possible.

OCULOMOTOR NERVE (III)

Because of the intensive contact of the oculomotor nerve with the sphenoid bone, lateral transverse movements, which change the oculomotor nerve, dura and cavernous sinus, are suggested primarily. Addition of temporal bone techniques can also be useful because this bone is a part of the neural container of the cavernous sinus.

Starting position and method

Examination of the sphenoid takes place by grasping the sphenoid bone using the left index finger and thumb on the right-hand side of the greater wings. This has already been described under the test for the optic nerve. To test the temporal bone as a part of this neurodynamic test, four fingers of the right hand touch the temporal area as described in the standard technique for this region (Chapter 15).

When eye movements are to be examined, the tips of the index and middle fingers of the right hand touch the cranial or medial side of the eyeball to test the superior and inferior part of the oculomotor nerve by a caudal or lateral passive eye movement (Fig. 17.53).

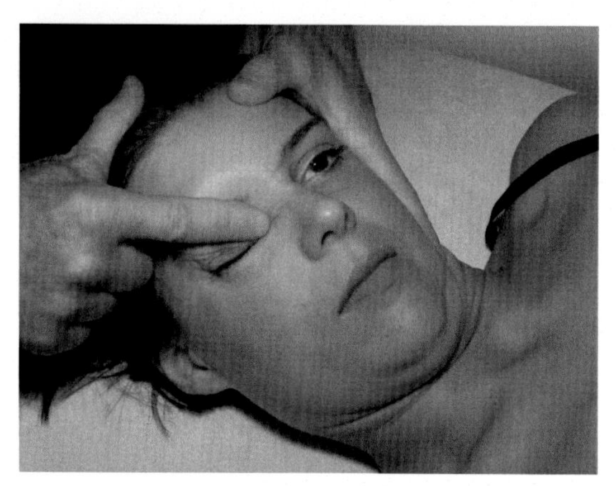

Fig. 17.53 Neurodynamic test of the oculomotor nerve (III).

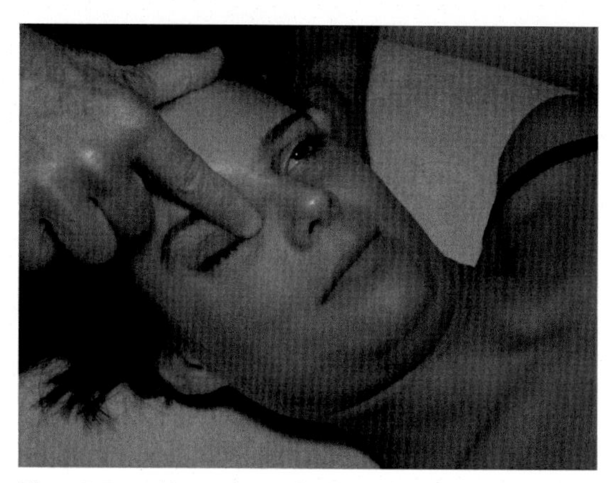

Fig. 17.54 Neurodynamic test of the trochlear nerve (III).

During the test the left hand performs an upper cervical flexion and lateroflexion away; the right hand, which contacts the sphenoid bone, guides this movement. Ensure a good body movement and avoid increased pressure of the left hand and of the fingers on the sphenoid bone. Now the movement can easily be performed. During temporal bone movement ensure that the pressure of the fingers contacting the temporal bone does not increase. For the eye movement, the right hand is slowly moved to the orbital region. It is essential to maintain the upper cervical flexion without increasing the pressure on the dorsal side of the cranium.

TROCHLEAR NERVE (IV)

A combination of movements in the lateral–caudal direction of the eye can challenge the branches that run to the medial cranial corner at the eye orbit. Cranial movements are performed to the sphenoid and temporal bones in order to change the cavernous sinus environment.

Starting position and method

The therapist's left hand cups the occiput bone so that the forearm is at 90° to the lateral side of the head and rests on the table. The manoeuvre can be executed with the right hand emphasizing eye or cranium movements of the sphenoid or temporal bones.

- For the sphenoid, the thumb and index finger of the left hand contact the lateral border of the greater wing of the sphenoid as already described. The left hand still holds the flexion and lateroflexion position of the head.
- To test the temporal bone as a part of this neurodynamic test the hand position is the same as described during the oculomotor neurodynamic test.
- When eye movements are examined, the tips of the index and middle fingers of the right hand touch the mediocranial corner of the orbit and contact the eyeball minimally. A laterocaudal movement of the eye using the index and middle fingers of the right hand can be performed as described during the oculomotor neurodynamic test. Ensure a good body movement during the manoeuvre and do not lose the upper cervical flexion when moving the left hand to the orbital region. The movement of the eye is a small movement of the interphalangeal joints of the left index and middle fingers (Fig. 17.54).

Table 17.10 Movements of different structures of the proposed neurodynamic test of the oculomotor nerves

	Cervical spine	Cranium	Eyes
Oculomotor (III)	Upper cervical flexion and lateroflexion	Orbit (general) Sphenoid Temporal	Caudal or lateral
Trochlear (IV)	Upper cervical flexion and lateroflexion	Orbit (general) Sphenoid Temporal	Caudal-lateral
Abducens (VI)	Upper cervical flexion and lateroflexion	Orbit (general) Sphenoid Temporal	Medial

ABDUCENS NERVE (VI)

Medial transversal movement of the eye tends to load the lateral branches; accessory movements of sphenoid, temporal and petrosal bones influence the dura and cavernous sinus.

Starting position and method

The left hand maintains the position of upper cervical flexion and lateroflexion while the right hand adds cranial bone movement (sphenoid, right temporal or petrosal bone) or eye movement.

- The cranial bone movements are the same as described above.
- The right index finger is pointed at the lateral side of the corner of the eye and the rest of the hand contacts posterior to the right ear. With an interphalangeal extension a medial movement of the eyeball is initiated.

Table 17.10 summarizes movements of different structures of the proposed neurodynamic test of the oculomotor nerves.

Palpation

Small infraorbital branches of these cranial nerves, which lie on the wall of the orbit, are sometimes very sensitive and can contribute to the hypothesis of an oculomotor nerve dysfunction. With the tip of the index finger the therapist tries to twang these branches and compares the quality and intensity of the response with those of the orbit and the other side (Fig. 17.55).

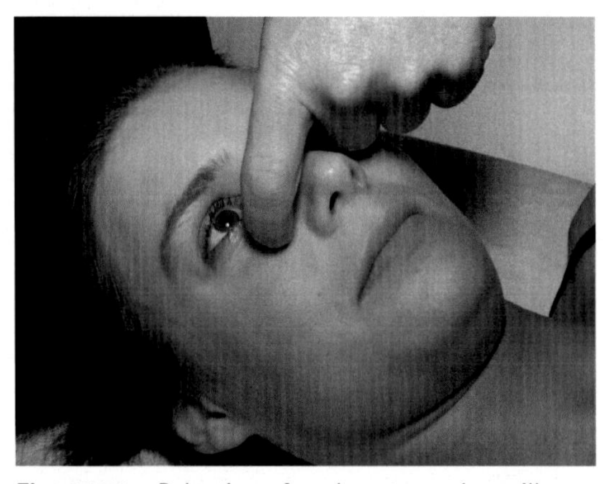

Fig. 17.55 Palpation of oculomotor and maxillary branches on the orbit.

Conduction test

Here the oculomotor, trochlear and abducens nerves will be tested together because they all innervate the extrinsic muscles of the eyeball. The oculomotor nerve also carries autonomic motor (parasympathetic) fibres to the pupil and ciliary muscles of the eye (Lang 2000). Therefore it is important to test pupillary function by constriction and dilatation (inspection) and also for nystagmus.

Inspection of the pupils

PUPILLARY LIGHT REFLEX

Pupillary reaction to light is assessed as above for the optic nerve. The direct reaction (pupillary constriction in the eye tested) as well as the consensual reaction (pupillary constriction in the eye not tested) should be inspected. A lack of consensual reaction, which is normal, can often be seen in unilateral optic nerve compression or neuritis (Spillane 1996). Such abnormal responses may indicate dysfunction of the optic nerve (afferent fibres) as well as the oculomotor nerve (efferent fibres).

ACCOMMODATION

Accommodation latency can be examined by holding a newspaper in front of the face at a distance where problems occur. This will depend on the problem, for instance a long distance (divergence) or short distance (convergence) problem. Move the paper forwards or backwards to test distance problems, noting the accommodation time. This can also be done with a small cord with a small ball on it which can be moved easily (Fig. 17.56) (Wilson-Pauwels et al 2002).

If accommodation deteriorates over several repeats, endurance and coordination of the eye musculature is poor, which may be related to pathology of the oculomotor system. This pattern may often be observed during repetitive eye movements in the same direction, such as in computer workers or tennis spectators (Radanov et al 1999, Keller et al 2000). Therefore, not only must eye function be investigated using the accommodation test, but standardized long-term eye movements must also be challenged, and the quality of movement and time until onset of symptoms should be assessed.

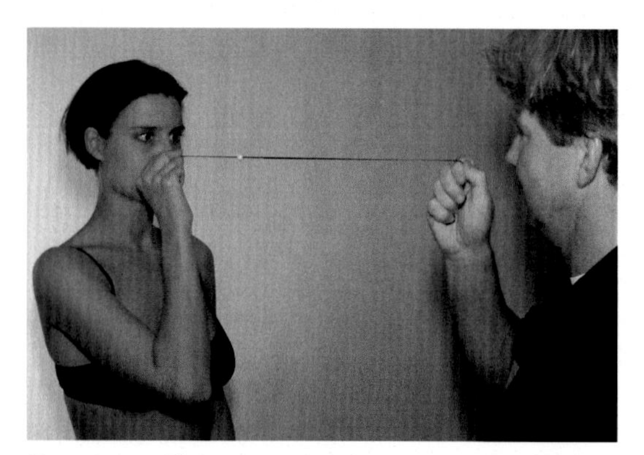

Fig. 17.56 The accommodation test using a cord with a ball on it which moves easily. The therapist judges the accommodation time and the distance that can still be accommodated.

Examining extraocular movements

The aim of the so-called cover test is to observe if one eye is lagging during movement, and also if there is any diplopia and/or nystagmus. It is impossible to understand the tests of oculomotor movement without knowledge of muscle function. As a summary, the eye movements are described related to their innervation in Table 17.11.

THE EYE-FOLLOWING TEST

Hold a pencil 10–15 cm in front of the patient's face and move it quickly in each of the nine directions, instructing the patient to follow the pencil with their eyes (Fig. 17.57). Each deviation has to be held for at least 5 seconds to detect nystagmus (Spillane 1996). A few beats of nystagmus in extreme lateral gaze are quite normal. A pair of Frenzel glasses can help detect the nystagmus better but be aware that most pathological nystagmus has to be diagnosed by an electronystagmogram (ENG).

Table 17.11 The oculomotor nerves and their main eye movement directions

Cranial nerve	Main eye movement direction(s)
Oculomotor (III)	Adduction, cranial, cranial-medial, cranial-lateral, caudal-medial
Trochlear (IV)	Endotorsion
Abducens (VI)	Abduction

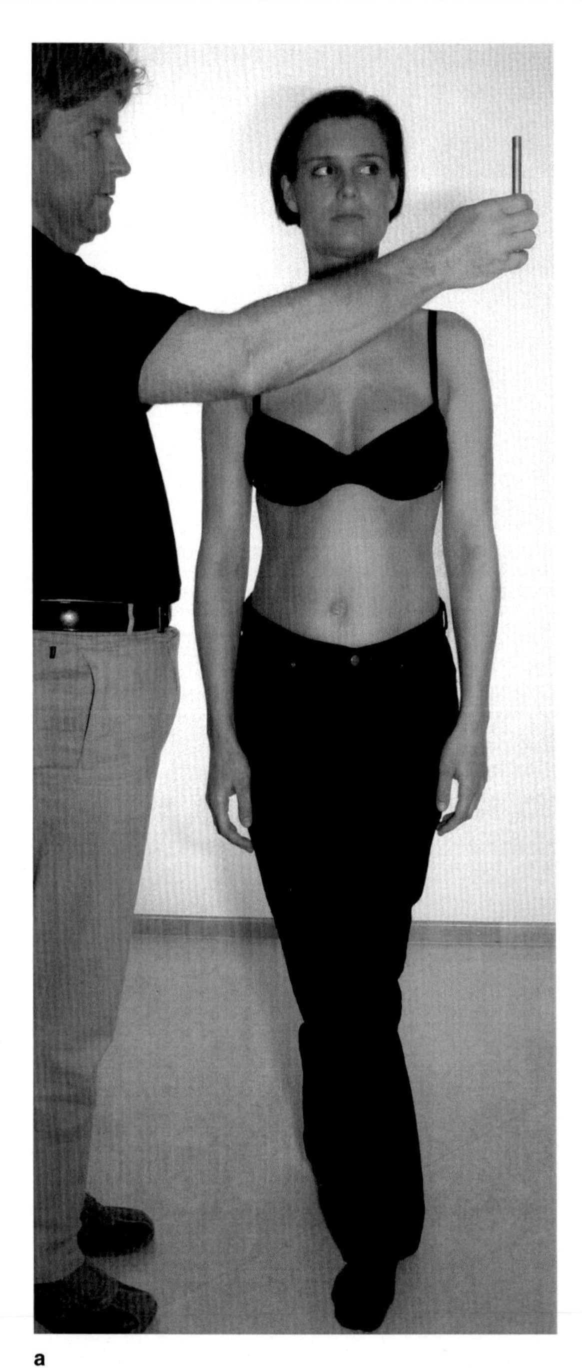

a

Fig. 17.57
a The eye-following test. Nine directions of eye movement are tested. The schematic shows which muscles are dominantly active for each movement. Table 17.11 shows oculomotor nerve involvement.
b Dominant muscle activities during the eye-following test.

Finally ask the patient to follow the pencil as it is moved toward the bridge of the nose. Note the normal convergence of the eyes to within 5–8 cm before visual acuity is lost – this is normal.

Performing the eye-following test in the neurodynamic positions with or without a pair of Frenzel glasses for each of the different nerves, or carrying out a short neurodynamic mobilization followed by reassessment of the cover test, can support a hypothesis of dysfunction of these cranial nerves.

This test also has therapeutic values. The movements can be challenged during active oculomotor rehabilitation as described below.

MEASUREMENT OF EYE DYSFUNCTIONS

The Maddox rod is an instrument that measures possible ocular deviations from the ideal position (Campos 1994, Sharifi Milani et al 1998). It is considered to be a reliable tool and is usually used in the (neuro)ophthalmologic field; nowadays it is applied more and more in 'posturology'. It can be an excellent tool to use during and after craniofacial–cervical and neural treatment. For this purpose, it is particularly indicated in association with the Maddox cross.

Before discussing measurement, a brief overview is given of the oculomotor dysfunctions that can be measured.

The ideal position for measurement (orthoposition)

The ideal position of the eyes, also called 'orthoposition', can be defined as the position of fusion where 'both main visual lines intersect at the staring point' (Bredemeyer & Bullock 1986). Eye deviation is often a functional adaptation to maintain the orthoposition. All six extraocular muscles are active and are orchestrated by the brain using the three cranial nerves. When one or more muscles are weak, an intermittent (Sharifi Milani et al 1998), latent (Kommerell & Kromeier 2002) or manifest strabismus occurs. This deviation from the orthoposition is defined as heterophoria or heterotropia according to its features.

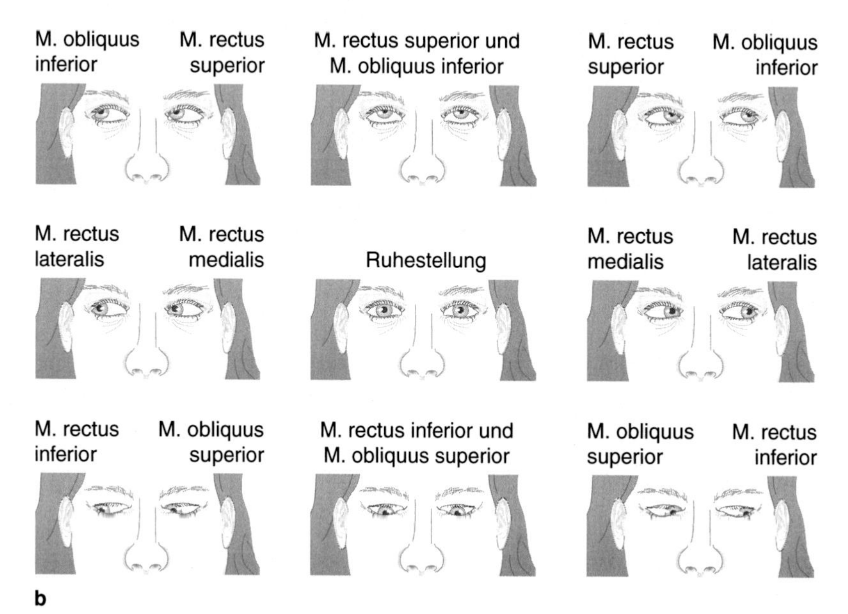

Fig. 17.57—cont'd

Heterophoria (latent strabismus)

Heterophoria occurs when, after interrupting the fusion through the covering of one eye, the free eye deviates from the orthoposition (Bredemeyer & Bullock 1986, Campos 1994, Kromier et al 2002). Various types of heterophoria are classified according to the direction taken by the covered eye with respect to the orthoposition. We are concerned in particular with the following horizontal deviations:

- Exophoria: After the covering of one eye, each eye turns out towards the forehead.
- Esophoria: After the covering of one eye, each eye turns in towards the nose (Bredemeyer & Bullock 1986).

Heterotropia (manifest strabismus)

Heterotropia, on the contrary, is a kind of deviation from the orthoposition that cannot be counterbalanced by the fusion reflex. It is a constant deviation, easily noticeable through a simple observation of the patient (Bredemeyer & Bullock 1986) (Fig. 17.58).

In particular, we see two main patterns:

- Esotropia: One eye is convergent with respect to the orthoposition.

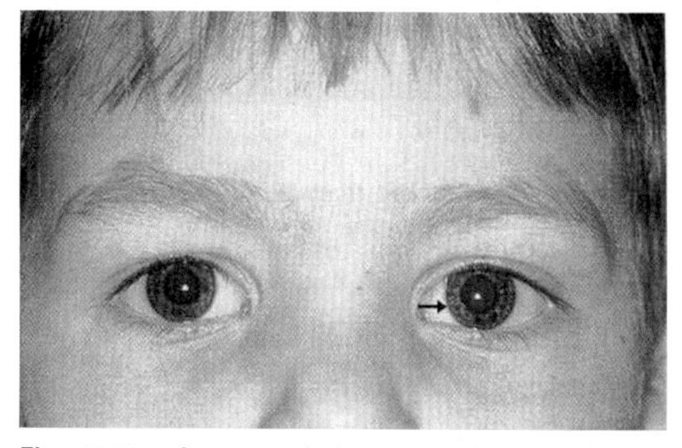

Fig. 17.58 Accommodative esotropia of the left eye during close fixation (arrow) (reproduced with permission from Lang 2000).

- Exotropia: One eye is divergent with respect to the orthoposition (Bredemeyer & Bullock 1986).

In only a small percentage of people do the eyes maintain the orthoposition after the fusion has been interrupted, for example, by covering one eye (Kommerell & Kromeier 2002). This happens during *orthophoria*, which is the particular position of the eyes when the main visual lines meet at the staring point; the position is reached and maintained without the help of the fusion reflex (Bredemeyer & Bullock 1986).

PATHOGENESIS OF HETEROPHORIAS AND HETEROTROPHIAS

The position of each ocular bulb depends on two factors:

- The anatomical structures connected to the bulb
- The extraocular muscle innervation.

The various structures and tissues connected to the ocular bulb (e.g. extraocular muscles, connective tissues, nerves and blood vessels) maintain the eye in its correct position within the eye socket. This position, not dependent on any innervation, is called the 'mechanically determined position' (Sharifi Milani et al 1998). Therefore heterotropia (manifest strabismus), and heterophoria (latent strabismus) are not primarily existing conditions but reactions to an interruption of the sensory–motor feedback control system. The reaction consists of a deviation from the vergence position (eye movements on both sides towards nasal or temporal). Binocular vision causes a continuous calibration of the vergence position. This 'orthophorization' explains why, in most persons, heterophoria differs only slightly from zero. Nevertheless, a small heterophoria is common (70–80% of the population) (Ellis et al 1998). The need to compensate for heterophoria by sensory–motor fusion can cause complaints such as headaches, concentration disturbances and neck pain from prolonged reading. Since a variety of other defects can lead to similar symptoms, a causal relationship with heterophoria can be assumed only after a thorough differential diagnosis (Kommerell & Kromeier 2002).

THE MADDOX ROD

The Maddox rod, a circular lens just a few centimetres wide (Fig. 17.59), is made up of a series of parallel glass cylinders (with a very short wavelength) that produce a linear image of a bright dot (Campos 1994, Sharifi Milani et al 1998). When a patient, looking through the Maddox rod, is shown a bright dot, they perceive a line of the same colour as the lens used (Garber 1995, Vibert et al 1999). This line will be perpendicular to the axes of the cylinders (Bricot 1996). If the axes are placed in a horizontal position, the line seen by the patient will appear vertical; if they are placed in a vertical position the line will appear horizontal.

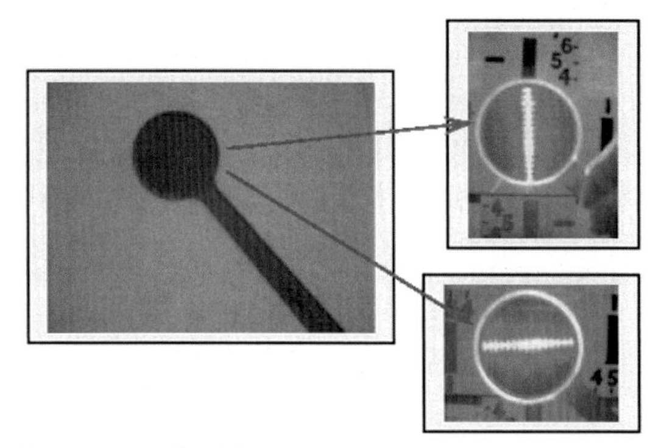

Fig. 17.59 The Maddox rod.

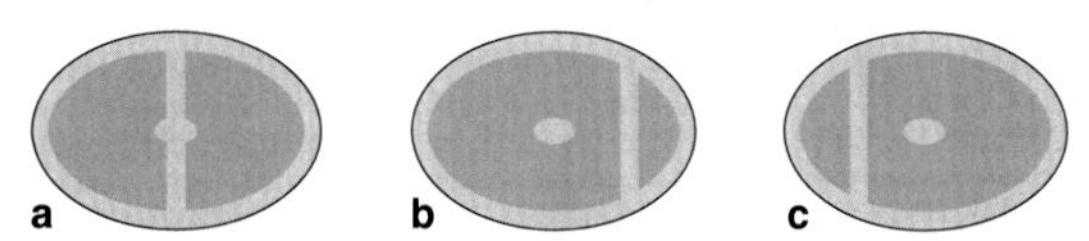

Fig. 17.60 Evaluation of results: **a** no abnormality; **b** esotropia or esophoria; **c** exotropia or exophoria.

The Maddox rod, generally used in association with a prism bar (Bricot 1996), allows the measurement of a patient's possible ocular deviations from the ideal position (Garber 1995).

Method of measurement

At the beginning of the test, a red Maddox rod is placed in front of the patient's right eye with its cylinders in the horizontal position. The patient is asked to look at a light dot, with both eyes opened. The patient will see a vertical red line and a bright spot.

- If the line and the bright spot coincide there is no deviation (= orthoposition) (Vibert 1995; Fig. 17.60a).
- If the patient has esotropia (ET) or esophoria (E) they will see the red line to the right side of the bright spot, i.e. the right eye is turned toward the nose (Bredemeyer & Bullock 1986; Fig. 17.60b).

- If the patient has exotropia (XT) or exophoria (X) they will see the red line to the left side of the bright spot, i.e. the right eye is turned toward the forehead (Fig. 17.60c).

The test is then repeated placing the Maddox rod in front of the left eye.

To quantify a patient's eye deviation, a prism bar that provides a measurement in dioptres is generally used (Campos 1994). This will be done by an eye specialist or optometrist.

USE OF THE MADDOX CROSS

An instrument that can be used in association with the rod is the Maddox cross (Toselli & Miglior 1979) (Fig. 17.61). It is formed by four equal branches, two of which are horizontal and two vertical. On each branch there are two graduate scales covering the distance from the centre to the extremity of the branch. The first scale, of large dimensions, reports numbers from 1 to 7, the other, with smaller and closer numbers, goes from 4 to 32. In the centre of the cross where the branches meet, there is a bright dot at which the patient will gaze.

Method

In our test we use a Maddox cross (without prism) and a Maddox rod fixed on a plastic structure. Before the start of the test, the patient must be placed at the right distance from the light source according to their functionality and problems. Sometimes 'phoric problems' are revealed only when the patient's head is in a particular position or when they are placed at a specific distance from the light source (Roll et al 1989). The various trials can therefore be compared only if they have been performed at the same distance. The next proposed distances are described in the medical literature.

- Heterophorias/tropias at close optical range, when the test is performed at a distance of 30–33 cm.
- Heterophorias/tropias at long optical range, when the test is performed at a distance of 5–6 m (Toselli & Miglior 1979).

The patient is asked to look at the light in the centre of the cross, with both eyes open, looking through the rod placed with the cylinders in horizontal position, first with one eye and then with the other. If the patient is not in the orthoposition, they are asked to identify which number (big or small) on the horizontal branch of the cross is touched by the vertical red line. It is also necessary to specify if the number is on the right or left side with regard to the light source and, for this purpose, it can be useful to specify the colour of the observed numbers (which are red on one side and black on the other). In this way phorias and/or tropias will be revealed and classified as esophorias (E)/tropias (ET) or exophorias (X)/tropias (XT) according to the position of the red line with regard to the light.

Disadvantages of using the Maddox rod and the Maddox cross

By using this procedure, we cannot quantify the patient's deviation from the orthoposition as precisely as with the prism's system.

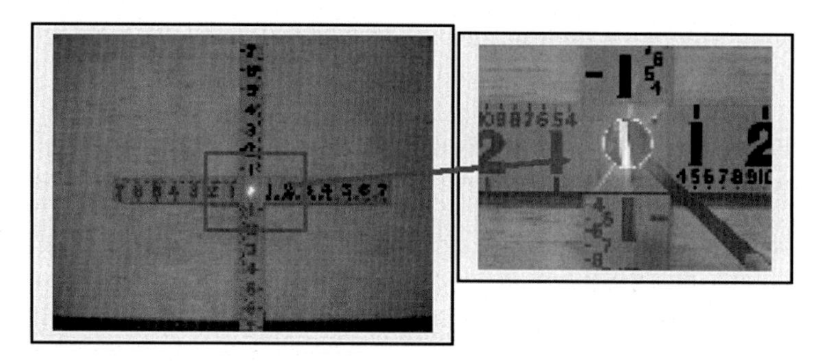

Fig. 17.61 The Maddox cross.

However, we obtain some useful data for reassessment carried out during and at the end of the craniofacial management. It is always the patient who judges the position of the red line.

Indications

The Maddox test can be applied to a single eye (monocular test) (Vibert et al 1999, Vibert & Häusler 2000) or to both eyes ('double Maddox rod' test) (Brazis & Lee 1998, Ellis et al 1998). The Maddox cross is often used to measure horizontal phorias at close optical range (Brautaset & Jennings 1999, Howarth & Heron 2000). However the Maddox rod is more reliable for measuring horizontal phorias (Howarth & Heron 2000).

The Maddox test is mentioned in different studies presented in the literature. It is generally used for evaluating ocular alignment and for measuring both tropias and phorias (Brautaset & Jennings 1999), either as separate tests or together with other measurements (Kromier et al 2002).

It has been proven in association with other tests that the Maddox rod provides reliable parameters (Brazis 1993, Capdepon et al 1994, Gwiazda et al 1999, Hyman et al 2001, Freedman et al 2002, Wong et al 2002):

- Diplopia
- Horizontal and vertical strabismus
- Progressions of myopia
- Subjective visual vertical perception in relation to inner ear lesions
- Brainstem lesions
- Unilateral paralyses of the fourth cranial nerve and of the vestibular nerve
- Surgery on oblique muscles of the eye
- Relationship between occlusion and visual focusing
- Paralysis of the superior oblique muscle of the eye
- Palsies of the trochlear nerve
- Eye interference on general body posture.

In summary, the Maddox rod is considered a reliable test in the ophthalmic field, providing data about patients with heterotropia or heterophoria which can be used for assessment and reassessment (Capdepon et al 1994).

The relationship between craniofacial assessment and posture

The Maddox rod is a useful instrument for therapists who assess the relationship between posture and oculomotor dysfunctions as described in this chapter. Ocular movements can be related via simple observation with postures, painful positions and functional movements of head, superior girdle or spine. The literature has frequently reported the actual link between eye work and body posture, proprioceptive systems, head posture and inner ear functionality (Roll et al 1989).

For example:

- It has been shown that dental occlusion influences visual focusing and how movements of the first few cervical vertebrae modify a person's visual field (Stephens et al 1996, 1999).
- It has also been established that some traumatic events can indirectly influence some parameters of ocular function, as, for example, in the case of whiplash (Wenngren et al 2002).
- In some research it is hypothesized that ocular imbalance plays a relevant role in cases of scoliosis (Safran et al 1994).
- Minor disturbances concerning the visual zone (e.g. strabismus in peripheral vestibular neuritis) are rarely diagnosed. Diplopia presents either with dizziness and nausea or with neurovegetative impairment (Safran et al 1994).
- A well-known phenomenon (in both the neuro-ophthalmologic and neuro-otologic field) is the ocular tilt reaction (OTR). This term means that lateroflexion of the head is associated with ocular torsion (inward rotation) (Vibert et al 1996), vertical strabismus and a possible compensation expressed in a thoracic and/or lumbar scoliosis. Although this dysfunction is considered a consequence of brainstem lesions, in the last few years it has also been found in patients with peripheral lesions of the otolithic organs in

the inner ear or in the vestibular nerve (Vibert & Häusler 2003).

Assessment and treatment of the patient with a craniofacial and cranioneural approach, together with oculomotor rehabilitation and a muscle balance approach integrated with (re)assessment by the Maddox test can help to understand the patient's presentation of oculomotor dysfunction in combination with clinical patterns that often have an unclear diagnosis.

How to integrate the Maddox rod test during assessment

This is always a part of an overall assessment and the data must be interpreted in light of other information that has been gathered.

- First collect *subjective data* that supports oculomotor dysfunction.
- Assessment of *conduction tests* such as inspection, accommodation, cover and the Maddox rod test.
- Assessment of *oculomotor function and equilibrium.* These specific tests are described below in the paragraph about oculomotor function and rehabilitation. They will set the basic level of further oculomotor rehabilitation
- Assessment of *posture.* Is there a correlation between the eye dysfunction and craniocervical position and/or scoliosis of the patient?
- Assessment of the *craniofacial region.* Make a choice as to which of the regions (craniocervical, craniofacial and cranioneural) is most related to the patient's oculomotor dysfunction. In most cases assessment of the cranioneurodynamics and the conduction tests for the oculomotor, trochlear and abducens nerves are included.
- A *clinical test treatment* of the most prevalent craniofacial dysfunction and *reassessment* of the measured dysfunction, including the Maddox test, are important in the ensuing decisions about treatment choices, explaining to the patient, etc. (see Case study 4).

Case study 4

Tanja, who is 8 years old, has a crossbite (Fig. 17.62a), a minor right convex scoliosis (Fig. 17.62b), a flat dorsal spine and minor headache in the right temporofrontal region. She was not considered for orthodontic treatment because of her young age and the orthodontist referred her for craniofacial asessement.

During inspection her head was examined in extension and then flexion to the left and rotation to the right.The sternocleidomastoid muscle was tight and sensitive (an early diagnosis of her paediatrician was 'torticollis') (Fig. 17.62c). Covering her right eye with an eye-patch for 20 minutes corrects her head to the midline. During correction of her head Tanja felt that her head was oblique on her trunk and the right eye moved and stayed cranial (Fig. 17.62d). During the cover test (covering the left eye; Fig. 17.62e) there was a clear movement dysfunction in the caudal and caudal-medial directions. The conclusion using the Maddox cross and rod was a right ocular deviation to medial (esotropia) and to cranial (hypertropia).

Tanja was treated once every 2–3 weeks for 9 months. Treatment consisted of neurodynamics, especially of the trochlear and oculomotor nerves, oculomotor rehabilitation and viscerocranial mobilization with emphasis on the maxilla-orbital region. After 9 months her scoliosis (measured with a scoliosis measure; Fig. 17.62f), flat dorsal spine and her crossbite (Fig. 17.62g) were reduced. The headache and the torticollis were gone, the sensitivity of both sternocleidomastoid muscles was the same and there was no difference in eye movements to the right in comparison to the left (Fig. 17.62h).

Table 17.12 gives a general overview of the physical examination options for the oculomotor system.

Oculomotor function and rehabilitation

Oculomotor rehabilitation is based on improvement of eye movements, positions and endur-

Table 17.12 Overview of the physical examination options for the oculomotor system

	Neurodynamic tests	Palpation	Conduction tests
Oculomotor nerve (III)	Craniocervical: Upper cervical flexion Contralateral lateroflexion Craniofacial: Orbit (general) Sphenoid Temporal Eyes: Caudal Lateral	Cranial and cranial region of the orbit (supra- and infraorbital branches)	Inspection: Pupillary light reflex Motor function Accommodation test: Maddox cylinder and cross
Trochlear nerve (IV)	Craniocervical: Upper cervical flexion Contralateral lateroflexion Craniofacial: Orbit Sphenoid Temporal Eyes: Caudal Lateral		
Abducens nerve (VI)	Craniocervical: Upper cervical flexion Contralateral lateroflexion Craniofacial: Orbit Sphenoid		

ance lacking during the cover, accommodation and Maddox tests. They will be integrated with passive craniofacial treatment and can be divided into *local* and *general* oculomotor rehabilitation.

LOCAL REHABILITATION

The training is focused primarily on the oculomotor system without influences of external factors such as posture changes or body movements. Parameters which can challenge the training are:

- The starting position of the test: For example, the abduction endurance of the left eye is less in sitting than in lying. The training can be performed first in lying and the endurance challenged. The next step is to build up the same movement in sitting and challenge the endurance.
- Duration: If nystagmus, strabismus or another non-symmetrical eye movement is noted, observe when the eye dysfunction appears. In general the recovery of motor fatigue of the eye muscles is fast. Training should be in series with short breaks (Thömke & Hopf 2001). One method is to start with an eye movement and reduce the duration to 40–50% of the test result. During the training first try to increase the number of series of good qualitative eye movement.

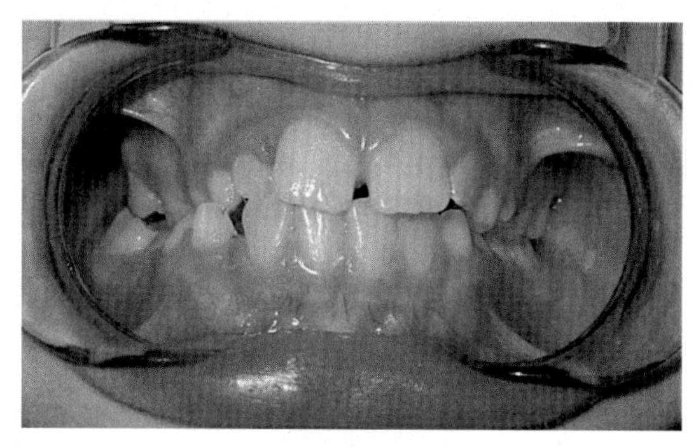

a

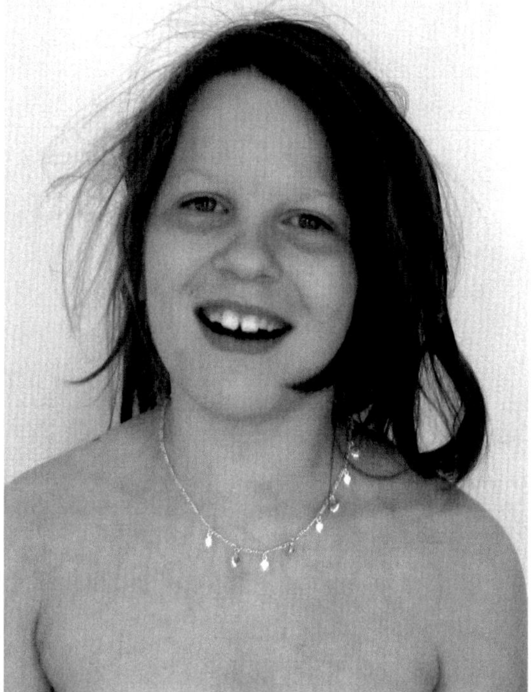

c

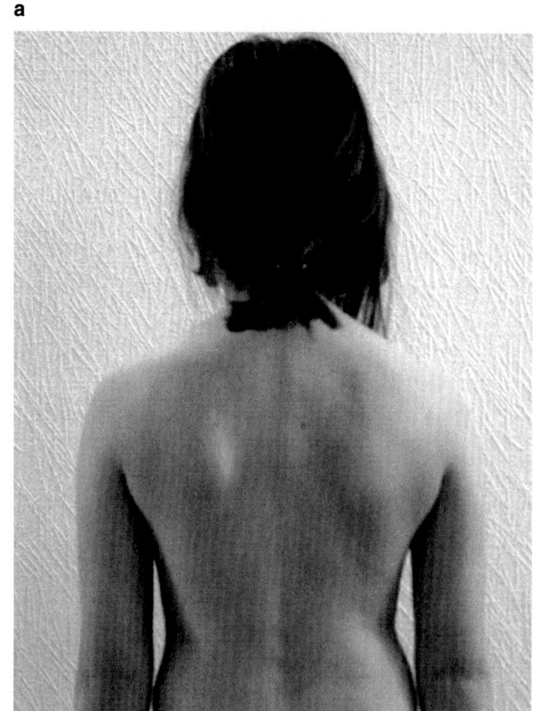

b

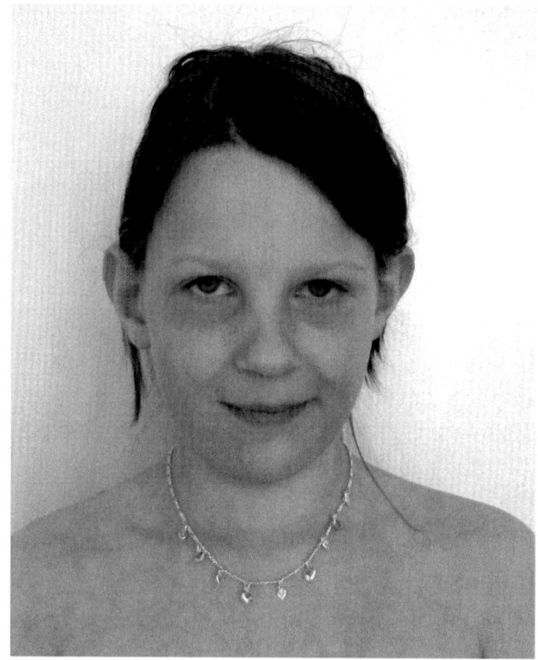

d

Fig. 17.62a–h An 8-year-old girl with eye dysfunctions and scoliosis.

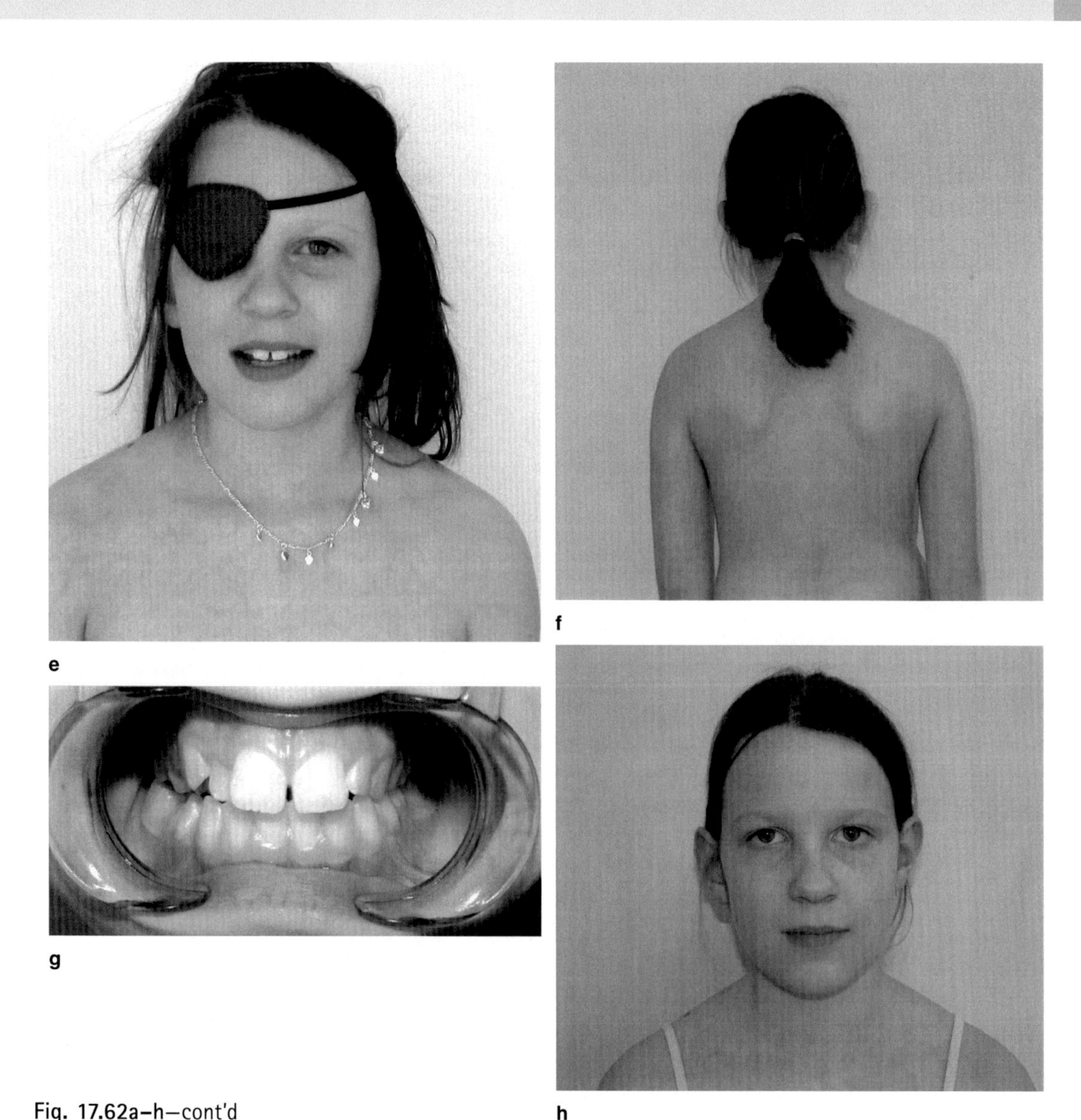

Fig. 17.62a–h—cont'd

At a later stage, try to increase the duration of every exercise by about 10–20% each time.

- Speed and variation of directions: To make the exercise more difficult, challenge the speed of the eye movement and add another movement direction, progressively combining both.
- With or without neurodynamic mobilization: If the therapist is convinced of the hypothesis that pathodynamic changes of the oculomotor nerves influence the target tissue (eye movements), combine neurodynamic treatment with eye movement rehabilitation. Reassessment of the cover test has to be undertaken to judge if cranioneurodynamic treatment is relevant for this patient's problem.
- With or without imagination: Before the active treatment starts, the patient has to imagine the eye movement to be performed. Demonstrate this by showing it on paper

or performing it yourself. A good support during this mental imagination is movement of the eyeball passively in the required direction.

GENERAL OCULOMOTOR REHABILITATION

Posture and body movements will be combined with local oculomotor rehabilitation. One requirement is that the quality and duration of the eye movements that will be used are progressed during the local rehabilitation. This type of exercise is closely related to daily life activities and can be used by a patient with:

- Dizziness during standing
- Vertigo and/or vertigo during accommodation function such as reading or looking around
- Diplopia while writing
- Balance problems during shopping
- Eye pain or fatigue during accommodation and long-term eye positions
- Changing of neck position and movements such as driving a car or watching tennis.

One or more of the following variations may be chosen:

- Changing of functional positions: The local rehabilitation will be performed from functional positions with a lot of contact to less contact, such as starting in lying to half sitting to sitting and standing on two legs progressing to one leg (Fig. 17.63).
- Transfers: Local eye rehabilitation will be trained before and after the transfers from one body position to another. For example, in a patient with dizziness from lying to sitting, eye movements can be trained in lying and directly after the sitting manoeuvre.
- Changes in neck position: The craniocervical position can influence oculomotor behaviour by the cervicovestibular (CVR) and ocular reflexes (Oosterveld & van der Laarse 1969, Peeters et al 2001). Here the functional craniocervical position that most provokes the patient's symptoms and most influences the quality of the oculomotor activities can be chosen. Start with local rehabilitation (Fig. 17.64).

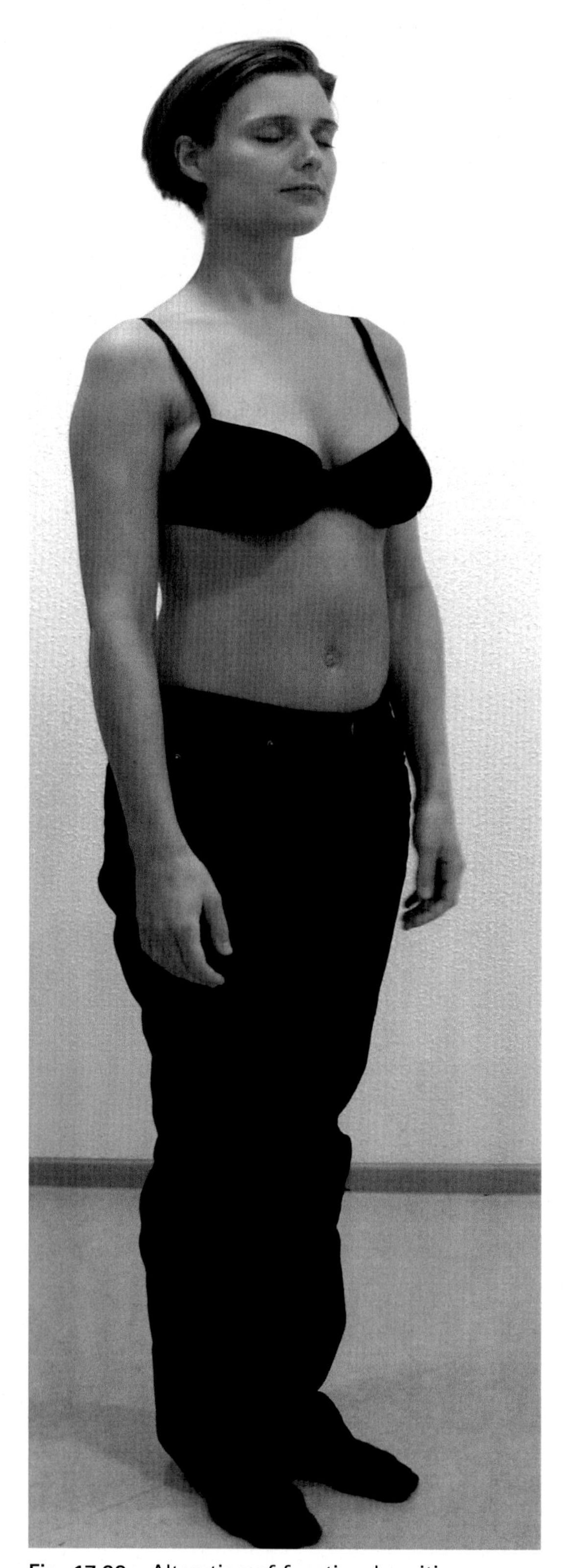

Fig. 17.63 Alteration of functional position.

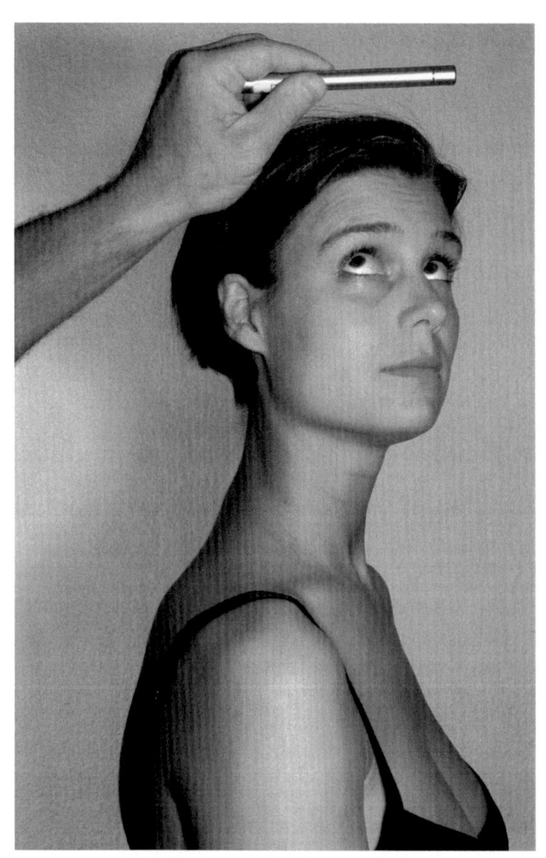

Fig. 17.64 Exercise of eye movements in the cranial direction in 45° right rotation.

- Uncoupling of craniocervical and eye movements: During this exercise, natural eye movements which are coupled with the craniocervical physiological movement will be switched off. For example, during craniocervical flexion, have the patient perform eye movements in a cranial direction instead of caudal, or craniocervical rotation to the right with eye movement towards the left (Fig. 17.65).
- With eyes open or closed: If the eyes are closed, there is less feedback to the brain which can influence the general balance, coordination and the quality of eye movements (Kavounoudias et al 1999). Eye movements with closed eyes are good exercises as an introduction to eye movement with open eyes in tinnitus and vertigo patients where the symptoms are provoked with the eyes open (Fig. 17.66). A disadvantage is that

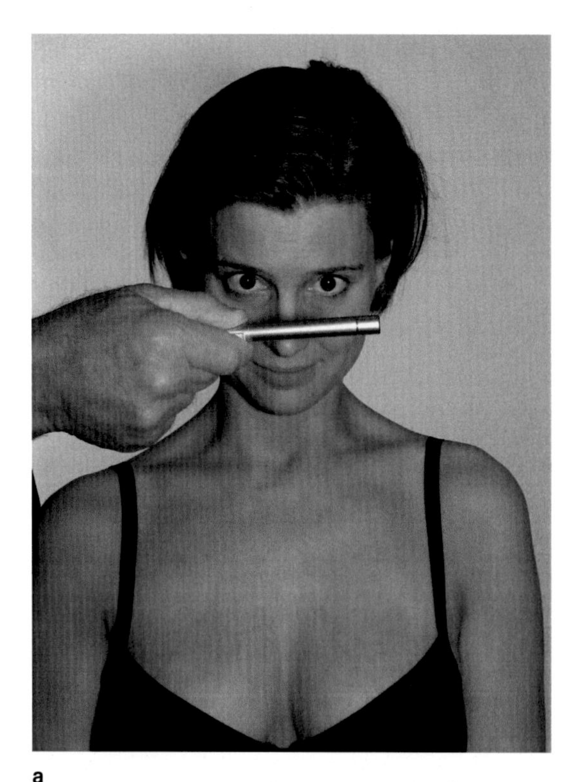

a

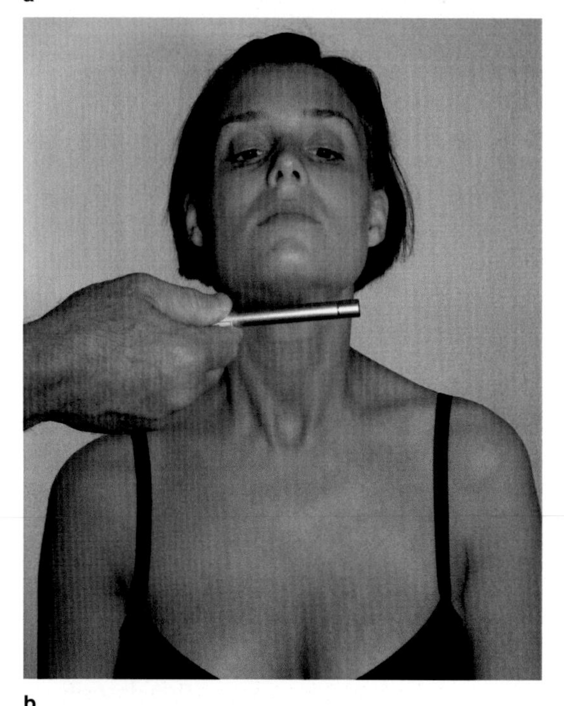

b

Fig. 17.65 Eye movement exercises: (a) Craniocervical flexion and extension with movement in the opposite direction in cranial or (b) caudal direction.

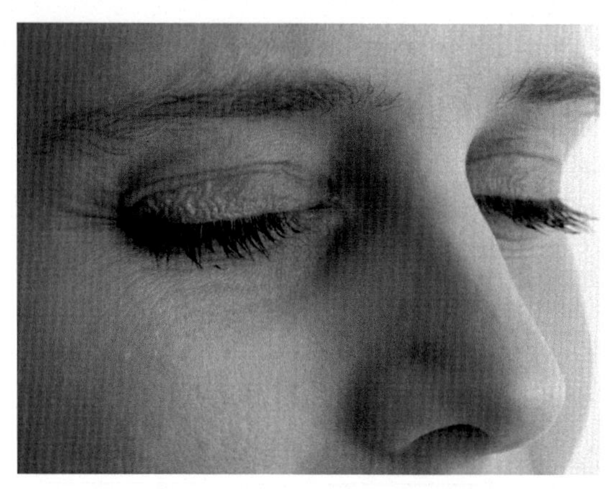

Fig. 17.66 Eye movements in horizontal direction to the right with closed eyes in standing.

assessment during closed eyes is more difficult than with open eyes.

- Combinations and variations: When two separate types of exercise improve, these can be combined. For example:
  - During rotation of the neck the training of eye movements
  - Disconnection of eye movements with craniocervical movements with closed eyes.

In summary it has to be mentioned that modern oculomotor rehabilitation is an integrated approach from manual therapeutic assessment of dysfunctions of the craniofacial, cervical and cranioneural region together with a constant assessment and training of oculomotor functions separate from or integrated with activities of daily living.

The effect of manual techniques will be evaluated by reassessment of the tests and exercises which are also used during oculomotor rehabilitation.

Comment

OCULOMOTOR NERVE

Diseases and dysfunction

In the neurological and ophthalmological literature the oculomotor nerve is often described as a cranial nerve that may be involved in intra- and/or extracranial pathologies and can contribute to oculomotor nerve palsies of variable intensity. Minor ocular paresis can be seen, mostly of the third and fourth pair of cranial nerves. The most common complaint is diplopia (>90%), more common in patients over 50 years of age. In this age group the most usual aetiologies are vascular and traumatic pathologies. In younger patients the most frequent pathologies are trauma and tumours.

The prognosis is better in the vascular group, the paresis recovery being more than 50% in comparison to all other pathologies except for tumours (McAvoy et al 2002, Kiratli et al 2003). Oculomotor dysfunction is also seen in young people after surgery and non-invasive facial trauma.

Schievink et al (1993) described oculomotor changes after general suboccipital surgery to intracranial structures. They noticed a common deficit in blood flow to the cervical internal carotid in all cases. One of the consequences is that the oculomotor nerve is more adrenaline sensitive than the others and is predisposed to dysfunctions (Keane & Ahmadi 1998). This nerve also appears to be sensitive to bacterial infections such as neurosyphilis (Holland et al 1986, Vogl et al 1992) or viral causes such as chronic active hepatopathy (Gastineau 1989, Pacifici et al 1992) which leads to a third cranial nerve palsy (ophthalmoplegia). Symptoms often present before clear diagnosis because of the frequent non-specific clinical presentation of the seronegative form of these diseases (Hooshman et al 1972). When a patient presents with diplopia, retro-orbital pain, (in)complete ptosis and pupil dilatation together with other neurological emotional changes, referral to a neurologist or ophthalmologist is advised. During diabetic neuropathy the most common cranial nerve affected is the third (El Mansouri et al 2000). The initial signs are lateral eye deviation and slight ptosis (Keane & Ahmadi 1998). The oculomotor and abducens nerves lie in the supralateral wall of the cavernous sinus (Castillo 2002) and are anatomically predisposed to adapt strongly to pressure during mechanical interface changes such as aneurysm of the internal carotid artery or meningioma (Kapoor et al 1991).

Patients with minor symptoms as described above can also exhibit responses during testing. The main symptoms are strabismus and consequent diplopia, ptosis, pupil dilatation due to decreased tone of the constrictor pupillae, downward, abducted eye position and accommodation problems (Lang 2000).

Clinical experience has shown that sphenoid movements into neurodynamic positions in particular may change symptoms dramatically. Exercises for the eye, eyebrow and forehead muscles in neurodynamic test positions may also result in a different afferent input and may be useful in therapy (Case study 5).

Case study 5

Ellen, who is 8 years old, has 'unclear' strabismus and diplopia. She complains about double vision during concentration activities such as reading and writing. Her parents noticed the double vision and extreme rotation movement of the neck when she wanted to look around (Fig. 17.67a). She was treated initially using cranial neurodynamics to the oculomotor (III), trochlear (IV) and abducens (IV) nerves, together with sphenoid mobilization and rehabilitation exercises for the eye movements that were lacking as well as with active neurodynamic position or movements of the cervical spine into flexion and lateroflexion. She was taught some home exercises related to the therapy and was stimulated to position herself in situations which provoked the symptoms. After 4 months her complaints had vanished. Neck movements were no longer directly coupled with eye movements. A little double vision and diplopia was evident only when she was tired (Fig. 17.67b).

Minor oculomotor dysfunction such as temporal asymmetrical positions or movement of the eyes during stress, tiredness and general sickness are often seen in patients after traumatic brain and/or neck injuries (Gimse et al 1996, Fischer et al 1997). During this period of stress, tiredness or sickness, the author ascertained that the ipsilateral eye is mostly positioned in a slight lateral and cranial position. Certain neck movements such as flexion to extension and rotations can produce extremely inconsistent coupled eye movements (mostly towards cranial and ipsilateral abduction) that can give clues for further examination and treatment.

TROCHLEAR NERVE (IV)

Trauma and dysfunction

Because of the long intracranial course and its position (just inferior to the free edge of the tentorium cerebelli), the trochlear nerve is predisposed to injury, especially due to compression in the dorsolateral brain, cavernous sinus and supraorbital fissure (Remulla et al 1995, Wilson-Pauwels et al 2002). Blunt head injury is the most common cause of unilateral but more particularly bilateral, fourth nerve injury. It occurs during violent confrontation and is seen most commonly in male youths (Hoya & Kirino 2000). Traumatological studies show that the incidence of trochlear nerve palsy due to trauma is three times that of the third or sixth cranial nerves although each of these is injured more often than the trochlear nerve (Keane & Baloh 1992). This is supported by limited pathological evidence (Heinze 1969) and imaging studies (Keane 1986). It is suggested that neural container changes in the form of lateral ventricle haemorrhage are a useful clue for dorsolateral midbrain contusion. Pathodynamics of the trochlear nerve can play an important role in this onset of pathology (Lang 1995, Remulla et al 1995). From these studies it is suggested that by (minor) pathodynamics of these nerves, upper cervical flexion and contralateral lateroflexion can be a good means of treatment to change the neural container of the trochlear nerve in the dorsolateral brain region.

The best guide to prognosis is provided by Mayo Clinic studies (Rush & Young 1981, Halmagyi et al 2003). Overall recovery from trochlear nerve deficits (at 53.5%) was at least as good as those of the other ocular motor nerves (Teller et al 1988). Patients with minor head trauma also attained 75% resolution. Many therapists see patients several years after an injury with symptoms that are related to old trauma. These patients often do not have a major neurological deficit but complain about craniofacial pain or eye dysfunction (diplopia, accommoda-

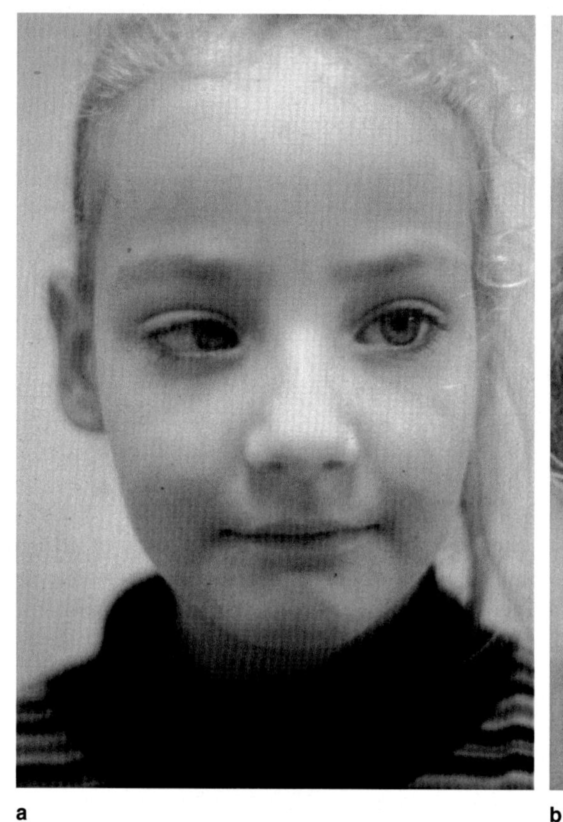
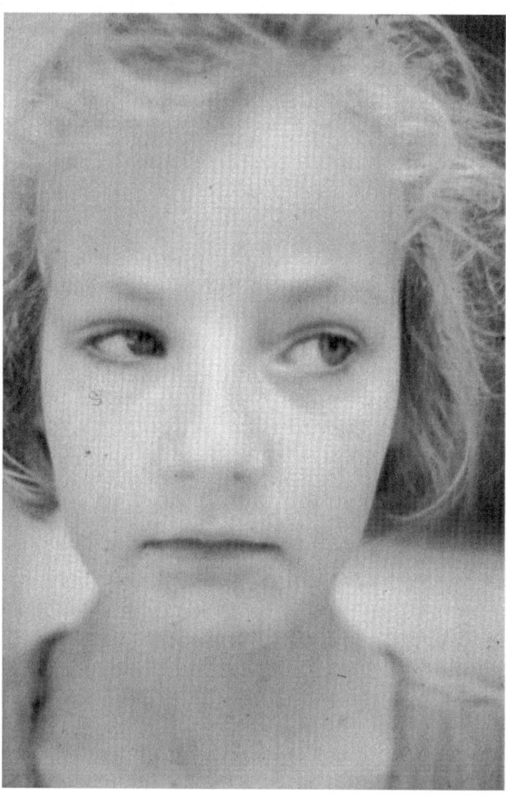

a b

Fig. 17.67
a Clinical example: an 8-year-old girl with strabismus.
b After 4 months' treatment.

tion dysfunction, etc.). Cranial nerve treatment together with cranial techniques may be one way of changing these symptoms.

Ocular torticollis

This minor trochlear nerve dysfunction, which is not uncommon, results in outward rotation (extortion) of the affected eye, diplopia and weakness of downward gaze which is most pronounced during attempted medial gaze. The extortion is often compensated through a torticollis (ocular torticollis) to the non-affected side (Wijnen 1993, Halmagyi et al 2003).

Differential diagnosis between an ocular and myogenic torticollis is possible using the occlusion test (Mein & Harcourt 1986, Gunter & Noorden 1990). By covering one eye for 20–30 minutes with a plaster, the cooperation between the two eyes is broken, enabling the therapist to differentiate the type of torticollis. When the dysfunction is ocular the torticollis should disappear after therapy.

In the absence of a definitive description of a neurogenic torticollis, many questions arise: we might ask if it really exists, and could it be neurodynamic in origin? We might ask ourselves if cranial neurodynamics might be responsible for creating a torticollis and how this could be proven. Clinically it is seen that, in patients with a minor torticollis, upper cervical flexion and ipsilateral rotation of the neck stimulate the affected eye in outward rotation. Upper limb neurodynamic tests (mainly in the region of 90° abduction of the shoulder) and SLR often change with eye and neck movements in pathological situations (Butler 2000).

It is important to be aware of such pathophysiological phenomena and to be able to use this awareness in examination and treatment. Remember too that long-term neck and headache problems, as well as post-traumatic neck problems such as whiplash, can cause dysfunction of the ocular nerves (Burke et al 1992, Brown 1995). Therefore, in cases of (minor) nerve pathophysiology such as meningitis, diabetes and postcervical syndromes, the trochlear neurodynamic test can be relevant. Muscle training of the eye with or without neurodynamic load positions may also prove to be valuable.

Intracranial connections and clinical consequences

In most anatomical studies of the trochlear nerve, the close relationship between the trochlear nerve, the dura mater and the cavernous sinus is described (Sinelmkov 1958, Wolff 1958, Romanes 1981, Engle et al 1997) and in some studies between the trochlear nerve and the trigeminal nerve. Recent studies showed that in 77.5% of 40 cadavers the trochlear nerve ran between the superficial and deep layers of the dura and was often directly connected with this layer. In these cases the nerve thickness in the posterior cranial fossa and the cavernous sinuses increased (80%) (Umansky & Nathan 1982, Bisaria 1988). This work suggests that the nerve has enormous design capacity for loading in the thickness of connective tissue and for movement in the dural layers. This has clinical consequences for examination and treatment of these nerves, particularly with regard to this dominance during elongation and sliding.

ABDUCENS NERVE (VI)

Neural container changes

Strabismus with diplopia as a consequence is not always seen after compression lesions of the abducens nerve but may occur because of minor changes of the mechanical interface and/or through tiredness (Koos et al 1993, Wutthiphan & Poonyathalang 2002). Post-inflammatory processes of the meninges, post-fracture situations of the floor of the posterior cranial fossa, increased intracranial pressure such as cranial growth during adolescence or sinusitis and/or middle ear infection (petrous, temporal bones) can change the neurodynamics of the abducens nerve (Hunt et al 1959). Neurodynamic tests combined with mobilizing of the petrous and temporal bones can often give spectacular changes in eye position or pain response and can be the first opportunity to assess and to treat.

Sympathetic responses after neck trauma

Strabismus, blurred vision, double vision (Fite 1970), sore tired eyes, spots before the eyes (Billig 1953), pupil anomalies (Duke-Elder & McFaul 1972) and defective accommodation (visual focusing mechanism) (Burke et al 1992) have been reported from neck contusion and whiplash injury. Because of the close anatomical relationship between the neck and the pathway of the sympathetic system supplying the eye, it has been postulated that the most common cause of ocular signs and symptoms would be damage to the cervical spine resulting in extreme interruption to the stimulation of the ocular sympathetic pathway (Burke et al 1992, Wutthiphan & Poonyathalang 2002). Prolonged disturbance of the sympathetic nervous system decreases blood flow to the cranial nerves and creates pathodynamics (Okeson 1995). The abducens nerve and the trigeminal nerve are two of the most richly sympathetically innervated cranial nerves (Wilson-Pauwels et al 2002). This could be an explanation for the fact that during upper cervical flexion (the first manoeuvre for most cranial nerves), and especially by the trigeminal neurodynamic test, pain and ocular dysfunction such as short nystagmus, double vision, pupil abnormalities and divergence have been seen.

Paresis

Isolated paresis of the abducens nerve may be caused by trauma (Baker & Epstein 1991, Holmes et al 2001). It develops slowly and may persist for more than 6 months (Galetta & Smith 1989). Neurodynamics may have a positive contribution to normal tissue healing in the neural container and connective tissue of the nerve itself (Butler & Gifford 1998). If the pathodynamics do not change or the paresis does not resolve as expected, the therapist must consider the possibility of neural container abnormalities such as intracranial tumours, aneurysms, etc. In such cases, the patient should be referred on for further investigation and diagnosis (Currie et al 1983, Chrousos 1993, Lang 2000).

GLOSSOPHARYNGEAL NERVE (IX)

Relevant functional anatomy

The glossopharyngeal nerve leaves the posterior lateral sulcus of the medulla oblongata above the branches of cranial nerves X and XI (Fig. 17.68). It consists of five superimposed bundles for different components (for specific anatomical details, see Chapter 2).

The motor component runs through the jugular foramen together with cranial nerves IX, X and XI. From the jugular foramen the axons descend in the neck deep to the styloid process and then curve forward around the posterior border of the stylopharyngeus muscle where the nerve supplies the muscle. The visceral motor component runs together with the mandibular nerve through the foramen ovale and synapses in the otic ganglion. From here postganglionic fibres form the auriculotemporal nerve (branch from V_3) to supply the secretomotor fibres to the parotid gland.

General sensory components start from the skin, the external ear, the inner surface of the tympanic membrane, posterior third of the tongue and upper larynx and have their nerve cell bodies in the superior–inferior glossopharyngeal ganglion which makes contact with the sphenoid and the falx cerebri (Koos et al 1993, Lang 1995). From here it runs further in the spinal trigeminal tract to the brainstem. Neurones from the sensory components pass through the jugular foramen and then run to the medulla (Patten 1995, Wilson-Pauwels et al 2002).

Neurodynamic test

Upper cervical flexion and lateroflexion away from the examined side loads the glossopharyngeal nerve generally. Motor and especially sensory components can be tested more specifically by moving the sphenoid and occipital bones.

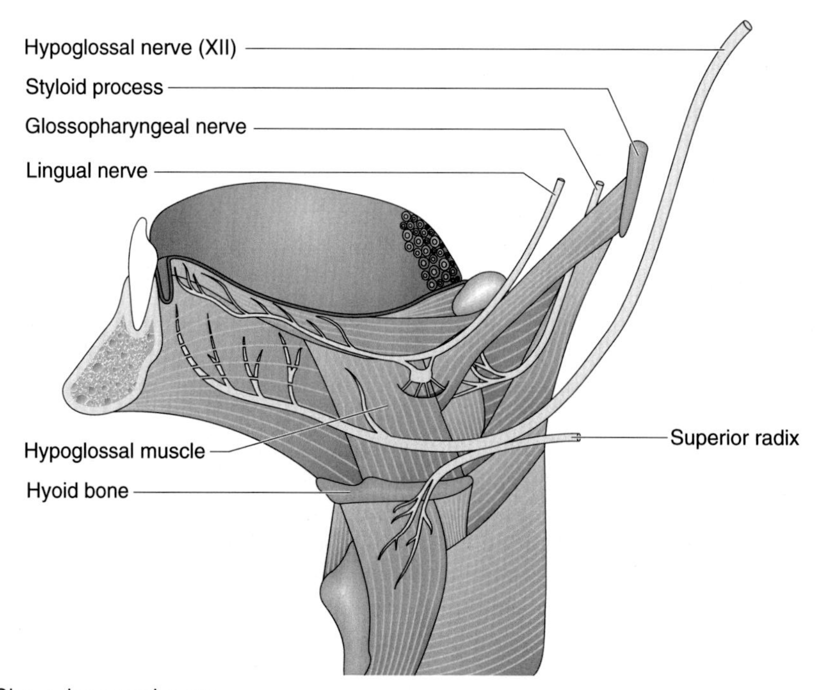

Fig. 17.68 Glossopharyngeal nerve.

Motor branches are emphasized by making a medial transverse movement of the styloid process. General sensory components can be influenced by sphenoid movements and the branches that innervate the tongue by posterior and anterior movements of the tongue. The addition of mandible movements such as laterotrusion, combined with protrusion, towards the other side also influence the extracranial branches of the glossopharyngeal nerve (Shankland 1995).

STARTING POSITION AND METHOD

The patient lies supine and comfortable in a relaxed position. The therapist sits behind the patient opposite the head. The left hand cups the occipital bone so that the forearm is perpendicular on the lateral side of the head and rests on the table. The manoeuvre can be executed emphasizing movements of the sphenoid or the temporal bone.

- Upper cervical flexion and lateroflexion away from the cervical spine with both hands can be carried out. The left hand always stays on the occiput, but the right hand is on the sphenoid or temporal bone depending upon which movement is examined after the neck movements (Fig. 17.69a).
- For the sphenoid, the thumb and index finger of the right hand contact the lateral border of the greater wing of the sphenoid.
- To test the temporal bone as a part of this neurodynamic test, four fingers of the right hand touch the temporal area. The ring and little fingers touch the mastoid part, the tip of the middle finger is in the external auditory canal and the index finger touches the zygomatic process of the temporal bone.
- For tongue movements, the frontal bone can be held in the palm of the right hand with index finger and thumb grasping the lateral edge of the sphenoid bone. This position is ideal for holding the head and sphenoid bone in any position required for neurodynamic tests. The patient can be asked to protrude the tongue not only to look at the quality of movement but also to assess abnormal responses such as pain (Fig. 17.69b). The head should stay in the same position during the craniocervical and tongue movements.

Palpation

Using the tip of the left index finger, it is possible to locate the superficial motor branch which lies ventral to the styloid process. The mechanical sensitivity of this branch can be strongly influenced by performing this palpation in lateroflexion. Relaxation of the superficial structures in lateroflexion towards the

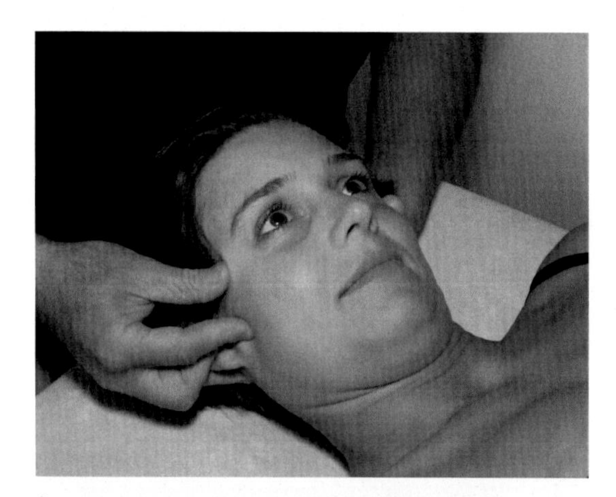

a

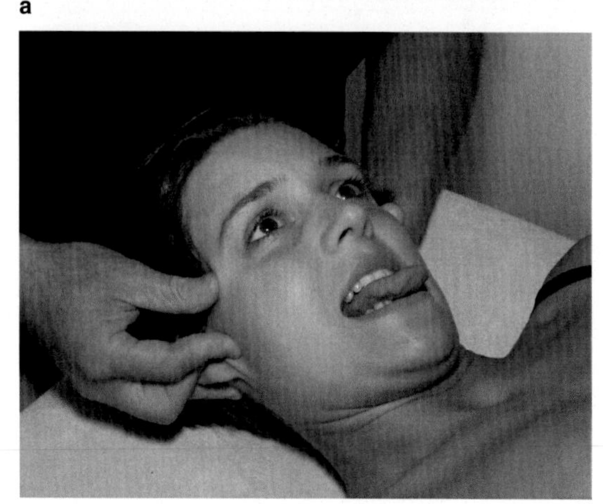

b

Fig. 17.69

a Neurodynamic test of the glossopharyngeal nerve (in upper cervical flexion and lateroflexion towards the other side, together with temporal movement).

b Protrusion and laterotrusion of the tongue, propulsion and laterotrusion to the opposite side to that being tested.

therapist enables localization of the styloid process and is sometimes needed to localize the glossopharyngeal branches. Twanging this nerve is not possible; only light sustained pressure provokes symptoms (Fig. 17.70).

Conduction tests

Clinically the functional conduction tests are not sufficiently clear to differentiate for the vagus nerve (X). Therefore these tests are described together with the vagus nerve (see below).

Table 17.13 gives a general overview of the physical examination options for the glossopharyngeal nerve.

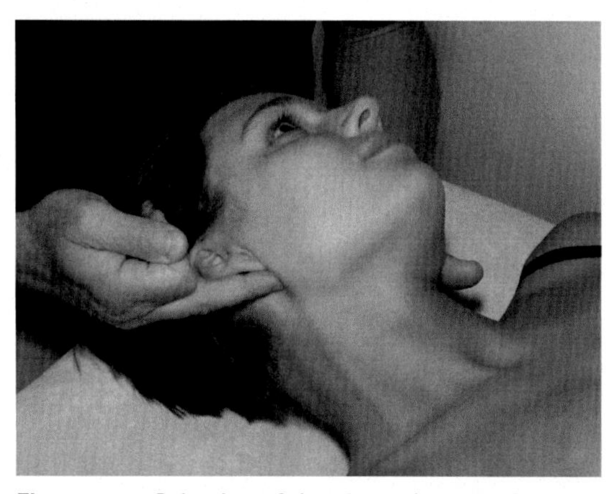

Fig. 17.70 Palpation of the glossopharyngeal nerve above the styloid process.

Comment

Be aware of the gag reflex if the fingers go too far down the patient's throat! Be ready to move quickly, especially in the case of patients with neurological dysfunctions such as paresis. Occasionally, lesions in this nerve or intracranial neurodynamic changes can lead to glossopharyngeal neuralgia, in turn provoking sudden pain of unknown cause (Wilson-Pauwels et al 1988). Arterial anomalies and arterioscleroses (e.g. elongated arterial loops in the CPA) can cause such changes (Jannetta 1977, Shiroyama et al 1988, Wilson-Pauwels et al 1988). Symptoms that appear to originate from this nerve, such as throat, ventral ear, dorsal lower jaw pain and swallowing problems, may be influenced by the above neurodynamic test. Clinically it is noted that tongue exercises in the glossopharyngeal tension test position produce beneficial results, especially for patients with neurological linguistic deficiency and undiagnosed throat pain.

NEUROMAS: NEUROPATHY AND SYMPTOMS

It is known from neurosurgical studies that glossopharyngeal neuromas develop slowly and can be progressive (Mountjoy et al 1974, Fink et al 1978, Quester et al 1993, Gupta et al 2002). The progressive symptoms increase over a number of years, and include unilateral headaches, vomiting, progressive hearing loss,

Table 17.13 Overview of the physical examination options for the glossopharyngeal nerve (IX)

Neurodynamic tests	Palpation	Conduction tests (together with vagus nerve)
Craniocervical:	Styloid process	Sensory functions:
Upper cervical flexion		Gag reflex
Contralateral lateroflexion		Taste (dorsal side of tongue)
Craniofacial:		Motor functions:
Sphenoid		Phonation test
Occiput		Speaking
Temporal (styloid process)		
Mandible:		
Contralateral laterotrusion		
Propulsion		

Case study 6

Maud, who is 8 years old, presented for treatment with an unknown neurological disease. This manifested itself as a clear case of tetraplegia with the head resting in upper cervical extension and right lateroflexion (Fig. 17.71a,b). Although there was no sign of mental deficiency she had speech problems and a regular chronic infection in both maxillary sinuses. Her tongue pressed against her palate more than it should, but she was able to move it up and down. On physical examination a higher than normal position of the hyoid was noted.

Correction of the neurodynamic loading of the hyoid or upper cervical spine was given in flexion, lateroflexion and contralateroflexion to increase the pressure of the tongue on her palate. Four sessions of treatment of the craniofacial mobilization together with dominantly glossopharyngeal and hypoglossal neurodynamic exercises supported by speech therapy changed her tongue tone. There have been clear positive changes in her ability to speak and reduction of sinusitis for the past 6 months (Fig. 17.71c,d). Antibiotics were no longer needed. Her parents described her as a 'new child with more energy and *joie de vivre*'. Her neurological disease remains unknown and her tetraplegia remains unchanged.

tinnitus, dizziness, hoarseness, swallowing or vocal problems with clear abnormalities (Naunton et al 1968, Crumley & Wilson 1984, Kaye et al 1984, Horn et al 1985, Quester et al 1993).

Some case reports describe clear pathological–mechanical interactions: minor symptoms caused by neurodynamic changes such as a change in upper spine position after acute wry neck or hyoid displacement during craniofacial growth (Rocabado 1983, Maitland 1986, Dibbets & Carlson 1995, Ozenci et al 2003) or scar tissue in the bottom of the mouth after radiotherapy for treatment of throat cancer (Leonetti et al 2001). The swelling or oedema which is extensive during hyperthyroidism is often seen in practice by many therapists but is not mentioned in the literature. In this case, neurodynamic examination and management is useful if signs and symptoms are found. Tongue exercises in neurodynamic positions have particularly sound empirical results (see Case study 6).

STYLOID PROCESS SYNDROME (EAGLE'S SYNDROME)

This syndrome is characterized by pain following mandibular or neck trauma in the region of a calcified and/or elongated stylohyoid ligament (Okeson 1995, Mortellaro et al 2002). The anatomy of the styloid process has great clinical significance due to its relationship to the following:

- Blood vessels: It lies between the internal and external carotid arteries and near the internal jugular vein.
- The local muscles: Three muscles originate from the styloid process, each innervated by a different nerve: the styloglossus innervated by the hypoglossal nerve, the stylopharyngeal innervated by the glossopharyngeal nerve and the stylohyoid innervated by the facial nerve.
- The cranial nerves: The styloid process lies close to five nerves: the facial, glossopharyngeal, vagus, spinal accessory and hypoglossal (Shankland 1995, Renzi et al 2005). This region is particularly predisposed to glossopharyngeal neuritis and carotodynia (Eagle 1948, Okeson 1995). Constant dull pharyngeal ache, sometimes sharp and stabbing pain (particularly when swallowing or during head rotation towards the symptomatic side), otalgia, dysphagia, temporal/parietal headache and the sensation of having a foreign object lodged in the throat are all classic symptoms of glossopharyngeal neuritis (Merskey & Bogduk 1994, Okeson 1995, Shankland 1995). Methods like palpation and radiography can differentiate glossopharyngeal neuritis from carotid artery and styloid process

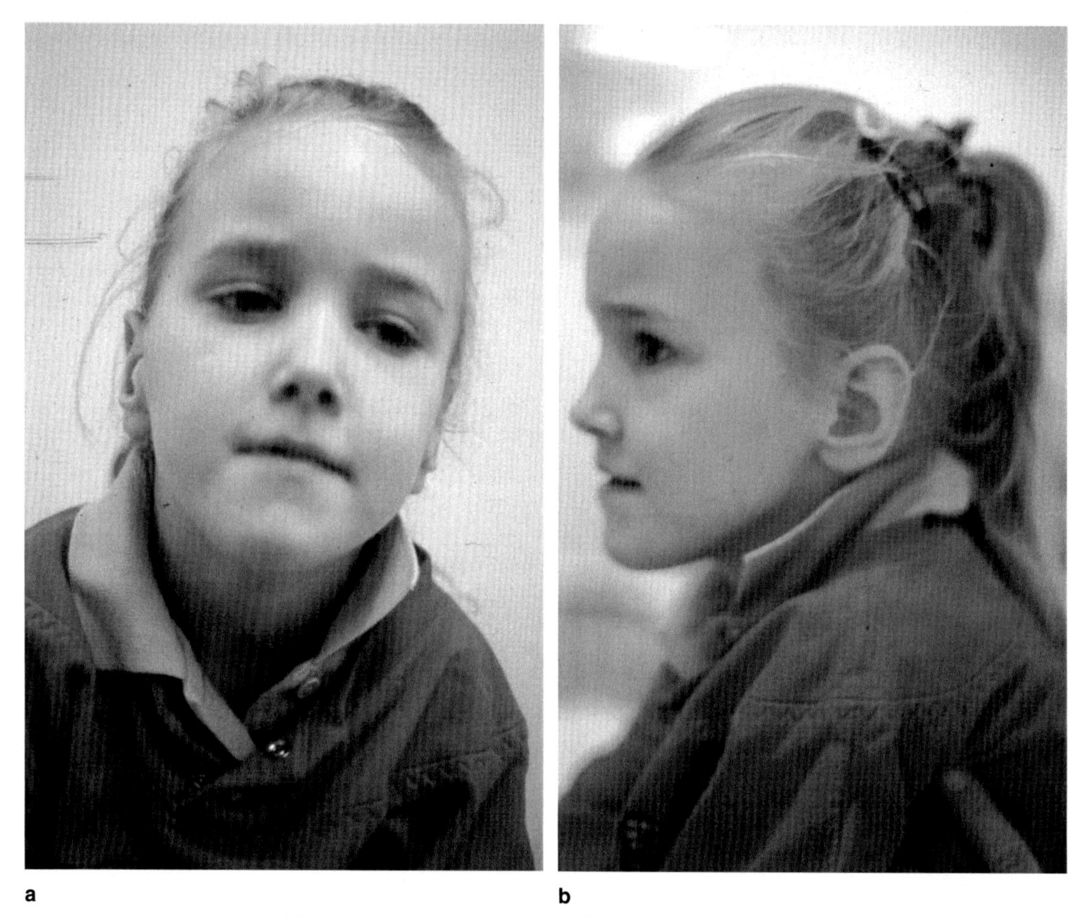

a b

Fig. 17.71a–d An 8-year-old girl with chronic sinusitis and cranial nerve dysfunction of the glossopharyngeal and hypoglossal nerves.

artery syndrome (Gossman & Tarsitano 1977, Karlan et al 1979, Dolan et al 1984, Yoshimura & Oka 1989). It has been stated that stretching of the complex of the five cranial nerves may reproduce pain and the other classic symptoms that fit in with Eagle syndrome (Gossman & Tarsitano 1977, Dolan et al 1984; Fig. 17.72).

Conservative treatment is advocated in the clinic more often than surgery and injection therapy, involving a mixture of local anaesthetic and cortisone, is recommended (Steinmann 1968, Shankland 1995). Yoshimura and Oka (1989) suggest sedatives, antidepressants drugs and physiotherapy. Craniofacial and cranioneurodynamic techniques, in the author's opinion, particularly those for the glossopharyngeal nerve, are worthwhile in the prevention of surgery and the reduction of symptoms. Often a combination of craniofacial mobilization of the petrosal, temporal or hyoid bones where the hypoglossal nerve is loaded to a greater or lesser extent has been beneficial in alleviating pain and allowing easier swallowing. Local techniques for the styloid process often reproduce the patient's symptoms but do not appear to provide good results.

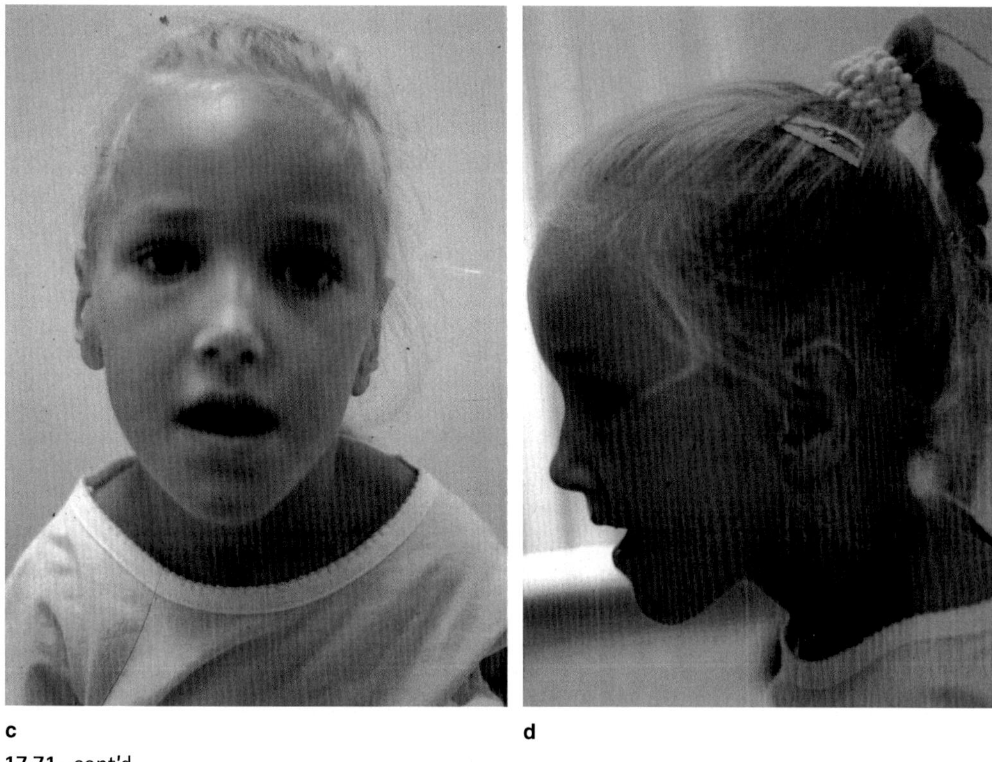

Fig. 17.71—cont'd

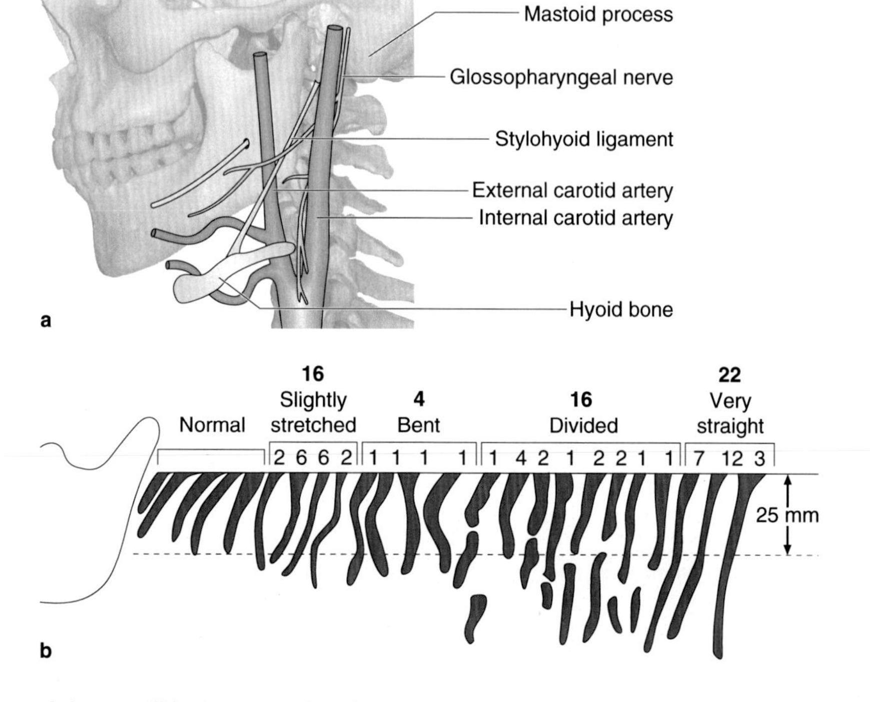

Fig. 17.72

a Medial view of the mandible demonstrating the glossopharyngeal nerve medial from the styloid process.

b Summary of panoramic x-rays revealing various degrees of elongation of the styloid process (n = 1771) (reproduced with permission from Correll & Wescott 1982).

Example of a patient with Eagle syndrome

Structural differentiation of a patient with the diagnosis 'unclear face–neck pain' is discussed in Case study 7. The result of the differentiation is a possible Eagle syndrome as discussed in Chapter 14 (temporal bone).

Case study 7

A 32-year-old man presents complaining of a pulling and sometimes burning sensation in his right suboccipital mandibular angle region. The symptoms are mostly provoked during or after work at his computer or desk, holding the phone between his head and left shoulder while talking on the telephone, yawning, chewing and swallowing. Sometimes he is woken by the pain and notices that if he moves his head or jaw the pain worsens. His wife indicates that he often sleeps on his left side, slightly bent to the left. He sleeps with a pillow between his head and shoulder and his mouth is open. The symptoms are inconsistent, and he is not conscious of them being cumulative or latent. Clear clues implicating structures such as craniocervical, craniomandibular, craniofacial or cranial nervous tissue are not obvious. In this case, differentiation in the position described above by the patient as his sleeping position is a reasonable starting point. It is a provocative position and it allows several structures to be stressed.

C0–C2

It is possible to examine this area using accessory movements such as transverse movements on C1 and then changing the mandibular position in several ways, including depression and/or laterotrusion. If these movements provoke symptoms, yet the craniomandibular movements fail to change the symptoms, it is probably a dominant C0–C2 problem. If craniomandibular movements change the symptoms during accessory movements on C1 there may also be a craniomandibular component.

Craniomandibular region

Accessory movements to the uppermost part of the mandible, especially in transverse to medial and posterior to anterior directions will reveal any relevant stiffness and/or pain. Different upper cervical spine positions, such as flexion and extension, during accessory movements of the craniomandibular region provide useful clues as to possible craniomandibular involvement.

Craniofacial region

Accessory movements, in this case temporal or petrosal bone movements and/or palpation of the styloid process, can once again be applied to ascertain symptom changes. Bear in mind that pressure changes in this area may also affect several small branches of cranial nerves contributing to the region. Bone, dura or cranial nerves may also provide a source of symptoms which can be influenced by specific therapeutic movements.

AURICULOTEMPORAL NERVE (TRIGEMINAL NERVE)

Cranial nervous system

It is possible to palpate the branches of the facial and vagus nerves on the mastoid process by 'twanging' them (Butler 2000). This can also be done with the trigeminal nerve above the head of the mandible. Just above the angle of the mandible and hypoglossal nerves, medial to the styloid process and lateral to the hyoid, it is possible to palpate the mandibular branch of the facial nerve in various neurodynamic positions to determine physical dysfunction of the nervous system in this region.

In this case, results of examination of the craniomandibular and craniocervical region were unremarkable. Temporal and petrosal bone movements diminished the pain; however, with upper flexion and slight contralateral flexion it increased. Palpation of the right petrosal bone provoked a severe local pain, caused by the glossopharyngeal nerve.

> **!** Where palpation of the glossopharyngeal nerve produces a burning pain and the pain increases during upper flexion or side bending of the upper cervical spine, a standard glossopharyngeal neurodynamic test should be used to detect a possible case of Eagle's syndrome.

VAGUS NERVE (X)

Relevant functional anatomy

The vagus nerve is the longest cranial nerve and is the parasympathetic nerve in the body (Patten 1995, Wilson-Pauwels et al 2002; Fig. 17.73). It has an extensive distribution from the visceral tissues of the neck to the thorax and abdomen. Wilson-Pauwels et al (2002) state that several roots emerge from the medulla of the brainstem and run ventrolaterally, exiting the skull through the jugular foramen along with the accessory nerve (XI). In the neck it lies between the jugular vein and the internal carotid artery, then descends vertically surrounded by the carotid sheath which is connected to the hyoid and cricothyroid via connective tissue. From the base of the neck downwards, the vagus takes a different path on each side of the body to reach the oesophageal plexus and the cardiac and pulmonary plexus in the thorax (Wilson-Pauwels et al 2002).

Neurodynamic test

For loading of the intracranial tissue, upper cervical flexion and lateroflexion away from the examined side is needed. In this position mid- and low cervical spine extension (neck-on-neck and neck-on-trunk movement) influence the branches lateral to the hyoid and cricohyoid.

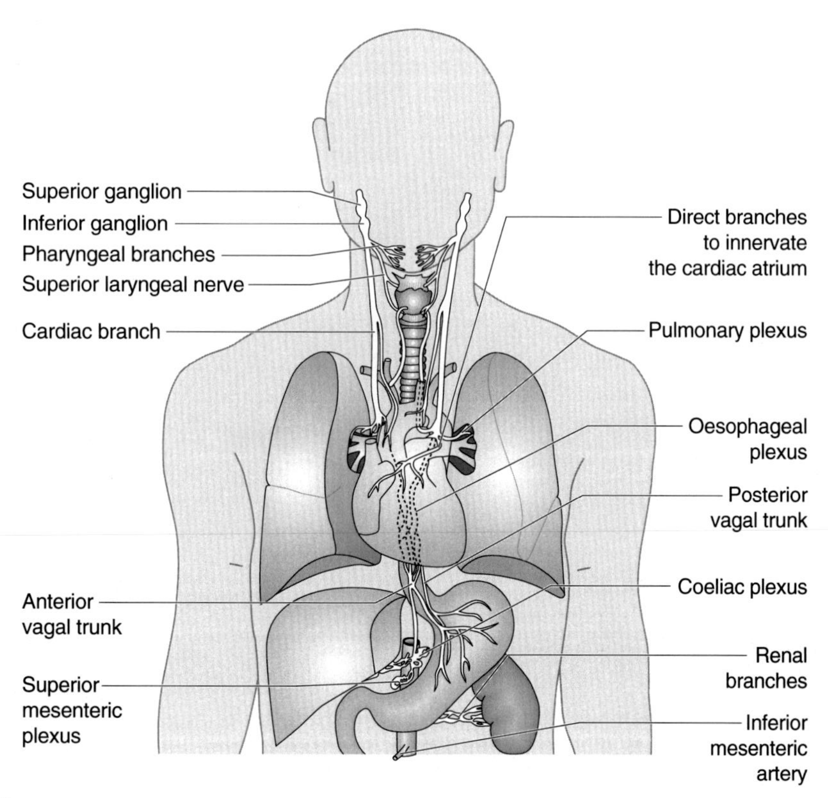

Fig. 17.73 Vagus nerve.

Sphenoid, occipital and temporal bone movement can be used for changing the jugular foramen as a mechanical interface.

Lateral movement of the hyoid for the pharyngeal branches of the visceral motor component is possible and the cricohyoid can be moved longitudinal to caudally for the bronchial motor component. A longitudinal to caudal movement investigates the visceral sensory and general sensory components.

The thorax can be moved from anterior to posterior with an angular movement, which is required for investigation of the cardiac and pulmonary plexi.

STARTING POSITION AND METHOD

Adjust the treatment couch down at the head end about 20° for the midcervical extension movement. If this is uncomfortable for the patient, return it to the flat position and use a rolled up towel to support the forearm.

- The therapist cups the lateral side of the occiput with both hands. Upper cervical flexion, lateroflexion away and mid–low cervical extension can be performed. If it is not possible to produce a good flexion position, it may be better to initiate the upper cervical spine movement by contacting the right thumb on the right mandibular angle and the other fingers on the right clavicular region.
- The hyoid and cricothyroid are now grasped between the radial part of the right index finger and the pad of the right thumb (Fig. 17.74a). In some patients this region is hypersensitive (e.g. after radiotherapy). It is then wise to use a full handgrip whereby the thenar and hypothenar eminences grasp around the hyoid and cricothyroid. Transverse and longitudinal movements are easy to perform and are often a good standard technique for treatment (Fig. 17.74b).
- For the thorax, the thenar and hypothenar eminences of the right hand contact the manubrium of the patient's sternum with the forearm in pronation (Fig. 17.74c).
- If craniofacial movements are executed, the therapist grasps both greater wings of the sphenoid or the temporal bone with the

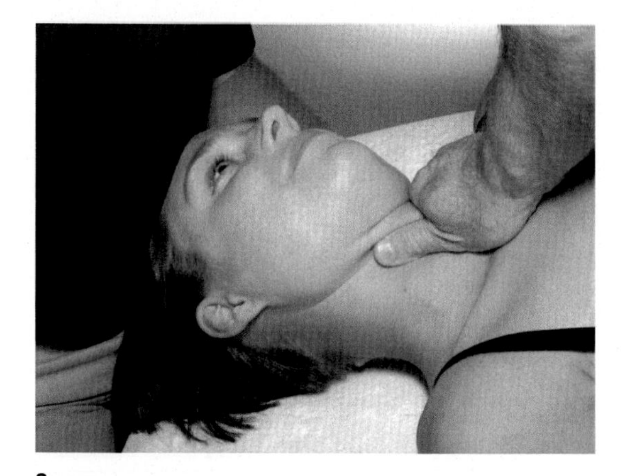

a

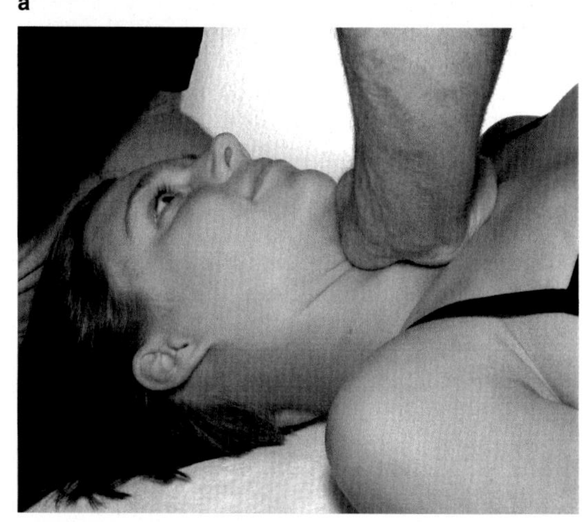

b

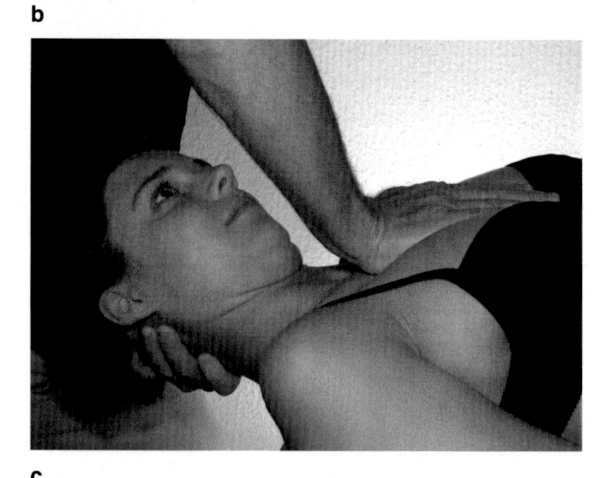

c

Fig. 17.74 Neurodynamic test for the vagus nerve.
a Movement of the hyoid and cricothyroid laterally.
b Full handgrip of cricothyroid.
c Anterior/posterior movement of the sternum.

right thumb and index finger. The tips of all five fingers of the right hand are in contact with the temporal bone with the forearm in supination. During addition of cranial movements of the sphenoid or temporal bone with the right hand, the therapist should ensure that the patient's head does not move and that the pressure of the left hand in the occipital region is not increased.

Palpation

The vagus nerve is palpable in the carotid sheath, medial to the sternocleidomastoid muscle, using the thumb or index finger of the left hand. Differentiation of symptoms is possible. It is difficult to 'twang' the nerve due to lack of hard surfaces to twang against (Butler & Gifford 1998, Butler 2000; Fig. 17.75a). Surgeons often use this palpation to make a decision about where they have to incise in order to perform a laryngoscopy (Procacciante et al 2001). Auricular branches are usually palpable laterally on the mastoid process (Fig. 17.75b).

Conduction tests for the glossopharyngeal (IX) and vagus (X) nerves

Clinically and even anatomically it is difficult to separate the activities of these two nerves. Subtle and relative conduction tests have to be performed so that both nerves are indeed being tested. The purpose of these tests is to determine:

- The quality of the gag reflex
- Abnormal sensation and abnormal motor responses from the larynx and palate.

THE GAG REFLEX

Using a cotton wool ball, touch the soft palate, posterior tongue or pharyngeal wall. If the soft palate raises asymmetrically, the afferent (IX) or efferent (X) branch of the reflex may be involved (Pertes & Gross 1996).

OTHER SENSORY FUNCTIONS

A dental probe may be used to test tactile discrimination of the back of the tongue. Taste can also be tested by focal application of bitter, sweet and sour substances (e.g. vinegar, sugar, syrup and lemon) to the back of the tongue. Often patients will have already described this sensation during subjective examination.

MOTOR FUNCTIONS

Ask the patient to open the mouth wide with the tongue resting on the floor of the mouth so that the palate can be observed. Have the patient say 'AH' while breathing out and 'UH' while breathing in. If this verbal expression is difficult, instruct the patient to breathe nor-

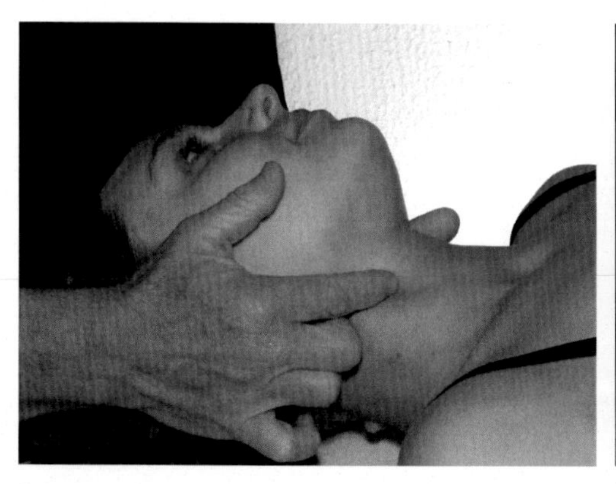

a

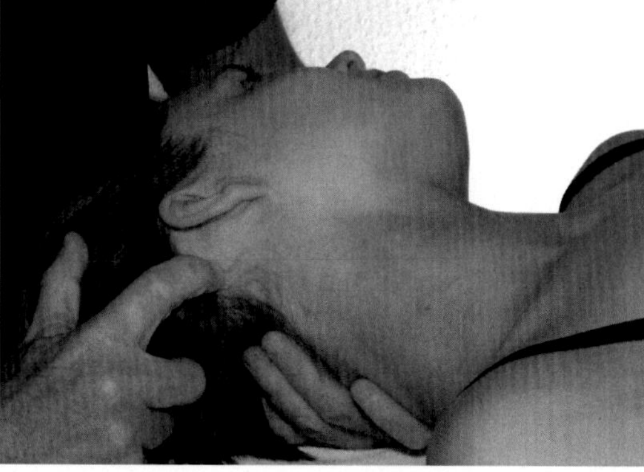

b

Fig. 17.75
a Palpation of the pharyngeal branches of the vagus nerve.
b Palpation of the auricular branches of the vagus nerve.

mally and inspect the palate on every change during the manoeuvre. The palate should move symmetrically up and back, the uvula remaining in the middle and the two sides of the pharynx should touch symmetrically (Patten 1995, Spillane 1996). The neurodynamic component used for the glossopharyngeal and vagus nerve can be added and the test can be repeated if there is any uncertainty about the physical findings.

PHONATION, SPEAKING CHANGES

Where there is less movement of the palate, dysphagia is likely, as is nasal regurgitation and nasal speech. Asking the patient to make a high pitched sound and to hold it, then a low sound for a few seconds provides a quick test to inspect the vocal cords. This gives an immediate impression of the function of the glossopharyngeal and vagus nerves and can also be used for reassessment.

Table 17.14 gives a general overview of the physical examination options for the vagus nerve.

Comment

THE VAGUS NERVE AND ITS MECHANICAL INTERFACE

A combination of occipital and sphenoid bone movements in 'loaded' positions of the vagus nerve will often cause signs and symptoms that are useful to test if a problem is suspected in the neural container of the jugular foramen.

These signs and symptoms may originate from three cranial nerves – the glossopharyngeal (IX), vagus (X) and accessory (XI) – whose clinical patterns do not manifest separately (Jannetta 1981). Changes in feeling in the tongue, pressure in the throat, increase in muscle tone in the sternocleidomastoid, heart palpitations, digestive disorders and bowel problems may present as part of the clinical pattern.

It should be borne in mind that testing may bring on increases in visceral sensation. Among these are stomach ache (due to heightened secretions of acidic gastric fluid), arrhythmia and pressure on the thorax which causes peripheral input to baro- and chemoreceptors of the viscera (Williams et al 1989). Stimulation of the tympanic membrane and the auricular branch around the auditory meatus can cause reflex coughing, vomiting and even fainting due to reflex activation in an irritable phase of the pathology.

Local techniques for cricoid and hyoid cartilage in neurodynamic positions can have rapid positive effects on neuralgia of the superior laryngeal nerve. The neuralgia presents as a unilateral stabbing pain lateral to the neck region with possible associated symptoms such as local tenderness when palpated, and possible autonomic phenomena, for example

Table 17.14 Overview of the physical examination options for the vagus nerve (X)

Neurodynamic tests	Conduction tests (together with glossopharyngeal nerve)
Craniocervical: Sensory functions:	Sensory functions:
Upper cervical flexion	Gag reflex
Contralateral lateroflexion	Taste (dorsal side of tongue)
Craniofacial:	Motor functions:
Sphenoid	Phonation tests
Occiput	Speaking
Temporal	
Cricohyoid:	
Lateral longitudinal to caudal	
Thorax:	
Anterior posterior	

salivation, flushing, possible tinnitus and vertigo (Merskey & Bogduk 1994).

VASOMOTOR HEADACHES

The vagus nerve, along with the trigeminal and upper cervical spinal nerves, supplies the pain-sensitive meninges (Levine 1991, Wilson-Pauwels et al 2002). Arteries and veins that supply the intracranial pain-sensitive structures often run with these nerves (Levine 1991, Emanuilov et al 2005). For example, the trigeminal nerve accompanies the middle meningeal artery which passes through the foramen spinosum of the sphenoid bone. The vagus nerve runs together with the glossopharyngeal and accessory nerves, as well as the inferior petrosal sinus and jugular vein, through the jugular foramen. Connective tissue changes, such as contractions in muscles and connective tissue of fascia, can cause an increase in pressure in the ventral craniocervical area, and the vagus nerve and jugular vein can suffer as a result of these contractions (Leblanc 1995, Netterville et al 2002).

These anatomical predisposing factors may explain why headaches such as migraines are often associated with symptoms such as gastrointestinal dysfunction. Some clinicians have long believed that migraines may be associated with the vagus nerve. The 'unknown neurogenic factor' of migraine is frequently cited (Shuaib et al 1997, Sadler et al 2002, Mauskop 2005). Clinically then, it makes sense to consider the vagus nerve as a starting point for treating vasomotor headaches.

This is especially true for children between the ages of 5 and 15 years presenting with vasomotor headache that does not respond to treatment. These children often have mild mental or physical retardation and/or heritable factors predisposing to headache. The following section gives an adequate (albeit incomplete) overview of the clinical pattern that emerged in our practice between 1996 and 2003 in a patient population of 48 individuals. Inclusion criteria were four affirmative answers to the parents' questionnaire (Box 17.2). The following physical parameters were measured:

Box 17.2 Questionnaire for parents (yes/no answers)

- Were there problems during the birth? (For example, premature delivery (before 37 weeks), extended labour, caesarean section, vacuum extraction or forceps delivery?)
- Have mental or physical developmental impairments been diagnosed by a specialist psychologist, school doctor or paediatric physiotherapist?
- Is orthodontic splint therapy required for faciomaxillary dysfunction?
- Did the parents, siblings or other family members also suffer from headaches at the same age?
- Does the patient take medicine for headaches? (For example, painkillers or drugs for vasomotor headache?)

- Posture
- Craniofacial asymmetry
- Abnormal neurodynamic features
- Passive intervertebral physiological movement of the craniocervical transit.

Posture found on physical examination of these patients concurred with the requirements and values of Kendall et al (1971) and Sahrmann (1998). Craniofacial asymmetry was recorded photographically. A control photograph was taken after six treatment sessions.

Abnormal neurodynamic features of the cranial nerves were diagnosed by reproduction of the symptoms in comparison with the other side, combined with neurodynamic manoeuvres such as the SLR, long sitting slump (LSS) and the slump tests. Of the 48 patients examined, 39 were restricted and had vegetative symptoms such as sweating, dizziness and/or headache in two or more of these tests. The most common pathological cranioneurodynamic findings were observed during passive neck flexion (NF)

Case study 8

An example of this patient population is an 11-year-old boy who has suffered from headaches from unknown causes since he was 6 years old. Results of neurological examinations were negative. He was prescribed medication for his migraine (sumatriptan).

He had had a prolonged birth without complications. At school his reading, writing and concentration were all below average, according to his mother and teacher. His main problem at the time of examination was two to three bilateral, throbbing headaches a week, which could be reduced with medication. Together with the associated symptoms such as sweating, nausea, vertigo and sometimes 'bellyache', his symptoms were clearly reproduced by the active LSS test and the neurodynamic test of the vagus nerve (Fig. 17.76e). He had undergone orthodontic treatment for malocclusion and a badly developed mandible (retrognathic mandible and asymmetric growth of the rami of the mandible) and had a clear anteroposition of his head (Fig. 17.76a,b). Splints had no effect on the headache pattern.

Relief of his symptoms after neurodynamic treatment, especially to the vagus nerve together with cranium and occiput–atlas mobilization, was clearly perceptible. After 10 treatments over a 21-week period (once every 2–3 weeks), his headaches had been substantially reduced in severity, and he was able to take medication only as needed. The other symptoms were also reduced by more than 75%, and his posture more balanced. His mother feels he is happier than before, he laughs more and he has more energy and has now really started to grow!

The treatment applied was upper cervical spine and cranial mobilization, with particular focus on the sphenoid–occipital joint and the joint around the temporal bone. Neurodynamic techniques with focus on the vagus nerve and active exercises were given to improve his posture. The retrognathic mandible and malocclusion can still be minimally observed following the splint therapy but asymmetry of the mandible was no longer present and the craniocervical anteroposition was reduced (Fig. 17.76c,d).

Retrospectively it is noted that a craniofacial and cranioneural approach was a contributing factor to reducing the patient's symptoms in his prepubertal phase.

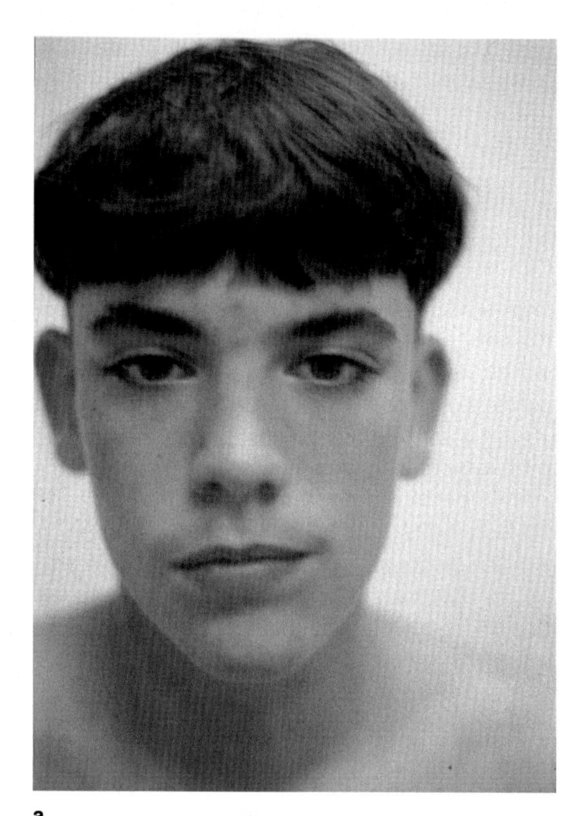

a

Fig. 17.76a An 11-year-old patient with migraine and dominantly autonomic symptoms.

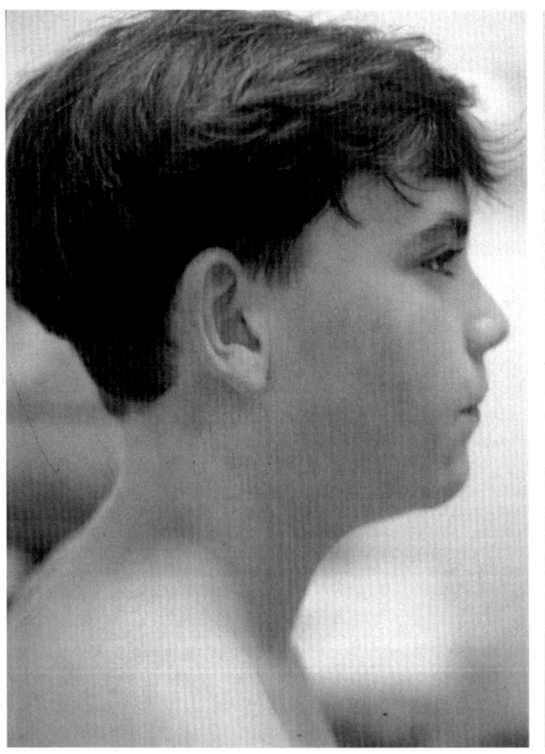

b

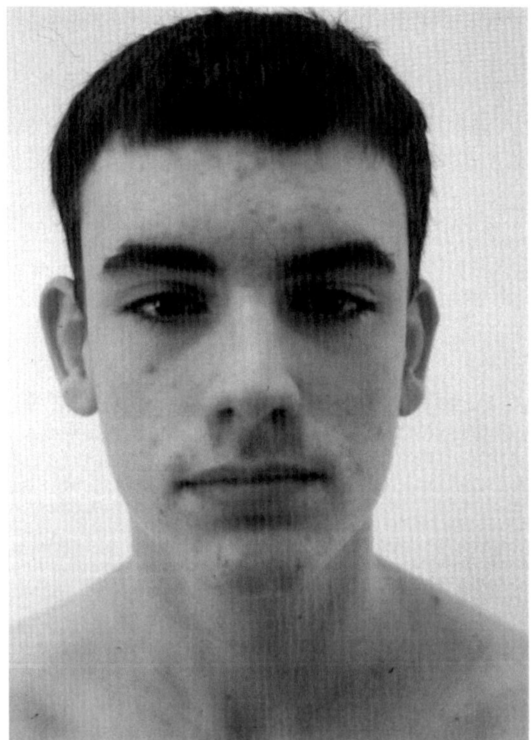

c

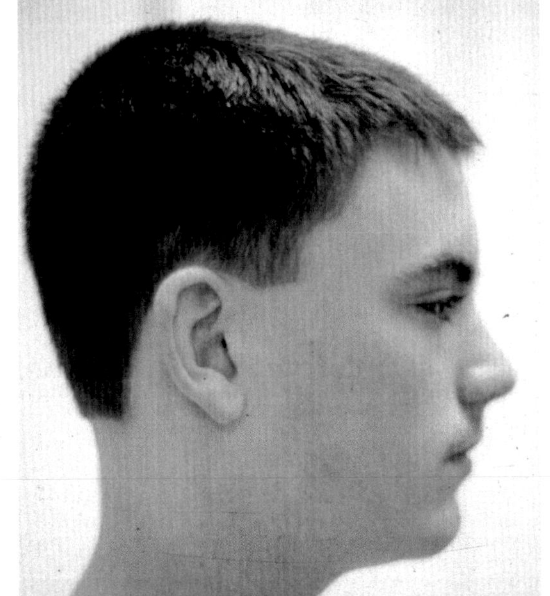

d

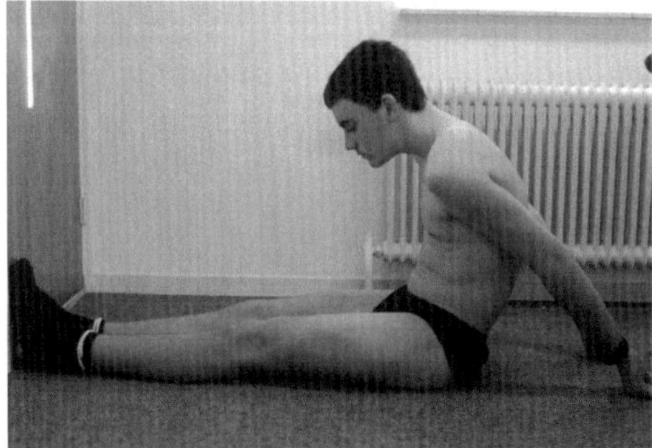

e

Fig. 17.76—cont'd
b Anteroposition of the head.
c Reduced mandibular asymmetry.
d Reduction of anteroposition.
e Long sitting slump (LSS).

and the trigeminal, facial, accessory and vagus tests.

Maitland et al (2001) described how to test abnormal intervertebral movements manually. The most common hypomobilities and immobilities (32 out of 48 cases) were observed at occiput–C1, normally on the side where the occipital bone was prominent.

It should be mentioned that the collection of these data, which is relatively straightforward in practice, is not a basis for more standardized research but to enable new clinical patterns to be recognized. The unproven correlations between these data which give the therapist clues for new investigation and management strategies are interesting (Case study 8).

SUMMARY

- In the third part of this chapter physical examination and different clinical patterns of the third category (specific cranial tissue) were discussed.
- In particular, cranial nerves with a specific function are discussed in this chapter, which also react with a typical clinical pattern in disease.
- Abnormal signs found during cranioneurodynamics can easily be integrated during passive and active rehabilitation programmes.
- When it is felt that the clinical pattern is unclear and the results are not what was expected, treatment must be stopped and the patient referred to a specialist for further diagnosis.

References

Abel M D, Levine R A 2004 Muscle contractions and auditory perception in tinnitus patients and nonclinical subjects. Cranio 22(3):181–191

Adams R, Victor M 1985 Principles of neurology, 3rd edn. McGraw-Hill, Berkshire

Agerberg G, Carlsson G 1972 Functional disorder of the masticatory system. I. Distribution of symptoms according to age and sex judged from investigation by questionnaire. Acta Odontologica Scandinavica 30:597

Aizawa S, Tsukiyama Y, Koyano K, Clark G T 2002 Reperfusion response changes induced by repeated, sustained contractions in normal human masseter muscle. Archives of Oral Biology 47(7):537–543

Alcantara J, Plaugher G, Klemp D, Salem C 2002 Chiropractic care of a patient with temporomandibular disorder and atlas subluxation. Journal of Manipulative and Physiological Therapeutics 25:63

Amyes E, Anderson F 1956 Fractures of the odontoid process. Archives of Surgery 72:377

Anderson R 1975 Shoulder disability and neck dissection. In: Anderson R, Hoopes J (eds) Symposium on malignancies of the head and neck. Mosby, St Louis

Aramideh M, Ongerboer de Visser B 2002 Brainstem reflexes: electrodiagnostic techniques, physiology, normative data, and clinical applications. Muscle and Nerve 26:14

Armon C, Daube J 1989 Electrophysiological signs of arterio-venous malformation of the spinal cord. Journal of Neurology, Neurosurgery and Psychiatry 52:1176–1181

Arzouman M, Otis L, Kipnis V, Levine D 1993 Observation of the anterior loop of the inferior alveolar canal. International Journal of Oral and Maxillofacial Implants 8:295

Ash C, Pinto O 1991 The TMJ and the middle ear: structural and functional correlates for aural symptoms associated with temporomandibular joint dysfunction. International Journal of Prosthodontics 4:51–57

Aspinall W 1989 Clinical testing for cervical mechanical disorders which produce ischemic vertigo. Journal of Orthopaedic and Sports Physical Therapy 11:176

Atkinson W 1949 The anterior inferior cerebellar artery. Its variations, pontine distribution, and significance in the surgery of cerebello-pontine angle tumours. Journal of Neurology, Neurosurgery and Psychiatry 12:137–151

Aurbach G, Ullrich D, Mihm B 1991 Chirurgische Anatomie des Nervus opticus und der Arteria carotis interna in der lateralen Keilbeinhöhlenwand. Eine anatomische Studie am Schädel–Basis–Präparat. HNO 39:467

Badia L, Parikh A, Brookes G 1994 Management of middle ear myoclonus. Journal of Laryngology and Otology 108:380

Badwin M, Singh Sahni K, Jensen M et al 1991 Association of vascular compression in trigeminal neuralgia versus other facial pain syndromes by magnetic resonance imaging. Surgical Neurology 36:447

Baguley D, Beynon G, Grey P, Hardy D, Moffat D 1997 Audio-vestibular findings in meningioma of the cerebello-pontine angle: a retrospective review. Journal of Laryngology and Otology 111:1022

Baker R, Epstein A 1991 Ocular motor abnormalities from head trauma. Surveys in Ophthalmology 35:245

Baloh R, Sakala S, Yee R, Langhofer L, Honrubia V 1984 Quantitative vestibular testing. Otolaryngology Head and Neck Surgery 92:145

Barat M 1983 Principles of rehabilitation in facial paralysis. In: Portmann M (ed.) Facial nerve. Proceedings of the Fifth International Symposium of the Facial Nerve. Masson, New York, p 66

Barba D, Alksne J 1984 Success of microvascular decompression with and without prior surgical therapy for trigeminal neuralgia. Journal of Neurosurgery 60:104

Barrett A, Hopper C, Landon G 2002 Intra-osseous soft tissue perineurioma of the inferior alveolar nerve. Oral Oncology 38:793–796

Bederson J, von Ammon K, Wichmann W et al 1991 Conservative treatment of patients with acoustic tumors. Neurosurgery 28:646

Begall K, Marggraff G, Schüler S, Freigang B 1994 Klinische und katamnestische Untersuchungen nach oto- und rhinobasalen Schädelfrakturen. HNO 42:405

Benecke R, Jost W H, Kanovsky P, Ruzicka E, Comes G, Grafe S 2005 A new botulinum toxin type A free of complexing proteins for treatment of cervical dystonia. Neurology 64(11):1949–1951

Berghaus A, Rettinger G, Böhme G 1996 Hals-Nasen-Ohren-Heilkunde. Hippokrates, Stuttgart

Beurskens C 1990 The functional rehabilitation of facial muscles and facial expression. Facial Nerve 2:509–514

Beurskens C, Burger-Bots I 1995 Mimetherapie helpt patiënten met perifere facialisverlamming. Fysiopraxis 4:38

Beurskens C, Bots I, Devriese P 1987 Resultaten van mimetherapie bij patiënten met een perifere facialisverlamming. Nederlands Tijdschrift voor Fysiotherapie 97:140

Beurskens C, Elvers J, Oosterhof J et al 1994a Fysiotherapie en de perifere facialisverlamming. Nederlands Tijdschrift voor Fysiotherapie 104:96

Beurskens C, Oosterhof J, Elvers J, Oostendorp R, Herraets M 1994b The role of physical therapy in patients with facial paralysis: state of the art. European Archives of Otorhinolaryngology Dec: S125–126

Billig H 1953 Traumatic neck, head, eye syndrome. Journal of the International College of Surgeons 20:558

Bisaria K 1988 Cavernous portion of the trochlear nerve with especial reference to its site of entrance. Journal of Anatomy 159:29

Bischoff C, Klingelhoefer J, Conrad B 1989 Decay and recovery of the stapedial reflex by prolonged stimulation in the diagnosis of myasthenia gravis. Journal of Neurology 236:343–348

Bocca E, Pignataro O 1967 A conservation technique in radical neck dissection. Annals of Otology, Rhinology and Laryngology 76:975

Bodner G, Harpf C, Gardetto A et al 2002 Ultrasonography of the accessory nerve: normal and pathologic findings in cadavers and patients with iatrogenic accessory nerve palsy. Journal of Ultrasound Medicine 21:1159

Boero R 1989 The physiology of splint therapy: a literature review. Angle Orthodontics 59:165

Bogduk N 1981 An anatomical basis for the neck–tongue syndrome. Journal of Neurology, Neurosurgery and Psychiatry 44(3):202–208

Bogduk N 1982 The clinical anatomy of the cervical dorsal rami. Spine 7:319

Bolton P, Stick P, Lord R 1990 Failure of clinical tests to predict cerebral ischemia before neck manipulation. Journal of Manipulative and Physiological Therapeutics 12:304

Born J 2002 Trigeminal neuralgia and hemifacial spasm. Vessel–nerve antagonism. Bulletin et Mémoires de l'Académie Royale de Médecine de Belgique 157:178

Borucki L, Wierzbicka M, Szyfter W 2002 Anastomosis of hypoglossal–facial nerves by modified May technique. Otolaryngologia Polska 56:39

Boussons J, Voisin P 1984 La reeducation faciale. Revue de Laryngologie 105:69

Brain A 1992 Laryngeal mask misplacement – causes, consequences and solutions. Anaesthesia 47:531

Brandenburg J, Lee C 1981 The eleventh nerve in radical neck surgery. Laryngoscope 91:1851

Brautaset R, Jennings J 1999 The influence of heterophoria measurements on subsequent associated phoria measurement in a refractive routine. Ophthalmic and Physiological Optics 19:347

Brazis P 1993 Palsies of the trochlear nerve: diagnosis and localization: recent concepts. Mayo Clinic Proceedings 68:501

Brazis P, Lee A 1998 Binocular vertical diplopia. Mayo Clinic Proceedings 73:55

Brazis P, Masdue J, Biller J 1990 Localisation in clinical neurology, 2nd edn. Little Brown, Boston

Bredemeyer H, Bullock K 1986 Ortottica teoria e pratica. Piccin, Padova

Breig A 1960 Biomechanics of the central nervous system. Almqvist and Wiksell, Stockholm
Breig A 1976 Adverse mechanical tension in the central nervous system. An analysis of cause and effect. Relief by functional neurosurgery. Almqvist and Wiksell, Stockholm
Bricot B 1996 La riprogrammazione posturale globale. Sauramps Medical, Montpellier
Brown B, Tatlow W 1963 Radiographic studies of the vertebral arteries in cadavers. Radiology 81:80
Brown S 1995 Ocular dysfunction associated with whiplash injury. Australian Journal of Physiotherapy 41:55
Brown W, Veitch J 1984 AAEM minimonograph: intraoperative monitoring of peripheral and cranial nerves. Muscle and Nerve 17:371
Bullit E, Tew J, Boyd J 1987 Intracranial tumors in patients with facial pain. Journal of Neurosurgery 64:865
Burchiel K, Clarke H, Haglund M, Loeser J 1988 Long term efficacy of microvascular decompression in trigeminal neuralgia. Journal of Neurosurgery 69:35
Burke J, Orton H, West J et al 1992 Whiplash and its effects on the visual system. Graefe's Archive for Clinical and Experimental Ophthalmology 230:335
Bush F 1987 Tinnitus and otalgia in temporomandibular disorders. Journal of Prosthetic Dentistry 58:495
Butler D 1991 Mobilisation of the nervous system. Churchill Livingstone, Edinburgh
Butler D 2000 The sensitive nervous system. Noigroup Publications, Adelaide
Butler D, Gifford L 1998 The dynamic nervous system: coursebook. NOI Press., Adelaide
Campos E 1994 Manuale di strabismo. Ed Ghedini, Milano
Capdepon E, Klainguti G, Strickler J, van Melle G 1994 Superior oblique muscle paralysis and ocular torsion. What is the effect of measuring method on the results? Klinische Monatsblätter fur Augenheilkunde 204:370
Capps F 1962 Temporomandibular joint syndrome of Costen. Proceedings of the Royal Society of Medicine 55:792
Casala B, Deutschl I 1994 Kraniozervikale Dystonien. Pragmatischer Sammelbegriff oder nosologische Einheit? Nervenarzt 65:75–94
Castillo M 2002 Imaging of the upper cranial nerves I, III–VIII, and the cavernous sinuses. Magnetic Resonance Imaging Clinics of North America 10(3):415–431
Chan S, Reade P 1994 Tinnitus and temporomandibular pain–dysfunction disorder. Clinical Otolaryngology 19:370
Chatelier G, Degoulet P, Devries C, Vu H, Plouin P, Menard J 1982 Symptom prevalence in hypersensitive patients. European Heart Journal 3:45
Chaunu M, Ratinahirana H, Raphael M et al 1989 The spectrum of changes in 20 nerve biopsies in patients with HIV infection. Muscle and Nerve 12:452–459
Chole R, Parker W 1992 Tinnitus and vertigo in patients with temporomandibular disorder. Archives of Otolaryngology, Head and Neck Surgery 4:118–126
Chong M, Bajwa Z 2003 Diagnosis and treatment of neuropathic pain. Journal of Pain and Symptom Management 25:4
Chrousos G 1993 Paresis of the abducens nerve after trivial head injury. American Journal of Ophthalmology 116:387
Ciftci E, Anik Y, Arslan A, Akansel G, Sarisoy T, Demirci A 2004 Driven equilibrium (drive) MR imaging of the cranial nerves V–VIII: comparison with the T2-weighted 3D TSE sequence. European Journal of Radiology 51(3):234–240
Cohen D, Perez R 2003 Bilateral myoclonus of the tensor tympani: a case report. Otolaryngology Head and Neck Surgery 128:441
Cohen N, Hammerschlag P, Berg H et al 1986 Acoustic neuroma surgery: with emphasis on preservation of hearing. The New York University Bellevue Approach. An electric approach. Annals of Otology, Rhinology and Laryngology 95:21
Coman W 1986 Dizziness related to ENT conditions. In: Grieve G (ed.) Manual therapy of the vertebral column. Churchill Livingstone, Edinburgh
Connor J 1985 Neural pacemakers and rhythmicity. Annual Review of Physiology 47:17
Cooper B, Alleva M, Cooper D, Lucente F 1986 Myofacial pain dysfunction analysis of 467 patients. Laryngoscope 96:1099
Corboy J, Galetta S 1989 Familiar cavernous angiomas manifestating with an acute chiasmal syndrome. American Journal of Ophthalmology 108:245
Correll R, Wescott W 1982 Eagle's syndrome diagnosed after history of headache, dysphasia, otalgia, and limited neck movement. Journal of the American Dental Association 104:491–492
Costen J 1934 Syndrome of ear and sinus symptoms dependent upon disturbed function of the temporomandibular joint. Annals of Otology, Rhinology and Laryngology 43:1–15
Costen J 1937 Some factors of the mandibular articulation as it pertains to medical diagnosis, especially in otolaryngology. Journal of American Dental Association 24:1507
Costen J 1956 Recognition of mandibular joint symptoms and treatment of their sources. Annals of Dentistry 15:90
Crile G 1906 Excision of cancer of the head and neck. Journal of American Medical Association 47:1780

Cross S 1993 Autonomic disorders of the pupil, ciliary body and the lacrimal apparatus. In: Low P P A (ed.). Clinical autonomic disorders. Little Brown, Boston
Crumley R, Wilson C 1984 Schwannomas of the jugular foramen. Laryngoscope 94:772
Csala B, Deuschl G 1994 Kraniozervikale Dystonien. Pragmatischer Sammelbegriff oder nosologische Einheit? Nervenarzt 65:75
Currie J, Lubin J, Lessell S 1983 Chronic isolated abducens paresis from tumors at the bone of the brain. Archives of Ophthalmology 40:226
Cusimano M, Sekhar L 1994 Partial hypoglossal to facial nerve anastomosis for reinnervation of the paralyzed face in patients with lower cranial nerve palsies: technical note. Neurosurgery 35:532
Daniel B, Guitar B 1978 EMG feedback and recovery of facial and speech gestures following neural anastomosis. Journal of Speech and Hearing Disorders 43:9
Davies P 1994 Starting again: early rehabilitation after traumatic brain injury or other severe brain lesion. Springer, Berlin
Davis L 1993 Viruses and vestibular neuritis: review of human and animal studies. Acta Otolaryngologica Suppl 503:70
De Souza C, Karnad D, De Souza R et al 1994 The stapedial reflex in cephalic tetanus. Journal of Laryngology and Otology 108:736
Devor M 1994 The pathophysiology of damaged peripheral nerve. In: Wall P, Melzack R (eds) Textbook of pain. Churchill Livingstone, Edinburgh, p 79
Devor M 1996 Pain mechanisms and pain syndromes. In: Campell J (ed.) Pain: an update review. IASP Press, Seattle
Devor M, Govrin-Lippmann R, Angelides K 1993 Na^+ channel immunolocalization in peripheral mammalian axons and changes following nerve injury and neuroma formation. Journal of Neuroscience 13:1976
Devor M, Govrin-Lippmann R, Rappaport Z H, Tasker R R, Dostrovsky J O 2002 Cranial root injury in glossopharyngeal neuralgia: electron microscopic observations. Case report. Journal of Neurosurgery 96(3):603–606
Devriese P 1986 Facialisverlammingen, Nederlandse Vereniging van K.N.O.-heelkunde en Heelkunde van het Hoofd- en Halsgebied. Mdbl. Revalid 15–18
Devriese P, Bronk J 1977 Revalidatie van de mimiek. Maandblad voor Revalidatie 8(4):34–47
Dibbets J, Carlson D S 1995 Implications of temporomandibular disorders for facial growth and orthodontic treatment. Seminars in Orthodontics 1(4):258–272
Dietz J 1981 Rehabilitation oncology. Wiley, New York
Dolan E, Mullen J, Papayoanou J 1984 Styloid–stylohyoid syndrome in the differential diagnosis of atypical facial pain. Surgical Neurology 21:291
Dolowitz D, Ward J, Fingerle C, Smith C 1964 The role of muscular incoordination in the pathogenesis of the temporomandibular joint syndrome. Laryngoscope 74:790
Donzelli R, Maiuri F, Peca C et al 2005 Microsurgical repair of the facial nerve. Zentralblatt für Neurochirurgie 66(2):63–69
Douglas F 1993 The dizzy patient: strategic approach to history, examination, diagnosis, and treatment. Chiropractic Techniques 5:171–186
Doursonian L, Alfonso J, Iba-Zizen M et al 1989 Dynamics of the junction between the medulla and the cervical spinal cord: an in vivo study in the sagittal plane by magnetic resonance imaging. Surgical and Radiological Anatomy 11:313
Downie P 1978 Cancer rehabilitation. Faber & Faber, London, p 98
Duke-Elder S, McFaul P 1972 Injuries in travel and sport. In: Duke-Elder S (ed.) System of ophthalmology. Henry Kimpton, London, 28:716
Dunn M, Seljeskog E 1986 Experience in the management of odontoid process injuries: an analysis of 128 cases. Neurosurgery 18:306
Eagle W 1948 Elongated styloid processes: further observations and a new syndrome. Archives of Otolaryngology 47:630
Eisele D, Schwartz A, Hari A et al 1995 The effects of selective nerve stimulation on upper airway airflow mechanics. Archives of Otolaryngology, Head and Neck Surgery 121:1361
Eisen A, Danon J 1974 The orbicularis oculi reflex in acoustic neuromas: a clinical and electrodiagnostic evaluation. Neurology 24:306–311
El Mansouri Y, Zaghloul K, Amraoui A 2000 Oculomotor paralyses in the course of diabetes: concerning 12 cases. Journal Français d'Ophtalmologie 23(1):14–18
Ellies L G 1992 Altered sensation following mandibular implant surgery: a retrospective study. Journal of Prosthetic Dentostry 68:664–671
Ellis F, Stein L, Guyton D 1998 Masked bilateral superior oblique muscle paresis: a simple overcorrection phenomenon? Ophthalmology 105:544
Elvey R 1986 Treatment of arm pain associated with abnormal branchial plexus tension. Australian Journal of Physiotherapy 32:225
Emanuilov A I, Shilkin V V, Nozdrachev A D, Masliukov P M 2005 Afferent innervation of the trachea during postnatal development. Autonomic Neuroscience 31:232
Engle E C, Goumernov B, McKeown C A et al 1997 Oculomotor nerve and muscle abnormalities in congenital fibrosis of the extraocular muscles. Annals of Neurology 41:314

Enlow D H 1986 The human face. Harper and Row, New York
Ertekin C, Aydogdu I, Secil Y et al 2002 Oropharyngeal swallowing in craniocervical dystonia. Journal of Neurology, Neurosurgery and Psychiatry 73(4):406–411
Evarts C 1970 Traumatic atlanto-occipital dislocation. Joint Surgery 52a:1653
Ewing M, Martin H 1952 Disability following radical neck dissection. Cancer 5:873
Fahn S 1988 Blepharospasm: a form of focal dystonia. Advances in Neurology 50:1
Feinmann C 1990 The medical management of facial pain. Annals of the Academy of Medicine, Singapore 15:409
Fetter M, Dichgans J 1996 Vestibular neuritis spares the inferior division of the vestibular nerve. Brain 119:755
Fields H 1990 Pain syndromes in neurology. Butterworth-Heinemann, Oxford
Fink L, Early C, Bryan R 1978 Glossopharyngeal schwannomas. Surgical Neurology 9:239
Fischer A, Verhagen W, Huygen P 1997 Whiplash injury. A clinical review with emphasis on neuro-otological aspects. Clinical Otolaryngology 22:192
Fischer G, Constantini J, Mercier P 1980 Improvement of hearing after microsurgical removal of acoustic neurinoma. Neurosurgery 7:154–159
Fischer G, Fischer C, Rémond J 1992 Hearing preservation in acoustic neurinoma surgery. Journal of Neurosurgery 76:910
Fite J 1970 Neuro-ophthalmologic syndromes in automobile accidents. Southern Medical Journal 63:57
Flickinger J, Lunsford L, Kondziolka D 1992 Dose prescription and dose-volume effects in radiosurgery. Neurosurgical Clinics of North America 3:51
Forssell C, Kitzing P, Bergqvist D 1995 Cranial nerve injuries after carotid artery surgery. A prospective study of 663 operations. European Journal of Vascular and Endovascular Surgery 10:445
Fowler T, May R 1985 Neurology. PSG Publishing, Littleton, MA
Franz B, Altidis P, Altidis B, Collis-Brown G 1999 The cervogenic oto-ocular syndrome: a suspected forerunner of Ménière's disease. International Tinnitus Journal 5:125
Freedman S, Rojas M, Toth C 2002 Strabismus surgery for large-angle cyclotorsion after macular translocation surgery. Journal of AAPOS 6:154
Frumker S, Kyle M 1987 Tinnitus as a symptom of temporomandibular joint dysfunction. Seminars in Hearing 8:21
Fukui S, Ohseto K, Shiotani M et al 1996 Referred pain distribution of the cervical zygapophyseal joints and cervical dorsal rami. Pain 68:79
Fukuyama E, Fujita Y, Soma K 2000 Changes in jaw-jerk on different levels of jaw closure and teeth-clenching in humans. Journal of Oral Rehabilitation 27:967
Fuller G, Guiloff R, Scaravilli F, Harcourt-Webster J 1989 Combined HIV–CMV encephalitis presenting with brainstem signs. Journal of Neurology, Neurosurgery and Psychiatry 52:975
Galetta S, Smith J 1989 Chronic isolated sixth nerve palsies. Archives of Neurology 46:79
Ganz F 1989 Ohrgeräusche; Tinnitus-Sprechstunde. Trias, Stuttgart
Garber N 1995 Evaluating diplopia with the Maddox rod, Risley's prism, and red glass. Journal of Ophthalmic Nursing and Technology 14:224
Gardiner K, Irvine B, Murray A 2002 Anomalous relationship of the spinal accessory nerve to the internal jugular vein. Clinical Anatomy 15:62
Gardner W, Miklos M 1959 Response of trigeminal neuralgia to 'decompression' of sensory root. Discussion of cause of trigeminal neuralgia. Journal of the American Medical Association 170:1773
Gastineau D 1989 Severe neuropathy associated with low-dose recombinant interferon alpha. American Journal of Medicine 87:1
Gelson S, Abd El-Bary T, Dujovny M et al 1994 Microsurgical anatomy of the trigeminal nerve. Neurology Research 16:273
Gerschman J, Burrows G, Reade P 1979 Chronic orofacial pain. In: Bonica J, Liebeskind J, Albe-Fessard D (eds) Advances in pain research and therapy. Raven Press, Philadelphia, p 317
Gimse R, Tjell C, Bjorgen I, Saunte C 1996 Disturbed eye movements after whiplash due to injuries to the posture control system. Journal of Clinical and Experimental Neuropsychology 18:178
Glasscock M, Kveton J, Jackson C 1986 A systematic approach to the surgical management of acoustic neuroma. Laryngoscope 96:1088
Gluckman J L, Myer C M, Aseff J N, Donegan J O 1983 Rehabilitation following radical neck dissection. Laryngoscope 93:1083–1085
Göbel H 1997 Die Kopfschmerzen. Ursachen, Mechanismen, Diagnostik und Therapie in der Praxis. Springer, Berlin
Göbel H, Klostermann H, Lindner V 1990 Changes in cerebral haemodynamics in cases of post-lumbar puncture headache. A prospective transcranial Doppler ultrasound study. Cephalalgia 10:117–122
Goebel G 1997 Retraining – Therapie bei Tinnitus. Paradigmawechsel oder alter Wein in neuen Schläuchen. HNO 9:664
Goodfriend D 1947 Deafness, tinnitus, vertigo and neuralgia. Archives of Otolaryngology 46:1
Gorge H 2001 Operative treatment of trigeminal neuralgia. Schmerz 15(1):48–58

Gorman R 1995a Treatment of presumptive optic nerve ischemia by spinal manipulation. Journal of Manipulative and Physiological Therapeutics 18:172
Gorman R 1995b Monocular visual loss after closed head trauma: immediate resolution associated with spinal manipulation. Journal of Manipulative and Physiological Therapeutics 18:308
Gorman R 1996 Monocular scotomata and spinal manipulation: the step phenomenon. Journal of Manipulative and Physiological Therapeutics 19:344
Gossman J, Tarsitano J 1977 The styloid–stylohyoid syndrome. Journal of Oral Surgery 35:555
Grant R 1988 Physical therapy of the cervical and thoracic spine. Churchill Livingstone, Edinburgh
Grant R 1996 Vertebral artery testing – the Australian Physiotherapy Association Protocol after 6 years. Manual Therapy 1(3):149–153
Grimaldi L, Luzi L, Martino G et al 1993 Bilateral eighth cranial nerve neuropathy in human immunodeficiency virus infection. Journal of Neurology 240:363–366
Gunter K, Noorden von M 1990 Binocular vision and ocular motility. Mosby, St Louis
Guntinas-Lichius O, Streppel M, Stennert E 2006 Postoperative functional evaluation of different reanimation techniques for facial nerve repair. American Journal of Surgery 191(1):61–67
Gupta V, Kumar S, Singh A K, Tatke M 2002 Glossopharyngeal schwannoma: a case report and review of literature. Neurology India 50(2):190–193
Gutmann G 1983a Injuries to the vertebral artery caused by manual therapy. Manuelle Medizin 21:2
Gutmann G 1983b Die funktionanalytische Röntgendiagnostik der Halswirbelsäule. In: Gutmann G, Biedermann H (eds) Funktionelle Pathologie und Klinik der Wirbelsäule. Fischer Verlag, Stuttgart, p 68–72
Gwiazda J, Grice K, Thorn F 1999 Response AC/A ratios are elevated in myopic children. Ophthalmic and Physiological Optics 19:173
Haas M 1991 Statistical methodology for reliability studies. Journal of Manipulative and Physiological Therapeutics 141:19
Hadjikoutis S, Jayawant S, Stoodley N 2002 Isolated hypoglossal nerve palsy in a 14-year-old girl. European Journal of Paediatric Neurology 6(4):225–228
Hadley M, Browner C, Sonntag V 1985 Axis fractures: a comprehensive review of management and treatment in 107 cases. Neurosurgery 17:281
Halmagyi G M 2005 Diagnosis and management of vertigo. Clinical Medicine 5(2):159–165
Halmagyi G M, Yavor R, Colebatch J 1995 Tapping the head activates the vestibular system: a new use for the clinical reflex hammer. Neurology 45:1927
Halmagyi G M, McGarvie L A, Aw S T, Yavor R A, Todd M J 2003 The click-evoked vestibulo-ocular reflex in superior semicircular canal dehiscence. Neurology 60(7):1172–1175
Hamlyn P, King T 1992 Neurovascular compression in trigeminal neuralgia: a clinical and anatomical study. Journal of Neurosurgery 76:948
Hammer A 1991 Lower cranial nerve palsies. Potentially lethal in upper cervical fracture dislocations. Clinical Orthopaedics 266:64
Hammerschlag P, Brundy J, Cusamano R, Cohen N 1987 Hypoglossal–facial nerve anastomosis and electromyographic feedback rehabilitation. Laryngoscope 97:705
Hanson M 1989 The dizzy patient: a practical approach to the dizzy patient. Postgraduate Medicine 18:99
Hardell L, Hansson Mild K, Sandstrom M, Carlberg M, Hallquist A, Pahlson A 2003 Vestibular schwannoma, tinnitus and cellular telephones. Neuroepidemiology 22(2):124–129
Harner S, Daube J, Ebersold M 1986 Electrophysiologic monitoring of facial nerve during temporal bone surgery. Laryngoscope 96:65
Harner S, Daube J, Ebersold M, Beatty C 1987 Improved preservation of facial nerve function with use of electrical monitoring during removal of acoustic neuromas. Mayo Clinic Proceedings 62:92–102
Harris M 1996 Idiopathic orofascial pain. In: Campell J (ed.) Pain: an update review. IASP Press, Seattle, p 403
Hassler W, Zentner J, Peterson D 1989 Cavernous angioma of the optic nerve. Surgical Neurology 31:444
Hazell J 2001 The mechanisms of hyperacusis, misophonia, phonophobia and recruitment. Online. Available: www.tinnitus.org
Hazell J 2002 Tinnitus retraining therapy from the Jastreboff model. Online. Available: www.tinnitus.org
Hazell J W, Jastreboff P J, Meerton L E, Conway M J 1993 Electrical tinnitus suppression: frequency dependence of effects. Audiology 32(1):68–77
Heinze J 1969 Cranial nerve avulsion and other neural injuries in road accidents. Medical Journal of Australia 2:1246
Herring D, King A, Connelly M 1987 New rehabilitation concepts in management of radical neck dissection syndrome. Physical Therapy 67:1095–1099
Hida W, Kurosawa H, Okabe S et al 1995 Hypoglossal nerve stimulation affects the pressure-volume behavior of the upper airway. American Journal

of Respiratory and Critical Care Medicine 151:455
Hoaglund F, Duthie R 1966 Surgical reconstruction for shoulder pain after radical neck dissection. American Journal of Surgery 112(4):522–526
Holland B, Parett L, Mills C 1986 Meningovascular syphilis: CT and MR findings. Radiology 158:439
Holmes J M, Beck R W, Kip K E, Droste P J, Leske D A 2001 Pediatric Eye Disease Investigator Group. Predictors of nonrecovery in acute traumatic sixth nerve palsy and paresis. Ophthalmology 108(8):1457–1460
Hooshman H, Escobar M, Kopf S 1972 Neurosyphilis: a study of 241 patients. Journal of the American Medical Association 219:726
Horn K, House W, Hitselberger W 1985 Schwannomas of the jugular foramen. Laryngoscope 95:761
Howarth P, Heron G 2000 Repeated measures of horizontal heterophoria. Optometry and Visual Science 77:616
Howe J, Loeser J, Calvin W 1977 Mechanosensitivity of dorsal root ganglia and chronically injured axons: a physiological basis for the radicular pain of nerve root compression. Pain 3:25
Hoya K, Kirino T 2000 Traumatic trochlear nerve palsy following minor occipital impact – four case reports. Neurologia Medico-chirurgica 40(7):358–360
Hromada J 1963 On the nerve supply of the connective tissue of some peripheral nervous system components. Acta Anatomica 55:343
Hu J, Dostrovsky J O, Sessle B 1981 Functional properties of neurons in cat trigeminal subnucleus caudalis (medullary dorsal horn). I. Responses to oral-facial noxious and nonnoxious stimuli and projections to thalamus and subnucleus oralis. Journal of Neurophysiology 45(2):173–192
Huffmann G 1979 Zur Prognose und Therapie peripherer Fazialislähmungen. Fortschritte der Medizin 97:380
Hulse M 1994 Cervical hearing loss. HNO 42:604
Hunt W, Meagher J, LeFever H, Zeman W 1959 Painful ophthalmoplegia. Its relation to indolent inflammation of the cavernous sinus. Neurology 6:56
Hyman L, Gwiazda J, Marsh-Tootle W et al 2001 The Correction of Myopia Evaluation Trial (COMET): design and general baseline characteristics. Controlled Clinical Trials 22:573
Iriarte Ortabe J, Thauvoy C, Reychler H 1993 Orbito-fronto-temporal approach to tumors of the base of the skull. Our experience in the creation of an orbito-zygomato-malar flap. Annales de Chirurgie Plastique et Esthétique 38:525
Isberg A M, Isaacson G, Williams W N, Lougner B A 1987 Lingual numbness and speech articulation deviation associated with temporalis disk displacement. Oral Surgery, Oral Medicine and Oral Pathology 1:11–19
Ito J, Naito Y, Honjo I 1990 The influence of middle ear pressure on the vestibular nerve activity in cats. Acta Otolaryngology 110:203
Iwakuma T, Matsumoto A, Nakamura N 1982 Hemifacial spasm. Comparison of three different operative procedures in 110 patients. Journal of Neurosurgery 57:753
Jacobson G P, Pearlstein R, Henderson J, Calder J H, Rock J 1998 Recovery nystagmus revisited. Journal of the American Academy of Audiology 9(4):263–271
Jankovic J, Leder S, Warner D, Schwartz K 1991 Cervical dystonia: clinical findings and associated movement disorders. Neurology 41:1088
Jannetta P 1970 Microsurgical exploration and decompression of the facial nerve in hemifacial spasm. Current Topics in Surgical Research 2:217
Jannetta P 1976 Treatment of trigeminal neuralgia by suboccipital and transtentorial cranial operation. Clinical Neurosurgery 24:538–549
Jannetta P 1977 Observations on the etiology of trigeminal neuralgia, hemifacial spasm, acoustic nerve dysfunction and glossopharyngeal neuralgia. Definitive microsurgical treatment and results in 117 patients. Neurochirurgia 20:145
Jannetta P 1980a Hemifacial spasm. In: Ransohoff J (ed.) Modern techniques in surgery. Neurosurgery, instalment II. Futura Publishing, New York, 15:1–15
Jannetta P 1980b Neurovascular compression in cranial nerve and systematic disease. Annals of Surgery 192:518
Jannetta P 1981 Cranial nerve vascular compression syndromes (other than tic douloureux and hemifacial spasm). Clinical Neurosurgery 28:445–456
Jannetta P 1990 Microvascular decompression of the trigeminal nerve root entry zone. In: Rovit R, Murali R, Jannetta P (eds) Trigeminal neuralgia. Williams and Wilkins, Philadelphia, p 201
Jannetta P, Bissonette D J 1985 Management of failed patients with trigeminal neuralgia. Clinical Neurosurgery 32:324
Jannetta P J, Moller M B, Moller A R 1984 Disabling positional vertigo. New England Journal of Medicine 310(26):1700–1705
Jannsen H 2000 Sensibilitätsstörungen und Implantation im Unterkiefer. Eine retrospective Studie. Dissertation. Universität Regensburg, Germany
Jastreboff P 1990 Phantom auditory perception (tinnitus): mechanisms of generation and perception. Neuroscience Research 8(4):221–254
Jastreboff P J, Hazell J W (eds) 2004 The neurophysiological model of tinnitus and decreased sound tolerance. In: Tinnitus retraining

therapy. Implementing the neurophysiological model. Cambridge University Press, Cambridge, p 16–60
Jastreboff P J, Hazell J W, Graham R L 1994 Neurophysiological model of tinnitus: dependence of the minimal masking level on treatment outcome. Hearing Research 80(2):216–232
Jiang R S, Hsu C Y, Shen B H 2001 Endoscopic optic nerve decompression for the treatment of traumatic optic neuropathy. Rhinology 39(2):71–74
Johnson E, Aseff J, Saunders W 1978 Physical treatment of pain and weakness following radical neck dissection. Ohio State Medical Journal 74:711
Jones M, Edards I, Gifford L 2002 Conceptual models for implementing biopsychosocial theory in clinical practice. Manual Therapy 7:2–9
Kaltenbach J A, Zacharek M A, Zhang J, Frederick S 2004 Activity in the dorsal cochlear nucleus of hamsters previously tested for tinnitus following intense tone exposure. Neuroscience Letters 355(1–2):121–125
Kapoor R, Kendall B, Harrison M 1991 Permanent oculomotor palsy with occlusion of the internal carotid artery. Journal of Neurology, Neurosurgery and Psychiatry 54:745
Karlan M, Beroza L, Cassisi N 1979 Anterior cervical pain syndromes. Otolaryngology, Head and Neck Surgery 87:284
Kavounoudias A, Gilhodes J, Roll R, Roll J 1999 From balance regulation to body orientation: two goals for muscle proprioceptive information processing. Experimental Brain Research 124:80
Kaye A, Hahn J, Kinney S et al 1984 Jugular foramen schwannomas. Journal of Neurosurgery 60:1045
Keane J 1986 Trochlear nerve pareses with brainstem lesions. Journal of Clinical Neurology and Ophthalmology 6:242
Keane J 1996 Twelfth-nerve palsy. Analysis of 100 cases. Archives of Neurology 53:561
Keane J R, Ahmadi J 1998 Most diabetic third nerve palsies are peripheral. Neurology 51(5):1510
Keane J, Baloh R 1992 Posttraumatic cranial neuropathies. Neurologic Clinics 10:849
Keller M, Hiltbrunner B, Dill C, Kesselring J 2000 Reversible neuropsychological deficits after mild traumatic brain injury. Journal of Neurology, Neurosurgery and Psychiatry 68(6):761–764
Kendall H, Kendall F, Wadsworth G 1971 Muscles. Testing and function. Williams and Wilkins, Boston
Keneally M 1985 The upper limb tension test. Proceedings of the 4th Biennial Conference of the Manipulative Association of Australia, Brisbane
Kerber C, Mangolis M, Newton T 1972 Tortuous vertebrobasilar system: a cause for cranial nerve signs. Neuroradiology 4:74–77
Kern R C, Quinn B, Rosseau G, Farbman A I 2000 Post-traumatic olfactory dysfunction. Laryngoscope 110(12):2106–2109
Kerr F, Lysak W 1964 Somatotopic organization of trigeminal neurons. Archives of Neurology 11:593
Kessinger R, Boneva D 2000 Vertigo, tinnitus, and hearing loss in geriatric patients. Journal of Manipulative and Physiological Therapeutics 23:352
Kido T, Sekitani T, Okinaka Y et al 1994 A case of cerebellar infarction occurring with 8th cranial nerve symptoms. Auris, Nasus, Larynx 21:111–117
Kieser J, Kieser D, Hauman T 2005 The course and distribution of the inferior alveolar nerve in the edentulous mandible. Journal of Craniofacial Surgery 16(1):6–9
Kim C S, Chang S O, Oh S H, Ahn S H, Hwang C H, Lee H J 2003 Management of intratemporal facial nerve schwannoma. Otology and Neurotology 24(2):312–316
King C, Street M 1994 Twelfth cranial nerve paralysis following use of a laryngeal mask airway. Anaesthesia 49:786
Kiratli H, Bilgic S, Caglar M, Soylemezoglu F 2003 Intramuscular hemangiomas of extraocular muscles. Ophthalmology 110(3):564–568
Kitteringham C 1996 The effect of straight leg raise exercises after lumbar decompression surgery. A pilot study. Physiotherapy 82:115–123
Kobayashi S, Otsuka A, Tsunoda T, Inoue H 1996 Intracranial hypoglossal neurinoma without preoperative hypoglossal nerve paresis. Case report. Neurologia Medico-chirurgica 36:384
Kommerell G, Kromeier M 2002 Prism correction in heterophoria. Ophthalmologe 99:3
Koos W, Spetzler R, Lang J 1993 Color atlas of microneurosurgery. Thieme, Stuttgart
Kopp S 1979 Short term evaluation of counselling and occlusal adjustments in patients with mandibular dysfunction involving the temporomandibular joint. Journal of Oral Rehabilitation 6:101
Kromier M, Schmitt C, Bach M, Kommerell G 2002 Comparison between dissociated and associated heterophoria. Ophthalmologe 99:549–554
Krueger B R, Okazaki H 1980 Vertebral–basilar distribution infarction following chiropractic cervical manipulation. Mayo Clin Proceedings 55(5):322–332
Kruschinski C, Weber B P, Pabst R 2003 Clinical relevance of the distance between the cochlea and the facial nerve in cochlear implantation. Otology and Neurotology 24(5):823–827
Kruse JJ, Awasthi D 1998 Skull-base trauma: neurosurgical perspective. Journal of Craniomaxillofacial Trauma 4(2):8–14
Kushen M, Gulbahce H E, Lam C H 2005 Ewing's sarcoma of the cavernous sinus: case report. Neurosurgery 56(6):E1375; discussion E1375
Kvale A, Ljunggren A E, Johnsen T B 2003 Examination of movement in patients with long-

lasting musculoskeletal pain: reliability and validity. Physiotherapy Research International 8(1):36–52

Kwan M, Wall E, Massie J, Garfin S 1992 Strain, stress and stretch of peripheral nerve. Acta Orthopaedica Scandinavica 63:267

Lachman N, Acland R D, Rosse C 2002 Anatomical evidence for the absence of a morphologically distinct cranial root of the accessory nerve in man. Clinical Anatomy 15(1):4–10

Laine F J, Underhill T 2002 Imaging of the lower cranial nerves. Magnetic Resonance Imaging Clinics of North America 10(3):433–449

Lam D, Lawrence H, Tenenbaum H 2001 Aural symptoms in temporomandibular disorder patients attending a craniofacial pain unit. Journal of Orofacial Pain 15:146

Lang G K 2000 Ocular trauma in ophthalmology. Thieme, Stuttgart, p 497–525

Lang J 1983 Clinical anatomy of the head: neurocranium, orbit, craniocervical regions. Springer, Berlin

Lang J 1995 Skull base and related structures: atlas of clinical anatomy. Schattauer, Stuttgart

Lang J, Kessler B 1991 About the suboccipital part of the vertebral artery and the neighbouring bone–joint and nerve relationship. Skull Base Surgery 1:64

Langford-Wilson A 1982 New view of tunnel vision. The Star, Mt Isa, Queensland

Langman A, Jackler R, Althaus S 1990 Meningioma of the internal auditory canal. American Journal of Otology 11:201–204

Leblanc A 1995 The cranial nerves. Springer, Berlin

Leduc A, Decloedt V 1989 La kinésithérapie an O.R.L. Acta-Otorhinolaryngologica 43:381

Leipzig G, Suen J Y, English J L, Barnes J, Hooper M 1983 Functional evaluation of the spinal accessory nerve after neck dissection. American Journal of Surgery 146:526–530

Leonetti J P, Wachter B, Marzo S J, Petruzzelli G 2001 Extracranial lower cranial nerve sheath tumors. Otolaryngology Head and Neck Surgery 125(6):640–644

LePage E 1993 A model for cochlear origin of subjective tinnitus: excitatory drift in operating point of inner hair cells. In: Tinnitus mechanisms. W B Saunders, London, p 1

Levine H L 1991 Otorhinolaryngologic causes of headache. Medical Clinics of North America 75(3):677–692

Levine R A 1999 Somatic (craniocervical) tinnitus and the dorsal cochlear nucleus hypothesis. American Journal of Otolaryngology 20(6):351–362

Levine R A, Abel M, Cheng H 2003 CNS somatosensory–auditory interactions elicit or modulate tinnitus. Experimental Brain Research 153(4):643–648

Liebenstund I 1989 Die Fazialislähmungen und ihre krankengymnastische Behandlung. Krankengymnastik 3:226

Linnet J, Madsen F 1995 Hypoglosso-facial nerve anastomosis. Acta Neurochirurgica 133:112

Linskey M, Sekhar L 1993 Cavernous sinus hemangiomas: a series, a review, and an hypothesis. Neurosurgery 30:101

Loeser J 1984 Tic douloureux and atypical face pain. In: Wall P, Melzack R (eds). Textbook of pain, 3rd edn. Churchill Livingstone, Edinburgh, p 699–711

Loewenfeld I 1993 The pupil. Iowa State University Press, Amers

Mackinnon S, Dellon A 1988 Surgery of the peripheral nerve. Thieme, Stuttgart

Mafee M, Kumar A, Valvassori G et al 1984 CT in the evaluation of the vestibulocochlear nerves and their central pathways. Evaluation of neurotologic disorders. Radiologic Clinics of North America 22:45

Maigne R 1972 Orthopaedic medicine: a new approach to vertebral manipulation. C C Thomas, Springfield, IL

Maitland C, Abiko S, Hoyt W et al 1982 Chiasmal apoplexy. Journal of Neurosurgery 56:118

Maitland G 1986 Vertebral manipulation, 5th edn. Butterworth-Heinemann, Oxford

Maitland G, Hengeveld E, Banks K, English K 2001 Maitland's vertebral manipulation, 6th edn. Butterworth-Heinemann, Oxford

Malkin D 1987 The role of TMJ dysfunction in the etiology of middle ear disease. International Journal of Orthodontics 25:20

Manni A, Brunori P, Giulanie M et al 1996 Oto-vestibular symptoms in patients with temporomandibular joint dysfunction. Electromyographic study. Minerva Stomatologica 45:1

Manz H, Klein L, Fermaglich J et al 1979 Cavernous hemangioma of optic chiasm optic nerve and right optic tract. Virchow's Archives 383:225

Marchiando A, Per-Lee J, Jackson R 1983 Tinnitus due to idiopathic stapedial muscle spasm. Ear, Nose and Throat Journal 62:8

Matharu M S, Goadsby P J 2003 Persistence of attacks of cluster headache after trigeminal nerve root section. Headache 43(4):428–429

Matsuka Y, Fort E, Merrill R 2000 Trigeminal neuralgia due to an acoustic neuroma in the cerebellopontine angle. Orofacial Pain 14:147

Mauskop A 2005 Vagus nerve stimulation relieves chronic refractory migraine and cluster headaches. Cephalalgia 25(2):82–86

Maxwell R 1990 Clinical diagnosis of trigeminal neuralgia and differential diagnosis of facial pain. In: Rovit R, Murali R, Jannetta P (eds) Trigeminal neuralgia. William and Wilkins, Philadelphia, p 53

McAvoy C E, Kamalarajab S, Best R, Rankin S, Bryars J, Nelson K 2002 Bilateral third and unilateral sixth nerve palsies as early presenting signs of metastatic prostatic carcinoma. Eye 16(6):749–753

McClearly A 1993 A fracture of the odontoid process complicated by tenth and twelfth cranial nerve palsies. Spine 18:932

Meaney J, Miles J, Nixon T et al 1993 Trigeminal neuralgia: preoperative demonstration of neurovascular compression with MR angiography. Radiology 189:142

Meansy J, Miles J, Mackenzie I 1994 Imaging of neurovascular compression in tinnitus. Lancet 344:200

Mein J, Harcourt B 1986 Diagnosis and management of ocular motility disorder. Blackwell Scientific, Oxford

Merskey H, Bogduk N 1994 Classification of chronic pain: descriptions of chronic pain syndromes and definitions of pain terms. IASP Press, Seattle

Miehlke A, Stennert E, Chilla R 1979 New aspects in facial nerve surgery. Clinics in Plastic Surgery 16(3):451

Miller H 1967 Facial paralysis. British Medical Journal 3:815

Misoh C, Crawford E 1990 Predictable mandibular nerve location. A clinical zone of safety. Today 9:32

Miura J, Doita M, Miyata K et al 2003 Horner's syndrome caused by a thoracic dumbbell-shaped schwannoma: sympathetic chain reconstruction after a one-stage removal of the tumor. Spine 28(2):E33–36

Mock D, Frydman W, Gordon A 1985 Atypical facial pain: a retrospective study. Oral Surgery 59:472

Mokri B 1982 Ræder's paratrigeminal syndrome. Original concept and subsequent deviations. Archives of Neurology 39:395

Møller A 1988 Evoked potentials in intraoperative monitoring. Williams and Wilkins, Philadelphia

Møller A, Jannetta P 1985 Hemifacial spasm: results of eletrophysiologic recording during microvascular decompression operations. Neurology (Cleveland) 35:969

Møller A, Jannetta P 1986 Physiological abnormalities in hemifacial spasm studied during microvascular decompression operations. Experimental Neurology 93:584

Møller A, Jannetta P 1987 Monitoring facial EMG responses during microvascular decompression operations for hemifacial spasm. Journal of Neurosurgery 66:681

Morley T 1985 Case against microvascular decompression in the treatment of trigeminal neuralgia. Archives of Neurology 42:801

Mortellaro C, Biancucci P, Picciolo G, Vercellino V 2002 Eagle's syndrome: importance of a corrected diagnosis and adequate surgical treatment. Journal of Craniofacial Surgery 13(6):755–758

Mountjoy J, Dolan K, McCabe B 1974 Neurilemmoma of the ninth cranial nerve masquerading as an acoustic neuroma. Archives of Otolaryngology 100:65

Mumenthaler M, Schliack H 1991 Peripheral nerve lesions, diagnosis and therapy. Thieme, Stuttgart

Mündnich K, Nessel E 1973 Die Beurteilung der idiopathischen und posttraumatischen Facialislähmung in der HNO-Praxis: Objektive Grundlagen für die Operationsindikation. HNO 21:12

Muthukumar N 2002 Delayed hypoglossal palsy following occipital condyle fracture – case report. Journal of Clinical Neuroscience 9(5):580–582

Nager G 1985 Acoustic neurinomas. Acta Otolaryngologica 99:245–261

Nagy E, Pontracz E 1997 Complex therapy of neck-related tinnitus, hyperacusis and vertigo. International Tinnitus Journal 3:141

Nahum A, Mullally W, Marmor L 1961 A syndrome resulting from radical neck dissection. Archives of Otolaryngology 74:424

Naidich T, Kricheff I, George A et al 1976 The normal anterior inferior cerebellar artery. Anatomic–radiographic correlation with emphasis on the lateral projection. Radiology 119:355–373

Nakayama M, Inafuku S, Hori M et al 1989 Anterior inferior cerebellar artery syndrome and 'internal auditory artery syndrome [in Japanese]. Practical Otology (Kyoto) 83:1693–1700

Naunton R, Proctor L, Elpern B 1968 The audiologic signs of ninth nerve neurinoma. Archives of Otolaryngology 87:222

Neff B, Willcox T Jr, Sataloff R 2003 Intralabyrinthine schwannomas. Otology and Neurotology 24:299

Nelson K, Phillips L 1990 Neurophysiology monitoring during surgery of peripheral and cranial nerves, and in selective dorsal rhizotomy. Seminars in Neurology 10:141

Netterville J L, Fortune S, Stanziale S, Billante C R 2002 Palatal adhesion: the treatment of unilateral palatal paralysis after high vagus nerve injury. Head and Neck 24(8):721–730

Nguyen M, Maciewitz R, Bouchons A, Poletti B J 1986 Facial pain symptoms in patients with cerebellopontine angle tumors. A report of 44 cases of cerebellopontine angle meningioma and a review of the literature. Clinical Journal of Pain 2:3

Nisch G 1973 Ergebnisse bei fazialis-hypoglossus-anastomosen. Psychiatrie, Neurologie, und Medizinische Psychologie 25:488

Nook B 1985 Upper extremity dyskinesis: a case report. Journal of Manipulative and Physiological Therapeutics 8:181

Normand M, Daube J 1994 Cranial nerve conduction and needle electromyography in patients with acoustic neuromas: a model of compression neuropathy. Muscle and Nerve 17:1401–1406
Nukada H, Dick P 1984 Microsphere embolization of nerve capillaries and fiber degeneration. American Journal of Pathology 115:275–287
O'Connel J 1946 The clinical signs of meningeal irritation. Brain 9:69
Oge A E, Yayla V, Demir G A, Eraksoy M 2005 Excitability of facial nucleus and related brain-stem reflexes in hemifacial spasm, post-facial palsy synkinesis and facial myokymia. Clinical Neurophysiology 116(7):1542–1554
Ogunrinde O, Lunsford L, Flickinger J, Kondziolks D 1994 Stereotactic radiosurgery for acoustic nerve tumors in patients with useful preoperative hearing: results at 2-year follow-up examination. Journal of Neurosurgery 80:1011
Okeson J P 1995 Bell's orofacial pains. Quintessence, Chicago
Olesen J 1988 Headache Classification Committee of the International Headache Society: classification and diagnostic criteria for headache disorders, cranial neuralgia and facial pain. Cephalalgia 8:7
Oostendorp R 1988 Vertebrobasilar insufficiency. In: Proceedings of the International Federation of Orthopaedic Manipulative Therapists Congress, Cambridge, p 42
Oosterveld W J, van der Laarse W D 1969 Effect of gravity on vestibular nystagmus. Aerospace Medicine 40(4):382–385
Optic Neuritis Study Group 1991 The clinical profile of optic neuritis. Archives of Ophthalmology 109:1673
Ozenci M, Karaoguz R, Conkbayir C, Altin T, Kanpolat Y 2003 Glossopharyngeal neuralgia with cardiac syncope treated by glossopharyngeal rhizotomy and microvascular decompression. Europace 5(2):149–152
Pacifici L, Passarelli F, Papa G et al 1992 Active third cranial nerve ophthalmoplegia: possible pathogenesis from alpha interferon treatment. Italian Journal of Neurological Science 14:579
Paley M, Wood G 1995 Traumatic bilateral hypoglossal nerve palsy. British Journal of Oral and Maxillofacial Surgery 33:239
Palla S 1998 Myoarthropathien des Kausystems und orofaziale Schmerzen. Fotoplast, Zürich
Pareja J A, Baron M, Gili P et al 2002 Objective assessment of autonomic signs during triggered first division trigeminal neuralgia. Cephalalgia 22(4):251–255
Parker W, Chole R 1995 Tinnitus, vertigo and temporomandibular disorders. American Journal of Orthodontics and Dentofacial Orthopedics 107:153
Patten J 1995 Neurological differential diagnosis, 2nd edn. Springer, Berlin
Peeters G G, Verhagen A P, de Bie R A, Oostendorp R A 2001 The efficacy of conservative treatment in patients with whiplash injury: a systematic review of clinical trials. Spine 26(4):E64–73
Peitersen E, Andersen P 1966 Spontaneous course of 220 peripheral non-traumatic facial palsies. Acta Otolaryngologica Suppl 224:296
Penning L 1968 Functional pathology of the cervical spine. Excerpta Medica, Amsterdam
Pertes R, Gross S 1996 Clinical management of temporomandibular disorders and orofacial pain. Quintessence, Chicago
Peschen-Rosin R 2002 Chronic facial pain from a psychiatric point of view – differential diagnosis and therapeutic strategies. Schmerz 16(5):395–403
Pinto O 1962 A new structure related to the temporomandibular joint and the middle ear. Journal of Prosthetic Dentistry 12:95
Procacciante F, Picozzi P, Pacifici M et al 2001 Palpatory method used to identify the recurrent laryngeal nerve during thyroidectomy. World Journal of Surgery 25(2):252–253
Puca A, Meglio M, Vari R et al 1995 Evaluation of fifth nerve dysfunction in 136 patients with middle and posterior cranial fossa tumors. European Neurology 35:33
Purvin V, Kawasaki A, Jacobson D M 2001 Optic perineuritis: clinical and radiographic features. Archives of Ophthalmology 119(9):1299–1306
Quester R, Menzel J, Thumfart W 1993 Radical removal of a large glossopharyngeal neurinoma with preservation of cranial nerve function. Ear Nose and Throat Journal 72:600
Quinones-Hinojosa A, Chang E F, Khan S A, McDermott M W 2003 Isolated trigeminal nerve sarcoid granuloma mimicking trigeminal schwannoma: case report. Neurosurgery 52(3):700–705
Radanov B P, Bicik I, Dvorak J et al 1999 Relation between neuropsychological and neuroimaging findings in patients with late whiplash syndrome. Journal of Neurology, Neurosurgery and Psychiatry 66(4):485–489
Ramachandran V S, Blakesee S 1998 Phantoms in the brain. William Morrow, New York
Rappaport Z, Devor M 1994 Trigeminal neuralgia: the role of self sustaining discharge in the trigeminal ganglion. Pain 56:127
Reddy K, Hobson D E, Gomori A, Sutherland G R 1987 Painless glossopharyngeal 'neuralgia' with syncope: a case report and literature review. Neurosurgery 21(6):916–919
Remmler D, Byers R, Scheetz J et al 1986 A prospective study of shoulder disability resulting

from radical and modified neck dissection. Head and Neck Surgery 11:280–286
Remulla H, Bilyk J, Rubin P 1995 Pseudo-entrapment of extraocular muscles in patients with orbital fractures. Journal of Craniomaxillofacial Trauma 1(4):16–29
Renzi G, Mastellone P, Leonardi A, Becelli R, Bonamini M, Fini G 2005 Basicranium malformation with anterior dislocation of right styloid process causing stylalgia. Journal of Craniofacial Surgery 16(3):418–420
Roberts A, Person P, Clarksburg W, Brooklyn N 1979 Etiology and treatment of idiopathic trigeminal and atypical facial neuralgias. Oral Surgery 48:298
Robinson P P, Boissonade F M, Loescher A R et al 2004 Peripheral mechanisms for the initiation of pain following trigeminal nerve injury. Journal of Orofacial Pain 18(4):287–292
Robson S 2002 Tinnitus: a neurophysiological condition: can understanding it help us treat pain? PPA News 15
Rocabado M 1983 Biomechanical relationship of the cranial, cervical, and hyoid regions. Physical Therapy 1(3):62
Roll J, Vedel J, Roll R 1989 Eye, head and skeletal muscle spindle feedback in the elaboration of body references. Progress in Brain Research 80:113
Romanes G 1981 Cunningham's textbook of anatomy. Oxford University Press, London
Rowland L 1989 Merritt's textbook of neurology, 8th edn. Lea & Febiger, New York
Roy G 1994 The vertebral artery. Journal of Manual Manipulative Therapy 2:28
Rubenstein B 1993 Tinnitus and craniomandibular disorders – is there a link ? Swedish Dental Journal Suppl 95:1
Rush J, Young B 1981 Paralysis of cranial nerves III, IV and VI: causes and prognosis in 1000 cases. Archives of Ophthalmology 99:76
Saadat D, O'Leary D P, Pulec J L, Kitano H 1995 Comparison of vestibular autorotation and caloric testing. Otolaryngology Head and Neck Surgery 113(3):215–222
Sadiq Z, Monaghan A, Wake M J 2003 Modified retractor for use in sectioning the inferior alveolar nerve. British Journal of Oral and Maxillofacial Surgery 41(2):124
Sadler R M, Purdy R A, Rahey S 2002 Vagal nerve stimulation aborts migraine in patients with intractable epilepsy. Cephalalgia 22(6):482–484
Safran A, Vibert D, Issoua D, Häusler R 1994 Skew deviation after vestibular neuritis. American Journal of Ophthalmology 118:238
Sahrmann S 1998 Diagnosis and treatment of movement-related pain syndromes associated with muscle and movement imbalances. Course Workbook. Zarzach. Manuale Therapie. Maitland Course
Salame K, Ouaknine G E, Arensburg B, Rochkind S 2002 Microsurgical anatomy of the facial nerve trunk. Clinical Anatomy 15(2):93–99
Salerno G, Cavaliere M, Foglia A et al 2002 The 11th nerve syndrome in functional neck dissection. Laryngoscope 112:1299
Sanna M, Agarwal M, Jain Y, Russo A, Taibah A K 2003 Transapical extension in difficult cerebellopontine angle tumours: preliminary report. Journal of Laryngology and Otology 117(10):788–792
Saunders R, Krout R, Sachs E 1971 Masticator electromyography in trigeminal neuralgia. Neurology 21:1221
Saunders W, Johnson E 1975 Rehabilitation of the shoulder after radical neck dissection. Annals of Otology, Rhinology and Laryngology 84:812
Schievink W, Mohri B, Garrity J et al 1993 Ocular motor nerve palsies in spontaneous directions of the cervical internal carotid artery. Neurology 43:1938
Schlessel D, Rowed D, Nedzelski J, Feghali J 1993 Postoperative pain following excision of acoustic neuroma by the suboccipital approach: observations on possible cause and potential amelioration. American Journal of Otology 14:491
Schwaber M, Whetsell W 1992 Cochleovestibular nerve compression syndrome. II. Vestibular nerve histopathology and theory of pathophysiology. Laryngoscope 102:1030–1036
Schwartz-Arad D, Dolev E, Williams W 2004 Maxillary nerve block – a new approach using a computer-controlled anesthetic delivery system for maxillary sinus elevation procedure. A prospective study. Quintessence International 35(6):477–480
Sekiya T, Iwabuchi T, Hatayama T, Shinozaki N 1991 Vestibular nerve injury as a complication of microvascular decompression. Neurosurgery 29:773
Sens M, Higer H 1991 MRI of trigeminal neuralgia: initial clinical results in patients with vascular compression of the trigeminal nerve. Neurosurgical Review 14:69
Servodidio C, Abramson D, Romanella A 1991 Optic nerve meningioma. A case report. Journal of Ophthalmic Nursing and Technology 10:18
Sessle B 1993 Neural mechanisms implicated in the pathogenesis of trigeminal neuralgia and other neuropathic pain. American Pain Society Journal 2:17
Shankland W E 1995 Craniofacial pain syndromes that mimic temporomandibular joint disorders. Annals of the Academy of Medicine, Singapore 24:83

Shankland W E 2001a The trigeminal nerve. Part II: The ophthalmic division. Cranio 19(1):8–12

Shankland W E 2001b The trigeminal nerve. Part III: The maxillary division. Cranio 19(2):78–83

Shankland W E 2001c The trigeminal nerve. Part IV: the mandibular division. Cranio 19(3):153–161

Shapiro H, Truex R 1943 The temporomandibular joint and the auditory function. Journal of the American Dental Association 30:1147

Sharifi Milani R, Deville de Periere D, Micallef J 1998 Relationship between dental occlusion and visual focusing. Cranio 16:109

Shearer V, Jhaveri H, Cunningham F 1995 Puerperal seizures after post-dural puncture headache. Obstetrics and Gynecology 85:255

Shelton C, Brackmann D, House W et al 1989 Acoustic tumor surgery. Prognostic factors in hearing conversation. Archives of Otolaryngology, Head and Neck Surgery 115:1213

Shenouda E F, Moss T H, Coakham H B 2005 Cryptic cerebellopontine angle neuroglial cyst presenting with hemifacial spasm. Acta Neurochirurgica 147(7):787–789

Shiozawa Z, Koike G, Seguchi K et al 1996 Unilateral tongue atrophy due to an enlarged emissary vein in the hypoglossal canal. Surgical Neurology 45:477

Shiroyama Y, Inove S, Tsuha M et al 1988 Intracranial neurinomas of the jugular foramen and hypoglossal canal. No Shinkei Geka 16:313

Short O, Kaplan J N, Laramore G E, Cummings C W 1984 Shoulder pain and function after neck dissection with or without preservation of the spinal accessory nerve. American Journal of Surgery 184:478–482

Shuaib A, Klein G, Dear R 1987 Migraine headache and atrial fibrillation. Headache 27(5):252–253

Sicher H 1948 Temporomandibular articulation in mandibular overclosure. Journal of the American Dental Association 36:131

Sicher H 1955 Structural and functional basis for disorders of the temporomandibular articulation. Journal of Oral Surgery 13:275

Silverstein H, Jackson L E 2002 Vestibular nerve section. Otolaryngology Clinics of North America 35(3):655–673

Simpson D, Bender A 1988 Human immunodeficiency virus-associated myopathy: analysis of 11 patients. Annals of Neurology 24:79–84

Sinelmkov P 1958 Atlas of human anatomy. Izdatelstovo Meditsins, Moscow

Skolnik E M, Tenta L T, Wineigeer D M et al 1967 Preservation of XI cranial nerve in neck dissection. Laryngoscope 77:1304–1314

Skolnik E M, Yee K F, Friedman M, Golden T A 1976 The posterior triangle in radical neck surgery. Archives of Otolaryngology 102:1–4

Smith D 1990 Dizziness, a clinical perspective. Neurologic Clinics 8:199

Soeira G, Abd El-Bary T, Dujovny M et al 1994 Microsurgical anatomy of the trigeminal nerve. Neurology Research 16:273

Spillane J 1996 Bickerstaff's neurological examination in clinical practice, 6th edn. Blackwell Science, Oxford

Stefan H 1994 Mechanische Läsionen des peripheren Nervensystems. Fortschritte der Medizin 112:477

Steinmann E 1968 Styloid syndrome in absence of an elongated process. Acta Otolaryngologica 66:347

Stephens D, Gorman R 1996 Does 'normal' vision improve with spinal manipulation? Journal of Manipulative and Physiological Therapeutics 19:415

Stephens D, Pollard H, Bilton D, Thomson P, Gorman F 1999 Bilateral simultaneous optic nerve dysfunction after periorbital trauma: recovery of vision in association with chiropractic spinal manipulation therapy. Journal of Manipulative and Physiological Therapeutics 22:615

Stoll W 1993 Operative Versorgung frontobasaler Verletzungen (inklusive Orbita) durch den HNO-Chirurgen. European Archives of Otorhinolaryngology (Suppl.) 1:287

Sunderland S 1948 Neurovascular relations and anomalies at base of brain. Journal of Neurology, Neurosurgery and Psychiatry 11:243

Sweet W 1988 Percutaneous methods for the treatment of trigeminal neuralgia and other faciocephalic pain: comparison with microvascular decompression. Seminars in Neurology 8:272

Tarsy D 1998 Comparison of acute- and delayed-onset posttraumatic cervical dystonia. Movement Disorders 13(3):481–485

Teller J, Karmon G, Svir H 1988 Long term follow up of traumatic unilateral superior oblique palsy. American Ophthalmology 20:424

Terrett A 1983 Importance and interpretation of tests designed to predict susceptibility to neurocirculatory accidents from manipulation. Journal of the Australian Chiropractic Association 13:29

Thömke F, Hopf H C 2001 Abduction paresis with rostral pontine and/or mesencephalic lesions: pseudoabducens palsy and its relation to the so-called posterior internuclear ophthalmoplegia of Lutz. BMC Neurology 18(1):4

Thompsett C, Cundy J 1992 Use of the laryngeal mask airway in the presence of a bleeding diathesis. Anaesthesia 47:530

Thompson P, Carroll W 1983 Hemimasticatory spasm: a peripheral paroxysmal cranial neuropathy? Journal of Neurology, Neurosurgery and Psychiatry 46:274–6

Tikkakoski T, Bode M K, Siponen P, Siniluoto T 2003 Imaging techniques in the diagnostics of pulsating tinnitus. Duodecim 119(2):103–112
Toole J, Tucker S 1960 Influence of head position upon cerebral circulation. Studies on blood flow in cadavers. Archives of Neurology 2:616
Torok N, Kumar A 1978 Experimental evidence of etiology in postural vertigo. Journal of Otorhinolaryngology 40:32
Toselli C, Miglior M 1979 Oftalmologia clinica. Monduzzi, Bologna
Troost B T 1980 Dizziness and vertigo in vertebrobasilar disease. Part II. Central causes and vertebrobasilar disease. Stroke 11:413–415
Tucker S M, Tarlov E C 2005 Intraorbital surgery for trigeminal neuralgia. Ophthalmic Plastic and Reconstructive Surgery 21(1):11–15
Tyeler R 2000 Tinnitus. Singular (Thomson Learning), Chicago
Umansky F, Nathan H 1976 The lateral wall of the cavernous sinus. A micro surgical study. Journal of Neurosurgery 45:169
Umansky F, Nathan H 1982 The lateral wall of the cavernous sinus with special reference to the nerves related to it. Journal of Neurosurgery 56:228
Upton A, McComas A 1972 The double crush in nerve entrapment syndromes. Lancet 2:359
van Wilgen C P, Dijkstra P U, van der Laan B F, Plukker J T, Roodenburg J L 2003 Shoulder complaints after neck dissection: is the spinal accessory nerve involved? British Journal of Oral and Maxillofacial Surgery 41(1):7–11
Verberne A J, Saita M, Sartor D M 2003 Chemical stimulation of vagal afferent neurons and sympathetic vasomotor tone. Brain Research. Brain Research Reviews 41(2–3):288–305
Verjaal A 1955 Acute perifere facialisparalyse. Nederlands Tijdschrift voor Geneeskunde 99:3767
Vernon J, Griest S, Press L 1992 Attributes of tinnitus associated with the temporomandibular joint syndrome. European Archives of Otorhinolaryngology 249:93
Vibert D 1995 Ocular tilt reaction associated with a sudden idiopathic unilateral peripheral cochleovestibular loss. ORL 57:310
Vibert D, Häusler R 2000 Long-term evolution of subjective visual vertical after vestibular neurectomy and labyrinthectomy. Acta Oto-Laryngologica 120:620–622
Vibert D, Häusler R 2003 Acute peripheral vestibular deficits after whiplash injuries. Annals of Otology, Rhinology and Laryngology 112:246
Vibert D, Häusler R, Safran A, Koerner F 1996 Diplopia from skew deviation in unilateral peripheral vestibular lesions. Acta Oto-Laryngologica 116:170
Vibert D, Häusler R, Safran A 1999 Subjective visual vertical in peripheral unilateral vestibular diseases. Journal of Vestibular Research: Equilibrium and Orientation 9(2):145
Villanueva R 1977 The role of rehabilitation medicine in physical restoration of patients with head and neck cancer. Cancer Bulletin 29:46
Vogl T, Dresel S, Lochmüller H et al 1992 Third cranial nerve palsy caused by gummatous neurosyphilis: MR findings. American Journal of Neuroradiology 14:1329–1331
von Eck L 1989 Die Fazialislähmungen und ihre kranken-gymnastische Behandlung. Krankengymnastik 3:222
von Piekartz H, Coppieters M, De Weerdt W 2001 Vorschlag für einen neurodynamischen Test des N. mandibularis. Reliabilität und Referenzwerte. Manuelle Therapie 5:56
Voyvodic F, Whyte A, Slavotinek J 1995 The hypoglossal canal: normal MR enhancement pattern. American Journal of Neuroradiology 16:1707
Wagner P, Lang G 2000 Lacrimal system. In: Lang G (ed.) Ophthalmology. Thieme, Stuttgart, 2:49
Wall P 1999 Pain: the science of suffering. Weidenfield and Nicholson, London
Wall P, Melzack R 1994 Textbook of pain. Churchill Livingstone, Edinburgh
Wasicko M, Jutt D, Parisis R et al 1990 The role of vascular tone in the control of upper airway collapsibility. American Review of Respiratory Disease 141:1569
Wasicko M, Giering R, Knuth S, Leiter J 1993 Hypoglossal and phrenic nerve responses to carotid baroreceptor stimulation. Journal of Applied Physiology 75:1395
Watanabe K, Watanabe M 2001 Activity of jaw-opening and jaw-closing muscles and their influence on dentofacial morphological features in normal adults. Journal of Oral Rehabilitation 28(9):873–879
Watanabe I, Kamagami H, Tsuda Y 1974 Tinnitus due to abnormal contraction of stapedial muscle. Journal of Otorhinolaryngology 36:217
Wechsler A, Ho D 1989 Bilateral Bell's palsy at the time of HIV seroconversion. Neurology 39:747–748
Wenngren B, Pettersson K, Lowenhielm G, Hildingsson C 2002 Eye motility and auditory brainstem response dysfunction after whiplash injury. Acta Otolaryngologica 122:276
White J C, Sweet W 1969 Pain and the neurosurgeon: a 40 year experience. C C Thomas, Springfield, IL, p 123
Wiarda V, Wimmers R 1988 De nekdissectie en haar behandeling. Nederlands Tijdschrift voor Fysiotherapie 98:134
Wijnen, van-Segeren I 1993 Torticollis bij n. IV parese is oculair. Fysiopraxis 3:10

Willer J, Lamas G, Fligny I, Soudant J 1993 Hypoglossal–facial anastomosis alters excitability of hypoglossal motoneurones in man. Neuroscience Letters 155:212

Williams P, Warwick R, Dyson M, Bannister L 1989 Gray's anatomy, 37th edn. Churchill Livingstone, Edinburgh

Williamson E 1990 Interrelationship of internal derangements of the temporomandibular joint, headache, vertigo and tinnitus: a survey of 25 patients. Cranio 4:301–306

Wilson C, Yorke C, Prioleau G 1980 Microvascular decompression for trigeminal neuralgia and hemifacial spasm: experiences with 72 cases. Western Journal of Medicine 132:481–484

Wilson-Pauwels L, Akesson E, Stewart P 1988 Cranial nerves, anatomy and clinical comments. BC Decker, Hamilton, Ontario

Wilson-Pauwels L, Akesson E, Stewart P, Spacey S 2002 Cranial nerves in health and disease, 2nd edn. BC Decker, Hamilton, Ontario

Wolderberg D, Greenberg R, Lane E, Cinnamon J et al 1994 The cranial meninges: anatomic considerations. Seminars in Ultrasound, CT and MRI 15:454

Wolff E 1958 The anatomy of the eye and orbit. H K Lewis, London

Wong A, Tweed D, Sharpe J 2002 Vertical misalignment in unilateral sixth nerve palsy. Ophthalmology 109(7):1315

Woolf C J, Salter I 2000 Neural plasticity: increasing the gain in pain. Science 288:1765–1768

Wutthiphan S, Poonyathalang A 2002 Abducens-oculomotor synkinesis following acquired sixth nerve palsy. Journal of Pediatric Ophthalmology and Strabismus 39(6):362–364

Xu Z, Xiong Y 1999 Effect of decompression of blood vessels on vascular compressive tinnitus. Lin Chuang Er Bi Yan Hou Ke Za Zhi 13(4):155–156

Yamamoto E, Nishimura H, Iwanaga M 1985 Tinnitus and/or hearing loss elicited by facial mimetic movement. Laryngoscope 95:966–970

Ylikoski J, Morra B, Hernandez I 1981 Vestibular nerve compression in eighth-nerve tumors. Journal for Oto-rhino-laryngology and its Related Specialties 43:17–25

Yoshimura Y, Oka M 1989 Does Eagle's syndrome always require operative intervention for treatment? Two case reports. Journal of Craniomandibular Practice 7:235

Zakrzewska J 1995 Trigeminal neuralgia: major problems in neurology. W B Saunders, New York

Zakrzewska J 2002 Trigeminal neuralgia. Clinical Evidence 7:1221

Zakrzewska J, Feinmann C 1990 A standard way to measure pain and psychological morbidity in dental practice. British Dental Journal 169(10):337–339

Zakrzewska J, Nally F 1988 The role of cryotherapy (cryoanalgesia) in the management of paroxysmal trigeminal neuralgia: a six year experience. British Journal of Oral and Maxillofacial Surgery 26:18

Zarb G, Schmidtt A 1990 The longitudinal clinical effectiveness of osseointegrated dental implants in partially edentulous patients. International Journal of Prosthodontistry 6:189–196

Zimmerman A 1959 An evaluation of Costen's syndrome from an anatomic point of view. In: Sarnat C (ed.) The temporomandibular joint. C C Thomas, Springfield, IL

Zochodne D W, Theriault M, Sharkey K A et al 1997 Peptides and neuromas, calcitonin gene related peptide, substance P, and mast cells in a mechanosensitive human sural neuroma. Muscle and Nerve 20:875–880

Chapter 18

Treatment guidelines for neurodynamic techniques and palpation of the cranial nervous system

Harry von Piekartz

CHAPTER CONTENTS

INTEGRATING CRANIODYNAMIC MOBILIZATION INTO THE OVERALL MANAGEMENT

Butler emphasizes: 'Neurodynamics is not an isolated treatment approach but should be embedded into the overall management' (Butler 1991, Butler & Moseley 2003). This principle may be applied at different stages of the treatment and may influence movement in various ways.

Neurodynamics is often misunderstood as a 'neural stretching technique'. This is not quite correct; rather the emphasis should be on nerve movement and on influencing its physiology. The techniques aim to restore the most important quality of the nerve, i.e. its ability to move (Nathan & Keniston 1993, Butler 2000). Neurodynamics has also been integrated into the assessment and treatment within pain management approaches (Gifford 1998, Butler 2000), which additionally broadens the therapeutic horizon.

During the late 1980s and early 1990s neurodynamics was primarily viewed as a mechanical model for the evaluation of peripheral nociceptive clinical patterns. Today the results of neurodynamic tests are interpreted by applying knowledge from recent pain research. Hence neurodynamics is integrated into pain management approaches and may be an important component of explanatory pain models. Neurodynamics is a big topic.

For the purpose of this chapter we will focus on the neurodynamics of the craniofacial region, although the odd excursion into the field of pain management might be necessary.

There are four options for cranial neuromobilization:

- Passive influence
- Active influence
- Indirectly influencing the neural container
- Direct influence, neurodynamic movement and palpation.

DIFFERENT TYPES OF CRANIAL NEUROMOBILIZATION

Passive influence

Passive influencing techniques include:

- Physiological movements: neurodynamic tests or components of neurodynamic tests
- Palpation: mentioned later in this chapter as a 'directly influencing technique'.

Neurodynamic tests have very specific features and the effects are different when the tests are performed passively rather than actively. The most important features are listed below:

- Optimum evaluation of movement parameters: Passive testing and mobilization allow for the assessment of pain, resistance and muscle spasm (Maitland et al 2000). These components will guide the clinical decision making process by indicating the intensity, range and direction of the appropriate mobilization technique. An example is shown as a movement diagram in Figure 18.1. This shows mandibular lateral movement before and after a mobilization technique.
- Reassessment tool: Since three parameters (pain, resistance and spasm) are included, the passive movement is a valuable tool to assess behaviour pre- and post-test (Maitland et al 2000).
- Indicator of pain mechanisms: Combining the results of the subjective examination with the findings from a passive movement gives us some idea about the dominant pathobiological mechanisms.
- Explanations: Understanding pain mechanisms and the possible sources of the symptoms may be of major importance for adequate problem management. For example, a patient with unspecific otalgia (toothache without any visible reason) might have an increase of symptoms on upper cervical flexion and laterotrusion of the mandible. The hypothesis points towards a neuropathic component. This technique and the patient's reaction to it provide valuable information towards an explanation of the underlying pain mechanisms (Table 18.1).

Active influence

There are fewer variations for active influence than for passive influence, but active influence has other advantages.

CONTINUOUS PHYSIOLOGICAL INFLUENCE

Because the patient can perform the techniques themselves and as often as they like, they are given the chance to continuously influence the physiology of the nervous system, especially axonal transport, the vascular system and the connective tissue of the cranial nervous system. Studies have shown that early mobilization results in positive outcomes for the (neuro)physiology (Rosenfeld et al 2000).

Target tissue rehabilitation

Target tissue exercises may be integrated into the regime of active neuromobilization and neurodynamic positioning. Due to the active afferent–reafferent impact, the somatosensory cortex receives information about the affected structures (Ramachandran & Blakesee 1998). Since the orofacial area is largely projected onto the somatosensory cortex, active target tissue exercises may be integrated into the overall management at an early stage. Some examples are as follows:

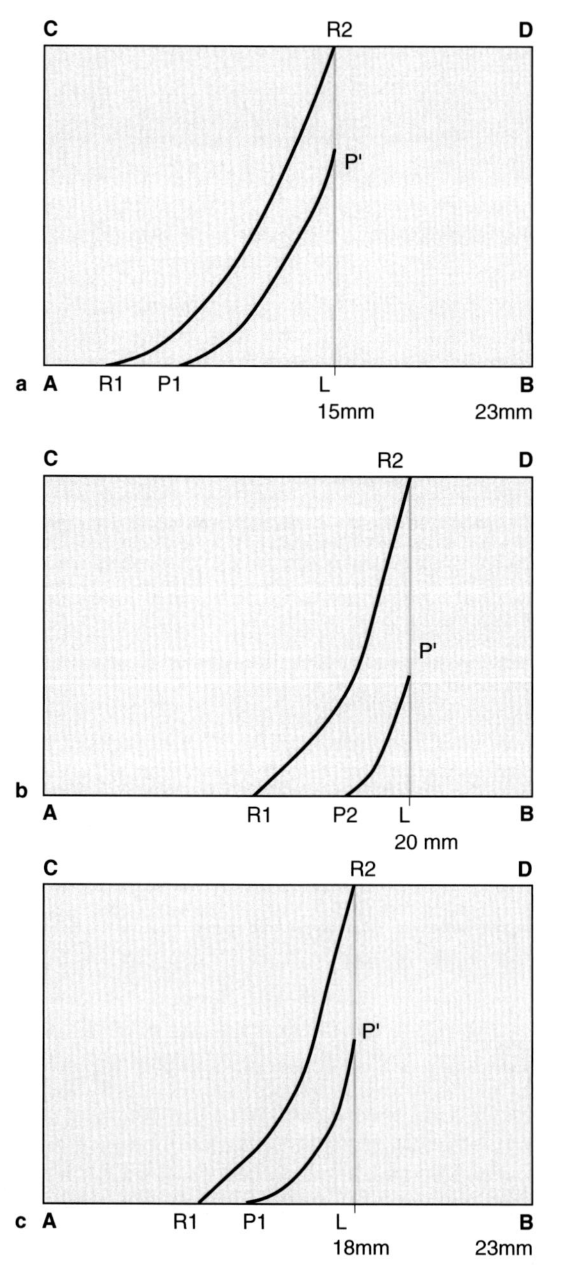

Fig. 18.1 Movement diagram showing resistance (R) and pain (P) on laterotrusion to the left with 2 cm of mouth opening in craniocervical flexion + lateroflexion to the left (test for the right mandibular nerve).

a Before the 'slider': Average laterotrusion (AB line is 23 mm; von Piekartz 2001). The resistance increases steadily and limits the movement at roughly 15 mm (R1–R2, L = limit = 15 mm); pain (P1–P′) is not dominant and shows a score of 7 on the visual analogue scale (VAS).

b Immediately after the 'slider': The onset of resistance (R1) and the onset of pain (P1) have moved further to the right of the diagram. The range of movement has increased: L has moved to the right in the diagram (20 mm), while P′ on the VAS is now 4.

c Assessment during the second session: The onset of R1 and P1 is earlier again. The limit is 18 mm and the pain intensity is described as 5 on the VAS.

- Patients with Bell's palsy may perform active neurodynamic movements of the head and also receive muscular facilitation in or out of neurodynamic tension.
- Patients with neck–tongue syndrome (Bogduk 1981) may experience mild dysphagia and paraesthesia of the tongue. It can be hypothesized that this is due to an irritation of the hypoglossal nerve (XII), and therefore neurodynamic movements may be effective, accompanied by functional target tissue exercises (for the tongue). The therapist may challenge somatosensory input by repeating the same exercise in various neurodynamic positions.

Table 18.1 Overview of clinical interpretations of patient responses based on pain mechanisms: this example shows passive shoulder depression on accessory nerve testing

Input dominant	Processing dominant	Output dominant
Stimulus response predictable	Stimulus response unpredictable	Stimulus response generally cumulative
Behaviour of pain and resistance consistent	Behaviour of pain and resistance inconsistent	Behaviour of pain and resistance variable
Resistance usually increases gradually towards the end of range	Pain may increase without an increase of resistance	Prolonged spasms and autonomic changes (e.g. sweating, temperature changes)
Anticipation pattern during test is known	Pain with accumulating and latent characteristics; coping, anxiety, modification of concentration and distraction modify the response	Increasing vegetative reactions (e.g. sweating, temperature changes) and affective influences largely determine the responses

- After whiplash injuries some patients might experience blurred vision and/or diplopia. Impaired accommodation of the eyes and diplopia may be symptoms of a dysfunction of the oculomotor nerve. In this case active and passive mobilization, combined with functional activities of the eyes, may be helpful.

Variations of active movements

There are many options for the integration of active craniodynamics into patient management and day-to-day activities.

Butler (2000) stated that the 'sequence of movements' and 'trick movements' may challenge the mechanical influence on the nervous system. If the homunculus receives a sufficient number of afferences, movement may no longer be interpreted as pain. This principle works whenever a pain has become chronic, i.e. when the central nervous system is sensitized, and may be useful for the management approach.

Sequence of movements and trick movements

Example of the sequence of movements

During a neurodynamic test the mandibular nerve becomes irritated on mouth opening with pain and trismus of the masticatory muscles. It is sensible here to assess mouth opening first followed by cranial flexion and lateroflexion. If the mouth can clearly be opened wider, it is sensible to first improve cranioneurodynamic movements with mouth activity.

Trick movements are closely connected to the sequence of movement components. They provide us with information about a movement and about the environment which is often used to challenge it.

Example of trick movements

This applies to gravity. If cervical flexion is more easily performed in side lying than in supine (fewer symptoms), it makes sense to incorporate side lying cervical flexion into the management of this patient. It is essential for the success of this exercise that the patient is conscious of these differences and understands what they mean.

Maximal mouth opening was 32 mm. Furthermore, unilateral increase in tone of the masseter muscle was noted. Admittedly, mouth opening is more than 32 mm when yawning or singing. The therapist now has the option to integrate functional activities such as singing or yawning, with or without neurodynamic positions, into therapy.

Part of pain management

The principle of distraction (physical and/or psychological distraction from the pain experience of a patient) can be easily integrated into the treatment by including neurodynamic exercises. If a patient suffers from atypical facial pain and fears to increase headache symptoms by moving the head, it might be useful to initiate the neurodynamic techniques in the long sitting slump position. The patient may move their legs or thoracic spine and keep the head static, while still achieving neurodynamic movement.

Cranioneurodynamic movements may also be applied as a pacing exercise. If, for example, craniocervical flexion triggers facial pain, the patient may be assessed and reassessed by a quota system with the onset of pain being the indicator for improvement (Harding 1997).

A disadvantage may be that neurodynamic movements are sometimes difficult to control. It is therefore sensible to wait for the effects of the passive techniques before starting on neurodynamic activities.

Indirectly influencing the neural container

'Neural container' stands for any tissue surrounding and potentially influencing the nervous system (Gifford 1998, Butler 2000). Depending on the location, these may be various types of tissue – blood vessels, bone, fascia, and, intracranially, other types of neural tissue (von Piekartz 2001, Austermann 2002). For example:

- The posterior cerebral artery within the cerebellopontine angle (CPA) that touches the trigeminal nerve (Lang 1995)
- The cranial foramina, e.g. the foramen jugulare with the vagus (X), glossopharyngeal (IX) and accessory (XII) nerves
- The lateral and medial pterygoid muscles contact the lingual nerve, a branch of the mandibular nerve
- The major occipital nerve within the superficial dorsal cranial fascia.

If the therapist becomes aware of a dysfunction in tissues surrounding the nerve during physical examination, a local technique should be attempted, followed by reassessment of the neurodynamic test that showed abnormal responses. In many cases an adequate answer will be found.

Direct influence: neurodynamic movement

Here the therapist performs specific manoeuvres designed to challenge nerve movement. The techniques are based on knowledge of the anatomy of peripheral nerves. The most common manoeuvre is the straight leg raise (SLR). Here dorsiflexion of the foot is the key movement to detect a neuropathic problem in the leg or the lumbosacral region. For treatment the therapist usually applies components of a neurodynamic test; sometimes the complete testing manoeuvre is used. The same principles apply for cranial nerves. Suggestions for neurodynamic testing of the cranial nerves based on the anatomical position are described in Chapter 17.

During the past 25 years various treatment strategies based on empirical data have been suggested. The following section gives an overview of the treatment choices:

- Distal techniques
- Proximal techniques
- Sliders and tensioners
- Neural palpation.

DISTAL TECHNIQUES

These techniques approach a problem from a remote site. For example, if the pathomechanic site of the accessory nerve is hypothesized to be near the jugular foramen, depression or retraction of the shoulder would be a distal technique.

The advantage of distal techniques is that they will not produce maximum stress and that painful sites do not have to be touched or moved (distraction).

One disadvantage is that the therapist will need thorough information about the neural container along the nerve. If a distal technique is applied, although dysfunctions along the neural container of the nerve exist, this may cause abnormal reactions at the dysfunctional site and possibly lead to pathodynamic changes (Breig 1978, Butler 2000). An example is scar tissue behind the ear after salivary gland surgery that might contribute to peripheral neuropathy. In this case the neural container (scar tissue) needs to be treated before approaching the facial nerve (VII). Afterwards the distal technique to influence the neurodynamics of the facial nerve could be a movement of the mandible that influences primarily the distal mandibular ramus of the facial nerve.

These days, distal techniques can no longer be viewed as purely mechanical influences on the nervous system; rather the effects may be viewed at the level of central processing mechanisms. Central neurones are stimulated at the same site of the brain that usually represents the previously experienced pain (Kaas et al 1999, Butler 2000).

PROXIMAL TECHNIQUES

These techniques apply movement near the neuraxis and therefore also near the trunk. For the peripheral arm nerves, these might be depression and elevation of the shoulder or midcervical sideglides (Elvey 1997). For the lower quadrant, proximal techniques are flexion + adduction of the hip. For the cranial nervous system craniocervical flexion and lateroflexion are proximal techniques biased towards the brainstem and the nerve exits at this region (Breig 1978). These proximal components are also part of the suggested cranioneurodynamic tests. The proximal components generally show a large range of movement and are therefore easily observed and controlled by the therapist. Clinically they not only influence peripheral processes but also the responses due to the close connection to the neuraxis, for example neural mobilization after acoustic neuroma surgery. The patient suffers from neck pain and stiffness on cervical flexion (proximal sign) and also frequently experiences fasciculations of the masseter muscle and toothache (distal sign). An appropriate treatment technique may be a proximal approach with craniocervical flexion/extension in combination with lateroflexion.

Furthermore, proximal techniques show fewer irritable reactions than distal techniques. Elvey (1986) observed this difference in reactions while testing the neurodynamics of the upper extremity. Because of the irritability of many shoulder problems he preferred shoulder movements rather than elbow or hand movements. If the pain behaviour varies in its duration and intensity it also makes sense to begin with a proximal technique. For example, if a patient complains of pain in the mandibular region, the problem is most likely irritable. If the therapist detects a clear mandibular dysfunction, treatment should begin with proximal mobilization techniques. Craniocervical mobilization should precede mandibular mobilization.

Viewed clinically, distal techniques show more disadvantages than proximal techniques. It should also be borne in mind that neurodynamic techniques not only approach neural tissue but also influence all other proximal structures. Systematic reassessment of neurocranial structures and surrounding muscles and joints is therefore essential after treatment.

SLIDERS

The concept of 'sliders/tensioners' was introduced in the mid 1990s by Butler et al (1994). The idea is to focus on the macroscopic function of the nervous system: on 'movement'. The choice of movement is directed by the anatomical position of the nerve and by knowledge from macroscopic movement studies (Breig 1978). In principle, the proximal end of the nervous system is relaxed while the distal end is put under tension and vice versa: the proximal component is under tension and therefore challenged while the distal component is relaxed. This procedure emphasizes the *movement* of these particular nervous structures.

Some examples for basic techniques for the cranial nervous system include:

- Mandibular nerve: During craniocervical extension the mandible is moved into laterotrusion with the mouth 2 cm opened. During the following craniocervical flexion the mandible is moved back to midline position (Fig. 18.2).
- Facial nerve: During craniocervical extension and lateroflexion towards the same side, the oral mimic muscles are activated. During the following craniocervical flexion and lateroflexion to the opposite side the facial muscles are relaxed.
- Hypoglossal nerve: During craniocervical flexion and lateroflexion to the contralateral side, the tongue is relaxed. During the following craniocervical extension and lateroflexion to the other side, the tongue is moved into laterotrusion to the contralateral side (a spatula may be used).
- Abducens nerve: During craniocervical extension the eye is moved towards medial. During the following craniocervical flexion the eye is moved back to the mid-position.

The great advantage of slider techniques is that they do not produce major stress for the peripheral nervous system and are therefore easily performed actively. The techniques should not hurt and generally are performed within a

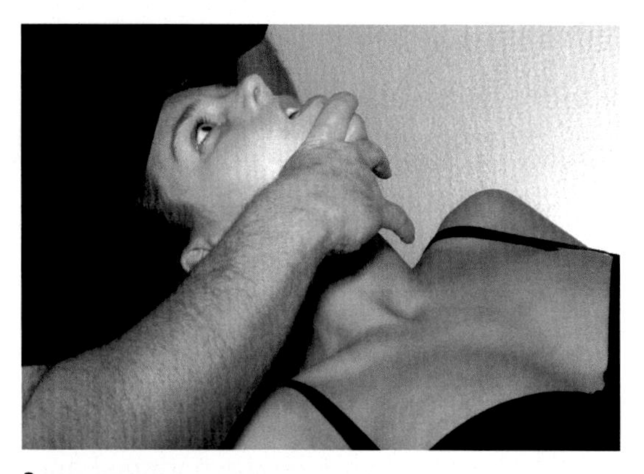

a

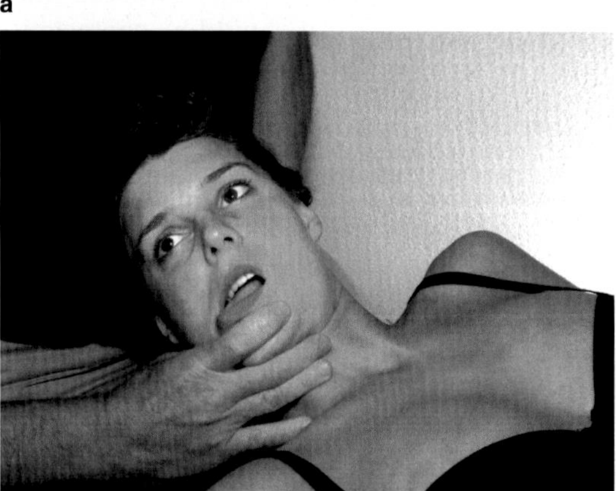

b

Fig. 18.2 Slider concept applied to the mandibular nerve.

a The mandible is moved into laterotrusion in craniocervical extension with the mouth open approximately 2 cm.

b The mandible is returned to the mid-position in upper cervical flexion.

slight amount of resistance. Sliders are good tools for pain management and may be used as 'distraction' and 'pacing' exercises. Furthermore, the therapist should make sure that the neural container does not cause any unnecessary stress and hence needs to be assessed prior to the slider techniques.

When does it make sense to work with sliders? Clinically there are some rules to support the clinician in the hypothesis-generating process which may point towards sliders as an effective treatment tool:

- Treating the neural container no longer influences neurodynamics.

- After applying a technique the neurodynamic test should have improved regarding range, resistance and symptoms.
- At the beginning of the follow-up session the signs and symptoms should not be worse than at the end of the previous session. After the second treatment they should be clearly improved (see Fig. 18.1).
- Conductive qualities of the nerve should not worsen after a technique. For example, if after a slider technique the size of a paraesthestic area at the chin has increased, the technique should be discontinued and a neurology specialist should be contacted.

TENSIONERS

Tensioners are the opposite of sliders; they produce an increase in tension in neural structures. Here, both ends – proximal and distal – are put under tension simultaneously. This technique focuses on loading the connective tissues along a peripheral nerve (Kwan et al 1992). It relies on the natural viscoelasticity of the nervous system and does not exceed the elastic limit. If it is performed gently, with constant assessment of the responses and the resistance that is felt during the manoeuvre, neural viscoelastic and physiological functions will improve (Shacklock 2005). In this case movement and the neural container are only of secondary interest.

Generally tensioners will not be a first choice technique. The following thoughts may need to be considered:

- The problem should not be irritable and has not been so in the recent past. Hence, the patient has not experienced any major variations in intensity and location of the symptoms during the past few weeks.
- For tensioners, the most positive results occur in situations that involve scar tissue around or within the nervous structures, for example scarring behind the ear at the facial nerve or at the cranial dura after craniocervical trauma.
- During protective muscle spasm one might want to try to move the patient from a neurodynamic position into a tensioner position and rest there for a few seconds, for example during trismus of the masticatory muscles.
- The conductive qualities of the nerve should not be affected negatively after any treatment technique but should be improved.
- If sliders no longer have the desired effect, or whenever treating the neural container does not improve the situation, tensioners may be attempted.

Craniofacial examples include tensioners at the hypoglossal nerve after submandibular scarring due to surgery at the mouth or radiotherapy, and tensioners at the auriculotemporal nerve after interneural scarring due to the pressure of glasses.

Direct influence: neural palpation

INTRODUCTION

As mentioned above, nerve palpation may be viewed as a direct passive technique that influences the peripheral nervous system. This is not a novelty. In medicine, especially among orthopaedic surgeons, this was described very early. Previously, during or after an operation, it was common practice to press, pull or move a nerve to confirm the condition of the structure. For example, before deciding on a tracheotomy, the main branches of the pharyngeal nerve (derived from the vagus nerve) needed to be palpated (Gavilán & Gavilán 1986).

With the new insights into the nervous system, palpation gained a new dimension. Butler (2000) suggested palpation in order to re-learn peripheral nerve anatomy, to decide upon a differential diagnosis and to detect anomalies, as well as to treat the nerve tissue. Nowadays nerve palpation has to be viewed in a larger context.

- Firstly, it is part of overall patient management and does not stand alone. Chronic craniomandibular and craniofacial dysfunctions generally involve many different structures. Mobilization of the cranial bones, cranioneurodynamics and palpation in mildly neurodynamic positions are key methods for the assessment and treatment of many head and facial complaints.

- Secondly, it may assist the therapist's understanding of the problem. Palpation of the lingual nerve may reproduce the patient's symptoms. If this is accompanied by a 'negative' MRI, it will be easier for the therapist to convince the patient that they are not suffering from a malignant tumour, a very common fear among patients.
- Thirdly, palpation can be considered within its wider context. For example, central sensitization and peripheral nerve tissue injuries in the past may change central modulation systems and cause unexpected reactions, including (secondary) hyperalgetic reactions.

It is strongly advised to integrate this knowledge when interpreting neurodynamic test results. The treatment of nervous tissue is not a purely mechanical business (Butler et al 1994). Clinical features regarding cranial tissues and testing/treatment procedures are discussed in the following section.

PATHOBIOLOGICAL CHANGES IN PERIPHERAL CRANIAL NERVES

Dysfunctions as we know them from the trunk and the upper and lower extremities are also common in the craniofacial and craniocervical regions. It should be borne in mind that the nerve endings in the face are extremely sensitive, more than comparable nerve endings of the upper and lower extremities. Motor responses of the facial and masticatory muscles are not uncommon. The following local dysfunctions are frequently seen in the cranial nerves:

- Adhesions around a nerve (a nerve might be 'glued together' at one site)
- Adhesions of the nervous connective tissue (intraneural adhesions)
- A combination of morphological changes of the neural container and the connective tissue.

Dysfunctions can be easily detected by the therapist and occur as swollen or hardened tissue with a loss of transverse mobility and abnormal mechanosensitivity (Jabre 1994, Butler 2000). When interpreting the clinical pattern, certain pathophysiological knowledge needs to be applied, for example the vascular system, axoplasmatic flow, abnormal 'pacemakers' (abnormal impulse generating sites, AIGS) and sensitization of the nervous system.

Adhesions around the nerve (nerve is 'glued together' at one site)

Stiff scar tissue affects the nerve, especially after injury, trauma or sustained abnormal function of the neural container. Examples include a trapped lingual nerve due to the lateral pterygoid muscle after sustained deviation on mouth opening, sustained compression of the hypoglossal and vagus nerves when the neck is swollen due to salivary gland problems, and scar tissue caused by a haematoma in the orbit that produces pressure on the lateral branches of the maxillary nerve.

Adhesions of the nervous connective tissue (intraneural adhesions)

The nerve demonstrates signs of intraneural connective tissue adhesions shown as swelling due to abnormal container movement or abnormal external pressure on gliding. Examples include the following:

- A long styloid process will produce pressure on the hypoglossal nerve on cervical flexion and ipsilateral lateroflexion.
- The auriculotemporal nerve needs to glide and extend excessively on mandibular subluxation when the mouth is opened.
- Scarring and the development of an abnormal 'pacemaker' (AIGS) at the inferior alveolar nerve of the mandible may occur after tooth extraction.
- Wearing ill-fitting glasses may cause pressure on the maxillary nerve near the orbital foramen.

Combination of morphological changes of the neural container and the connective tissue

This phenomenon is mainly seen when dysfunctions have started very slowly, have a long

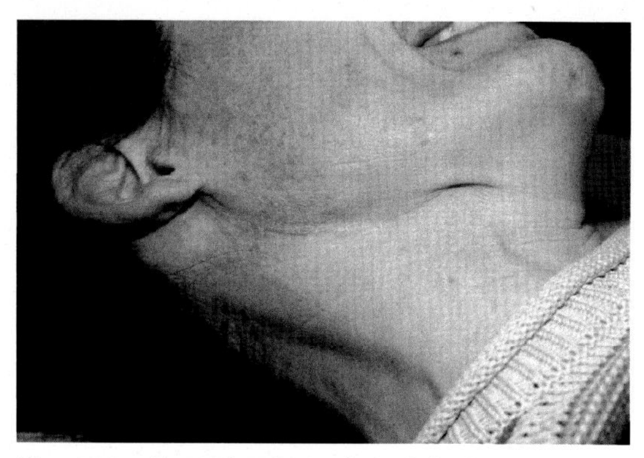

Fig. 18.3 Example of scarring of the hypoglossal and glossopharyngeal nerves at the ventral neck.

history and show multistructural changes. Okeson describes how reduced blood flow may risk the health of various structures in this region and emphasizes the effect on cranial neural connective tissue (Okeson 1995). Long-term vasomotor changes in the cranium as known in tension headaches and migraines may result in such multistructural changes. An example is the development of trigger points in the masticatory muscles. Trigger points are defined by various clinicians and scientists as the entrapments of peripheral nerve endings in hypertonic muscles (see also Chapter 8). Other examples are multistructural changes following craniofacial surgery (e.g. after salivary gland surgery) when abnormal swelling around the ear occurs (mainly ventrocaudally) accompanied by minimal trauma of the facial nerve (anastomosis of the buccal and mandibular branches). In particular, cancer surgery at the neck in combination with radiotherapy leads to multistructural changes of the skin, the muscles and the nerves (mainly the accessory nerve) (Lang 1995).

Assessment and treatment techniques

A number of assessment and treatment methods have been suggested. At present there is still a lack of efficacy studies. Jabre (1994) presented an efficacy study on the topic of 'nerve rubbing' in the cubital region. Twenty therapy-resistant men diagnosed with ulnar nerve neuropathy were treated with a certain nerve palpation technique; 50% improved in their subjective and objective reassessment. Unfortunately there was no placebo or control group in this study (Jabre 1994).

It is difficult to decide which technique to choose in which clinical situation. Some parameters such as mechanosensitivity, centralized data documentation, level of treatment and (meta-)cognition of the therapist play an important role in the clinical decision-making process. Some basic techniques, modifications of the 'twanging' described by Butler, may guide the therapist to find the appropriate intensity of stimulation.

- Starting position: The nerve is placed 'in tension' or 'out of tension'. This depends on the individual anatomy and the irritability of the problem.
- Position of the thumb or finger: The tip of the finger or thumb should touch the nerve laterally if the focus is on the nerve interface. If the emphasis is more on general local tension, the fingertip may be placed directly onto the nerve.
- Nerve movement: The palpatory movement may be performed in various directions. Nerve movement affects a large part of the nerve and may be a preparation for the following neurodynamic techniques. The advantage of choosing a position 'in neural tension' is that the head does not need to be moved, since headache, dizziness and tinnitus patients might prefer if their head remains in a position that they can control. The therapist's finger or thumb can remain at the same spot during palpation. This way the nerve receives more stimulation.

The basic principles for the progression of nerve stimuli and for the nerve's surrounding structures may be combined. In the following text the general methods for treatment and assessment are discussed and applied to craniofacial dysfunctions. Figure 18.4 illustrates a clinical example applied to the extracranial part of the accessory nerve.

- Transverse movement of the relaxed nerve: For this first step of the twanging, gentle movement on the ophthalmic foramen

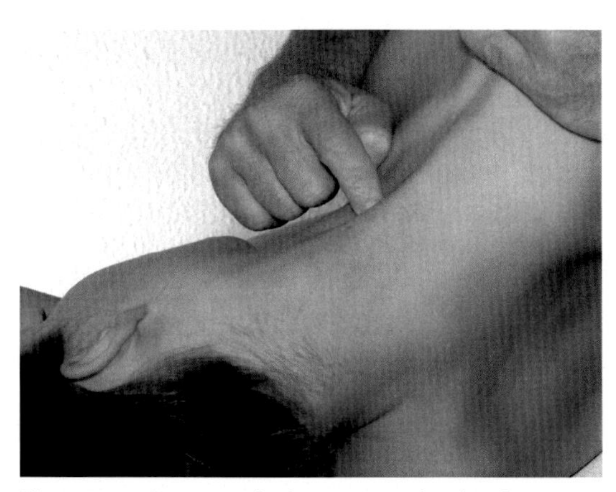

Fig. 18.4 An example for a manual palpation technique on a cranial nerve (extracranial branch of the accessory nerve).

reproduces slight unilateral headache and punctiform pain at the front. The advantage of this technique is that local scar tissue within and around those tiny nerve branches may be influenced.

- Transverse movement in optimal neurodynamic relaxation: Assessment and treatment of the buccal nerve (branch of the facial nerve) above the zygomatic bone in a position of upper cervical extension and lateroflexion away/rotation towards (optimum relaxation of the facial nerve). The transverse movement of the nerve can be observed easily since the nerve runs superficially over the zygomatic bone. Note also how the movement continues over a long distance of the nerve.
- Transverse movement in increased neurodynamic tension: If there is no hypersensitivity of the nervous system and the patient is able to tolerate the position for a few minutes, this might be an effective technique. The local stimulus is quite intensive and appropriate for local scar tissue. For example, a patient who suffered from headaches, tinnitus and neck pain for 2 years following an episode of mastoiditis shows scar tissue behind the ear on the mastoid process and on some small branches of the vagus nerve. The example shows a good position for examining and treating this patient.
- Transverse nerve movement combined with moving the whole nerve: Performed on the auriculotemporal nerve with jaw opening, this emphasizes the mobilization of local adhesions within and around this nerve branch, for example in dysfunction and pain after prolonged wearing of glasses or a stethoscope.
- Mobilization of the neural container in various neurodynamic positions: This enables information about adhesions around the nerve to be collected without directly pressing on the nerve. This can be helpful if the treatment technique is supposed to mainly influence the mechanical interface of the nerve. A good example is the accessory nerve: the trapezius muscle pars descendens may have an abnormal mechanical influence on the accessory nerve after long-term neck pain or ventral neck surgery. This may lead to adhesions and movement deficits of the nerve and the surrounding tissues. Palpating the nerve directly or placing it into neurodynamic tension might be painful. Therefore it is suggested that the therapist apply a little oil and influence the resistance of and around the nerve by applying vertical movements onto the nerve and the surrounding structures. This technique may be progressed by combining it with nerve movement, influencing a larger range than the palpation technique.
- Pressure on the nerve during neurodynamic movement: The emphasis here is on the neurodynamics of the nerve itself, for example moving the hyoid bone caudally and laterally while holding the thumb on a branch of the suprahyoid hypoglossal nerve (that is slightly swollen when palpating the styloid process). A potential hypothesis to explain this technique is that intraneural transmitter substances such as cell fluids, blood with proteins and neurotransmitter might be mobilized. This may contribute to better health of the neural tissue and its surroundings. Within a context of information and education it may lead to positive results. A logical progression would be to combine transverse local techniques with neurodynamic movements.

SUMMARY

- Palpation of cranial nervous tissue needs to be viewed as a regular part of the assessment and management, combined with the results of subjective data, conduction and neurodynamic tests of the cranium and the rest of the body.
- Based on the tests performed, the therapist will gain information about the relevance and health of the nervous tissue, and may use the assessment technique as the basic treatment technique. However, these tests are not useful for all patients.
- A general overview of the pathobiologic mechanisms is necessary to interpret the relevance of differentiation tests, peripheral sensitization and previous nerve injuries. This might contribute to additional care and precautions (Table 18.2).

Table 18.2 General overview of advantages and disadvantages of various treatment approaches to influence the cranial nervous system

Treatment approach	Advantage	Disadvantage
Indirect		
Neural container	Local technique Minimal neural stress Many variations in neurodynamic positions possible	Local (neural) stress might be intense
Direct		
Neurodynamic		
Distal technique	Low load Easy to integrate in pain management activities (e.g. mental distraction)	Little control over neural container deficiencies
Proximal technique	Low irritability Influences neuraxis and the peripheral system of the extremities	When performed in neurodynamic positions it might produce large loads on the nervous system
Sliders	Low load to the nervous system Easily performed actively Good integration into pain management programmes	Neural container needs to be clear
Tensioners	Focus on tension in and around the nerve Neural containers experience less load than during sliders	Sometimes difficult to identify the critical site
Palpation	Strong local influence of neural container and local nervous tissue	Do not perform when situation is irritable or central mechanisms dominate the problem

GUIDELINES FOR DETERMINING THE INITIAL TECHNIQUE

If the therapist has decided to treat the patient with cranioneuromobilization techniques, the following parameters may guide the decision for the initial technique:

- Starting position: The patient should be positioned 'out of neural tension' or with only minimal stress on the cranial nervous system.
- Direct or indirect influence: Usually an indirect technique is chosen (neural container). Once the neurodynamic tests have improved, direct cranioneural mobilization may be preferred.
- Location and order: Which cranioneurodynamic test is first priority? Which is second and which is third? Generally the primary site of compression is chosen. This will also help to decide whether the proximal or the distal component should be moved first.
- Amplitude of movement: Large amplitudes are helpful whenever the nerve runs through a 'tunnel', when the trophic situation is insufficient and to reduce fear of movement. Small amplitudes within the resistance zone are used to improve stiffness of the neural tissue and to influence scar tissue and intraneural oedema (van den Berg 1999, Abenhaim et al 2000).
- Time and duration.
- Passive or active: As mentioned above, a passive technique is preferred initially since the dosage and impact are more easily controlled by the therapist.
- Target tissue test and/or rehabilitation: The therapist needs to control the function of the target tissue of the treated nerve and might need to include its functional rehabilitation.

CASE STUDIES

In this part of the chapter, two case studies are presented that show dysfunction of the cranial nervous system: one is of a patient with acute tissue injury and cranial neuropathy (Case study 1); in the other the patient suffers from prolonged chronic pain and neurological changes resulting in relevant physical dysfunctions (Case study 2). The examples intentionally show peripheral neurogenic problems to demonstrate that cranioneurodynamics may also contribute to improvement in this group of patients. These examples might be used as general guidelines for the treatment of the most common cranial neuropathies that are accompanied by physical dysfunctions.

Case study 1

Previous history

A 68-year-old male patient suffers from a facial paresis after salivary gland surgery to remove a benign tumour. Two weeks after surgery he realizes that some oral activities such as speech and swallowing have become difficult to perform. The worst problem for him is that saliva flows out of his mouth in public. His right eye feels dry and he cannot close it properly. After 4 weeks the situation remains unchanged and he worries that he may not improve. His surgeon reassures him that the symptoms will eventually disappear but the patient is not convinced. After 6 weeks he is still the same and discusses the problem with his GP who refers him to a specialized physiotherapy and manual therapy clinic (Fig. 18.5a).

Following the subjective and physical examination a subacute peripheral neuropathy of the facial nerve is diagnosed. Additionally, the patient fears worsening of the symptoms and does not appear well informed. Therefore it was decided to use mainly cranioneurodynamic techniques accompanied with information and a thorough patient management with long and short appointments.

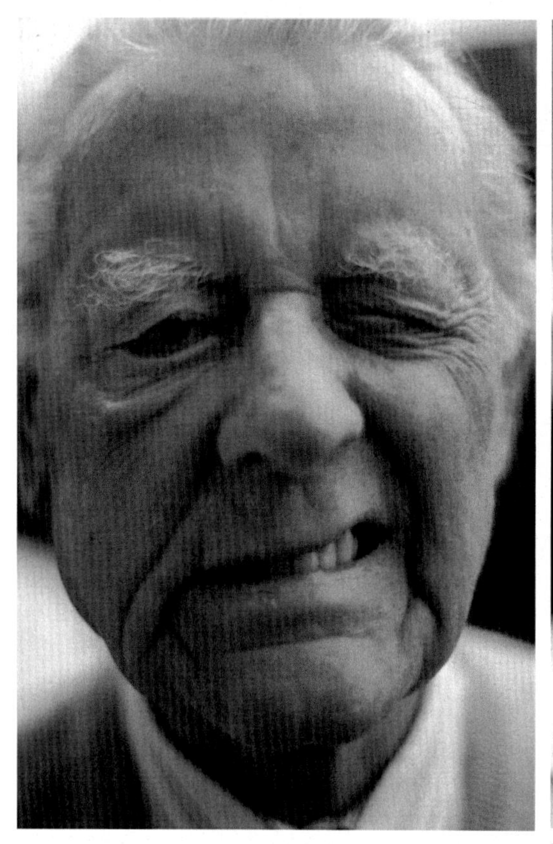

a

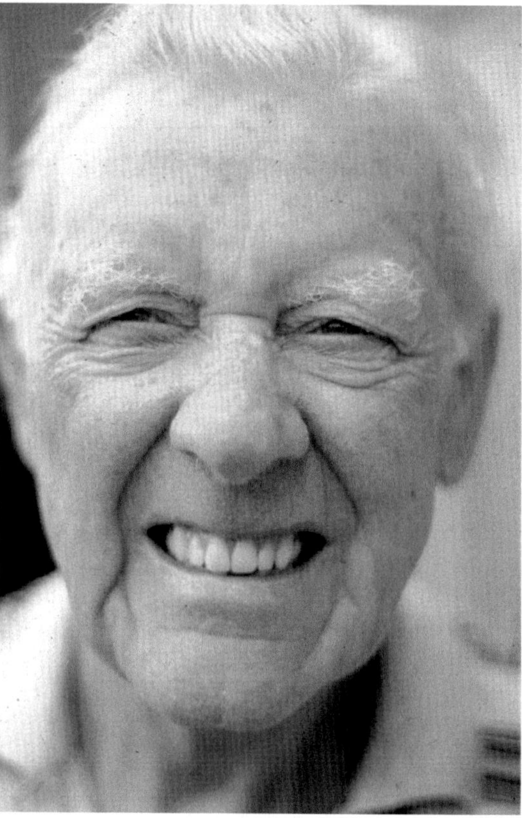

b

Fig. 18.5 A 68-year-old patient with a subacute peripheral neuropathy of the facial nerve.
a Stable condition during treatment.
b Six weeks after treatment.

Starting position

No matter which technique is used, a pain-free 'out of tension' position is chosen. For this patient craniocervical extension, ipsilateral lateroflexion and relaxed facial muscles are suggested.

Indirect passive techniques

The most important neural containers that might be the potential source of facial nerve dysfunction are assessed. In this case the temporal and petrous bones, potential scarring and the facial muscles are included. Which technique is applied depends entirely on the signs and symptoms and the clinical reasoning process of the therapist (wise action concept, see Chapter 1). In this case the main dysfunctions were found on rotation about the transverse axis of the right temporal bone and some scar tissue in front of the ear. These dysfunctions were treated by cranial mobilization of the temporal region and by stretching techniques around the scar tissue.

Direct techniques

- *Proximal component:* During the physical examination a minimal stiffness was found on craniocervical flexion and lateroflexion to the right. Proximal techniques were therefore not the first choice.

- *Sliders:* 'Distal' sliders without discomfort or pain and lateroflexion to the right alternated with activation of the facial muscles might be a good technique for this patient if the neural container techniques reduce the physical signs and symptoms. In this case the technique proved to be very helpful.
- *Order:* Initially the facial muscles are activated without neural tension (upper cervical extension, lateroflexion to the symptomatic side). During muscle relaxation the therapist gently moves the head into lateroflexion to the left.
- *Dosage:* In the subacute phase the technique is initially performed 'out of resistance' and without perceived discomfort. The duration is variable: it should not be performed for too long (minutes) but also for no less than 10 seconds. The position was chosen during the neurodynamic testing procedure. If the treatment duration was too long, even though it was performed pain-free, it may drastically change the symptoms immediately or cause neurogenic inflammation so that the symptoms will worsen over the following days. Only the optimum dosage of input will facilitate improvement during the subacute state (Rosen 1981, van den Berg 1999, Stelnicki et al 2000).
- *Other nerves:* Directly related nerves such as the trigeminal nerve (pain and facial muscles) and the vagus (X), glossopharyngeal (IX) and hypoglossal (XII) nerves should be assessed on both the affected and the unaffected side. Should they present any dysfunctions they may be integrated into the treatment. This patient did not show any dysfunctions.

Treatment by palpation

Transverse movement of the auricular posterior nerve and the proximal portion of the buccal nerve in a position of slight neurodynamic tension, plus slight pressure on the nerve while performing gentle neurodynamic mobilization of the facial nerve, improved oral muscle activity in various neurodynamic positions.

Target tissue re-education

The salivary glands can be exercised by dripping lemon juice onto the tongue. The patient is asked to note the amount of saliva production and to compare it before and after treatment with the non-affected side. The amount of lemon juice is increased with time and the resting time between stimulation is shortened.

In particular, the orofacial muscles can be facilitated in various neurodynamic positions. For example, craniocervical extension and ipsilateral lateroflexion helped this patient to pull up the right side of his mouth. However, as endurance training was required, he exercised this activity in frequent repetitions. Facilitation of the hypoglossal muscles and the tongue may also contribute to facial muscle activity improvement. The patient was taught to gently press his tongue against the roof of his mouth while practising, which immediately improved the activity of the orofacial muscles.

Home exercises

The described neurodynamic sliders and target tissue exercises were discussed and practised. The number of repetitions depended on the phase of the treatment and the effect of the exercises.

Results

The patient soon lost his feeling of hopelessness when he realized that after the first week his muscle function had clearly improved due to the neurodynamic unloading of the facial nerve and the tongue facilitation technique. Progression of the treatment included an increase of repetitions for each exercise: the neurodynamic mobilization and the palpation mobilization. After the third treatment the neurodynamic tension was increased and target tissue exercises enhanced.

The prognosis was good since this well-motivated patient reduced his fear and his physical dysfunctions after only two treatment sessions. After 6 weeks (two sessions per week) his situation was stable and he only retained some problems of muscle activity around his mouth when he felt tired (Fig. 18.5b).

Retrospectively it can be concluded that neurodynamic treatment within a biopsychosocial concept was what this patient needed for his pathology that usually shows a high percentage of self-healing (Honda et al 2002).

Case study 2

Previous history

A 38-year-old car mechanic had surgery 4 years ago to remove an acoustic neuroma in the cerebellopontine angle (CPA) that was detected because he suffered from headaches and toothache as well as hypertonic masticatory muscles, swallowing and balance dysfunctions and tinnitus. After the operation the symptoms were reduced significantly and he returned to work. Three years later, for no obvious reason, he experienced new symptoms such as diffuse deep headaches, deep toothache near the mandible and neck stiffness on flexion activities (e.g. getting into his car, reading, putting on his shoes). Furthermore he showed an involuntary muscle contraction ('tic') when his head was placed in a certain position. Acupuncture every 2 weeks helped initially but no longer has any effect, which is getting him worried. The neurologist claims that a second operation will not help and that medication is his only choice.

During the physical examination components of neurodynamic tests clearly provoked his symptoms. His head is constantly held in craniocervical extension and lateroflexion towards the symptomatic side (Fig. 18.6a). Correction of this position sets off his 'tic'.

The spontaneous contractions of the masticatory and facial muscles and the headaches occurred with delay (Fig.18.6b). Neck flexion is limited by a protective muscle spasm. During the standard slump test the same symptoms as when correcting the neck posture were provoked in an 'on/off' manner. Based on these results the clinical pattern matches 'tic douloureux' (Breig 1978). In this pathology the physical dysfunction of the cranioneural tissue including the trigeminal nerve plays an important role. The situation is stable and not irritable. The behaviour of the symptoms shows an 'input mechanism'. A suggested physiotherapy treatment focusing on neurodynamic techniques is described below.

Starting position

If an indirect technique is chosen and the signs do not change after the first session, the techniques in the second session may be performed in neurodynamic tension: craniocervical flexion and lateroflexion.

Indirect technique

The main neural containers – in this case the occipital bone, the craniocervical region (suboccipital scarring due to surgery), sphenoid bone and the mandible (neural container of the trigeminal nerve) – need to be assessed for dysfunction and treated if necessary.

Direct techniques

Sliders and tensioners

In this case a combination of 'sliders' and 'tensioners' is suggested, since intracranial scarring of the dura and other connective tissue structures (e.g. falx cerebri and tentorium) is suspected.

Proximal components

One might start immediately with the proximal components which include depression/elevation of the shoulder, sideglides (Elvey 1986) and/or mandibular depression/laterotrusion. If these techniques do not show the desired effect, cranial flexion and lateroflexion can be undertaken.

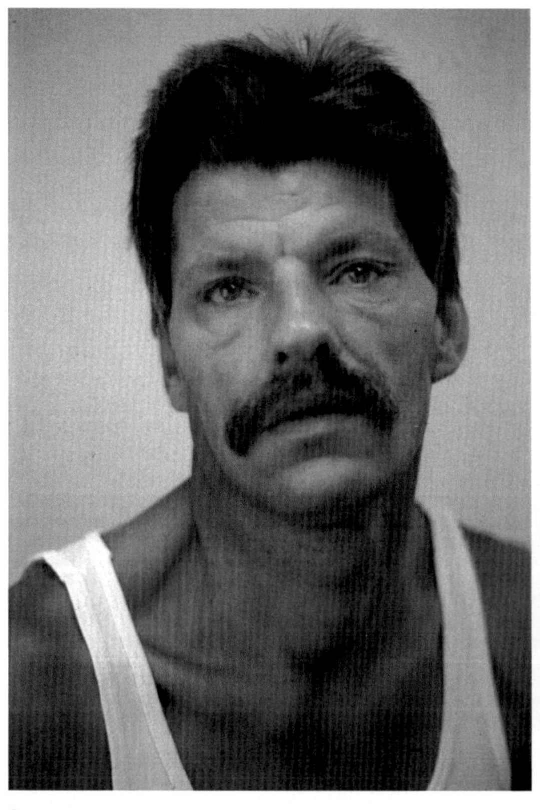
a

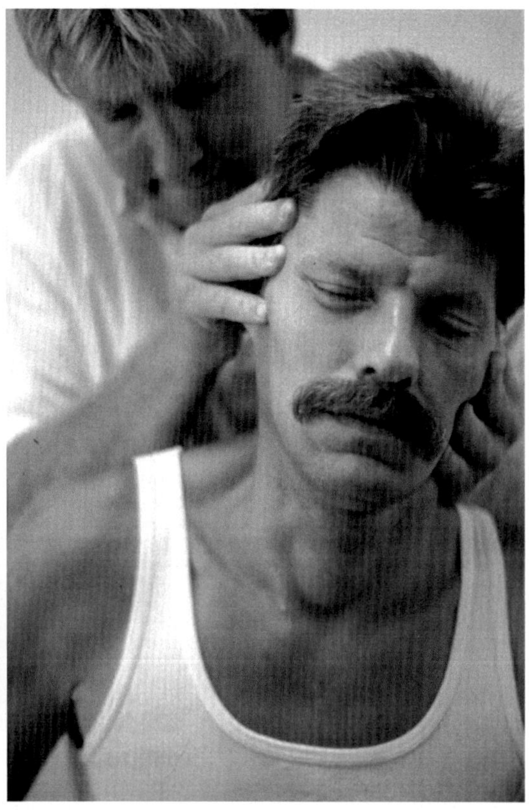
b

Fig. 18.6 A 38-year-old patient with physical dysfunction of the cranioneural tissue.
a Head position of the patient prior to treatment. Elevated tension of the neck and facial musculature is noteworthy.
b Correction of posture provokes tension and pain.

Sequence of movements

Since the problem appears to include cranioneurodynamic components, one should start with the proximal component, craniocervical flexion and lateroflexion. Combinations and order of sliders and tensioners that were applied in this case study were:

- Craniocervical flexion, lateroflexion and lumbar/thoracic flexion in sitting
- Craniocervical flexion, lateroflexion and shoulder depression in supine
- Craniocervical flexion, lateroflexion and long sitting slump (LSS)
- Mandibular laterotrusion, craniocervical flexion, lateroflexion and LSS.

Dosage

During the treatment the therapist has to be prepared to move into resistance but to also respect the patient's symptoms. Therefore the therapist needs to continuously communicate verbally or non-verbally with the patient to confirm that the symptoms are bearable for the patient. Neurological signs such as paraesthesia, numbness, cramping or fasciculations should not be provoked.

The frequency and duration depend on the patient's or the therapist's capacities. One would think in minutes rather than in

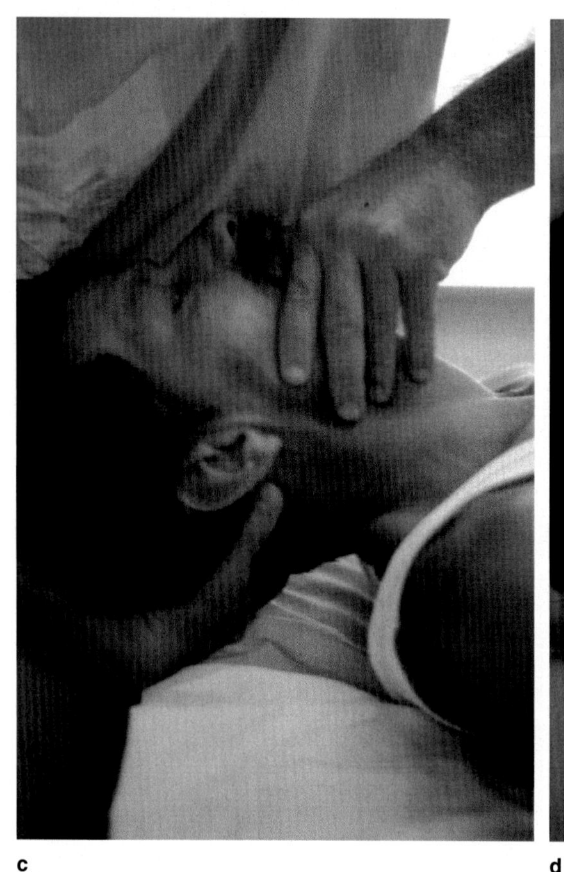

c

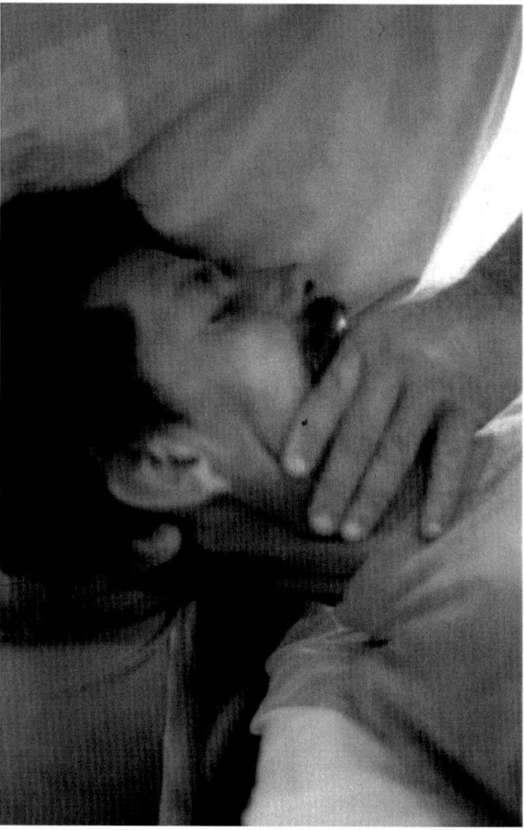

d

Fig. 18.6—cont'd
c Passive neck flexion prior to treatment.
d Passive neck flexion 6 weeks after treatment.

seconds, since a morphological change of a non-irritable situation is desired.

Other nervous tissue

Other cranial nerves that should be included are the facial nerve due to the patient's mimic expressions and the similar intracranial anatomical location with the trigeminal nerve; also the vestibulocochlear and hypoglossal nerves because of the previous history with the acoustic neuroma and the experienced symptoms (tinnitus and balance and swallowing dysfunctions).

Treatment technique: palpation

Palpation of the peripheral branches of the trigeminal (V), facial (VII) and hypoglossal (XII) nerves did not show any signs or symptoms. The intracranial tissue of the suboccipital region could obviously not be palpated.

Target tissue re-education

Static and dynamic coordination of the masticatory muscles (trigeminal nerve) and the facial muscles are assessed before and after neurodynamic treatment. If quality and endurance of the activity improves, the activity is automatically part of the home exercise regime.

Home exercises

If a neurodynamic technique results in an improvement that persists until the following session this neurodynamic technique is adapted as a home exercise. For this patient this included:

- Craniocervical flexion and lateroflexion in sitting; sliders alternated with tensioners
- Craniocervical flexion and knee flexion in LSS; sliders alternated with tensioners.

Target tissue exercises as described above are also integrated into the patient's home activities.

Results

After six sessions over 5 weeks the symptoms were reduced dramatically. Headaches and toothache showed reduced intensity and frequency after 3 weeks although the patient initially experienced exacerbated symptoms for 24 hours after the first two sessions. The perceived neck stiffness on flexion improved at the same time. Objectively, a greater range of movement was noted on craniocervical flexion (Fig. 18.6c,d). The 'tic' occurred less frequently but worsened in stressful situations. Nevertheless, the patient was looking forward to his return to work. Some sessions of acupuncture improved the 'tic' and 8 weeks after the initial treatment the patient returned to work full time.

SUMMARY

- **Various possibilities for cranioneurodynamic mobilizations are described and their advantages and disadvantages are discussed. Furthermore, active versus passive techniques and direct versus indirect techniques are presented.**
- **There is no 'recipe' for treatment method and dosage when treating cranioneurodynamic dysfunctions and pathologies.**
- **Due to the lack of scientific data in this relatively new field, the therapist needs to rely on open models of thinking such as clinical reasoning skills. Some treatment choices are presented in two case studies.**

References

Abenhaim L, Rossignol M, Valat J et al 2000 The role of activity in the therapeutic management of back pain. Spine 25:1

Austermann K 2002 Frakturen des Gesichtsschädels (Mittelgesichtsfrakturen) In: Schwenzer N, Ehrenfeld M (eds) Spezielle Chirurgie, Zahn-, Mund-, Kiefer-, Heilkunde, Bd. 2. Thieme, Stuttgart, p 339

Bogduk N 1981 An anatomical basis for the neck–tongue syndrome. Journal of Neurology, Neurosurgery and Psychiatry 44(3):202

Breig A 1978 Adverse mechanical tension in the central nervous system. Almqvist and Wiksell, Stockholm

Butler D 1991 Mobilisation of the nervous system. Churchill Livingstone, Melbourne

Butler D 2000 The sensitive nervous system. NOI Press, Adelaide

Butler D, Moseley L 2003 Explain pain. Noigroup Publications, Adelaide

Butler D, Shacklock M, Slater H 1994 Treatment of altered nervous system mechanisms. In: Boyling J, Palastanga M, Grieve S (eds) Modern manual therapy, 2nd edn. Churchill Livingstone, Edinburgh

Elvey R 1986 Treatment of arm pain associated with abnormal brachial plexus tension. Australian Journal of Physiotherapy 32:225

Elvey R 1997 Physical evaluation of the peripheral nervous system in disorders of pain and dysfunction. Journal of Hand Therapy 10:122

Gavilán J, Gavilán C 1986 Recurrent laryngeal nerve. Identification during thyroid and parathyroid surgery. Archives of Otolaryngology, Head and Neck Surgery 112:1286

Gifford L 1998 Neurodynamics. In: Pitt-Brooke J, Reid H, Lockwood J, Kerr K (eds) Rehabilitation of movement: theoretical basis of clinical practice. Saunders, London, p 159

Harding V 1997 Application of the cognitive-behavioural approach. In: Pitt-Brooke J, Reid H, Lockwood J, Kerr K (eds) Rehabilitation of movement: theoretical basis of clinical practice. Saunders, London, p 540

Honda N, Hato N, Takahashi H et al 2002 Pathophysiology of facial nerve paralysis induced by herpes simplex virus type 1 infection. Annals of Otology, Rhinology and Laryngology 111:616

Jabre J 1994 'Nerve rubbing' in symptomatic treatment of ulnar nerve paraesthesiae. Muscle and Nerve 17:1237

Kaas J, Florence S, Jain N 1999 Subcortical contributions to massive cortical reorganisations. Neuron 22:657

Kwan M, Wall E, Massie J, Garfin S 1992 Strain, stress and stretch of peripheral nerve. Rabbit experiments in vitro and in vivo. Acta Orthopaedica Scandinavica 63:267

Lang J 1995 Skull base and related structures: atlas of clinical anatomy. Schattauer, Stuttgart, p 31

Maitland G, Banks K, English K, Hengeveld E 2000 Vertebral manipulation, 6th edn. Butterworth-Heinemann, Oxford

Nathan P, Keniston R 1993 Carpal tunnel syndrome and its relation to the general physical condition. Hand Clinics 9:253

Okeson J 2005 Bell's orofacial pains, 6th edn. Quintessence, Chicago, p 435

Ramachandran V, Blakesee S 1998 Phantoms of the brain. William Morrow, New York

Rosen J M 1981 Concepts of peripheral nerve repair. Annals of Plastic Surgery 7(2): 165–171

Rosenfeld M, Gunnarson R, Borenstein P 2000 Early intervention in whiplash-associated disorders. Spine 25:1782

Shacklock M 2005 Clinical neurodynamics. A new system of musculoskeletal treatment. Elsevier, Edinburgh

Stelnicki E J, Doolabh V, Lee S et al 2000 Nerve dependency in scarless fetal wound healing. Plastic and Reconstructive Surgery 105(1): 140–147

Van den Berg F 1999 Angewandte Physiologie: Das Bindegewebe des Bewegungsapparats verstehen und beeinflussen. Thieme, Stuttgart, p 215

Von Piekartz H 2001 Neurodynamics of cranial nervous tissue (cranioneurodynamics). In: von Piekartz H, Bryden L (eds) Craniofacial dysfunction and pain, manual therapy, assessment and management. Butterworth-Heinemann, Oxford, p 116

Chapter 19

Headaches in children: the state of the art

Harry von Piekartz

CHAPTER CONTENTS

INTRODUCTION

Headaches are a growing problem in our society (Brna et al 2005). Therapists frequently find themselves stuck for an adequate answer to a seemingly simple syndrome such as juvenile headache. A detailed analysis has become necessary and frequent support from other medical disciplines is required. Some patients/ parents might turn to 'therapy shopping' as a consequence, which for many is a frustrating and unsatisfactory process (Überall 1999). This chapter aims to expand the knowledge of therapists about current research, epidemiological prevalence, pathophysiology and contributing factors to headaches in children. In Chapter 20, recommendations for the subjective and the physical examination as well as the management of this problem are discussed.

THE NATURE OF THE PROBLEM

Epidemiology

The prevalence of headache in children has increased considerably during the past 30 years. Between 10 and 20% of preschool children complain of headaches (Pothmann et al 2001). Frankenberg et al (1992) examined 7000 German pupils with headaches: they classified 60% as tension headaches and approximately 12% as migraines; 30% of the headaches could not be clearly classified.

Dutch researchers (Van Duin et al 2000) interviewed 2691 children under the age of 18 as well as their parents and concluded that:

- 46% of 6–16 year old children had headaches more than twice a year. However, these children did not perceive their headaches as a serious problem.
- 9% had disabling headaches and children as well as parents agreed that the medical profession was unable to give these children adequate attention.
- 10% had to discontinue sport or games; 2% took time off sport more than once a month.
- By applying the diagnostic criteria of the International Headache Society, 56% of these headaches could not be clearly classified and belong to the category 'normal' or 'unspecific' headaches.

Another Dutch study examining 2358 pupils between the ages of 10 and 17 years found that 21% of the boys and 26% of the girls in elementary schools and 14% of the boys and 28% of the girls in secondary schools had headaches at least once a week. Comparing these findings with a study from 1985, a 6% increase in the weekly complaints of headaches can be found (Bandell-Hoekstra et al 2001).

Most studies note a higher prevalence in girls (Deubner 1977, Linet & Stewart 1987, Wang et al 2005). An average age for the onset of migraines remains unknown. Sillanpää (1983) claims, after assessing and reassessing 2291 children from age 0 to age 7, that 20% of migraine headaches begin between these ages.

The occurrence of classic migraine is highest at the ages of 7–13 years (McGrath & Hiller 2001). Fifty per cent of juvenile migraine patients will continue to have migraines in adulthood (Bille 1981).

PAIN: DEFINITIONS AND CATEGORIES

Since we are discussing children with pain, the following are some thoughts on the phenomenon of pain itself. The International Association for the Study of Pain (IASP), a worldwide organization of experts from various disciplines, defined pain in 1994 as:

> 'an unpleasant sensory and emotional experience associated with actual or potential tissue damage or described in terms of such damage' (Classification of chronic pain, task force of taxonomy, IASP Press, 1994).

This definition underlines the importance of personal experience in the individual's pain perception. The following dimensions of pain have been described (Melzack & Katz 1994):

- The *sensory–discriminative* dimension, e.g. area, intensity, behaviour of pain
- The *affective–motivational* dimension, e.g. rage, anxiety, fear
- The *cognitive–evaluative* dimension, e.g. thoughts and beliefs.

These dimensions vary from person to person with regard to their individual interpretation and proportion. They reflect dynamic pathobiological processes. Children process their sensomotor inputs by applying the same dimensions but in a more straightforward and simple way (Skoyles 2006). There is evidence that children with migraines demonstrate a different affective–motivational dimension from children without migraines (McGrath & Hillier 2001). A summary of pain mechanism and pain perception categories is represented in the diagram by Melzack and Katz (1994) (Fig. 19.1).

In most cases it is helpful for the therapist to find out how the child describes its pain. For example, children under the age of 5 frequently identify their headaches as stomach ache.

Emotions and cognition of the child are sometimes expressed in dramatic drawings packed with expression. For example, Figure 19.2a is a drawing made by an 8-year-old girl who describes her headaches as being like a pony, which is tied firmly to a fence, that stamps with its hoofs. Another example shows

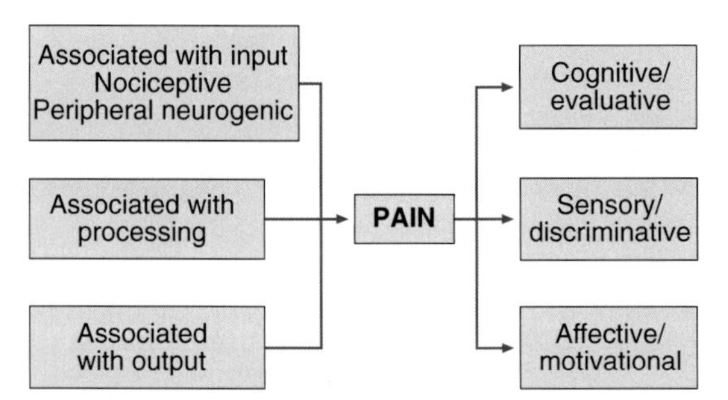

Fig. 19.1 Overview of pain mechanisms and individual pain experience (reproduced with permission from Melzack and Katz 1994).

how a 12-year-old boy perceives his headaches as being as if a knife stabbed into his brain. He also shows an unusual fear of weapons which could be due to the experience of his brother threatening him with a knife (Fig. 19.2b).

THE INTERNATIONAL CLASSIFICATION OF FUNCTION (ICF)

The World Health Organization (WHO) has proposed a classification of functions (ICF). Therefore the clinical examination of the child should also include a multidimensional functional examination.

The proposed model is based on the ICF and can easily be adapted for the examination of children with headaches. It is followed by an overview of the definitions found in the current literature (see also Chapter 1).

Impairment (tissue damage)

There is loss or deviation from the norm in the emotional, physiological or anatomical structure or function, for example skull asymmetry or divergence of the eyes.

Level of activity

This shows impairment of ability to perform a physical action, activity or task in a way that is efficient, typically expected or competent, for example lack of concentration and difficulties studying (Fig. 19.3).

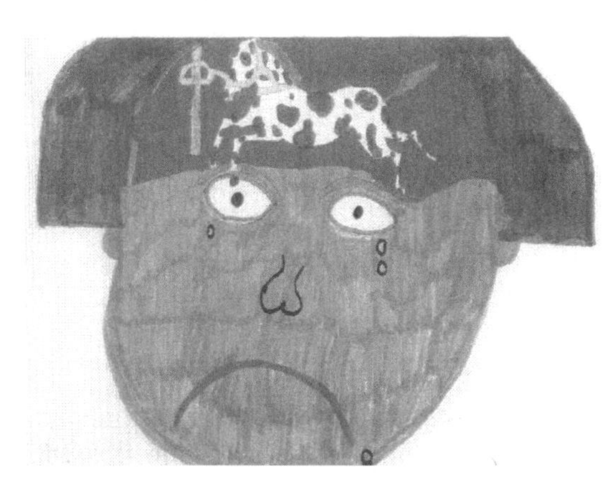

a

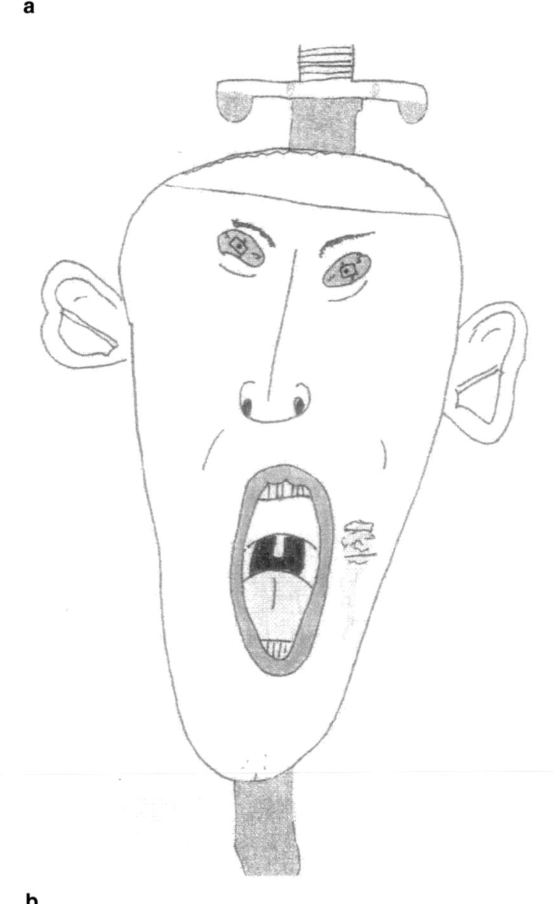

b

Fig. 19.2 Children's depiction of headache.
a Picture by an 8-year-old girl who describes her pain as a tethered pony stamping on the ground.
b A 12-year-old boy experiences pain as a knife being stabbed through his head.

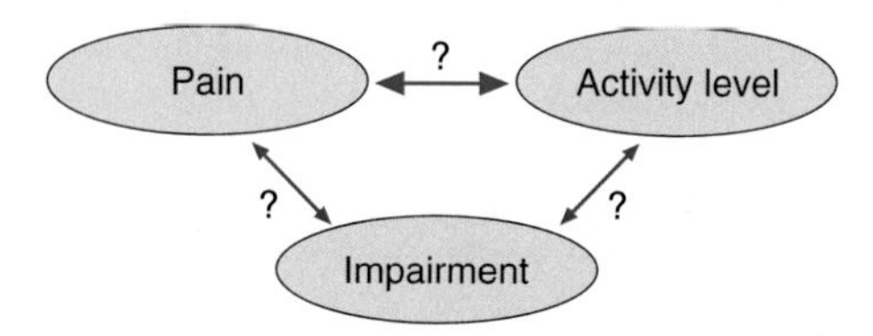

Fig. 19.3 With juvenile headaches there is frequently no direct relationship of pain, dysfunction/impairment and activity level.

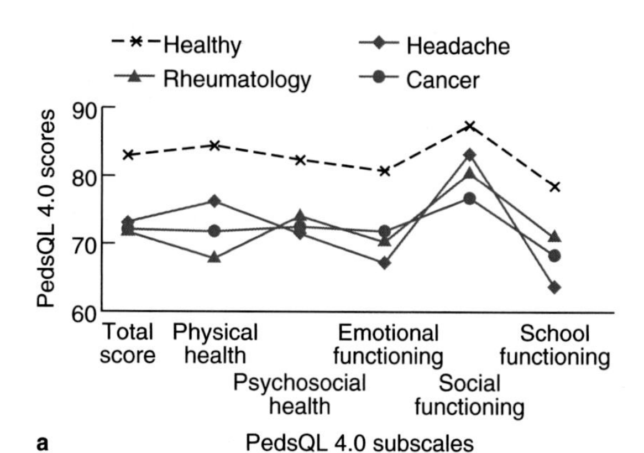

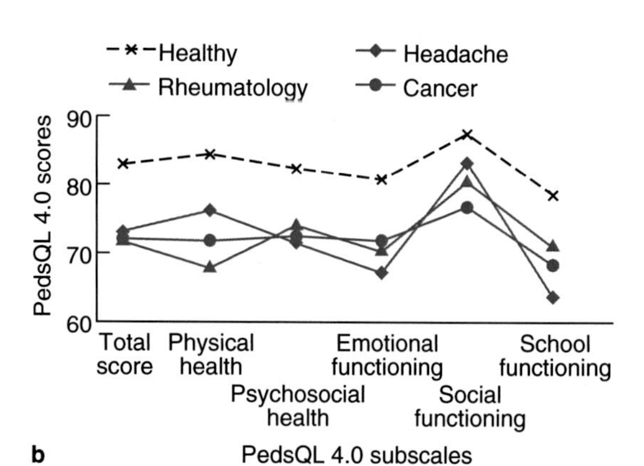

Fig. 19.4 Pedsol 4.0 child self-report scores across disease groups.

a Data presented for healthy children, children with headaches, and children with rheumatoid diseases and cancer. The full range of the PedsQL 4.0 is 0–100. This figure uses a more limited range presentation (reproduced with permission from Powers et al 2003).

b Pedsol 4.0 parent-report scores across disease groups with the same parameter as used in Figure 19.4a (reproduced with permission from Powers et al 2003).

Participation

Limitation of function within a certain social context and/or physical environment, for example the child backs away from sport activities and is happiest playing on its own.

The literature on chronic pain emphasizes that there is no proportional relation of pain, tissue damage and function in longstanding neuromusculoskeletal pain disorders (Waddell 1998). It is concluded from a survey study (Pediatric Quality of Life Inventory – PedsQL 4.0) conducted on 572 children with primary headache aged 8–15 years that headaches significantly affected their health (quality of life, QOL) (Powers et al 2003; Fig. 19.4). The impact of headaches on QOL appears to be similar to that found in other chronic illness conditions such as rheumatoid diseases and cancer. Of all impairments at school and in emotional functioning, headache is the most prominent (Powers et al 2003). This is also true for longstanding headaches in children. The consequence is that it can sometimes be difficult for the therapist to evaluate and to manage the pain and behaviour of the child (McGrath 2001) (see Fig. 19.3).

THE CHILD AND ITS EXPERIENCES WITH HEADACHES

Forty per cent of children and adolescents describe headaches as the main reason for suffering and disability in their day-to-day life, although the medical system classifies their symptoms as a dysfunction and not as a medical disease (McGrath 2001). Disability can be quantified by days off school and the amount of painkillers taken (Martin-Herz et al 1999). Girls seem to suffer more than boys (Bille 1981, Frankenberg et al 1992). Adolescents frequently claim that their social peers misunderstand their headache problems and this makes them feel isolated (McGrath 2001). For a better comprehension of the clinical features of juvenile headaches, the general characteristics of juvenile headache will be briefly discussed in the following paragraphs.

General characteristics of juvenile headaches

The properties of headache, including accompanying symptoms, vary from child to child. The most common characteristics of juvenile headache are described below.

PAIN PATTERN

- Time and intensity: Pain is usually experienced over several hours (1–6 hours). Intensity can be measured using a coloured analogue scale (CAS) and has an average value of 5.9 (McGrath & Koster 2001).
- Localization: Typical localization is frontal and temporal.
- Quality: Mostly throbbing, dull pain; booming and pulsating in younger children.

CONCOMITANT SYMPTOMS

Most children have typical concomitant symptoms such as nausea and vomiting, which are a criterion for migraine; nausea is often not present during an attack.

DISABILITY

The majority of children do not consider their headache to be a significant day-to-day problem. For this reason parents may also not seek help for a first mild attack of headache in their children. This can then become a contributing factor for chronic headache (McGrath 2001).

Diagnostic classification of juvenile headache

The classification of juvenile headache is based on the recommendations of the International Headache Society (IHS) (Soyka 1999). The majority of headaches belong to the two main categories: migraine and tension headaches.

Table 19.1 provides an outline of the diagnostic classification of the IHS (International Classification of Headache Disorders-II [ICHD-II], IHS 2004). Note that:

- Migraine and tension headaches are code numbers 1 and 2 of the ICHD-II, indicating that they the highest in the hierarchy of headache types.
- Migraine headache in childhood (code 1.3) is a separate entity.
- Migraine headache is promoted to stage 3 instead of stage 5 in the ICHD-I (IHS 1988).

SOME CRITICAL COMMENTS ON THE INTERNATIONAL HEADACHE SOCIETY (IHS) CLASSIFICATION

The current literature criticizes the International Classification of Headache Disorders (ICHD), published in 1988, as being outdated, claiming that the system does not account for all types of juvenile headache.

Some facts:

- Maytal stated that 92.4% (high sensitivity) of children without migraine were classified correctly but that this was only the case for 27.3% of migraine patients (low specificity). He concluded that the IHS criteria do not necessarily apply for children with headaches (Maytal et al 1997, Viswanathan et al 1998).
- Wöber-Bingöl et al (1996) evaluated the validity of the IHS classification in 156 children and adolescents who had been diagnosed as tension headache patients. They came to a similar result, with the IHS classification showing a high sensitivity and a low specificity (Wöber-Bingöl et al 1996).

It can be construed that the IHS and other classification systems do not give a clear indication of the aetiology of primary headache in children. At present, Olesen's (1997) modified recommended classification is used clinically, for which the intensity and number of symptoms present are adjusted (Table 19.2).

In 2004, the second edition of the International Classification of Headache Disorders (ICHD-II) was released. These criteria provided improved recognition of childhood

Table 19.1 ICHD-II classification code and WHO ICD-10 code

ICHD-II	Diagnosis	WHO ICD-10
1	**Migraine**	**G43.9**
1.1	Migraine without aura	G43.0
1.2	Migraine with aura	G43.1
1.2.1	Typical aura with migraine headache	G43.10
1.2.2	Typical aura with non-migraine headache	G43.10
1.2.3	Typical aura without headache	G43.104
1.2.4	Familial hemiplegic migraine	G43.105
1.2.5	Sporadic hemiplegic migraine	G43.105
1.2.6	Basilar-type migraine	G43.103
1.3	Childhood periodic syndromes that are commonly precursors of migraine	G43.82
1.3.1	Cyclical vomiting	G43.82
1.3.2	Abdominal migraine	G43.820
1.3.3	Benign paroxysmal vertigo of childhood	G43.821
1.4	Retinal migraine	G43.81
1.5	Complications of migraine	G43.3
1.5.1	Chronic migraine	G43.3
1.5.2	Status migrainous	G43.2
1.5.3	Persistent aura without infarction	G43.3
1.5.4	Migrainous infarction	G43.3
1.5.5	Migraine-triggered seizures	G43.3
1.6	Probable migraine	G43.83
1.6.1	Probable migraine without aura	G43.83
1.6.2	Probable migraine with aura	G43.83
1.6.5	Probable chronic migraine	G43.83
2	**Tension-type headache (TTH)**	**G44.2**
2.1	Infrequent episodic TTH	G44.2
2.1.1	Infrequent episodic TTH associated with pericranial tenderness	G44.20
2.1.2	Infrequent episodic TTH not associated with pericranial tenderness	G44.21
2.2	Frequent episodic TTH	G44.2
2.2.1	Frequent episodic TTH associated with pericranial tenderness	G44.20
2.2.2	Frequent episodic TTH not associated with pericranial tenderness	G44.21
2.3	Chronic TTH	G44.2
2.3.1	Chronic TTH associated with pericranial tenderness	G44.22
2.3.2	Chronic TTH not associated with pericranial tenderness	G44.23
2.4	Probable TTH	G44.28
2.4.1	Probable infrequent episodic TTH	G44.28
2.4.2	Probable frequent episodic TTH	G44.28
2.4.3	Probable chronic TTH	G44.28

headache in the migraine (primary headache) group. The important criteria are:

- Expanded duration of attacks from 1 to 72 hours, but still possessing the features of a throbbing or pulsating headache of moderate to severe intensity with exacerbation with physical activity.
- Pain localization can be bifrontal or bitemporal. Occipital pain requires further assessment.
- Migraine-associated symptoms include nausea or vomiting (or both), or light and sound sensitivity. Additionally, the criteria allowed for parental inference of these associated symptoms.

Table 19.2 International Headache Society diagnostic criteria for migraine in children younger than 15 years of age

Migraine without aura	Migraine with aura
At least five attacks Duration 4–72 hours At least two of the following: • Unilateral • Pulsating quality • Moderate to severe intensity • Exacerbation by activity At least one of the following: • Nausea, vomiting or both • Photophobia or phonophobia	At least two attacks At least three of the following: • At least one fully reversible aura • Symptoms indicating focal, cerebral, cortical or brainstem dysfunction • At least one aura symptom developing gradually for > 4 minutes or > 2 symptoms in succession • No aura > 60 minutes • Headache begins before, simultaneously, or within 60 minutes of aura

Adapted from Olesen (1997).

Recent reliability studies of the ICHD-II suggest that, in idiopathic headache in children under 6 years of age, the ICHD-II is too restrictive for migraine with aura and tension headache (Balottin et al 2005). The same conclusion is made in chronic headache in children under 16 years of age (Wiendels et al 2005). In addition, a recent study on the sensitivity of ICHD-II in paediatric migraine suggests further revisions and modifications (Hershey et al 2005).

PRIMARY AND SECONDARY HEADACHES

A headache is called a primary headache if the mechanisms and the nature of the problem are directly responsible for the symptoms. Examples of primary headaches are migraines and tension headaches (codes 1–4 of the ICHD-II).

Secondary headaches (code 5 of the ICHD-II – headache attributed to head and/or neck trauma – and above) are headaches due to indirect causes and mechanisms, suggesting that the IHS consider this to be a less common category of headaches. It has also been shown that classification of secondary headache using the IHS definitions is more difficult than for primary headache (Überall 1999).

There is evidence that secondary headaches might be caused by, for example, maxillary sinusitis or impaired vision. Otitis media (middle ear infection) or musculoskeletal dysfunctions are possible causes for migraines and tension headaches. Existing headache symptoms can be made worse by these impairments (Pothmann et al 1994, 2001).

A number of juvenile headache syndromes cannot be categorized by current classification systems. It has been observed clinically that many children with headaches also show accompanying symptoms such as motor, balance and psychosocial problems. Many of these disorders are associated with the craniocervical region and with scoliosis and hip displacements (Biedermann 1999, 2004).

In summary it can be concluded that the aetiology of juvenile headaches (primary, secondary and mixed) is not fully understood and there is to date no precise classification system. To fully comprehend children's pain experience and the resulting pain behaviour, multicausal and integrative clinical reasoning of the treating therapist is required. The so called 'onion-ring model' by Loeser (1980) that

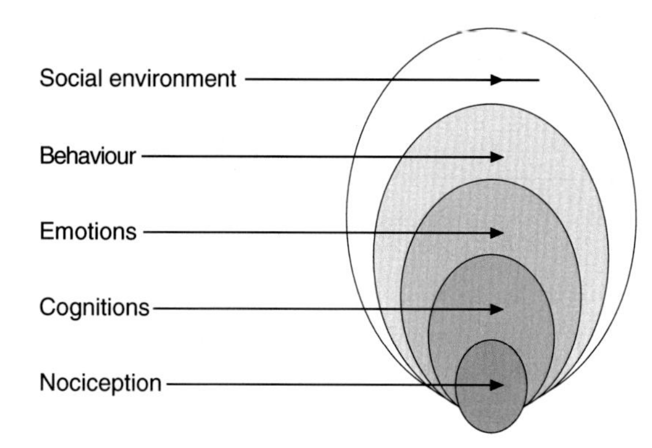

Fig. 19.5 Biopsychosocial levels of pain experience (according to Loeser 1980).

is frequently used to explain complicated longstanding pain, as found in fibromyalgia and non-specific low back pain, can also be helpful for the assessment of juvenile headache sufferers (Fig. 19.5).

The described headache dimensions can also be applied to juvenile headache syndromes. In order to completely understand and correctly assess an existing pain problem, the therapist needs to follow several hypotheses that represent the various aspects of the pain problem. Case study 1 explains this procedure.

Case study 1

Elena is a 16-year-old girl who suffered from recurrent ear infections (nociception) between the ages of 6 and 10 years. Her parents were told by the ENT doctor and by other parents to keep Elena away from water, noise and cold wind. Whenever she started to complain of ear pain they wrapped her up warm, worrying that the symptoms might otherwise get worse. She was not allowed to go horse riding or join her usual gymnastics class. Her parents made her stay at home whenever she was feeling ill. Usually the ear pain went away after a week and she did not need to take antibiotics. If the pain remained for longer, her family doctor prescribed antibiotics. Now, at 16 years of age, she still suffers from regular ear pain and headaches.

A year ago, the specialist undertook several diagnostic procedures including x-rays, computed tomography and clinical examination, but did not find any residual inflammation (nociception). Nevertheless, Elena claims that she suffers at least 10 acute episodes of head and ear pain each year. Her behaviour when she gets the pain is similar to that of her parents: she believes the problem will get worse (cognition) and feels anxious for that reason (emotion). She always wears warm jumpers during the painful episodes, even in summer, and tells everyone not to come too close because they might catch her germs (behaviour, social contacts). She usually stays at home for a couple of days because she believes this is essential to her recuperation. When at home, she stays up later than usual which she enjoys. When she does this, she knows that the pain will be gone within 2 days, so she does not need painkillers (cognition).

Clinical thoughts

This example shows that Elena has learned from her parents' behaviour and its positive consequences (freedom from pain). The positive effect is possibly that she continues to apply the same coping strategies as when she was aged between 6 and 10 years. She does not know any other strategy than this, and it has always been successful. Why should she change anything when it eases her pain? She probably still believes that her symptoms are caused by inflammation, because the pain is the same.

According to Loeser, the therapist will need to assess all levels of the pain experience. There is evidence that chronic ear infections at school age can cause morphological changes of the cranium leading to stress transducing dysfunctions. These are contributory factors for unilateral ear pain (Oudhof 2001, Spermon-Marijnen &

> Spermon 2001). The mucosa of ear and nose might also sensitize the nervous system without themselves being inflamed (Okeson 2005). A thorough manual therapy assessment is certainly indicated but coping strategies and emotional factors (fear) should also be considered, and management strategies for these applied if necessary.

HYPOTHESIS CATEGORIES AND RECURRENT JUVENILE HEADACHES

As mentioned above, the aetiology of juvenile headaches remains unknown (McGrath 2001). Multistructural and multicomponent influences are often difficult to identify. The logical consequence is that there is no commonly accepted plan for the diagnostic procedure in children with headaches. The only option for the therapist is to work in collaboration with the child and its parents, to include the parents' views in the therapeutic decision-making process, to aim for mutual goals and to agree on management strategies. This procedure is called 'collaborative clinical reasoning' (Jones & von Piekartz 2001). The therapist's role is one of a coach who guides the dynamic interaction between parent and child. The task is to categorize the information obtained, to consider clinical patterns and to evaluate its contents according to hypotheses formulated (Jones & von Piekartz 2001, Maitland et al 2001). This concept has been dealt with in greater detail in Chapter 1.

Contributing factors to recurrent headaches in children

One of the main topics in the literature about juvenile headaches is the role of contributing factors. To gain an insight into the aetiology of the symptoms, to develop management strategies and to be able to make prognostic decisions, the therapist needs to assess the contributing factors towards the individual headache syndrome.

Contributing factors have been defined as:

> 'any predisposing factor involved in or directly responsible for the development or persistence of a patient problem'. This includes psychosocial, genetic, anthropometric and ergonomic factors (Gifford 1998, Butler 2000).

These might be found in various different fields, for example in biomechanics, the environment or psychology. These factors are also called 'yellow flags' (Gifford 1999, McGrath & Koster 2001).

Some contributing factors have been described explicitly for juvenile headache patients. The most important are listed below. Contributing factors are categorized as:

- History
- Emotional and psychological influences
- Acquired factors
- Daily life activities
- Musculoskeletal factors
- Growth factors.

HISTORY

- Genetic: Prevalence rises by 64% if one parent suffers from headaches and by 98% if both parents suffer (Messinger et al 1991).
- Bad general health, depression, malnutrition and sleep disorders during childhood are predisposing factors for headaches later in life (Aromaa et al 1998).
- Children with a history of traumatic experiences such as sexual, verbal, physical abuse, recurrent illnesses, death of a family member or divorce of the parents, show a higher prevalence of (chronic) facial pain syndromes (Curran et al 1995, Goldberg et al 1999, Yucel et al 2002).

EMOTIONAL AND PSYCHOLOGICAL INFLUENCES

- Emotional factors such as anger caused by stressful situations at school and colds have an important role (Pothmann et al 1994).
- Daily hassles (Soyka 1999) and personality structures, such as hypersensitivity and anxious personalities, as well as depressive moods (Andrasik et al 1988).

- Neurovegetative instability, high ambitions and perfectionism have been shown to correlate with headaches (Vahlquist & Hucknell 1949, Bille 1981). Children with anxiety and depression have more frequent headaches (principally migraine) than children without these character traits; prevalence is higher among females than males (Rhee 2005).

ACQUIRED FACTORS

- Influence of parental care on increase or decrease of the symptoms. In the management of children with headaches the emphasis often lies more on external influences such as air quality, nutrition, etc rather than psycho-emotional factors like fear and aggression (Joffe et al 1983, Andrasik et al 1988).
- Model learning through copying the behaviour of family members is contentious and presumably not genetic (Überall 1999).

DAILY LIFE ACTIVITIES

- Sleeping habits can potentially influence headache symptoms. In particular, chronic sleep deficits, irregular sleep, restless sleep or frequent short sleep periods throughout the day have been shown to contribute to headache problems in adults and in children (Bruni et al 1997, Paiva et al 1997, Feikema 1999).
- Bright sunlight and high temperatures are better, changes in air pressure, noise, crowds, and excessive running during physical activities are worse (McGrath & Koster 2001).
- Greasy foods such as chocolate, eggs, nuts, cheese, as well as milk and wheat products, affect the neurobiology of the juvenile organism which might lead to headache symptoms (Dalton & Dalton 1979, Leviton et al 1984).
- Dehydration or caffeine intake in the evening (e.g. Coca-Cola, coffee) can potentially influence headaches (Feikema 1999).
- Children with parafunctions of the temporomandibular joint or with chewing habits (chewing gum, tongue biting, cheek biting, nail biting) and children who talk a lot or play a musical instrument might be at risk of developing bruxism, clenching of the jaws and headaches (Molina et al 2001).
- Atlanto-occipital dysfunctions in nursing children have been described as predisposing factors for the development of headaches later in life (KISS syndrome, Biedermann 2001a).
- Posture (i.e. head forward posture) or irregular breathing patterns combined with altered craniofacial morphology (Vig et al 1981, Linder-Aronson & Woodside 2000) have been put forward as 'triggering factors' for persistent headaches (see Chapter 21).

GROWTH

Juvenile headaches, especially migraines, can be accompanied by growth-dependent changes in the neurobiological processing of the brain. This becomes apparent if the response to a repeated stimulus is too strong or lasts for too long. Habituation is a protection from overstimulation of the brain that sometimes does not act adequately and produces headache symptoms in some children (Kropp 2000).

SLEEP DISORDERS – ONE OF THE MAIN CONTRIBUTING FACTORS

There are different patters of interaction between headaches and sleep disorders:

- Primary sleep disorder; headaches are usually secondary symptoms
- Primary headaches which lead to sleep disorders
- Both problems are present but have separate pathological causes
- Headaches and sleep disorders with a strong interactive correlation.

A study by Paiva et al (1997) found that 55% of juvenile headache patients showed a significant sleep disorder. It was striking that headache children on average show shorter night sleeping times and wake up more frequently than non-headache children. They also feel more tired in the mornings and do not settle to sleep as easily (Bruni et al 1997). Another study describes a correlation of headaches and sleep disorders with fear and depression (Kowal & Pritchard 1990, Passchier & Andrasik 1993, Miller et al 2003).

Caffeine intake late in the day, dehydration, long resting times during the daytime or watching television before going to bed might be directly responsible for sleep disorders (Feikema 1999). Accompanying symptoms can be (mainly for migraines): nightmares, sleep talking, restless sleep and bruxism (Bruni et al 1997).

THE INFLUENCE OF COGNITIVE-EMOTIONAL-BEHAVIOURAL FACTORS

In the literature it has been stated that emotional and cognitive factors strongly influence the behaviour of children with headaches.

Patricia McGrath, an American researcher and psychologist, has investigated this specialized area for years and published a descriptive study, stating exactly which cognitive and emotional factors can play a dominant role for recurrent headaches in children.

A summary of the study with the following topics is shown in Box 19.1:

- Cognitive factors
- Beliefs about pain control
- Emotional factors
- Behavioural factors.

Based on pain mechanism models a clear correlation between input, output and processing factors becomes obvious.

Box 19.1 Cognitive and affective factors that influence repetitive juvenile headaches

Cognitive factors
- Beliefs about ethology
- Patient and parents believe that the headaches have a certain cause
- Not understanding the primary and secondary causes
- Belief that the environment triggers the symptoms
- Expectation that the headaches will be maintained in the future

Lack of trust in pain control
- Little knowledge of possible medication
- Little knowledge of alternative therapies
- Belief that the child needs to rest or sleep during an attack
- Belief that no treatment will be successful
- Beliefs about the influence of stress
- Limited belief that stress might trigger the symptoms
- Limited knowledge of stress factors for the child
- Little appreciation of high achievement expectations

Emotional (affective) factors
- Specific stress situations (e.g. school, traffic, personal contacts)
- Emotional suppression or denial of pressures
- Fear of high achievement expectations
- Fear of a non-diagnosed condition
- Fear of a life-threatening condition
- Fear of increasing symptoms and disability
- Distress during a headache
- Frustration that symptoms are unpredictable
- Frustration that activities are limited (child and family)
- Not understanding why medicine cannot cure the headaches

Behavioural features
- Behaviour of child and parents during an attack
- Inconsequent behaviour of the parents
- Ineffective use of pain medication
- Withdrawal from school, sports and social activities
- Reduction of daily family activities
- Reactions of the parents that promote illness behaviour and stimulate limitations
- Reactions of the parents to the recurrence of headache symptoms
- Primary confidence in medication
- Diagnostic assessment
- Constant search for direct environmental factors influencing the condition

A model of factors influencing recurrent juvenile headache

The proposed model aims to represent the current paradigms of the individual therapist and the physiotherapy profession in general, including knowledge and evidence from other disciplines. It is designed to support therapists, parents and patients in the process of analysing the dominant influences that have contributed to the individual headache problem (Fig. 19.6).

Neuromusculoskeletal dysfunction and its relationship to juvenile headache

The neuromusculoskeletal system is a potential factor in headache which cannot be clearly diagnosed (around 30%) (Biedermann 2001b). Both clinical experience and the literature (Biedermann 1999, von Piekartz 2001) give some key indications as to why the musculoskeletal system should be considered as an important contributing factor to recurrent juvenile headache. In the author's opinion neuromusculoskeletal impairment should also be considered in this model.

When following this model the therapist is guided towards the applicable assessment and management strategies:

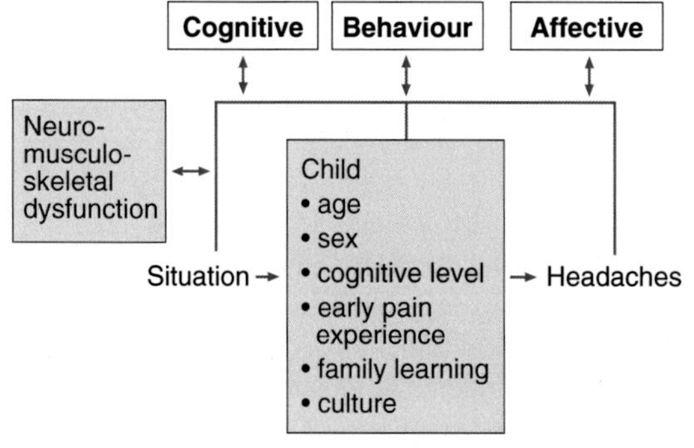

Fig. 19.6 Work model for possible influences on juvenile headaches (modified from McGrath 2001).

- Structured subjective assessment including pain measurements.
- Assessment and treatment of physical dysfunction of the musculoskeletal system. The changes seen in the reassessment are also helpful parameters for parents as it helps them to understand the treatment strategy.
- Proof that symptoms can be intentionally provoked and reproduced.
- Development of a consistent 'plan of action' for acute pain episodes.
- Identify and desensitize stress increasing/inducing situations.

The therapist needs to gain an insight into the multilayered components of the individual headache syndrome to ensure successful treatment and management.

SUMMARY

- Although the prevalence of juvenile headache is increasing, its aetiology remains unclear. The IHS does not appropriately classify juvenile headaches.
- Multifactorial influences such as posture, stress, fear, daily routines and diurnal habits are potential contributing factors for recurrent and ongoing headache syndromes.
- A thorough insight into the pathobiological mechanisms as well as the pain mechanisms, including emotional and cognitive factors of child and parents, are important for assessment, treatment and management.
- The neuromusculoskeletal system might be a powerful contributing factor and should be incorporated into the clinical reasoning model.

References

Andrasik F, Kabela E, Quinn S et al 1988 Psychological functioning of children who have recurrent migraine. Pain 34:43–52

Aromaa M, Sillanpää M L, Rautava P, Helenius H 1998 Childhood headache at school entry: a controlled clinical study. Neurology 50:1729–1736

Balottin U, Termine C, Nicoli F et al 2005 Idiopathic headache in children under six years of age: a follow-up study. Headache 45(6):705–715

Bandell-Hoekstra I, Abu-Saad H, Passchier J et al 2001 Prevalence and characteristics of headache in Dutch schoolchildren. European Journal of Pain 5:145

Biedermann H (ed.) 1999 Biomechanische Besonderheiten des occipito-cervicalen Überganges bei Kindern. In: Manualtherapie bei Kindern. Enke, Stuttgart, p 19

Biedermann H 2001a Primäre und sekundäre Schädelasymmetrie bei KISS-Kindern. In: von Piekartz H (ed.) Kraniofaziale Dysfunktion und Schmerzen: Untersuchung – Beurteilung – Management. Thieme, Stuttgart, p 45

Biedermann H 2001b Manual therapy in children: with special emphasis on the upper cervical spine. In: Vernon H (ed.) The craniocervical syndrome. Butterworth-Heinemann, Oxford, p 207–231

Biedermann H 2004 Manual therapy in children. Churchill Livingstone, Edinburgh

Bille B 1981 Migraine in childhood and its prognosis. Cephalalgia 1:71–75

Brna P, Dooley J, Gordon K, Dewan T 2005 The prognosis of childhood headache: a 20-year follow-up. Archives of Pediatric and Adolescent Medicine 159(12):1157–1160

Bruni O, Fabrizi P, Ottaviano S, Cortesi F 1997 Prevalence of sleep disorders in childhood and adolescence with headache: a case-control study. Cephalalgia 17:492–498

Butler D 2000 The sensitive nervous system. Noigroup Publications, Adelaide

Curran S, Sherman J, Cunningham L et al 1995 Physical and sexual abuse among orofacial pain patients: linkages with pain and psychological distress. Journal of Orofacial Pain 9:340

Dalton K, Dalton M E 1979 Food intake before migraine attacks in children. Journal of the Royal College of General Practitioners 29:662–665

Deubner D 1977 An epidemiologic study of migraine and headache in 10–20 year olds. Headache 17:173

Feikema W J 1999 Hoofdpijn en chronisch slaaptekort – een vaak miskende relatie bij kinderen en volwassenen. Nederlands Tijdschrift voor Geneeskunde 143(38):1897–1900

Frankenberg S, Pothmann R, Müller B et al 1992 Epidemiologie von Kopfschmerzen bei Schulkindern. In: Köhler B, Keimer R (eds) Aktuelle Neuropädiatrie. Springer, Berlin, p 433

Gifford L 1998 Pain, the tissues and the nervous system: a conceptual model. Physiotherapy 84:27

Gifford L 1999 Biopsychosocial assessment and management: relationships and pain. CNS Press, Falmouth

Goldberg R, Pachas W, Keith D 1999 Relationship between traumatic events in childhood and chronic pain. Disability and Rehabilitation 21:23–30

Hershey A D, Winner P, Kabbouche M A et al 2005 Use of the ICHD-II criteria in the diagnosis of pediatric migraine. Headache 45(10):1288–1297

International Headache Society 1988 Headache Classification Committee of the International Headache Society. Classification and diagnostic criteria for headache disorders, cranial neuralgias and facial pain. Cephalalgia (Suppl 7):1–96

International Headache Society 2004 Headache Classification Subcommittee of the International Headache Society. The International Classification of Headache Disorders. Cephalalgia (Suppl 1):9–160

Joffe R, Bakal D A, Kaganov J 1983 A self-observation study of headache symptoms in children. Headache 23:20–25

Jones M, von Piekartz H 2001 Clinical reasoning – a basis for examination and treatment in the cranial region. In: von Piekartz H (ed.) Craniofacial dysfunction and pain: manual therapy, assessment and management. Butterworth-Heinemann, Oxford

Kowal A, Pritchard D 1990 Psychological characteristics of children who suffer from headache: a research note. Child Psychology and Psychiatry 31:637–649

Kropp P 2000 Zur Psychobiologie von kindlichen Kopfschmerzen. Migräne – Störung zerebraler Reifung? Symposium Medical 30

Leviton A, Slack W V, Masek B, Bana D, Graham J R 1984 A computerized behavioral assessment for children with headaches. Headache 24:182–185

Linder-Aronson S, Woodside D G 2000 Excess face height malocclusion: etiology, diagnosis and treatment. Quintessence, Chicago

Linet M S, Stewart W F 1987 The epidemiology of migraine headache. In: Blau J N (ed.) Migraine: clinical and research aspects. Johns Hopkins University Press, Baltimore, p 451

Loeser J D 1980 Perspectives on pain. In: Turner P (ed.) Clinical pharmacy and therapeutics. Macmillan, London, p 313

Maitland G D, Hengeveld E, Banks K, English K 2001 Maitland's vertebral manipulation, 6th edn. Butterworth-Heinemann, Oxford

Martin-Herz S P, Smith M S, McMahon R J 1999 Psychosocial factors associated with headache in junior high school students. Journal of Pediatrics and Psychology 24:13–23

Maytal J, Young M, Shechter A, Lipton R 1997 Pediatric migraine and the International Headache Society. Neurology 48:607

McGrath P 2001 Headache in children: the nature of the problem. In: McGrath P, Hillier L (eds) The child with headache: diagnosis and treatment. IASP Press, Seattle, p 1

McGrath P, Hillier L (eds) 2001 Treatment of recurrent headache: an effective strategy for primary care providers. In: The child with headache: diagnosis and treatment. IASP Press, Seattle, p 159

McGrath P, Koster L 2001 Headache measures for children: a practical approach. In: McGrath P, Hillier L (eds) The child with headache: diagnosis and treatment. IASP Press, Seattle, p 29–56

Melzack R, Katz J 1994 Pain measurement in people in pain. In: Wall P D, Melzack R (eds) Textbook of pain, 3rd edn. Churchill Livingstone, Edinburgh, p 337

Messinger H B, Spierings E L, Vincent A J 1991 Overlap of migraine and tension-type headache in the International Headache Society classification. Cephalalgia 11:233–237

Miller V A, Palermo T M, Powers S W, Scher M S, Hershey A D 2003 Migraine headaches and sleep disturbances in children. Headache 43(4):362–368

Molina O M, Santos Dos J, Mazetto M et al 2001 Oral jaw behaviors in TMD and bruxism: a comparison study by severity and bruxism. Journal of Craniomandibular Practice 19(2):114–123

Okeson J 2005 Bell's orofacial pains, 6th edn. Quintessence, Chicago, p 435

Olesen J 1997 International Headache Society classification and diagnostic criteria in children: a proposal for revision. Developmental Medicine and Child Neurology 39(2):138

Oudhof H A J 2001 Skull growth in relation to mechanical stimulation. In: von Piekartz H J M, Bryden L (eds) Craniofacial dysfunction and pain. Butterworth Heinemann, Oxford

Paiva T, Farinha A, Martins A, Batista A, Guileminault C 1997 Chronic headaches and sleep disorders. Archives of Internal Medicine 157:1701

Passchier J, Andrasik F 1993 Migraine: psychological factors. In: Olesen J, Tfelt-Hansen P, Welch K M A (eds) The headaches. Raven Press, New York, p 233–240

Pothmann R, von Frankenberg S, Müller B, Sartory G, Heilmeier W 1994 Epidemiology of headache in children and adolescents: evidence of high prevalence of migraine among girls under 10. International Journal of Behavioral Medicine 1:76–89

Pothmann R, Luka-Krausgrillz U, Seemanns H, Naumann E 2001 Kopfschmerzbehandlung bei Kindern Schmerz. Schmerz 15:265–271

Powers S, Patton S, Hommel K, Hershey A 2003 Quality of life in childhood migraines: clinical impact and comparison to other chronic illnesses. Pediatrics 112:1–5

Rhee H 2005 Relationships between physical symptoms and pubertal development. Journal of Pediatric Health Care 19(2):95–103

Sillanpää M 1983 Changes in the prevalence of migraine and other headaches during the first seven school years. Headache 23:15–19

Skoyles J R 2006 Human balance, the evolution of bipedalism and dysequilibrium syndrome. Medical Hypotheses 66(6):1060–1068

Soyka D 1999 60 Jahre Migraineforschung. Retrospektive und Synopsis. Schmerz 13:87–96

Spermon-Marijnen H E M, Spermon J R 2001 Manual therapy movements of the craniofacial region as a therapeutic approach to children with long-term ear disease. In: von Piekartz H J M, Bryden L (eds) Craniofacial dysfunction and pain. Butterworth Heinemann, Oxford, p 22–45

Überall M A 1999 Pharmakologische Akuttherapie der migraine bei Kindern. Der Schmerz 13(Suppl 1):37–38

Van Duin N P, Brouwer H J, Gooskens R H J M 2000 Kinderen met Hoofdpijn. Een onderschat Probleem. Medisch Contact 55:26

Vig P S, Sarver D M, Hall D J, Warren D W 1981 Quantitative evaluation of nasal airflow in relation to facial morphology. American Journal of Orthodontics 79:263–272

Viswanathan V, Bridges S, Whitehouse W, Newton R 1998 Childhood headaches: discrete entities or continuum? Developmental Medicine and Child Neurology 40:544

von Piekartz H 2001 Kraniofaziale Dysfunktion und Schmerzen: Untersuchung – Beurteilung – Management. Thieme, Stuttgart

Waddell G (ed.) 1998 The problem. In: The back pain revolution, Churchill Livingstone, Edinburgh, p 1–8

Wang S J, Fuh J L, Juang K D, Lu S R 2005 Rising prevalence of migraine in Taiwanese adolescents aged 13–15 years. Cephalalgia 25(6):433–438

Wiendels N J, van der Geest M C, Neven A K, Ferrari M D, Laan L A 2005 Chronic daily headache in children and adolescents. Headache 45(6):678–683

Wöber-Bingöl C, Wober C, Karwautz A et al 1996 Tension-type headache in different age groups at two headache centers. Pain 67:53–58

Yucel B, Ozyalcin S, Sertel H O et al 2002 Childhood traumatic events and dissociative experiences in patients with chronic headache and low back pain. Clinical Journal of Pain 18(6):394–401

Chapter 20

Assessment, evaluation and management of juvenile headache patients

Harry von Piekartz

CHAPTER CONTENTS

INTRODUCTION

Based on Chapter 19, suggestions for subjective examination, pain measurement, physical examination and management strategies will be presented and discussed. As the ideas presented are the result of many years of clinical experience as well as a review of current literature, they should be easy to integrate into daily practice. The reader will probably recognize a number of the techniques described in this book. Please note how they have been adapted for the treatment of often very young children.

Subjective examination and pain measurement

INTERVIEWS AND QUESTIONNAIRES

The subjective examination is usually an interview with the child and its parents. It is essential to include the parents or at least one parent so that the therapist can gain an insight into the previous experiences, knowledge and behaviour of both the child and the parents. The initial therapy session is therefore of great importance since it usually provides the greatest informational content.

There are a variety of interview styles to choose from. One method favoured by many physiotherapists is an open dialogue with the child and its parents. Spontaneous information is collected and later categorized according to its content. The advantage of an open dialogue is that the headache patient and their carers can express their very personal experience of the situation and usually provide valuable 'directly to the point' information about impairment, function and participation (Maitland et al 2001), uninfluenced by the interviewer.

Another interview style is one that is based upon predesigned documentation forms such as questionnaires or pain diaries, a method providing detailed information on exactly the topics relevant to the therapist. The advantages of this procedure are that:

- It supports the diagnostic procedure of the headache type
- It collects and analyses potential contributing factors and therefore is helpful in management and prognostic procedures
- It provides an individual reassessment tool
- A number of questionnaires have been previously tested for reliability and validity
- The collected data may be used for research purposes.

The major disadvantage of this method is its rigidity. Spontaneous information cannot be included and important clinical information might be lost (Jones & von Piekartz 2001, Jones & Rivett 2004). The most important questions, which may be addressed either in a spontaneous interview or by questionnaire, are outlined below.

The questions are divided into sections as follows:

- Localization and type of juvenile headache
- Triggering situations and associated symptoms
- Contributing factors.
- Effect of headache on daily life.

Localization and type of juvenile headache

- How would you describe the headache?
- Do all headaches feel the same?
- Where do you usually feel the headache?

Body chart

Name:.. Profession:..........................

DOB: .... Hobbies:..........................

Diagnosis: ....

GP: ....

Date of first assessment: ....

Physiotherapist: ....

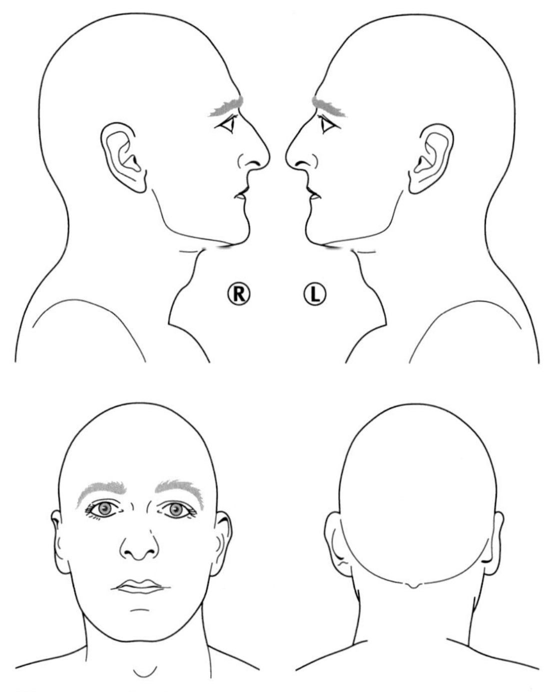

Fig. 20.1 Body chart.

A body chart of a head or a ball the size of a child's head is a helpful tool for the assessment of the site of the pain (Fig. 20.1).

The European Workgroup for Manual Medicine (EWMM) has developed a questionnaire especially for use with children suffering from complaints related to a craniocervical dysfunction caused during or after birth. This questionnaire enables the therapist to distinguish children with cervicogenic dysfunction and pain from those with other craniofacial dysfunctions (including juvenile headache). An overview of the EWMM questionnaire is provided in Appendix 1 (p. 612).

Pain measurement and documentation

Pain measurement tools have been researched in the literature over the past 10 years. Some have been evaluated for reliability and validity (McGrath et al 1995). There are three types of measurement tool:

- Biological measures (how the body reacts)
- Behavioural measures (what the child does)
- Self-documentation measures (what the child says).

BIOLOGICAL MEASURES

Neurobiological reactions such as pulse and vagus activity are recorded during a short intense pain stimulus (Porter et al 1988, McIntosh et al 1993). Even the release of cortisone can be measured during brief pain exposure (Gunnar et al 1981).

BEHAVIOURAL MEASURES

Tools for the measurement of behaviour are usually checklists of a variety of expected pain behaviours. They document the individual behavioural response of the patient and are useful protocols for the assessment of change, for example the effect of treatment (McGrath & Koster 2001). Behavioural measures may also provide information about the level of function; however, these tools do not necessarily correlate with self-documentation measures (Beyer et al 1990).

An example for a behaviour scale is the 'non-communication children's pain checklist' (McGrath & Koster 2001). This was designed for use with mentally and physically disabled children who are unable to communicate verbally. This tool can also be helpful for the assessment of juvenile headache patients and can be used by therapists as well as by parents (see Appendix 2, p. 614).

SELF-DOCUMENTATION MEASURES

There are a variety of self-documentation tools that can be useful for the measurement of juvenile headaches during or after the treatment. Which tool to use depends on the type of information that is relevant at the time, for example to explain or to gain insight into a problem, reassessment or data for evidence-based practice. The age and personality of the child will also influence the choice of assessment tool.

Examples of self-assessment tools include the following:

Pain scales

Research has shown that visual analogue scales (VAS) as well as numerical rating scales (NRS) and verbal rating scales are all reliable tools for the assessment of school-age children (Abu-Saad 1990, Tesler et al 1991). Verbal rating scales (the third scale in this text) can be applied as early as age 5.

Visual analogue scale

The patient is asked to mark their level of pain on a 10 cm line, for example: 'Draw a cross on the line to show me how much it hurts' (Fig. 20.2). The very left of the line represents very little or no pain at all; the further right, the more intense the pain.

Numerical rating scale

'Give me a number that says how bad your headache is' (Fig. 20.3).

Verbal rating scale

'Draw a line that shows how bad your pain is' (Fig. 20.4).

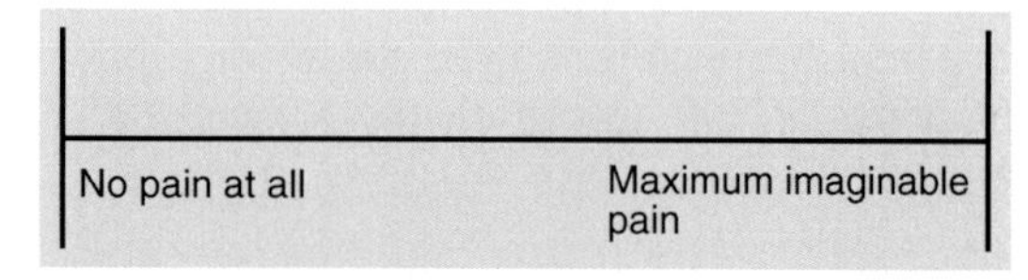

Fig. 20.2 Visual rating scale.

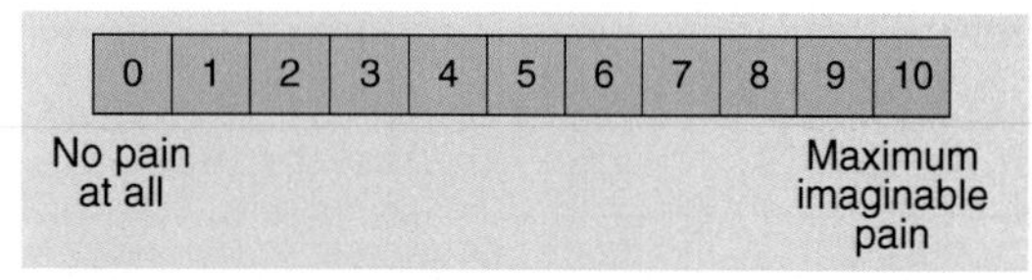

Fig. 20.3 Numerical rating scale.

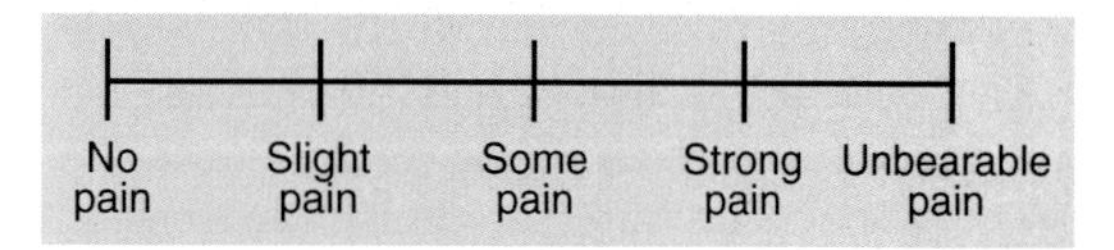

Fig. 20.4 Verbal rating scale.

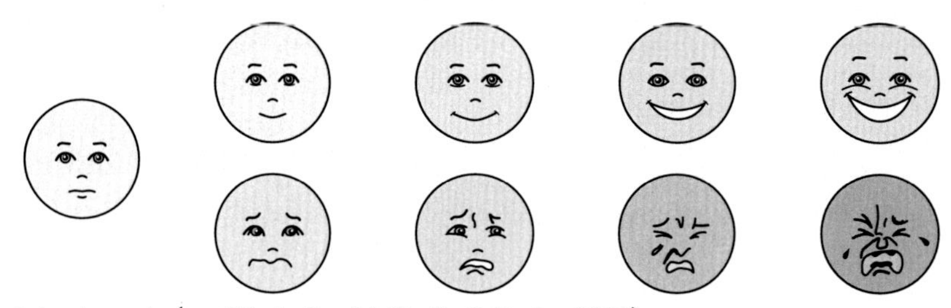

Fig. 20.5 Facial pain scale (modified after McGrath & Koster 2001).

Facial scale for pain measurement

This can be used for the assessment of children as young as 4 years of age (Hester 1979). Two versions are used: the original scale (Bieri et al 1990) and the reduced version with one face less. Both have shown a high level of reliability and validity at different pain intensities and syndromes in children (Hicks et al 2001). The faces express how badly something hurts: the face on the left represents 'no pain'; the face on the far right shows 'unbearable pain'.

'Show me the face that best expresses how much pain you feel' (Fig. 20.5)

Colour analogue scale

The colour analogue scale (CAS) is another method to measure pain intensity. The scale itself has a slider which shows a colour band on one side and a number on the other. The child indicates their level of pain using the colour scale. A clinical trial on children with recurrent headaches showed an average pain intensity of 6.5 (McGrath & Koster 2001) (Fig. 20.6).

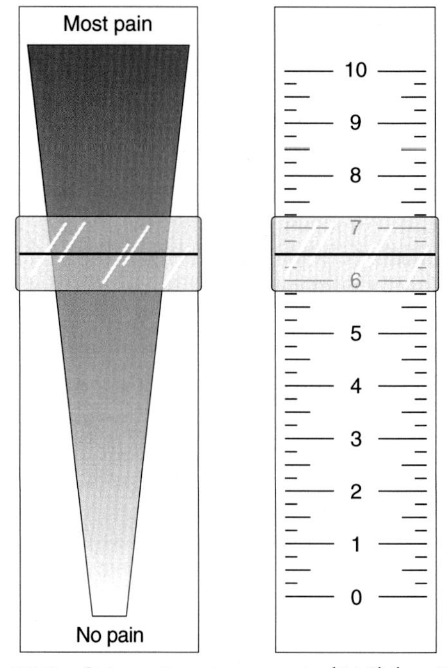

Fig. 20.6 Coloured analogue scale (CAS) (modified after McGrath & Koster 2001).

Facial affective scale

Children with headaches show significantly more psychological and emotional problems than children without headaches (McGrath & Hillier 2001). To gain an insight into the psychological components of the headache syndrome, this measurement tool can provide helpful information (Fig. 20.7).

'I am going to say some words that people use when talking about their headaches. Do you feel that any of these words describe your headaches: sad, anxious, distressed, angry, scared, worried.'

A number of drawn facial expressions are then shown to the patient who is encouraged to choose the one that represents best how they feel about the pain: 'Search deep down before you decide on one picture'.

DIARIES

With chronic headache syndromes it is sometimes useful to ask patients to complete pain diaries (see Appendix 3, p. 615). There is a diagnostic, a therapeutic and an evaluative dimension to pain diaries. This method is particularly useful to highlight experiences

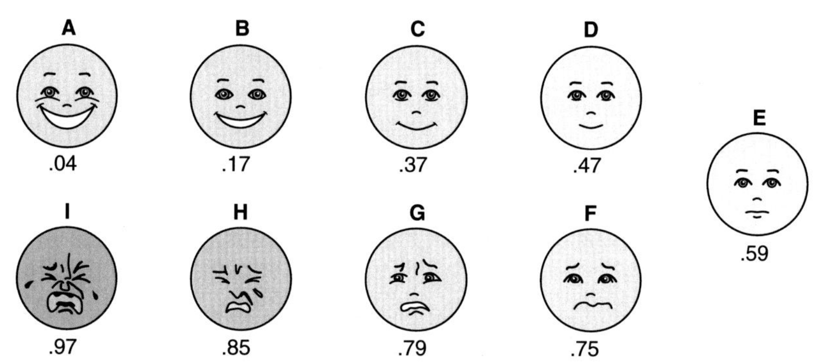

Fig. 20.7 The facial scale and correspondence with the VAS numerical scale.

the child might have forgotten or simply not mentioned. It enhances self-management strategies since changes in the daily routine become obvious as soon as they occur (Denecke & Kröner-Herwig 2000).

Advantages of diary use

The therapist will gain a thorough insight into the daily life activities of the child and can therefore evaluate the level of activity and participation (International Classification of Function categories). Since the information is provided over a longer stretch of time the therapist is in a position to assess the effect of treatment interventions retrospectively and can adapt the treatment plan if necessary.

Disadvantages of diary use

Children who do not normally keep a diary may find it a great effort to write up their experiences every day. An already structured day (school, homework, sports, hobbies) might become even more overloaded with such a new task. For a better overview the diary will need to be updated every day and it is asking a great deal of discipline from the child and its parents to do so. This method is not applicable for children under the age of 4 and children older than 14 tend to dislike 'childish things' like diaries. The measurement is restricted to pain intensity, duration and frequency of the headache episodes and does not measure disability (McGrath & Koster 2001). Therefore the therapist will need to assess whether to use a pain diary (see Appendix 3, p. 615) or one of the above-mentioned pain measurement tools.

THE CONTINUUM MODEL AS A BASIS FOR PHYSIOTHERAPEUTIC TREATMENT OF JUVENILE HEADACHE

The continuum model

Since longstanding headache syndromes are usually the result of a variety of causes and structures, it is important for the therapist to narrow down the potential causes. Olesen (1991) and Nelson (1994) have developed the continuum model for benign chronic headaches, which concurs with the current paradigms in physiotherapy. A detailed description for further reading can be found in Westerhuis (2001). The following is a brief summary of the most important aspects.

Following this model, headaches depend on the activity of the *nucleus trigeminus.* Its activity increases or decreases with:

- Nociceptive peripheral neurogenic input: This includes the neuromuscular system of craniocervical, mandibular and facial structures with dura mater and mucosa of the sinus cavities (Olesen 1991).
- Vascular impulses: The connective tissue surrounding the blood vessels is capable of transferring nociceptive information by the means of neurogenic inflammation which might set off the trigeminal nerve (Buzzi & Moskowitz 1991, 1992). This might serve as an explanation for the frequently described pulsating pain quality (Mongini 1999, Westerhuis 2001).

- The degree of inhibition of neuromodulators: Serotonin is important here.

The effect of serotonin on vascular sources of pain is not yet fully understood, particularly in the incompletely developed vascular system of children (McGrath 1990, Moskowitz 1990). Thinking and coping strategies for headache can channel emotions and determine the results in terms of the release of pain modulators such as opiates, serotonin and noradrenaline (Giesler et al 1994).

The clinical consequences are that headache in general is not determined solely by the input mechanisms, but that there is also a clear central processing component. These may, for example, include neurobiological changes in the brainstem, or in higher brain regions, influenced by affective and cognitive factors (Maytal et al 1995).

For the therapist, this means:

- Thorough examination, evaluation and individual treatment of the relevant structural craniocervical or craniofacial dysfunction to reduce peripheral nociceptive input
- Evaluation and reduction of contributing factors
- Cognitive-behavioural strategies to influence pain-modulating chemicals.

Figure 20.8 shows a model that includes the cognitive-behavioural approach.

Physiotherapy strategies for juvenile headache patients

The normal 'harmonic' and balanced development of a child implies optimum growth and progress of all structures and dimensions (biological, motor, intellectual and emotional). During the process of growing up, sensitive phases occur that indicate the development of new skills, which can be individually supported should an intervention be necessary (Kropp 2000, Zeltzer & Schlank 2004). These phases are necessary to progress to the next

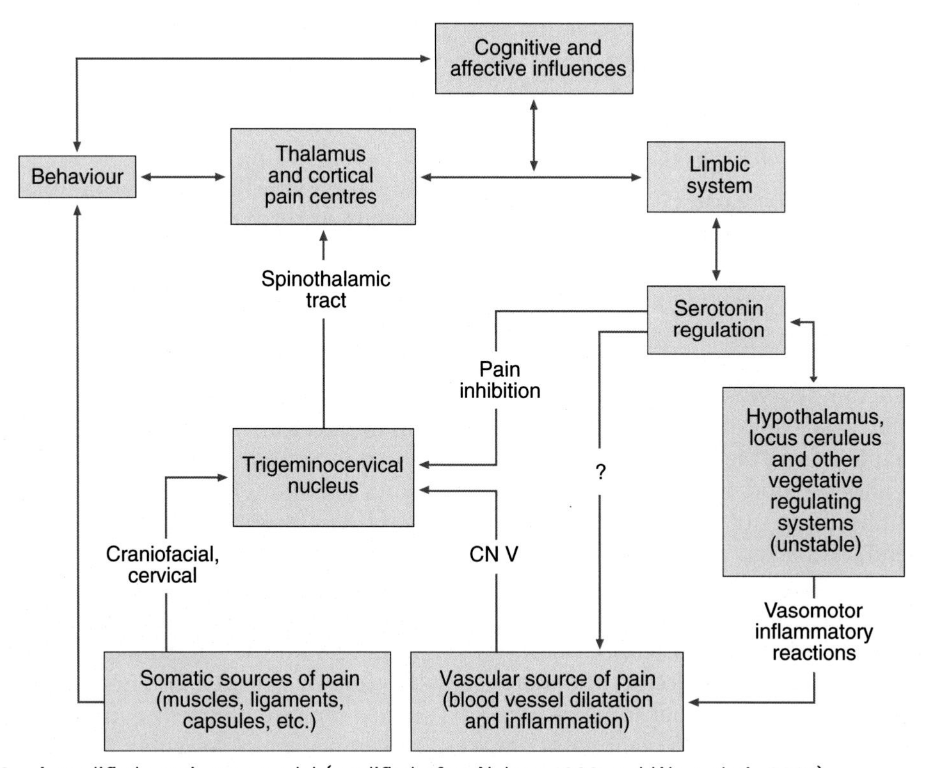

Fig. 20.8 A modified continuum model (modified after Nelson 1993 and Westerhuis 2001).

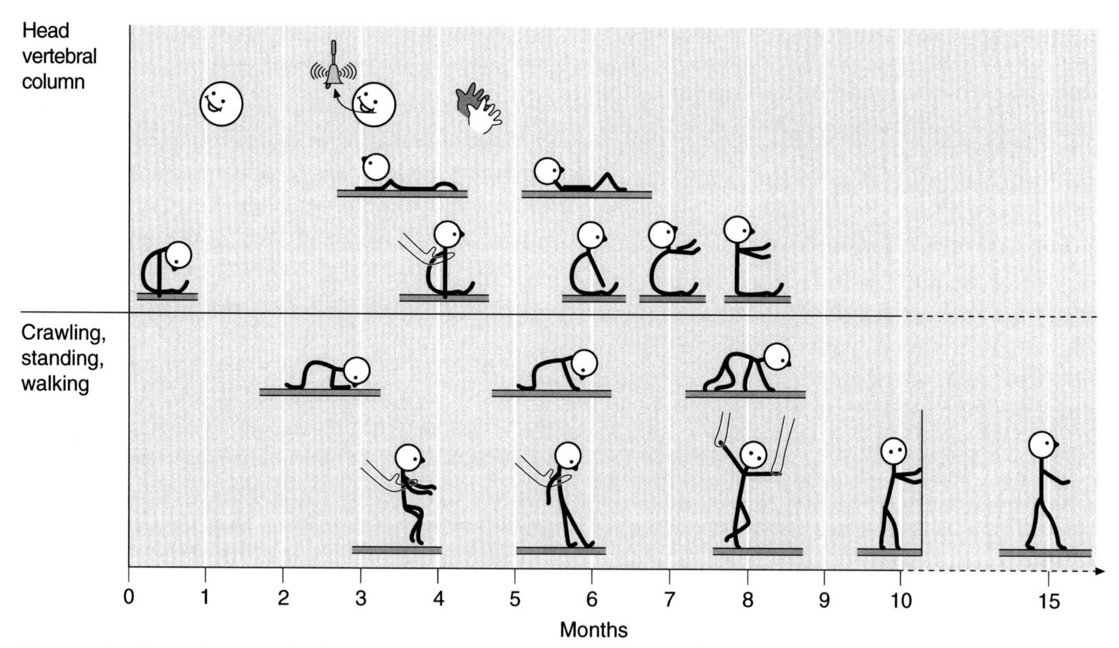

Fig. 20.9 Normal motor development in infants and small children (modified after Mumenthaler 1990).

stage of development, for example motor development (Fig. 20.9). This modified model by Mumenthaler (1990) presents an overview of the sensomotor development of a baby from 0 to 15 months. It is, for example, beneficial for the baby to begin its motor development in prone and supine positions before starting to crawl. Children who have skipped crawling and proceed straight to walking show a tendency towards static and dynamic coordinative retardation (Zukunft-Huber 1998).

COMMENT

The various paths of child development are well researched and documented. However, the author is not aware of any authors that describe the interaction of the development of the various body parts and sensomotor skills. For example, a number of authors have investigated craniofacial growth or the steps of sensomotor development, but there is very little basic literature on the effects of craniofacial dysfunction on sensomotor skills and vice versa. If a child skips crawling, will that potentially influence its craniofacial development? Are there any patterns emerging?

Furthermore, cognitive and behavioural aspects appear to play a dominant role in pain syndromes but whether cognitive and psychological development influences the prevalence of pain syndromes later in life is barely mentioned in the literature.

It might be due to the unclear aetiology of juvenile headaches that these specialized regions remain separated, which does not help in the search for adequate management of these problems (McGrath 2001).

Is there a solution?

The surprising conclusion of 10 years of pain science is that one can now prove that typical coping strategies, history, personality, suffering, etc. have an influence on the development and course of chronic pain (Gifford 1999). An increasing number of physiotherapists working in the neuromusculoskeletal field have started to integrate this current knowledge on chronic pain into practice, which in turn offers a new perspective on well-known problems.

Physiotherapists have started to adopt the new paradigms and have expressed the need for a different perspective on the management of children with chronic headaches. If you would like to look further into this topic, the books *Pediatric Chiropractic* (Anrig & Plaugher 1998), *Manual Therapy in Children* (Biedermann 1999, 2004), *Chiropractic Paediatrics* (Davies 2000) and *Craniofacial Dysfunction and Pain* (von Piekartz 2001) provide detailed information. In the author's opinion some headaches might be a strategy for the child to gain more attention. This can be challenging for the therapist who needs to assess the complex clinical picture by applying both clinical and theoretical knowledge. Due to the increasing interest in juvenile headaches and the knowledge gained from recent publications, there is now hope for a better understanding and treatment of children with headaches in the near future.

Physical examination

The following paragraphs outline the author's suggestions for a thorough physical examination. The results of the physical examination will be the treatment parameters for each individual headache problem and will guide clinical reasoning. The list of regions to be examined only covers the main primary structures that are possible sources of the symptoms. It is by no means an extensive list and cannot account for the wide variety of headache syndromes for each child's individual dysfunction.

The following regions will be covered:

- Craniocervical region
- Craniofacial region
- The nervous system: nerve conduction of cranial nerves/neurodynamics of craniocervical nerves
- Equilibrium.

CRANIOCERVICAL REGION

The craniocervical region is defined as the top three vertebrae and the occiput and their arthrokinematic influences (Pennings 1995). A dysfunction of these complex structures can potentially influence the weight-bearing function of the cranium during growth or even trigger the trigeminal nucleus, resulting in long-lasting nociceptive inputs (Biedermann 1999, 2004). The effects of this might be:

- Dysfunction of the craniocervical junction: Combined movements of extension, lateral flexion plus rotation to the same side have a direct influence on the neurodynamics of the dura mater (Gutmann 1983); overstimulation of the brainstem with sympathetic symptoms (Gutmann 1983).
- Stimulation of impulses: This can cause neurogenic inflammation of the intercranial blood vessels (Moskowitz 1990).
- A change in proprioceptive input to the sensomotor cortex: This can potentially cause problems in perception leading to movement disorders (Ramachandran & Blakesee 1998, Biedermann 1999).

Dysfunctional afferent inputs (e.g. C1–C2) to the 'homunculus' of the child also have the capacity to influence the motor reflexes that are directly connected with the cervical spine. This implies potential consequences for the motor, affective and cognitive development of the child (Coenen 1996, Knutson 2003).

Posture control system (PCS)

PCS is a reflex mechanism that is responsible for maintaining body balance, i.e. equilibrium, and is under continual adjustment (Gimse et al 1996). It is a complex of interacting vestibular, visual and proprioceptive reflexes, including the paramedian pontine reticular formation (PPRF) (see Fig. 20.5). Disturbances due to insufficient reflex mechanisms in, for example, whiplash-associated disorders (WAD) (Gimse et al 1996) or a vestibulopathy (Mierzwinski et al 2000) and tension headache (Carlsson & Rosenhall 1988) may lead to equilibrium disorders, vertigo, posture anomalies and nystagmus (see Fig. 20.7)

Figure 20.10 shows a model that summarizes the possible varieties of presentation of longstanding dysfunctional afferent inputs to the craniocervical region.

As a result of these longstanding nociceptive inputs, retardation of sensomotor development has been observed. It has been frequently stated that 'horizontal' development (from lying to sitting) occurs later or that children have difficulties during this phase. Many of these children appear normal after this barrier has been overcome but more than 50% suffer dysfunction or symptoms at school age (Biedermann 2003, 2004). One or more of the following symptoms may occur:

- Headaches
- Dysgnosia and dyslexia
- Secondary asymmetry of the skull (mostly plagiocephaly)
- Postural problems (scoliosis or head forward posture)
- Balance problems (Fig. 20.11).

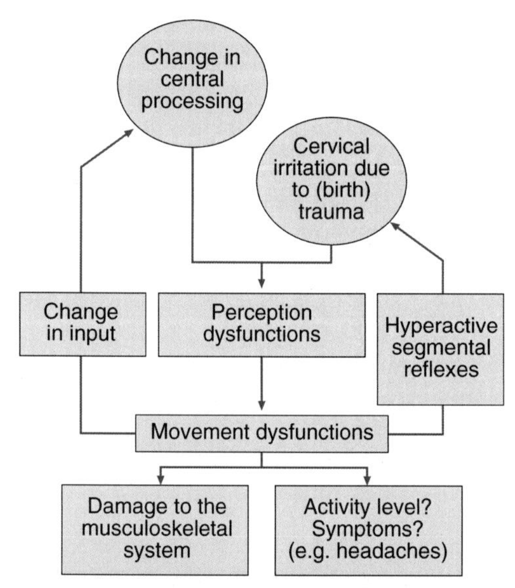

Fig. 20.10 Nociceptive information of the craniocervical region in children and its hypothetical influence on other systems (modified after Biedermann 1999).

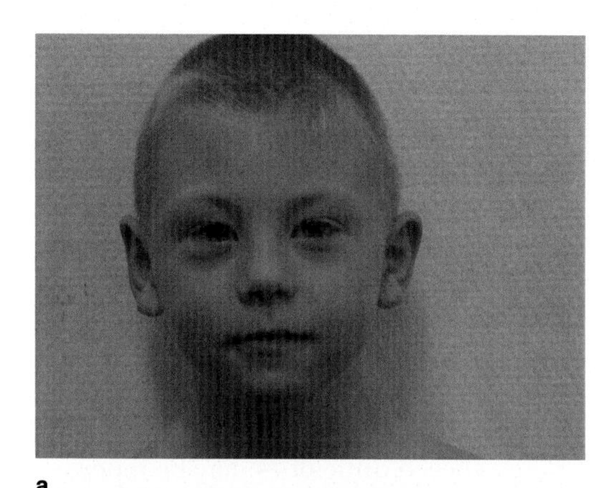

a

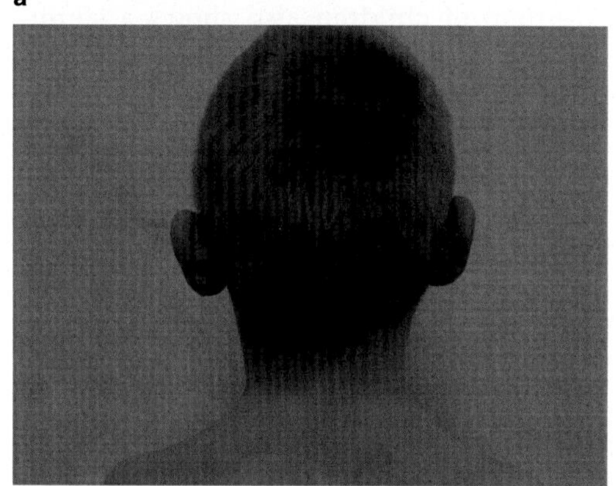

b

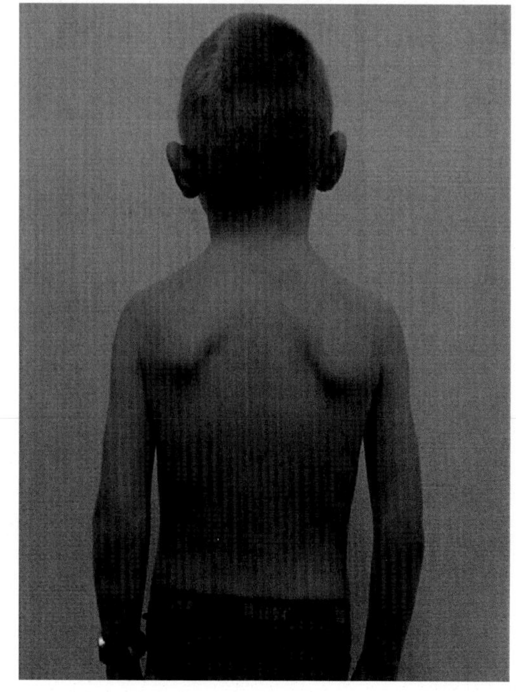

c

Fig. 20.11 Classic pattern of a 6-year-old boy with a history of KISS. His current complaints are headache, lack of concentration and equilibrium problems.
a Head ventral: left orbit smaller than the right with a prominent right frontal region.
b Head dorsal: light lateroflexion of the head towards the left and right ear slightly elevated.
c Posture dorsal: slight scoliosis: thoracal left convex and lumbar right convex with a winged left scapula.

The children we see as patients in physiotherapy clinics have usually been referred for manual therapy of headaches (Biedermann 2004). Children that show one or more of the associated symptoms mentioned above are often classified as kinematically induced dysgnosia and dyspraxia (KIDD) (Biedermann 1999).

Abnormal orofacial development might result in children breathing through their mouths and having problems with swallowing, eating and drinking as well as breathing; vocal and speech difficulties may be reported. This group of children also shows a significantly higher prevalence of other sensomotor dysfunction such as balance problems, distorted orientation in place and time, side-dominance related problems, impaired sensory perception and types of autism (Treuenfelds 1999).

Physical examination of the craniocervical region

Naturally this region needs to be examined with great care. This paragraph will focus on the most common dysfunctions and will suggest appropriate examination procedures. For an overview of the anatomy and function of the craniocervical region, see Chapter 6.

The following tests are recommended for the first therapy session:

- Occiput–atlas GS1:
  - Position of the atlas (C1)
  - Intervertebral movement in flexion and extension
- Atlas–axis GS1:
  - Rotation in supine and sitting positions

Clinical pattern

One or more of the following findings are frequently present:

- Palpation of the craniocervical junction (muscles and ligaments) is sensitive on one side.
- Atlas shift to one side.
- Occiput feels more prominent on one side, usually the side to which the atlas is shifted.
- Rotation C1–C2 is more limited towards the side to which the atlas is shifted.
- Increased range of motion in the midcervical spine in extension (especially in schoolchildren or older children) or slightly decreased flexion.

If one or more of these signs is found, a thorough examination of the spine and pelvis should be the logical next step.

Arthrokinematics of the craniocervical region of the young child

Clinical studies based on manual therapy and radiology findings confirm that movements in the upper cervical spine are different in young children (up to 5 years) compared to adults. The therapist needs to be aware of the biomechanics and include this knowledge in the clinical decision-making process.

- During cervical lateroflexion the atlas does not move towards concavity but towards convexity (Biedermann 2004).
- The instantaneous axis of rotation in the sagittal plane (lateroflexion) is at C2–C4, not C5–C6 (Hill et al 1984, Nitecki & Moir 1994).
- An increased atlas movement in the sagittal plane is found on extension and flexion (Biedermann 2004).

CRANIOFACIAL REGION

General

- Minimal craniosynostoses (prematurely closed sutures) can cause sensomotor retardation and personality changes, usually observed at school age (Fehlow 1993).
- If the volume of the skull is too small, the brain cannot develop into maturity, which can cause minimal dysfunction. It has been previously shown that incomplete growth can cause migraine-type headaches (Kropp 2000).
- Dysfunction of the atlas can cause abnormal growth of the neurocranium and consequently influence the cranial dura mater (Gutmann 1983, von Piekartz 2001). This phenomenon is called secondary skull asymmetry (Biedermann 2004).

The stress-transducer system of the cranium is best evaluated by passive movement. The following signs can be observed:

Inspection and palpation

- Inspection and palpation of the occiput in relation to the position of atlas:
  - Is the atlas shifted to one side?
  - Does the occiput appear prominent on the same side to which the atlas has drifted?
  - Is the occiput flat in the middle?
- Inspection and palpation of the frontal bone and orbit:
  - Does the diameter appear larger on one side?
  - Does the frontal bone feel more prominent on one side (commonly the same side on which the orbit seems enlarged; see Fig. 20.8).
- Inspection of the zygoma:
  - Does the zygoma appear more prominent on one side?

Manual examination of the craniofacial region/neurocranium

- *Occiput–frontal bone* (general technique): Evaluation of general tissue compliance: does one or more of the techniques provoke an unpleasant sensation?
- *Occiput–frontal bone* (diagonally): Evaluation of compression: left side of occiput onto right frontal bone compared to right side of occiput onto left frontal bone.

Even minimal asymmetry will show a difference in tissue resistance and reaction of the child. It might reproduce unpleasant sensations or even headaches (Fig. 20.12a).

- *Occiput* (bilateral transverse movement ('compression') and sagittal axis rotation): Evaluation: if there is a difference between left and right this may indicate a translation of the atlas.
- *Occiput–sphenoid bone* (transverse movement of the sphenoid bone): Evaluation: Compare movement to the right versus movement to the left and note tissue resistance and reaction of the child.
- *Zygoma* (anterior–posterior movement): Evaluation: Tissue compliance of the right versus the left side. This is usually easier to assess at early school age due to the growth of the facial bones (Fig. 20.12b).

Clinical note

A number of cases show the following pattern of dysfunction, which may form the basis of treatment:

- Transverse movement of the occiput is reduced towards the prominent side but

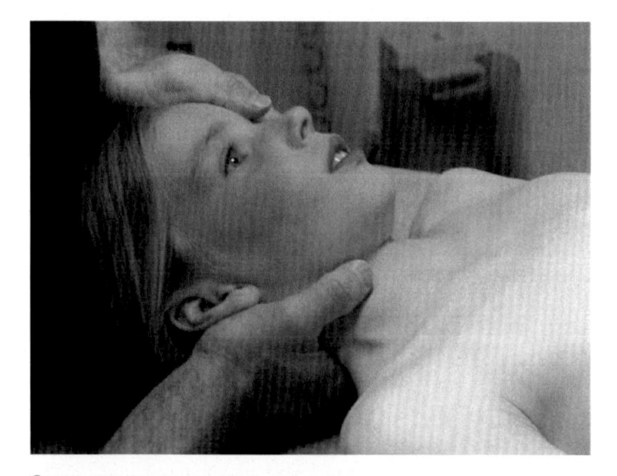

a

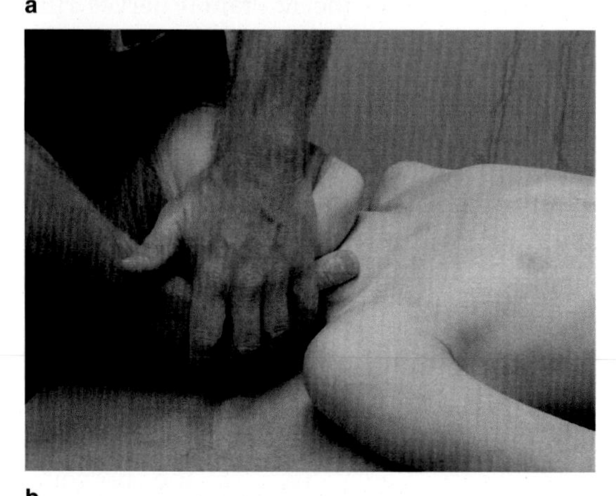

b

Fig. 20.12 Assessment of the craniofacial region by passive movements for compliance and sensory responses.
a Occiput/frontal (diagonal).
b Anterior/posterior examination of the zygoma region.

more sensitive to touch on the opposite side.

- If there is a clear dysfunction of the frontal bone, rotation (sagittal axis) will usually produce symptoms and show tissue resistance.
- Transverse movements of the sphenoid bone are dominantly stiff in the direction of the non-prominent side
- Anterior–posterior movement of the zygoma is usually stiffer on the prominent side. Symptoms can vary to either side.

THE JUVENILE NERVOUS SYSTEM

Overview

Impaired nerve conduction does not generally correlate with a dysfunction of neurodynamic capacities (Butler 2000). A child can therefore show significant signs during neurodynamic testing without suffering from nerve conduction problems. The nervous system forms both neurobiologically and neuroanatomically a continuum, which is designed to function in a moving body (Butler 2000). The following facts may be relevant:

- The atlas (C1) is not directly connected to the dura mater, unlike C2 and the occiput (Lang & Kehr 1983).
- The cranial dura is connected with the falx cerebri and cerebelli and with the cranial foramina. Ten of the 12 cranial nerves run through the cranial foramina.
- From maximum cervical flexion to maximum cervical extension the cervical nervous system adapts by 20% (Breig 1960). Adaptation from neutral to maximum flexion is about 10% (Yuan et al 1998). The sagittal diameter of the spinal cord reduces by 30% in maximum extension compared to flexion (Muhle et al 1998).
- The cranial dura mater shows a greater number of nociceptors per centimetre than the spinal dura mater (Kumar et al 1996).

Neurodynamic adaptation of the nervous system in the craniocervical and craniofacial regions is considerable.

The large number of anchorage points, relatively free mobility and rich innervation by nociceptors give rise to convergence at many places which may predispose towards possible pathodynamics. This can be an important accompanying factor for juvenile headache.

Furthermore, the condition of the dura appears to play an important role in the growth of the skull (Wagemans et al 1988).

Growth of the nervous system compared with the growth of other structures

Arthrogenic and myogenic structures generally show a later growth spurt than the nervous system (Scammon 1930) (Fig. 20.13).

Reidi and Pratt (1988) stated that girls between the ages of 13 and 14 years show a significantly smaller range of motion on slump testing. At later ages the stiffness is lost again and returns to an average value. Kendall and Kendall (1971) described long sitting slump as a mobility test for the hamstrings (Fig. 20.14). They noticed that children between the ages of 12 and 14 years have a lack of mobility and concluded that this must be due to a temporary shortening of the hamstrings.

The shortening of the hamstrings might be due to the still growing neuromusculoskeletal system. To determine if hamstring shortening or stiff active or passive neck flexion has a neuro-

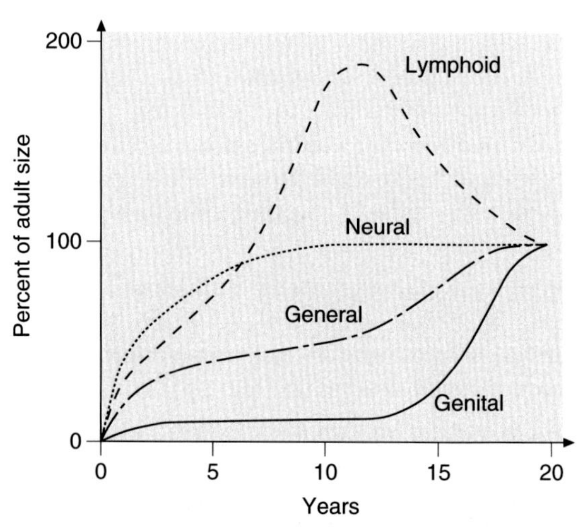

Fig. 20.13 Scammon's growth curve of the four major tissue systems (1930). Note that the neural tissue is almost fully developed at age 6–7 years. General body tissue such as muscle, bone and organs shows an S-curve with a delay at age 10–11 years and an increase during puberty.

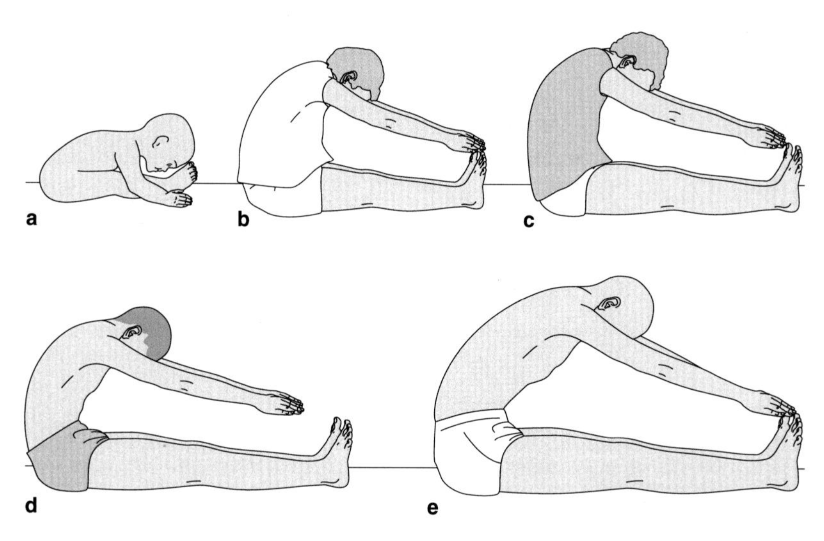

Fig. 20.14 Long sitting test according to Kendall and Kendall (1971) at five different ages:
a 1–3 years.
b 4–7 years.
c 8–10 years.
d 11–14 years.
e 15 years and over.

dynamic component, the so-called 'distance techniques' can be helpful: the test is performed up to the point where symptoms are produced. Passive neck flexion is added and the child is asked for any change in symptoms. If there is a change in symptoms (usually resistance and local pulling pain) the conclusion is that there might be a neurodynamic contribution to the problem. One might also reverse the test by starting off with passive neck flexion and using a leg distance technique (knee extension, hip adduction). The long sitting slump is therefore a very neurodynamic test for structural differentiation. Poor condition of the cranial dura can be a contributory factor for juvenile headache. Although often noted clinically, these facts have not been rigorously researched.

Neurodynamic tests

The two most useful tests in the assessment of headache children are passive neck flexion (PNF) – as described in Chapter 18 – and long sitting slump (LSS) (Fig. 20.15).

The standard test procedure by Butler (2000) needs to be adapted slightly for the assessment of children since a number of them experience a strong and unpleasant pulling at the back of their legs. Slight knee flexion is therefore recommended as a starting position. This position also provides a good impression of the quality, responses and mobility of neck flexion.

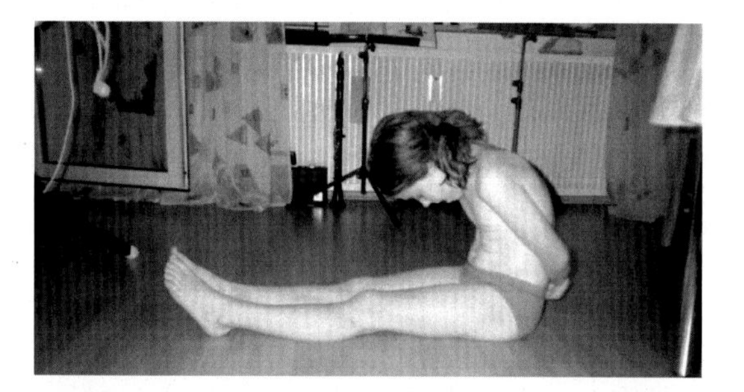

a

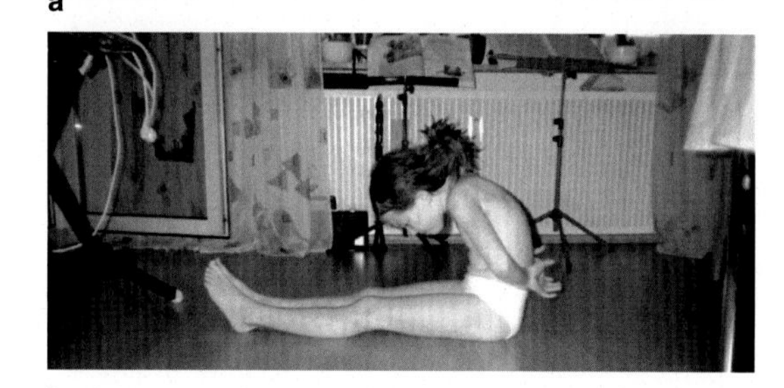

b

Fig. 20.15 Long sitting slump (LSS) in 7-year-old identical twins.
a The first girl is an average student and has no complaints.
b Her sister was a 'crying baby' and has a delay in her neuromotor development and needs a lot of attention at school. She complains of headache at least twice a week. Note the minimal difference in knee flexion and reduced craniocervical flexion in the second girl.

Research report 1

This study (von Piekartz et al 2006a) investigates the difference in craniocervical flexion and sensory responses (intensity and localization) during the LSS tests in children (n = 141) aged 6–12 years, between a migraine group (n = 45) (primary headache group), a cervicogenic headache group (n = 43) (secondary headache group) and a control group (n = 53).

The results show that the reproducibility of the modified LSS test was an interclass correlation coefficient (ICC) of 0.96 (95% CI 0.89–0.99). The standard error of the mean (SEM) was 2.83° and the smallest detectable difference was 7.9°. Significant differences in sacrum positions (in degrees) were noted during the execution of the test in both of the headache groups as compared to the control group. There was, however, no significant difference between the migraine and cervicogenic headache groups.

The results show a statistically significant difference in craniocervical flexion between the migraine group and the cervicogenic headache group in both the knee extension and flexion phases of the LSS position. The sensory responses in the migraine group were predominantly in the legs whereas in the cervicogenic headache group they were mainly located in the spinal column, with a significantly higher intensity than in the control group. This suggests different pathophysiological mechanisms in both headache groups. From animal studies and through mechanisms of nociception and neurogenic inflammation, it is thought that movement of the dura may evoke pain (Groen et al 1988, Bove & Moskowitz 1997). In addition, neurogenically inflamed (craniocervical) dura may result in changes of the contractile state of the blood vessels in the head which may lead to headache (Moskowitz 1993).

During the study it was interesting to note that craniocervical flexion in the cervicogenic headache group during the knee flexion phase improved less than it did in either the control group or the migraine group. This may be explained by anatomical differences. It has been postulated that most cervical flexion (even in children) takes place between the atlas and axis (Gutmann 1983, Biedermann 1999). The atlas is not attached to the dura as a rule, which means that the neurodynamic positions have less influence on the arthrokinematics of the atlas (Gutmann 1983, Lang & Kehr 1983). This does not mean that neurodynamic effects on cervical flexion in the cervicogenic headache group can be excluded. Clear differences in the intensity of the local responses measured using the colour analogue scale were observed in the control group on the one hand and in both headache groups on the other (Fig. 20.16). This confirms reports in the literature that children with recurrent headaches have generally increased levels of sensitivity (McGrath & Koster 2001), but it may also be related to changed neurodynamics which contributes to elevated neural sensitivity (Groen et al 1988, Bove & Moskowitz 1997).

In summary, this study shows clear differences between measurements (neck flexion, localization and intensity of sensory responses) of a modified LSS in a cervicogenic headache group, a migraine group and a control group of children between the ages of 6 and 12 years. These results suggest: 1) different pathophysiological mechanisms of headache, and 2) different biomechanical patterns of the craniocervical region.

Cranial nerves

The cranial nerves need to be assessed for any neurological and neurodynamic deficits since they might influence the development of the child and are a potential source of headaches.

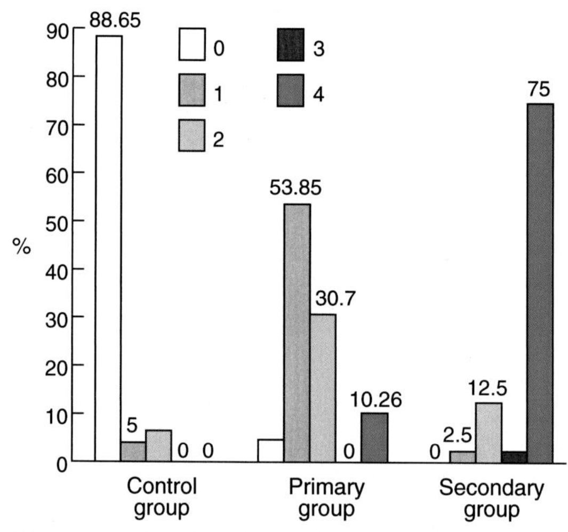

Fig. 20.16 Results of static/dynamic tests in the three headache groups.

Okeson (2005) found significantly more dysfunction of the cranial nerves in children with migraine-type headaches than in children without headaches.

Screening an older child for dysfunction of the cranial nerves is easier than assessing a younger child (4 years and younger). With very young children the tests should be modified and one sometimes needs to become very creative.

For a detailed description of these tests, see Chapter 17.

Equilibrium/balance

As previously stated, children with headaches frequently show insufficient motor balance skills (static and dynamic). In particular, children whose symptoms are classified as being primary headaches seem to struggle with vestibular functions (equilibrium and vertigo) (Szirmai & Farkas 2000, D'Amico et al 2003). For secondary headaches no literature was available, but since dysfunction concerns/affects the neuromusculoskeletal system, a clinical correlation of headaches and equilibrium seems very likely and has been observed clinically.

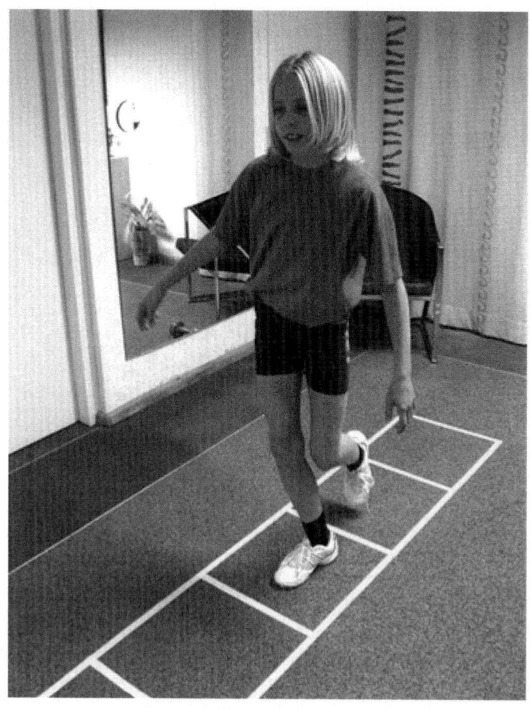

Fig. 20.17 Dynamic balance test. Hopping in six squares on one leg (category 9–10 years).

BALANCE TESTS

There are a range of possibilities to test balance but one of the most detailed and reliable tools is the Movement Assessment Battery for Children (Movement ABC). This test is a revised version of the Test of Motor Impairment (TOMI) (Stott et al 1984). The psychologists Henderson and Sugden (1992) revised the TOMI test and renamed it 'Movement ABC'. It is now a worldwide testing procedure for psychologists and physiotherapists specializing in paediatrics. This battery of tests consists of a checklist and motor tests. The result aims to represent the motor function of the child in daily life. The test is designed for the age groups 4–6 years, 7–8 years, 9–10 years and 10–12+ years. All the groups are guided through eight test categories. The final three categories consist of standardized balance tests differentiating static and dynamic balance skills.

An example of a dynamic balance test for the 9–10 years age group is shown in Figure 20.17.

Table 20.1 Test with scores from the Movement ABC test battery

Balancing on a board (record time in seconds, Refused, Inadequate)

Preferred leg			Non-preferred leg	
Attempt 1			Attempt 1	
Attempt 2			Attempt 2	
9 years	10 years	Points	9 years	10 years
6–20 s	9–20 s	0	6–20 s	8–20 s
5 s	6–8 s	1	5 s	6–7 s
4 s	5 s	2	4 s	5 s
3 s	4 s	3	3 s	4 s
2 s	3 s	4	2 s	3 s
0–1 s	0–2 s	5	0–1 s	0–2 s

Total points (preferred leg + non-preferred leg)/2

Jumping in squares (six squares of 45 × 45 cm, using one leg only. Record the number of correct jumps; Failed, Refused, Inadequate)

Preferred leg			Non-preferred leg	
Attempt 1			Attempt 1	
Attempt 2			Attempt 2	
Attempt 3			Attempt 3	
9 years	10 years	Points	9 years	10 years
5	5	0	5	5
–	–	1	–	–
–	–	2	4	4
4	4	3	3	3
1-3	3	4	1–2	2
0	0–2	5	0	0–1

Total points (preferred leg + non-preferred leg)/2

Balancing a ball on a board (walking to the right of a 2.5 metre long line and back on the left of the line, turn around and stand still, do not touch the line. Either hand can be used, the whole hand should be under the board. Record how often the ball is dropped to the floor; Failed, Refused, Inadequate)

Attempt 1	Attempt 2	Attempt 3
How often was the hand used:		
Points	9 years	10 years
0	0	0
1	–	–
2	1	1
3	2	2
4	3–4	3–4
5	5+	5+

Total points

Material

Six squares measuring 45 × 45 cm are stuck on the floor using coloured tape. The total length should be 2.7 metres.

Task

'Jump on one leg from one square to the next until you reach the last square.'

The test is failed if the subject:

- Touches the lines
- Touches the ground with the free leg
- Jumps into one square more than once
- Fails to stop in the last square.

Method

The examiner demonstrates the task and the child is asked to do a trial run. The actual test includes three runs; if a maximum score is achieved in the first run, the child proceeds to the next test.

Evaluation

The scores are divided into quantitative and qualitative data. The quantitative results scored by each leg are counted separately on an ordinate scale from 0 to 5, the highest score being 0. The final score (item score) for this test item is reached by adding up the highest scores of the right and the left leg and dividing the result by 2.

The qualitative results are descriptive data and are categorized into 13 common compensatory reactions (Table 20.1).

Why use balance tests in children with headache?

The therapist who chooses this standardized form of balance testing should be aware that only some of the Movement ABCs are tested. This means that no general conclusions about the child's level of motor development can be drawn. Nevertheless, these tests provide a good opportunity for assessment and reassessment during craniofacial and (cranio)neurodynamic treatment. If a clinical relationship is discovered in a child, the therapist may also use these tests for the purpose of rehabilitation if the level is not sufficient for the child's age group. The impression given is that these balance exercises together with diagnostic work and treatment of the craniofacial dysfunction can clearly reduce the rate of headache attacks.

Balance training as part of rehabilitation for some tinnitus patients can reduce the experience of tinnitus (Berry et al 2002), although whether there is any relationship to juvenile headache is unknown. The investigation of this is an enormous challenge for the future.

Research report 2

The quantitative data of the statistical and dynamic coordination of the Movement ABC test is investigated in the same group of children (n = 141) as in Research report 1 (see p. 600) (von Piekartz et al 2006b). An analysis of the scores of the three tests (one static and two dynamic tests) were distributed on an ordinal scale from A to E. Score A was given when all three tests were sufficient (0 points), score B when the static test was insufficient and the two dynamic tests were sufficient, score C when one dynamic test was sufficient and the other dynamic test and the static test were insufficient, score D when the static test was sufficient but none of the dynamic tests was sufficient and score E when none of the tests was sufficient (Fig. 20.18). The results show that 88.6% of the control group had all three tests sufficient (score A) and 75% of the cervicogenic headache group had all three tests insufficient (score E; see Fig. 20.16). This suggests that there is a clear difference in balance between the cervicogenic headache and control groups and confirms the reliability and the construct validity of this part of the Movement ABC test (Croce et al 2001, Chow & Henderson 2003).

It is interesting that, in the migraine group, 53.9% are insufficient on the static coordination test but had the full score on both dynamic coordination tests (see Fig. 20.16). This may be related to different mechanisms of the reduced equilibrium in the migraine and cervicogenic headache groups. The relationship with the craniocervical region as a possible hypothesis is outlined in Figure 20.10. A powerful hypothesis is that juvenile migraine may be strongly related to vestibular disorders (Mierzwinski et al 2000, Uneri & Turkdogan 2003). In complete otolaryngological assessment – audiometry, electro- and videonystagmography, Dix–Hallpike test for benign paroxysmal positional vertigo (BPPV) and Romberg and Unterberger–Fukuda tests for static coordination (vestibulospinal reflexes) – in children with migraine it is seen that peripheral vestibular problems present in a wide spectrum which varies from fluctuating sensory hearing loss to short episodes of dizziness and vertigo (Parker 1989, Mierzwinski et al 2000, Uneri & Turkdogan 2003). This suggests that the vestibular system may have a contributory role in juvenile migraine. Clinical questions – such as how much balance and coordination training (e.g. parts of the Movement ABC test), as well as BPPV training, affects the headache in a positive sense – still await answers.

GUIDELINES FOR THE MANAGEMENT OF RECURRENT JUVENILE HEADACHE

The physiotherapy intervention consists of 'hands on' and 'hands off' components. 'Hands on' are any techniques requiring direct physical contact with the child. 'Hands off' components (i.e. no physical contact) usually include management strategies based on any clinical finding from the subjective and physical examinations.

MCGRATH'S MODIFIED IDEAS OF COGNITIVE-BEHAVIOURAL THERAPY (MCGRATH 1990)

Pamela McGrath – a Canadian psychologist and head of a large childhood pain clinic in Ontario – has acquired years of clinical experience with this patient group. Some of her ideas are sufficiently straightforward to integrate into daily practice. Broadly speaking, hands-off management can be divided into three different activities. The therapist has to decide when each activity is introduced into the treatment plan:

Score	Stat. test	Dyn. test 1	Dyn. test 2
A	+	+	+
B	–	+	+
C	–	+ ⟷	–
D	+	–	–
E	–	–	–

Fig. 20.18 Movement ABC test.

- Informing the child and parents about pain models and contributing factors, and explaining them as far as possible.
- Formulating a treatment plan based on the subjective and objective findings.
- Identifying, evaluating and setting the short- and long-term goals of the child and its parents.

INFORMATION AND EXPLANATION OF PAIN MECHANISMS

With the help of a pain mechanism model, the therapist can explain the mechanisms of recurrent headaches to both child and parents. Our suggestion is to use a modified version of the 'mature organism model' (MOM) (Gifford 1998, Butler 2000, Butler & Moseley 2003).

Pain mechanism models have the great advantage of clarifying the dominant influence from the choice of pain mechanisms for the therapist and in helping both the child and its parents visualize pain mechanisms. Further advantages include the three-dimensional aspects of pain in general (sensory–discriminative, affective–motivational, cognitive–evaluative) (Melzack & Katz 1994) and experience (McGrath & Hillier 2001) which can easily be integrated.

Behaviour guidelines for parents and children

It is essential to provide the parents with detailed information about the causes and aetiology of their child's headache problem, especially since research has shown a correlation between the behaviour of the parents before and after the headache episode and the frequency and intensity of the headache attacks (McGrath 2001). Behaviour guidelines should, if necessary, be discussed with the parents early on in the course of treatment.

CAUSES OF RECURRENT HEADACHE

Headaches (tension headaches and migraines) are a common occurrence in children.

- Headaches are usually caused by more than one factor. There are some factors that all headache children have in common, others that are individual for the child. The physiotherapy assessment supported by information from the parents will help identify the factors that are dominant as a cause for the particular headache syndrome in an individual child.
- Manual therapy is an important part of the treatment but not the most important.
- Common causes for headaches are stress and fear/pressure associated with normal day-to-day activities such as school, homework, sports, family. Most children do not realize that these factors influence their headaches.

CONTENTS OF THE TREATMENT SESSION

The following points can generally be discussed with the child and parents during or after the treatment session, if management strategies are clear to the therapist:

- The treatment goal is to reduce the headache symptoms and to influence the identified contributing factors positively.
- As soon as slight headache symptoms arise, it is advisable to try distraction strategies. Distraction is a powerful method in reducing the severity of the symptoms. For example, when the headache symptoms begin the child is allowed to do something they enjoy before returning to the interrupted activity.
- A child with headaches needs to feel the empathy of the therapist but should nevertheless strictly follow the treatment regime. The regime ought to include as many non-medication components as possible and the child needs to be informed of the benefits of this plan.
- It might be helpful to arrange a therapy session for the day after the headache attack while at school, playing sport or with friends, so this can be discussed while fresh in the memory. There might be unnecessary stress, perceived pressure or fears and to talk about these will help the child to recognize and control similar situations in the future.

CLINICAL RECOMMENDATIONS – FORMING THE TREATMENT PLAN

Based on the results of the subjective and physical examinations, it is recommended that the therapist formulate treatment guidelines that reflect information and explanations given to child and parents. Short-term goals should also be discussed.

The following examples give an indication of how management guidelines can be constructed.

- Short-term (sessions 1–3):
  - Manual therapy – dysfunction of the craniocervical and craniofacial regions
  - Explanation of pain mechanisms with emphasis on the cognitive and contributing factors (lifestyle, stress).
- Long-term (after three or more sessions):
  - Detailed information on the individual stress factors based on pain scales and diary
  - Identifying unnecessary attention to symptoms and developing a plan for distraction techniques
  - Implementing a pacing programme.

Manual therapy for dysfunctions of the craniocervical, facial and neural regions (short term)

During the first three therapy sessions a thorough manual therapy assessment and (if necessary) treatment should be performed. The following are some suggestions for the first sessions:

- Influencing the craniocervical region
- The sustained atlas technique (Fig. 20.19).

This technique is described in detail since it is gentle, safe and can result in rapid subjective and physical improvement in younger children (under 12 years of age) with headache and suspected atlantal craniocervical dysfunction.

INDICATION

This technique is indicated when stiffness is detected during intervertebral movements of the atlas and occiput (during lateroflexion occiput–atlas). Usually the head is held in a position of minimal lateral flexion and in slight upper cervical extension away from the stiff side. In the following the technique is described for the case of a head held in extension and lateral flexion to the left. The therapist has diagnosed upper cervical stiffness to the right and restricted mobility of the atlas to the left. The reader is reminded of the altered arthrokinematics of the craniocervical transition in children, already described in this chapter. For further information on craniocervical biomechanics, see Chapter 6.

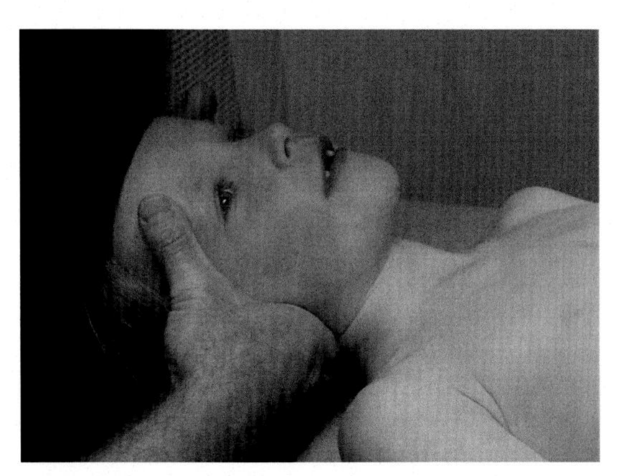

Fig. 20.19 Sustained atlas technique. In this example the atlas is sustained in craniocervical lateroflexion to the right.

STARTING POSITION AND METHOD

The patient lies relaxed on the plinth with the therapist sitting behind the patient. The therapist grasps the patient's head with both hands and makes contact with the tip of the right transverse process of the atlas with the proximal radial side of the right index finger. The head is now moved carefully into maximal lateral flexion to the right. The movement causes the pressure of the atlas against the finger to increase minimally. If pressure increases considerably, the therapist attempts to hold the position for a few seconds. Depending on the reaction of the child, this manoeuvre can be repeated a few times, followed by a reassessment of craniocervical intervertebral movements.

A variation of the index finger position – holding the atlas with the right index finger and mobilizing the cranium to the right around the sagittal axis – is also possible if the first option is ineffective.

INFLUENCING THE STRESS TRANSDUCER SYSTEM OF THE CRANIOFACIAL REGION

Often one or two of the examination techniques described in this chapter are used during the initial examination. One should decide on the technique that reproduces stiffness rather than headache symptoms to allow the child to gain confidence in the therapist and because stiffness is easier to reassess than perceived pain symptoms. Re-examination of upper cervical intervertebral movements and of neurodynamics is advisable because of the continuity of these structures.

INFLUENCING NEURODYNAMICS

On neurodynamic testing of young children the therapist might be surprised by the rapidly increasing tissue resistance and strong symptom responses. 'Pulling in the neck' and/or the hamstrings and rapidly increasing resistance are examples of typical symptoms.

The 'slider' principle recommended by Butler (2000) is therefore often appropriate for the child's neuromusculoskeletal system, which is not fully developed. 'Sliders' highlight movement of the nervous system in which two parts of the body are moved from distance, avoiding loading of the nervous system.

Principles that can often be used with children are:

- Long sitting slump: Neck flexion with flexion of the knee joints, alternated with extension of the neck and extension of the knee.
- Upper cervical neck flexion and lower cervical neck extension: These movements are alternated with upper cervical neck extension and lower cervical neck flexion.

These techniques can be performed passively, and later actively at home. Ergonomic recommendations can also be derived from relevant tests, for example not to read or study for long while sitting in bed. When sitting on a chair, neck flexion provokes the headache, but the child sits too much in lumbar and thoracic flexion (slump). The starting position and methods of the tests described above are given in Chapter 17.

Attention, distraction and pacing (long-term therapy)

ATTENTION AND DISTRACTION

This is a simple method for pain control and can be very effective for the treatment of juvenile headache patients (Ross & Ross 1988, McGrath 1990). As soon as the child notices any headache symptoms, they are asked to change their current activity and do something they enjoy. This can reduce the neurogenic response to a stimulus. One property of this method is that the child does not ignore the headaches but can actively reduce the symptoms (McGrath 2001). For example, a 7-year-old child returns home from school with a headache. Rather than eating immediately the child is allowed a few minutes on a swing or any other activity they enjoy. Another clinical example is a 13-year-old child with headaches while doing homework. The child is allowed to interrupt homework and listen to their favourite music for a while. The headaches usually disappear before they can reach their climax. It is important to limit the favoured activity to a specified length of time so that the homework still gets done.

PACING

Pacing is a systematic approach to increase the strength of loading which can be momentarily tolerated by using a quota system. It permits classification and stepwise increase of daily activities and positions with concomitant prevention of an increase in pain. Pacing gives the patient control over their painful daily activities (Gifford 1998, Butler 2000, Butler & Moseley 2003).

The time until the onset of pain during a particular activity is measured, and the average value from three attempts is calculated. This average value, less 20%, is then the basic time for the activity, which should be carried out every day at home. If headache during this activity persists for a week, the duration can be reduced by a further 10–20%, and another activity can be performed if necessary. In children it can be difficult to measure the time, in which case estimates will suffice.

Other principles that can easily be integrated in the pacing programme include:

- Movement breakdowns: Movements or activities that usually trigger pain are performed with other body parts in different positions. For example, turning the head is painful but turning the head with flexed elbows and slightly elevated shoulders reduces the pain.
- Trick activities: The same movement that usually triggers the pain is performed in a different setting, with a different goal or in a different position. For example, if the child always has headaches while reading, and the head's flexion position influences the pain, exercises involving head circling or curl-ups are selected.

These two suggestions imply that no serious physical impairment of the craniocervical region exists. Their aim is to change the input on the 'homunculus' (receptor field in the sensory cortex) and therefore reduce the correlation of an activity with the sensation of pain (Ramachandran & Blakesee 1998, Butler 2000). This retraining of the brain can potentially reduce recurrences of headache symptoms even in very young children.

SHORT- AND LONG-TERM GOAL SETTING

Together with the child and its parents, short- and long-term goals and realistic time schedules are agreed upon. These goals should reflect the hypothesis of pathobiological processes underlying the individual syndrome and should correlate with therapeutic guidelines.

This requires close collaboration of the therapist with the whole family, sharing the same long-term goal of control over the headache symptoms or even a pain-free status. Sometimes it can be a lengthy journey to reach that long-term goal but an intense discussion about when and how to reach short-term goals is effective and motivating for everybody involved. This procedure is called 'collaborative reasoning' (Jones et al 2002).

Case study 1

Consider the example of an 8-year-old child with headache for over 2 years, with four intermediate targets.

Intermediate target 1: What does therapy achieve?

- Expectations. What does it achieve and what does it not achieve?
- This is in support of the ultimate aim and is not the ultimate aim in itself.

Intermediate target 2: What is pain?

- Which pain mechanisms are present?
- Affective and cognitive influences.

Intermediate target 3: Types of headache

- Different types of headache that correlate with one another.
- Natural history.
- Control.

Intermediate target 4: How can the headaches be controlled?

- Changes in lifestyle.
- Analysis of pain tables.
- What can I do myself?

SUMMARY

- Recurrent juvenile headaches require a thorough and time-consuming analysis of all potentially involved components.
- They also require an interdisciplinary approach, with the combination of medication and physiotherapy (management of neuromusculoskeletal components) having the best prognosis.
- Manual therapy is a valuable tool for the assessment and therapy of the craniocervical and craniofacial regions as well as for the neurodynamic aspects.
- Affective and cognitive coping strategies as described in this chapter can easily be integrated into the management procedure and positively influence the behaviour of the symptoms. In some cases it might be advisable to involve a psychologist to support the child and parents during the time of treatment.

References

Abu-Saad H H 1990 Toward the development of an instrument to assess pain in children. Dutch study. In: Tyler D C, Krane E (eds) Advances in pain research and therapy: pediatric pain. Raven Press, New York, p 101

Anrig P, Plaugher G 1996 Pediatric chiropractic. William and Wilkins, Baltimore

Berry J, Gold S, Frederick E, Gray W, Staecker H 2002 Patient-based outcomes in patients with primary tinnitus undergoing tinnitus retraining therapy. Archives of Otolaryngology, Head and Neck Surgery 128:1153

Beyer J E, McGrath P, Berde C 1990 Discordance between self-report and behavioral pain measures in children aged 3–7 years after surgery. Journal of Pain and Symptom Management 5(6):350

Biedermann H 1999 Biomechanische Besonderheiten des occipito-cervicalen Überganges bei Kindern. In: Biedermann H (ed.) Manualtherapie bei Kindern. Enke, Stuttgart, p 19

Biedermann H 2001 Primäre und sekundäre Schädelasymmetrie bei KISS-Kindern. In: von Piekartz H (ed.) Kraniofaziale Dysfunktion und Schmerzen: Untersuchung – Beurteilung – Management. Thieme, Stuttgart, p 45

Biedermann H 2003 Personal communication.

Biedermann H 2004 Manual therapy in children. Churchill Livingstone, Edinburgh

Bieri D, Reeve R A, Champion G D, Addicoat L, Ziegler J B 1990 The Faces Pain Scale for the self-assessment of the severity of pain experienced by children: development, initial validation, and preliminary investigation for ratio scale properties. Pain 41(2):139

Bove G M, Moskowitz M A 1997 Primary afferent neurons innervating guinea pig dura. Journal of Neurophysiology 77(1):299–308

Breig A 1960 Biomechanics of the central nervous system. Almqvist and Wiksell, Stockholm

Butler D 2000 The sensitive nervous system. Noigroup Publications, Adelaide

Butler D, Moseley L 2003 Explain pain. Noigroup Publications, Adelaide

Buzzi M G, Moskowitz M A 1991 Evidence for 5H/1B/1D receptors mediating the antimigraine effect of sumatriptan and dihydroergotamine. Cephalalgia 11:165

Buzzi M G, Moskowitz M A 1992 The trigenovascular system and migraine. Pathologie-Biologie 40:313

Carlsson J, Rosenhall U 1988 Oculomotor disturbances in patients with tension headache. Acta Otolaryngologica 106(5–6):354–360

Chow S, Henderson S 2003 Interrater and test-retest reliability of Movement Assessment Battery for Chinese preschool children. American Journal of Occupational Therapy 57(5):574–577

Coenen W 1996 Die sensomotorische Integrationsstörung. Manuelle Medizin 34:141

Croce R, Horvat M, McCarthy E 2001 Reliability and concurrent validity of movement assessment battery for children. Perceptual and Motor Skills 93(1):275–280

D'Amico D, Grazzi L, Usai S et al 2003 Use of the migraine disability assessment questionnaire in children and adolescents with headache: an Italian pilot study. Headache 43:767

Davies N 2000 Chiropractic paediatrics: a clinical handbook. Churchill Livingstone, Edinburgh

Denecke H, Kröner-Herwig B 2000 Kopfschmerztherapie mit Kindern und Jugendlichen. Hogrefe, Göttingen

Fehlow P 1993 Craniosynostosis as a risk factor. Child's Nervous System 9:325

Giesler G I, Katter K T, Dado R J 1994 Direct spinal pathways to the limbic system for non-nociceptive information. Trends in Neuroscience 17:244

Gifford L 1998 Pain, the tissues and the nervous system: a conceptual model. Physiotherapy 84:27

Gifford L 1999 Biopsychosocial assessment and management: relationships and pain. CNS Press, Falmouth

Gimse R, Tjell C, Bjorgen I, Saunte C 1996 Disturbed eye movements after whiplash due to injuries to the posture control system. Journal of Clinical and Experimental Neuropsychology 18:178

Groen G J, Baljet B, Drukker J 1988 The innervation of the spinal dura mater: anatomy and clinical implications. Acta Neurochirurgica 92(1–4):39–46

Gunnar M R, Fisch R O, Korsvik S, Donhowe J M 1981 The effects of circumcision on serum cortisol and behavior. Psychoneuroendocrinology 6(3):269

Gutmann G 1983 Die funktionanalytische Röntgendiagnostik der Halswirbelsäule. In: Gutmann G, Biedermann H (eds) Funktionelle Pathologie und Klinik der Wirbelsäule. Fischer Verlag, Stuttgart, p 68–72

Henderson S E, Sugden D A 1992 Movement assessment battery for children: manual. Psychological Corporation, London

Hester N O 1979 The preoperational child's reaction in immunization. Nursing Research 28:250

Hicks C L, von Baeyer C L, Spafford P A, van Korlaar I, Goodenough B 2001 The faces pain scale – revised: toward a common metric in pediatric measurement. Pain 93:173

Hill S, Miller C, Kosnik E, Hunt W 1984 Pediatric neck injuries: a clinical study. Neurosurgery 60:700

Jones M, von Piekartz H 2001 Clinical reasoning – Grundlage für die Untersuchung und Behandlung in der kranialen Region. In: von Piekartz H (ed.) Kraniofaziale Dysfunktion und Schmerzen: Untersuchung – Beurteilung – Management. Thieme, Stuttgart

Jones M, Rivett D 2004 Clinical reasoning for manual therapists. Butterworth-Heinemann, Edinburgh
Jones M, Edwards I, Gifford L 2002 Conceptual models for implementing biopsychosocial theory in clinical practice. Manual Therapy 7:2
Kendall H, Kendall G 1971 Muscles: testing and function, 2nd edn. Williams and Wilkins, Baltimore
Knutson G 2003 Vectored upper cervical manipulation for chronic sleep bruxism, headache, and cervical spine pain in a child. Journal of Manipulative and Physiological Therapeutics 26:E16
Kropp P 2000 Zur Psychobiologie von kindlichen Kopfschmerzen. Migräne – Störung zerebraler Reifung? Symposium Medical 30
Kumar R, Berger R, Dunsker S, Keller J 1996 Innervation of the spinal dura: myth or reality? Spine 21:18
Lang G, Kehr P 1983 Vertebragene Insuffizienz der Arteria vertebralis. In: Hohmann D, Kügelgen B, Liebig K (eds) Neuroorthopädie. Springer, Berlin, p 251
Maitland G D, Hengeveld E, Banks K, English K 2001 Maitland's vertebral manipulation, 6th edn. Butterworth-Heinemann, Oxford
Maytal J, Bienkowski R D, Patel M, Eviater L 1995 The value of brain imaging in children with headaches. Pediatrics 96:413–416
McGrath P J 1990 Pain in children: nature, assessment and treatment. Guilford Publications, New York
McGrath P 2001 Headache in children: the nature of the problem. In: McGrath P, Hillier L (eds) The child with headache: diagnosis and treatment. IASP Press, Seattle, p 1
McGrath P, Hillier L 2001 Treatment of recurrent headache: an effective strategy for primary care providers. In: McGrath P, Hillier L (eds) The child with headache: diagnosis and treatment. IASP Press, Seattle, p 159
McGrath P, Koster L 2001 Headache measures for children: a practical approach. In: McGrath P, Hillier L (eds) The child with headache: diagnosis and treatment. IASP Press, Seattle, p 29–56
McGrath P, Unruh M, Finley A 1995 Pain measurement in children. Pain Clinical Updates Vol. III, Issue 2. IASP Press, Seattle
McIntosh N, Van Veen L, Brameye H 1993 The pain of a heel prick and its measurements in preterm infants. Pain 52:71
Melzack R, Katz J 1994 Pain measurement in people in pain. In: Wall P D, Melzack R (eds) Textbook of pain, 3rd edn. Churchill Livingstone, Edinburgh, p 337
Mierzwinski J, Kazmierczak H, Pawlak-Osinska K et al 2000 The vestibular system and migraine in children. Otolaryngologia Polska 54(5):537–540
Mongini M D (ed.) 1999 Classification and pathophysiology. In: Headache and facial pain. Thieme, Stuttgart, p 2
Moskowitz M A 1990 Basic mechanisms in vascular headache. Neurologic Clinics 8:801
Moskowitz M A 1993 Neurogenic inflammation in the pathophysiology and treatment of migraine. Neurology 43(3):16–20
Muhle C C, Wiskirchen J, Weinert D et al 1998 Biomechanical aspects of the subarachnoid space and cervical cord in healthy individuals examined with kinematic magnetic resonance imaging. Spine 23:556
Mumenthaler M 1990 Neurology, 3rd edn. Thieme, New York, p 2
Nelson C F 1994 The tension headache. Migraine headache continuum: a hypothesis. Journal of Manipulative and Physiological Therapeutics 17:156
Nitecki S, Moir C 1994 Predictive factors of the outcome of traumatic cervical spine fracture in children. Journal of Pediatric Surgery 29:1409
Okeson J 2005 Bell's orofacial pains, 6th edn. Quintessence, Chicago
Olesen J 1991 Clinical and pathophysiological observations in migraine and tension-type headache, explained by integration of vascular, supraspinal and myofascial inputs. Pain 46:125
Parker W 1989 Migraine and the vestibular system in childhood and adolescence. American Journal of Otology 10(5):364–371
Pennings L 1995 Craniovertebral kinematics in man and some quadrupedal mammals. An anatomico-radiological comparison. Neuro-orthopedics 17:3
Porter F L, Porges S W, Marshall T E 1988 Newborn pain cries and vagal tone: parallel changes in response to circumcision. Child Development 59:495
Ramachandran V S, Blakesee S 1998 Phantoms in the brain. William Morrow, New York
Reidi H, Pratt S 1988 Slump test in female children between 12–15 years. Thesis. Queensland University, Brisbane
Ross D M, Ross S A 1988 Childhood in pain: current issues, research and management. Urban and Schwarzenberg, Baltimore
Scammon R E 1930 The measurement of the body in childhood. In: Harris J (ed.) The measurement of man. University of Minnesota Press, Minneapolis
Stott D H, Moyes F A, Henderson S E 1984 Manual. Test of motor impairment – Henderson Revision. Book Educational, Guelph
Szirmai A, Farkas S 2000 Vestibular disorders in migrainous children and adolescents. Journal of Headache and Pain 1:39
Tesler M D, Savedra M C, Holzemer W L, Wilkie D J 1991 The word graphic rating scale as a measure

of children's and adolescent's pain intensity. Research in Nursing and Health 14:361
Treuenfelds H 1999 Der Bionator als orthopädischer Vermittler zwischen Gebiss und Wirbelsäule. In: Biedermann H (ed.) Manualtherapie bei Kindern. Enke, Stuttgart, p 133
Uneri A, Turkdogan D 2003 Evaluation of vestibular functions in children with vertigo attacks. Archives of Disease in Childhood 88(6):510–511
Von Piekartz H 2001 Kraniofaziale Dysfunktion und Schmerzen: Untersuchung – Beurteilung – Management. Thieme, Stuttgart
Von Piekartz H, Schouten S, Aufdemkampe G 2006a Neurodynamic responses in children with primary or craniocervical headache versus a control group. A comparative study. Manual Therapy (submitted)
Von Piekartz H, Schouten S, Aufdemkampe G 2006b Static and dynamic coordination in juvenile migraine, cervical headache and a control group. Manual Therapy (submitted)
Wagemans P A H M, Velde van de J P, Kuipers-Jaghtman A 1988 Sutures and forces: a review. American Journal of Orthodontics and Dentofacial Orthopedics 94:129–141
Westerhuis P 2001 Cervical headache: a clinical perspective. In: Von Piekartz H J M, Bryden L (eds) Craniofacial dysfunction and pain: manual therapy, assessment and management. Butterworth-Heinemann, Oxford, p 83
Yuan G, Dougherty L, Margulies S S 1998 In vivo human spinal cord deformation and displacement in flexion. Spine 23:1677
Zeltzer L, Schlank C 2004 Conquering your child's chronic pain. A pediatrian's guide for reclaiming a normal childhood. HarperResource, Los Angeles
Zukunft-Huber B 1998 Die ungestörte Entwicklung ihres Babys. Trias, Stuttgart

APPENDIX 20.1 ANAMNESTIC QUESTIONNAIRE (EWMM)

Dear parents

To complete the subjective examination, there are a number of questions that will help us to design an individual assessment and treatment for your child. You may not be able to answer all of these questions; some may not even apply to your child.
The more you know, the better; please circle the correct answers. If you are not sure, mark it with a question mark or you may leave the question out. If you should have any additional comments, please make a note, so we can talk about them in the next session.

1. Your family:

Are there any known spinal diseases (e.g. scoliosis, deformities, one leg shorter)	Yes / No	Who?
Are there any cervical and/or lumbar dysfunctions (e.g. neck pain/headaches, migraine)	Yes / No	Who?

2. Pregnancies: number......... age of the mother at birth:..........years

Duration of pregnancy..........weeks   Weight at birth..........g   Length..........cm

Breech delivery or other abnormal positions	Yes / No	Which?

3. Birth: Multiple pregnancy   Yes / No

Duration of labour..........hours

Forceps, vacuum extractor	Yes / No	Which?
Caesarean	Yes / No	Why?
Birth trauma	Yes / No	Which?

4. Particulars:

The child had problems going to sleep	Yes / No	
How long did it take on average?	..........hours	
The child woke up frequently	Yes / No	How often?
A certain sleeping position was preferred	Yes / No	Which?
Breast feeding was difficult on one side	Yes / No	Which side?
The baby did not feed well	Yes / No	
It was dribbling and spitting a lot	Yes / No	
It was screaming a lot	Yes / No	
It suffered from 3 month colic	Yes / No	
Our child has a sensitive neck (e.g. when getting dressed)	Yes / No	
It keeps pulling its hair	Yes / No	

5. Other health problems:

Our child suffers from:		
Throat infections	Yes / No	
Neurodermatitis	Yes / No	Since when?
Allergies	Yes / No	Which?
Headaches	Yes / No	How often per week?
Neurological diseases	Yes / No	Which?
Our child needs glasses	Yes / No	Since when?
It keeps its mouth open	Yes / No	

6. Retarded development: How?

Posture and movement	Yes / No	
Speech and understanding	Yes / No	
Concentration/social competence	Yes / No	

7. Asymmetry, posture dysfunctions:

We noticed it immediately after birth	Yes / No	
It took a while until we noticed it	Yes / No	How long?
Somebody pointed it out to us (doctor, midwife, physiotherapist)	Yes / No	Who?
We particularly noticed: (head asymmetry, trunk, leg or arm position, etc.)	....	
The baby: looks only to the	Right / Left	Yes / No
moves only to the	Right / Left	Yes / No
moves both arms symmetrically	Yes / No	Which arm less?
moves both legs symmetrically	Yes / No	Which leg less?
The face is smaller on one side	Yes / No	Right / Left?
The back of the head seems flat on one side	Yes / No	Right / Left?
The back of the head is bald on one side	Yes / No	Right / Left?

8. Therapy until today:

APPENDIX 20.2
CHECKLIST FOR NON-COMMUNICATING CHILDREN WITH PAIN

Vocal
- Groaning, crying, whimpering
- Shouting, screaming
- A certain noise or sound for pain, a 'word', crying or a type of 'laughing'

Eating/sleeping
- Eats less, not interested in food
- Sleeps more
- Sleeps less

Social/personality
- Not cooperative, whining, irritable, unhappy
- Little interaction, secluded
- Seeks comfort and physical contact
- Difficult to distract, impossible to be calmed or to be content

Facial expression for pain (pulling a face, grimacing)
- Frowning
- Changes of the eyes, blinking, eyes widened
- Corners of the mouth pulled down, no smiling
- Mouth shaking, sulking, tight lips
- Clenching/grinding of the teeth, chewing, sticking the tongue out

Activities
- Does not move, less active, quiet
- Jumps around, restless

Trunk and extremities
- Floppy
- Stiff, spastic, tensed, rigid
- Detailed description of body parts
- Points to or touches aching body parts
- Draws back body parts, sensitive to touch
- Moves the body in a certain way to show that it hurts (pulling the head back, arms down, etc.)

Physiological
- Trembling
- Changes in colour, pale
- Sweating, perspiring
- Crying, tears
- Drawing in air, gasping for air
- Holding the breath

After McGrath & Koster (2001).

APPENDIX 20.3
OVERVIEW OF A PAIN DIARY FOR CHILDREN, ACCORDING TO DENECKE & KRÖNER-HERWIG (2000)

Diary

....

No more pain!

Wednesday	Thursday	Friday	Saturday	Sunday
No ☐	No ☐	No ☐	No ☐	No ☐
Yes ☺ Yes ☹	Yes ☺ Yes ☹	Yes ☺ Yes ☹	Yes ☺ Yes ☹	Yes ☺ Yes ☹
What?	What?	What?	What?	What? ....
No ☐ STOP	No ☐ STOP	No ☐ STOP	No ☐ STOP	No ☐ STOP
Yes ☐ What	Yes ☐ What	Yes ☐ What	Yes ☐ What	Yes ☐ What
Please continue	Please continue	Please continue	Please continue	Please continue
0 – 10	0 – 10	0 – 10	0 – 10	0 – 10
12, 3, 6, 9 during the day; 12, 3, 6, 9 at night	12, 3, 6, 9 during the day; 12, 3, 6, 9 at night	12, 3, 6, 9 during the day; 12, 3, 6, 9 at night	12, 3, 6, 9 during the day; 12, 3, 6, 9 at night	12, 3, 6, 9 during the day; 12, 3, 6, 9 at night
Yes ☐ No ☐	Yes ☐ No ☐	Yes ☐ No ☐	Yes ☐ No ☐	Yes ☐ No ☐
Yes ☐ No ☐	Yes ☐ No ☐	Yes ☐ No ☐	Yes ☐ No ☐	Yes ☐ No ☐
Yes ☐ No ☐	Yes ☐ No ☐	Yes ☐ No ☐	Yes ☐ No ☐	Yes ☐ No ☐
Place your sticker here	Place your sticker here	Place your sticker here	Place your sticker here	Place your sticker here

Chapter 21

Postural changes in the craniofacial and craniocervical regions as a result of changed breathing patterns

Ronel Jordaan

CHAPTER CONTENTS

INTRODUCTION

In 1861, a well-known American artist, George Catlin, wrote about the noxious effects of mouth breathing. The title of this publication, *The Breath of Life*, was subsequently changed to *Shut Your Mouth and Save Your Life*. He stated that this infernal habit causes the teeth to take different and unnatural directions and often, to sadly disfigure the human face for life (Fig. 21.1). According to him, these changes affect confidence and an open mouth could even weaken a person to the end of their fingers and toes. Catlin was the first to direct attention to the fact that mouth breathing can lead to facial deformity and malocclusion (abnormal alignment) of the teeth (Goldsmith & Stool 1994).

The role of impaired nasorespiratory function as an aetiological factor in the development of certain dentofacial characteristics has been argued since 1872, when Tomes described the changes associated with nasal airway blockage (Venetikidou 1993). Numerous studies have been conducted to indicate the close association between obstruction of the nasal airway and craniocervical posture. These studies clearly show that obstruction or decreased adequacy of the nasopharyngeal airway results in an increased craniocervical angulation

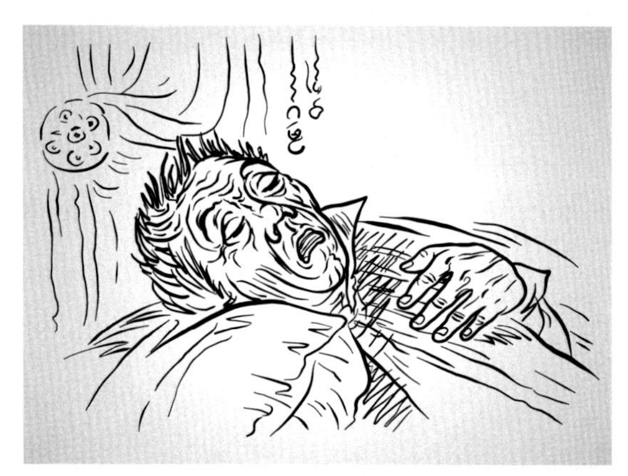

Fig. 21.1 Appearance of the face due to habitual mouth breathing, as described by George Catlin in 1861.

(Linder-Aronson 1979, Wenzel et al 1983, Hellsing et al 1986, Tourne & Schweiger 1996).

An important concept in the field of craniofacial research is the adaptability and plasticity of the craniofacial bones (Miller et al 1984). Solow and Kreiborg (1977) suggested a chain of interactions after a change in airway adequacy. The effects of changed airway adequacy on the growth and development of craniofacial structures have been extensively studied for several decades (Solow & Kreiborg 1977, Solow et al 1984, Wenzel et al 1985, Ono et al 1998, Tadao & Kenji 2003, Sousa et al 2005). The detrimental influence of abnormal breathing patterns on craniocervical development during the adolescent growth spurt has not yet been determined. Little or no research has been done on the resultant effect of growth on an abnormally aligned craniocervical posture.

The aim of this chapter is to renew and stimulate an interest in the interaction between form and function in the orocraniofacial and cervical regions, particularly focusing on altered breathing patterns and the resultant postural alignment.

BREATHING PATTERNS

Respiration is an important life-sustaining function involving numerous structures. The mandible and tongue are intimately associated with respiration, as respiratory needs are the primary determinant of the posture of the mandible, tongue and head (Proffit & Fields 1993, Wiltshire 1996). The axial musculature of the spinal vertebrae is also involved in respiration, contributing to the maintenance of the airway (Rocabado & Iglash 1991, Wiltshire 1996). As the physiological maintenance of the airway is essential to life it must be sufficiently dynamic to accommodate the growth and development of the musculoskeletal system and its response to physiological activity (Rocabado & Iglash 1991).

No two persons breathe in exactly the same manner, and no single person breathes in exactly the same way under all conditions (Proffit & Fields 1993). A variety of normal breathing patterns is used under different conditions. To understand and recognize altered breathing patterns, it is important to define normal breathing patterns and the relevant biomechanics of the orocraniofacial and oropharyngeal structures involved in breathing.

NORMAL BREATHING PATTERNS

According to Ricketts (1968), normal breathing takes place through the nasal cavity with little or no strain, while the mouth is closed (Fig. 21.2). The function of the tortuous nasal passages is not only to warm and humidify the inspired air, but also to create an element of resistance to air flow (Proffit & Fields 1993, Kraus 1994, Jankelson 1995). Nasal breathing will ensure a more ideal use of the diaphragm, the principal driver of respiration, and proper ventilation of the lungs, promoting general relaxation of the body (Kraus 1994).

Although humans are primarily nasal breathers, everyone breathes partially through the mouth under certain physiological conditions (Ricketts 1968, Proffit & Fields 1993). For the average individual, there is a transition to partial oral breathing when ventilatory exchange rates above 40–45 litres per minute are reached. This can happen during exercise, heavy mental concentration or even normal conversation, all leading to an increase in air flow (Proffit & Fields 1993).

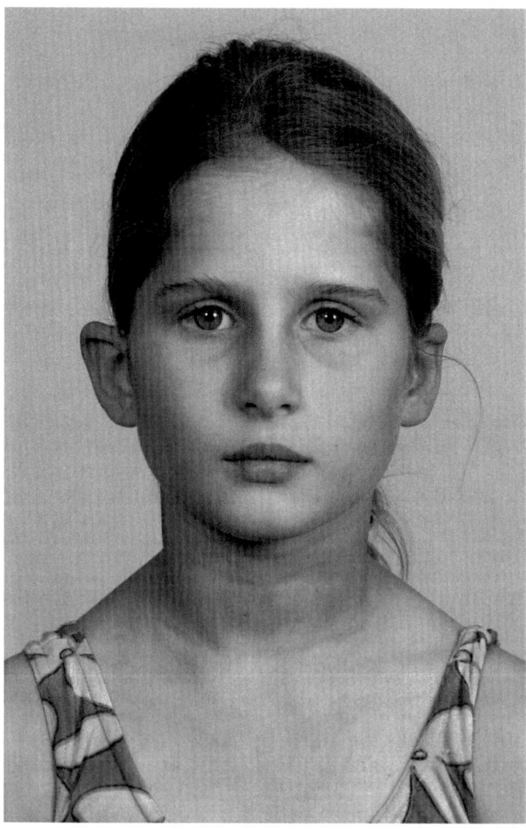

Fig. 21.2 A child with a normal nasal breathing pattern.

The mandibular resting position

In the natural resting position of the mandible, a nasal breathing pattern is present, preventing breathing through the mouth (Rocabado & Iglash 1991). This position has been described as a relatively static posture maintained by a delicate balance of muscle forces. This balance is determined by the muscle tone of the masticatory muscles pulling from above and the force of gravity, as well as the tone of the hyoid muscles pulling from below (Kraus 1988, 1994a, Jankelson 1995) (see Fig. 21.2). The mandible is suspended from the cranium by passive myotonic activity of the masticatory muscles, and the position of the mandible is dictated by the muscles of mastication and the anterior cervical muscles (Lawrence & Samson 1988).

The muscular equilibrium that determines the rest position of the mandible is a function of the maintenance of head posture (Ayub et al 1984). A more appropriate term for the mandibular resting position is probably the upright postural position of the mandible, as this implies the essential interrelationship of the mandible, head and neck in the upright position (Kraus 1994). In this position, the head is held in an upright or orthostatic position, with the malar bone of the craniofacial region vertically aligned with the sternum, and the cranium in 15° of anterior rotation (Rocabado & Iglash 1991). No occlusal contact occurs between the upper and lower teeth in this position, and an interocclusal or free space of 2–5 mm exists between the maxillary and mandibular central incisors (Kraus 1988, 1994a, Rocabado & Iglash 1991).

The significance of the mandibular resting position lies in the fact that all stomatognathic structures are in balance. This entails light lip contact or lips slightly apart, opposing teeth separated, jaw muscles at rest from function, mandible passively suspended against gravity and the tongue at rest. The position of the mandible impacts on the position of the head on the neck, and indirectly on the entire upper body posture (Ayub et al 1984, Rocabado & Iglash 1991). It is a position at which all functional movements of the mandible start and end (Kraus 1994). It permits tissues of the stomatognathic system to rest and repair (Kraus 1988).

The resting position of the tongue

The resting position of the tongue against the palate occurs when the anterior part of the tongue is in contact with the rugae of the palate, just posterior to the upper central incisors. The lateral margins of the tongue are contained within the lingual aspects of the maxillary bone, and the base of the tongue is in contact with the soft palate. The dorsum of the tongue is held against the hard palate by the space of negative air pressure created by the vacuum system of the tongue against the palate. This triple seal during lip closure enables the tongue to overcome the force of gravity (Ricketts 1968, Rocabado & Iglash 1991, Kraus 1994).

When the tongue assumes its normal resting position, the musculature of the craniomandibular system (temporal, masseter and pterygoid muscles) enters a reflex relaxation stage and the mandible descends into its rest position to create the free space. The lips, cheeks and tongue exert a balanced internal and external force against the teeth. Therefore, normal lip seal and tongue position promote normal development of the dental alveolar region by equalizing forces applied to the teeth (Fig. 21.3). A correct resting position of the tongue forces nasal–diaphragmatic breathing (Rocabado & Iglash 1991, Kraus 1994).

Normal nasal breathing depends on a balanced, interactive relationship between all the components of the head, neck and shoulder region (Fig. 21.4). An imbalance of one component will have an effect on all the other components, causing an altered breathing pattern.

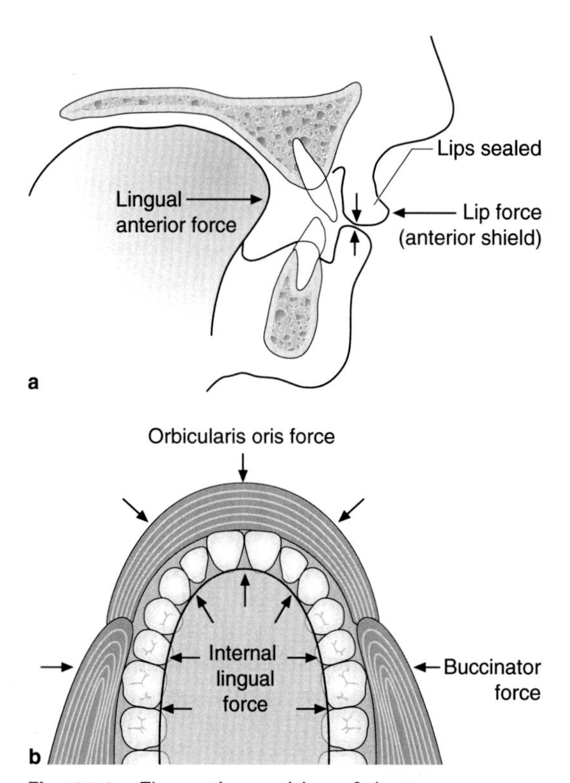

Fig. 21.3 The resting position of the tongue promotes normal development of the dental alveolar region by equalizing the internal and external forces applied to the teeth.

ABNORMAL BREATHING PATTERNS

Wenzel et al (1983) describe increased oral involvement in respiration with obstruction of the nasal airway as an abnormal breathing pattern. According to Wiltshire (1996), when the nasal passageways prove ineffective in performing the life-sustaining breathing function, the mouth exists as an emergency alternative breathing route. Rocabado and Iglash (1991) define the mouth breathing syndrome as a habitual pattern through the mouth instead of the nose. They also mention that a combination of nasal and oral breathing is often observed, but this is not a normal breathing pattern.

Respiration is most efficient with modest resistance present in the respiratory system, but increased work for nasal respiration is physiologically acceptable only to a point. With partial nasal obstruction, the work associated with nasal breathing increases and, at a certain level of resistance to nasal airflow, the individual switches to partial mouth breathing. This crossover point varies among individuals.

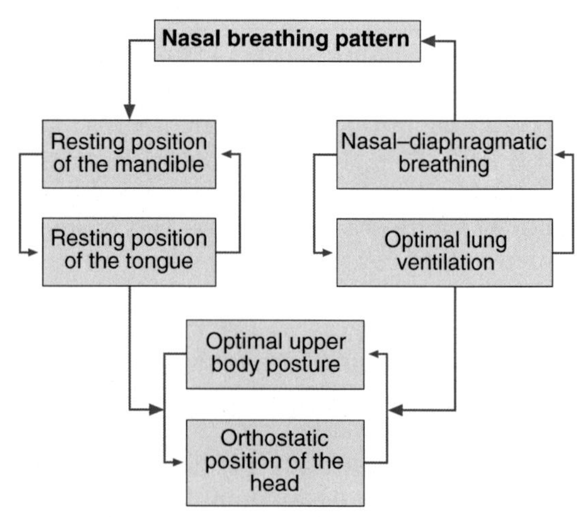

Fig. 21.4 A normal nasal breathing pattern and its relationship to function of all parts of the head, throat and shoulder region.

Total obstruction in humans is rare, but partial nasal obstruction can occur occasionally for a period of time, or in some children chronically (Proffit & Fields 1993). In some cases, extremely obstructed individuals continue to force air through the nose, using more effort to breathe. On the other hand, some people with clear nasopharyngeal passages are habitual mouth breathers. There are, however, some individuals with total blockage of the nasal airways who may be described as pure mouth breathers. In all other cases a combination of nasal and oral respiration is found (Linder-Aronson & Woodside 2000).

Certain neuromuscular adjustments are required to maintain adequate respiratory function when nasal resistance increases (Miller et al 1984). Therefore, because the respiratory need is the primary determinant of the posture of the jaw, tongue and head, it seems reasonable that an altered respiratory pattern can change the posture of the jaw, tongue and head (Proffit & Fields 1993). When the equilibrium position of the tongue and jaw changes, a chain of body adaptations is triggered. This could lead to dysfunctional patterns and could also have a significant deleterious effect on craniofacial growth and tooth positions (Rocabado & Iglash 1991, Wiltshire 1996). Breathing through the mouth also decreases the effects of diaphragmatic breathing and increases the use of the accessory muscles of breathing (Kraus 1994).

Causative factors of changed breathing patterns

There are numerous factors that can contribute to obstruction or partial obstruction of the nasal airways, changing normal breathing patterns to physiologically abnormal breathing patterns.

Chronic respiratory obstruction can be produced by prolonged inflammation of the nasal mucosa associated with allergies, chronic respiratory infection and asthma. Nasal allergies and respiratory infections in early childhood are common causes of adenoidal hypertrophy (enlargement of the adenoids that can cause obstruction and restricted respiratory flow through the nasal passages). Symptoms associated with adenoidal hypertrophy are blocked nose, mouth breathing, snoring or rhinitis (Solow et al 1993, Haapaniemi 1995). For example, an 11-year-old boy with nasal allergy and recurrent respiratory infections presents with nasal obstruction and mouth breathing. This boy is also an orthodontic patient, and is being treated for dental malocclusion (Fig. 21.5).

The size of the posterior nasopharyngeal soft tissue, or adenoids, increases rapidly after birth. Maximum size is attained between 4 and 6 years, after which it stays the same until 8–9 years of age. Thereafter this lymphoid tissue gradually begins to involute (Haapaniemi 1995). Any condition that causes hypertrophy of the adenoids can cause respiratory obstruc-

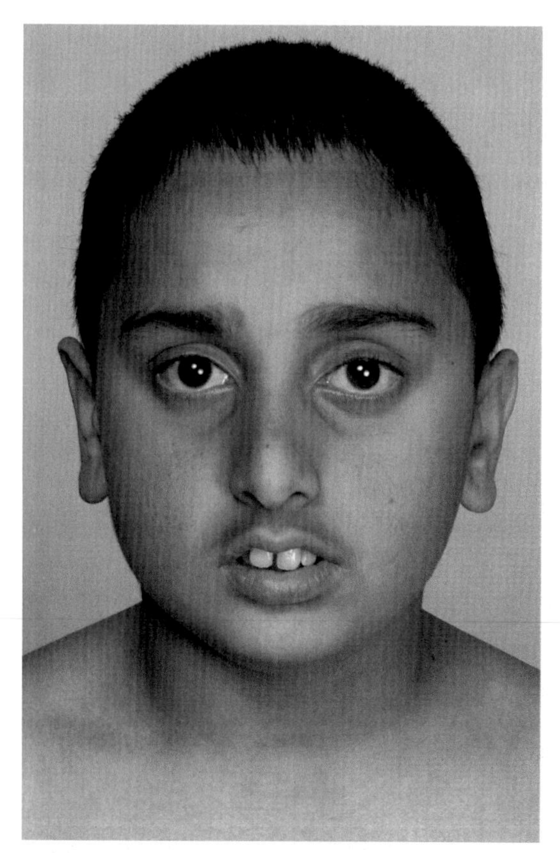

Fig. 21.5 An 11-year-old boy with a mouth breathing pattern.

tion in the nasopharynx (Garry 1992, Linder-Aronson & Woodside 2000). The oropharyngeal space, situated dorsal to the tongue, can be obstructed by enlarged tonsils as a result of chronic or recurrent acute tonsillitis (Linder-Aronson & Woodside 2000). One reason for reduced nasal resistance in older children and transiently increased nasal resistance in prepubertal children (Crouse et al 2000) may be hypertrophy of the adenoid glands in prepubertal children, a phenomenon that is well described in the literature. Another possible reason could be swelling of the nasal mucosa in response to increased gonadotrophin secretion in early puberty.

Developmental deficiencies in the facial skeleton may predispose a patient to mouth breathing, for example a maxilla deficient in vertical height or mandibular growth deficiencies in the mandibular head, impairing nasopharyngeal function. Other causes could be deviation of the nasal septum or narrowing of the external nares (Rocabado & Iglash 1991, Garry 1992, Kraus 1994). Extreme obesity could cause a dorsal position of the tongue with a short posterior airway space between the tongue and the posterior pharyngeal wall, causing airway obstruction in adults (Solow et al 1993). Other interesting trigger factors for changed breathing patterns are disturbances in the visual or proprioceptive system as well as cervical spine anomalies (Solow et al 1984).

FUNCTIONAL ADAPTATIONS AS A RESULT OF ALTERED BREATHING PATTERNS

Changed breathing patterns necessitate changes in the biomechanics of respiration. Due to the fact that all the orocraniofacial and craniocervical structures are biomechanically intimately linked, respiratory changes will have an impact on all these structures. The chain of reactions entails a change in mandibular posture, changing the forces in the oral and craniofacial regions and consequently affecting the craniocervical posture (Ricketts 1968, Miller et al 1984).

CHANGED BIOMECHANICS OF RESPIRATION

Nasal obstruction induces a change in respiratory function involving the anterior portion of the upper respiratory tract. Nasal obstruction initiates a change in which the oral cavity must then serve as the major or perhaps the only pathway for periodic airflow during all respiratory demands. In adapting the oral passages for chronic respiratory work, the anterior portal is achieved by two mechanisms: raising the upper lip and lowering the mandible (Miller et al 1984, Lawrence & Razook 1994). A proprioceptive response at the dorsum of the tongue resulting from hypertrophied lymphoid tissue leads to a non-physiological lowered position of the tongue involving a lowered mandible. In this position the protrusive action of the tongue can widen the posterior cavity to increase oral breathing (Miller et al 1984, Garry 1992).

In contrast to this proposed mechanism to achieve oral breathing, Ricketts (1968) suggests that by lifting the head into extension, away from the hyomandibular complex, the transition from nose to mouth breathing is facilitated. The increased craniocervical angulation associated with obstruction of the upper airway could possibly reduce the airway resistance by increasing the diameter of the oropharyngeal and nasopharyngeal airways (Solow et al 1993, Lawrence & Razook 1994).

With mouth breathing a higher inspiratory effort is demanded of the accessory muscles of respiration (sternocleidomastoid, upper trapezius, scalene and pectoral), the resultant hyperactivity of which leads to poor postural alignment. The decreased activity of the diaphragm and hypotonicity of the abdominal musculature will perpetuate the faulty posture, characterized by protrusion of the abdominal region and an increased lumbar lordosis. The postural changes include a forward head posture, protracted shoulders, depressed sternum, abnormal development of the upper thoracic region and an anterior pelvic tilt with an increased lumbar lordosis (Rocabado & Iglash 1991, Kraus 1994, Ribeiro et al 2004) (Fig. 21.6).

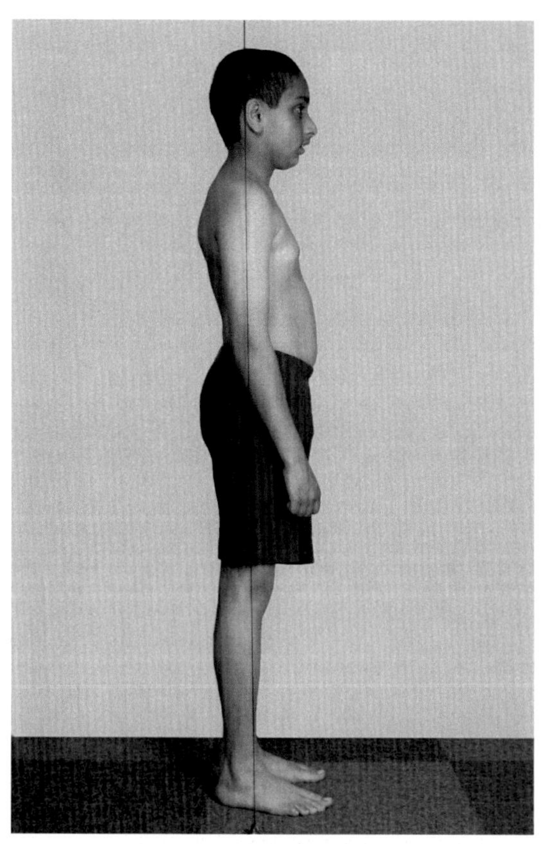

Fig. 21.6 Mouth breathing impacts on the whole body posture as seen in this 11-year-old boy with nasal obstruction. Note the protracted shoulders, the forward head posture and the retrognathic mandible.

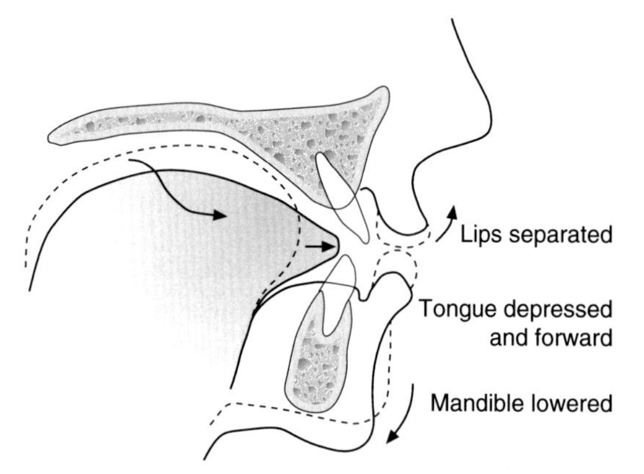

Fig. 21.7 Functional adaptation in the oral region resulting from nasal obstruction. The mandible adopts a lower functional position, the lips are separated and the tongue is displaced inferior and forward.

Although there are different opinions on the exact mechanism involved in oral respiration, it is clear that the mandible is lowered, the head tilted into extension and that the total body posture changes as a result.

CHANGES IN THE ORAL AND CRANIOFACIAL REGIONS

To maintain adequate respiratory function when the nasal airway becomes obstructed, neuromuscular adjustments are required, resulting in postural changes in the oral and craniofacial structures.

The neuromuscular suspension of the mandible is a highly sensitive mechanism that responds with an altered mandibular position during nasopharyngeal obstruction (Linder-Aronson & Woodside 2000). The mandible adopts a lower functional postural position, separating the lips, displacing the tongue inferiorly and the hyoid bone caudally (Fig. 21.7). In the presence of enlarged tonsils or adenoids, the tongue will be displaced inferiorly and forward (Ricketts 1968, Miller et al 1984, Lawrence & Razook 1994). Misalignment of the mandible in relation to the craniomaxillary complex predisposes the temporomandibular joint to dysfunction, as the optimal position of the joint is disturbed (Garry 1992, Kritsineli & Shim 1992, Okeson 1998).

Altered respiratory mode from the nasal to the oral passage is associated with neuromuscular adaptations, inducing changes in electromyographic (EMG) activity of various muscles (Miller et al 1984, Ono et al 1998). A lowered mandibular position inhibits the activity in the masseter and anterior temporal muscles (Hellsing et al 1986, Ono et al 1998). Nasal obstruction is associated with increased activity in the suprahyoid area, generated by several muscles. The anterior digastric muscle depresses the mandible and maintains it in this position. The geniohyoid muscle helps to maintain the position of the hyoid bone as well as airway adequacy with the mandible in the depressed position. Adaptation of the oral cavity for respiratory function is mediated by a change in tongue position, to a position inferior and anterior, increasing the activity in the genioglossus muscle (Miller et al 1984, Hellsing et al 1986, Ono et al 1998).

Other muscles showing increased EMG activity are the lateral pterygoids (sustaining the open mouth position), the nasal dilator muscles (dilating the external nares), superior orbicularis oris and the lip elevator muscles (Miller et al 1984, Williams et al 2000).

All these changes in the oral and craniofacial structures indicate the intimate functional relationships, stressing the fact that a change in one component will have an effect on all the other components (Fig. 21.8).

CHANGES IN ORAL AND CRANIOFACIAL MORPHOLOGY

Impaired breathing is a significant factor contributing to the aetiology of dentofacial deformities and malocclusion during childhood growth (Cheng et al 1988, Hideharu & Kenji 2003, Tecco et al 2005). It is generally accepted that chronic mouth breathing influences craniofacial growth and development (Sousa et al 2005). The changed posture of the head, jaw and tongue with mouth breathing could alter the equilibrium of pressures on the jaw and teeth and affect jaw growth and tooth positions (Huggare & Cooke 1994, Weinstein 1994, Turner et al 1997). There is no effect on craniofacial growth in subjects who convert to mouth breathing for a short time. However,

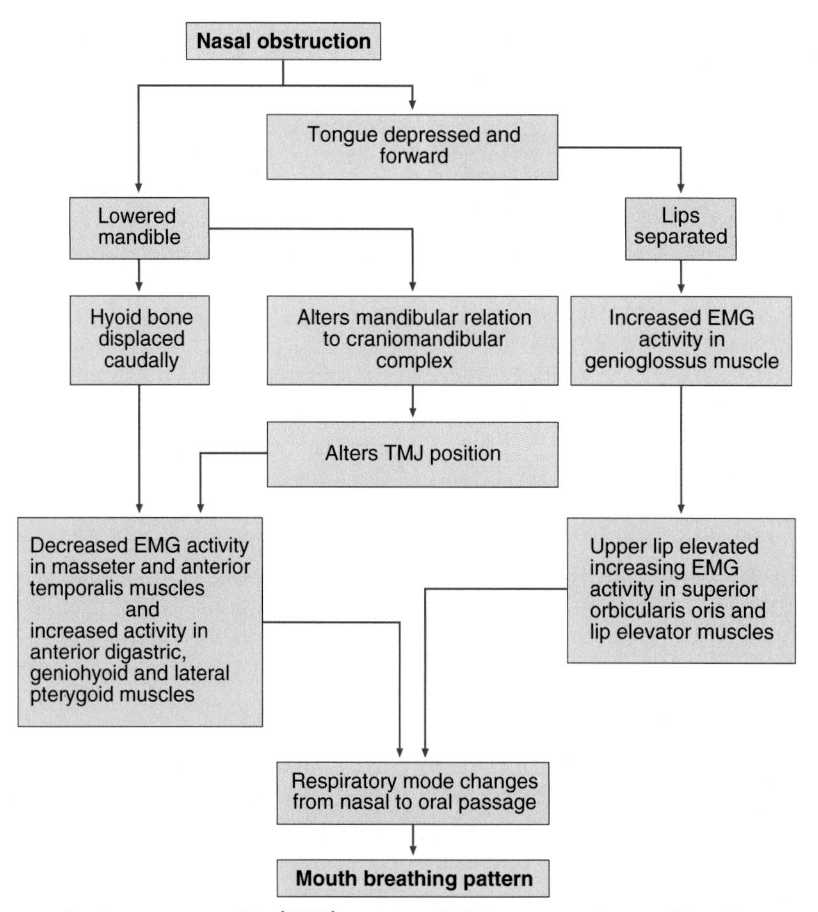

Fig. 21.8 Changes in electromyographic (EMG) activity of different muscles resulting from nasal obstruction (modified after Linder-Aronson & Woodside 2000). TMJ, temporomandibular joint.

chronic respiratory obstruction and maintained postural changes could have a definite effect on the stress-reducing system of the neuro- and viscerocranium, causing abnormal craniofacial growth in the growing child (Özbek & Köklü 1993, Huggare 1998, Schlenker et al 2000, Oudhof 2001, von Piekartz 2001). The relationship between mouth breathing, changed posture and the development of malocclusions is not clearly defined and experimental studies have only attempted to partially clarify the enigma (Proffit & Fields 1993, Wiltshire 1996).

With changed breathing and a lowered mandible, a steep mandible plane angle and a dolichocephalic face (long and narrow) develop (Cheng et al 1988, Garry 1992). 'Adenoid face' is the popular term associated with mouth breathing, consisting of narrow facial dimensions, protruding teeth and narrowed dental arches, as well as non-functional lips that are separated at rest. The changed position of the tongue causes a decrease in lingual pressure on the maxillary arches, consequently losing the tongue's expansion force that promotes normal growth and development (Rocabado & Iglash 1991). With the increased pressure from the stretched cheeks due to an open mouth position, a narrowed maxillary dental arch will result, as well as lingualization of the teeth (Garry 1992, Proffit & Fields 1993, Linder-Aronson & Woodside 2000) (Fig. 21.9). The transverse compression of the maxillary arch causes a crossbite and a high arched or deep palate. With crossbite, the maxillary incisors are crowded or protruded. The lips become shortened, hypertonic and non-functional, with less pressure on the anterior teeth that would tend to procline. A downward and backward rotation of the mandible and tongue protrusion will occur with mouth breathing, with an increased overjet and development of an anterior open bite. The increased activity of the genioglossus muscle exerts a definite influence on incisor position (Rocabado & Iglash 1991, Proffit & Fields 1993, Turner et al 1997, Schlenker et al 2000). The characteristics of an adenoid face are:

- Mouth breathing
- Long, narrow dimensions of the face
- Flat mandibular angle
- Protruded teeth
- Narrowed dental arches
- Non-functional, hypertonic lips
- Lips separated in the resting position
- Depressed and swollen tongue
- Lingualization of the teeth
- Crossbite
- Anterior open bite
- High arched or deep palate
- Downward and backward rotation of the mandible
- Abnormal stress-reducing forces in the neurocranium and viscerocranium.

A typical adenoid face is shown in Figure 21.10.

In the search for determinants of craniofacial development, a clear pattern of association

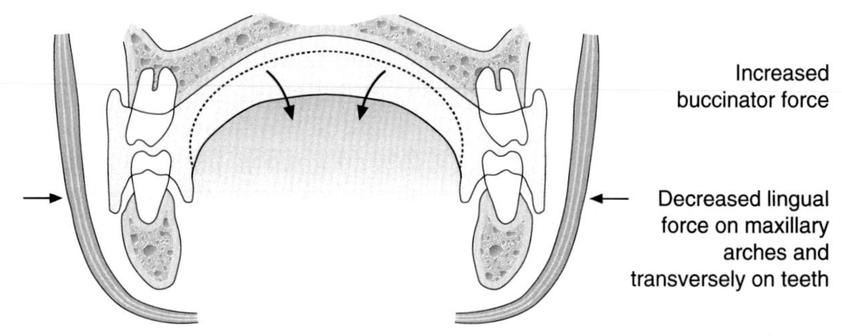

Fig. 21.9 Intra- and extraoral forces resulting from mouth breathing and a changed resting position of the tongue.

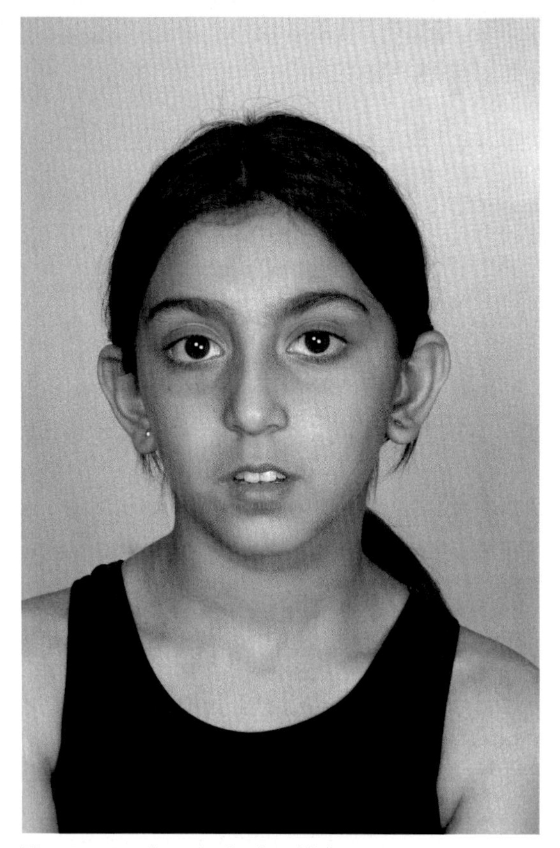

Fig. 21.10 A typical adenoid face.

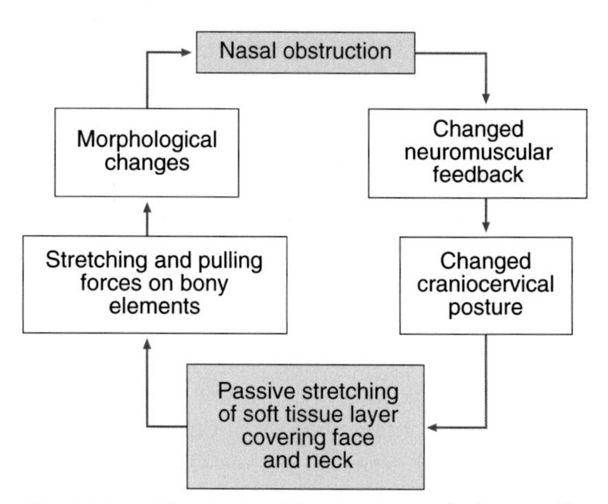

Fig. 21.11 The chain of interactions relating nasal obstruction to craniofacial morphology and posture (modified after Solow & Kreiborg 1977).

between craniocervical posture and craniofacial morphology was noticed. Among the characteristics were reduced facial prognathism, a large mandibular plane inclination and a large lower anterior facial height (Solow & Sonnesen 1998, Schlenker et al 2000). Solow and Kreiborg (1977) proposed a soft tissue stretch hypothesis to account for the association between airway obstruction, head posture and craniofacial morphology. They suggested that head extension causes an increase in tension, or stretching of the soft tissue layer covering the face, continuing into the investing fascia of the neck. A subsequent retrusive force on facial morphology will result. According to Buchman et al (1994), determinants of skeletal development reside in the surrounding soft tissues and not in the bone. Properties such as pressure and muscle pull and tension have been implicated as possible factors that could regulate bone growth.

Further consideration of the mechanism relating head posture to craniofacial morphology leads to a chain of interactions (Fig. 21.11). Any link in this sequence of events could be the site of the primary symptoms. In children, an example of triggering factors could be enlarged adenoid tissue or asthma, causing airway obstruction, changed biomechanics of respiration, changed neuromuscular feedback and changed craniocervical posture. This will lead to passive stretching forces on the soft tissue layer comprising skin, muscles and fascia that covers the head and neck. Stretching of this convex tissue layer creates a dorsally directed force on the bony elements to which they attach, impeding normal growth of the face in a forward direction, resulting in morphologic changes (Solow & Kreiborg 1977, Solow et al 1984, Sandham 1988, Solow & Sonnesen 1998).

It is clear that there are a number of interrelated factors that could produce orocraniofacial changes in chronic mouth breathing cases. However, according to Linder-Aronson and Woodside (2000), for malocclusion and altered skeletal relationships to occur, one or all of the following neuromuscular responses must be present:

- Altered mandibular posture
- Altered tongue posture
- Extended head posture.

Diagnostic factors such as nasal obstruction may be relatively unimportant in an individual. The important point is the individual's neuromuscular response to the initial stimulus. If a person with airway obstruction responds in one or all of the stated ways, malocclusion will occur. If not, the individual may respond by breathing with increased chest activity to overcome the obstruction (Linder-Aronson & Woodside 2000).

Many malocclusions previously thought to be of genetic origin are in reality neuromuscular imitations of genetically based problems. This is an important concept because, if it is true, it implies that such malocclusions could be partially reversed by removal of the neuromuscular impact (Linder-Aronson & Woodside 2000).

CHANGES IN CRANIOCERVICAL POSTURE

The head posture is maintained by a series of paired agonistic and antagonistic muscles that provide stability, dynamic balance and function. The posterior cervical muscles pull the head posterior and inferior, whereas the muscles of the anterior region of the head (muscles of mastication, hyoid muscles and anterior cervical muscles) exert a counterbalance by pulling the head anteriorly and slightly inferior (Fig. 21.12). The resulting forces of these interacting muscles maintain the head in the orthostatic or upright position (Rocabado & Iglash 1991). According to Brodie (1950) and Okeson (1998), the muscles act as elastic bands to maintain a balanced head position. If the tension in one elastic band or muscle increases or changes, it will result in a change in all the others, altering head posture.

Many studies have demonstrated the correlation between nasal obstruction and head posture. Hellsing et al (1986) induced oral respiration in human subjects, and an immediate response observed was head extension and a lowered mandible. Tourne and Schweiger (1996) conducted a similar study, inducing nasal obstruction, but used radiographic techniques to examine the head posture, which

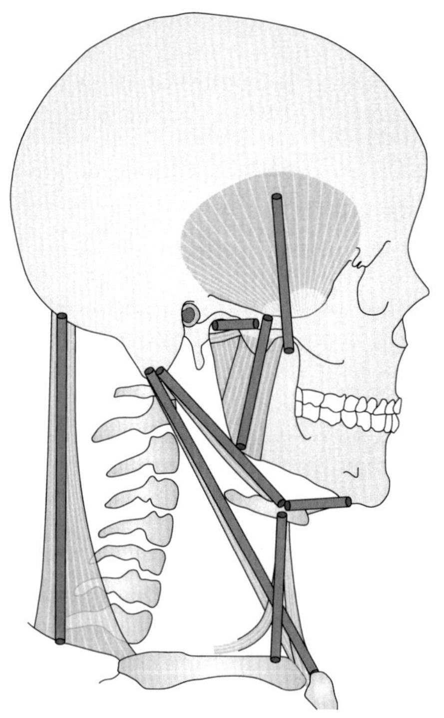

Fig. 21.12 The resulting forces of a series of interacting muscles maintain the head in the orthostatic or upright position. The posterior cervical muscles pull the head posteroinferior and the muscles of the anterior region exert a counterbalance by pulling the head anteroinferior. At the same time, there is a balance between the craniomandibular or masticatory muscles and the hyoid muscles (adapted from Okeson 1998).

also indicated head extension in response to nasal obstruction. Wenzel et al (1985) treated children with chronic asthma and rhinitis with intranasal corticosteroids and after 1 month the nasal resistance decreased, which was associated with a significant decrease in craniocervical angulation. A study by Solow et al (1984) showed marked correlations between airway obstruction and craniocervical angulation with cervical inclination. Children with adenoidal obstruction presented with an increase in craniocervical angulation or forward head posture, which decreased after adenoidectomy (Solow et al 1993).

If the head posture is changed by extending the head from the lower cervical region, the nasopharynx will be obstructed. However, if the head is extended from the upper cervical vertebrae, the nasopharynx will be widened (Hellsing 1989). It is clear that airway obstruction triggers an increase in head extension via the upper cervical vertebrae (Linder-Aronson & Woodside 2000) as the occiput extends on the atlas and the atlas extends on the axis (Kraus 1988). This facilitates oral breathing by enlargement of the nasopharyngeal and oropharyngeal airway space (Linder-Aronson & Woodside 2000). The increased craniocervical angulation is described by Ricketts (1968) as a lift of the head away from the hyomandibular complex to facilitate mouth breathing. This head extension entails a posterior roll and anterior glide of the occipital condyles on the atlantal facets (White & Panjabi 1990, Hanten et al 1991).

To sustain this altered head posture resulting from mouth breathing, the EMG activity in all the associated muscles will change as these muscles are closely functionally linked in a kinetic chain. Head extension will cause an increase in activity in the following muscles:

- Suprahyoid and infrahyoid muscles: The activity will increase, possibly due to an increased stretch in the suprahyoid muscles which causes displacement of the hyoid bone; the infrahyoid muscles will respond by increasing the activity to stabilize the hyoid bone (Forsberg et al 1985). Another reason could be that the sustained position of the mandible in a depressed posture generates an increase in activity (Rocabado 1983, Hellsing et al 1986, Lawrence & Samson 1988).
- Masseter muscle (Forsberg et al 1985, Hellsing et al 1986, Kraus 1994).
- Sternocleidomastoid (Forsberg et al 1985).
- Lateral pterygoid muscle: To sustain the depressed position of the mandible (Lawrence & Samson 1988).
- Anterior cervical muscles: To sustain the mandible position (Lawrence & Samson 1988).
- Temporalis and anterior digastric muscles (Kraus 1994).

Muscles that show a decrease in EMG activity are:

- Posterior cervical muscles: As the centre of gravity moves closer to the supporting occipital condyles with the changed head posture, lower muscle activity is needed to balance the head (Forsberg et al 1985, Hellsing et al 1986, 1987).
- Anterior temporal muscle: Activity decreases as the mandible is lowered beyond the clinically established rest position (Hellsing et al 1986). Forsberg et al (1985) mentioned in their study that activity in this muscle varied and no significant association between a changed head posture and EMG activity could be established.

The individual will protract their head in this extended head posture as the visual axis needs to be maintained in its original horizontal position. Protraction of the head entails an anterior gliding or translation movement of the cervical spine to lower the visual axis. This will result in a forward head posture (Darlow et al 1987, Rocabado & Iglash 1991, Bogduk 1994, Grimmer 1997). This forward displacement of the head is associated with a lowered mandible, disrupted lip seal and loss of tongue rest position; the malar bone is positioned anterior to the sternum. In addition, the accessory respiratory muscles (sternocleidomastoid, scaleni and pectoralis major) could be hyperactive, producing shoulder protraction and depression of the sternum (Ayub et al 1984, Rocabado & Iglash 1991).

The resultant effects of a forward head posture are excessive compression forces on the cervical apophyseal joints and the posterior part of the vertebral bodies (Ayub et al 1984). The anterior vertebral muscles on the convex side of the curvature– neck flexors and infrahyoid muscles – are stretched and subsequently become lengthened and weakened, elevating the hyoid bone. The posterior muscles on the concave side of the curvature – the suboccipital, rectus capitis posterior and oblique capitis muscles – will shorten, as will the suprahyoid muscles (Ayub et al 1984, Darling et al 1984, Enwemeka et al 1986, Darlow et al 1987, White & Sahrman 1994).

Box 21. 1 Clinical implications of altered craniocervical posture associated with mouth breathing

The therapist should consider the following structures when assessing and treating the patient:

- Cervical apophyseal joint compression
- Anterior cervical muscles stretched and weakened
- Posterior cervical muscles shortened
- Changed craniocervical posture impacting on alignment of total body posture
- Altered proprioceptive input
- Increased tension in certain soft tissue structures and decreased tension in others
- Changed joint loading – increasing/decreasing compressive forces on bony structures together with their impact on morphology of the craniofacial and craniocervical regions.

According to Janda (1994), muscle imbalance patterns will not remain limited to the cervical region, but will gradually involve the entire muscular system. As a result, movement patterns will change and dysfunction of the spinal column may elicit symptoms of the neuromusculoskeletal system (Box 21.1).

THE EFFECT OF ALTERED BREATHING PATTERNS ON CRANIONEURODYNAMICS

When assessing patients with abnormal breathing patterns, the therapist will most probably find musculoskeletal dysfunction. The primary structures that should be examined as a possible cause for symptoms are the bony structures and the neuromuscular tissue. But what about the peripheral nervous system? Could changes in the craniofacial region over a long period of time (months or longer) cause alterations in cranioneurodynamics? The structures of the nervous system that could possibly be influenced during altered breathing patterns are the brainstem and the dura, cranial nerves such as the buccal, lingual and inferior alveolar divisions of the trigeminal nerve (V), as well as the facial (VII), accessory (XI) and hypoglossal (XII) nerves (von Piekartz 2001). For neuroanatomy, neurodynamics, pathodynamics and discussion of the tests, see Chapters 17 and 18.

THE IMPORTANCE OF ALTERED BREATHING PATTERNS DURING THE ADOLESCENT GROWTH SPURT

Puberty can be defined as the transitional period between the juvenile stage and adulthood. It starts with a marked increase in the general growth rate and ends with the termination of growth. Every muscular and skeletal dimension appears to be involved in this growth spurt (Taranger & Hägg 1980, Rocabado & Iglash 1991, Proffit & Fields 1993).

In 1998, Hensinger and Arbor made an important statement. According to them, growth is that which sets paediatric orthopaedics apart from adult orthopaedics. In paediatric orthopaedics the three dimensions are presented by the frontal, sagittal and coronal axes. The fourth dimension is growth, or change over time. It is this concept of growth that creates the challenge, as growth is a continuum and, as a consequence, in paediatric orthopaedics there is no 'end of case' until growth is completed (Hensinger & Arbor 1998).

The processes of growth and development are usually accepted as facts of everyday life. However, when one considers the powerful forces at work and the many harmoniously intermingled regulators that harness them, the emergence of a mature adult human being is a source of wonder (Proffit & Fields 1993).

THE PRINCIPLES OF GROWTH

Growth is defined as the increase in the number of cells and size. But growth is not just about growing bigger, it is also about maturing. It is a dynamic process of change over time (McGowan et al 1995, Hensinger & Arbor 1998).

Growth is strongly influenced by genetic factors, but is also significantly affected by the environment, in the form of nutritional status, degree of physical activity, health or illness and other similar factors. Exactly what determines growth remains unclear, and different theories have attempted to explain the determinants of growth (LeVeau & Bernhardt 1984, Proffit & Fields 1993). According to Moss' 'functional matrix theory' of growth (which is the most widely accepted theory concerning determinants of growth control), the growth of the spinal and craniofacial skeleton lies in the adjacent soft tissues (Proffit & Fields 1993, Moss 1997, Oudhof 2001).

The importance of mechanical influences constantly acting on the body is extraordinary, and can affect the shape and size of the body parts, especially those of the musculoskeletal system (LeVeau & Bernhardt 1984, Hensinger & Arbor 1998). According to LeVeau and Bernhardt (1984), almost all tissues are sensitive to the tension, compression, shearing, torsional and bending loads that are placed on them in such a manner that these forces contribute to their progressive differentiation. An imbalance in muscle forces or a lack of muscle forces may lead to skeletal deformation and malformation of the discretely articulated segments of the spine, especially if these abnormal forces are applied over a long period of time (LeVeau & Bernhardt 1984, Proffit & Fields 1993). Rocabado and Iglash (1991) state that soft tissue plays a significant role in the process of growth and development of the craniofacial and vertebral regions, because bones grow and remodel in response to the application of external forces exerted by soft tissues.

On a cellular level, cells adjust to forces and even molecules respond to changes in mechanical forces by altering enzymatic function (Khan & Sheetz 1997, Matsumoto et al 1999). The effect of mechanical deformation is mediated by a series of cell responses, causing an effect on cellular metabolism. The consequent production and release of chemical substances results in the remodelling of structures (Turner & Pavalko 1998).

THE INFLUENCE OF ALTERED BREATHING PATTERNS ON ADOLESCENT GROWTH

There is a great deal of variation in the timing of puberty, but the adolescent growth spurt occurs on average nearly 2 years earlier in girls than in boys as illustrated in Figure 21.13. The onset of the adolescent growth spurt in girls is at 10 or 11 years, with peak growth velocity at 12 years; growth finishes at 14 years when the epiphyseal plates close. In boys, puberty starts at 12 years, but extends over a longer period (about 5 years in comparison to 3.5 years in girls). Peak growth in boys is at 14 years and finishes at 16 or 17 years (Taylor & Twomey 1986, Proffit & Fields 1993, Jacobson 1995).

One of the most obvious features of the adolescent spine is that it is growing actively. Growth applies forces to the neuromusculoskeletal system, the magnitude of which varies with the rate of growth. Since the growth velocity is highest in the infant and the adolescent, it could be expected that the resulting forces applied to the neuromusculoskeletal system are greatest at these ages. Although the forces that result from growth are of small magnitude, they may result in changes in the skeletal structure, as light forces applied for longer periods have a far greater effect than heavy forces sustained over a short period of time (LeVeau & Bernhardt 1984, Weinstein 1994, Turner et al 1997). During peak growth velocity, the rapidly growing spine can be considered unstable, and phases

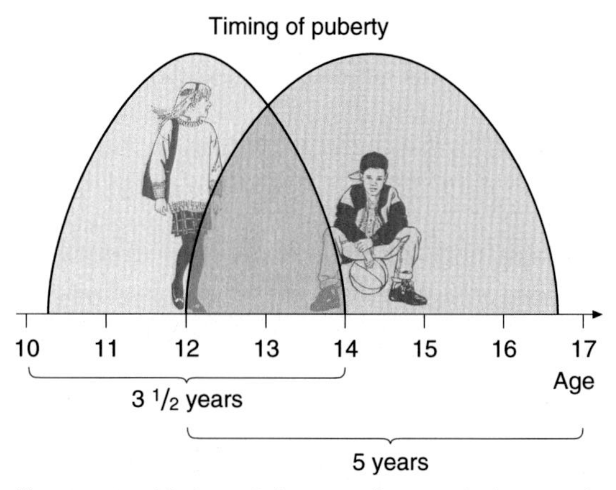

Fig. 21.13 Timing of the growth spurt in boys and girls.

of rapid growth are known to be susceptible to development instabilities (McGowan et al 1995, Nissinen et al 2000). The effect of load on growth is directly proportional to the speed of growth. Any load applied even for a short time during the period of rapid growth may result in permanent deformity of a bone (LeVeau & Bernhardt 1984).

The paediatric spine can adapt to applied stresses much more readily than the aged spine, due to its growth potential, intrinsic tissue plasticity and prominent remodelling capabilities. The result of this adaptability is that the child can often maintain a functional level in the presence of significant pathology. Although immature musculoskeletal tissue has a considerable capacity to adapt and remodel, neurological tissue does not have the same capacity (LeVeau & Bernhardt 1984, Weinstein 1994). Muscle imbalances, abnormal muscle tone, persistent abnormal positioning and lack of normal weight bearing can all contribute to abnormal growth and development of the neuromusculoskeletal system (LeVeau & Bernhardt 1984).

Growth is a dynamic force that we can use to the patient's advantage. If unchecked, it can be a force for increased deformity, muscle imbalances, misalignment and abnormal craniocervical loading (LeVeau & Bernhardt 1984, Hensinger & Arbor 1998). In general, the modification of tissues is achieved more easily when they are more adaptable in periods of rapid growth. Early correction yields the best corrective results (LeVeau & Bernhardt 1984). In orthodontics, whenever a mandibular discrepancy exists, the ideal solution is to correct it by modifying growth, so that the skeletal problem literally grows out. The ideal time for growth modification is the period of rapid growth associated with puberty. With appropriate management of the deforming forces, the adaptive changes may be reversed or completely avoided (LeVeau & Bernhardt 1984, Proffit & Fields 1993, Bishara 2000).

It is clear that the nasally obstructed child is very susceptible to abnormal growth and development, especially during the adolescent growth spurt. The malalignment of segments resulting from the changed posture and the abnormal loading on bony structures resulting from muscle imbalances and altered muscle tone, combined with the forces of rapid growth, could cause abnormal growth of the neuromusculoskeletal system.

Therefore, if any changes are to be made, either to soft tissue or to skeletal alignment, they should be done before or during the final growth spurt. A study by Harreby et al (1995) suggests that low back pain in the growth period is an important risk factor for low back pain in later life. Low back pain in the growth period also demonstrates a trend toward aggravation as time passes, emphasizing the importance of implementing preventative measures at an early age.

It is clear that growth influences our diagnosis and treatment. In planning the clinical intervention for children with altered breathing patterns and associated neuromusculoskeletal adaptations, the forces and timing of the growth spurt should be considered. Early screening, management and intervention by the therapist might prevent dysfunction and symptoms developing in adult life.

Change over time is the true fourth dimension of paediatric orthopaedics.

SUMMARY

- In this chapter an overview was given of the possible changes and clinical patterns associated with altered breathing patterns.
- The discussions were based partly on evidence-based literature and partly on clinical experiences and observations.
- Not all the dysfunctions discussed will be represented in a single patient, and therefore individualized assessment and management is essential. This should be done in a framework of clinical reasoning that will be discussed in Chapter 22.
- A summary of all the possible changes in the neuromusculoskeletal system as a result of mouth breathing is given in Table 21.1.

Table 21.1 Summary of changes in the neuromusculoskeletal system as a result of a mouth breathing pattern

Region	Adaptation/change	Function /reason
	Altered biomechanics of respiration	
Anterior portal of the upper respiratory tract (nose)	Changes to the mouth by raising the upper lip and lowering the mandible	Anterior portal/entrance to the upper airway obstructed, change to maintain adequate air entry for respiratory demands
Tongue	Lowered and protruded	Proprioceptive response to hypertrophy of lymphoid tissue at dorsum of tongue, widened posterior oral cavity to facilitate breathing
Head	Lifts away from the hyomandibular complex into extension, increasing the craniocervical angle	Decreased airway resistance by increased diameter of oro- and nasopharyngeal airways
Accessory respiratory muscles (sternocleidomastoid, scalene and pectoralis major muscles)	Hyperactive, resulting in poor postural alignment with shoulder protraction and sternum depressed	Increased effort required to breathe against increased resistance to air flow
Diaphragm	Decreased activity associated with hypotonicity of the abdominal muscles Patient presents with increased lumbar lordosis and protruding abdomen, contributing to faulty postural alignment of the shoulder girdle	Resting position of tongue forces nasal–diaphragmatic breathing, but an increase in resistance in upper airway and mouth breathing facilitates accessory muscles of respiration

References

Ayub E, Glasheen-Wray M, Kraus S 1984 Head posture: a case study of the effects on the rest position of the mandible. Journal of Orthopaedic and Sports Physical Therapy 5(4):179

Bishara S E 2000 Facial and dental changes in adolescents and their clinical implications. Angle Orthodontist 70(6):471

Bogduk N 1994 Biomechanics of the cervical spine. In: Grant R (ed.) Clinics in physical therapy. Physical therapy for the cervical and thoracic spine. Churchill Livingstone, Oxford

Brodie A G 1950 Anatomy and physiology of head and neck musculature. American Journal of Orthodontics 36:831

Buchman S R, Bartlett S P, Wornom I L, Whitaker L A 1994 The role of pressure on regulation of craniofacial bone growth. Journal of Craniofacial Surgery 5(1):2

Cheng M-C, Enlow D H, Papsidero M et al 1988 Developmental effects of impaired breathing in the face of the growing child. Angle Orthodontist 58(4):309–320

Crouse U, Laine-Alava M T, Warren D W 2000 Nasal impairment in prepubertal children. American Journal of Orthodontic and Dentofacial Orthopedics 118(1):69

Darling D W, Kraus S, Glasheen-Wray M B 1984 Relationship of head posture and the rest position

of the mandible. Journal of Prosthetic Dentistry 52(1):111
Darlow L A, Pesco J, Greenberg M S 1987 The relationship of posture to myofascial pain dysfunction syndrome. Journal of the American Dental Association 114:73
Enwemeka C S, Bonet I M, Ingle J A et al 1986 Postural correction in persons with neck pain: I survey of neck positions recommended by physical therapists. Journal of Sport and Physical Therapy 8(5):235
Forsberg C M, Hellsing E, Linder-Aronson S, Sheikholeslam A 1985 EMG activity in neck and masticatory muscles in relation to extension and flexion of the head. European Journal of Orthodontics 7:177
Garry J F 1992 Upper airway obstruction and TMJD/ MPD. In: Coy R E (ed.) Anthology of craniomandibular orthopedics, Vol. I. Buchanan, Baltimore
Goldsmith J L, Stool S E 1994 George Catlin's concepts on mouth-breathing, as presented by Dr. Edward H. Angle. Angle Orthodontist 64(1):75
Grimmer K 1997 An investigation of poor cervical resting posture. Australian Physiotherapy 43(1):7
Haapaniemi J J 1995 Adenoids in school-aged children. Journal of Laryngology and Otology 109:196
Hanten W P, Lucio R M, Russel J L, Brunt D 1991 Assessment of total head excursion and resting head posture. Archives of Physical and Medical Rehabilitation 72:877
Harreby M, Neergaard K, Hesselsøe G, Kjer J 1995 Are radiologic changes in the thoracic and lumbar spine of adolescents risk factors for low back pain in adults? A 25-year prospective cohort study of 640 school children. Spine 20(21):2298
Hellsing E 1989 Changes in the pharyngeal airway in relation to extension of the head. European Journal of Orthodontics 11:359
Hellsing E, Forsberg C M, Linder-Aronson S, Sheikholeslam A 1986 Changes in postural EMG activity in the neck and masticatory muscles following obstruction of the nasal airways. European Journal of Orthodontics 8:247
Hellsing E, McWilliam J, Reigo T, Spangfort E 1987 The relationship between craniofacial morphology, head posture and spinal curvature in 8, 11 and 15-year-old children. European Journal of Orthodontics 9:254
Hensinger R N, Arbor A 1998 The challenge of growth: the fourth dimension of pediatric care. Journal of Pediatric Orthopedics 18(2):141
Hideharu Y, Kenji S 2003 Malocclusion associated with abnormal posture. Bulletin of Tokyo Dental College 44(2):43
Huggare J 1998 Postural disorders and dentofacial morphology. Acta Odontologica Scandinavica 56:383
Huggare J A V, Cooke M S 1994 Head posture and cervicovertebral anatomy as mandibular growth predictors. European Journal of Orthodontics 16:175
Jacobson A 1995 Radiographic cephalometry: from basics to videoimaging. Quintessence, Copenhagen
Janda V 1994 Muscles and motor control in cervicogenic disorders: assessment and management. In: Grant R (ed.) Clinics in physical therapy. Physical therapy for the cervical and thoracic spine. Churchill Livingstone, Oxford
Jankelson R R 1995 Neuromuscular dental diagnosis and treatment. Ishiyaku EuroAmerica, St Louis
Khan S, Sheetz M P 1997 Force effects on biochemical kinetics. Annual Review of Biochemistry 66:785
Kraus S L (ed.) 1988 Cervical spine influences on the craniomandibular region. In: Clinics in physical therapy: TMJ disorders. Management of the craniomandibular complex. Churchill Livingstone, New York
Kraus S L (ed.) 1994a Cervical spine influences on the management of TMD. In: Clinics in physical therapy: temporomandibular disorders, 2nd edn. Churchill Livingstone, New York
Kraus S L (ed.) 1994b Physical therapy management of TMD. In: Clinics in physical therapy: temporomandibular disorders, 2nd edn. Churchill Livingstone, New York
Kritsineli M, Shim Y S 1992 Malocclusion, body posture, and temporomandibular disorder in children with primary and mixed dentition. Journal of Clinical Pediatric Dentistry 16(2):86
Lawrence E S, Razook S J 1994 Nonsurgical management of mandibular disorders. In: Kraus S L (ed.) Clinics in physical therapy: temporomandibular disorders, 2nd edn. Churchill Livingstone, New York
Lawrence E S, Samson G S 1988 Growth and development influences on the craniomandibular region. In: Kraus S L (ed.) Clinics in physical therapy: TMJ disorders. Churchill Livingstone, New York
LeVeau B F, Bernhardt D B 1984 Developmental biomechanics. Effect of forces on growth, development, and maintenance of the human body. Physical Therapy 64(12):1874
Linder-Aronson S 1979 Respiratory function in relation to facial morphology and dentition. British Journal of Orthodontics 6:59
Linder-Aronson S, Woodside D G 2000 Excess face height malocclusion: etiology, diagnosis and treatment. Quintessence, Chicago
Matsumoto T, Kawakami M, Takenaka T, Tamaki T 1999 Cyclic mechanical stretch stress increases the

growth rate and collagen synthesis of nucleus pulposus cells in vitro. Spine 24(4):315

McGowan D P, Bernhardt M, White A A 1995 Biomechanics of the juvenile spine. In: Pang D (ed.) Disorders of the pediatric spine. Raven Press, Stratford-on-Avon

Miller A J, Vargervik K, Chierici G 1984 Experimentally induced neuromuscular changes during and after nasal airway obstruction. American Journal of Orthodontics 85(5):385

Moss M L 1997The functional matrix hypothesis revisited. 1. The role of mechanotransduction. American Journal of Orthodontics and Dentofacial Orthopedics 112(1):8

Nissinen M J, Heliövaara M M, Seitsamo J T et al 2000 Development of trunk asymmetry in a cohort of children aged 11 to 22 years. Spine 25(5):570

Okeson J P 1998 Management of temporomandibular disorders and occlusion, 4th edn. Mosby, St Louis

Ono T, Ishiwata Y, Kuroda T 1998 Inhibition of masseteric electromyographic activity during oral respiration. American Journal of Orthodontics and Dentofacial Orthopedics 113(5):518

Oudhof H A J 2001 Skull growth in relation to mechanical stimulation. In: von Piekartz H J M, Bryden L (eds) Craniofacial dysfunction and pain. Manual therapy, assessment and management. Butterworth-Heinemann, Oxford

Özbek M M, Köklü A 1993 Natural cervical inclination and craniofacial structure. American Journal of Orthodontics and Dentofacial Orthopedics 104(6):584

Proffit W R, Fields H W 1993 Contemporary orthodontics, 2nd edn. Mosby Year Book, St Louis

Ribeiro E C, Marchiori S C, Da Silva A M T 2004 Electromyographic muscle EMG activity in mouth and nasal breathing children. Cranio 22(2):145

Ricketts R M 1968 Respiratory obstruction syndrome. American Journal of Orthodontics 54(7):495

Rocabado M 1983 Biomechanical relationship of the cranial, cervical and hyoid regions. Journal of Craniomandibular Practice 1(3):62

Rocabado M, Iglash Z A 1991 Musculoskeletal approach to maxillofacial pain. J B Lippincott, Philadelphia

Sandham A 1988 Repeatability of head posture recordings from lateral cephalometric radiographs. British Journal of Orthodontics 15:157

Schlenker W L, Jennings B D, Jeiroudi M T, Caruso J M 2000 The effects of chronic absence of active nasal respiration on the growth of the skull: a pilot study. American Journal of Orthodontics and Dentofacial Orthopedics 117(6):706

Solow B, Kreiborg S 1977 Soft-tissue stretching: a possible control factor in craniofacial morphogenesis. Scandinavian Journal of Dental Research 85:505

Solow B, Sonnesen L 1998 Head posture and malocclusions. European Journal of Orthodontics 20:685

Solow B, Siersbaek-Nielsen S, Greve E 1984 Airway adequacy, head posture, and craniofacial morphology. American Journal of Orthodontics 86(3):214

Solow B, Oveson J, Nielsen P W, Wildschiødtz G, Tallgren A 1993 Head posture in obstructive sleep apnoea. European Journal of Orthodontics 15:107

Sousa J B R, Anselmo-Lima W T, Valera F C P, Gallego A J, Matsumoto M A N 2005 Cephalometric assessment of the mandibular growth pattern in mouth-breathing children. International Journal of Pediatric Otorhinolaryngology 69(3):311

Tadao N, Kenji S 2003 Anatomy of oral respiration: morphology of the oral cavity and pharynx. Acta Otolaryngology Supplement 550:25

Taranger J, Hägg U 1980 The timing and duration of adolescent growth. Acta Odontologica Scandinavica 38:57

Taylor J R, Twomey L T 1986 Factors influencing growth of the vertebral column. In: Grieve G P (ed.) Modern manual therapy of the vertebral column. Churchill Livingstone, Edinburgh

Tecco S, Festa F, Tete S, Longhi V, D'Attillio M 2005 Changes in head posture after rapid maxillary expansion in mouth-breathing girls: a controlled study. Angle Orthodontics 75(2):171

Tourne L P M, Schweiger J 1996 Immediate postural responses to total nasal obstruction. American Journal of Orthodontics and Dentofacial Orthopedics 110(6):606

Turner C H, Pavalko F M 1998 Mechanotransduction and functional response of the skeleton to physical stress: the mechanisms and mechanics of bone adaptation. Journal of Orthopaedic Science 3(6):346

Turner S, Nattrass C, Sandy J R 1997 The role of soft tissues in the aetiology of malocclusion. Dental Update 24:209

Venetikidou A 1993 Incidence of malocclusion in asthmatic children. Journal of Clinical Pediatric Dentistry 17(2):89

von Piekartz H J M 2001 Neurodynamics of cranial nervous tissue (cranioneurodynamics). In: von Piekartz H J M, Bryden L (eds) Craniofacial dysfunction and pain. Manual therapy, assessment and management. Butterworth-Heinemann, Oxford

Weinstein S L 1994 The pediatric spine: principles and practice, Vol. I. Raven Press, New York

Wenzel A, Henriksen J, Melsen B 1983 Nasal respiratory resistance and head posture: effect of intranasal corticosteroid (Budesonide) in children

with asthma and perennial rhinitis. American Journal of Orthodontics 84(5):422
Wenzel A, Höjensgaard E, Henriksen J M 1985 Craniofacial morphology and head posture in children with asthma and perennial rhinitis. European Journal of Orthodontics 7:83
White A A, Panjabi M M 1990 Clinical biomechanics of the spine, 2nd edn. J B Lippincott, Philadelphia
White S G, Sahrman S A 1994 A movement system balance approach to management of musculoskeletal pain. In: Grant R (ed.) Clinics in physical therapy. Physical therapy for the cervical and thoracic spine. Churchill Livingstone, New York
Williams J S, Janssen P L, Fuller D D, Fregosi R F 2000 Influence of posture and breathing route on neural drive to upper airway dilator muscles during exercise. Journal of Applied Physiology 89:590
Wiltshire W A 1996 Orthodontics and chronic nasal obstruction. Current Allergy and Clinical Immunology 7(2):16

Chapter 22

Management of craniofacial and cervical postural changes in children with altered breathing patterns

Ronel Jordaan, Harry von Piekartz

CHAPTER CONTENTS

INTRODUCTION

Altered breathing patterns associated with nasal obstruction are often seen in children, and especially in the orthodontics department, as many of them also present with malocclusions in need of orthodontic treatment. According to Kritsineli and Shim (1992), children with temporomandibular dysfunction often have no symptoms, and this is also the case with children with altered postures resulting from nasal obstruction. However, inefficient skeletal alignment and muscle imbalances, maintained for a long time, will eventually result in spasm, pain and dysfunction and, in advanced cases, degenerative changes will gradually encroach on the joints (Darlow et al 1987, Braun & Amundson 1989, Bryden & Fitzgerald 2001).

According to Janda (1994), it is a well-recognized fact that effective protection of joints depends largely on the appropriate functioning of the muscle system. It has also been recognized that the dysfunctions of muscles and joints are so closely related that the two should be considered as a single, inseparable functional unit, and should be assessed, analysed and treated together.

A thorough systematic examination of the patient is essential to plan suitable treatment.

It is important to keep in mind that a young patient with an altered breathing pattern will often not present with any symptoms. However, a complete examination is still necessary as it will enable the therapist to plan treatment that will prevent symptoms from developing in later life, prevent morphological abnormalities that could predispose the patient to the development of symptoms and enhance the outcome of orthodontic treatment. Appropriate treatment and further management, properly timed, might contribute to an optimal period of growth and development during the adolescent growth spurt.

In this chapter the examination and treatment of patients with an altered breathing pattern will be discussed.

SUBJECTIVE ASSESSMENT

A complete medical history should be taken. It should include general health, illnesses, surgery (especially adenoidectomy and tonsillectomy or similar operations), respiratory infections, asthma, allergies and the use of medication. Partial or total nasal obstruction should be determined, as well as parafunctional habits such as nail or pen biting, thumb sucking, gum chewing and lip biting. The area and type of symptoms, intensity, aggravating factors and activities that provide relief should be included. The therapist should be aware of 'red flag' signs and symptoms, indicating serious pathology, as this would indicate the referral to another member of the medical team (Rocabado & Iglash 1991, Proffit & Fields 1993, Magee 1997, Butler 2000, Lee 2000, Petty & Moore 2000) (see also Chapter 3).

PHYSICAL EXAMINATION

The objective or physical examination aims to determine which structure(s) and/or factor(s) are responsible for producing the patient's symptoms or dysfunction. The objective examination is an extension of the subjective examination (Magee 1997, Petty & Moore 2000).

ASSESSMENT OF THE POSTURAL ALIGNMENT OF THE BODY AS A WHOLE

Postural analysis in relation to the sagittal, coronal and transverse planes of the body is essential. Careful observation of muscle form and tone, symmetry and, in particular, of the alignment of segments in relation to a vertical line is essential. The ideal skeletal alignment used as a standard when evaluating posture is described as the posture conducive to maximal efficiency of the body with a minimal amount of stress and strain (Kendall et al 1993):

- Anterior view: The head should be positioned straight on the shoulders, the nose in line with the manubrium of sternum, the clavicles should be level and equal, the iliac crest height and the anterior superior iliac spines should be on the same level on the right and left side, the lower limb should be straight with the patellae and medial malleoli level on the left and right and depression of the sternum and ribs should also be noted (Magee 1997, Lee 2000).
- Lateral view: Ideally, if the body is viewed from the lateral aspect, a vertical line should pass through the following points: the external auditory meatus, bodies of the cervical vertebrae, the glenohumeral joint, slightly anterior to the bodies of the thoracic vertebrae, transecting the vertebrae at the thoracolumbar junction, the bodies of the lumbar vertebrae, the sacral promontory, slightly posterior to the coronal axis of the hip joint, slightly anterior to the axis of the knee joint and through the calcanocuboid joint (Kendall et al 1993, Lee 2000).
- Posterior view: Straight head posture with the head in the midline, level shoulders, inferior angles and medial borders of the scapulae equidistant from the spine without rotation or winging, a straight spine without lateral curves, arms equidistant from the body and equally rotated, posterior superior iliac spines are level, gluteal folds and knee joint lines level, Achilles tendons and heels straight (Magee 1997).

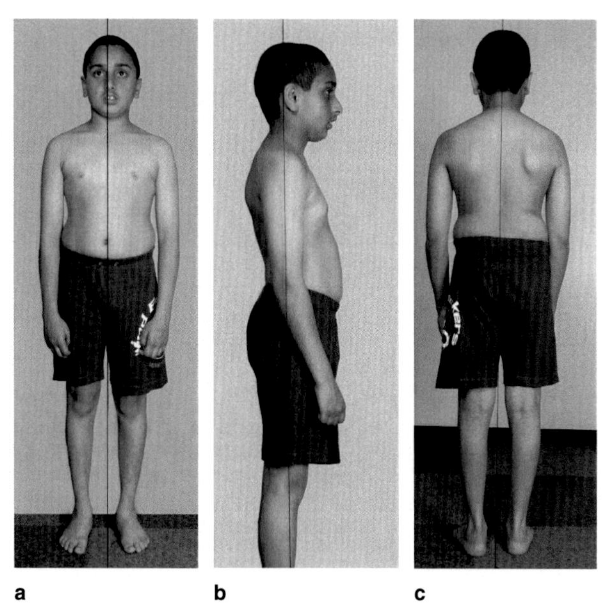

Fig. 22.1 Posture of a child with nasal obstruction.
a Anterior view.
b Lateral view.
c Posterior view.

The child with nasal obstruction and an altered breathing pattern presents with a typical posture (Rocabado & Iglash 1991). The assessment of the alignment of the different segments will give the therapist an indication of structures that should be examined. The posture of a child with nasal obstruction is shown in Figure 22.1.

Postural alignment in a child with nasal shift (nasal obstruction)

- Extension of the head with increased craniocervical angle
- Craned neck
- Shoulders displaced forwards
- Depressed sternum
- Hyperactivity of the accessory respiratory muscles and reduced activity of the diaphragm with shoulder elevation
- Hypotonic and protruded abdominal muscles
- Pelvis tipped forwards
- Increased lumbar lordosis
- Retrognathic (dorsally displaced) mandible (Rocabado & Iglash 1991, Kraus 1994).

OROFACIAL FINDINGS

Patients with modified breathing patterns may have the following characteristic changes in the oral and craniofacial regions:

- Adenoid face/long face (Cheng et al 1988, Rocabado & Iglash 1991, Gary 1992)
- Mouth or nasal/mouth breathing pattern (Rocabado & Iglash 1991, Wiltshire 1996, Linder-Aronson & Woodside 2000)
- Short upper lip (Rocabado & Iglash 1991, Proffit & Fields 1993)
- Open or non-functional lips (Rocabado & Iglash 1991, Proffit & Fields 1993)
- Ventrally displaced and depressed mandible (Linder-Aronson & Woodside 2000)
- Tongue anteriorly and caudally displaced (Ricketts 1968, Miller et al 1984)
- Protruded upper incisors (Cheng et al 1988, Proffit & Fields 1993, Linder-Aronson & Woodside 2000)
- Changed EMG activity in particular muscles (Miller et al 1984, Ono et al 1998)
- High and narrow tooth alignment (Garry 1992, Proffit & Fields 1993)

- Temporomandibular dysfunction (Garry 1992, Hackney et al 1993).

Investigation of the orocraniofacial region includes three main components:

- Anatomical components
- Functional components
- Neuromuscular components (Rocabado & Iglash 1991).

Anatomical

- Facial dimensions: Aspects that should be included in the observation are the facial expression and the face from all perspectives, assessing symmetry, muscle tone and mandibular posture to determine if it is in a resting or a lowered position. Observe the shape of the face, looking for a narrow and long face, known as an 'adenoid' face (see Fig. 21.10), which is typical in a chronic mouth breather (Rocabado & Iglash 1991, Wiltshire 1996).
- Nostrils: The patency of the superior airway space should be assessed, together with flaring/dilatation of the external nares which can indicate an increased effort of breathing (Rocabado & Iglash 1991).
- Upper lip: Determine if the upper lip is elevated, if a normal functional length is present or if it is shortened with an increased activity in the lip elevators (Rocabado & Iglash 1991, Proffit & Field 1993). The upper lip should cover at least three-quarters of the surface of the upper front teeth. Inability of the upper lip to assume this position is referred to as a short anatomical upper lip (Rocabado & Iglash 1991).
- Lower lip: Observe the position and length of the lower lip. Normally, the lower lip should not cover more than the inferior quarter of the upper teeth (Rocabado & Iglash 1991, Proffit & Fields 1993).
- Position of incisors: Observe crowding or protrusion of the incisors or any other malocclusion that might be present (Rocabado & Iglash 1991, Proffit & Fields 1993, Wiltshire 1996).

Functional activity

Lip closure and the functional relationship of the upper and lower lips at rest should be determined. Assess the ability of the upper lip to descend actively over the surfaces of the upper teeth. With normal functional length, the cupid line (red line of the upper lip) disappears under the edges of the upper teeth. It may appear that the lip is anatomically short, but the patient can actively lower the lip so that the cupid line disappears under the edges of the upper teeth. This is referred to as a short, functional upper lip. A short, non-functional lip will actively descend, but will not completely cover the surfaces of the teeth and the cupid line will not disappear under the edges of the teeth. This patient will use extra effort to maintain lip closure, and the lower lip must be excessively elevated to try to make contact with the upper lip. The elevated lower lip will elongate, and in time the elongated lip at rest will become everted with increased activity of the mentalis muscle (Rocabado & Iglash 1991).

Assess the resting position of the tongue by using the ring finger to palpate the hyoid bone. The thumb and index finger of the same hand apply gentle downward pressure below the lower lip on the mental protuberance of the mandible. The thumb and index finger of the other hand apply gentle upward pressure above the upper lip. After a normal swallowing action, palpate the descending hyoid bone to its normal resting position. Now gently open the lips to observe the resting position of the tongue (Rocabado & Iglash 1991). Is the tongue up against the palate (i.e. the normal resting position), is it on the floor of the mouth or is there an anterior thrusting movement? Then evaluate the upper airway space for normal breathing patterns. A nose, nose–mouth or mouth breathing pattern can be determined by placing a piece of cotton in front of the nostrils or the opened mouth. Observe in which position the cotton moves (Rocabado & Iglash 1991).

Temporomandibular joint movement should be assessed actively and passively. Note the quality of movement, including symmetry, deviation and joint sounds (crepitus and clicking) during opening and closing, indicating abnormal muscle activity or joint dysfunction. Other aspects that should be noted are range of movement, behaviour of pain through the range, resistance through and at the end of range, and provocation of muscle spasm. Active and passive physiological movements that should be tested are depression (opening), elevation (closing), protraction, retraction, depression in the retracted position and left and right lateral deviation. Careful testing is essential, as abnormal joint irritation will cause reflex muscle contraction, increasing the intra-joint pressure (Rocabado & Iglash 1991, Magee 1997, Petty & Moore 2000).

Accessory movements of the joint should also be assessed, noting quality of movement, resistance, pain, spasm and range of movement (Rocabado & Iglash 1991, Magee 1997, Petty & Moore 2000). Clinically it has been observed that the posteroanterior movement with protrusion and longitudinal caudal movement are often hypomobile and provoke muscle spasm.

Parafunctional habits (bad oral habits, e.g. pencil or nail biting and chewing gum) should be evaluated as these could cause an abnormal resting position of the tongue, abnormal craniomandibular relationship and a forward head posture (Rocabado & Iglash 1991).

Neuromuscular

The neuromuscular evaluation is divided into palpation of the relevant structures and muscle testing.

- Palpate the joint to assess temperature, oedema, mobility of the superficial tissues, position of the mandible and temporomandibular joint, tenderness of bone, ligament and muscle, and note any pain or muscle spasm elicited.
- Palpate the craniomandibular region to determine local or radiating pain, fibrous adhesions, trigger points, swelling and muscle activity. The muscles should be palpated by gentle pressure parallel or perpendicular to the muscle fibres to elicit any intramuscular changes or changed muscle activity. Muscle activity should also be assessed at the insertion because excessive muscle activity can cause a traction force at the muscle–periosteum junction, provoking an inflammatory response and muscle spasm (Rocabado & Iglash 1991) (see also Chapters 7 and 8).
- Palpation of specific muscles:
  - Mandibular elevators: Temporalis, masseter and medial pterygoid muscles. The activity in these muscles will be decreased if the mandible is maintained in a depressed position, and the mandibular elevators are easy to palpate under these conditions (Rocabado & Iglash 1991, Lawrence & Razook 1994).
  - Mandibular depressors: Lateral pterygoid, supra- and infrahyoid muscles. These muscles are active in maintaining the mandible in a lowered position, and an increase in tone or even tenderness might be palpated (Rocabado & Iglash 1991, Lawrence & Razook 1994).

On palpation, the masseter and medial pterygoid muscles have the highest tone and the greatest number of trigger points. Palpation of the other craniofacial muscles is illustrated in Chapter 9.

The supra- and infrahyoid muscles are the most affected of the mandibular depressors. These muscles are often very sensitive on palpation with an increased tone (Fig. 22.2). This is probably caused by the increased activity of the tongue and the elevated hyoid bone.

CRANIOCERVICAL ASSESSMENT

The craniocervical adaptations seen in a child with an altered breathing pattern as a result of nasal obstruction present with a characteristic clinical pattern:

- Increased craniocervical extension (Solow et al 1984, Wenzel et al 1985, Hellsing et al 1986, Tourne & Schweiger 1996)
- Extension of the upper cervical spine (Hellsing 1989, Hanten et al 1991)
- Forward tilt of the cervical spine (Solow et al 1984, 1993)
- Protraction of the head resulting in a ventrally displaced head posture (Rocabado & Iglash 1991, Grimmer 1997, Solow & Sonnesen 1998)

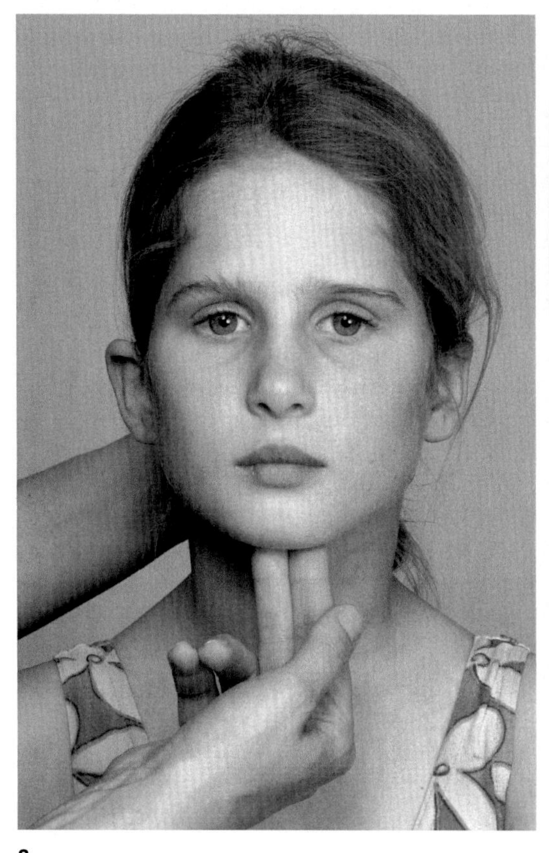

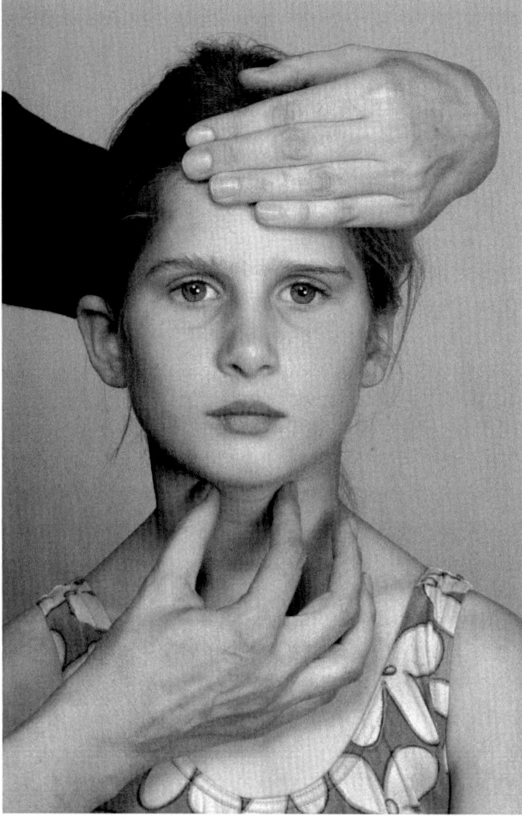

a b

Fig. 22.2 Palpation of the suprahyoid and infrahyoid muscles (reproduced with permission from Rocabado & Iglash 1991).

a Suprahyoid muscle: This muscle can be palpated extraorally at the floor of the mouth. Intraorally, the suprahyoid, mylohyoid and geniohyoid can also be palpated as they run from the anterior part of the hyoid bone to the anterior corpus mandibulae.

b Infrahyoid muscle: The patient flexes her head on her neck to around 15° anterior cervical rotation. The therapist's thumb and index finger are placed laterally to the thyroid cartilage. Gentle resistance to head flexion will produce an isometric muscle contraction of the infrahyoid muscle, which is an accessory neck flexor.

- Shortened dorsal neck muscles (Ayub et al 1984, Forsberg et al 1985, Janda 1994)
- Lengthened and weakened ventral neck muscles (Ayub et al 1984, Forsberg et al 1985)
- Raised hyoid bone (Rocabado 1983, Ayub et al 1984, Lawrence & Razook 1994)
- Altered proprioceptive input (Janda 1994).

Posture

- The craniocervical posture or head-on-neck position should be observed from different angles. In the child with nasal obstruction, the cranium is usually rotated posteriorly about the transverse axis, resulting in an increased craniocervical angulation, indicating that the head is in extension in relation to the upper cervical spine (Solow et al 1984, Wenzel et al 1985, Hellsing et al 1986, Tourne & Schweiger 1996).
- The inclination of the cervical spine is usually displaced forward in relation to the vertical reference line in mouth breathers. The lower cervical spine might present with a loss of the normal lordosis, whereas the

upper cervical spine will probably be in hyperextension (Hellsing 1989, Solow et al 1993, Linder-Aronson & Woodside 2000). This forward displacement will ensure that the visual axis is restored to the normal horizontal line (Darlow et al 1987, Rocabado & Iglash 1991, Solow & Sonnesen 1998).

- The resultant effect of upper cervical extension and a forward inclination of the lower cervical spine will be a typical forward head posture (Rocabado & Iglash 1991, Grimmer 1997, Solow & Sonnesen 1998).

Functional activity

Active movements of the craniocervical region and cervical spine should be observed to assess the quality of movement and motor patterning, range of movement and pain. With the patient in sitting, the following should be tested:

- Cervical flexion and extension
- Upper cervical flexion and extension
- Lateral flexion and rotation (Magee 1997, Petty & Moore 2000).

Observe the deep neck flexors initiating the active flexion movement, giving an indication that the deep stabilizing muscles are not inhibited and are of a normal muscle recruitment pattern. The patient might present with decreased active craniocervical flexion and lower cervical extension.

Neuromuscular

- Palpate the muscles and soft tissues of the craniocervical region for any changes, mobility, local and referred pain, spasm, adhesions, trigger points, swelling and muscle activity. The posterior muscles of the upper cervical region might be tender, have trigger points, decreased mobility and increased muscle activity or muscle tone.
- Muscle strength testing of the deep neck flexors is very important, as a forward head posture will inhibit these muscles. The therapist can test these muscles by observing the pattern of movement that occurs when the patient flexes the head from a supine position. This flexion is upper cervical flexion, or head-on-neck flexion. The patient is instructed to do a small nodding movement to initiate the movement (Jull 2001). When the deep neck flexors are weak, the sternocleidomastoid muscle initiates the movement, causing the jaw to lead the movement and the upper cervical spine to hyperextend. This weakness is clearly demonstrated in Figure 22.3. Upper cervical flexion will only start further into the range, after about 10° of flexion (Petty & Moore 2000).
- The mid- and lower cervical extensor muscles should be tested for strength. This can be done with the patient in a prone position, supported on the elbows. The patient is asked to relax the head into flexion, assisted by the force of gravity. The patient must then flex the upper cervical spine by tucking the chin in. While maintaining upper cervical flexion, the mid and lower cervical spine is lifted into an extended or posteriorly translated position, with the head and neck in line with the spinal column. A patient with weak cervical extensors will not be able to perform this activity, and might use substitution mechanisms such as shoulder girdle elevation, increased activity of the interscapular muscles or even a loss of upper cervical flexion (Bryden & Fitzgerald 2001).
- Test the length of the posterior upper cervical muscles. These muscles maintain the

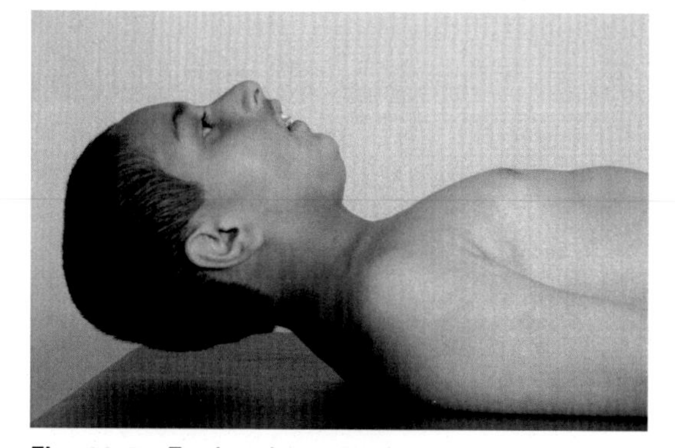

Fig. 22.3 Testing the strength of the deep neck flexors in upper extension. The chin leads the movement, indicating weak deep neck flexors.

head in a posteriorly rotated position and are probably shortened. This can be done by passively flexing the head on the neck.
- Passive physiological and accessory joint movements can be valuable in examining the movement at each segmental level of the cervical spine for hypo- or hypermobility. The patient will most likely present with restricted upper cervical flexion (especially flexion of the occiput in relation to C1 and C1 in relation to C2) and possibly also restricted lower cervical extension (Magee 1997, Petty & Moore 2000) (see also Chapters 5 and 6).

CRANIOFACIAL REGION

Dysfunctions are often found during passive movements of the neuro- and viscerocranium:

- Firstly, assess the five general movements of the neurocranium: occipital–frontal, temporal–temporal, occipital, frontal and parietal–parietal techniques, giving gentle pressure into resistance as described in Chapter 14.
- Secondly, test the general movements of the viscerocranium: the orbital, zygomatic and maxillary regions.
- Determine which responses (stiffness, discomfort and/or other symptoms) were provoked in which region, and then follow up with specific techniques for this region.
- The specific techniques that are most provocative are predominantly located in the midface of the viscerocranium, and include transverse maxilla–sphenoid, nasofrontal, frontal–maxilla, zygomatic and the palate techniques.

SHOULDER GIRDLE AND THORACIC SPINE

There is a typical clinical pattern in the shoulder girdle and thoracic spine in the patient with nasal obstruction. This is as a result of the dysfunctional breathing pattern, use of accessory respiratory muscles, and the altered mandible, tongue and craniocervical posture (Ayub et al 1984, Rocabado & Iglash 1991).

Clinical pattern of the shoulder girdle and chest area in nasal obstruction (Rocabado & Iglash 1991, Kraus 1994):

- Shoulders pulled forwards
- Raised shoulder girdle
- Depressed sternum
- Abduction, rotation and winging of the shoulder blades
- Increased thoracic kyphosis
- Reduced diaphragmatic breathing and increased upper rib cage breathing.

Posture

- The posture of the scapulae should be observed. This is best done from a posterior view. Note the scapular abduction and/or rotation, as well as winging (Fig. 22.4). These

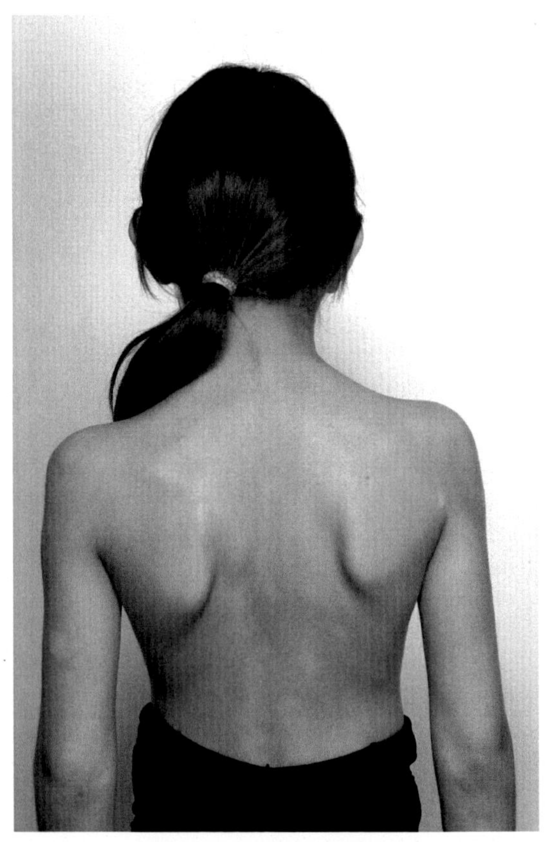

Fig. 22.4 Posterior view of a typical shoulder girdle posture in a patient with nasal obstruction (reproduced with permission from von Piekartz 2001).

findings indicate weakness of the stabilizing muscles of the shoulder girdle – a common problem in these patients.

- The shoulder girdle is typically in protraction and elevation, rotating the humerus medially and depressing the sternum (Rocabado & Iglash 1991, Kraus 1994). If the patient experiences symptoms, the symptomatic side might present with slight shoulder elevation and more protraction on that side when compared to the asymptomatic side.
- The thoracic spine should be observed for an increased kyphotic curvature.
- The patient will probably present with a typical crossed shoulder syndrome as described by Janda (1994), which entails elevation and protraction of the shoulders, rotation and abduction of the scapulae and a forward head posture.

Functional activity

- Test for scapula control and muscle imbalance around the scapula by observation of two upper limb movements:
  - Firstly, the patient performs a slow push-up from the prone position. Note excessive or abnormal movement of the scapula. Muscle weakness will cause the scapula to rotate and glide laterally and/or move superiorly. A weak serratus anterior muscle will result in scapular winging (scapula alata).
  - Secondly, shoulder abduction, with the elbow in flexion, is performed in sitting. Observe the quality of movement of the glenohumeral joint and control of the scapula. Note any abnormal movements which might indicate that the synergistic function of the scapular muscles (mid- and lower fibres of trapezius, rhomboids and serratus anterior) are not functioning optimally. An example is an imbalance between the upper fibres of trapezius and the lower fibres of trapezius and serratus anterior, where an overactive upper portion of the trapezius pulls the scapula into elevation, inhibiting the stabilizing function of the other muscles (Petty & Moore 2000, Bryden & Fitzgerald 2001).
- Observe the breathing pattern. Normally a diaphragmatic pattern is present with the expansion of the lateral costal border of the rib cage. In a patient with nasal obstruction, the diaphragm activity might be decreased, moving the breathing to the upper thoracic area, increasing the activity of the upper trapezius, levator scapulae and scalene muscles. The inferior and lateral part of the rib cage might even move inward (depression of the rib cage), indicating that the spinal stabilizers are not functioning optimally, particularly the transverse abdominal muscle.
- Determine the mobility of the thoracic region by actively moving into flexion, extension, rotation and lateral flexion. It is possible that some of the movements are limited.

Neuromuscular

- Palpate the muscles and soft tissue structures of the shoulder girdle and thoracic spine for local or referred pain, spasm, trigger points, muscle activity and mobility. The pectoral, trapezius (pars descendens), levator scapulae and scalene muscles are often tender on palpation, with increased muscle activity and trigger points. The palpation of the fascia of the superior shoulder region and the pectoral area might reveal shortening and decreased mobility.
- The strength of the stabilizing muscles of the scapula should be tested. This includes the mid- and lower fibres of trapezius, rhomboids and serratus anterior muscles.
- Assess the mobility and muscle length of pectoralis major, upper fibres of trapezius, levator scapulae and the scalene muscles.
- Passive physiological and accessory movements should be used to test joint mobility of the thoracic spine. The mid-thoracic region is often stiff, especially in the direction of extension. The passive physiological and accessory movements might also be more restricted into the direction of extension than the direction of flexion, as the

patient is in a sustained thoracic flexion posture.

- Scapulothoracic movement should also be examined to determine the amount of hypo- or hypermobility present. With the patient in side lying, the arm resting behind the back, the uppermost scapula is tested. With one hand along the medial border of the scapula and the other hand holding the upper dorsal surface of the scapula, the therapist uses their body to push the shoulder posteriorly to obtain a better hold. The scapula is moved medially, laterally, caudally, cranially and away from the thorax (distraction) (Magee 1997). The scapulothoracic movements are often relatively hypermobile, especially distraction.

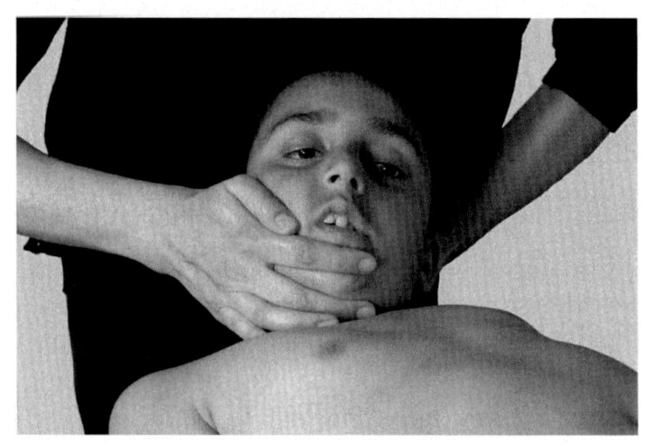

Fig. 22.5 Testing the neurodynamics of the mandibular nerve (V_3) of a mouth-breathing child (von Piekartz 2001). The patient presented with decreased lateral deviation that also caused significant discomfort.

CRANIONEURODYNAMIC TESTING

In this patient population, the most relevant cranioneurodynamic tests are the trigeminal, facial, accessory and hypoglossal nerves (see Chapter 17).

The following clinical patterns are often seen:

- Increased tone in the muscles innervated by the above nerves, resulting in upper cervical stiffness. These muscles include the masticatory, facial, infra- and suprahyoid, trapezius and sternocleidomastoid. During cranioneurodynamic testing, the motor reactions are particularly increased in the masseter, orbicularis oris and trapezius (pars descendens) muscles.
- The subjective response of the patient is often described as an intense 'pulling' or 'pressure' sensation, and less often as a 'burning' or 'pinching' sensation.
- The last movement of the test provokes in most cases an increase in subjective responses as well as muscle spasm. For example, during the mandibular nerve test, the last movement is laterotrusion of the mandible (Fig. 22.5), depression and retraction of the shoulder during the accessorius neurodynamic nerve test, and the transverse movement of the hyoid bone during the hypoglossus neurodynamic test (von Piekartz 2001).
- On palpation, the nerves are, in most cases, thicker than normal and very mechanosensitive.
- During accumulative neurodynamic testing (one movement after another) the subjective responses often increase.

TREATMENT

In planning a treatment programme, it is essential that the aetiological factors should be reduced before a physiotherapeutic rehabilitation programme can be introduced successfully. If the patient presents with chronic nasal obstruction, they should be referred to an otorhinolaryngologist or allergist, as the case might be acute (Wiltshire 1996). If the patient presents with dental problems or malocclusion, this demands the skills of an orthodontist. It is essential that a multidisciplinary approach is followed (Rocabado & Iglash 1991).

According to Jull and Janda (1987) and Jull and Moore (2002), the importance of adequate sensory input, proprioceptive control and proper function of sensorimotor integration has been underestimated in the pathogenesis of muscle imbalances and the pathogenesis of pain. With good knowledge and application of these principles, clinicians can help to direct the normal growth and development of the musculoskeletal system (LeVeau & Bernhardt 1984, Jull & Janda 1987).

If the patient experiences any symptoms or pain, which in children is not often the case, this should be addressed before any neuromusculoskeletal rehabilitation can be initiated (Jull & Janda 1987). There are a variety of techniques or approaches to choose from when treating pain or other symptoms. Some manipulative therapy approaches are based on a biomechanical analysis of articular dysfunction, whereas others rely more on analysis of pain response to movement. According to Jull and Moore (2002), within the broader definition of manual musculoskeletal therapy, evidence is suggesting that a multimodal approach – including for example manipulative therapy, exercise and education – seems to provide better outcomes than a single therapy approach.

According to Lee (2000), the ultimate goal of therapeutic intervention is to restore the biomechanics of the dysfunctional region. Other important factors are the re-education of postural control and to create kinaesthetic awareness of optimal postural alignment (Bryden & Fitzgerald 2001).

A biopsychosocial approach should be followed with the assessment, as it includes consideration of the patient's attitudes and beliefs related to the problem and symptoms experienced, and how these interact with social, cultural and other influences (Butler 2000).

OROCRANIOFACIAL REHABILITATION

Nasal obstruction

The first step in the nasally obstructed patient toward restoring the biomechanics of the orocraniofacial and cervical regions is to reduce the number of aetiological factors. This could, for example, include surgery to remove hypertrophied adenoids or tonsils, or the use of medication to reduce the inflammatory response as a result of allergies. Once the obstruction is reduced, the tongue and mandibular resting position can be re-educated in order to achieve a normal nasal–diaphragmatic breathing pattern (Wiltshire 1996).

Lingual re-education

PROPRIOCEPTION AND STEREOGNOSIS

Initially the therapist introduces the concept of proprioception and stereognosis to the patient by rubbing the rugae of the palate with a finger. The patient repeats this by rubbing the tongue over the rugae. Once this is accomplished, the patient can compare this sensation with other tissues of the mouth such as the teeth, cheeks and gums. This process enables the patient to differentiate hard from soft tissues. Now the patient should be able to recognize the incorrect tissue contact with the tongue and be able to reposition the tongue against the hard palate in the normal resting position (Rocabado & Iglash 1991).

NORMAL RESTING POSITION OF THE TONGUE AND MANDIBLE

The resting position of the tongue is maintained by negative air pressure causing a suction effect in the oral cavity, rather than by muscular force. The patient can be advised to make a 'clucking' sound to feel the correct position, and then should be taught to maintain the anterior third of the tongue against the palate with a slight pressure to ensure normal swallowing and a resting posture with the least amount of muscle activity (Rocabado & Iglash 1991).

The resting position of the tongue is also related to the resting position of the mandible and the maintenance of a certain 'freeway space' between the teeth. As the patient learns to place the tongue against the palate, mouth breathing ceases and nasal breathing occurs as patency shifts from the inferior to the superior airway space. Simultaneously the masticatory muscles will relax (Rocabado & Iglash 1991).

RESTORING THE NORMAL POSITION AND MOTION OF THE HYOID BONE

The hyoid bone moves in response to changes in the tongue position. If the hyoid bone is elevated, it will ascend excessively with swallowing, increasing the activity in the tongue in its dysfunctional resting position. It is therefore essential for the therapist to re-educate the hyoid musculature to rest in a normal descended position and ascend appropriately during function. To retrain the hyoid muscles, the patient is instructed to elevate the tongue against the palate, while the therapist flexes the head approximately 15° anteriorly. The patient now performs an isometric contraction of 6 seconds by pressing anteriorly while the therapist stabilizes the frontal bone (Fig. 22.6).

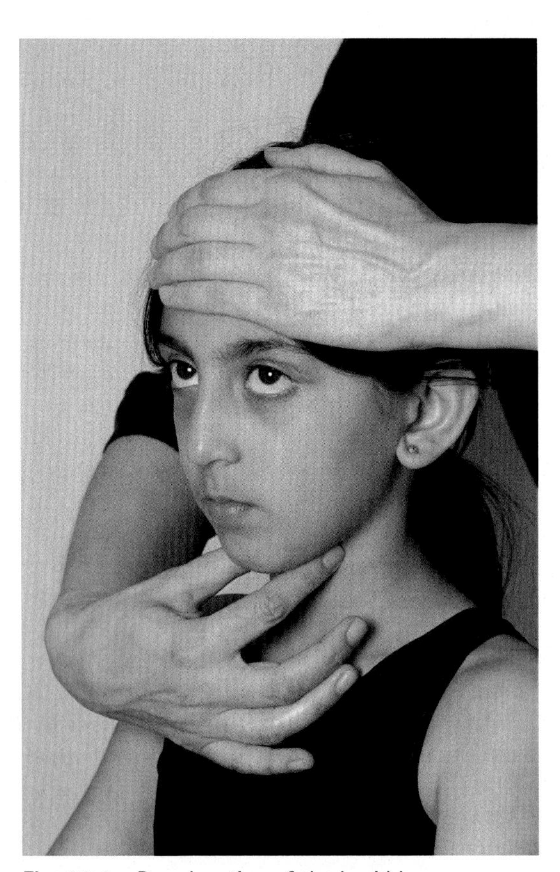

Fig. 22.6 Re-education of the hyoid bone movement (reproduced with permission from Rocabado & Iglash 1991).

This contraction activates the infrahyoid muscles bilaterally and brings the hyoid bone downward, causing a slight, effective contraction (Rocabado & Iglash 1991).

LINGUAL COORDINATION

To enhance lingual coordination, the patient can perform functional movements of the tongue, maintaining the tongue against the palate within the borders of the upper teeth. The tongue can be moved in circular, triangular or posterior and lateral patterns, always returning to the rugae. The tongue must move against the palate, avoiding tooth contact (Rocabado & Iglash 1991).

For more information on the rehabilitation of orofacial function, see Chapters 9, 12 and 13.

Re-education of nasal–diaphragmatic breathing

Diaphragmatic breathing is the normal mode of breathing, using the diaphragm and external intercostal muscles for inspiration. The patient should be instructed to relax the accessory respiratory muscles by proper use of the diaphragm. With the patient sitting in a chair, the purpose of the technique should be explained and demonstrated. The therapist's hands are placed on the costophrenic angle and the patient is asked to breathe in against the hands. There should be no resistance to inspiration, but a gentle inward and downward squeeze on expiration can be given. This will facilitate the next inspiratory effort (Frownfelter 1987).

Habit awareness and oral modification

Parafunctional habits such as nail or pencil biting, gum chewing or resting the chin on the hand should be discouraged by patient awareness (Rocabado & Iglash 1991, Kraus 1994).

Craniomandibular dysfunction

If the temporomandibular joint is dysfunctional, passive mobilization techniques can be used to address the articular component, for relieving pain or restoring range of motion. The soft tissues surrounding the joint should also be treated for muscle spasm, trigger points, tightness or any other problems detected on assessment. The muscles should be re-educated by using isometric contractions to restore joint stability and muscle balance.

CRANIOCERVICAL REHABILITATION

Articular dysfunction

Various passive mobilization techniques or mobilization with movement techniques can be used to restore articular dysfunction.

CRANIOCERVICAL JOINTS

The joints between the occiput and the third cervical vertebrae are hypomobile. The most limited movement will be flexion as a result of the extended position of the upper cervical region associated with nasal obstruction.

MID- AND LOWER CERVICAL JOINTS

The patient with nasal obstruction presents with a forward head posture, indicating that the mid- and lower cervical regions are in an anteriorly inclined alignment. The extension needed for the normal slight lordotic curvature of this region is probably stiff, and this is the main movement that should be restored in the area.

Muscular dysfunction

Tight muscles can affect the mobility of joints of the craniocervical region. Specific muscle lengthening can be effective in restoring the osteokinematics. These techniques are often referred to as 'muscle energy' techniques or active mobilization techniques. They facilitate and restore motion at the joint and can be used in conjunction with passive mobilization techniques (Lee 2000).

POSTERIOR UPPER CERVICAL MUSCLES

The posterior muscles of the upper cervical region are shortened as a result of the sustained craniocervical extension. These muscles must be lengthened to restore normal function in this region. With the patient in supine, the therapist stabilizes the mid- and lower cervical spine with one hand posteriorly. The other hand supports the occiput. The head is flexed on the neck (upper cervical flexion) to the point of resistance. The patient is then instructed to resist further motion while the therapist applies a gentle flexion force to the head to build up a strong isometric contraction. This isometric contraction is followed by a period of complete relaxation. The head is then passively taken further into flexion into the new physiological range. The technique is repeated a few times and then followed by re-evaluation of the osteokinematic function.

ANTERIOR CERVICAL MUSCLES

The deep neck flexors on the anterior aspect of the neck are most probably weak as a result of the abnormal postural alignment of the patient. Re-education of the deep neck flexors will also ensure better cervical stability. This is done with the patient in crook lying. The craniocervical and cervical spine are in a midrange neutral position (the face line must be horizontal as should the longitudinal axis of the neck). The head can be supported with a small folded towel under the base of the occiput, if required.

Instruct the patient to place the tongue on the roof of the mouth, keep the teeth separated and the lips gently touching. The patient is instructed to gently nod the head (as if saying 'yes'). Ensure that the patient is performing a pure nod, no head retraction or lifting of the head. Slow, controlled movement must be performed. Check that the hyoid musculature is relaxed by a gentle mobilization of the trachea from side to side. Start the holding time with 5 seconds, increasing this gradually to 10 seconds and increase the number of repetitions to 10 before progressing to the next exercise. Slowly progress to a prone position supported on the elbows, with control of the scapular position. This should be incorporated into scapular stability training as well as postural retraining, progressing to weight bearing and eventually standing and functional activities. Always ensure that the patient uses a correct pattern of movement from extension to neutral and neutral to flexion by leading the movement with upper cervical flexion. Correct recruitment and sequencing are more important than strengthening (Jull 2001).

POSTERIOR MID- AND LOWER CERVICAL MUSCLES

These muscles need to be strengthened to retrain proper postural alignment. This is done in a similar way as the testing of these muscles. The patient is in prone, supported on the elbows. The patient relaxes the head with gravity into flexion. The patient is instructed to tuck the chin in by head-on-neck flexion, activating the deep neck flexors, and then to lift the head into extension while maintaining the chin tuck. The head and neck should be in line with the spine. Scapular stability should be maintained throughout, as should the correct position of the tongue. This should be restored before the postural rehabilitation begins.

SHOULDER GIRDLE AND THORACIC SPINE REHABILITATION

Articular dysfunction

The mid-thoracic region is probably in a slightly increased kyphotic posture, indicating that the intervertebral joints are hypomobile. These joints should be mobilized with passive mobilization techniques to increase the range of motion, especially extension range. To enhance the improved articular function, the relevant muscles should be re-educated.

Muscular dysfunction

SCALENUS MUSCLES

To decrease activity in the muscles, a correct nasal–diaphragmatic breathing pattern must be restored. If the muscle is shortened, active mobilization can be used to improve the muscle length. With the patient in supine, stabilize the first rib with one hand, and with the other hand supporting under the occiput, laterally flex the head to the opposite side to the point of resistance. An isometric contraction is obtained by instructing the patient to resist further side flexion, maintain the contraction, relax and then take the head further into lateral flexion. Repeat three times and re-evaluate the range.

LEVATOR SCAPULAE

This muscle can also be stretched with active mobilization techniques, similar to the scalenes. The only differences are that the one hand stabilizes the scapula into depression, while the head is taken into lateral flexion and rotation away from the side to be treated.

PECTORALIS MAJOR

Lengthen this muscle by active mobilization, using the arm as a lever. Move the arm into flexion, abduction and external rotation, obtain an isometric contraction of the pectoralis major muscle and lift the arm further into the range on relaxation.

MOTOR CONTROL OF THE SHOULDER GIRDLE

Poor patterns of neuromuscular control in the shoulder girdle muscles have the potential to create or prolong symptomatic dysfunction in the cervical spine as well as the glenohumeral complex (Jull & Janda 1987).

SHOULDER GIRDLE STABILITY

It is usually the force couple of serratus anterior and the trapezius muscle controlling lateral (upward) rotation of the scapula that requires rehabilitation. Overactivity in other muscles such as levator scapulae, pectoralis minor or upper trapezius must be addressed first, before scapula control can be re-educated (Jull & Moore 2002).

The serratus anterior can be activated by using variations of the classic grade III muscle test of scapula protraction with lateral rotation. It can be done in supine, side lying or sitting with the arm supported, or even with the hand against the wall.

> **!** The pectoralis major should not be excessively active!

As soon as possible, retraining should progress to weight bearing through the arm to facilitate the stabilization function of the muscle and co-contraction of trapezius. Initial weight bearing may be trained by leaning against a wall, maintaining scapular position while shifting weight from one arm to the other. Progression may include static positioning in four point kneeling, weight shift in this position, slow controlled wall push-ups and half push-ups prone on elbows. Progress to free glenohumeral movement while maintaining scapular position against the thorax, focusing on eccentric control (Jull & Janda 1987).

Lower trapezius activation starts in non-weight bearing positions, such as prone with the arm by the side, side lying or with the arm supported. Palpate the coracoid process anteriorly. Perform a very gentle retraction, depression action (Jull & Janda 1987). Once this is achieved the inferior angles of the scapulae can be palpated, and the patient is instructed to abduct the arm a few degrees without moving the scapular angles away from the therapist's fingers. The degree of abduction can be increased until the inferior angles can be controlled in every position.

Tapping is another method that can be used to facilitate appropriate muscle patterning and activation within all stages of rehabilitation.

Rehabilitation of the shoulder girdle and the thoracic spine will in most cases be combined with assessment of the musculoskeletal system of the craniofacial region. For further information on this specific topic, see Chapter 12.

POSTURAL RETRAINING

Successful rehabilitation of the orocraniofacial–cervical complex requires not only the restoration of articular and myofascial function, but also postural alignment and the restoration of normal movement patterns. Strength, endurance and especially timing of recruitment of the inner and outer muscle units must be rehabilitated to restore the ability of the deep stabilizing muscles to protect the craniocervical region. Stability training is the first step towards postural re-education. The main aim is to isolate the appropriate muscles, retrain their holding capacity and their ability to automatically contract appropriately with other synergists to support and protect the spine under various functional loads. Optimal postural alignment and awareness must be re-educated in all static and dynamic activities, such as sitting, standing, walking and eventually also in sport.

ACTIVITY PROGRAMME AT HOME

Successful rehabilitation includes an activity programme at home to reinforce the clinical treatment regime and also to modify the patient's lifestyle. Exercises extinguish parafunctional habits and reinforce new postures and functions. This should impact not only on the orthostatic equilibrium of the entire upper body, but also on the body as a whole (Rocabado & Iglash 1991, Lee 2000).

The objectives of a home programme are to:

- Learn a new postural position
- Facilitate the new position of the soft tissues
- Restore muscles to their original length and strength
- Restore normal joint movement
- Prevent symptoms from developing and recurrence of the problem
- Provide an ongoing activity programme for incorporation into the patient's daily activities (Rocabado & Iglash 1991).

The techniques that are described in this chapter can easily be transformed into activities at home. When the therapist reassess these activities with the patient and adapts them over time, the patient's compliance will increase (Van de Sluis 1991).

SUMMARY

- From the literature it is a known fact that altered breathing patterns can influence the neuromusculoskeletal system and that this is recognized by specific clinical patterns. This functional adaptation reflects not only in the craniofacial and craniocervical regions, but also in the rest of the body, and can contribute to the development of further dysfunction and pain in later years.
- Although the effect of the forces of growth on an abnormally aligned spine is not clear, perhaps these forces could be directed and used to ensure optimal growth and development of the neuromusculoskeletal system. This includes the child with altered breathing patterns and abnormal orofacial development, as they are more vulnerable for abnormal growth.
- The importance of early intervention and prevention cannot be overemphasized, especially in the prepubertal child who is on the brink of the final and most important growth spurt. The child may not present with any symptoms, but early intervention may ensure that this child does not turn into an adult seeking treatment a decade or two later (Proffit & Fields 1993, Linder-Aronson & Woodside 2000).
- Suggestions for assessment and management of the neuromusculoskeletal system, based on recent clinical evidence, have been described. This will hopefully stimulate an interest and guide the therapist in the management of this specific group of patients.

References

Ayub E, Glasheen-Wray M, Kraus S 1984 Head posture: a case study of the effects on the rest position of the mandible. Journal of Orthopaedic and Sports Physical Therapy 5(4):179

Braun B L, Amundson L R. Quantitative Assessment of Head and Shoulder Posture. Archives of Physical and Medical Rehabilitation. 1989; 70:322

Bryden L, Fitzgerald D 2001 The influence of posture and alteration of function upon the craniocervical and craniofacial regions. In: von Piekartz H J M, Bryden L (eds) Craniofacial dysfunction and pain. Manual therapy, assessment and management. Butterworth-Heinemann, Oxford

Butler D S 2000 The sensitive nervous system. NOI Publications, Adelaide

Cheng M-C, Enlow D H, Papsidero M et al 1988 Developmental effects of impaired breathing in the face of the growing child. Angle Orthodontist 58(4):309–320

Darlow L A, Pesco J, Greenberg M S 1987 The relationship of posture to myofascial pain dysfunction syndrome. Journal of the American Dental Association 114:73

Forsberg C M, Hellsing E, Linder-Aronson S, Sheikholeslam A 1985 EMG activity in neck and masticatory muscles in relation to extension and flexion of the head. European Journal of Orthodontics 7:177

Frownfelter D L 1987 Chest physical therapy and pulmonary rehabilitation. An interdisciplinary approach, 2nd edn. Year Book, Chicago

Garry J F 1992 Upper airway obstruction and TMJD/MPD. In: Coy R E (ed.) Anthology of craniomandibular orthopedics, Vol. I. Buchanan, Baltimore

Grimmer K 1997 An investigation of poor cervical resting posture. Australian Physiotherapy 43(1):7

Hackney J, Bade D, Clawson A 1993 Relationship between forward head posture and diagnosed internal derangement of the temporomandibular joint. Journal of Orofacial Pain 7(4):386

Hanten W P, Lucio R M, Russel J L, Brunt D 1991 Assessment of total head excursion and resting head posture. Archives of Physical and Medical Rehabilitation 72:877

Hellsing E 1989 Changes in the pharyngeal airway in relation to extension of the head. European Journal of Orthodontics 11:359

Hellsing E, Forsberg C M, Linder-Aronson S, Sheikholeslam A 1986 Changes in postural EMG activity in the neck and masticatory muscles following obstruction of the nasal airways. European Journal of Orthodontics 8:247

Janda V 1994 Muscles and motor control in cervicogenic disorders: assessment and management. In: Grant R (ed.) Clinics in physical

therapy. Physical therapy for the cervical and thoracic spine. Churchill Livingstone, Edinburgh
Jull G 2001 The physiotherapy management of neck disorders. Course notes, Antwerp. Cervical Spine and Whiplash Research Unit, Department of Physiotherapy, University of Queensland, Brisbane
Jull G A, Janda V 1987 Muscles and motor control in low back pain: assessment and management. In: Twomey L T, Taylor J R (eds) Physical therapy of the low back, 2nd edn. Churchill Livingstone, Melbourne
Jull G, Moore A 2002 Are manipulative therapy approaches the same? Manual Therapy 7(2):63
Kendall F P, McCreary E K, Provance P G 1993 Muscles. Testing and function, 4th edn. Williams and Wilkins, Philadelphia
Kraus S L (ed.) 1994 Physical therapy management of TMD. In: Clinics in physical therapy: temporomandibular disorders, 2nd edn. Churchill Livingstone, New York
Kritsineli M, Shim Y S 1992 Malocclusion, body posture, and temporomandibular disorder in children with primary and mixed dentition. Journal of Clinical Pediatric Dentistry 16(2):86
Lawrence E S, Razook S J 1994 Nonsurgical management of mandibular disorders. In: Kraus S L (ed). Clinics in physical therapy: temporomandibular disorders, 2nd edn. Churchill Livingstone, New York
Lee D 2000 The pelvic girdle. An approach to the examination and treatment of the lumbo-pelvic-hip region, 2nd edn. Churchill Livingstone, Oxford
LeVeau B F, Bernhardt D B 1984 Developmental biomechanics. Effect of forces on growth, development, and maintenance of the human body. Physical Therapy 64(12):1874
Linder-Aronson S, Woodside D G 2000 Excess face height malocclusion: etiology, diagnosis and treatment. Quintessence, Chicago
Magee D J 1997 Orthopedic physical assessment, 3rd edn. W B Saunders, Los Angeles
Miller A J, Vargervik K, Chierici G 1984 Experimentally induced neuromuscular changes during and after nasal airway obstruction. American Journal of Orthodontics 85(5):385
Ono T, Ishiwata Y, Kuroda T 1998 Inhibition of masseteric electromyographic activity during oral respiration. American Journal of Orthodontic and Dentofacial Orthopedics 113(5):518
Petty N J, Moore A P 2000 Neuromusculoskeletal examination and assessment. Churchill Livingstone, Oxford
Proffit W R, Fields H W 1993 Contemporary orthodontics, 2nd edn. Mosby Year Book, St Louis
Ricketts R M 1968 Respiratory obstruction syndrome. American Journal of Orthodontics 54(7):495
Rocabado M 1983 Biomechanical relationship of the cranial, cervical and hyoid regions. Journal of Craniomandibular Practice 1(3):62
Rocabado M, Iglash Z A 1991 Musculoskeletal approach to maxillofacial pain. J B Lippincott, Philadelphia
Solow B, Sonnesen L 1998 Head posture and malocclusions. European Journal of Orthodontics 20:685
Solow B, Siersbaek-Nielsen S, Greve E 1984 Airway adequacy, head posture, and craniofacial morphology. American Journal of Orthodontics 86(3):214
Solow B, Oveson J, Nielsen P W, Wildschiødtz G, Tallgren A 1993 Head posture in obstructive sleep apnoea. European Journal of Orthodontics 15:107
Tourne L P M, Schweiger J 1996 Immediate postural responses to total nasal obstruction. American Journal of Orthodontics and Dentofacial Orthopedics 110(6):606
Van de Sluis E M 1991 Patient education in physical therapy. Thesis. Rijksuniversiteit Limburg, Maastricht
Von Piekartz H J M 2001 Neurodynamics of cranial nervous tissue (cranioneurodynamics). In: von Piekartz H J M, Bryden L (eds) Craniofacial dysfunction and pain. Manual therapy, assessment and management. Butterworth-Heinemann, Oxford
Wenzel A, Höjensgaard E, Henriksen J M 1985 Craniofacial morphology and head posture in children with asthma and perennial rhinitis. European Journal of Orthodontics 7:83
Wiltshire W A 1996 Orthodontics and chronic nasal obstruction. Current Allergy and Clinical Immunology 7(2):16

Chapter 23

Clinical presentations from daily practice: how would you deal with these cases?

Harry von Piekartz

CHAPTER CONTENTS

INTRODUCTION

Five different case studies of patients with dysfunctions and pain in the head, face and neck regions are presented and discussed in this chapter. All five patients were treated according to the approach upon which this book is based. However, do not be misguided into thinking that the chosen techniques are the only options for these multidimensional syndromes. They are only suggested approaches that are based on thorough biomedical knowledge in this area and clinical decision-making processes which retrospectively led to the desired results.

The following examples were documented by colleagues of the author. The case studies are structured into:

- Subjective examination and history
- Physical examination
- Therapeutic procedure
- Clinical course
- Conclusions.

Only the relevant information is mentioned; these reports are by no means exhaustive.

As a theoretical exercise the reader might want to take a break after reading the section on physical examination and, in line with the guidance given in Chapters 1 and 3, form their own thoughts about potential hypotheses (including categories such as potential sources or precautions), management and prognosis before reading the rest of the case report.

Case study 1: Female, 27 years old

Thomas Horre, Osnabrück, Germany

Diagnosis: Craniomandibular dysfunction

Subjective examination and history

A 27-year-old physiotherapist complained of problems in the jaw region. She had noticed a clicking in the right temporomandibular joint (TMJ) for the past 5 years when she was eating. On maximum mouth opening (e.g. when yawning) she felt as if the jaw would dislocate. This affected her daily life activities and she was embarrassed to speak in public. Two years ago she had a root resection of a right lower molar tooth. Following the procedure the dentist recommended isometric exercises to improve the jaw movements. The patient exercised for 6 weeks without success. The dentist then recommended manual therapy and she came to our practice for treatment.

She did not experience any pain in the head, neck or face regions. The only problem was the clicking noise and the fear of jaw dislocation when opening the mouth wide. Because she felt uncomfortable when she heard the clicking she avoided maximum mouth opening. Although she did not feel any pain, the problem affected her quality of life at participation level.

The subjective examination did not indicate any reasons for caution during the physical examination.

Physical examination

On inspection a slightly increased thoracic kyphosis and a head forward position was noted. Correction and excessive correction of the head position were asymptomatic. Face measurement according to the method by Trott resulted in a ratio of 1.4. The head of the mandible was palpated in a central position with the jaw closed. Active testing resulted in a swinging opening pattern to the right (Fig. 23.1a) that was easily corrected passively. She was able to open her mouth by 20 mm without any compensatory activities. The laterotrusion to the left was reduced by 4 mm compared to laterotrusion to the right. She achieved 3 points on the Helkimo Index (clinical dysfunction index) which classified her problem as a 'slight craniomandibular dysfunction' (Di I; see Chapter 3 for details of the Helkimo Index).

Therapeutic procedure

In the first treatment session the patient learned to palpate the head of the mandible. Sitting in front of a mirror, she learned how to open her mouth as far as possible without compensatory movements controlled by palpation and the reflection in the mirror (Fig. 23.1b).

On the second day of treatment the range of motion had increased to 24 mm without deviations and the patient had gained confidence. She was now hoping to gain control of the problem. Since the left mandibular head showed a palpable translation to the left on depression beyond 24 mm, accessory movements (transverse medial) were applied. The jaw was placed into a position of depression where the onset of translation was felt. In the reassessment, depression had increased to 27 mm.

The patient was asked to continue the controlled opening exercise but to reduce the visual and tactile control gradually.

Clinical course

During the following four treatment sessions mouth opening increased to 46 mm without visible or palpable compensatory movements. The clicking during chewing activities had decreased significantly. The patient no longer feared dislocating her jaw due to the learned control mechanisms. The Helkimo Index was down to 1 point, indicating that she still had a slight dysfunction but with a good prognosis towards complete healing.

It was agreed that the patient would continue her exercises daily for the next 4–6

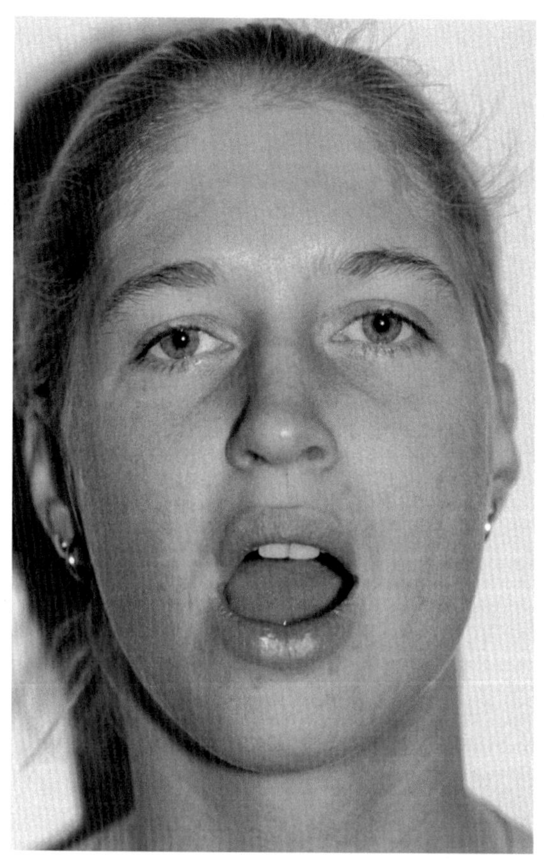

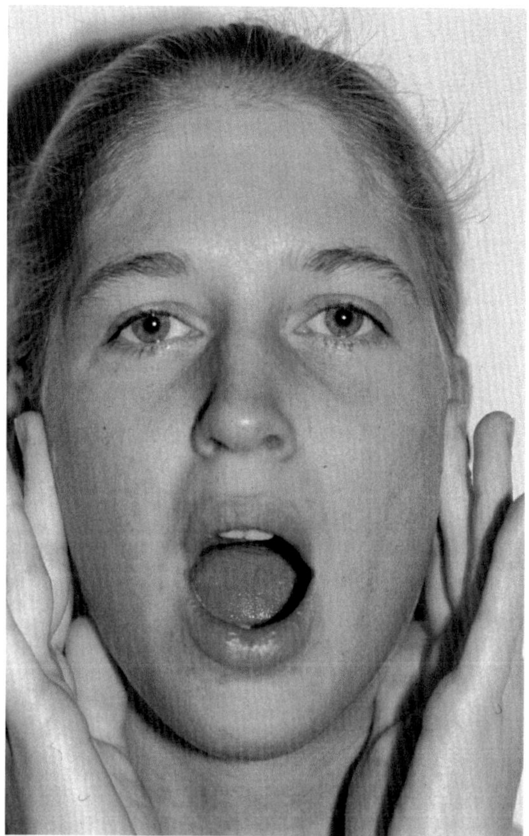

Fig. 23.1 A 27-year-old female with craniomandibular dysfunction (Helkimo Index Di I).
a On active depression the jaw deviates to the right.
b Self-palpation of the head of the mandible to control deviation during depression.

weeks. After that time she rang to say that she was well, that the clicking hardly ever occurred now and that she was able to almost completely open her mouth without symptoms.

Conclusions

This case study shows that a minimal craniomandibular dysfunction (Helkimo Index Di I) with a slow onset may affect a patient's daily life regarding function, participation and even emotionally. It also shows that minimal intervention and simple techniques (passive mobilization, information and home exercises) may quickly improve the dysfunction as well as the emotional and cognitive aspects.

Case study 2: Martijn, 13 years

Cara Raaijmakers, Schaijk,
The Netherlands

Diagnosis: Facial asymmetry with regressed right zygoma and shortening of the right sternocleidomastoid muscle

Subjective examination and history

Martijn initially came for treatment 2 and a half years ago. His parents were worried about his worsening facial asymmetry and the head position that was tilted to the right. This was particularly affecting him when he had to sit for a long time at school and also in the evenings. Parents, family members and friends had started to point out this problem. They asked his GP to refer him for plastic surgery. The boy himself noticed his asymmetrical face and suffered because of it. The GP asked me to assess the situation and to treat the patient if possible.

Physical examination

The examination showed a significantly regressed right zygoma and a severe shortening of the sternocleidomastoid muscle on the right side associated with an elevated position of the right shoulder (Fig. 23.2a). The neck was held in lateroflexion to the right. Even in a supine position the neck was kept tilted to the right. Martijn is an active, sporty child and is doing well at school. The mother advised that he used to be a 'cry baby' with a torticollis to the right. This was treated by a paediatric physiotherapist without success. The crying eventually stopped and further motor development continued normally, if a little slowly. He was screened for hip dysplasia that could not be confirmed (the mother did not remember which side). When he was 8 months old, a surgical splitting of the right sternocleidomastoid showed a positive result.

Active testing showed a decreased lateroflexion to the left with stretching pain in the right sternocleidomastoid. The local manual examination showed a disturbed atlas–occiput relation with a decreased transverse movement of the atlas to the right. Palpation of the atlas, C2 and C3 was painful. Further findings included a significantly shortened right sternocleidomastoid, right shoulder high, head forward position, slight C-scoliosis right convex (culmination point T5) and both zygoma painful on pressure (Fig. 23.2c).

Hypotheses

The preliminary hypothesis regarding the source of the symptoms was a shortness of the right sternocleidomastoid based on an upper cervical dysfunction.

The long-term abnormal craniocervical afference might be the result of a previous history of kinematic imbalance due to suboccipital strain (KISS) syndrome. A secondary cranial asymmetry might be the result of an abnormal stress transducer. During the critical phase of viscerocranial development, facial asymmetry became more obvious.

At the age of 13, an x-ray of the craniocervical junction was taken to decide upon further treatment. The findings from this investigation were a high atlas arch in relation to the teeth and normal atlas–occiput position. This was not considered a radiologically abnormal result.

Therapeutic procedure

Based on the findings in the craniocervical junction and the previous history, the initial treatment technique was a unilateral passive mobilization of the atlas in anteroposterior and transverse (to the right) directions. This was followed by transverse occiput techniques and, in sessions 2–4, occiput–sphenoid mobilizations dominated the treatment. A further evaluation of the facial structures, as noted in the treatment plan, showed a small upper jaw with canine teeth that were positioned ventrocranially of the other upper jaw teeth. Mobility of the occipital bone relative to the sphenoid bone to the left was painful and limited, dorsal rotation of the right temporal bone was painful, anteroposterior movement of the right zygomatic bone was painful and restricted locally and was incorporated into the treatment plan.

Mouth opening was performed with a deviation to the right. The laterotrusion of the jaw to the right was reduced. Mobilizing techniques such as transverse lateral and laterotrusion were chosen to achieve normal mouth opening. Besides the hands-on techniques, proprioceptive training was performed: Martijn was asked to guess his head position after it was placed into various cervical angles. When he was wrong he was asked to correct the position. As a home

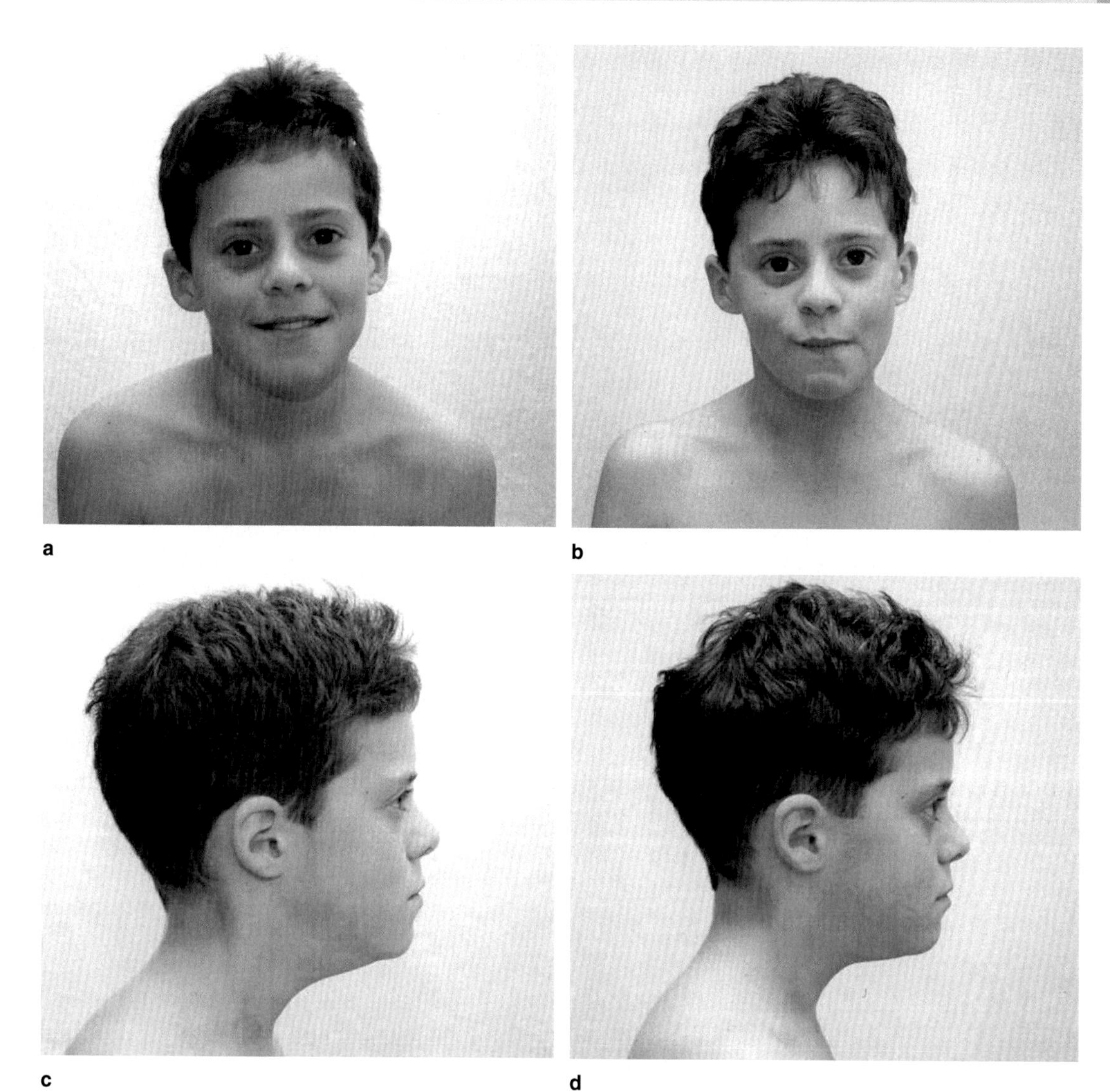

Fig. 23.2 A 13-year-old boy with facial asymmetry and shortness of the right sternocleidomastoid (torticollis).
a Posture pre-therapy.
b Corrected posture post-therapy of the craniocervical and craniofacial regions.
c Lateral view showing head forward position.
d Lateral view post-therapy with less head forward position.

exercise palate mobilization techniques were taught. In consultation with the orthodontist a brace was planned later on in the treatment.

Clinical course

After four sessions, Martijn was able to lie supine with his head straight and to keep his head upright when sitting. His parents still had to remind him a few times a week to keep his head straight. The scoliosis and his capability to correct his own posture were improved. The right zygoma was less prominent (Fig. 23.2b,d) and the head forward posture was reduced. The pressure on his shoulder, which Martijn had described as 'someone pushing onto his shoulder', was gone.

The facial asymmetry had improved significantly by the end of the treatment (after 8 weeks) and the deviation on mouth opening was gone. The muscle tone of the right sternocleidomastoid had improved vastly but was not completely absent.

Conclusions

Retrospectively the hypothesis about the sources of the symptoms was more accurate than may have been expected. Treatment of the craniocervical dysfunction and improved proprioception resulted in a reduction of the secondary craniofacial dysfunction and of the thoracic scoliosis. In the following 8 weeks the face became more symmetrical due to neural and viscerocranial techniques.

This example appears to confirm the theory that an untreated KISS syndrome will result in long-term dysfunctions later in life. In this case it was not pain that was the main problem but the shape of the face, and this could be treated successfully by specific craniocervical and craniofacial techniques and by providing appropriate advice to the child and parents.

Case study 3: Female, 52 years

Cara Raaijmakers, Schaijk,
The Netherlands

Diagnosis: Facial pain after resection of a right frontal/temporal meningioma with infiltration along the optic nerve

Subjective examination and history

The patient had undergone surgery 4 years ago and the tumour was resected completely. To access the tumour, the surgeon had to remove a piece of the temporal and the sphenoid bones ventrally of the right ear. These bone pieces were not replaced. The trigeminal and facial nerves were held permanently in the artificial space by a small sling. Due to the affected right optic nerve, the patient had blurred vision in the right eye and difficulties in focusing. Reading had become difficult for her. She could only read for 30 minutes and perceived this as very disabling since reading used to be one of her favourite hobbies. Furthermore, she had to give up working as a secretary. She now did secretarial work for her husband which gave her the opportunity to organize her workload depending on the variation in her capabilities.

Immediately after the operation, fluids began to collect at her right eye near the zygomatic bone. As the patient had had a glass tear duct implanted prior to this surgery, it was suspected that this was the reason for the disturbed flow of fluids. However, the problem persisted over the years. The neurosurgeon did not diagnose any treatable components and explained that she had to be satisfied with the results.

Six months ago she started to experience fasciculation around the lateral side of the eye and the collection of fluids increased. The upper eyelid was slack and her vision deteriorated. Reading became impossible, she had to concentrate hard and got tired quickly; the maximum was now 5 minutes. The trembling around her eye worried her. Her GP referred her to our practice for physiotherapy, wondering whether there was anything that could be done for the fasciculation.

Physical examination

On inspection a clear swelling in the right orbit was observed and in supine the right eye seemed more prominent than the left (Fig. 23.3a,b). Assessment of the craniocervical region showed that upper cervical rotation was restricted to both sides, masseter and temporal muscles on the right were hypertonic and the right TMJ showed crepitation on mouth opening due to effects of radiotherapy around the mandibular nerve. Laterotrusion to the left was restricted and provoked pain on the right side in the same region. Examination of the cranium showed an early resistance on sphenoid transverse

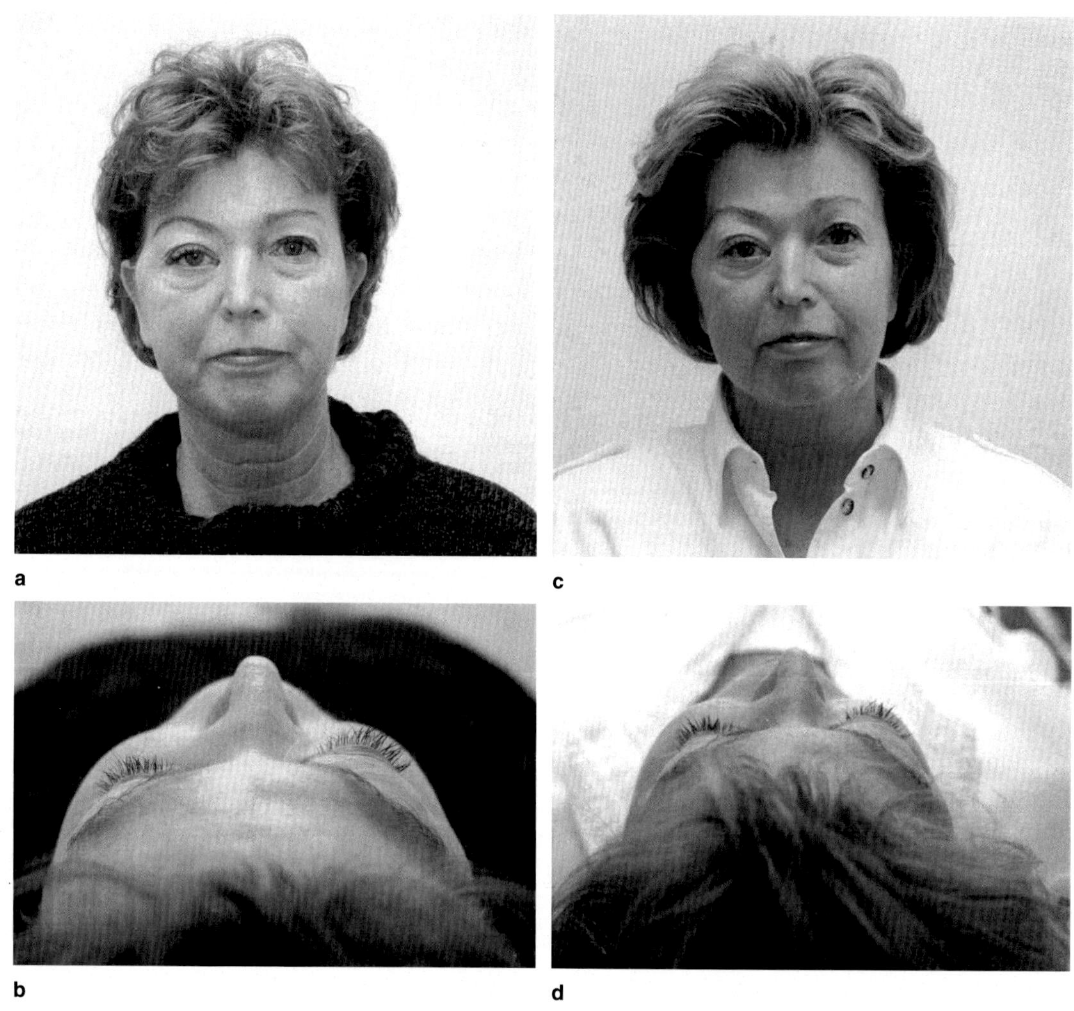

Fig. 23.3 A 52-year-old female with chronic orbital dysfunction and pain following surgical resection of a frontotemporal meningioma on the right with associated facial and mandibular nerve dysfunction.
a Clear swelling of the right orbit.
b Cranial view of the patient lying in supine showing a prominent right eye.
c Reduced swelling of the right eye post-therapy.
d Reduced swelling post-therapy in supine.

movement to either side that gave some symptomatic relief. Accessory movement of the temporal and zygomatic bones resulted in pain in the zygomatic region. On palpation the bony gap on the right side of the skull could be felt. This not only provoked local pain but symptoms were referred towards the ear and the TMJ. A great amount of fluid was found intra- and extraorbitally, medially caudal and laterally.

Testing the right mandibular nerve for pain with pre-stressing of the cervical region was positive. A possible hypothesis was minimal neuropathic dysfunction of the right orbital and mandibular region, potentially influenced by a craniofacial dysfunction. Various pain mechanisms may be important in chronic pain. The assessment showed a clear input component but due to the long-term symptoms central mechanisms were also expected. The long-term swelling indicated the influence of the autonomic nervous system and the fasciculation pointed towards an abnormal output of the motor system.

Therapeutic procedure

The initial, experimental treatment session consisted of local mobilization of the right trigeminal and facial nerves.

This resulted in a clear improvement of the pain and the fasciculation. To reduce the swelling, the eye and cheek were treated with soft tissue techniques. In addition, cranial techniques – particularly of the occiput in relation to the sphenoid, zygomatic and temporal bones – were applied.

The treatment continued for 4 months with a low frequency (once every 2 weeks).

Clinical course

The swelling around the eye decreased significantly after the orbital distraction technique and soft tissue mobilization during the first two treatment sessions (Fig. 23.3c,d).

After 4 months and eight treatment sessions the facial swelling had diminished and the fasciculation was gone. The patient was able to read for 1–1.5 hours. She felt physically fitter and went for walks to improve her condition. She was especially pleased that her quality of life had improved so much despite the neurosurgeon telling her not to expect any improvements.

Conclusions

Retrospectively it can be assumed that the dysfunction of the functional unit of the cranium had a larger effect on her nervous system than was initially anticipated. By influencing the craniofacial dysfunction with passive movements and facial soft tissue techniques, regulation of the autonomous nervous system was supported and thereby pain reduced and function improved.

Case study 4: Male, 56 years

Alfonds Ulbrich, Schweich, Germany

Diagnosis: Adenocystic carcinoma in the left maxilla

Subjective examination and history

Four months prior to coming to our physiotherapy practice the patient had undergone the following surgical interventions: hemimaxillectomy on the left with resection of the orbital floor, including the infraorbital rim and parts of the zygomatic bone. The orbital floor was reconstructed with titanium mesh and the temporal muscle for cushioning. The oral cavity was covered with a split skin graft taken from the right upper thigh. A fixation plate was inserted and fixed to the three remaining teeth (canine I and both premolars I) on the left and held at the zygomatic bone. Further pulmonary tumours were detected and remain under close observation.

At the activity level, the patient was severely restricted in eating, speaking and yawning. Physiotherapy treatment started at the hospital 3 weeks after the operation and was continued for 3 months during his stay at the hospital. Daily treatment consisted of extraoral passive mobilization techniques, supported by cryotherapy and active automobilization exercises.

He was asked to perform mobilization of the craniomandibular region several times a day without provoking pain aggravation. This was extremely difficult because the temporal region was very irritable at that time and he suffered from severe sickness due to the radiotherapy.

Mouth opening after 3 months had increased to five spatulas, equivalent to a depression of 9 mm (Fig. 23.4a). The severe bilateral temporal pain on speaking, chewing, yawning, etc. had reduced slightly but still greatly affected the patient's activity levels. The patient perceives the pain during such

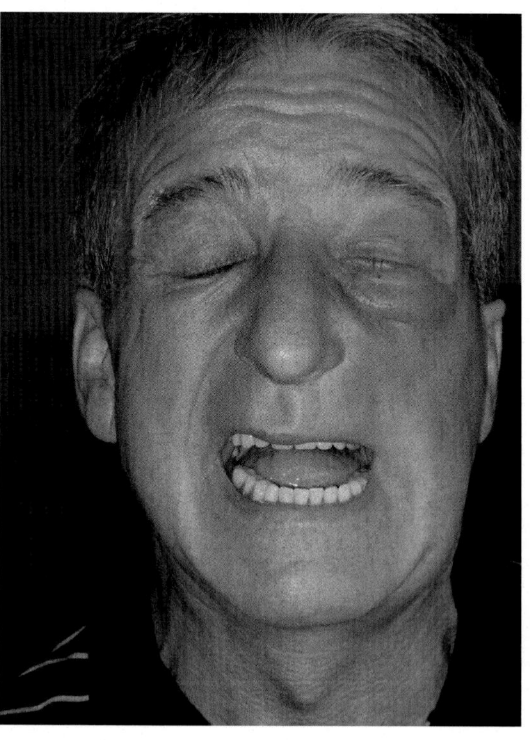
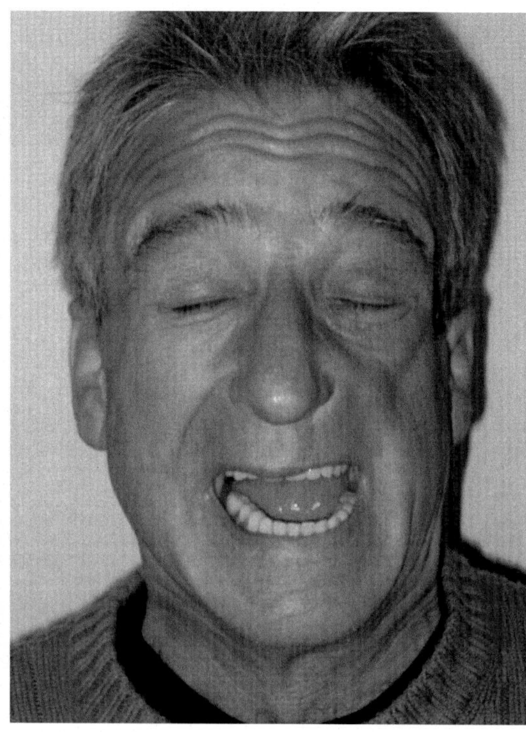

a b

Fig. 23.4 A 56-year-old male following surgical resection of an adenocystic carcinoma in the left upper jaw.
a 3 months post-surgery. Active mandibular depression 11 mm, slightly increased by cervical extension.
b 5 months post-surgery. Isolated active mandibular depression post-therapy 25 mm.

activities as 7.8–8.2 on the visual analogue scale (VAS). The parotid gland reacts with swelling to activities and therapy. The patient can control these reactions by gentle stroking movements in supine.

The patient is worried about his health status: he fears that he may not be able to open his mouth again, that the pain may remain, and he is naturally worried about the prospect of relapses and metastases. Nevertheless, he was motivated and showed a strong willpower when he presented at our clinic.

Physical examination

On inspection, redness, swelling and heat in the temporal and infraorbital regions were the most noteworthy characteristics. The scar, running from the upper lip paranasally to the left corner of the eye, was slightly hardened. The patient showed a very kyphotic cervicothoracic junction and hyperextension of the upper cervical spine. The cervical extensor muscle and the trapezius/levator scapulae muscles were hypertonic.

Assessment of the active physiological movements of the craniomandibular region showed the following results:

- Depression: 11 mm, laterotrusion to the right/left: 4 mm each, protrusion 3 mm, retraction 1 mm. Apart from the laterotrusion to the left all movements were associated with severe pain in the left temporal region.
- Isometric testing of the craniomandibular region was normal. Static depression showed a tendency to deviate to the left. On palpation, the temporal and masseter muscles were bilaterally hypertonic.

- Cervical flexion and extension were reduced to 50%, rotation to the left was reduced by 60°, to the right by 30° and lateroflexion bilaterally by 10°.
- Rotation to the left provoked severe pain while all other end-range movements were accompanied by moderate to severe craniocervical pain.
- Craniofacial assessment with occipito/frontal compression and temporal/temporal rotations in the transverse plane were very painful and therefore impossible at this stage.
- The general techniques for the parietal region (parietal/parietal compression and distraction) showed stiffness on the left (operated) side.
- Temporal techniques (temporal/zygoma and temporal/parietal) provoked typical pain in the temporal region and were stiff.

Hypothetically it could be concluded that trismus after radiotherapy and a craniocervical dysfunction were the main sources of the patient's symptoms: limited mouth opening and pain in the temporal region. Passive craniomandibular mobilization would be too intense at this stage and might further contribute to the trismus.

Therapeutic procedure

The first treatment sessions were intended to reduce the pain in the temporal region and to increase the range of mouth opening. To achieve this, general craniofacial techniques were applied followed by specific techniques for the temporal and occipital regions. These were dominantly sustained techniques at the temporal bone and sustained temporal/occipital techniques once the mobility had improved, combined with active mouth opening.

Clinical course

The pain was significantly reduced after six treatment sessions (VAS 4.9). The patient was able to chew bread for the first time since the operation. After the sixth treatment session the craniomandibular region was incorporated into the treatment. The most limited accessory movements of the TMJ were mobilized into resistance (R) but before the onset of symptoms (P1).

The active physiological movements improved within 3 months, as follows:

- Depression improved from 11 mm to 25 mm
- Protrusion improved from 3 mm to 4 mm
- Laterotrusion to the right = 5 mm
- Laterotrusion to the left = 10 mm (Fig. 23.4b).

The heat and the swelling were gone and there was only a little redness remaining. The craniofacial and craniomandibular techniques described above were continued for the following 2 months with progressing duration, intensity and reduced treatment frequency (once a week). This resulted in further pain reduction (to VAS 2.1).

The treatment intervals were therefore reduced from three times a week initially to once a week (60 minutes per session). The aim was now to maintain the achieved results. The patient was very pleased with the treatment; he was also motivated and trusted the therapy. This was a great advantage since it reduced his fear which progressively diminished with increasing range of motion and pain reduction.

Conclusions

Retrospectively it can be assumed that the trismus, possibly aggravated by the radiotherapy, could not be effectively reduced by craniomandibular techniques. The pain-free craniofacial techniques were more successful. They not only achieved a reduction in pain but also an improvement of the active physiological craniomandibular movements. Regular treatment intervals and home exercises (coordination and mobilization of the craniomandibular and craniofacial regions) resulted in optimal results, in this particular case improved speech, chewing, yawning and an improved quality of life with reduced fear of relapses.

Case study 5: Jana, 6 years old

Michaela Bulling, Stuttgart, Germany

Diagnosis: Recurrent juvenile headaches

Subjective examination and history

Six-year-old Jana suffered from headaches. Her parents were extremely worried since the symptoms had increased significantly in intensity and frequency, requiring medication, and it was only a few months before Jana was due to start school. Besides the headaches Jana also described symptoms in her arms and legs, which her mother called 'growing pains'.

The pain, which was mainly felt in the area of the frontal bone, was described by Jana as 'scary' and perceived as 7.5 on the colour analogue scale (CAS). When the pain occurred, Jana did not want to play or have company but preferred to lie down in a dark room. This meant that she could not fully participate in birthday parties, sports and family activities. For example, she missed most of her grandfather's birthday party and was instead bedded on chairs for most of the time. Without medication she could not have attended the occasion at all, her mother claimed.

Jana's pain did not occur in patterns. It occurred at various times of the day, as well as in the evenings and even woke her during the night. During the day only lying down, quiet and darkness reduced the symptoms.

The headaches initially started in her early childhood. She always complained of headaches. Until now, however, she never had to stop playing or take medication. Six months ago the symptoms had increased to an extent that Jana suffered from headaches daily. Over the past 3 months Jana was given fever syrup and eventually tablets for her pain. Other treatment methods were not suggested by her doctor. It was the idea of a pharmacist to try craniocervical/craniofacial manual therapy and the mother was grateful for any suggestions.

The information Jana's mother gave about her development indicates that it is highly likely that she is a KISS child. She is a second child; pregnancy and birth were normal. Over the first 3 months as a baby she was very restless, cried a lot, and was always hungry but drank very little at a time, dribbled and threw up a lot and suffered from 3-month colic. Her posture was very asymmetrical with her head placed into lateroflexion to the left and rotation to the right. This was noted during the routine check-ups but never treated. Jana's behaviour was noted by her mother since she could only go to sleep in her mother's or father's arms in a certain position and woke up frequently during the night. Breast feeding on the right was difficult. Additionally Jana had severe neurodermatitis, allergies and later on allergic asthma that continues to be treated. Jana often keeps her mouth open and frequently suffers from sore throats.

Social development (speech, understanding, concentration, social capacities) were normal, as was motor development according to her mother (who is a professional child minder). The balance tasks required for the Movement Assessment Battery for Children (Movement ABC) test for 7–8 year old children were performed faultlessly shortly after her 6th birthday. Her mother further stated that Jana was ambitious to keep up with her brother (4 years older) and generally succeeded in that.

Physical examination

Assessment during the first session showed a hypotonic posture in standing: the feet were wide apart, the arches of the feet were reduced, knees were bilaterally in hyperextension, knock-knee on both sides, lumbar lordosis was increased, thoracic kyphosis, scapulae in depression and anterior, cervical spine in lateroflexion to the left, face scoliosis right convex with prominent right zygomatic bone, a smaller sloping left eye and clear divergence of the connecting line of the eyes and the corners of the mouth as well as a prominent occiput (Fig. 23.5a,b).

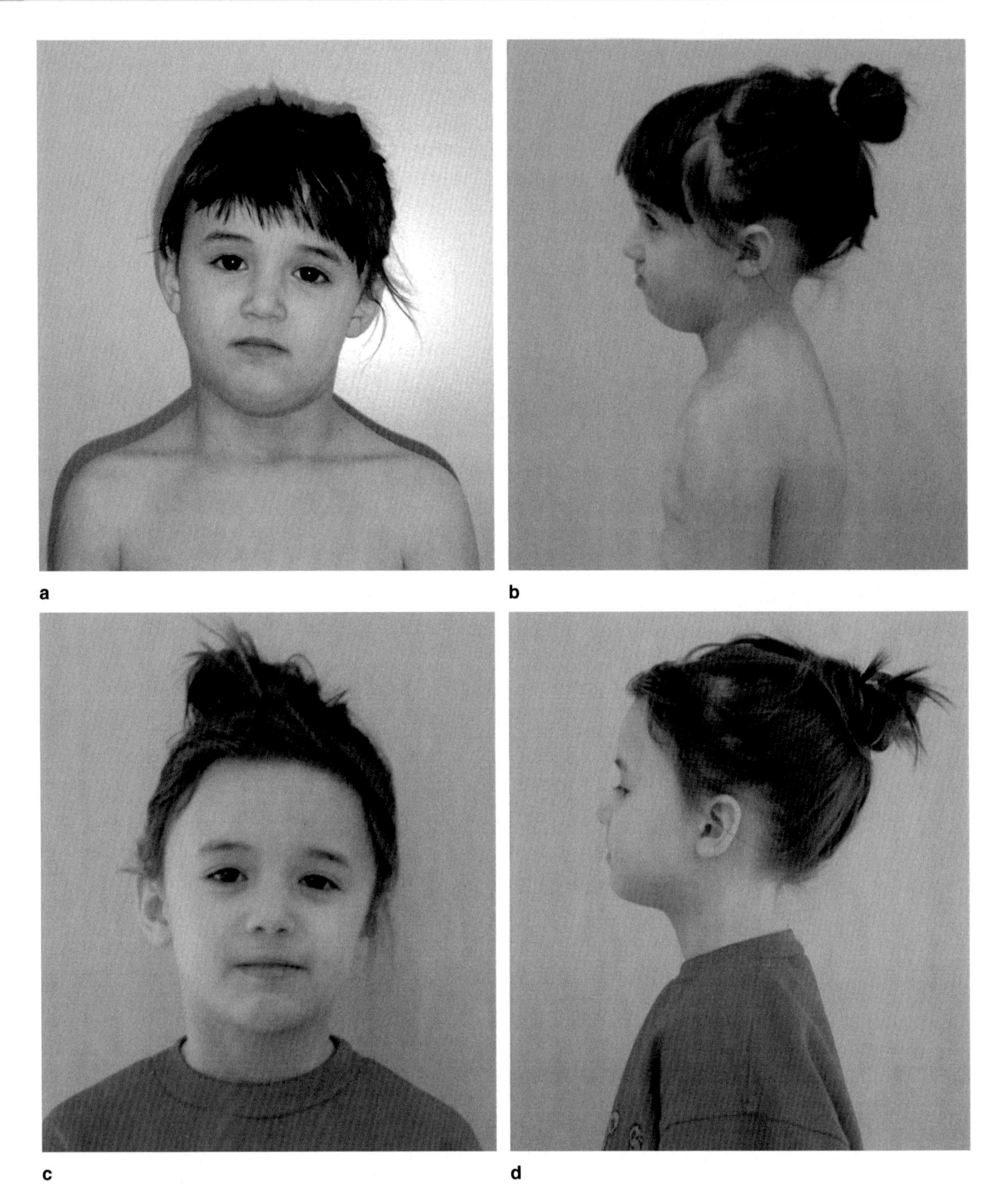

Fig. 23.5 A 6-year-old girl with recurrent juvenile headaches. Note the changes of the craniocervical junction and the facial asymmetry before (a+b) and after (c+d) treatment within 2 months.
a Posture pre-therapy.
b Lateral view with increased thoracic kyphosis and abnormal head position.
c Significantly improved posture and reduced facial asymmetry.
d Reduced thoracic kyphosis and improved head position.

Manual assessment of the craniocervical region showed that the atlas was positioned to the right and hypomobile. Upper cervical rotation to the left between occiput and C2 was reduced by 75%; lateroflexion was bilaterally reduced but more so to the right.

Regarding the craniofacial region, the right occiput and the left frontal bone were prominent and the cranium felt tight on occiput/frontal (O/F) compression. The mobility of the sphenoid bone in relation to the occiput showed increased resistance on transverse lateral movement (left > right). Neurodynamic mobility (passive neck flexion in long sitting slump) was normal.

Therapeutic procedure

Occipital/frontal compression provoked Jana's headaches in the initial sessions after 5 minutes (later the symptoms no longer occurred on O/F compression) and remained for 1 minute after the technique was stopped. Reassessment showed that upper cervical rotation to the right had improved by one-third and was therefore now reduced by only 50%.

The following sessions included the following craniofacial techniques: occipital/frontal compression (also diagonally), occipital/sphenoid transverse/lateral and zygoma compression. In the craniocervical region a sustained atlas technique was applied. Motor balance was normal. The thoracic spine also showed hypermobile segments that were mobilized throughout the course of treatments.

Jana's mother was informed about contributing factors such as sleeping habits and drinking habits, and about the KISS syndrome.

Clinical course

The physical findings (reduced upper cervical and craniofacial mobility) improved quickly and the achieved results were maintained to the following treatment session. After the initial treatment Jana complained of a symptom aggravation, but this did not affect her motivation to come for treatment. Jana liked coming for therapy and showed good compliance. It almost seemed as if she enjoyed the techniques. From the second session on, the intensity and frequency of the symptoms slowly but progressively diminished. In the sixth session the mother stated that, according to the pain diary, Jana had only suffered from headaches once during that week (previously she had experienced daily headaches for 3 months!). She also did not stop playing this time and did not require medication. For 3 weeks Jana did not have any more problems going to sleep and was not wakened by pain. Jana returned to kindergarten and now seems more lively, talkative and awake at home. The parents only realized once they saw the improvements how quiet, tired and inactive Jana had become in the previous months.

To stabilize the treatment effects, six more treatments were planned with intervals of 2–4 weeks.

Compared with the initial assessment 8 weeks ago the craniocervical and craniofacial dysfunctions are now clearly reduced (Fig. 23.5c,d). One can assume that Jana will be able to start school this summer and will experience no problems but a lively, positive and childhood full of normal curiosity.

Postscript: Jana and her mother told me at a later stage that she had experienced headaches only once since the treatment and that was associated with a bad cold.

Conclusions

Retrospectively the craniofacial therapeutic approach was an effective, low cost and low effort physiotherapeutic intervention for Jana that led to many positive changes (and might have done so a lot earlier!). The return to a normal physiological upper cervical mobility that allowed a symmetrical head position as well as the increased cranial mobility enabled the patient to move without pain and to continue a normal physical and emotional–affective development.

Appendix 1

Craniomandibular and craniofacial dysfunctions and pain

This questionnaire and record covers most of the screening questions and tests suggested in this book and is suitable for craniofacial, craniomandibular and cranioneural dysfunctions.

The contents are identical to the digital record developed by the Craniofacial Therapy Academy (CRAFTA®). The tests have proved to be useful tools to gain helpful information from the physical examination and to evaluate outcomes in a research setting. Naturally, further questions or tests may be added at any time.

1. Subjective examination

• Main problem

Location of symptoms/quality — VAS

1. ______________ [ ]
2. ______________ [ ]
3. ______________ [ ]
4. ______________ [ ]

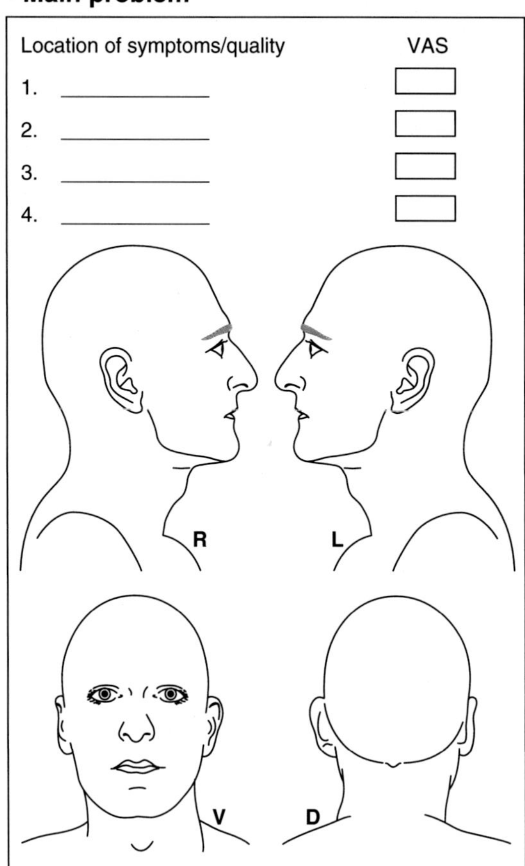

• Behaviour of the symptoms

• Specific mouth activities — yes/no
If yes, which activity? ______________
Which behaviour? ______________

• Accumulating — yes/no

• Cranium — yes/no
If yes, which part? ______________
Which behaviour? ______________

• Accumulating — yes/no

• Previous history

	Yes	No
• Orthodontic treatment (brace)	[ ]	[ ]
• Birth		
– birth trauma	[ ]	[ ]
– long duration	[ ]	[ ]
– forceps/suction	[ ]	[ ]
• Trauma		
– sports	[ ]	[ ]
– accident	[ ]	[ ]
– dental treatment	[ ]	[ ]
– cerebral commotion	[ ]	[ ]
– cerebral contusion	[ ]	[ ]
– date	______	
• Diseases	[ ]	[ ]
– encephalitis	[ ]	[ ]
– meningitis	[ ]	[ ]
– rheumatoid arthritis (RA)	[ ]	[ ]
• Orthodontist	[ ]	[ ]
– date	______	
• Influence on symptoms	[ ]	[ ]

Comments
____
____
____
____
____
____
____

• Special questions

	Yes	No
• Doctor, dentist, orthodontist	☐	☐
• Medication	☐	☐
• Specific functions	☐	☐
– chewing	☐	☐
– swallowing	☐	☐
– speaking	☐	☐
• Extraoral functions (parafunctions)	☐	☐
– bruxism	☐	☐
– trismus	☐	☐
– chewing on one side	☐	☐
– cheek or tongue biting	☐	☐
– lip biting	☐	☐
• Grinding, locking	☐	☐
• Juvenile rheumatoid arthritis (RA)	☐	☐
• Social field	☐	☐
– work situation	☐	☐
– home situation	☐	☐
– stress	☐	☐
– processing problems	☐	☐
• Other headaches	☐	☐
– If yes, what type?	________	
• Inflammations	☐	☐
– nose	☐	☐
– sinuses	☐	☐
– ears	☐	☐
• Operations	☐	☐
Eyes	☐	☐
– diplopia	☐	☐
– ptosis	☐	☐
Nose	☐	☐
– septum (vomer)	☐	☐
Ears	☐	☐
Cervical spine	☐	☐
• Behaviour	☐	☐
– concentration	☐	☐
– memory	☐	☐
– social contacts	☐	☐
– stress	☐	☐
– work/home situation	☐	☐
– processing problems	☐	☐
• Dental or orthodontic treatments	☐	☐
• Comforter (dummy)	☐	☐

	Yes	No
• Associated symptoms	☐	☐
– dizziness	☐	☐
– tinnitus	☐	☐
– clicking in ear	☐	☐
– dysarthria	☐	☐
– diplopia	☐	☐
– dysphagia	☐	☐
– drop attacks	☐	☐

Comments

____
____
____
____
____
____
____

2. Physical examination of the craniomandibular region

• Current pain Yes | No

Inspection

Extraoral	Yes	No
• Method by Trott $\frac{AB}{CD}$	☐	☐
• Orbital, nasal, oral line	☐	☐
– abnormal	☐	☐
• Mandibular length	left ___mm right ___mm	
• Hyoid position	normal high low	☐ ☐ ☐

Intraoral

- Tongue position
  - upper incisors ☐
  - lower incisors ☐
  - mid-palatinum ☐
  - other ☐

	Yes	No
• Impressions	☐	☐
• Abrasions	☐	☐
• Habitual occlusion stable ☐ unstable ☐		
– front teeth in contact	☐	☐
– side teeth without contact	☐	☐
• Non-physiological occlusion contacts		
– habitual	☐	☐
– centric	☐	☐
– protrusion	☐	☐
– laterotrusion right	☐	☐
– laterotrusion left	☐	☐

	Right	Left
• Condyle position		
– cranial	☐	☐
– caudad	☐	☐
– medial	☐	☐
– lateral	☐	☐
– posterior	☐	☐
– anterior	☐	☐

Functional demonstration

	Yes	No
• Performed	☐	☐

– dominant structure

- Differentiation test craniomandibular/ craniocervical region

• Craniocervical		Spatula/brace		Test
– flexion	☐	☐	☐	☐
– extension	☐	☐	☐	☐
– rotation right	☐	☐	☐	☐
– rotation left	☐	☐	☐	☐
– lateroflexion right	☐	☐	☐	☐
– lateroflexion left	☐	☐	☐	☐
• Hip				
– static flexion in 90° hip flexion	☐	☐	☐	☐
– Patrick–Kubis test	☐	☐	☐	☐

Active tests

VROM (from ventral) profile

right left ventral dorsal

	Sympton Range (mm) Stable	Unstable
• Movement direction		
– depression (DE)	☐	☐
– elevation (EL)	☐	☐
– retropulsion (RE)	☐	☐
– protrusion (PRO)	☐	☐
– laterotrusion (LT) right	☐	☐
– laterotrusion (LT) left	☐	☐
• Overjet (horizontal)	☐	
• Overbite (vertical)	☐	

Static tests

	Symptom	Force	Comments
• Direction			
– depression (DE)	☐	☐	________
– elevation (EL)	☐	☐	________
– retropulsion (RE)	☐	☐	________
– protrusion (PRO)	☐	☐	________
– laterotrusion (LT) right	☐	☐	________
– laterotrusion (LT) left	☐	☐	________

Other regions and structures (hypothetical)

	Tests
• Craniocervical region	________
• Nervous system (general)	________
• Cranial nervous system	________
• Craniofacial region	________
• Other	________

- Trial treatment and reassessment

____

____

- Evaluation

____

____

Passive tests of the craniomandibular region (accessory movements)

	Right Symptom	Right Range	Left Symptom	Left Range
• Longitudinal caudad	☐	☐	☐	☐
• Transverse lateral	☐	☐	☐	☐
• Transverse medial	☐	☐	☐	☐
• Posterior–anterior	☐	☐	☐	☐
• Anterior–posterior	☐	☐	☐	☐

• Evaluation

____

____

	Right	Left	Important signs
• Hypothesis intra-articular dysfunction	☐	☐	________
– degeneration	☐	☐	________
– perforation	☐	☐	________
– disc derangement anterior			
with reduction (VMR)	☐	☐	________
without reduction (VOR)	☐	☐	________
– disc derangement anteromedial	☐	☐	________
– disc derangement medial	☐	☐	________
– disc derangement dorsal	☐	☐	________

Palpation

Trigger points right			Trigger points left	
		Masseter superficialis muscle		
		Masseter profundus muscle		
		Lateral temporomandibular artery		
		Dorsal temporomandibular artery		
		Anterior temporal muscle		
		Medial/posterior temporal muscle		
		Suboccipital/nuchal muscles		
		Trapezius muscle		
		Sternocleidomastoid muscle		
		Infrahyoid muscle		
		Suprahyoid muscle		
		Digastric muscle, posterior belly		
		Medial pterygoid muscle		
		Lateral pterygoid muscle/isometric		

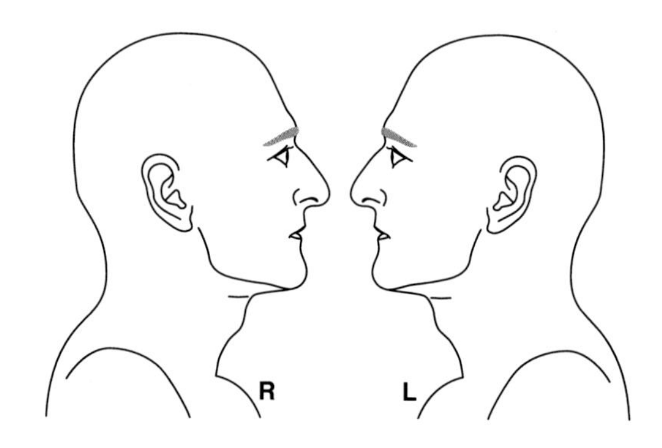

Hypotheses

____

____

____

____

3. Physical examination of the craniofacial region

Inspection

	Yes	No
• Asymmetry	☐	☐
– neurocranium	☐	☐
– viscerocranium	☐	☐

• Anthropometric measurements
(see heads V, D, p. 670)

Evaluation

____
____
____

Functional demonstration

Tests	Yes	No	Dominant structure
________	☐	☐	________
________	☐	☐	________
________	☐	☐	________

Passive tests

• Neurocranium

	Symptom	Sign	Comment
• General			
–occiput/frontal (O/F)	☐	☐	______
–temporal/temporal (T/T)	☐	☐	______
–occiput (compression) (O)	☐	☐	______
–frontal (distraction) (F)	☐	☐	______
–parietal/parietal (P/P)	☐	☐	______

• Specific techniques

____
____
____

Evaluation

____
____
____

• Viscerocranium

	Right Symptom	Right Range	Left Symptom	Left Range
• General				
–orbit	☐	☐	☐	☐
–zygoma	☐	☐	☐	☐
–maxilla	☐	☐	☐	☐

• Specific techniques

____
____
____

Evaluation

____
____
____

4. Physical examination of the cranial nervous system

Inspection

	Yes	No
• Clear indications for cranioneural dysfunction	☐	☐

– if yes, which

____
____
____

• Conduction tests – abnormal		
– upper limb	☐	☐
– lower limb	☐	☐

– if yes, which

____
____
____

First category

General neurodynamic tests for the craniocervical region

Cervical spine

	Symptom	Sign	Comments
– neck flexion			
• upper	☐	☐	________
• lower	☐	☐	________
• combination	☐	☐	________
– additional lateroflexion			
• left	☐	☐	________
• right	☐	☐	________
– neck extension			
• upper	☐	☐	________
• lower	☐	☐	________
• combination	☐	☐	________

Second category

Physical examination of the cranial nerves (I)

Trigeminal nerve (V)

- Conduction tests
  - sensitivity
    - surface sensitivity
    - temperature
  - corneal reflex
  - jaw reflex
  - isometric masticatory muscles
    - depression
    - elevation
    - protrusion
    - laterotrusion right/left

Ophthalmic nerve (V_1)

- Neurodynamic tests (Right / Left)
  - cervical spine
    - neck flexion
    - lateroflexion
  - eyes
    - caudad
    - medial
    - lateral
  - cranium
    - F
    - S
    - La
  - palpation
    - supraorbital fossa

Maxillary nerve (V_2)

- Neurodynamic tests (Right / Left)
  - cervical spine
    - neck flexion
    - lateroflexion
  - eyes
    - medial
    - cranial
  - cranium
    - Z
    - M
    - Pa
    - S
  - palpation
    - infraorbital fossa
    - major palatinum fossa

Mandibular nerve (V_3)

- Neurodynamic tests (Right / Left)
  - cervical spine
    - neck flexion
    - lateroflexion
  - mandible
    - depression
    - laterotrusion
  - cranium
    - S
  - palpation
    - medial angle
    - intraoral (incisiva 3.1, 4.1)
    - chin

Facial nerve (VII)

- Conduction tests
  - mimic muscles
    - teeth
    - mouth
    - eyes
    - forehead
    - teeth/forehead
    - taste sweet salty sour bitter
    - salivary glands
    - lacrimal glands
- Neurodynamic tests (Right / Left)
  - cervical spine
    - neck flexion
    - lateroflexion
    - rotation (opposite side)
  - cranium
    - T
    - Pe
    - hyoid longitudinal caudad/lateral
  - palpation
    - masticatory nerve
    - buccinator nerve
    - zygomatic nerve
    - mandibular nerve
    - auricular nerve

Vestibulocochlear nerve (VIII)

- Conduction tests (Right / Left)
  - hearing
    - finger snapping ☐ ☐
    - Weber test ☐ ☐
    - Rinne test ☐ ☐
  - balance
    - Rhomberg test ☐
    - rope walk ☐
    - Stern test ☐
    - fingertip to nose test ☐
  - nystagmus Yes ☐ No ☐

	Right	Left	Comments
– rotation test	☐	☐	________
– temperature test			________
– Hallpike manoeuvre			________

- Neurodynamic tests
  - cervical spine (Right / Left)
    - upper flexion ☐ ☐
    - lateroflexion ☐ ☐
  - cranium
    - O ☐ ☐
    - Pe ☐ ☐
    - S ☐ ☐
    - T ☐ ☐

Accessory nerve (XI)

- Conduction tests (Right / Left)
  - force
    - trapezius muscle ☐ ☐
    - sternocleidomastoid ☐ ☐
  - length
    - trapezius ☐ ☐
    - sternocleidomastoid ☐ ☐
- Neurodynamic tests
  - cervical spine (Right / Left)
    - upper flexion ☐ ☐
    - lateroflexion ☐ ☐
  - cranium
    - O ☐ ☐
    - S ☐ ☐
  - shoulder
    - depression ☐ ☐
    - retraction ☐ ☐
  - palpation
    - supraclavicular triangle ☐ ☐

Hypoglossal nerve (XII)

- Conduction tests
  - tongue
    - inspection ☐
  - movements
    - protrusion ☐
    - laterotrusion right ☐
    - laterotrusion left ☐
  - static tests
    - protrusion ☐
    - laterotrusion right ☐
    - laterotrusion left ☐
- Neurodynamic tests
  - cervical spine (Right / Left)
    - upper flexion ☐ ☐
    - lateroflexion ☐ ☐
  - cranium
    - O ☐ ☐
  - hyoid
    - longitudinal caudad movement ☐ ☐
    - transverse lateral movment ☐ ☐
  - palpation
    - cranial of the hyoid ☐ ☐

Third category

Physical examination of the cranial nerves (II)

Olfactory nerve (I)

- Conduction tests
  - smelling (VAS) Yes ☐ No ☐

left 0________________________10

right 0________________________10

- Neurodynamic tests
  - cervical spine (Right / Left)
    - upper flexion ☐ ☐
    - lateroflexion ☐ ☐
  - cranium
    - ethmoid ☐ ☐
    - nasal/frontal ☐ ☐
    - Pa ☐ ☐

Optic nerve (II)

- Conduction tests — Right / Left
  - visual field ☐ ☐ / ☐ ☐ ; ☐ ☐ / ☐ ☐
- Neurodynamic tests

	Right	Left
– cervical spine		
• upper flexion	☐	☐
• lateroflexion	☐	☐
– cranium		
• S	☐	☐
– eyes		
• anterior–posterior	☐	☐
• lateral	☐	☐
• medial	☐	☐

Oculomotor system (III,IV,VI)

• Conduction tests	Right	Left	Comments
– inspection pupil	☐	☐	________
• direct	☐	☐	________
• consensual	☐	☐	________
– accommodation	☐	☐	________
• quality	☐	☐	________
• speed	☐	☐	________
• symmetry	☐	☐	________
• fatigue	☐	☐	________
– cover test	☐	☐	
• both eyes	☐	☐	________
• one eye covered	☐	☐	________

- Neurodynamic tests

	Right	Left
– cervical spine		
• upper flexion	☐	☐
• lateroflexion	☐	☐
– cranium	Right	Left
• S	☐	☐
• T	☐	☐

Oculomotor nerve (III)

- Neurodynamic tests

	Right	Left
– eye		
• caudad	☐	☐
• lateral	☐	☐

Trochlear nerve (IV)

- Neurodynamic tests

	Right	Left
– eye		
• caudad/lateral	☐	☐

Abducen nerve (VI)

- Neurodynamic tests

	Right	Left
– eye		
• medial	☐	☐

Glossopharyngeal nerve (IX)

• Conduction tests	Yes	No	Comments
– gag reflex	☐	☐	________
– motor (sounds)			
• 'Ah'	☐	☐	________
• 'Uh'	☐	☐	________
– high sounds	☐	☐	________
– low sounds	☐	☐	________
– phonation	☐	☐	________

- Neurodynamic tests

	Right	Left
– cervical spine		
• neck flexion	☐	☐
• lateroflexion	☐	☐
– cranium		
• styloid process	☐	☐
• S	☐	☐
• Pe/T	☐	☐
– mandible		
• protrusion	☐	☐
• laterotrusion	☐	☐
– palpation		
• styloid process (dorsal)	☐	☐

Vagus nerve (X)

- Conduction tests Yes No Comments
  - – gag reflex ☐ ☐ ______
  - – motor (sounds)
    - • 'Ah' ☐ ☐ ______
    - • 'Uh' ☐ ☐ ______
  - – high sounds ☐ ☐ ______
  - – low sounds ☐ ☐ ______
  - – phonation ☐ ☐ ______
- Neurodynamic tests
  - – cervical spine Right Left
    - • upper neck flexion ☐ ☐
    - • lateroflexion ☐ ☐
  - – cranium
    - • S ☐ ☐
    - • O ☐ ☐
    - • T ☐ ☐
  - – hyoid
    - • transverse–lateral ☐ ☐
  - – cricoid
    - • transverse–lateral ☐ ☐
  - – thorax
    - • anterior–posterior ☐ ☐
  - –palpation Right Left
    - • cranial of the hyoid ☐ ☐
    - • ventral of the mastoid ☐ ☐

Comments

Index

Notes: Entries in **boldface** refer to boxes, figures and tables.
Common names for bones, muscles and nerves have been used throughout.

A

B

C

D

F

G

H

I

J

K

L

M

N

O

P

S

T

U

V

W

X

Y

Z

Printed in the United States
By Bookmasters